The Handbook of Child and Adolescent Clinical Psychology

A Contextual Approach

Second Edition

Alan Carr

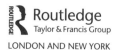 Routledge
Taylor & Francis Group

LONDON AND NEW YORK

First edition published 1999
by Routledge
11 New Fetter Lane, London EC4P 4EE

Second edition published 2006
by Routledge
27 Church Road, Hove, East Sussex BN3 2FA
Simultaneously published in the USA and Canada
by Taylor & Francis Inc
270 Madison Ave, New York, NY 10016

Routledge is an imprint of the Taylor & Francis Group

© 2006 Alan Carr

Typeset in Times by RefineCatch Ltd, Bungay, Suffolk
Printed and bound in Great Britain by
TJ International Ltd, Padstow, Cornwall
Paperback cover design by Sandra Heath

This publication has been produced with paper manufactured to
strict environmental standards and with pulp derived from
sustainable forests.

British Library Cataloguing in Publication Data
A catalogue record for this book is available from the British Library

Library of Congress Cataloging in Publication Data
Carr, Alan, Dr.
    The handbook of child and adolescent clinical psychology: a contextual
approach/ Alan Carr.—2nd ed.
    p. cm.
Includes bibliographical references and index.
ISBN 1-58391-830-2—ISBN 1-58391-831-0 (pbk.)
    1. Child psychology—Handbooks, manuals, etc.   2. Adolescent
psychology—Handbooks, manuals, etc.   I. Title.
RJ503.3.C37 2006
618.92'89—dc22   2005044758

ISBN 10: 1-58391-830-2
ISBN 10: 1-58391-831-0
ISBN 13: 9-78-1-58391-830-2
ISBN 13: 9-78-1-58391-831-0

Author Notes

Professor Alan Carr is the director of the Doctoral Programme in Clinical Psychology at University College Dublin and Consultant Psychologist and Family Therapist at the Clanwilliam Institute Dublin. His other publications with Brunner Routledge include *The Handbook of Adult Clinical Psychology* (co-edited with Muireann McNulty), *The Handbook of Intellectual Disability and Clinical Psychology Practice* (co-edited with Gary O'Reilly, Patricia Noonan Walsh and John McEvoy), *The Handbook of Clinical Intervention with Young People who Sexually Abuse* (co-edited with Gary O'Reilly, Bill Marshall and Richard Beckett), *What Works With Children and Adolescents?*, *Prevention: What Works with Children and Adolescents?*, *Positive Psychology* and *Abnormal Psychology*. His other books include *Family Therapy: Concepts, Process and Practice* (Wiley, 2000) and *Clinical Psychology in Ireland, Volumes 1–5* (Edwin Mellen Press). He has worked in the fields of clinical psychology and family therapy in the UK, Ireland and Canada.

Foreword to the First Edition

Alan Carr has pulled off, with this textbook, an unusual and extraordinary feat: unusual in managing singlehandedly to produce a guide to clinical theory and practice with such a comprehensive range; extraordinary in formulating multi-system and developmental conceptual frameworks that succeed convincingly in integrating many of the themes and 'loose ends' in child and adolescent clinical psychology. The author combines impressive scholarship and clinical knowledge in a reader-friendly book which should be of inestimable value to post-graduate clinical trainees and, indeed, to experienced practitioners.

Martin Herbert
Emeritus Professor of Clinical Child Psychology,
University of Exeter

Acknowledgements

I am grateful to the many people who have helped me develop the ideas presented in this book. A particular debt of gratitude is due to Thérèse Brady, who inspired me to begin the project, and to all of the clinical psychology post-graduates who have challenged me to articulate my ideas on the nuts and bolts of case management in clinical practice. I am grateful to the many colleagues who have offered support in various ways while I was writing both editions of this book. In particular, my thanks to Professor Martin Herbert, Professor Ciarán Benson, Professor Patrick Clancy, Dr Muireann McNulty, Dr Gary O'Reilly, Dr Barbara Dooley, Dr Teresa Burke, Muriel Keegan, Dr Suzanne Guerin, Dr Eilis Hennessy, Dr Patrick Walsh, Professor Patricia Noonan Walsh, Donna McGinley, Dr Michael Byrne, Dr Mairi Keenleyside, Fiona Kelly Meldon, Frances Osborne, Dr Imelda McCarthy, Dr Ed McHale, Phil Kearney, Clive Garland, Declan Roche, Rob Pethebridge, Dr Jim Sheehan, Dr Mark O'Reilly, Dr Tony Bates, Dr Richard Booth, Dr Kevin Tierney, Professor Mike Wang, Dr Jan Aldridge, Professor Neil Frude, Dr Jenny Ashcroft, Professor Peter Stratton, Dr Evan Eisler, Professor Dave Hemsley, Dr David Green, Dr Bob Woods, Dr Mike O'Driscoll and Dr Mike Hills. Thanks also to all of the graduates of the doctoral programme in clinical psychology at UCD and the many post-grads who have e-mailed me or buttonholed me at conferences over the past few years to comment on aspects of the first edition. Insofar as it was possible, I have tried to incorporate their feedback into this second edition. Some of the more important insights into child and adolescent psychology have arisen within the context of my family, and so to them I am particularly grateful.

We are grateful to the American Psychiatric Association for permission to reproduce diagnostic criteria previously published in 2000 in the Text Revision of the Fourth Edition of the *Diagnostic and Statistical Manual of Mental Disorders* and to the World Health Organization for permission to reproduce diagnostic criteria previously published in 1992 in *The ICD-10 Classification of Mental and Behavioural Disorders. Clinical Descriptions and Diagnostic Guidelines*.

Alan Carr
February 2005

Preface to the Second Edition

When a dog barks late at night and then retires again to bed he punctuates and gives majesty to the serial enigma of the dark, laying it more evenly and heavily upon the fabric of the mind. King Sweeney in the trees hears the sad baying as he sits listening on a branch, a huddle between earth and heaven; and he hears also the answering mastiff that is counting the watches in the next parish. Bark answers bark till the call spreads like fire through all Erin. Soon the moon comes forth from behind her curtains riding full tilt across the sky, lightsome and unperturbed in her immemorial calm. The eyes of the mad king upon the branch are upturned, whiter eyeballs in a white face, upturned in fear and supplication. Was he mad? The more one studies the problem the more fascinated one becomes.

Flann O'Brien (1939) *At Swim Two Birds* (pp. 216–217).
London: Penguin.

The current edition of this volume, like its predecessor, has been written as a core textbook in the *practice* of clinical child and adolescent psychology for post-graduate psychology students who are undertaking a professional training programme in clinical psychology.

The second edition of this handbook differs from the first in a number of ways. Here are some of the revisions that have been included in this second edition: throughout the book, references have been updated to reflect important developments since the publication the first edition. At the end of each chapter, addresses of relevant websites are given; these are largely for clinician and client resources. In Chapter 1, new sections on emotional intelligence, a new table on the development of emotional competence and a new section on gay and lesbian identity formation have been added. In Chapter 2, tables and sections on defence mechanisms and coping strategies have been revised; the section on attachment has been rewritten and there is a new figure on attachment styles. In Chapter 3, information on the Zero to Three (1994) diagnostic classification system has been included. There is also a new table based on Meltzer et al.'s (2000) national epidemiological study of child psychological disorders in the UK. Information has also been added on new structured interviews and screening instruments for use in epidemiological research. In Chapter 4, there is a new intake form, which includes a section on consent. Also, details of the Health of the Nation Outcome Scales for Children and Adolescents (HoNOSCA; Gowers et al., 1998), Achenbach's System for Empirically Based Assessment (ASEBA; Achenbach & Rescorla, 2000, 2001) and the Strengths and Difficulties Questionnaire assessment system (SDQ; Goodman, 2001) are given. In Chapter 5, information on programmes for making genograms, software for report writing and website addresses for resources for clients have been added. In Chapter 6, information on new child sleep assessment instruments has been added. There is also a new figure containing the Goodlin-Jones and Anders (2004) classification and diagnostic criteria for sleep onset and night-waking disorders in young children. In Chapter 7, details of the ERIC website for incontinence information in the UK is given. In Chapter 8, reference is made to the new, tenth, revision of the American Association for Mental Retardation's manual (AAMR 10; Luckasson et al., 2002) and to the World Health Organization's International Classification of Functioning, Disability and Health (ICF; WHO, 2001). The section on assessment of intellectual disability has been revised to include material on differential diagnosis and needs assessment as recommended in AAMR 10. Reference is made to new revisions of widely used psychological tests, such as the UK fourth edition of the Wechsler Intelligence Scale for Children (WISC-IV UK; Wechsler, 2005) and the second edition of the Wechsler Individual Achievement Tests (WIAT-II; Wechsler, 2001). In Chapter 9, selective reference is made to the explosion of new literature on autistic spectrum disorders and the chapter has been extensively revised. Noteworthy references are made to the MRC review on the aetiology and epidemiology of autism (Johnstone & MRC Autism Review Group, 2001), the major US report by the National Research Council on educating children with autism (Lord & National Research Council, 2001) and new assessment instruments including the Diagnostic Interview for Social and Communication Disorders (DISCO; Wing et al., 2002) and the Revised Autistic Diagnostic Interview (ADI-R; LeCoutier et al., 2003). In Chapter 10, on conduct problems, reference is made to the new ASEBA syndrome scales for aggressive and rule-breaking behaviour, to recent neurobiological research on the aetiology of aggression and to important recent treatment outcome reviews of parent training, family therapy, multi-systemic therapy and treatment foster care. Guidelines for consulting to high support units are also given. In Chapter 11, on ADHD, reference is made to new ASEBA syndrome scales for inattention, to Gillberg's (2003) Disorder of Attention, Motor control and Perception (DAMP), to Barkley's (2003) new executive function deficit theory of ADHD, to recent neurobiological research on the aetiology of ADHD and to important recent treatment outcome reviews and major studies including the MTA trial (MTA Cooperative Group, 1999). In Chapter

12, on anxiety disorders, a new section on elective mutism, now considered to be a childhood precursor of social phobia, has been added. The section on PTSD has been completely revised in light of recent developments. New assessment instruments, specifically for DSM IV anxiety disorders, have been added. Reference is made to therapy resources for evidence-based intervention for children with anxiety disorders, notably the FRIENDS programme (Barrett & Shortt, 2003). In Chapter 13, the assessment and treatment protocols for OCD (Barrett et al., 2004; March & Mulle, 1998) and Tourette's syndrome (Chowdhury, 2004) have been modified to take account of recent developments. In Chapter 14, on somatic conditions, a new section has been added on chronic fatigue syndrome. In Chapter 15, data from new national epidemiological surveys of drug abuse in Ireland and the UK are given and new references to advances in family-based intervention for drug abuse have been added. In Chapter 16, on mood disorders, a new section on bipolar disorder has been added and the section on suicide risk assessment has been completely revised. In Chapter 17, on eating disorders, Jim Lock's (Lock et al., 2001) manualized family therapy programme for adolescent anorexia is described and a new section on cognitive behaviour therapy for bulimia has been added. In Chapter 18, on schizophrenia, account is taken of recent UK and US guidelines for evidence-based practice, which involve combining psychological and pharmacological interventions in the treatment of schizophrenia (American Academy of Child and Adolescent Psychiatry, 2001; National Collaborating Centre for Mental Health, 2003). A section on cognitive behavioural approaches to relapse prevention in schizophrenia has been added. Chapters 19, 20 and 21, on child abuse and neglect, have been revised in light of new data on abuse and its effects and the many recent developments in this field outlined in the second edition of the *APSAC Handbook on Child Maltreatment* (Myers et al., 2002). A new section on parent alienation syndrome has been added to Chapter 23, on divorce. References to quality-of-life scales for use in paediatric psychooncology have been added to Chapter 24.

Despite these extensive revisions and additions, the original structure of the handbook has been retained. A set of conceptual frameworks for practice is given at the outset, and then problems commonly encountered in clinical work with children and adolescents are considered.

I have used the term *contextual* to describe the broad approach taken in this handbook, although I was tempted to describe it as multi-systemic, developmental and pan-theoretically integrative, since it is all of these things. The approach is multi-systemic, insofar as it rests on the assumption that children's psychological problems are most usefully conceptualized as being nested within multiple systems, including the child, the family, the school and the wider social network. It is also multi-systemic insofar as it assumes that assessment and intervention must address the systems relevant to the aetiology and maintenance of the particular problem with which the child presents. Ecological models of child development and family-based intervention strategies have been a particularly strong influence on the development of this approach. The approach is developmental because it takes account of the literature on individual lifespan development, developmental psychopathology and the family lifecycle. The approach is pan-theoretical insofar as it rests on an acceptance that useful solutions to youngsters' difficulties may be developed by considering them in light of a number of different theoretical perspectives rather than invariably attempting to conceptualize them from within a single framework or theoretical model. Biological, behavioural, cognitive, psychodynamic, stress and coping, family systems, ecological and sociological theories are the main conceptual frameworks considered within this approach. The approach is integrative, insofar as it attempts, through a commitment to rigorous case formulation, to help clinicians link together useful ideas from different theories in a coherent and logical way when dealing with particular problems. A piece-meal, eclectic approach is thereby avoided.

The over-arching framework that has guided the development of this approach is social constructionism. That is, an assumption that, for children, families and clinical psychologists, problem definitions and solutions are socially negotiated within the constraints of the physical world and physiological limitations of the body. Thus we can never ask if a particular diagnostic category (like DSM IV depression) or construct (like Minuchin's triangulation) is really true. All we can say is that, for the time being, making distinctions entailed by these categories fit with observations made by communities of scientists and clinicians and is useful in understanding and managing particular problems. The challenge is to develop integrative models or methods for conceptualizing clinical problems that closely fit with our scientist–practitioner community's rigorous observations and requirements for workable and ethical solutions.

The book is divided into six sections. In the first section, a number of frameworks for practice are given. These frameworks offer the reader a way of thinking about both clinical problems and the process of psychological consultation. In Sections II, III and IV, problems that commonly occur in early childhood, middle childhood and adolescence, respectively, are discussed. Coverage of problems in these sections is not even handed. Problems which are commonly referred for consultation are given greatest attention, with the exception of intellectual disabilities and neuropsychological problems. This is because in most clinical psychology training programmes (and indeed in our own programme at University College Dublin), these areas are covered by specialist courses and are touched upon only briefly in the main clinical child psychology course. In Section V the focus is on child abuse and in Section VI clinical problems associated with major life transitions, such as entering foster care, divorce and bereavement, are considered. These topics are given special attention because managing cases where these transitions have occurred is increasingly becoming a central part of the remit of clinical child psychologists in Ireland, the UK and elsewhere.

Within each of the chapters on specific clinical problems, case examples are given at the outset. This is followed in most instances by a consideration of diagnosis, classification, epidemiology and clinical features. Reference is made to the tenth edition of World Health Organization's *International Classification of Diseases* (ICD-10; WHO, 1992, 1996) and text revision of the fourth edition of the American Psychiatric Association's *Diagnostic and Statistical Manual of Mental Disorders* (DSM IV TR; APA, 2000a). These systems, despite their many faults, are widely used and, in my view, developing a familiarity with them and their shortcomings is an important part of training in clinical psychology. Theoretical explanations are considered after diagnosis and classification. Reference is made to available evidence and its bearing on various theoretical positions. However, extensive critical reviews of evidence are not given, since the central focus of this textbook is on practice rather than research. A summary of the empirical evidence on which much of the practice in this handbook is based is given in two companion volumes: *What Works with Children and Adolescents? A Critical Review of Psychological Interventions for Children, Adolescents and their Families* (Carr, 2000a) and *Prevention: What Works with Children and Adolescents? A Critical Review of Psychological Prevention Programmes for Children, Adolescents and their Families?* (Carr, 2002a). Frameworks for assessment and case management are given in light of available theories and research conclusions.

In offering frameworks for assessment, an attempt has been made wherever possible to delineate important pre-disposing, precipitating, maintaining and protective factors deserving evaluation for the particular problem in question. Also, reference is made to available psychometric instruments. In offering options for intervention, wherever possible, interventions for which there is evidence of efficacy are described. Where research evidence is lacking, best practice based on available clinical literature and experience is offered. For most problems, multi-systemic intervention approaches are described. These incorporate psychoeducational, child-focused, family-focused and broader network-focused elements.

Summaries are given at the end of each chapter, along with exercises to help post-graduates develop their formulation and case-planning skills on the one hand and their interviewing and consultation skills on the other. I have attempted, wherever it seemed useful, to offer diagrammatic summaries of material presented within the text and also to list practice manuals, resources for clients and websites at the end of each chapter.

This text, in my view, has five main shortcomings. First, I have over-emphasized problems and deficits and under-emphasized the extraordinary resourcefulness that characterizes most children and families. This is probably because the entire field is dominated by a deficit discourse. My book, *Positive Psychology* (Carr, 2004a), offers a more resource-oriented perspective and may be read as a useful balance to the deficit dominated perspective of this handbook. Second, I have over-emphasized technical aspects of the consultation process and probably paid insufficient attention to relationship factors in clinical practice. My hope is that through live supervision on placement and through experiential work or personal psychotherapy, students will develop interpersonal sensitivity and enhanced relationship skills. Third, the book is under-referenced. I took a decision to make a few references, in the opening sentences of each section, to major texts or significant papers to substantiate assertions made throughout the section. I hoped that this would enhance the readability of the material and prevent the lack of fluency that occurs when all assertions are multiply referenced. Fourth, many issues have not been covered or have been dealt with only briefly. This is because I wished to keep the book to manageable proportions. Finally, this book is far too long. I began with the intention of writing a very short practical clinical text, but conversations with students and clinical placement supervisors repeatedly alerted me to other areas requiring coverage. Hence this over-sized pocket book.

The *Handbook of Child and Adolescent Clinical Psychology* is one of a set of three texts which cover the lion's share of the curriculum for clinical psychologists in training in the UK and Ireland. The other two volumes are: *The Handbook of Adult Clinical Psychology: An Evidence Based Practice Approach* (Carr & McNulty, in press) and *The Handbook of Intellectual Disability and Clinical Psychology Practice* (O'Reilly, Walsh, Carr & McEvoy, in press).

Alan Carr, University College Dublin
February 2005

Contents

List of figures

List of tables

List of boxes

Section I

Frameworks
for practice

Chapter 1

Normal development

This book is primarily concerned with psychological problems that occur during the first eighteen years of life. The first eighteen years is a period during which the most profound changes occur in physical, cognitive and social development. A summary of important normative findings from the fields of developmental psychology and psychopathology will be presented in this chapter. However, the development of the individual child is primarily a social process and the family is the central social context within which this development occurs. We will therefore begin with a consideration of the family lifecycle.

THE FAMILY LIFECYCLE

Families are unique social systems insofar as membership is based on combinations of biological, legal, affectional, geographic and historical ties. In contrast to other social systems, entry into family systems is through birth, adoption, fostering or marriage and members can leave only by death. Severing all family connections is never possible. Furthermore, while family members fulfil certain roles that entail specific definable tasks such as the provision of food and shelter, it is the relationships within families that are primary and irreplaceable.

With single-parenthood, divorce, separation and remarriage as common events, a narrow and traditional definition of the family is no longer useful for the practising clinical psychologist (Walsh, 2003). It is more expedient to think of the child's family as a network of people in the child's immediate psychosocial field. This may include members of the child's household and others who, although not members of the household, play a significant role in the child's life. For example, a separated parent and spouse living elsewhere with whom the child has regular contact, foster parents who provide respite care periodically, a grandmother who provides informal day care and so forth. In clinical practice the primary concern is the extent to which this network meets the child's developmental needs.

Having noted the limitations of a traditional model of the family structure, paradoxically, the most useful available models of the family lifecycle are based on the norm of the traditional nuclear family, with other family forms being conceptualized as deviations from this norm (Carter & McGoldrick, 1999; Walsh 2003). One such model is presented in Table 1.1. This model delineates the main developmental tasks to be completed by the family at each stage of development. In the first two stages of family development, the principal concerns are with differentiating from the family of origin by completing school, developing relationships outside the family, completing one's education and beginning a career. In the third stage, the principal tasks are those associated with selecting a partner and deciding to marry. In the fourth stage, the childless couple must develop routines for living together that are based on a realistic appraisal of the others strengths, weaknesses and idiosyncrasies rather than on the idealized views (or mutual projections) that formed the basis of their relationship during the initial period of infatuation. Coming to terms with the dissolution of the mutual projective system that characterizes the infatuation so common in the early stages of intimate relationships is a particularly stressful task for many couples. However, it is usually easier for individuals to manage this process if they have experienced secure attachments to their own parents in early life (Johnson & Denton, 2002).

In the fifth stage, the main task is for couples to adjust their roles as marital partners to make space for young children. This involves the development of parenting roles, which entail routines for meeting children's needs for:

- safety
- care
- control
- intellectual stimulation.

Developing these routines is a complex process, and often difficulties in doing so leads to a referral for psychological consultation. Routines for meeting children's needs for safety include protecting children from accidents by, for example, not leaving young children unsupervised, and also developing skills for managing the frustration and anger that the demands of parenting young children often elicit. Failure to develop such routines can lead to accidental injuries or child abuse. Routines for providing children with food and shelter, attachment, empathy, understanding and emotional support need to be developed to meet children's needs for care in these various areas. Failure to develop such routines can lead to a variety of emotional difficulties. Routines for setting clear rules and limits; for providing supervision to ensure that children conform to these expectations; and for offering appropriate rewards and sanctions for rule following and rule violations meet children's need for control. Conduct problems may occur if such routines are not developed.

Table 1.1 Stages of the family lifecycle

Stage	Tasks
1. Family of origin experiences	• Maintaining relationships with parents, siblings and peers • Completing school
2. Leaving home	• Differentiation of self from family of origin and developing adult to adult relationship with parents • Developing intimate peer relationships • Beginning a career
3. Premarriage stage	• Selecting partners • Developing a relationship • Deciding to marry
4. Childless couple stage	• Developing a way to live together based on reality rather than mutual projection • Realigning relationships with families of origin and peers to include spouses
5. Family with young children	• Adjusting marital system to make space for children • Adopting parenting roles • Realigning relationships with families of origin to include parenting and grandparenting roles • Children developing peer relationships
6. Family with adolescents	• Adjusting parent–child relationships to allow adolescents more autonomy • Adjusting marital relationships to focus on midlife marital and career issues • Taking on responsibility of caring for families of origin
7. Launching children	• Resolving midlife issues • Negotiating adult to adult relationships with children • Adjusting to living as a couple again • Adjusting to including in-laws and grandchildren within the family circle • Dealing with disabilities and death in the family of origin
8. Later life	• Coping with physiological decline • Adjusting to the children taking a more central role in family maintenance • Making room for the wisdom and experience of the elderly • Dealing with loss of spouse and peers • Preparation for death, life review and integration

Note: Based on Carter & McGoldrick (1999).

Parent–child play and communication routines for meeting children's needs for age-appropriate intellectual stimulation also need to be developed if the child is to avoid developmental delays in emotional, language and intellectual development. In addition to developing parental roles and routines for meeting children's needs, a further task of this stage is the development of grandparental roles and the realignment of family relationships that this entails.

In the sixth stage, which is marked by children's entry into adolescence, parent–child relationships require realignment to allow adolescents to develop more autonomy. Good parent–child communication and joint problem-solving skills facilitate this process, and skills deficits in these areas underpin many adolescent referrals for psychological consultation. However, parents who find their families at this stage of development must contend not only with changes in their relationships with their maturing children but also with the increased dependency of the grandparents upon them and also with a midlife re-evaluation of their marital relationship and career aspirations. The demands of grandparental dependency and midlife re-evaluation may compromise parents' abilities to meet their adolescents' needs for the negotiation of increasing autonomy.

The seventh stage is concerned with the transition of young adult children out of the parental home. Ideally, this transition entails the development of a less hierarchical relationship between parents and children. During this stage, the parents are faced with the task of adjusting to living as a couple again, to dealing with disabilities and death in their families of origin and of adjusting to the expansion of the family, if their children marry and procreate. In the final stage of this lifecycle model, the family must cope with the parents' physiological decline and approaching death, while at the same time developing routines for benefiting from the wisdom and experience of the elderly.

This lifecycle model draws attention to the ways in which the family meets the developing child's needs, and also the way in which the family places demands on children and other members at different stages of the lifecycle. For example, the parents of a teenager may meet her needs for increasing autonomy by allowing greater freedom and unsupervised travel, and she may meet her grandparents' needs for continued connectedness by visiting regularly. Family lifecycle models also focus attention on the transitions that the child and other family members must make as one stage is left behind and another stage is entered. For example, the transition from being a family with young children to being a family with teenage children requires a renegotiation of family rules and roles.

The hierarchical relationship between the parents and children must be renegotiated and, in some families, women may concurrently decrease their focus on homemaking while increasing their focus on their career. This may coincide with men taking a more active role within the household. Families require some degree of flexibility to adapt the way relationships are organized as each of these transitions is negotiated. They also require the capacity to maintain stable roles and routines during each of the stages.

A third important requirement is the capacity to permit children to move from dependency towards autonomy as development progresses. This is as true for the transition into adolescence as it is for the launching stage where children are leaving home. A further feature of family lifecycle models is that they point to certain junctures where there may be a build-up of family stress with many individual transitions occurring simultaneously. For example, in the launching stage it is not uncommon for older children to be leaving home and having their first children while their grandparents may be succumbing to late life illnesses or death. Psychological difficulties often occur during such periods of transition. Data on changes in family members perception of strains and well-being, drawn from Olson's (1993) major study are set out in Figure 1.1, which shows that well-being is greatest during the early and later stages of the family lifecycle, whereas the childrearing years (which are of central concern in this text) are associated with the highest level of stress.

It is within the context of the family lifecycle that physical, cognitive and social development occurs and it is to these that we now turn. The distinctions between physical, cognitive and social development are to some degree arbitrary as, for example, the development of moral reasoning, one aspect

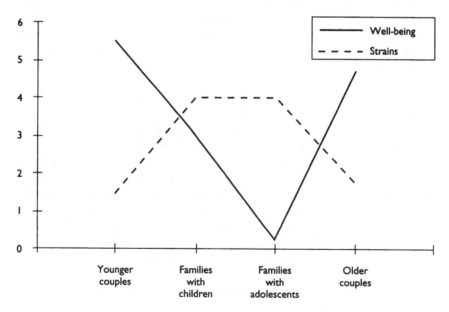

Figure 1.1 Well-being and strains across the family lifecycle

Note. Adapted from Olson (1993).

of social development, depends to some extent on the development of intelligence, an aspect of cognitive development. However, the distinctions provide a useful framework for summarizing those aspects of available research that are of particular relevance to the practice of clinical psychology.

PHYSICAL DEVELOPMENT

Reviews of research on physical development paint the following picture of the infant's growth (Illingworth, 1987; Rutter & Rutter, 1993; Vasta, Haith & Miller, 2003). At birth, infants can distinguish good and bad smells and sweet, sour and salt flavours. Even before birth, babies can respond to tactile stimulation and recognize their mother's voice. The skill of localizing a sound is also present at birth. In the first weeks of life infants can only focus on objects about a foot away and show a particular interest in dark–light contrasts. By three months they have relatively well-developed peripheral vision and depth perception and a major interest in faces. Visual acuity is usually fully developed by twelve months. Sensory stimulation is important for the development of the nervous system and inadequate stimulation may prevent normal neurological and sensory development. For example, children born with a strabismus (squint), which goes uncorrected, may fail to develop binocular vision.

When considering motor development, a distinction is usually made between locomotion and postural development on the one hand, and prehension or manipulative skills on the other. The former concerns the development of control over the trunk, arms and legs for moving around. The latter refers to the ability to use the hands to manipulate objects. Some of the milestones of motor development are set out in Table 1.2. Also included here for convenience are some sensory skills, which have already been discussed. The development of motor skills follow proximodistal (from trunk to extremities) and cephalocaudal (from head to tail) progressions. So infants first learn to control their arms before their fingers and their heads before their legs. After infancy, motor development entails increased co-ordination of locomotion and manipulative skills. The development of effective motor skills in childhood, including those required for sports, gives the child a sense of mastery and engenders self-efficacy and self-esteem. Failure to develop motor skills places children at a disadvantage and may lead to adjustment difficulties.

Different parts of the body develop at different rates following a cephalocaudal progression. The head and brain develop early but the limbs develop later. From birth until the onset of adolescence, the rate of growth slows. With adolescence, a growth spurt occurs which concludes at the end of adolescence. Until adolescence the rates of growth for boys and girls are comparable. With the onset of adolescence, girls enter the growth spurt between one and two years earlier than boys. Height, muscle mass and shoulder width are

Table 1.2 The development of motor and sensory skills

Age	Motor and sensory skills
0 months	• Turns head to one side when lying on stomach • Legs make crawling movements when placed on stomach • Holds a ring in a reflex grasp • Can focus on objects 9 inches away • Can distinguish mother's voice • Can distinguish sweet, sour and salt tastes
3 months	• Sits with support • Pushes head and shoulders up when lying on stomach • Grasps a rattle and reaches with two hands • Breast-fed children can distinguish their mother's odour • Shows interest in faces • Depth perception emerges
6 months	• Sits briefly unaided • Rolls from back to stomach • Transfers cube between hands
9 months	• Walks holding furniture • Crawls • Sits alone • Picks up button with thumb and forefinger
12 months	• Walks unaided • Into everything • Holds crayon and makes mark
18 months	• Climbs stairs • Throws a ball into a box • Builds a tower with three cubes
24 months	• Runs • Walks backwards • Puts square peg in square hole • Builds a tower with six cubes
3 years	• Can stand on one foot for five seconds • Pedals a tricycle • Draws a circle
4 years	• Hops on one foot • Buttons clothes • Draws a square
5 years	• Hops on both feet • Ties shoelaces • Draws triangle
6 years	• Copies diamond
7 years	• Can learn new motor skills like throwing, riding a bicycle

Note: Adapted from Illingworth (1987).

the main areas of development during the adolescent growth spurt for boys. Girls add more overall fat and hip-width than boys.

In adolescence, youngsters develop primary sexual characteristics (menstruation in women and the capacity to ejaculate in men) and secondary sexual characteristics (auxiliary hair, breasts and voice changes). The average age for the emergence of primary sexual characteristics in the US and the UK for girls is ten to eleven years and for boys is 11.5–12.5 years (Coleman, 1995). In a review of the literature on the impact of puberty, Alsaker (1996) drew the following conclusions: Hormonal changes in adolescence have effects on some boys and girls, with raised testosterone levels contributing to male aggression and dominance. In girls, higher oestrogen levels are associated with positive moods and increased activity, while lower levels are associated with poorer moods. Physical changes in adolescence, notably height and weight, affect body-image satisfaction. Short boys and heavy girls tend to be dissatisfied with their body image, whereas satisfaction with body image is expressed by tall boys and slim girls. The timing of the onset of puberty also affects satisfaction with body image, although this association is probably mediated by associated changes in height and weight. Early-maturing boys are more satisfied with their bodies and feel more attractive, whereas early-maturing girls tend to be dissatisfied with their bodies because maturation is associated with weight gain (early-maturing adolescents constitute 10–20% of the population). Early-maturing girls develop more conduct problems than late-maturing girls because of involvement in networks of older deviant peers. In the long term, these conduct problems abate. However, for girls, early maturity may leave a legacy in the form of being less educationally advantaged than their later-maturing counterparts. Early-maturing girls also show greater heterosexual behaviour than their female peers but early-maturing boys do not show this increased level of sexual behaviour.

Mild concern about body shape is common among adolescents. In clinical work, *anorexia nervosa* (self-starvation) and *bulimia* (binge–purge syndrome) are two common disorders associated with a dissatisfaction with body shape. They will be discussed more fully in Chapter 17.

Although genetics play a major role in physical development, environmental factors also contribute significantly to physical development. In particular nutrition, disease, trauma and (indirectly) socioeconomic status all contribute to physical development. A century ago, the average age for the onset of puberty was about five years later than is currently the case. This secular trend probably reflects a change in nutrition, health care and living conditions. Vigorous exercise and dieting may retard the onset of puberty in girls and these activities characterize some young girls with anorexia nervosa. Because of rapid muscular and skeletal growth, and the high energy usage of adolescents, a diet including much protein and minerals is optimal.

COGNITIVE DEVELOPMENT

A distinction between language development and the development of intelligence has traditionally been made by researchers in the field of cognitive development. This distinction will be used in summarizing findings of relevance to the practice of clinical psychology below. Most of the research on intelligence that is relevant to the practice of clinical psychology has been conducted within three traditions (Sternberg, 2000):

- psychometric intelligence testing movement
- Piagetian cognitive development tradition
- information-processing approach.

Findings from these three fields will be summarized separately.

The psychometric study of intelligence

The psychometric study of intelligence began with Binet's attempt in the first decade of the twentieth century to develop a method for assessing children's abilities so that they could be placed in appropriate educational settings (Deary, 2000). He devised a series of puzzles and tasks that he believed tapped the full range of verbal and non-verbal abilities and administered these to samples of children of different ages. He determined, at each age level, what group of tasks 50% of children of that age could complete and subsequently used this normative data to assign *mental ages* to children about whom he wished to make educational placement decisions.

William Stern subsequently noted that a clinically more useful index of ability would express the child's mental age as a proportion of their chronological age, since a ten-year-old with a mental age of five would require different educational placement than a five-year-old with a mental age of five. The index he developed was the intelligence quotient or IQ, which is calculated using the following formula.

Intelligence quotient = (Mental age/Chronological age) × 100

While this quotient was useful for children, with adults over 18 years, it yielded increasingly declining IQs as people aged. Wechsler solved this problem by replacing the ratio IQ with the deviation IQ. For each age group, he defined an IQ of 100 as the mean score of the standardization sample. A score that fell one standard deviation (15 IQ points) above the mean was given an IQ value of 115 and a score that fell one standard deviation below the mean was given an IQ value of 85. Other IQ values were given in a similar fashion on the basis of the degree to which they deviated from the mean. The Stanford–Binet intelligence test and the Wechsler intelligence scales for pre-schoolers, children and adults have become the most widely used measures of intelligence in the world and have undergone numerous revisions and restandardizations over the past 80 years. They are still routinely used in clinical practice by psychologists to evaluate specific and general learning difficulties and to make placement decisions similar to those faced by Binet almost a century ago. The psychometric movement and the tests developed within this tradition have also spawned a great deal of research, which has addressed the following questions:

- Is intelligence most usefully conceptualized as a single trait, multiple independent traits or a hierarchically organized pyramid of related traits?
- Does intelligence (and the constellation of abilities that make up intelligence) remain stable over time?
- How is intelligence distributed within the population?
- What are the relative contributions of heredity and environment to the development of intelligence?
- Can environmental changes improve intelligence?
- What are the relationships between intelligence and scholastic attainment, vocational adjustment, and social competence?

Factor-analytic studies show that most tests of ability are positively correlated, but these correlations are only moderate. Such studies suggest that there is a trait of general intelligence, which influences performances on many problem-solving tasks. However, there is also a range of specific abilities that affect the performance of particular types of tasks. Many psychometric theorists argue that general intelligence and specific abilities are most usefully conceptualized as being hierarchically organized. Hierarchical models of abilities propose a broad general intelligence factor at the top of the hierarchy and a range of specific abilities underneath (Deary, 2000). For example, the Wechsler tests of intelligence are based on a model that places the full-scale IQ as an index of overall intelligence at the top of the hierarchy. Beneath this are verbal and performance IQs, which reflect specific verbal and visuo-spatial abilities. Neuropsychological investigations broadly indicate that verbal functions in adult males may be subserved largely by the left side of the brain, whereas visuo-spatial abilities are subserved by the right side. With females and children, lateralization of function is less clearly defined (Goodman, 2002).

The second question of interest to the psychometric movement concerns the stability of intelligence over time. Broadly speaking, intelligence measurements taken at two separate times in a person's life will be positively correlated. However, population studies of this type show that the correlations are far from perfect and are probably influenced by a variety of environmental factors and by the tasks used to assess intelligence. For example, Bornstein and Sigman (1986) have shown that curiosity about new stimuli in infants under six months correlates .5 with IQ as measured on standard intelligence tests at school entry. Curiosity was assessed by noting the speed with which infants lose interest in a stimulus and show renewed interest when presented with a novel stimulus. These findings are important because traditional psychometric measures of infant development, such as the Bayley scales, do not predict later IQ (Lipsitt, 1992). Unfortunately, well-standardized inspection time tests for assessing infant intelligence have not yet been developed for use in clinical practice.

A second example of temporal changes in the contribution of different abilities to overall intelligence comes from the work of Cattell (1963), who distinguished between *crystallized intelligence* and *fluid intelligence*. Fluid intelligence is reflected in cognitive abilities that do not depend on experience, such as attention, short-term memory and reasoning, and these reach their peak in early adult life. Crystallized intelligence is reflected in vocabulary, general information and experiential evaluation. This form of intelligence is highly dependent on experience and gradually increases across the entire lifespan. Peak years for creativity for pursuits involving crystallized intelligence are usually in the middle adult years, included here are creative writing and social sciences. Peak years for production in pursuits requiring fluid intelligence occur before the forties; included here are the natural sciences and mathematics. This information is valuable for clinical psychologists involved in career guidance.

The third question addressed within the psychometric tradition is the way in which intelligence is distributed within the population. Most studies show that intelligence test scores approximate a normal (bell-shaped) distribution. That is, very few people obtain either extremely high or extremely low scores and the majority obtain moderate scores. Clinical psychologists may use this knowledge of the distribution of intelligence in service planning.

While there continues to be controversy about the fourth question concerning the contribution of heredity and environment to the development of intelligence, more balanced considerations of the evidence conclude that both heredity and environment make roughly equal contributions (Deary, 2000). In view of this, it is not surprising that the level of intellectual stimulation provided by parents and environmental enrichment programmes for disadvantaged children have been shown to enhance intelligence and subsequent school performance and both social and vocational adjustment (Lange & Carr, 2002).

While traditional psychometric conceptions of intelligence have focused largely on verbal, visuo-spatial, and mathematical abilities, Gardner (2000) has argued that a far broader conception of intelligence is warranted and has proposed that there are at least eight different intelligences, with work on the specification of others in progress. The eight intelligences are: linguistic, logical–mathematical, spatial, bodily–kinesthetic, musical, interpersonal, intrapersonal and naturalist. Only the first three of Gardner's intelligences are addressed within the psychometric tradition. Goleman (1995) has argued that interpersonal and intrapersonal intelligence are the most important for successful psychological adaptation in life. Together, these constitute what Goleman refers to as emotional intelligence; that is, the capacity to recognize and manage one's own emotions and those of others in significant interpersonal relationships (Carr, 2004a). Within developmental psychology, these types of skills are traditionally covered under the rubric of social and emotional development, and so a fuller discussion of them will be reserved until that section of this chapter.

The Piagetian tradition and stages of cognitive development

In contrast to the psychometric movement with its emphasis on individual differences in levels of intelligence and stability of intelligence over time, the Piagetian movement has concerned itself with commonalties across children in their cognitive styles as they progress through stages of cognitive growth. A useful critical appraisal of Piaget's work in the light of recent research is contained in Vasta et al. (2003). Piaget conceived of the growth of intelligence as dependent on the child actively attempting to adapt to the world, assimilating new knowledge into available schemas or accommodating to new knowledge and experiences by altering schemas. The main questions addressed by Piaget and members of this tradition have been:

- What are the stages of cognitive development?
- Are there qualitatively different cognitive structures that underpin intelligent problem solving in each of these stages?
- Is progression through the stages invariant?
- Can progression through stages be accelerated by training?

In answer to the first question Piaget posited the existence of four main stages. In the first of these – the sensorimotor period – which extends from birth until about two years of age, the child's approach to problem solving and knowledge acquisition is based on manipulating objects and trial-and-error learning. The main achievements of this stage are the development of cause and effect sensorimotor schemas and the concept of object permanence. That is, the realization that objects have a permanent existence independent of our perception of them.

The second stage of development in Piagetian theory is the pre-operational period. During this stage the child moves from the use of sensorimotor schemas as the main problem-solving tool to the formation of internal representations of the external world. The ability to use internal representations of the world to solve problems under-pins a number of important achievements readily observable in pre-schoolers. These include increasingly sophisticated language usage, engagement in make-believe or symbolic play, the ability to distinguish between appearance and reality and the ability to infer what other people are thinking. This ability to infer what others are thinking has been referred to as theory-of-mind and deficits in this ability typify children with autism; a fuller discussion of this issue will be given in Chapter 9. Reasoning in the pre-operational period is largely intuitive, with the child linking one particular instance to another rather than reasoning from general to particular. For example, a pre-operational child will say 'I'm tired so it must be night time' rather than 'It's getting dark so it must be night time'. The pre-operational child's attempts to solve problems are influenced to a marked degree by what is perceived rather than by what is remembered. The main limitations of the pre-operational period are an inability to take the visual perspective of another person, difficulty in retelling a story coherently (egocentric speech), a belief that inanimate objects can think and feel like people (animism), and an inability to focus on more than one dimension of a problem at a time. For example, if liquid is poured from a short, wide glass into a tall, narrow glass, the pre-operational child will say that there is now more liquid because the level is higher, without making reference to the decreased width of the second glass. Piaget referred to the capacity to take account of two dimensions simultaneously as conservation of quantity.

Conservation of quantity is one of the primary achievements of the concrete operational period, which extends from between five and seven years up until about twelve years. The concrete operational period is the third of Piaget's developmental stages. During this period the child develops the ability to classify objects, place objects in series, engage in rule-governed games, adopt the geographic perspective of another person, and manipulate numbers using addition, subtraction, multiplication and division. These abilities involve the use of logic (rather than intuition) to solve concrete problems.

At about the age of twelve the child begins to use logic to solve abstract problems. That is, the child can develop hypotheses about what might be true and then make plans to test these hypotheses out. This is the primary characteristic of the formal operational period. This is Piaget's fourth and final developmental stage. Many achievements occur during this period. The adolescent can manipulate two or more logical categories, such as speed and distance when planning a trip. Time-related changes can be projected so the adolescent can predict that her relationship with her parents will be different in ten years. The logical consequences of actions can be predicted, so career options related to certain courses of study can be anticipated. The adolescent can detect logical inconsistencies, such as those that occur when parents do not practice what they preach. A final achievement of the formal operational period is the capacity for relativistic thought. Teenagers can see that their own behaviour and that of their parents is influenced by situational factors.

Alongside these extraordinary achievements, there are limitations that characterize the formal operational period. Just as egocentric pre-schoolers cannot take another person's perspective because they do not realize that others occupy a different geographical location than themselves, young adolescents do not realize that others occupy different (and less logical) philosophical positions than themselves. This cognitive egocentricism compromises the adolescent's capacity to solve interpersonal problems that entail logical conflicts and contradictions. Riegel (1973) has suggested that this limitation of the formal operational period is overcome in a final stage of cognitive development, which he refers to as dialectical thinking. Logical reasoning, a sensitivity to practical and ethical considerations, the ability to reframe apparently insoluble problems in solvable terms and the capacity to tolerate ambiguity characterize this period, which occurs in early adulthood.

Riegel's (1973) work is a good example of later research, which showed that Piaget's account of the stages of cognitive development was incomplete. The other main criticism of Piaget's work concerns the boundaries between the stages. Many tests of Piaget's theory have shown that under certain simplified experimental conditions or following certain enriching developmental experiences or training programmes, children at a given stage can perform tasks that require the cognitive capacities which Piaget's theory attributes to a later stage (Vasta et al., 2003). The limitations of children at each stage of cognitive development are important to keep in mind when interviewing them alone or in family sessions. Complex questions or elaborate interpretations or reframings which may routinely be used with adults are often inappropriate when working with children.

The information-processing approach and the acquisition of skills and strategies

Information-processing approaches to the study of intelligence look to the computer as the main metaphor for studying the growth of problem-solving abilities. This approach is concerned with four main questions:

- Can models of sequences of steps and processes that intervene between posing a problem and the child performing a solution be developed for specific domains?
- What strategies are used to solve memory problems?
- What role do scripts and schemas play in problem solving?
- What conditions under-pin cognitive change?

In answer to the first question, numerous models of processes that intervene between input and output have been developed (Deary, 2000). Most information-processing models distinguish between: (1) sensory registers where, for example, images of visual and auditory stimuli are held for less than a second; (2) short-term memory where information is retained for a few seconds; (3) temporary working memory where information from the short-term memory is processed by using control strategies including rehearsal, organization and elaboration; (4) long-term memory; and (5) retrieval.

Regardless of age, the child's information-processing capacity is limited. In teenagers and adults the limits are seven bits (±2). However, older children remember more than younger children. This is probably because they use more effective control strategies for remembering material. Three commonly used strategies are rehearsal (repetition), organization (chunking or group-ing) and elaboration (using a device like imagery to link together items to be remembered). However, these strategies are not used indiscriminately. Rather, they are informed by youngsters' knowledge about the impact of these strat-egies on recall, recognition and reconstruction of material the child wishes to remember. This knowledge about memory is called metamemory. For example, if there are more than five items on a shopping list, some people will consciously use chunking to help them recall the list.

Automatization and strategy construction are two of the main processes by which cognitive change occurs. In the early stages of learning a new skill, much information-processing capacity is taken up with attention to each component of the skill. With rehearsal, sequences of components become automatic and spare capacity becomes available for developing strategies for refining the skill or using it to develop further skills or expertise. For example, a child whose bicycle-riding skills have become automatic may use the available spare capacity to learn new cycle routes.

When children have little knowledge of a topic, they rely largely on recall memory. However, reconstructive memory is an alternative to recall. Here, the child rebuilds the material he or she has remembered on the basis of information coded as schemas and scripts. The greater the child's expertise (or knowledge base in a particular domain) the more effective the use of reconstructive memory, because there is a rich network of associations through which to reconstruct the new material he or she has learned. Knowl-edge bases contain both schemas and scripts. Schemas are representations of the typical structure of familiar experiences. For example, the way furniture is laid out in a dining room. Scripts are representations of typical sequences of events. For example, the routine used to make a cup of tea. Schemas and scripts aid the learning of new material.

The information-processing approach has demonstrated that short-term memory capacity, the amount of information encoded in a problem-solving situation, the rate of automatization, the strategies employed, and the use of metacognitive skills evolve with age. However, performance is also greatly influenced by familiarity with the content of any problem-solving task and the context within which the problem occurs. For example, children engaged in street vending may perform complex mathematical calculations when selling their wares, yet perform poorly in a classroom situation.

Autobiographical memory constitutes a special collection of scripts in which aspects of self and identity are represented. Autobiographical memory probably emerges in conversations with parents where personal memories are retrieved and rehearsed. Infantile amnesia (the inability to remember the first two years of life), from an information-processing perspective, may be conceptualized as the lack of autobiographical memory for this period, which may in turn be attributed to the absence of parent–child conversations in this prelinguistic period. This is quite a different account of infantile amnesia than that given by Freud (1905), who attributed it to repressed memories of sexual desires for parents.

The information-processing approach is a particularly valuable framework for clinical psychologists to use when coaching parents and children in the development of new communication and problem-solving skills. It is also a useful framework from which to interpret the burgeoning literature on the accuracy of children's testimony in court (Ceci, 2002; Jones, 2003).

Vygotsky and the social context of intellectual development

The three main traditions within which intelligence has been studied have relied predominantly on an individualistic approach to the development of skills and problem-solving capabilities. Vygotsky (1934/1962) is unique in conceptualizing the development of intelligence in fundamentally social terms. He observed that children who displayed similar levels of individual problem-solving skills when operating in isolation often showed marked individual differences when coached by an adult or peer. This discrepancy between aided and unaided performance Vygotsky referred to as the *zone of proximal development*. Within this zone of proximal development optimal learning occurs if the parent, teacher or peer adjusts her level of input to take account of the child's actual ability level. With this teaching method, which Vygotsky called *scaffolding*, the teacher gives just enough help to ensure that the pupil has a mastery experience. In clinical practice, helping parents and children define the zone of proximal development and employ scaffolding may be useful in empowering parents to help their children deal with learning difficulties or social adjustment difficulties.

Language development

Some children show normal intellectual development but delayed language development (Bishop, 2002). In contrast, some individuals with intellectual disabilities show particularly well-developed language skills once they reach between two and four years (Yamada, 1990). These two observations suggest that language development is to some degree independent of intellectual development. For this reason, language development is best considered separately from cognitive development. However, cognitive developmentalists following in the Piagetian tradition have continued to point out the ways in which linguistic and cognitive development interact. For example, the statement 'all-gone' depends on the child having developed the concept of object permanence (Gopnik & Meltzoff, 1987).

The milestones of language development and exceptions to these have been well documented in many longitudinal studies (Bates, Bretherton & Snyder 1988). In utero, the fetus can recognize the mother's voice and at birth infants orient to voices differently than sounds. Babbling begins at three to four months and at seven months is used for both social interaction and personal amusement. By six months, babbling is affected by sensory input. Evidence for this comes from the fact that deaf children show a gradual cessation of babbling from this age. Children with language problems do not show the characteristic speech-like cadences that characterize babble at the end of the first year, and do not show any signs of comprehension or communicative pointing in the way that normal children do. The use of single words begins between twelve and eighteen months. By two years, most children know 200 words, and before their third birthday the vast majority of children use two word sentences and grammatical morphemes such as '-ed' and '-ing'. Between three and five years, vocabulary, grammar and the accuracy with which words are used to denote concepts increase. Over-extensions (e.g. calling a horse a dog) and under-extensions (e.g. not calling a poodle a dog) of the meanings of words and the coining of new words, where the child has a vocabulary gap, are all common during this period. So too are grammatical inaccuracies such as over-regularization (e.g. house, houses; mouse, mouses).

Delays in the development of linguistic comprehension and expression tend to be associated with poorer outcomes than simple expressive language delays. And those that are more prolonged have a poorer prognosis than transient developmental language delays. They are also associated with greater psychosocial and scholastic difficulties (Bishop, 2002). Developmental language delays will be discussed in Chapter 8.

The debate about the relative influences of heredity and environment on language development, exemplified by the exchange in the 1950s between Skinner and Chomsky, has reached a partial resolution (Vasta et al., 2003). The rapidity of language development and the creativity shown by children in their use of language suggests that the capacity to derive and apply linguistic rules is subserved by some set of genetically based mechanisms. Psycholinguistic theorists have focused their efforts on clarifying the characteristics of these mechanisms, although they are more complex than originally proposed in Chomsky's original language acquisition device (LAD; Rosenberg, 1993). However, the finding that severe environmental deprivation, such as being locked in an attic throughout infancy, can completely arrest language development while subsequent placement in a normal environment can lead to normal levels of linguistic development within a few years points to the importance of the environment in the development of language (Skuse, 1984).

Environmentalists have focused attention on the way in which parent–child interactions facilitate language development. During their first four months, babies cycle between states of attention and inattention. Mothers gradually learn to concentrate their emotional face-to-face interactions with their babies during the infants' periods of attention. This interactional synchrony gives way to turn-taking, which may represent the infant's first conversations (Kaye, 1982). Infants of depressed mothers have difficulty establishing interactional synchrony and it may be this that compromises their later adjustment (Field et al., 1990).

A further finding that under-pins the important role of environmental factors in language development is the observation that adults in all cultures speak to their children in a unique idiom that has been termed 'motherese' (Snow & Ferguson, 1977). Motherese has the following attributes:

- it is simpler than adult speech
- shorter sentences than adult speech are used
- it is more concrete than adult speech
- it involves repetition of what the child said
- the adult expands on what the child said
- the adult's voice is pitched at a higher than normal frequency
- the adult's pattern of intonation is more meaningful.

A third important aspect of parent–child interaction in the development of language is the provision of a series of formats or structured social interactions in which verbal communication occurs. These include looking at books, naming things and playing word and action games and rhymes. Simplification, repetition and correction of errors characterize the parents behaviour within these formatted interactions. Taken together, these formats comprise the language support system (LASS; Bruner, 1983).

Language is used by children to both control their own behaviour and to engage in speech acts that may be intended to influence others in their social world. Vygotsky (1962) distinguished between private speech, internal speech and social speech. Private speech is used to control the child's own behaviour but is spoken aloud. For example saying 'up-down, up-down' when playing ball. Internal speech or self-talk is silent. It is used to guide and control the child's own behaviour and appears after the age of seven. Self-instructional training, a procedure where children are coached in the use of internal speech to improve academic or social skills, is commonly used as part of a multimodal programme involving home and school-based behavioural management and stimulant medication in the treatment of attention deficit disorder with hyperactivity (Nolan & Carr, 2000); this will be discussed more fully in Chapter 11. Social speech is used for controlling interactions with others and appears by three years. Social speech is made up of speech acts such as 'Daddy bobo', which is a request to Daddy for a bottle.

SOCIAL DEVELOPMENT

The focus in the following sections will be on the social development of the child, including emotional development, moral development, the development of identity, sex-role development and the development of friendships and peer group relationships.

Development of emotional intelligence

Research on emotional competence offers insights into probable developmental precursors of what is now referred to as emotional intelligence (Bar-On & Parker, 2000; Carr, 2004). Emotional regulation skills, the skills for expressing emotions and the skills for managing relationships involving emotional give-and-take develop gradually from infancy to adolescence, as can be seen from Table 1.3 (Saarni, 1999).

Infancy

During the first year of life, infants develop rudimentary self-soothing skills, such as rocking and feeding, for regulating their emotions. They also develop skills for regulating their attention to allow themselves and their caretakers to co-ordinate their actions to sooth them in distressing situations. They rely on their caretakers to provide emotional support or 'scaffolding' during such stress. During the first year of life there is a gradual increase in non-verbal emotional expression in response to all classes of stimuli, including those under the infant's control and those under the control of others. At birth, infants can express interest, as indicated by sustained attention and disgust in response to foul tastes and odours. Smiling, reflecting a sense of pleasure, in response to the human voice appears at four weeks; sadness and anger in response to removing a teething toy are first evident at four months; facial expressions reflecting fear following separation become apparent at nine months. Infants also show an increasingly sophisticated capacity to discriminate positive and negative emotions expressed by others over the course of their first year of life. The capacity for turn-taking in games such as peek-a-boo develops once children have the appropriate cognitive skills for understanding object constancy. Social referencing also occurs towards the end of the first year, when children learn the appropriate emotions to express in a particular situation by attending to the emotional expressions of their caretakers (Feinman, 1992).

The second year

During the second year of life, toddlers show increased awareness of their own emotional responses. They show irritability when parents place limits on

Table 1.3 Development of emotional competence

Age	Regulation of emotions	Expression of emotions	Managing emotional relationships
Infancy 0–1 year	• Self-soothing • Regulation of attention to allow co-ordinated action • Reliance on 'scaffolding' from caregivers during stress	• Increased non-verbal emotional expression in response to stimuli under own control and control of others	• Increased discrimination of emotions expressed by others • Turn-taking (peek a boo) • Social referencing
Toddlerhood 1–2 years	• Increased awareness of own emotional responses • Irritability when parents place limits on expression of need for autonomy	• Increased verbal expression of emotional states • Increased expression of emotions involving self-consciousness and self-evaluation such as shame, pride or coyness	• Anticipation of feelings towards others • Rudimentary empathy • Altruistic behaviour
Pre-school 2–5 years	• Language (self-talk and communication with others) used for regulating emotions	• Increased pretending to express emotions in play and teasing	• Increased insight into others' emotions • Awareness that false expression of emotions can mislead others about one's emotional state
Kindergarten 5–7 years	• Regulating self-conscious emotions, e.g. embarrassment • Increased autonomy from caregivers in regulating emotions	• Presents 'cool' emotional front to peers	• Increased use of social skills to deal with emotions of self and others • Understanding of consensually agreed emotional scripts
Middle childhood 7–10 years	• Autonomous regulation of emotions is preferred to involving caregivers	• Increased use of emotional expression to regulate relationships	• Awareness of feeling multiple emotions about the same person

	• Distancing strategies used to manage emotions if child has little control over situation		• Use of information about emotions of self and others in multiple contexts as aids to making and maintaining friendships
Pre-adolescence 10–13 years	• Increased efficiency in identifying and using multiple strategies for autonomously regulating emotions and managing stress	• Distinction made between genuine emotional expression with close friends and managed display with others	• Increase understanding of social roles and emotional scripts in making and maintaining friendships
Adolescence 13 + years	• Increased awareness of emotional cycles (feeling guilty about feeling angry) • Increased use of complex strategies to autonomously regulate emotions • Self-regulation strategies are increasingly informed by moral principles	• Self-presentation strategies are used for impression management	• Awareness of importance of mutual and reciprocal emotional self-disclosure in making and maintaining friendships

Note: Adapted from Saarni (1999).

the expression of their needs for autonomy and exploration. This irritability is often referred to as the 'terrible twos'. In their second year, infants show increased verbal expression of emotional states and increased expression of emotions involving self-consciousness and self-evaluation such as shame, pride or coyness. This occurs because their cognitive skills allow them to begin to think about themselves from the perspective of others. In relationships they can increasingly anticipate feelings they will have towards others in particular situations. They show rudimentary empathy and altruistic behaviour.

Pre-schoolers

Pre-schoolers between the ages of two and five years increasingly use language for regulating emotions. They use both internal speech and conversations with others to modulate their affective experience. During this period, children increasingly pretend to express emotions in play when teasing or being teased by other children. There is increased insight into the emotions being experienced by others. During this period there is an increased awareness that we can mislead others about what we are feeling by falsely expressing emotions. More sophisticated empathy and altruistic behaviour also develops during the pre-school years.

Kindergarten

Children in kindergarten between the ages of five and seven years increasingly regulate emotions involving self-consciousness such as embarrassment. There is also increased autonomy from caregivers in regulating emotions. Children at this age present a 'cool' emotional front to peers. There is also an increased use of social skills to deal with emotions of self and others. During this period children develop an understanding of consensually agreed emotional scripts and their roles in such scripts.

Middle childhood

Children in middle childhood, between the ages of seven and ten years, prefer to autonomously regulate their emotional states rather than involving caregivers in this process, as they would have done earlier in their lives. Distancing strategies are used to manage emotions if children have little control over emotionally demanding situations. There is increased use of emotional expression to regulate closeness and distance within relationships. Children become aware that they can feel multiple conflicting emotions about the same person, that they can be angry with someone they like. They use information and memories about the emotions of self and others in multiple contexts as aids to making and maintaining friendships.

Pre-adolescence

During pre-adolescence, between the ages of ten and thirteen years, children show increased efficiency in using multiple strategies for autonomously regulating emotions and managing stress. They make distinctions between genuine emotional expression with close friends and managed emotional displays with others. They develop an increasingly sophisticated understanding of the place of social roles and emotional scripts in making and maintaining friendships.

Adolescence

During adolescence, from thirteen to twenty years, there is an increased awareness of complex emotional cycles, for example feeling guilty about feeling angry or feeling ashamed for feeling frightened. In adolescence, youngsters increasingly use complex strategies to autonomously regulate emotions. These self-regulation strategies are increasingly informed by moral principles, beliefs about what is right and good and what is wrong and evil. However, alongside this concern with morality, self-presentation strategies are increasingly used for impression management. Adolescents gradually become aware of the importance of mutual and reciprocal emotional self-disclosure in making and maintaining friendships.

Difficulties with the regulation of anger, fear and sadness may lead to referral to a clinical psychologist. Anger is the principal emotion associated with conduct disorder (discussed in Chapter 10). Anxiety and depression are discussed in Chapters 12 and 16 respectively.

Throughout middle childhood and up until adolescence, the awareness that actions may lead to approval or disapproval by parents and other important attachment figures leads to the internalization of standards of conduct (Kochanska, 1993). This process of internalizing standards permits the experience of complex emotions such as pride, shame and guilt. These emotions have particular implications for moral development.

Moral development

Research based on both Piaget's (1932) and Kohlberg's (Colby & Kohlberg, 1987) stage theories of moral development confirm that the basis on which children make moral judgements changes as they become older and more cognitively mature (Kagan & Lamb, 1987). Up until the age of five or six (during the pre-operational period) children evaluate the wrongness of an action in terms of the amount of damage it caused. Children at this age believe that apparently immoral acts may be carried out justifiably if there is no chance of detection and punishment. When children progress to the concrete operational period at about seven years they judge the wrongness of an action on the basis of both the amount of damage caused by the act and the actor's intentions. The morality of an act is judged against the degree to which the actor conformed to rules of good conduct. However, rules are seen as rigid and absolute rather than an arbitrary negotiated social contract. At about the age of ten, as they move into the period of formal operations, it is the actor's motives that is the primary criterion used to evaluate the wrongness of a particular action. Rules are seen as a basis for judging the morality of an act and these rules are seen as useful social conventions.

Children's concept of fairness in allocating rewards also evolves with increasing cognitive maturity. Up until about four, when children complete a team task they tend to keep the majority of the reward given to the team for themselves if they are given a team reward and asked to divide it. At five or six years they tend to give equal rewards to all team members and after seven years of age, they link rewards to output.

There are sex differences in reasoning about moral dilemmas. Males tend to base their judgements about the morality of an act on the degree to which it conforms to agreed societal rules, whereas females tend to view the moral course of action as that which fulfils their obligations within a personal relationship (Gilligan, 1982).

The capacity to make mature moral judgements does not necessarily imply that these judgements will find expression in moral conduct and prosocial behaviour, such as co-operation, sharing and helping. Moral behaviour appears to depend on the internalization of standards of good conduct (Kochanska, 1993). Optimal parenting conditions for internalizing standards and developing moral behaviour involves the following components (Hoffman, 1970):

- secure attachment between parents and children involving warmth and communication
- clear rules operationalizing moral standards
- consistent use of sanctions
- withdrawal of approval to provoke anxiety rather than physical punishment to provoke anger
- use of reasoning and explanation
- giving age-appropriate responsibility
- tolerance for self-expression.

The absence of these conditions, along with a variety of other factors, contributes to the development of conduct problems, which are discussed in Chapter 10.

Development of identity

Harter (1999) tackles the complex problem of personal identity by conceptualizing the functions of self-knowledge, self-evaluation and self-regulation as the three primary components of the self-system. Self-knowledge refers to all that the child knows about herself but particularly to autobiographical memory, which was referred to when we discussed information-processing models of intelligence. Self-knowledge also includes insights about how the child functions in her social world. Self-evaluation refers to the way in which the child judges herself against others and against herself at other developmental stages. Self-regulation refers to the capacity to persist in independent, focused goal-directed behaviour despite distractions posed by competing internal impulses or external stimuli.

Self-evaluation

Self-esteem, which incorporates self-evaluative opinions and related emotions, tend to be high in pre-schoolers and during the pre-adolescent years. At about twelve there is a drop in self-esteem and it then increases gradually over the course of adolescence (Harter, 1999). The drop in self-esteem may be due to the child evaluating the physical changes that accompany the transition to adolescence negatively. Alternatively, it may be a reflection of their increased capacity to imagine how others judge them: an ability that emerges in the formal operational period.

In addition to global self-evaluations, children make evaluations of the self within specific domains such as the family, the school or the peer group. These evaluations lead to domain-specific experiences of self-esteem such as parental self-esteem, social self-esteem or academic self-esteem. Self-report questionnaires such as the Battle (2002) Culture-free Self-esteem Inventory are useful for assessing domain specific self-esteem profiles. A ubiquitous finding in developmental psychopathology is the relationship between high self-esteem and positive adjustment (Carr, 2004a).

Self-regulation

The degree to which children can regulate their emotions and focus on solving specific problems in effective ways depends on their beliefs about their capacity to control their situation and the specific defence mechanisms and coping strategies that they have at their disposal. A discussion of self-regulatory beliefs systems and skills will be reserved for Chapter 2.

Self-knowledge

Self-recognition, a rudimentary form of self-knowledge, emerges at about two years when children recognize their reflection in a mirror. Self-recognition is associated with secure attachment and abused children show deficits in this area of self-knowledge (Cicchetti, 1991). Children who show self-recognition are more likely to help another child in distress. As children develop through Piagetian stages, their self-descriptions evolve in sophistication (Damon & Hart, 1988). Pre-operational children describe themselves in terms of physical characteristics, possessions and preferences. For example, 'I have blond hair, a scooter and like sausages'. Concrete operational children describe themselves in terms of class membership and personal traits. For example, 'I'm a member of Sutton Dinghy Club and I'm a good sailor'. More complex abstract or hypothetical self-descriptions are given by adolescents who have entered the formal operational period. 'I'm an idealist at heart but that doesn't mean I shouldn't be able to come up with a practical solution to any problem' is the type of self-description that typifies this period of cognitive development.

The particular issues about which important self-descriptions are made at different stages in the development of identity have been extensively described by Erikson (1968). Newman & Newman's (2003) modification of Erikson's model of psychosocial development is presented in Table 1.4. At each stage of social development, according to this model, the individual must face a personal dilemma. The way in which each dilemma is resolved influences the way in which individuals describe themselves, and the type of resolution that is reached is dependent on the youngster's social context. The main psychosocial dilemma to be resolved during the first two years of life is trust versus mistrust. If parents are responsive to infants' needs in a predictable and sensitive way, the infant develops a sense of trust. In the long term, this underpins a capacity to have hope in the face of adversity and to trust, as adults, that difficult challenges can be resolved. If the child does not experience the parent as a secure base from which to explore the world, the child learns to mistrust others and this underpins a view of the world as threatening. This may lead the child to adopt a detached position during later years and difficulties with making and maintaining peer relationships may occur.

The main psychosocial dilemma in the pre-school years is autonomy versus shame and doubt. During this period children become aware of their separateness and strive to establish a sense of personal agency and impose their will on the world. Of course, sometimes this is possible but at other times their parents will prohibit them from doing certain things. There is a gradual moving from the battles of the terrible twos to the ritual orderliness that many children show as they approach school-going age. Routines develop for going to bed or getting up, mealtimes and playtimes. The phrase 'I can do it myself' for tying shoelaces or doing their buttons is an example of their appropriate channelling of the desire to be autonomous. If parents patiently provide the framework for children to master tasks and routines, autonomy and a sense of self-esteem develop. As adults, such children are patient with themselves and have confidence in their abilities to master the challenges of life. They have high self-esteem and a strong sense of will and self-efficacy. If parents are unable to be patient with the child's evolving wilfulness and need for mastery, and criticize or humiliate failed attempts at mastery, the child will develop a sense of self-doubt and shame. The lack of patience and parental criticism will become internalized and children will evolve into adults who criticize themselves excessively and who lack confidence in their abilities. In some instances, this may lead to the compulsive need to repeat their efforts at problem solving so that they can undo the mess they have made and so cope with the shame of not succeeding.

At the beginning of the school-going years, the main psychosocial dilemma is initiative versus guilt. When children have developed a sense of autonomy in the pre-school years, they turn their attention outwards to the physical and social world and use their initiative to investigate and explore its

Table 1.4 Newman's revision of Erikson's psychosocial stage model

Stage	Dilemma and main process	Virtue and positive self-description	Pathology and negative self-description
Infancy 0–2 years	**Trust v. mistrust** Mutuality with caregiver	**Hope** I can attain my wishes	**Detachment** I will not trust others
Early childhood 2–4 years	**Autonomy v. shame and doubt** Imitation	**Will** I can control events	**Compulsion** I will repeat this act to undo the mess that I have made and I doubt that I can control events and I am ashamed of this
Middle childhood 4–6 years	**Initiative v. guilt** Identification	**Purpose** I can plan and achieve goals	**Inhibition** I can't plan or achieve goals so I don't act
Late childhood 7–11 years	**Industry v. inferiority** Education	**Competence** I can use skills to achieve goals	**Inertia** I have no skills so I won't try
Early adolescence 12–18 years	**Group identity v. alienation** Peer pressure	**Affiliation** I can be loyal to the group	**Isolation** I cannot be accepted into a group
Adolescence 19–22 years	**Identity v. role confusion** Role experimentation	**Fidelity** I can be true to my values	**Confusion** I don't know what my role is or what my values are
Young adulthood 23–34 years	**Intimacy v. isolation** Mutuality with peers	**Love** I can be intimate with another	**Exclusivity** I have no time for others so I will shut them out
Middle age 34–60 years	**Productivity v. stagnation** Person–environment fit and creativity	**Care** I am committed to making the world a better place	**Rejectivity** I do not care about the future of others, only my own future
Old age 60–75 years	**Integrity v. despair** Introspection	**Wisdom** I am committed to life but I know I will die soon	**Despair** I am disgusted at my frailty and my failures
Very old age 75–death	**Immortality v. extinction** Social support	**Confidence** I know that my life has meaning	**Diffidence** I can find no meaning in my life so I doubt that I can act

Note: Adapted from Erikson (1968) and Newman & Newman (2003).

regularities with a view to establishing a cognitive map of it. The child finds out what is allowed and what is not allowed at home and at school. Many questions about how the world works are asked. Children conduct various experiments and investigations, for example by lighting matches, taking toys apart, or playing doctors and nurses. The initiative versus guilt dilemma is resolved when the child learns how to channel the need for investigation into socially appropriate courses of action. This occurs when parents empathize with the child's curiosity but establish the limits of experimentation clearly and with warmth. Children who resolve the dilemma of initiative versus guilt, act with a sense of purpose and vision as adults. Where parents have difficulty empathizing with the child's need for curiosity and curtail experimentation unduly, children may develop a reluctance to explore untried options as adults because such curiosity arouses a sense of guilt.

At the close of middle childhood, and during the transition to adolescence, the main psychosocial dilemma is industry versus inferiority. Having established a sense of trust, of autonomy and of initiative, the child's need to develop skills and engage in meaningful work emerges. The motivation for industry may stem from the fact that learning new skills is intrinsically rewarding and many tasks and jobs open to the child may be rewarded. Children who have the aptitude to master skills that are rewarded by parents, teachers and peers emerge from this stage of development with new skills and a sense of competence and self-efficacy about these. Unfortunately, not all children have the aptitude for skills that are valued by society. So youngsters who have low aptitudes for literacy skills, sports and social conformity are disadvantaged from the start. This is compounded by the fact that Western culture makes social comparisons through, for example, streaming in schools and sports. In our society, failure is ridiculed. Youngsters who fail and are ridiculed or humiliated develop a sense of inferiority and in adulthood lack the motivation to achieve.

The young adolescent faces a dilemma of group identity versus alienation. There is a requirement to find a peer group with which to become affiliated so that the need for belonging will be met. Joining such a group, however, must not lead to sacrificing one's individuality and personal goals and aspirations. If young adolescents are not accepted by a peer group they will experience alienation. In the longer term, they may find themselves unaffiliated and have difficulty developing the social support networks that are particularly important for health and well-being. To achieve group identity, their parents and school need to avoid over-restriction of opportunities for making and maintaining peer relationship. This has to be balanced against the dangers of overpermissiveness, as lack of supervision is associated with conduct problems and drug dependence. While the concern of early adolescence is group membership and affiliation, the establishment of a clear sense of identity – that is, a sense of who I am – is the major concern in late adolescence.

Marcia (1981) has found that adolescents may achieve one of four identity states. With identity diffusion there is no firm commitment to personal, social, political or vocational beliefs or plans. Such individuals are either fun-seekers or people with adjustment difficulties and low self-esteem. With foreclosure, vocational, political or religious decisions are made for the adolescent by parents or elders in the community and are accepted without a prolonged decision-making process. These adolescents tend to adhere to authoritarian values. In cases where a moratorium is reached, the adolescent experiments with a number of roles before settling on an identity. Some of these roles may be negative (delinquent) or non-conventional (drop-out/ commune dweller). However, they are staging posts in a prolonged decision-making process on the way to a stable identity. Where adolescents achieve a clear identity following a successful moratorium, they develop a strong commitment to vocational, social, political and religious values and usually have good psychosocial adjustment in adulthood. They have high self-esteem, realistic goals, a stronger sense of independence and are more resilient in the face of stress. Where a sense of identity is achieved following a moratorium in which many roles have been explored, the adolescent avoids the problems of being aimless, as in the case of identity diffusion, or trapped, which may occur with foreclosure. Parents may find allowing adolescents the time and space to enter a moratorium before achieving a stable sense of identity difficult, and referral for psychological consultation may occur.

The major psychosocial dilemma for people who have left adolescence is whether to develop an intimate relationship with another or whether to move to an isolated position. People who do not achieve intimacy experience isolation. Isolated individuals have unique characteristics (Newman & Newman, 2003). Specifically, they overvalue social contact and suspect that all social encounters will end negatively. They also lack the social skills, such as empathy or affective self-disclosure, necessary for forming intimate relationships. These difficulties typically emerge from experiences of mistrust, shame, doubt, guilt, inferiority, alienation and role-confusion associated with failure to resolve earlier developmental dilemmas and crises in a positive manner. A variety of social and contextual forces contribute to isolation. Western culture's emphasis on individuality gives an enhanced sense of separateness and loneliness and our valuing of competitiveness (particularly among males) may deter people from engaging in self-disclosure. Men have been found to self-disclose less than women, to be more competitive in conversations and to show less empathy.

Parents of very young children referred for consultation may struggle with the dilemma of intimacy versus isolation and parents of older children often face the midlife dilemma of productivity versus stagnation. Parents who select and shape a home and work environment that fits with their needs and talents are more likely to resolve this dilemma by becoming productive. Productivity may involve procreation, work-based productivity or artistic creativity. Those who become productive focus their energy into making the world a better place for further generations. Those who fail to select and shape their environment to meet their needs and talents may become overwhelmed with stress and become burnt out, depressed or cynical on the one hand, or greedy and narcissistic on the other.

In later adulthood the dilemma faced is integrity versus despair and this issue is often of concern to grandparents of children referred for psychological consultation. A sense of personal integrity is achieved by those who accept the events that make up their lives and integrate these into a meaningful personal narrative in a way that allows them to face death without fear. Those who avoid this introspective process, or who engage in it and find that they cannot accept the events of their lives or integrate them into a meaningful personal narrative that allows them to face death without fear, develop a sense of despair. The process of integrating failures, disappointments, conflicts, growing incompetencies and frailty into a coherent life story is very challenging and is difficult to do unless the first psychosocial crisis of trust versus mistrust was resolved in favour of trust. The positive resolution of this dilemma in favour of integrity rather than despair leads to the development of a capacity for wisdom. In the final months of life the dilemma faced by the very old is immortality versus extinction. A sense of immortality can be achieved by living on through one's children, through a belief in an afterlife, by the permanence of one's achievements (either material monuments or the way one has influenced others), by viewing the self as being part of the chain of nature (the decomposed body becomes part of the earth that brings forth new life) or by achieving a sense of experiential transcendence (a mystical sense of continual presence). When a sense of immortality is achieved, the acceptance of death and the enjoyment of life, despite frailty, becomes possible. This is greatly facilitated when people have good social support networks to help them deal with frailty, growing incompetence and the possibility of isolation. Those who lack social support and have failed to integrate their lives into a meaningful story may fear extinction and find no way to accept their physical mortality while at the same time evolving a sense of immortality.

Erikson's model has received some support from a major longitudinal study (Valliant, 1977). However, it appears that the stages do not always occur in the stated order and often later life events can lead to changes in the way in which psychosocial dilemmas are resolved.

Sex-role development

One particularly important facet of identity is the sex role (Vasta et al., 2003). From birth to five, children go through a process of learning the concept of gender. They first distinguish between the sexes and categorize themselves as male or female. Then they realize that gender is stable and does not change from day to day. Finally, they realize that there are critical differences (such as genitals) and incidental differences (such as clothing) that have no effect on gender. It is probable that during this period they develop gender scripts, which are representations of the routines associated with their gender roles. On the basis of these scripts they develop gender schemas, which are cognitive structures used to organize information about the categories male and female (Levy & Fivush, 1993).

Extensive research has shown that in Western culture, sex-role toy preferences, play, peer-group behaviour and cognitive development are different for boys and girls (Serbin, Powlishta & Gulko, 1993). Boys prefer trucks and guns; girls prefer dolls and dishes. Boys do more outdoor play with more rough and tumble, and less relationship-oriented speech. They pretend to fulfil adult male roles such as warriors, heroes and firemen. Girls show more nurturent play involving much relationship conversation and pretend to fulfil stereotypic adult female roles such as homemakers. As children approach the age of five they are less likely to engage in play that is outside their sex role. A tolerance for cross-gender play evolves in middle childhood and diminishes again at adolescence. Boys play in larger groups whereas girls tend to limit their group size to two or three.

There are some well-established gender differences in the abilities of boys and girls (Halpern, 2000). Girls show more rapid language development than boys and earlier competence at maths. In adolescence, boys' competence in maths exceeds that of girls and their language differences even out. Males perform better on spatial tasks than girls throughout their lives.

Although an adequate explanation for gender differences on cognitive tasks cannot be given, it is clear that sex-role behaviour is influenced by parental treatment of children (differential expectations and reinforcement) and by children's response to parents (identification and imitation) (Serbin et al., 1993). Numerous studies show that parents expect different sex-role behaviour from their children and reward children for engaging in these behaviours. Boys are encouraged to be competitive and activity oriented. Girls are encouraged to be co-operative and relationship oriented. A problem with traditional sex roles in adulthood is that they have the potential to lead to a power imbalance within marriage, an increase in marital dissatisfaction, a sense of isolation in both partners and a decrease in father involvement in childcare tasks (Gelles, 1995).

However, rigid sex roles are now being challenged and the ideal of androgyny is gaining in popularity. The androgynous youngster develops both male and female role-specific skills. Gender stereotyping is less marked in families where parental behaviour is less sex-typed, where both parents work outside the home and in single-parent families. Gender stereotyping is also less marked in families with high socioeconomic status (Vasta et al., 2003).

Gay and lesbian identity formation

For gay and lesbian adolescents, self-definition and 'coming out' are two significant transitional processes (Laird & Green, 1996). The first process – self-definition as a gay or lesbian person – occurs initially in response to experiences of being different or estranged from same-sex heterosexual peers and later in response to attraction to and/or intimacy with peers of the same gender. The adolescent typically faces a dilemma of whether to accept or deny the homoerotic feelings he or she experiences. The way in which this dilemma is resolved is in part influenced by the perceived risks and benefits of denial and acceptance. Where adolescents feel that homophobic attitudes within their families, peer groups and society will have severe negative consequences for them, they may be reluctant to accept their gay or lesbian identities. Attempts to deny homoerotic experiences and adopt a heterosexual identity may lead to a wide variety of psychological difficulties including depression, substance abuse, running away and suicide attempts, all of which may become a focus for therapy. By contrast, where the family and society are supportive and tolerant of diverse sexual orientations, and where there is an easily accessible supportive gay or lesbian community, then the benefits of accepting a gay or lesbian identity may outweigh the risks, and the adolescent may begin to form a gay or lesbian self-definition. Once the process of self-definition as gay or lesbian occurs, the possibility of 'coming out' to others is opened up. This process of coming out involves coming out to other lesbian and gay people, to heterosexual peers and to members of the family. The more supportive the responses of members of these three systems, the better the adjustment of the individual.

In response to the process of 'coming out', families undergo a process of destabilization. They progress from subliminal awareness of the young person's sexual orientation, to absorbing the impact of this realization and adjusting to it. Resolution and integration of the reality of the youngster's sexual identity into the family belief system depends on the flexibility of the family system, the degree of family cohesion and the capacity of core themes within the family belief system to be reconciled with the youngster's sexual identity. Therapy conducted within this frame of reference aims to facilitate the processes of owning homoerotic experiences, establishing a gay or lesbian identity and mobilizing support within the family, heterosexual peer group and gay or lesbian peer group for the individual.

Peer group

Research on the development of friendships and peer-group behaviour has led to a number of findings of relevance to the practice of clinical psychology (Dunn & McGuire, 1992; Malik & Furman, 1993; Williams & Gilmore, 1994). Over the first five years, with increasing opportunities for interaction with others and the development of language, interaction with other children increases. Co-operative play premised on an empathic understanding of other children's viewpoints gradually emerges and is usually fully established by middle childhood. Competitive rivalry (often involving physical or verbal aggression or joking) is an important part of peer interactions, particularly among boys. This allows youngsters to establish their position of dominance within the peer-group hierarchy. It has already been mentioned that there are important sex differences in styles of play adopted, with girls being more co-operative and relationship focused and boys being more competitive and activity focused. Boys tend to play in larger peer groups whereas girls tend to play within small groups characterized by emotionally intimate, exclusive friendships. Sex-segregated play is almost universal in middle childhood.

Peer friendships are important because they constitute an important source of social support and a context within which to learn about the management of networks of relationships. Children who are unable to make and maintain friendships, particularly during middle childhood and early adolescence, are at risk for the development of psychological difficulties. Children who have developed secure attachments to their parents are more likely to develop good peer friendships. This is probably because their experience with their parents provides them with a useful cognitive model on which to base their interactions with their peers. Children reared in institutions have particular difficulty with peer relationships in their teens.

At all developmental stages, popular children are described by their peers as helpful, friendly, considerate and capable of following rules in games and imaginative play. They also tend to be more intelligent and physically attractive than average. They accurately interpret social situations and have the social skills necessary for engaging in peer-group activities. About 10–15% of children are rejected by their peer group. In middle childhood two main types of unpopular child may be distinguished: the aggressive youngster and the victim. Victims tend to be sensitive, anxious, have low self-esteem and lack the skills required to defend themselves and establish dominance within the peer-group hierarchy; they are often the targets for bullies (Olweus, 1993). Unpopular aggressive children are described by peers as disruptive, hyperactive, impulsive and unable to follow rules in games and play. Their aggression tends to be used less for establishing dominance or a hierarchical position in the peer group and more for achieving certain instrumental goals. For example, taking a toy from another child.

Popular children are effective in joining in peer-group activities. They hover on the edge, tune-in to the group's activities and carefully select a time to become integrated into the group's activities. Unpopular children, particularly the aggressive type, do not tune-in to group activities. They tend to criticize other children and talk about themselves rather than listening to others. Warmth, a sense of humour and sensitivity to social cues are important features of socially skilled children. Unpopular children, particularly the aggressive type, are predisposed to interpreting ambiguous social cues negatively and becoming involved in escalating spirals of negative social interaction.

Unpopularity is relatively stable over time. A child who is unpopular this year is likely to remain so next year and this unpopularity is not wholly based on reputation. For the aggressive unpopular child, inadequate cognitive models for relationships, difficulties in interpreting ambiguous social situations and poor social skills appear to be the main factors underpinning this stability of unpopularity. For the unpopular victim the continued unpopularity is probably mediated by low self-esteem, avoidance of opportunities for social interaction and a lack of pro-social skills. Also, both types of unpopular children miss out on important opportunities for learning about co-operation, team work and the management of networks of friendships. Although unpopularity is not uniformly associated with long-term difficulties, it appears to put such youngsters at risk for developing academic problems, dropping out of school, conduct problems in adolescence, mental health problems in adulthood and criminality.

Unpopular children may benefit from social skills training. The central features of effective social skills programmes have been described by Malik and Furman (1993). First, they are offered in a group format, which has the advantage of providing participants with a ready-made social laboratory within which to rehearse and obtain feedback on the skills learned. Second, successful programmes focus on broad social competencies such as listening skills, self-disclosing skills, turn-taking and handling teasing rather than discrete behavioural skills such as maintaining eye contact. Third, it has also been found that effective social skills programmes for unpopular aggressive children include anger-management training. Here youngsters learn to interpret ambiguous social situations in less threatening ways and to manage their aggressive impulses in ways that do not lead to escalating violent exchanges. Programmes that require unpopular children and their natural peer group at school to engage co-operatively in structured games or activities have been found to decrease unpopularity and so may supplement the benefits of social skills training, by creating opportunities within which newly acquired social skills may be deployed.

Effective bullying-prevention programmes address some of the problems faced by unpopular victims and unpopular aggressive bullies (McCarthy & Carr, 2002). Olweus's (1993) approach, described in *Bullying at school – what we know and what we can do*, is a particularly good example of such a programme. The approach aims to create a social context in which adults (school staff and parents) show positive interest and warmth towards pupils and use consistent non-aggressive sanctions for aggressive behaviour in a highly consistent way. The programme involves a high level of surveillance of children's activities and a high level of communication between parents and teachers.

SUMMARY

Child development, with its physical, cognitive and social facets, occurs within the context of the family lifecycle. The family lifecycle can be conceptualized as a series of stages, each characterized by a set of tasks family members must complete to progress to the next stage. With respect to physical development, children progress through an ordered sequence of milestones. Environmental factors such as socioeconomic status and nutrition, in addition to genetic factors, can alter the rate of progression through these milestones and this may have consequences for social adjustment. For example, at adolescence, early-maturing girls show adjustment problems whereas early-maturing boys do not.

Three different approaches have been taken to the study of cognitive development. Piaget's stage-based cognitive developmental theory shows how problem solving at different stages of development is based on different representational cognitive structures. The information-processing approach to cognition highlights the way different strategies are used to solve problems so that the output of a limited information-processing capacity is maximised. The psychometric approach to intelligence focuses on how abilities are organized and how individual differences in these abilities are distributed within populations.

A minimum level of cognitive development is essential for language acquisition but once this level is reached language and cognition develop relatively independently. While language acquisition depends in part on a genetically furnished physiological substrate, finely tuned social interaction is the critical environmental condition for its optimal linguistic development.

Various aspects of social development, such as the development of emotional competence, morality, identity, sex-role and peer relationships are all paced to some degree by the cognitive development of the child. Complex emotions like embarrassment, moral judgements based on abstract principles, sophisticated self-knowledge and self-regulatory strategies all require cognitive maturity. However, moral conduct is relatively independent of advanced moral reasoning capabilities and is determined in large part by an authoritative parenting style. Adaptive peer relations depend to a large degree on the prior experience of secure attachment. The functions of self-knowledge, self-evaluation and self-regulation are the three primary components of the self-system. Accurate self-knowledge, high self-esteem, and self-regulatory beliefs, defences and coping strategies all contribute to positive adjustment.

EXERCISE 1.1

Work in pairs. One person take the role of interviewer and the other take the role of interviewee. The interviewer should take twenty minutes to ask the interviewee about their physical, cognitive and social development within the overall context of their family's lifecycle:

- List the particular events that the interviewee says stand out in his or her memory about his or her physical and intellectual growth.
- Specify how particular physical and intellectual strengths have helped the interviewee's social development.
- Specify how the interviewee resolved the various psychosocial dilemmas listed in Table 1.4.
- Specify if the interviewee was socialized into a traditional or a non-traditional sex role.
- Specify any special role peers played in the interviewee's development.
- List any unusual events that have happened within the family lifecycle to affect the interviewee's development.

The interviewer should then check the accuracy of his or her conclusions with the interviewee. Reverse roles and repeat the exercise.

FURTHER READING

Carter, B. & McGoldrick, M. (1999). *The Expanded Family Lifecycle. Individual, Family and Social Perspectives* (Third Edition). Boston: Allyn & Bacon.
Smith, P., Cowie, H. & Blades, M. (2003). *Understanding Children's Development* (Fourth Edition). Oxford: Blackwell.

WEBSITES

Developmental psychology websites

APA Division 7: Developmental Psychology http://classweb.gmu.edu/awinsler/div7/links.shtml
Online developmental psychology library: http://www.questia.com

Psychological association websites

American Psychological Association: http://www.apa.org
Australian Psychological Society: http://www.aps.psychsociety.com.au/
British Psychological Society: http://www.bps.org.uk/
Canadian Psychological Association: http://www.cpa.ca/

European Federation of Psychologist's Associations (EFPA): http://www.efpa.be/
International Union of Psychological Science (IUPsyS): http://www.iupsys.org/
New Zealand Psychological Society: http://www.psychology.org.nz/
Psychological Society of Ireland: http://www.psihq.ie/
World Health Organization: http://www.who.int/en/

Chapter 2

Influences on problem development

The development of psychological problems in children and adolescents is influenced by many factors. A distinction may be made between risk factors that pre-dispose children to developing psychological problems, precipitating factors that trigger the onset or marked exacerbation of psychological difficulties, maintaining factors that perpetuate psychological problems once they have developed, and protective factors that prevent further deterioration and have implications for prognosis and response to treatment. Pre-disposing risk factors, protective factors and maintaining factors may be subclassified as falling into the personal or contextual domains, with personal factors referring to biological and psychological characteristics of the child and contextual factors referring to features of the child's psychosocial environment including the family, the school, the peer group and involved treatment agencies. A framework within which some of the more important variables in each these categories are classified is presented in Figure 2.1. This chapter describes the variables listed in this framework.

PERSONAL PRE-DISPOSING FACTORS

Genetic vulnerabilities, the consequences of pre-natal and peri-natal complications and the sequelae of early insults, injuries and illnesses may pre-dispose youngsters to developing problems in later life (McGuffin, Owen & Gottesman, 2002; Rutter & Casaer, 1991). In addition to these biological pre-disposing factors, a number of psychological characteristics, traits and relatively enduring belief systems may also pre-dispose youngsters to developing psychological difficulties. Low intelligence, difficult temperament, low self-esteem and an external locus of control are some of the more important variables in this category (Luthar, 2003). These biological and psychological pre-disposing factors are addressed in the following sections.

Genetic factors

Twin and adoption studies show that the development of many psychological characteristics, such as temperament and intelligence, is in part influenced by genetic factors (Deary, 2000; Matthews, Deary & Whiteman, 2003; McGuffin et al., 2002). The size of this influence is of the order of 30–60% of overall variation within a population for most such characteristics. The mechanism of influence is usually polygenetic. With the possible exceptions of conditions such as autism, Down syndrome and bipolar affective disorder, genetic factors determine the development of specific psychological problems through their influence on broader psychological characteristics such as temperament. Current evidence does not support the view that childhood psychological problems are unalterably genetically determined.

Pre-natal and peri-natal complications

The intrauterine environment may contain hazards that compromise the healthy development of the fetus (Rutter & Casaer, 1991). Maternal age, blood-type incompatibility, malnutrition, smoking, alcohol use and drug use are among the factors that may negatively impact on the intrauterine environment. For example, the progeny of women who abuse alcohol while pregnant may develop *fetal alcohol syndrome*, a condition characterized by microcephaly, mental handicap and craniofacial anomalies (Steinhausen, Williams & Spohr, 1994). Infections such as rubella, syphilis and AIDS may also be transmitted from the mother to the fetus. Often, infants who have developed in a hazardous intrauterine environment have *low birth weight* (less than 4.5 lbs or 2000 grammes) or their size in relation to their gestation period is sufficiently below average to be described clinically as *small-for-dates*. In comparison with brain damage in later life, pre-natal brain damage is less likely to result in specific deficits and more likely to result in a general lowering of academic and intellectual abilities because specialization of function does not occur until later in the development of the central nervous system.

Peri-natal brain insults associated with anoxia or cortical tissue damage can lead to later cognitive impairment. Various birth complications are associated with such neurological damage, including forceps delivery, breech delivery (where the head is last to emerge), a difficult passage through the birth canal and accidental twisting of the umbilical cord. The infant's post-natal medical status is typically expressed as an Apgar score. Apgar scores range from 0 to 10, with scores below 4 reflecting sufficient difficulties to warrant intensive care. The score is based on an evaluation of the infant's skin colour (with blue suggesting anoxia), respiration, heart rate, respiration, muscle tone and response to stimulation.

Premature infants are particularly susceptible to brain injury during birth.

PRE-DISPOSING FACTORS

PERSONAL PRE-DISPOSING FACTORS

Biological factors
- Genetic vulnerabilities
- Pre- and peri-natal complications
- Early insults, injuries and illnesses

Psychological factors
- Low intelligence
- Difficult temperament
- Low self-esteem
- External locus of control

CONTEXTUAL PRE-DISPOSING FACTORS

Parent–child factors in early life
- Attachment problems
- Lack of intellectual stimulation
- Authoritarian parenting
- Permissive parenting
- Neglectful parenting
- Inconsistent parental discipline

Exposure to family problems in early life
- Parental psychological problems
- Parental alcohol and substance abuse
- Parental criminality
- Marital discord or violence
- Family disorganization
- Deviant siblings

Stresses in early life
- Bereavements
- Separations
- Child abuse
- Social disadvantage
- Institutional upbringing

PERSONAL MAINTAINING FACTORS

Biological factors
- Dysregulation of various physiological systems

Psychological factors
- Low self-efficacy
- Dysfunctional attributional style
- Negative cognitive distortions
- Immature defence mechanisms
- Dysfunctional coping strategies

PERSONAL PROTECTIVE FACTORS

Biological factors
- Good physical health

Psychological factors
- High IQ
- Easy temperament
- High self-esteem
- Internal locus of control
- High self-efficacy
- Optimistic attributional style

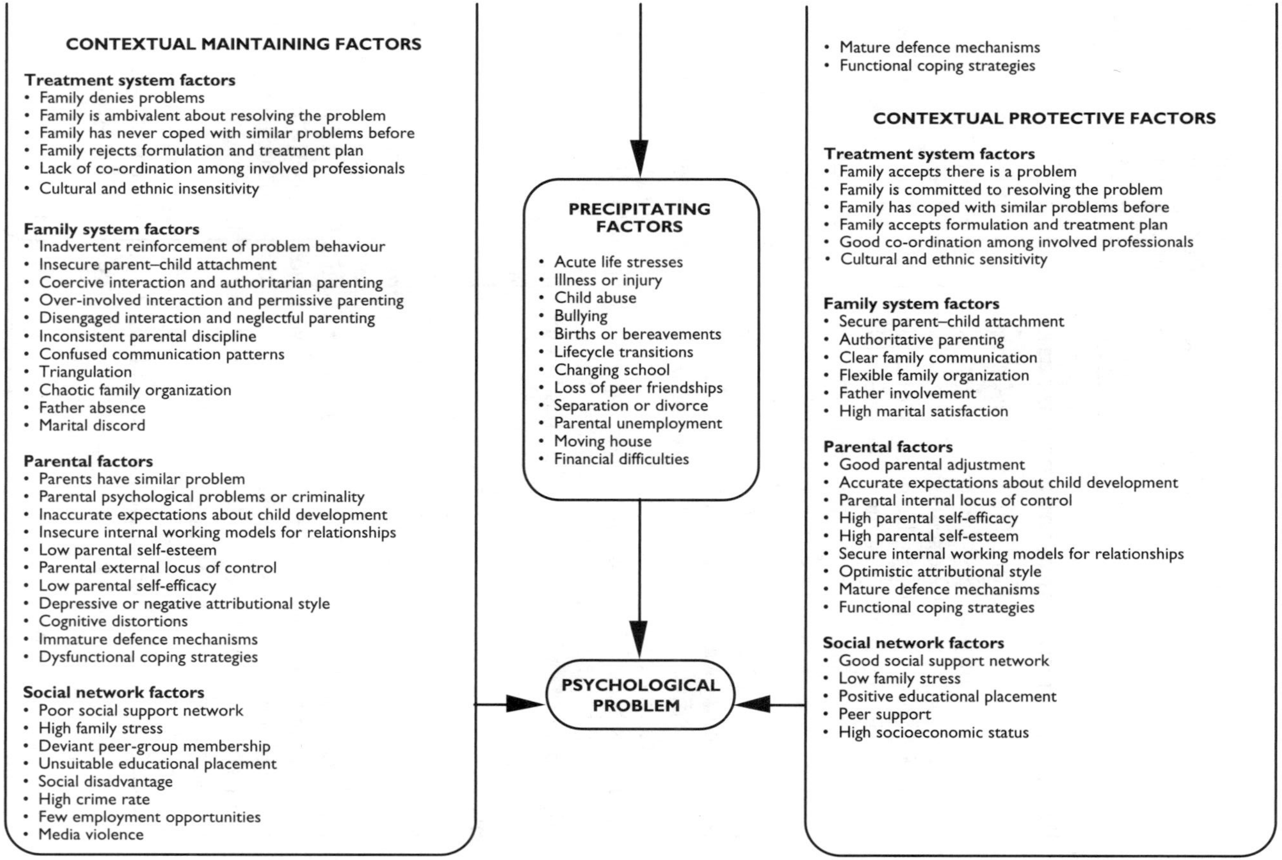

CONTEXTUAL MAINTAINING FACTORS

Treatment system factors
- Family denies problems
- Family is ambivalent about resolving the problem
- Family has never coped with similar problems before
- Family rejects formulation and treatment plan
- Lack of co-ordination among involved professionals
- Cultural and ethnic insensitivity

Family system factors
- Inadvertent reinforcement of problem behaviour
- Insecure parent–child attachment
- Coercive interaction and authoritarian parenting
- Over-involved interaction and permissive parenting
- Disengaged interaction and neglectful parenting
- Inconsistent parental discipline
- Confused communication patterns
- Triangulation
- Chaotic family organization
- Father absence
- Marital discord

Parental factors
- Parents have similar problem
- Parental psychological problems or criminality
- Inaccurate expectations about child development
- Insecure internal working models for relationships
- Low parental self-esteem
- Parental external locus of control
- Low parental self-efficacy
- Depressive or negative attributional style
- Cognitive distortions
- Immature defence mechanisms
- Dysfunctional coping strategies

Social network factors
- Poor social support network
- High family stress
- Deviant peer-group membership
- Unsuitable educational placement
- Social disadvantage
- High crime rate
- Few employment opportunities
- Media violence

PRECIPITATING FACTORS
- Acute life stresses
- Illness or injury
- Child abuse
- Bullying
- Births or bereavements
- Lifecycle transitions
- Changing school
- Loss of peer friendships
- Separation or divorce
- Parental unemployment
- Moving house
- Financial difficulties

PSYCHOLOGICAL PROBLEM

- Mature defence mechanisms
- Functional coping strategies

CONTEXTUAL PROTECTIVE FACTORS

Treatment system factors
- Family accepts there is a problem
- Family is committed to resolving the problem
- Family has coped with similar problems before
- Family accepts formulation and treatment plan
- Good co-ordination among involved professionals
- Cultural and ethnic sensitivity

Family system factors
- Secure parent–child attachment
- Authoritative parenting
- Clear family communication
- Flexible family organization
- Father involvement
- High marital satisfaction

Parental factors
- Good parental adjustment
- Accurate expectations about child development
- Parental internal locus of control
- High parental self-efficacy
- High parental self-esteem
- Secure internal working models for relationships
- Optimistic attributional style
- Mature defence mechanisms
- Functional coping strategies

Social network factors
- Good social support network
- Low family stress
- Positive educational placement
- Peer support
- High socioeconomic status

Figure 2.1 Pre-disposing, precipitating, maintaining and protective factors for psychological problems of children and adolescents

The skull of the premature infant, because it is not sufficiently developed, does not provide the protection offered by that of the full-term infant. Neurological damage sustained during the peri-natal period by premature infants is most commonly associated in later life with attention problems and hyperactivity (Goodman, 2002). While most premature infants suffer some developmental delay, with adequate medical care, maternal care and stimulation, they catch up with their full-term counterparts before starting school.

Physical insults, injuries and diseases

Head injuries later in childhood are associated with the development of cognitive impairment, disinhibition and behavioural problems, although the nature and extent of these sequelae depend on both the severity and location of the injury and the social context within which the injury and recovery occur (Goodman, 2002; Snow & Hooper, 1994). For example, the overall psychological consequences for a child who sustains a head injury as a result of abuse which leads to a multiplacement experience will be quite different from that of a child who sustains a similar injury through a road traffic accident and who recovers within a stable family context. A fuller discussion of head injury will be presented in Chapter 8.

Chronic diseases such as asthma or diabetes, and life-threatening illnesses such as cancer or cystic fibrosis, will all impact on psychological adjustment insofar as they are biopsychosocial stresses which place chronic demands on the child and family (Roberts, 2003). Chapters 14 and 24 discuss the adjustment of children and their families to such conditions.

Temperament

In their 25-year longitudinal study of 133 children, Chess and Thomas (1995) classified infants into three sub-groups. *Easy-temperament children* constituted 40% of the sample. They established regular patterns for feeding, toileting and sleeping. They approached new situations and adapted easily to such environmental changes while showing positive mood responses of mild or moderate intensity. Easy-temperament children had a good prognosis. They attracted adults and peers to form a supportive network around them. Easy temperament is therefore a protective factor.

Difficult-temperament children constituted 10% of the group studied. They had difficulty establishing regular routines for eating, toileting and sleeping. They tended to avoid new situations and responded to change with intense negative emotions. Difficult-temperament children were found to be at risk for developing psychological difficulties. This finding has been replicated in a number of other subsequent studies (Chess & Thomas, 1995). Thomas and Chess found that difficult-temperament children had more conflict with parents, peers and teachers. They elicited negative reactions from caretakers and tended to choose a peer group later in life that engaged in deviant, risky activities. They also developed more conduct and adjustment problems. Difficult-temperament children adjust better when there is a *goodness-of-fit* between their temperament and parental expectations. Difficult-temperament children need tolerant, responsive parents.

Fifteen per cent of Thomas and Chess's sample were classified as *slow to warm up* and showed mild negative emotional responses to new situations. After repeated contact, adaptation occurred. These children were also characterized by moderate levels of regularity in feeding, toileting and sleeping. The prognosis for this group was halfway between that of the easy and difficult temperament groups. The remainder of the sample were not classifiable into one of these three categories.

Using a different framework, Kagan has classified children into those with inhibited and uninhibited temperaments. About one in six children may be classified as having inhibited temperament. Such children are shy, timid and withdrawn in new situations (Kagan, Reznick & Gibbons, 1989). A higher proportion of youngsters with an inhibited temperamental style have parents with anxiety and mood disorders. It is therefore probable that this temperamental style is a risk factor for anxiety and mood disorders in childhood.

Intelligence, self-esteem and locus of control

A number of personal psychological characteristics, which have been discussed in Chapter 1, have been found to pre-dispose children to developing psychological difficulties (Friedman & Chase-Lansdale, 2002; Haggerty, Sherrod, Garmezy & Rutter, 1994; Luthar, 2003; Rutter, 2002a). Low intelligence, as measured by IQ tests, is a risk factor for conduct disorders in particular. Low self-esteem places children at risk for both conduct and emotional disorders. Entrenched beliefs about having little control over important sources or reinforcement and significant aspects of one's situation are also associated with conduct and emotional problems. Such beliefs are reflected in an external locus of control (Rotter, 1966).

PERSONAL MAINTAINING FACTORS

Once psychological problems have developed, they may be maintained, at a personal level, by both psychological and biological factors. Beliefs about self-regulation and self-regulatory skills are important psychological maintaining factors. In particular youngsters' psychological problems may be maintained by self-efficacy beliefs, dysfunctional attributions, cognitive distortions; immature defence mechanisms and dysfunctional coping strategies (Abramson, Seligman & Teasdale, 1978; Bandura, 1997; Conte & Pultchik, 1995; Friedberg & McClure, 2002; Stallard, 2002; Zeider & Endler, 1996).

Self-regulatory beliefs

When children are successful at completing a task and when they attribute their successes to their abilities, they develop a sense of self-efficacy (Bandura, 1997). That is, a belief that they will be effective at similar tasks in the future. High levels of self-efficacy are associated with more effective task completion, but children with low self-efficacy tend not to persist in trying to solve their problems and so low self-efficacy may maintain psychological difficulties.

When youngsters fail at academic, social or chronic illness management tasks and receive feedback from their parents or teachers that their failure was due to lack of ability or an uncontrollable disease process (rather than effort), they develop a sense of learned helplessness and a depressive attributional style. That is, a belief that no matter how hard they try they can never succeed, and a tendency to attribute failure to internal, global, stable factors such as lack of ability or physiological factors beyond their control. In contrast, successes are attributed to external, specific and transient factors such as luck (Abramson et al., 1978). Such a depressive attributional style may lead to inactivity, which may maintain psychological problems, particularly low mood, school failure and lack of adherence to medical regimes.

School-based learned helplessness does not usually appear until middle childhood and is more common in girls than boys. Fortunately, it is reversible if learning tasks are carefully matched to the child's ability level, if positive feedback is given for all successes and corrective feedback attributes errors to effort rather than ability (Dweck, 1975).

The opposite to learned helplessness is learned optimism and is under-pinned by an attributional style where successes are attributed to internal, global, stable factors (such as ability or skill) and failures to external, specific and unstable factors such as chance. Learned optimism is associated with better adjustment (Carr, 2004a).

Where parents inconsistently and unpredictably use verbal or physical aggression to discipline children, these youngsters learn to expect unpredictable aggression (like that shown by their parents) from others, unless there are very clear indications to suggest otherwise (Crick & Dodge, 1994). That is, these youngsters attribute hostile intentions to others, especially where their behaviour is ambiguous. This hostile attributional bias leads to provocative behaviour, which in turn engenders retaliation or rejection. In this way a dysfunctional hostile attributional bias may maintain persistent problems in regulating aggression.

A variety of other cognitive distortions (other than depressive attributional style or hostile attributional bias), which entail problematic interpretations of situations, may maintain youngsters' problems (Friedberg & McClure, 2002; Stallard, 2002). For example, cognitive distortions which highlight the threat potential of situations may maintain anxiety.

Defence mechanisms

Defence mechanisms are used to regulate the negative emotional states that accompany conflict (Conte & Plutchik, 1995). Conflict usually arises when a person wishes to pursue one course of action but fears the consequences of doing so. These consequences may be negative external events, such as the angry reactions of parents, or internal events, such as the experience of guilt. For example, a youngster who is angry at his mother may wish to express his anger directly but fear the mother's retaliation or the personal experience of guilt. If he uses the primitive defence mechanism of passive aggression he may regulate the negative emotions associated with this conflict by agreeing to do certain household chores but doing them slowly or inefficiently. If he uses a neurotic defence mechanism, he may deal with the conflict by displacing his anger onto siblings and fighting with them. If he uses a mature defence mechanism like sublimation, he may play football after doing chores to physically release the tension associated with the negative emotional state.

Appendix B of *DSM IV TR* (American Psychiatric Association, 2000a) presents a defensive functioning scale that organizes defence mechanisms into seven levels. This scale is summarized in Table 2.1. On this scale, less adaptive or immature defences have greater potential to maintain psychological problems than more mature defences. At the action level, conflict-related negative affect is regulated by expressing it through behaviour, be it aggressive or promiscuous sexual behaviour or social withdrawal. Where major image distortion is used to regulate negative affect associated with conflict, splitting is the prototypical defence. Here, negative affect is regulated by viewing some people as 'all bad' and directing all unacceptable aggressive impulses towards them. Concurrently, a subset of people are viewed as 'all good' and revered for this. Traditionally, these defences are referred to as borderline since they typify the borderline personality. At the next level, negative affect associated with conflict between unacceptable impulses and pro-social wishes is regulated by disavowal through denial, projection or rationalization. Minor image distortion of the self or others, through devaluation, idealization or omnipotence occurs at the next level. Defences at this level regulate self-esteem by enhancing or exaggerating positive aspects of the image of the self and one's allies and exaggerating negative attributes of others. Traditionally, these defences are referred to as narcissistic since they typify the narcissistic personality. At the next level – the level of mental inhibitions or compromise formation – defences regulate negative affect by keeping unacceptable wishes out of consciousness. Of these, repression is the prototypical defence. Other defences at this level include displacement, dissociation, intellectualisation, isolation of affect, reaction formation and undoing. At the adaptive level defences regulate negative affect by allowing a balance to be achieved between unacceptable impulses and pro-social

Table 2.1 Defence mechanisms at different levels of maturity

Level	Features of defences	Defence	The individual regulates emotional discomfort associated with conflicting wishes and impulses or external stress by . . .
High adaptive level	Promote an optimal balance among unacceptable impulses and pro-social wishes to maximize gratification and permit conscious awareness of conflicting impulses and wishes	**Anticipation**	considering emotional reactions and consequences of these before the conflict or stress occurs and exploring the pros and cons of various solutions to these problematic emotional states
		Affiliation	seeking social support from others, sharing problems with them without making them responsible for them or for relieving the distress they entail
		Altruism	dedication to meeting the needs of others and receiving gratification from this (without excessive self-sacrificing)
		Humour	reframing the situation which gives rise to conflict or stress in an ironic or amusing way
		Self-assertion	expressing conflict-related thoughts or feelings in a direct yet non-coercive way
		Self-observation	monitoring how situations lead to conflict or stress and using this new understanding to modify negative affect
		Sublimation	channelling negative emotions arising from conflict or stress into socially acceptable activities such as work or sports
		Suppression	intentionally avoiding thinking about conflict or stress

Mental inhibitions compromise formation level	Keep unacceptable impulses, out of awareness	**Displacement**	transferring negative feelings about one person onto another less threatening person
		Dissociation	experiencing a breakdown in the integrated functions of consciousness, memory, perception or motor behaviour
		Intellectualization	the excessive use of abstract thinking or generalizations to minimise disturbing feelings arising from conflict
		Isolation of affect	losing touch with the feelings associated with descriptive details of the conflict, trauma or stress
		Reaction formation	substituting acceptable behaviours, thoughts or feelings which are the opposite of unacceptable or unwanted behaviours thoughts or feelings that arise from a conflict
		Repression	expelling unwanted thoughts, emotions or wishes from awareness
		undoing	using ritualistic or magical words or behaviour to symbolically negate or make amends for unacceptable impulses
Minor image distorting level	Distort image of self and others to regulate self-esteem	**Devaluation**	attributing exaggerated negative characteristic to the self or others
		Idealization	attributing exaggerated positive characteristics to the others

Continued

Table 2.1 Continued

Level	Features of defences	Defence	The individual regulates emotional discomfort associated with conflicting wishes and impulses or external stress by . . .
		Omnipotence	attributing exaggerated positive characteristics or special abilities and powers to the self which make oneself superior to others
Disavowal level	Keep unacceptable impulses and ideas out of consciousness with or without misattribution of these to external causes	**Denial**	refusing to acknowledge the painful features of the situation or experiences which are apparent to others
		Projection	attributing to others one's own unacceptable thoughts, feelings and wishes
		Rationalization	providing an elaborate self-serving or self-justifying explanation to conceal unacceptable thoughts, actions or impulses
Major image distorting level	Gross distortion or misattribution of aspects of the self or others	**Autistic fantasy**	engaging in excessive daydreaming or wishful thinking as a substitute for using problem solving or social support to deal with emotional distress
		Projective identification	attributing to others one's own unacceptable aggressive impulses. Then inducing others to feel these by reacting aggressively to them. Then using the other person's aggressive reactions as justification for acting out unacceptable aggressive impulses.

		Splitting of self-image or image of others	failing to integrate the positive and negative qualities of self and others and viewing self and others as either all good or all bad
Action level	Action or withdrawal from action	**Acting out**	acting unacceptably to give expression to the experience of emotional distress associated with conflict or stress
		Apathetic withdrawal	not engaging with others
		Help-rejecting complaining	making repeated requests for help and then rejecting help when offered as a way of expressing unacceptable aggressive impulses
		Passive aggression	unassertively expressing unacceptable aggression towards others in authority by overtly complying with their wishes while covertly resisting these
Level of defensive dysregulation	Failure of defences to regulate conflict related feelings leading to a breakdown in reality testing	**Delusional projection**	attributing to others one's own unacceptable thoughts, feelings and wishes to an extreme degree
		Psychotic denial	refusing to acknowledge the painful features of the situation or experiences which are apparent to others to an extreme degree
		Psychotic distortion	viewing reality in an extremely distorted way

Note: Based on DSM IV Defensive Functioning Scale (American Psychiatric Association, 2000a, pp. 807–813).

wishes or between demands and coping resources. This balance maximizes the possibilities of gratification. Also, while the balance is being achieved, the conflicting impulses and wishes, demands and personal resources and related emotions are all held in consciousness. Anticipation, affiliation, altruism, humour, self-assertion, self-observation, sublimation and suppression are adaptive defences. These adaptive defences are protective, rather than problem-maintaining factors.

Coping strategies

The construct of defence mechanisms evolved within the psychodynamic tradition and it is assumed that these methods for regulating negative emotions usually operate unconsciously. Coping strategies, on the other hand, are assumed to be consciously and deliberately used. The construct of coping strategies has developed within the cognitive-behavioural tradition (Zeider & Endler, 1996). Coping strategies are used to manage situations in which there is a perceived discrepancy between stressful demands and available resources for meeting these demands. Distinctions may be made between problem-focused, emotion-focused and avoidant coping strategies. Emotion-focused coping strategies are appropriate for managing affective states associated with uncontrollable stresses such as bereavement. For controllable stresses such as examinations, problem-focused coping strategies, which aim to directly modify the source of stress, are more appropriate. In some situations where time-out from active coping is required to marshal personal resources before returning to active coping, avoidant coping may be appropriate. For all three coping styles, a distinction may be made between functional and dysfunctional strategies. Some commonly used functional and dysfunctional coping strategies are listed in Table 2.2.

Dysfunctional coping strategies may lead to short-term relief but, in the long term, they tend to maintain rather than resolve stress-related problems. Dysfunctional problem-focused coping strategies include: accepting little responsibility for solving the problem, seeking inaccurate or irrelevant information, seeking support and advice from inappropriate sources (such as fortune tellers), developing unrealistic plans (such as winning the lotto), not following through on problem-solving plans, procrastination and holding a pessimistic view of one's capacity to solve the problem. Dysfunctional emotion-focused coping strategies include: making destructive rather than supportive relationships, seeking spiritual support that is not personally meaningful, engaging in long-term denial rather than catharsis, engaging in wishful thinking rather than constructive reframing, taking oneself too seriously rather than looking at stresses in a humorous light, abusing drugs and alcohol rather than using relaxation routines and engaging in aggression rather than physical exercise. Psychologically disengaging from a stressful situation and the judicious short-term involvement in distracting activities and relationship are functional avoidant coping strategies. Avoidant coping strategies become dysfunctional when they are used as a long-term solution to stress management. The adolescent version of the Coping Inventory for Stressful Situations inventory (CISS; Endler & Parker, 1996) may be used to assess task-focused, emotion-focused coping and avoidant coping.

Table 2.2 Functional and dysfunctional, problem-, emotion- and avoidance-focused coping strategies

Type	Aim	Functional	Dysfunctional
Problem focused	Problem solving	• Accepting responsibility for solving the problem • Seeking accurate information • Seeking dependable advice and help • Developing a realistic action plan • Following through on the plan • Postponing competing activities • Maintaining an optimistic view of one's capacity to solve the problem	• Taking little responsibility for solving the problem • Seeking inaccurate information • Seeking questionable advice • Developing unrealistic plans • Not following through on plans • Procrastination • Holding a pessimistic view of one's capacity to solve the problem
Emotion focused	Mood regulation	• Making and maintaining socially supportive and empathic friendships • Seeking meaningful spiritual support • Catharsis and emotional processing • Reframing and cognitive restructuring • Seeing the stress in a humorous way • Relaxation routines • Physical exercise	• Making and maintaining destructive relationships • Seeking meaningless spiritual support • Unproductive wishful thinking • Long-term denial • Taking the stress too seriously • Drug and alcohol abuse • Aggression
Avoidance focused	Avoiding source of stress	• Temporarily mentally disengaging from the problem • Temporally engaging in distracting activities • Temporally engaging in distracting relationships	• Mentally disengaging from the problem for the long term • Long-term engagement in distracting activities • Long-term engagement in distracting relationships

Note: Based on Zeider & Endler (1996).

Biological maintaining factors

In addition to personal psychological characteristics, biological factors may in some instances maintain psychological problems. Abnormal levels of physiological arousal, dysregulation of neurotransmitter systems, dysregulation of neuroendocrine systems, abnormal circadian rhythms and a variety of abnormalities in other bodily systems have been implicated (with varying degrees of empirical support) in the maintenance of some psychological problems (Roberts, 2003; Rutter, 2002a). Typically, specific biological maintaining factors are associated with specific conditions. For example, megacolon (an enlarged colon) is associated specifically with the maintenance of encopresis (see Chapter 7) and the neuroendocrine consequences of starvation are associated specifically with the maintenance of anorexia nervosa (see Chapter 17). Because of the specificity of biological factors further discussion of them will be reserved for Chapters 6 to 18, in which specific problems are discussed in detail.

CONTEXTUAL PRE-DISPOSING FACTORS

While personal characteristics may pre-dispose youngsters to develop psychological problems and maintain them once they emerge, a variety of contextual factors also make youngsters vulnerable to developing psychological difficulties and play a significant role in perpetuating such problems. Environmental factors account for about 50% of the variance in most psychological characteristics (Deary, 2000; Matthews et al., 2003; McGuffin et al., 2002). Youngsters' vulnerability to developing psychological problems is influenced by specific features of the parent–child relationship, exposure to various ongoing family problems and specific stresses (Friedman & Chase-Lansdale, 2002).

Parent–child factors in early life

The quality of parent–child attachment, the degree to which parents offer their children age-appropriate intellectual stimulation and the way in which control and warmth are combined to form a parenting style have been shown to have highly significant effects on children's later psychological adjustment (Bradley & Caldwell, 1989; Cassidy & Shaver, 1999; Darling & Steinberg, 1993). However, it is important to preface a summary of key findings on these three areas with a brief discussion of bonding, since this concept has given rise to many misconceptions within the field.

Bonding

Klaus and Kennell (1976) argued that for close mother–child relationships to develop, the mother and child must have skin-to-skin contact in a critical period immediately following the birth of the child. Bonding theory has not been supported by the results of well-controlled research studies (e.g. Sluckin, Herbert & Sluckin, 1983). Secure mother–infant attachments can develop in the absence of post-natal skin-to-skin contact. Despite the lack of empirical support, bonding theory has had a strong influence on the way mothers and new-borns are treated in hospitals in many parts of Europe and the US. Close and frequent mother–infant contact is encouraged, often in inappropriate circumstances where the mother's or infant's health make such contact onerous. This is because bonding theory entails the view that failure to bond puts children at risk for neglect, failure to thrive and physical child abuse, a view unsupported by many studies (e.g. Gaines, Sandgrund, Green & Power, 1978). While immediate post-natal contact may not be critical for later adjustment, the quality of attachment that develops between the child and primary caregivers, particularly the mother and father, during the first two years of life is of particular significance for healthy psychological development.

Attachment

Children who develop secure attachments to their caregivers develop emotional competence and children who fail to do so may be at risk for developing psychological problems. Children develop secure emotional attachments if their parents are attuned to their needs for safety, security and being physically cared for and if their parents are responsive to children's signals that they require their needs to be met. When this occurs, children learn that their parents are a secure base from which they can explore the world. John Bowlby (1988), who developed attachment theory, argued that attachment behaviour, which is genetically programmed and essential for survival of the species, is elicited in children between six months and three years when faced with danger. In such instances children seek proximity with their caretakers. When comforted they return to the activity of exploring the immediate environment around the caretaker. The cycle repeats each time the child perceives a threat and his or her attachment needs for satisfaction, safety and security are activated. Over multiple repetitions, the child builds an internal working model of attachment relationships based on the way these episodes are managed by the caregiver in response to the child's needs for proximity, comfort and security. Internal working models are cognitive relationship maps based on early attachment experiences, which serve as a template for the development of later intimate relationships. Internal working models allow people to make predictions about how the self and significant others will behave within the relationship. In their ground-breaking text, *Patterns of attachment*, Mary Ainsworth and colleagues (1978) described three patterns of mother–infant interaction following a brief episode of experimentally contrived separation, and further empirical research with mothers and children led to the identification of a fourth category (Cassidy & Shaver, 1999). A summary of these four attachment styles is given in Figure 2.2. Later work on intimate relationships in adulthood confirms that these four relational styles show continuity over the lifecycle. Significant adult relationships and patterns of family organization may be classified into four equivalent categories, which are also outlined in Figure 2.2.

Securely attached children react to their parents as if they were a secure base from which to explore the world. Parents in such relationships are attuned and responsive to the children's or partner's needs. While a secure

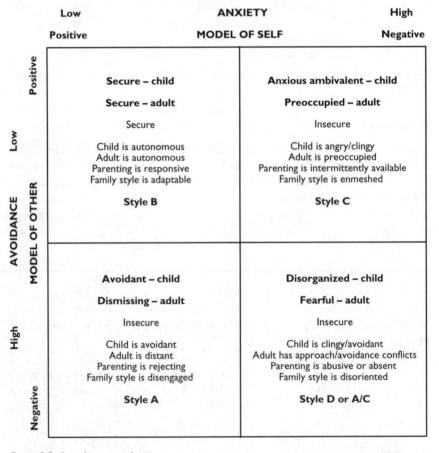

Figure 2.2 Attachment styles

Note: Based on Cassidy and Shaver (1999) and Carr (2000b, p. 167).

attachment style is associated with autonomy, the other three attachment styles are associated with a sense of insecurity. Anxiously attached children seek contact with their parents following separation but are unable to derive comfort from it. They cling and cry or have tantrums. Avoidantly attached children avoid contact with their parents after separation; they sulk. Children with a disorganized attachment style following separation show aspects of both the anxious and avoidant patterns. Disorganized attachment is a common correlate of child abuse and neglect and early parental absence, loss or bereavement.

Intellectual stimulation

The level of sensorimotor and intellectual stimulation that parents provide for infants is critical for their intellectual development. A series of studies by Bradley and Caldwell have shown that the variety of play materials in the home and the number of opportunities used by the parents to intellectually stimulate the child are associated with current intellectual level and future IQ (Bradley, 1994). Bradley and Caldwell used the Home Observation for Measurement of the Environment rating scale (HOME; Caldwell & Bradley, 2001) in their studies. The scale can be completed during a one-hour home visit and measures among other factors maternal responsivity to the child, punitiveness, availability of play materials, and opportunities for stimulation. Versions are currently available for infants, toddlers, children and young adolescents.

Parenting styles

Reviews of the extensive literature on parenting suggest that by combining the two orthogonal dimensions of warmth and control, four parenting styles may be identified and each of these is associated with particular developmental outcomes for the child (Darling & Steinberg, 1993). These four styles are presented in Figure 2.3. *Authoritative parents* who adopt a warm, child-centred approach coupled with a moderate degree of control which allows children to take age-appropriate responsibility, provide a context which is maximally beneficial for children's development as autonomous confident individuals. Children of parents who use an authoritative style learn that conflicts are most effectively managed by taking the other person's viewpoint into account within the context of an amicable negotiation. This set of skills is conducive to efficient joint problem solving and the development of good peer relationships and consequently the development of a good social support network. Children of *authoritarian parents* who are warm but controlling tend to develop into shy adults who are reluctant to take initiative. The parents' disciplinary style teaches them that unquestioning obedience is the best way to manage interpersonal differences and to solve problems.

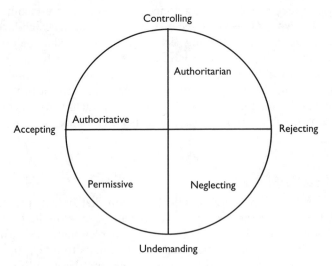

Figure 2.3 Patterns of parenting

Children of *permissive parents*, who are warm but lax in discipline, in later life lack the competence to follow through on plans and show poor impulse control. Children who have experienced little warmth from their parents and who have been either harshly disciplined or had little or inconsistent supervision develop adjustment problems. This is particularly the case with corporal punishment. When children experience corporal punishment, they learn that the use of aggression is an appropriate way to resolve conflicts and tend to use such aggression in managing conflicts with their peers. In this way children who have been physically punished are at risk for developing conduct problems and becoming involved in bullying (Olweus, 1993). This parenting pattern is referred to as *neglecting*.

Children who reported being disciplined once a month or more with corporal punishment were found in the National Youth Victimization Study to be three times more likely to develop a major depressive disorder (Turner & Finkelhor, 1996). A representative national sample of over 2000 children were interviewed for this study and the findings were independent of children's age, gender or socioeconomic status. Furthermore, it was also found that parental support did little to reduce the psychological distress experienced by youngsters who received corporal punishment more than once per month. Figure 2.4 illustrates this point and also shows that parental support greatly reduces the negative impact of corporal punishment on youngsters who received such punishment between three and eleven times a year.

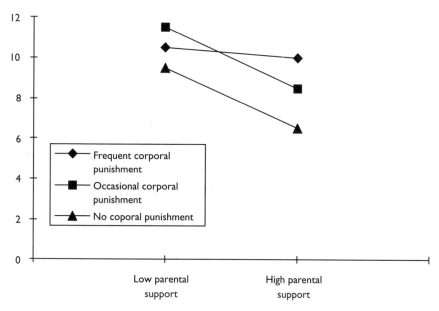

Figure 2.4 The modifying effect of parental support on the psychological distress of children who receive regular, occasional and no corporal punishment

Note: Adapted from Turner and Finkelhor (1996). Scores are adjusted for age, gender and socioeconomic status. Occasional punishment = 3–11 times per year. Frequent punishment = more than 12 times per year.

Exposure to family problems in early life

Children whose parents have significant personal adjustment problems, who grow up in families characterized by disorganization and marital discord and in which there are deviant siblings are at risk for developing psychological difficulties (Friedman & Chase-Lansdale, 2002).

Parental problems

Parental adjustment problems such as depression, alcohol abuse or criminality may render children vulnerable to psychological difficulties for two main reasons. First, such problems may compromise parents' capacity to offer their children a secure attachment relationship, adequate intellectual stimulation and an authoritative parenting environment. For example, depressed mothers find it difficult to interpret their infant's distress signals and to respond appropriately and quickly so as to foster secure attachment. Fathers with alcohol problems often play a very peripheral role in family life, making little input to the child's parenting environment. The second reason why parental adjustment difficulties may pre-dispose youngsters to developing psychological problems is because, through a process of modelling and inadvertent shaping and reinforcement, such children may learn belief systems, behavioural patterns, defence mechanisms and coping strategies similar to their parents.

Marital discord

Figure 2.5 shows that marital satisfaction varies over the course of the family llifecycle, with high levels of satisfaction occurring prior to the birth of children and after they have left home, and lowest levels of satisfaction being associated with the period where families contain school-going children. These data underline the demands children place on parents and their potential to reduce marital satisfaction. In families where marital dissatisfaction and discord are present, psychological difficulties – notably conduct problems – often occur. Exposure to marital discord and violence may pre-dispose youngsters to developing psychological problems in a number of ways (Moffit & Caspi, 1998). First, witnessing quarrelling, conflict and violence of any sort is stressful, but particularly so when those engaged in the conflict are

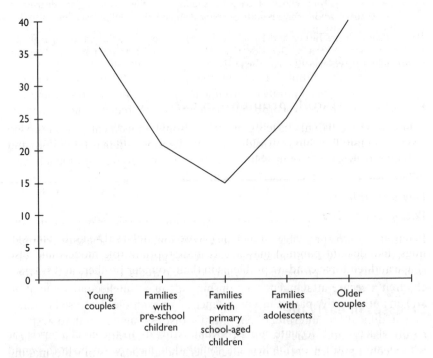

Figure 2.5 Marital satisfaction across the lifespan

Note: Adapted from Rollins and Feldman (1970).

the main sources of safety, care and control in the child's life. Second, children feel strong loyalty to both parents and fear that a positive gesture made towards one parent may be interpreted as a disloyalty to the other and result in being abandoned or abused by the offended parent. Third, children may believe that they were responsible for the marital discord and so are responsible for resolving the parents' difficulties or preventing the parents from engaging in conflict or violence. Fourth, marital discord may prevent parents from working co-operatively together to provide their children with an optimal parenting environment.

Parental co-operation is particularly important in cases where separation or divorce has occurred (Hetherington & Kelly, 2002). Two years following divorce, 20% of children show clinically significant emotional and behavioural problems. Continued parental acrimony and detouring parental conflict through children is one of the most significant factors contributing to this sub-group's adjustment problems. Co-operative parenting, on the other hand is associated with good post-divorce adjustment. Adjustment to divorce is discussed in Chapter 23.

Family disorganization

A chaotic family environment characterized by inconsistent rules, unclear roles and the absence of regular routines may pre-dispose youngsters to developing psychological problems, particularly conduct problems. Such disorganized families tend to lack communication skills and problem-solving skills. Often, these families have multiple problems and progress from one crisis to the next. Such family environments probably pre-dispose youngsters to develop psychological problems because the unpredictability associated with such environments is highly stressful and these family environments fail to offer children secure attachments and the authoritative parenting they require for their needs to be met.

Deviant siblings

Having older brothers or sisters who have conduct problems may pre-dispose youngsters to developing conduct problems themselves. Deviant older siblings (like deviant parents) may act as inappropriate role models and also shape and reinforce conduct problems in their younger brothers and sisters.

Stresses in early life

In the absence of adequate supports, major threats to the child's needs for safety, care, control or intellectual stimulation may pre-dispose the child to developing psychological problems in later life. Chief among these early life stresses are bereavements, parent–child separations, child abuse, social disadvantage and institutional upbringing (Friedman & Chase-Lansdale, 2002; Sandberg & Rutter, 2002). Virtually all of these early life stresses disrupt the child's relationship with their attachment figures.

Separation and bereavement

Significant loss experiences such as separations from a parent or loss of a parent through bereavement may place children at risk for a variety of problems particularly depression (Goodyer, 2001a,b). Children who have suffered losses in early life tend to be vulnerable to depression when faced with loss experiences in later life.

Child abuse

Physical, sexual and emotional abuse in early childhood may make youngsters vulnerable to developing later emotional and conduct problems (Myers et al., 2002). Children who have been abused are also at risk for becoming involved in relationships in which they are repeatedly abused. They also are at risk for abusing others.

Social disadvantage

Chronic social disadvantage and poverty in early life is a risk factor for later psychological problems (Friedman & Chase-Lansdale, 2002). A variety of mechanisms may be involved. An inadequate physical environment and inadequate nutrition may adversely affect children's health and this in turn may adversely affect children's psychological well-being. In addition, parents coping with the multiple stresses associated with social disadvantage may have few personal resources available for meeting their children's needs for safety, care, control and intellectual stimulation.

Institutional upbringing

Where children are brought up in an institution and have multiple caretakers, they are at risk for later psychological difficulties particularly making and maintaining relationships (O'Connor, 2002). These children, who have had no stable attachment experience themselves, lack a model on which to base later socially supportive relationships.

CONTEXTUAL MAINTAINING FACTORS

Once children develop psychological problems, they may persist because of the way in which members of the child's social network respond to the difficulties. Children's problems may be maintained by patterns of interaction within the family, by ongoing parental adjustment problems, by factors within the wider culture and social network, including the school, and by the way in which the family engage with treatment agencies (Friedman & Chase-Lansdale, 2002; Imber-Black, 1991; Nikapota, 2002; Rutter, 2002a; Rutter & Nikapota, 2002).

Family system factors

Within the family, parents and siblings may maintain psychological difficulties by engaging in problem-maintaining interaction patterns with the child who has psychological problems. There are many such interaction patterns, but a number deserve particular mention. These include interaction patterns characterized by inadvertent reinforcement, insecure attachment, coercion, over-involvement, disengagement, inconsistent parental discipline, confused communication and triangulation (Carr, 2000b). Problem-maintaining interaction patterns are more common in family systems characterized by chaotic organization, marital discord and father absence.

Inadvertent reinforcement

Children's psychological problems may be maintained if parents or siblings continuously or intermittently interact with the child when it occurs in ways that entail some pay-off or reinforcement for the child (Herbert, 2002). This pay-off may be as simple as offering attention. Typically, parents and siblings do not intend to reinforce problematic behaviour, but nevertheless do so inadvertently by, for example, repeatedly inquiring about a child's mood or commenting on his or her negative conduct. Furthermore, in many instances, children are unaware that their problem behaviour is being maintained by inadvertent parental reinforcement. Inadvertent reinforcement is a particularly powerful problem-maintaining factor when it is offered intermittently rather than continuously.

Insecure attachment

Where children do not experience their parents as a secure base from which to explore the world, they may engage in a variety of problematic proximity-seeking behaviours such as clinging, crying on separation or at bed time and so forth. Where parents respond on some occasions by comforting the child while on others pushing the child away, the child is more likely to continue to engage in intensive proximity-seeking behaviour. This is the hallmark of anxious attachment (Cassidy & Shaver, 1999).

Coercive interaction

Coercive interaction patterns, which involve mutual negative reinforcement, are central to the maintenance of children's conduct difficulties (Patterson, 1982). Children with conduct problems may become involved in escalating patterns of negative interaction with their parents. Within such patterns the child responds to parental criticism and reprimands with increasingly aggressive or destructive behaviour. Eventually, on some occasions parents withdraw from these exchanges. This withdrawal leads both the child and the parent to experience relief. This experience of relief negatively reinforces the behaviour of both the child and the parent that immediately preceded it. For the child, a high level of aggressive and destructive behaviour is reinforced. For the parent, withdrawal from the child in the face of escalating conduct difficulties is reinforced. Coercive interaction patterns may evolve from an extremely authoritarian parenting style characterized by a high level of control and a low level of warmth.

Over-involvement

Parental criticism and parental emotional over-involvement are the two main components that make up the construct of expressed emotion (EE) which was originally shown to be associated with relapse rates in schizophrenia and subsequently has been shown to influence the course of childhood psychological disorders (Rosenbaum Asarnow, Tompson, Woo & Cantwell, 2001). Both the criticism and over-involvement components of EE probably reflect aspects of family members' attempts to cope with their children's difficult behaviour. Parents may respond to psychological difficulties by construing them as disobedience, and cope with this by being critical of the child. Alternatively they may respond by construing the child as an invalid and responding to the child's problems in an over-protective or emotionally over-involved manner. Children may interpret over-involvement as a sign that their parents believe them to have particularly serious problems and this belief, along with related expectations, may maintain their problems. In addition, over-involvement may be associated with parents inadvertently reinforcing problem behaviours. Over-involvement may reflect a form of permissive parenting characterized by a high level of warmth and intrusiveness and a low level of control.

Disengagement

Psychological difficulties may be maintained by infrequent parent–child interaction. In some infants and young children, delays in language and cognitive development may be maintained by low-frequency, disengaged parent–child interaction patterns (Iwaniec, 1995; Smith & Fong, 2004). During middle childhood and adolescence, disengaged parent–child relationships may maintain conduct problems (Behan & Carr, 2000; Brosnan & Carr, 2000). With a low level of supervision, youngsters are free to become involved with a deviant peer group and engage in socialized delinquency. Disengaged parent–child relationships at any age may maintain a low sense of self-esteem, since low rates of parent–child interaction may be interpreted by the child as indicating that he or she is not valued by the parent.

Inconsistent discipline

Where the rules governing acceptable and unacceptable behaviour and the consequences associated with adherence to rules or rule violations are either unclear, or clear but inconsistently enforced, problem-maintaining parent–child interaction patterns may emerge (Behan & Carr, 2000; Brosnan & Carr, 2000). Children may refuse to comply with parental requests, because it is unclear what the consequences for compliance or defiance will be. In such situations, the child finds it difficult to internalize the rules for acceptable behaviour and so may continue to show problem behaviours.

Confused communication patterns

Children's psychological problems may be maintained by confused communication patterns (Carr, 2000a,b). Confused communication patterns may be characterized by problematic parental listening or by giving unclear and indirect messages. Low self-esteem and related difficulties may be maintained by parent–child interaction patterns in which parents are unable to listen to the child and give the child clear and direct feedback that their position has been heard and understood. A wide variety of conduct and emotional problems may be maintained by parent–child communication patterns in which parents and children fail to communicate directly with each other. For example, a parent who wants a child to tell the truth, rather than instructing the child directly may say 'Sometimes I wish people would tell the truth.' This type of indirect communication is far less effective than a direct communication such as: 'If we are going to trust each other, then we need to tell each other the truth. Now, what happened?' Many psychological problems may be maintained by parent–child communication patterns in which the parent's message to the child is unclear. For example, a parent may give a child a vague message, two conflicting verbal messages or a clear verbal message which conflicts with the non-verbal message. With all of these unclear messages, their negative impact on the child may be exacerbated if the child is unable to or prevented from either requesting clarification or escaping from the ambiguous situation. From the child's perspective, this type of situation is very stressful when the conflicting messages are commands and disobedience will lead to punishment or loss of parental approval. This is because the child knows that if she carries out either instruction she will be disobeying the parent and there is no way of escaping or clarifying which is the right instruction to follow. This type of communication was first observed in families of people with schizophrenia, although subsequent research showed that it does not play an aetiological role in the psychoses. However, clinical experience shows that this type of double-binding communication is quite a common maintaining factor in conduct and emotional disorders.

Triangulation

Children's psychological difficulties may be maintained by three-person interactional patterns where there is a secretive cross-generational coalition between one parent and the child and the other parent is peripheral to this parent–child alliance (Carr, 2000a). Typically this pattern involves a close mother–child coalition to which the father is peripheral. With separation anxiety or conduct problems, the mother may inadvertently reinforce the problem behaviour and either intentionally or inadvertently undermine the father's attempt to contribute to the resolution of the child's difficulties. Where parents have unresolved or unacknowledged marital difficulties, a child's difficulties may be maintained by the parents engaging in conflict about the management of the child's difficulties. This type of detouring may be particularly pronounced in families where parents are separated or divorced. While triangulation may maintain children's problems in some instances, a word of caution is in order since triangulation is not always a problem-maintaining factor. Jenkins and Smith (1990) have shown that children with particularly close positive relationships with a parent are less adversely affected by marital discord and show fewer signs of psychological distress than their siblings who share the stress of exposure to marital discord but who do not reap the benefits of a close parent–child relationship.

Father absence

Father absence and poor identification with the father, in boys, is associated in particular with conduct disorders (Lamb, 2004). This may be because there are fewer parenting resources in families in which the father is absent and also because mothers and absent fathers may involve their children in problem-maintaining triangulation patterns discussed in the previous section. The greater the quantity and quality of time the father spends with children, the better the overall adjustment of children in the long term. Children from families with high levels of father involvement show greater instrumental and interpersonal competence and higher self-esteem. Research in family therapy has shown that father involvement in therapy is an important predicator of successful outcome (Carr, 2000a,b).

Parental factors

Certain parental characteristics make it more likely that they will engage in problem-maintaining interaction patterns with their children (Reder et al., 2000, 2004; Reder & Lucey, 1995). Where parents have a similar problem to their children they may act as a role model and so maintain their youngsters behaviour in this way. Where parents have other psychological problems, or criminality, their personal resources for coping with the demands of parenting may be compromised or they may be unavailable due to hospitalization or incarceration. Where parents have inaccurate knowledge of child development, they may misinterpret children's problem behaviour and engage in problem-maintaining interaction patterns. For example, a child crying in distress may be interpreted as intentionally punishing the parents and they may respond with criticism, or unsocialized aggression may be misinterpreted as a sign of depression and lead the parents to respond with over-involvement. Parents who did not experience secure attachment to their own primary caregivers may lack internal working models for secure attachments and so be unable to offer their children this type of relationship. As a result, patterns of interaction based on insecure attachment may evolve and maintain children's psychological difficulties. Where parents lack the beliefs and skills necessary for emotional self-regulation, they may find it difficult to provide an authoritative parenting environment and find that their treatment of their children is fuelled by their immediate emotional reactions rather than a planned response. Thus low self-esteem, an external locus of control, low self-efficacy, a problematic attributional style, cognitive distortions, immature defences and dysfunctional coping strategies are parental characteristics that may underpin parents' involvement in problem-maintaining interaction patterns.

Social network factors

Certain features of the family's social network make it more likely that problem-maintaining patterns of interaction will develop and be sustained. These include the family's levels of stress and social support, children's school placements and peer relations, the family's ethnic origin and the type of community in which the family lives (Carr, 2000a; Friedman & Chase-Lansdale, 2002; Garmezy & Masten, 1994; Nikapota, 2002; Rutter, 1985a,b, 2002a; Rutter & Nikapota, 2002; Uchino Cacioppo & Kiecolt-Glaser, 1996).

Lack of social support

In socially isolated families that have poorly developed social support networks, with little positive contact with the extended family and few friends, parents and children are more likely to become involved in problem-maintaining interaction patterns (Friedman & Chase-Lansdale, 2002;

Garmezy & Masten, 1994). For parents and children, social support increases a personal sense of well-being and provides a forum for receiving advice on managing problems. Social support has also been shown to facilitate endocrine, cardiovascular and immune system functioning (Uchino et al., 1996). In the absence of social support, parents and children have fewer personal resources for coping with problems and so are more likely to drift into problem-maintaining interaction patterns.

Chronic life stress

Major stressful life events such as parental unemployment, serious illness or bereavement, or an accumulation of minor stressful events such as transport problems or quarrels, are examples of stresses that erode parents' and children's coping resources and promote problem-maintaining patterns of family interaction (Friedman & Chase-Lansdale, 2002; Garmezy & Masten, 1994). These types of stress are more common where families are socially disadvantaged.

The parents' work contexts may entail both stresses and supports which influence the degree to which they meet their children's needs. Parents who work are less likely than those who do not to develop mental health problems such as depression (Warr, 1987). Along with meeting financial needs, work may meet parents' needs for social support, a purpose in life, achievement and status. However, work may also be a source of stress. Within the work context stress has been found to be consistently associated with jobs where there is a low level of control over responsibilities, resources and the working environment. Both excessive and minimal work loads are stressful, with the latter leading to boredom and the former to burnout. Stress is also associated with work situations where an individual's responsibilities are unclear or ambiguous, where there is considerable time pressure and where the work-related tasks are overly complex or extremely monotonous. Physically uncomfortable work environments and work situations where supportive relationships with co-workers, management and subordinates are absent are also stressful. For women, particularly, role strain associated with homemaking and working outside the home may be a significant source of stress. Work transitions which involve geographic relocation are particularly stressful if they involve the loss of the family's social support network. Promotion beyond the limits of a person's abilities may also prove stressful, as may the lack of promotion if such advancement is expected.

Unsuitable educational placement

Unsupportive, poorly resourced educational placements with inadequate staffing and staff training or dealing with children with psychological problems may maintain children's psychological problems (Rutter, 1985a,b,

2002a). Children with learning difficulties may fall further and further behind in their attainments, due to the lack of appropriate remedial tuition. They may also develop negative self-evaluative beliefs as a result of failure experiences or being labelled as lazy or educationally inadequate. They may also become involved in problem-maintaining interaction patterns with teachers and fellow pupils.

Deviant peer-group membership

Where youngsters with conduct or substance-abuse problems are members of a delinquent or drug-abusing peer group, then interactions with these peers may maintain the youngster's problem behaviour through modelling and reinforcement (Brosnan & Carr, 2000).

Community problems

Children's conduct and school-based psychological difficulties may be maintained by a variety of community problems, including social disadvantage, racism, social exclusion, living in a high-crime area, having few employment opportunities and being exposed to community violence (Carr, 2000a; Friedman & Chase-Lansdale, 2002; Garmezy & Masten, 1994; Nikapota, 2002; Rutter, 2002a).

Problem-maintaining treatment system factors

Children's psychological problems may be maintained by the way in which they and their families engage with treatment agencies and professionals within the healthcare, educational, juvenile justice and other relevant systems (Carr, 2000b; Imber-Black, 1991; Nikapota, 2002). Serious psychological adjustment problems are more likely to persist if they are denied by the child or significant family members or if family members are ambivalent about resolving the child's problems. This is a common problem where the referral is initiated by someone outside the family such as a teacher, a social worker or a probation officer. Denial of the problem or ambivalence about engaging in treatment leads children and families to develop problem-maintaining rather than problem-resolving interaction patterns. Problems are more likely to persist in situations where families have not successfully coped with similar problems before. Parents and children have no grounds on which to believe that they have the resources to solve their problems or any problem-solving routines with which to tackle them. Nor do they have the experience of making and maintaining a good working alliance with a clinical psychologist or treatment team. Children's difficulties are more likely to persistent in situations where the child and parents reject the treatment team's formulation of the problem and the treatment plan based on the formulation. A lack of co-ordination among professionals on a multi-disciplinary treatment team or in an interagency network may also maintain a child's problems, especially where different professionals have conflicting formulations and treatment plans. Families from ethnic minorities may have difficulty engaging with services which are insensitive to the needs, expectations, norms, beliefs and values of the ethnic minority culture. In such circumstances there may be difficulty in establishing a therapeutic alliance and clients may drop out of treatment. This cultural insensitivity of service provision may maintain children's problems.

PRECIPITATING FACTORS

Some psychological problems, such as autism are present at birth. Others, such as primary enuresis, reflect a delay in development. Here the child fails to develop a particular competency at the appropriate age. In some instances, the onset of psychological difficulties is quite gradual. For example, some youngsters with eating disorders become gradually anorexic over a period of months. In other instances, the onset of psychological problems is very sudden and in response to a clear stressor, as in the case of post-traumatic stress disorder. Despite these variations, it is conceptually useful to distinguish precipitating factors from pre-disposing and maintaining factors, while recognizing that precipitating factors may not be identifiable in all instances (Sandberg & Rutter, 2002). Children's psychological problems may be precipitated by acute life stresses such as illness or injury, child abuse, bullying and births or bereavements. They may also be precipitated by lifecycle transitions such as entry into adolescence, changing schools, loss of peer friendships and parental separation or divorce. Family stresses such as parental unemployment, moving house or financial difficulties may also precipitate the onset of psychological problems. Once an episode of a problem has been precipitated and then resolved, there is considerable variability in whether youngsters become 'sensitized' or 'steeled' to the next build-up of stressful life events (Rutter, 2002a). Some youngsters become more resilient and are better able to cope with future stresses having successfully resolved a problem once. Others are rendered more vulnerable and require less stress to develop future problems.

PROTECTIVE FACTORS

The presence of personal and contextual protective factors that have been found to characterize children who show resilience in the face of stress and which typify cases that respond positively to psychological interventions may be used as a basis for judging the prognosis for a particular child referred for psychological consultation (Carr, 2000a,b, 2002, 2004; Fonagy, Target, Cottrell, Phillips & Kurtz, 2002; Haggerty et al., 1994; Kazdin & Weisz, 2003; Luthar, 2003; McNeish, Newman & Roberts, 2002; Rolf et al., 1990; Rutter, 2002a; Rutter & Casaer, 1991; Sexton Weeks & Robbins, 2003; Sprenkle, 2002; Weisz & Weiss, 1993).

Personal protective factors

At a personal level both biological and psychological protective factors have been identified.

Biological protective factors

Children are more likely to show good adjustment if they have good physical health (Carr, 2004a; Rutter & Casaer, 1991). The absence of genetic vulner-abilities, an adequate intrauterine environment, an uncomplicated birth, no history of serious illnesses and injuries, adequate nutrition and regular exercise all contribute to robust physical health. Gender and age may also affect adjustment positively. Before puberty, girls manage stress better than boys, but after puberty it is boys who have the advantage. Young children are less adversely affected by trauma and stress than older children.

Psychological protective factors

An easy temperament, a high level of intellectual ability and high self-esteem are all associated with positive adjustment (Carr, 2004a; Rolf et al., 1990; Rutter, 2002a). Well-developed self-regulation skills and confidence in the use of these skills are also protective factors. Thus, positive adjustment is associated with an internal locus of control, high self-efficacy beliefs and an optimistic attributional style where successes are attributed to internal, global stable factors such as ability and failures to external, specific, unstable factors like luck. With respect to self-regulatory skills, mature defence mechanisms and functional coping strategies such as those listed in Tables 2.1 and 2.2 are protective factors.

Anticipation, affiliation, altruism, humour, self-assertion, self-observation, sublimation and suppression are adaptive defences (Vaillant, 2000). Anticipation involves considering and partially experiencing emotional reactions and the consequences of these before the conflict or stress occurs and exploring various solutions to these problematic emotional states. Affiliation involves seeking social support from others, sharing problems with them and doing this without making them responsible for the problem or for relieving the distress it entails. Altruism is dedication to meeting the needs of others and receiving gratification from this without engaging in excessive self-sacrifice. When humour is used as a defence, we reframe situations that give rise to conflict or stress in an ironic or amusing way. Self-assertion involves expressing conflict-related thoughts or feelings in a direct yet non-coercive way. Self-observation involves monitoring how situations lead to conflict or stress and using this new understanding to modify negative affect. Sublimation is the channelling of negative emotions arising from conflict or stress into socially acceptable activities such as work, sports or art. Suppression is the intentional avoidance of thinking about conflict or stress.

Functional problem-focused, emotion-focused and avoidant coping strategies are listed in Table 2.2 (Zeider & Endler, 1996). Where stresses are controllable, functional, problem-focused coping strategies, are appropriate to use. These include accepting responsibility for solving the problem, seeking accurate information about the problem, seeking dependable advice and help, developing realistic action plans, carrying out plans either alone or with the help of other people, staying focused by postponing engaging in competing activities and maintaining an optimistic view of one's capacity to solve the problem. Where stresses are uncontrollable, emotion-focused coping strategies such as making and maintaining socially supportive friendships, particularly those in which it is possible to confide deeply felt emotions and beliefs, are appropriate. An emotion-focused coping strategy related to seeking social support is catharsis. That is the process of verbally expressing in detail intense emotional experiences and engaging in processing of emotionally charged thoughts and memories within the context of a confiding relationship. Seeking meaningful spiritual support is another emotion-focused coping strategy. Re-framing, cognitive restructuring and looking at stresses from a humorous perspective are emotion-focused coping strategies where the aim is to reduce distress by thinking about a situation in a different way. Relaxation routines and physical exercise are other functional emotion-focused coping strategies used to regulate mood in a highly deliberate way. These emotion-focused coping strategies permit the regulation of negative mood states that arise from exposure to stress. Psychologically disengaging from a stressful situation and the judicious short-term involvement in distracting activities and relationships are functional avoidant coping strategies.

CONTEXTUAL PROTECTIVE FACTORS

Within the child's social context, features of the treatment system, aspects of the family system, individual characteristics of the child's parents or primary caregivers and features of the wider social network including the child's school may all have positive prognostic implications.

Protective treatment system factors

When children and parents engage positively with treatment agencies and professionals within the healthcare, social welfare, educational, juvenile justice and other relevant systems, a positive prognosis may usually be made (Carr, 2000b, 2002a, Fonagy et al., 2002; Nikapota, 2002; Kazdin & Weisz, 2003; Sexton et al., 2003; Sprenkle, 2002). Children are more likely to benefit from treatment if they and their families accept that there is a problem, are committed to resolving it, have coped with similar problems before and accept the formulation and treatment plan of the psychologist and treatment team. Children are also more likely to benefit from treatment where there is good co-ordination among professionals on a multi-disciplinary treatment team or in an interagency network that is sensitive to children's cultural and ethnic context.

Protective family system factors

A positive prognosis is associated with certain aspects of the family system (Carr, 2000b; Lamb, 2004; Rutter, 2002a). Better long-term adjustment may be expected in cases where the child has a secure attachment to a parent or primary caregiver and where parents adopt a warm and moderately controlling authoritative parenting style. Clear and direct communication within the family and a flexible pattern of family organization characterized by explicit rules, roles and routines facilitate a positive response to treatment. Where fathers are involved in the care of the child and where parents have a high level of marital satisfaction, a positive prognosis is more likely.

Protective parental factors

A number of protective parental characteristics have consistently been identified in research studies and clinical practice (Reder et al., 2000, 2004; Reder & Lucey, 1995). A positive response to treatment is probable when parents with high self-esteem who are well psychologically adjusted have an internal working model for secure attachment relationships and accurate knowledge and expectations about their children's development. Self-regulatory beliefs and skills including internal locus of control, high self-efficacy, an optimistic attributional style, mature defences and functional coping strategies are other important parental protective factors. This combination of attributes equips parents particularly well for providing their children with secure attachment relationships; an authoritative parenting environment and for meeting children's needs for safety, care, control and intellectual stimulation. This type of parental profile is typical of parents who have had secure attachments to their own parents as children and who have not been exposed to high levels of life stress without adequate social support. Parents who have faced major challenges in their childhood, including child abuse, major trauma and bereavement, but who have been supported through them by parents, peers, teachers or other significant support figures often develop the protective parenting profile outlined above.

Protective social network factors

Within the child and family's wider social network, the higher the level of social support and the lower the level of stress, the more probable it is that the child will respond positively to treatment (Carr, 2000b; Fonagy et al., 2002; Kazdin & Weisz, 2003; Sexton et al., 2003; Sprenkle, 2002). Better treatment response occurs when children have higher socioeconomic status, probably because high socioeconomic status is associated with a lower level of stress. For children, day care, pre-school placements, school placements and peer-group membership may be particularly important sources of social support and a forum within which children learn important self-regulatory skills and coping strategies.

Protective day-care placements

High-quality day care is characterized by a continuity in the relationship between the infant and the staff; a responsivity in staffs' reactions to infants' signals and needs; a low ratio of infants to staff; and a safe, spacious and well-equipped physical facility (McGurk, Caplan, Hennessy & Moss, 1993). Children who receive high-quality day care and whose parents adopt a responsive style in their interactions with them develop secure attachments to their parents. Where parents have difficulty in meeting their youngster's needs, high-quality day care may be an important source of social support for the children. Furthermore, such day-care placements may provide parents with an opportunity to work outside the home and receive the social support that work-based relationships can provide.

Protective pre-school placements

Pre-school early intervention educational programmes for socially disadvantaged and handicapped children can have long-lasting effects on psychosocial adjustment, cognitive development and school attainment, particularly if certain conditions prevail (Lange & Carr, 2002; NESS, 2004). A central factor is a good working relationship between the parents and the pre-school staff. Children and parents must also have access to positive role models who, by their example and success, show the value of schooling. Finally, a teaching method which incorporates the elements of planning activities, doing these activities and reviewing performance is vital to success. This *plan–do–review* cycle is premised on Vygotsky's (1934/1962) analysis of effective instruction. Four life skills, the foundations of which are laid by successful pre-school programmes, distinguish those children who have positive outcomes. The first is the development of a goal-oriented and planful approach to solving scholastic and social problems. The second is the development of aspirations for education and employment. The third is the development of a sense of responsibility for one's own actions. The fourth is a sense of duty and responsibility towards others.

Protective school placements

In their ground-breaking study of secondary schools, Rutter, Maughan, Mortimore & Ouston (1979) found that a series of features of the secondary school environment had a favourable influence on behaviour and attainment, and that these factors were independent of child and family characteristics. These features are:

- Firm authoritative leadership of the staff team by the principal.
- Firm authoritative management of classes by teachers with high expectations of success, clear rules and regular homework, which was graded routinely.
- A participative approach to decision making among the staff about curriculum planning and school management which fostered cohesion among the staff and the principal.
- Many opportunities for pupils to participate in the running of the school, which fostered pupil loyalty to the school.
- A balance of emphasis on both academic attainment and excellence in other fields such as sport.
- Teachers modelled good behaviour.
- Teachers regularly appreciated, rewarded and praised academic and non-academic achievements.
- A balance between intellectually able and less able pupils.
- An attractive, comfortable and pleasant school environment.

Subsequent research on both primary and secondary schools has supported and extended Rutter's original findings and shown that the following attributes are also associated with high attainment: presenting pupils with clear pre-determined goals or standards, creating an expectation of success, structuring material so that it is easily interpretable, using sufficient repetition to keep the pupils on task, presenting information clearly, providing extra help if necessary to ensure that goals are reached and providing feedback. This type of approach to teaching requires moderate class sizes, a variable which has been consistently associated with pupil performance (Sylva, 1994).

Protective peer-group membership

Peer friendships are important because they constitute a significant source of social support and a context within which to learn about the management of networks of relationships (Dunn & McGuire, 1992; Malik & Furman, 1993; Willams & Gilmore, 1994). Emotionally expressive children who have developed secure attachments to their parents and whose parents adopt an authoritative parenting style are more likely to develop good peer friendships. This is probably because their experience with their parents provides them with a useful cognitive model on which to base their interactions with their peers. Surveys of children referred to clinics for psychological consultation show that, in comparison with non-referred children, they have fewer stable friendships and their understanding of the reciprocities involved in friendship are less well developed. Children reared in institutions or whose parents use harsh or physical punishment have particular difficulty with peer relationships in their teens. This is unfortunate since it is precisely these children who need the social support provided by positive peer relationships.

IMPLICATIONS FOR PRACTICE

This cursory review of factors that influence problem development has clear implications for clinical practice. When children and their families are referred for psychological consultation, their status on relevant personal and contextual pre-disposing, precipitating, maintaining and protective factors reviewed here, and summarized in Figure 2.1, deserve assessment. Salient points from these investigations may then be integrated into a concise formulation which explains how the problem developed and suggests how the child's and family's problems may be treated. Effective psychological treatment and case management typically involves modifying personal and contextual problem-maintaining factors. Often, this entails enhancing personal and contextual protective factors. Thus, some psychological interventions may aim to improve children's self-regulatory beliefs and skills through individual or group therapy and training. Other interventions aim to enhance parenting skills and the quality of the family environment through parent training and family therapy. Still other interventions may address the wider social system and aim to reduce stress and enhance extra-familial support through working with the child's school, peer group, extended family or other involved agencies. The decision about which multi-systemic package of interventions to employ in a particular case should be determined by the formulation and available treatment resources. A fuller general discussion of assessment, formulation and treatment planning will be given in Chapter 4. Guidelines for managing specific problems are given in Chapters 6 to 24.

SUMMARY

The development of psychological problems may be conceptualized as arising from risk factors, which predispose children to developing psychological problems, precipitating factors, which trigger the onset or marked exacerbation of psychological difficulties, maintaining factors, which perpetuate psychological problems once they have developed, and protective factors, which prevent further deterioration and have implications for prognosis and response to treatment. Most of these factors may be subclassified as falling into the personal or contextual domains, with personal factors referring to biological and psychological characteristics of the child and contextual factors referring to features of the child's psychosocial environment including the family, the school and peer group. When children and their families are referred for psychological consultation, factors in each of these domains require assessment and salient points from these investigations are integrated into a concise formulation which explains how the problem developed. Treatment typically involves modifying personal and contextual problem maintaining factors by enhancing personal and contextual protective factors.

EXERCISE 2.1

Work in pairs. One person take the role of interviewer and the other take the role of interviewee. The interviewer should take twenty minutes to ask the interviewee about influences on an episode of low mood (or some other minor problem) that they have experienced. The various factors mentioned in the chapter should be covered in this interview. The interviewer should then list the pre-disposing, precipitating, maintaining and protective factors associated with the problem. Then check with the interviewee for accuracy. Reverse roles and repeat the exercise.

EXERCISE 2.2

This exercise may be completed by an individual or a team. Read the following case and identify pre-disposing, precipitating, maintaining and protective factors using the framework set out in Figure 2.1.

Carla, aged twelve, is an only child whose parents brought her for treatment because she has not been sleeping recently and is persistently tearful. She has been seen by the family doctor and the school counsellor and it was her teacher who suggested the referral to your service. Her developmental history is relatively normal. She has always had a good relationship with both parents. Her parents take her viewpoint seriously but have clear rules about homework, house chores and pocket money. She also has a few very close friends and plays hockey for the school team. Carla is a determined student and does very well at school. The main problems in her life centre on her mother's illness. Her mother has been repeatedly hospitalized for depression since Carla was born. During these hospitalizations Carla normally stays with her grandmother. In the two years prior to the referral the grandmother has developed dementia and moved into a residential centre three months go. Shortly afterwards, Carla's mother was hospitalized and Carla was cared for by a live-in au pair. Carla's father is very worried about her and has tried to cut down on the amount of time he spends at work. He is a supervisor in a factory and works a shift-work schedule where he is on nights one week in three. Carla's father has been trying to follow the family doctor's advice of cheering her up by taking her out more and avoiding talking about the mother's depression or the grandmother's dementia. However, the school counsellor has advised that he should spend more time at home talking with her about the sadness she feels about her mother's and grandmother's problems.

FURTHER READING

Carr, A. (2004). *Positive Psychology. The Science of Happiness and Human Strengths*. London: Brunner Routledge.

Rutter, M. & Taylor, E. (2002). *Child and Adolescent Psychiatry (Fourth Edition)*. Oxford: Blackwell.

Chapter 3

Classification, epidemiology and treatment effectiveness

The classification of children and adolescents' psychological problems, their prevalence, and the effectiveness of psychological treatment in ameliorating these problems are considered in this chapter. There will be a particular focus on Chapter 5 from the tenth edition of the World Health Organization's *International classification of diseases* (ICD-10; WHO, 1992, 1996), a clinical version of which is widely used in day-to-day practice in Europe, and on the text revision of the fourth edition of the American Psychiatric Association's (APA) *Diagnostic and statistical manual of mental disorders* (DSM IV TR; APA, 2000a), which is widely used clinically in North America. The reliability and validity of these classification systems will be considered and their shortcomings outlined. Reference will also be made to the increasingly influential *Diagnostic classification of mental health and developmental disorders of infancy and early childhood* (DC 0–3; Zero to Three, 1994). The results of some epidemiological studies of childhood psychological disorders will then be reviewed. Finally, research on the effectiveness of the psychological treatment of children and adolescents' problems will be summarized.

FUNCTIONS OF CLASSIFICATION

In clinical psychology, classification has three main functions. First, it permits information about particular types of problems to be ordered in ways that facilitate the growth of a body of expert knowledge. This information typically includes the accurate clinical description of a problem and the identification of factors associated with the aetiology, maintenance, course and possible management plans effective in solving the problem. Such expert information constitutes the basis for sound clinical practice. Second, classification systems allow for the development of epidemiological information about the incidence and prevalence of various problems. This sort of information is particularly useful in planning services and deciding how to prioritize the allocation of sparse resources. Third, classification systems provide a language through which clinicians and researchers communicate with each other.

Currently the two major classification systems in widespread use are the ICD 10 and the DSM IV TR. The DSM IV TR is the text revision of the fourth edition of the *Diagnostic and statistical manual of the mental disorders* of the American Psychiatric Association (APA, 2000a). The ICD 10 is the tenth edition of the *International classification of diseases*. Psychological problems are classified in Chapter 5 of this system (WHO, 1992) and a multi-axial version of it is available for the classification of child and adolescent psychological problems (WHO, 1996). Where ICD 10 is mentioned below, it is to this multi-axial version that reference is being made, since it is this version, based on the pioneering work of Rutter, Shaffer & Shepherd (1975), that is most influential in the field of child and family mental health in the UK and parts of Europe. It should be highlighted that although, in clinical practice, the DSM IV TR is viewed as the US alternative to the European ICD 10, in fact the ICD 10 is not exclusively European. It is the instrument through which the World Health Organization, a United Nations Agency, collects data and compiles statistics on all diseases in all UN countries.

Both DSM IV TR and ICD 10 are premised on a medical model of psychological difficulties. For this reason, they may be ideologically unacceptable to clinical psychologists who adopt systemic, constructivist, cognitive-behavioural, psychodynamic, humanistic or other such frameworks as a basis for practice. However, the administration and funding of clinical services and research programmes is predominantly framed in terms of the ICD and DSM systems and so it is important for clinical psychologists to be familiar with them. What follows is a cursory summary of the main advantages and problems of both systems.

ADVANTAGES OF ICD 10 AND DSM IV TR

Both systems are multi-axial; the main features of each system are set out in Table 3.1. As multi-axial systems, they allow for complex information about important facets of a case to be coded simply and briefly without the drawback of over-simplification, which characterizes single-axis categorical systems. In both ICD 10 and DSM IV TR, the principal diagnoses are given on axis I and other facets of the case are described on the remaining axes. In both systems a case may receive more than one diagnosis on the first axis. This provides both the clinician and the researcher with a way of dealing with the problem of co-morbidity. In both systems, the diagnoses on axis I are given in categorical rather than dimensional terms, although both systems contain dimensional axes on which to code aspects of psychosocial stress and overall level of psychosocial functioning. There has been an emphasis, within both systems, on hierarchical organization of axis I categories, with a few broadband categories subsuming many narrowband categories. In both systems each axis I diagnostic category is defined in atheoretical terms. For

Table 3.1 DSM IV TR, ICD 10 and DC 0–3 multi-axial classification systems

DSM IV TR	ICD 10	DC 0–3
Axis I. Clinical disorders Disorders usually first diagnosed in infancy, childhood or adolescence Learning disorders (e.g. reading disorder) Motor skills development disorder Communication disorders (e.g. expressive language disorder) Pervasive developmental disorder (e.g. autistic disorder) Attention deficit and disruptive behaviour disorders (e.g. conduct disorder) Feeding and eating disorders of infancy and early childhood (e.g. Pica) Tic disorders (e.g. Tourette's disorder) Elimination disorders (e.g. encopresis) Other childhood disorders	**Axis I. Clinical psychiatric syndromes Behavioural and emotional disorders with onset usually occurring in childhood and adolescence** Hyperkinetic disorders (e.g. disturbance of activity and attention) Conduct disorders Mixed disorders of conduct and emotion (e.g. depressive conduct disorder) Emotional disorders with onset specific to childhood (e.g. separation anxiety disorder) Disorders of social functioning with onset specific to childhood (e.g. elective mutism) Tic disorders (e.g. de la Tourette's syndrome) Other childhood disorders (e.g. encopresis and pica)	**Axis I. Primary diagnosis** Traumatic stress disorder Disorders of affect (anxiety, grief reaction, childhood depression, mixed emotional disorder, identity disorder, reactive attachment disorder) Adjustment disorder Regulatory disorder (hypersensitive, under-reactive, impulsive, other) Sleep behaviour disorder Eating behaviour disorder Multi-system and pervasive developmental disorders
Delirium, dementia, amnestic and other cognitive disorders Mental disorders due to a general medical condition Substance-related disorders Schizophrenia and other psychotic disorders Mood disorders Anxiety disorders Somatoform disorders Factitious disorders Dissociative disorders Sexual and gender identity disorders Eating disorders Sleep disorders Impulse control disorders Adjustment disorders Other conditions	**Organic mental disorders Mental and behavioural disorders due to psychoactive substance use Schizophrenia, schizotypal and delusional disorders Mood disorders Neurotic, stress-related and somatoform disorders Behavioural syndromes associated with physiological disturbances and physical factors Disorders of adult personality and behaviour**	

Continued

Table 3.1 continued

DSM IV TR	ICD 10	DC 0–3
Axis II. Personality disorders and mental retardation Paranoid Schizoid Schizotypal Anti-social Borderline Histrionic Narcissistic Avoidant Dependent Obsessive compulsive	**Axis II. Specific delays in development** Specific developmental disorders of speech and language (e.g. expressive language disorder) Specific developmental disorders of scholastic skills (e.g. specific reading disorder) Specific developmental disorder of motor function Pervasive developmental disorders (e.g. childhood autism, Rett's syndrome) **Axis III. Intellectual level**	**Axis II. Relationship disorder classification** Over-involved Under-involved Anxious Angry Mixed Abusive (verbally, physically, sexually)
Axis III. General medical conditions	**Axis IV. Medical conditions**	**Axis III. Medical and developmental disorders and conditions**
Axis IV. Psychosocial and environmental problems Problems with primary support group Problems related to the social environment Educational problems Occupational problems Housing problems Economic problems Problems with access to health-care services Problems related to interaction with the legal system	**Axis V. Abnormal psychosocial situations** Abnormal intrafamilial relationships Familial mental disorder deviance or handicap Inadequate or distorted intrafamilial communication Abnormal qualities of upbringing Abnormal immediate environment Acute life events Societal stressors Chronic interpersonal stress associated with school work Stress resulting from the child's disorder	**Axis IV. Psychosocial stressors** Examples include abduction, abuse adoption, hospitalization, illness, loss, separation, violence Rate effects from 1 = no effect to 7 = severe effect

Axis V. Global assessment of functioning
A score between 1 and 100 is given, e.g.
    10: Danger to self and others
	Axis VI. Global assessment of functioning
	A score between 0 and 8 is given, e.g.
	    8: Profound and pervasive social disability
		Axis V. Functional emotional developmental level
		Mutual attention
		Mutual engagement
		Interactive intentionality and reciprocity

| 50: Serious symptoms and impairment of social functioning
75: Transient impairment of social functioning
100: Superior functioning | 5: Serious and pervasive social disability
2: Slight social disability
0: Superior social functioning | Representational/affective communication
Representational elaboration
Representational differentiation
Rate from 1 = has reached expected levels to 5 = has not mastered prior levels |

Note: Based on APA (2000a), WHO (1996), Zero to Three (1994).

the most part, diagnostic categories are based on observable clusters of symptoms. This strategy was adopted to avoid the unreliability of diagnoses based on inferred intrapsychic variables which characterized DSM I and DSM II. However, in some instances organic or psychosocial aetiological factors are used to define disorders. For example, substance-related disorders are defined by the substances abused and exposure to a major stressor is one of the criteria for post-traumatic stress disorder. Both systems attempt to address the complexity of the difficulties with which children and families present by providing an axis on which to code psychosocial and contextual adversity. A facility for assessing adaptive social functioning on a dimensional axis is also provided by both systems. Both systems include an axis on which to code general medical conditions and an axis on which to code general intellectual functioning. The ICD 10 multi-axial system also provides a separate axis for coding specific developmental delays whereas these are coded as co-morbid disorders on the first axis of the DSM IV TR. While not of relevance to children, it should be mentioned that DSM IV TR codes personality disorders on the second axis.

Both the DSM and ICD systems are open to revision in the light of new information. So, for example, in ICD 10 a distinction is made between oppositional defiant disorder and conduct disorder, whereas its precursor ICD 9 did not make this distinction. The differentiation of the two disorders is based on research that shows that the two disorders have different correlates and prognoses. Conduct disorder is associated with more pervasive family- and school-based difficulties and has a worse prognosis. In an appendix of DSM IV TR, diagnostic criteria and axes for further study are included. Among these a defensive functioning axis and a global assessment of relational functioning axis are outlined. The latter is of particular relevance to childhood disorders, since it provides an overall index of family functioning. Research on this axis is promising (Dausch, Miklowitz & Richards, 1996; GAP, 1996).

TECHNICAL PROBLEMS WITH DSM IV TR AND ICD 10

Both ICD 10 and DSM IV TR have serious short-comings. Their technical problems can be distinguished from ethical and pragmatic concerns, which will be discussed later. The main technical problems include low reliability, poor coverage, high co-morbidity and low validity.

Reliability

In the past, a major problem with the ICD and DSM systems was their poor inter-rater reliability. Clinicians who interviewed the same cases frequently reached different conclusions about the most appropriate diagnosis. It was hoped that the use of diagnostic criteria based on atheoretical observable symptoms would improve the unacceptably low reliability co-efficients obtained for many of the DSM II categories. No such improvement was observed in carefully controlled studies comparing the DSM II (in which no diagnostic criteria were given) and DSM III (in which diagnostic criteria were first introduced) (e.g. Kirk & Kutchins, 1992; Mattison, Cantweell, Russell & Will, 1979). However, in later studies that coupled the use of diagnostic criteria with standardized approaches to interviewing, it was found that diagnoses could be made with a fair degree of reliability for a small number of relatively common psychological disorders. Reliability data for conduct disorder, attention deficit disorder, major depression and anxiety disorders (including over-anxious disorder and separation anxiety disorder) are presented in Table 3.2. The data come from Hodges' review of seven major clinic-based studies involving structured interviews with 750 children (Hodges, Cools & Mcknew, 1989). The most striking feature of these results is the fact that, even with the use of highly structured interviews, diagnostic

Table 3.2 The reliability of diagnoses of four childhood psychological disorders

Disorder	Mean kappa reliability co-efficient	Range of kappa reliability co-efficients
Conduct disorder	.62	.31 to 1.00
Attention deficit disorder	.52	.21 to 1.00
Major depression	.62	.36 to .90
Anxiety disorders	.52	.24 to .84

Note: Reliability co-efficients in this table are based on data presented in Table 1 of Hodges (1993). This review covers seven major studies involving 750 clinical cases (Bird et al., 1988; Chambers et al., 1985; Costello et al., 1984; Hodges et al., 1989; Last, 1987; Shaffer et al., 1988; Welner et al., 1987). The reliability of DSM III R diagnoses are based on information drawn from structured interviews for children such as the Diagnostic Interview for Children (DISC; Costello et al., 1984). In all studies children were interviewed twice by different interviews and the test–retest interval varied from 2 hours to 3 weeks. Kappa values of .9 are good; of .7 are satisfactory; .5 to .6 are fair; and those below .4 indicate unreliability (Spitzer & Fleiss, 1974).

criteria and in some instances computer algorithms to reach diagnoses, reliability co-efficients still fall within the .5 to .6 range, which Spitzer and Fleiss (1974), in their seminal article, describe as 'fair'. Kappa reliability co-efficients must be above .7 to be classified as 'satisfactory'. More recently, Jensen et al. (1995) found that when data from parallel, structured parent and child interviews were combined, in clinical samples satisfactory levels of reliability were recorded for conduct disorder (.71) and depression (.70). However, only fair levels of reliability were obtained for anxiety and attention deficit disorders in clinical samples and only fair levels of reliability were obtained for all four categories in community samples. Currently, for both DSM IV TR and ICD 10, the demonstration of satisfactory reliability remains a central problem.

Studies which address this issue employ the structured interview schedules. Reliability data from Angold (2002) on the test–retest reliability of four common diagnostic categories from some of the more widely used structured interviews are listed in Table 3.3. The data show that some interviews are more reliable than others for some or all diagnostic categories. A distinction is made between interviewer- and respondent-based structured interviews. With the former, expert clinicians have latitude to phrase questions and probes in ways that they see fit and to make complex judgements about the presence and severity of symptoms. In contrast, respondent-based interviews such as the DISC IV are designed to be administered by lay interviewers. Questions are read verbatim by interviewers and responses coded with a minimum latitude for clinical judgement. From Table 3.3 it appears that interviewer-based interviews are a little more reliable. (See Table 3.11 at the end of the chapter for information and contact addresses for widely used structured interviews.)

Table 3.3 The test–retest reliability of four diagnostic categories from structured interviews

Disorder	CAPA	CAS	DICA	ISCA	K SADS	DISC IV
Conduct disorder	.55	–	.90	–	.83	.55
Attention deficit hyperactivity disorder	–	.43	1.0	–	.69	.62
Major depression	.90	1.0	–	–	.80	.65
Anxiety disorders	.64	.72	.76	.82	.59	.59

Note: Based on averaged data from Table 3.1 of Angold (2002). CAPA, Child and Adolescent Psychiatric Assessment; CAS, Child Assessment Schedule; DICA, Diagnostic Interview for Children and Adolescents; ISCA, Interview schedule for children and adolescents; KSADS, Schedule for Affective Disorders and Schizophrenia for School-age Children; DISC, Diagnostic Interview Schedule for children.

Coverage

Along with the use of diagnostic criteria, there has been a gradual narrowing of definitions of disorders to reduce within-category heterogeneity and improve reliability. This effort to improve within-category homogeneity has led to a problem of poor coverage. That is, many cases typically referred for consultation cannot be classified into clearly defined categories using either system. Two strategies have been adopted to deal with the poor coverage problem. The first is to include an undefined subcategory for many disorders to accommodate individuals who show constellations of symptoms which fall between two clearly defined clinical syndromes. In the DSM such categories are labelled *not otherwise specified* (NOS) and in the ICD the term *unspecified* is used, for example, *conduct disorder, unspecified*. The second solution to the coverage problem has been to include a list of problems, concerns and factors that may lead to referral but which fall outside the overall diagnostic framework. In the ICD system these are termed Z codes and in the DSM, they are referred to as V codes. For example, in the ICD 10, code Z64.0 is used when a person has *problems related to unwanted pregnancy*. In DSM IV TR, code V61.20 is used if there is a *parent–child relational problem*.

Co-morbidity

Co-morbidity refers to situations where more than one diagnosis may be given. Co-morbidity rates for four major DSM categories are presented in Table 3.4. These are based on aggregated data from four major international community-based non-clinical studies involving a total of 2662 cases (Anderson, Williams, McGee & Silva, 1987; Bird et al., 1988; Kashani et al., 1987; McGee et al., 1990). In each of the studies, structured interviews with

Table 3.4 Co-morbidity in community populations for four major DSM diagnostic categories

	Conduct disorder	Attention deficit disorder	Major depression
Attention deficit disorder	23.3%		
Major depression	16.9%	10.5%	
Anxiety disorders	14.8%	11.8%	16.2%

Note: Figures in this table are based on aggregated data from four international studies involving 2662 cases abstracted from Table 2 in McConaughy and Achenbach (1994). These studies include Anderson et al.'s (1987) investigation of 792 11-year-olds and McGee et al.'s (1990) study of 943 15-year-olds in New Zealand; Bird et al.'s (1988) study of 777 4- to 16-year-olds in Puerto Rico and Kashani et al.'s (1987) study of 150 14- to 16-year-olds in Missouri. In all studies the DISC (Costello et al., 1984) was used except Kashani's where the DICA (Herjanic & Reich, 1982) was employed. Bidirectional co-morbidity in all cells = Cases Da, Db / CasesDa, Db+ Cases Da, not Db+ Cases Db, not Da, where Da is diagnosis a and Db is diagnosis b.

the child were employed to gather data and diagnoses were made according to DSM III criteria. From these data it is clear that between approximately 10 and 20% of cases in the community exhibit symptoms consistent with the diagnosis of two of the four most common childhood disorders: conduct disorder, depression, anxiety disorder and attention deficit hyperactivity disorder.

Further co-morbidity data are presented in Table 3.5, and are drawn from McConaughy and Achenbach's (1994) study of 2600 community and 2707 clinical cases in the US, aged 4–16. Parents completed the Child Behaviour Checklists and youngsters over 11 completed the Youth Self-Report Form. Cases were given a positive diagnosis if they scored above the 95th percentile on the syndrome scales. These scales hold much in common with DSM diagnostic categories contained in Table 3.4 and are discussed more fully below when dimensional alternatives to categorical systems are considered. The aggressive behaviour scale overlaps considerably with the DSM diagnosis of conduct disorder. The attention problem scale holds much in common with the DSM attention deficit hyperactivity disorder. Symptoms of both depressive and anxiety disorders are contained in the anxious-depressed scale. The somatic complaints scale contains items that are common in cases of both separation anxiety and somatization disorder. From Table 3.5, it may be seen that co-morbidity is far more common in clinical compared with community

Table 3.5 Co-morbidity in community and clinic populations for four ASEBA syndromes

	Aggressive behaviour	Attention problems	Anxious depressed
Attention problems	Comm. Parent rep 28% Comm. Child rep 26%		
	Clinic Parent rep 47% Clinic Child rep 40%		
Anxious depressed	Comm. Parent rep 26% Comm. Child rep 20%	Comm. Parent rep 28% Comm. Child rep 25%	
	Clinic Parent rep 41% Clinic Child rep 34%	Clinic Parent rep 43% Clinic Child rep 43%	
Somatic complaints	Comm. Parent rep 14% Comm. Child rep 16%	Comm. Parent rep 12% Comm. Child rep 16%	Comm. Parent rep 15% Comm. Child rep 20%
	Clinic Parent rep 23% Clinic Child rep 25%	Clinic Parent rep 23% Clinic Child rep 25%	Clinic Parent rep 30% Clinic Child rep 32%

Note: Figures in this table are abstracted from Tables 3 and 5 in McConaughy and Achenbach (1994) and are based on 2600 community and 2707 clinical cases in the US, aged 4–16. Parents completed Child Behaviour Checklists and youngsters over 11 completed the Youth Self-Report Form. Cases were given a positive diagnosis if they scored above the 95th percentile on the syndrome scale. Bidirectional co-morbidity in all cells = Cases Da, Db / CasesDa, Db+ Cases Da, not Db+ Cases Db, not Da, where Da is diagnosis a and Db is diagnosis b. Comm., community; Clinic, clinical; rep, report.

samples. Co-morbidity is also more commonly reported by parents for aggressive behaviour coupled with either attention problems or anxious depression. Co-morbidity is more commonly reported by children for somatic complaints coupled with aggressive behaviour, attention problems or anxious depression. These data on co-morbidity suggest that children who meet the criteria for more than one disorder are more likely to be referred to clinics, that parents are more likely to notice attention and mood problems when they occur in conjunction with aggression and that young-sters are more likely to have problems with aggression, attention and mood when they also experience somatic complaints.

Validity

The validation of diagnostic categories within the DSM and ICD systems involves demonstrating that cases which meet the diagnostic criteria for a particular category share common critical characteristics. These include pre-disposing risk factors, precipitating factors that trigger the onset of the disorder, maintaining factors that lead to persistence or exacerbation of the disorder and protective factors that modify the impact of aetiological factors. The course of the disorder over time and the response of cases to specific treatments should also be shared to a fairly marked degree by cases falling within the same valid diagnostic category. Despite extensive research on many disorders, it is difficult to point to any one condition where validity on all of these criteria has been established. There is not a high level of specificity in the links between aetiological factors and the psychological problems of children and adolescents. Indeed, the literature reviewed in Chapter 2 under-lines the degree to which many of the same pre-disposing, precipitating and maintaining factors are shared by different types of psychological problems. Furthermore, the course of any disorder and its response to treatment is highly variable and is strongly influenced for most disorders by co-morbidity and the number of risk factors present (Clark, Watson & Reynolds, 1995; Friedman & Chase-Lansdale, 2002; Luthar, 2003; Rolf et al., 1990).

Developmental relevance

Dissatisfaction among clinicians about the applicability of the DSM and ICD to children under the age of three inspired the National Association for Children and Toddlers to develop the Diagnostic Classification of Mental Health and Developmental Disorders in Infancy and early Childhood, known as DC: 0–3 (Zero to Three, 1994). DC: 0–3 is a multi-axial system, like the current ICD and DSM systems, but cast in a way to take greater account of the developmental psychology of children under three than the ICD or DSM. For convenience, key features of DC: 0–3 have been included in Table 3.1. The list of possible diagnoses on axis I reflects an extension of those available in the ICD and DSM systems, and the diagnostic criteria have been refined for use with young children. On the second axis, the quality of the relationship that the child has with the primary caregiver is coded and this reflects the importance accorded to attachment and exposure to abuse in child development. Medical problems are coded on the third axis and exposure to psychosocial stresses on the fourth axis. On the fifth axis functional emotional developmental level is coded. This axis has been included in recognition of the importance of achieving milestones in emotional competence during the first three years for overall long-term adjustment. The Preschool Age Psychiatric Assessment (PAPA; Egger & Angold, 2004) listed in Table 3.11 (p. 103) is one of the very few structured interviews for making DC: 0–3 diagnoses. The DC: 0–3 is a useful attempt to develop a diagnostic classification system of relevance to children under three, but because it rests on a categorical framework, it will probably be shown to have many of the difficulties entailed by the DSM and ICD systems.

DIMENSIONAL MODELS OF PSYCHOLOGICAL PROBLEMS

The reason both the ICD and DSM systems have reliability, coverage and co-morbidity difficulties which compromise their validity is because most psychological difficulties are not distributed within the population as disease-like categorical entities. Rather, they occur as either complex interactional problems involving children and members of their social networks or as dimensional psychological characteristics or combinations of both (Sonuga-Barke, 1998; Volkmar & Schwab-Stone, 1996). It is therefore expedient for clinical psychologists to make use of dimensional and systemic frameworks in assessing many categorically defined childhood problems. It is to these that we now turn.

The Achenbach System of Empirically Based Assessment (ASEBA; Achenbach & Rescorla, 2000, 2001), a dimensional approach to conceptualizing children's problems, is a recent example drawn from a tradition which includes Eysenck (1967) in the UK and Quay (1983) in the US (Sonuga-Barke, 1998). Achenbach's (Achenbach & Rescorla, 2000, 2001) analysis of standardization data for the Child Behaviour Checklist (and related ASEBA instruments) gathered from over 2000 parents, teachers and youngsters on children aged 1.5–18 years has shown that many of the behavioural difficulties which lead to referral are most parsimoniously conceptualized as reflecting extreme scores on two major behavioural dimensions. The first of these dimensions contains items that inquire about *emotional* behaviours such as crying, worrying and withdrawal. Items on this dimension have been termed *internalizing behaviour problems* and are most acutely problematic for the child rather than for parents or teachers, although it goes without saying that parents and teachers are invariably concerned about such youngsters when they realize the level of internal distress that these children experience. The second dimension contains items which focus on aggressive and delinquent *conduct* problems. These have been termed *externalizing behaviour problems* and include difficulties such as fighting, disobedience, drug abuse and delinquent gang membership.

Cases which obtain extreme scores on these internalizing and externalizing dimensions typically receive ICD and DSM diagnoses. Inevitably, however, many children who do not score at the outer extremities of these dimensions, but who nevertheless are referred for clinical consultation, are unclassifiable within categorical systems such as the DSM or the ICD. This is one explanation for the coverage difficulties both systems exhibit. Because internalizing and externalizing dimensions are normally distributed within the population, it is understandable that most children show some problems associated with both dimensions and a significant minority of youngsters score extremely on both. This way of conceptualizing children's behavioural problems offers a parsimonious explanation for the co-morbidity problem discussed above.

Underlying the two broad-band dimensions of internalizing and externalizing behaviour problems are a small number of narrow-band syndrome scales which emerged from factor analyses of checklists completed by parents, teachers and youngsters. These syndrome scales are summarized in Table 3.6. (Co-morbidity data derived from four of these narrow-band scales have already been presented in Table 3.5.) It is notable just how few syndromes emerged from these factor analyses in comparison to the proliferation of categories and subcategories in the DSM and ICD systems, both of which contain more than 50 diagnostic categories or subcategories relevant to children. Indeed, even fewer empirically based factors emerged from factor analyses of the Strengths and Difficulties Questionnaire (SDQ; Goodman, 2001) a

Table 3.6 Empirically derived syndromes assessed by the child behaviour checklist and related ASEBA instruments

	Age 1.5–5	Age 6–18
Internalizing syndromes	Anxious/depressed Withdrawn Somatic complaints Emotionally reactive	Anxious-depressed Withdrawn-depressed Somatic complaints
Externalizing syndromes	Aggressive behaviour Attention problems	Aggressive behaviour Rule-breaking behaviour
Mixed syndromes	Sleep problems	Attention problems Thought problems Social problems

Note: Based on Achenbach and Rescorla (2000, 2001).

widely used, UK-based screening instrument. The SDQ yields scores for conduct, emotional, peer and ADHD problems only. (Websites for SDQ and ASEBA instruments are listed in Table 3.11.) The proliferation of categories in DSM IV TR and ICD 10 in many instances is based on insubstantial evidence. Both systems were evolved by committee consensus following literature reviews, and may reflect committee biases (Clark et al., 1995).

However, it is important to mention that multi-variate methods, such as those used by Achenbach, while particularly good at identifying frequently occurring syndromes which contain many symptoms, are poor at identifying rare syndromes which are more parsimoniously conceptualized in categorical rather than dimensional terms, such as bipolar disorder, or those involving a single symptom, such as encopresis (Cantwell & Rutter, 1994; Taylor & Rutter, 2002). Thus, the DSM and ICD systems are particularly useful for conceptualizing some pervasive developmental disorders, tic disorders, and single-symptom presentations such as pica or night terrors.

Specific learning disabilities, such as dyslexia, and extreme general learning problems such as profound intellectual disability are also distributed within the population as categorical disease-like entities. In contrast, mild and moderate mental handicap appear to be distributed as the tail of a normal distribution of cognitive ability conceptualized in dimensional terms (Cantwell & Rutter, 1994; Taylor & Rutter, 2002).

Dimensional conceptualizations of behavioural and learning problems offer a useful framework for assessment in many instances. The use of reliable and valid behaviour checklists and ability tests can readily be incorporated into routine clinical practice to provide assessments of the status of children on such dimensions. Furthermore, cut-off scores can be used, when administratively necessary, to translate dimensional scores into diagnoses (Kasius, Ferdinand, van den Berg & Verhulst, 1997). Finally, improvement or deterioration may be assessed in terms of changes in scores along dimensions. Manuals for most tests and checklists give rules for interpreting change scores which take into account the psychometric properties of the instrument.

However, with any assessment system, account must be taken of the impact of the situation in which observations are made and the status of the observer. Achenbach (1991) found that the degree of agreement between parents, teachers and youngsters about the severity of internalizing and externalizing behavioural problems varied substantially in the 1991 standardization sample of the ASEBA instruments. This variation was due to the context in which the behaviour was observed (home, or school or both) and the respondent (parent, teacher or youngster). Mothers' and fathers' scores from the standardization sample showed high correlations (r = .77); scores of parents and teachers showed a moderate correlation (r = .44); those between parents and youths were also moderate (r = .41); but those between teachers and youths had the lowest correlation of all (r = .31) (Achenbach, 1991).

INTERACTIONAL MODELS OF PSYCHOLOGICAL PROBLEMS

Both categorical and dimensional approaches for conceptualizing childhood problems entail the assumption that behavioural and learning problems are inherent characteristics of the child. Of course, to some degree this is a useful way to think about such difficulties, particularly with disorders such as autism. However, children's problems are typically part of patterns of inter-action that involve family members and members of the wider social and professional networks in which families are embedded (Carr, 2000b). For example, many conduct problems evolve as part of a chaotic family system characterized by marital discord and parenting skills deficits within a social context where the parents experience little social support and considerable stress. Similarly, separation anxiety is described in the ICD and DSM sys-tems as if it were an inherent characteristic of the child, when the evidence suggests that it is one part of an interactional pattern usually involving mutual concerns for safety expressed by both mother and child, which the father and occasionally involved medical and educational professionals criti-cize as inappropriate or deviant. It is common for this type of system to evolve following some threat to the family's integrity such as a loss or bereavement. The results of research on conduct disorders and separation anxiety which support these views are presented in Chapters 10 and 12, respectively.

Categorical individualistic models, such as the DSM and ICD, run the risk of obscuring the interactional embeddedness of most childhood problems. In both the ICD and DSM systems there is a facility for coding psychosocial and contextual factors. However, this occurs on the second last axis, a pos-ition which is not likely to command a busy clinician's attention. This may be unhelpful for clinical psychologists, since often it is the characteristics of the system of relationships around the child which has the greatest implica-tions for management and prognosis. For example, the treatment resources required for multi-problem reconstituted families are greater than those needed for focal problem intact families (Carr, 2000b).

Families whose children are referred for psychological consultation may differ along a variety of contextual parameters which allow therapeutically useful distinctions to be made (Carr, 2000b). These distinctions include:

- focal problem families versus multi-problem families
- simple/traditional family structure versus complex/alternative family structure
- adaptively organized families versus rigidly or chaotically organized families
- emotionally close enmeshed families versus emotionally distant dis-engaged families
- families at different lifecycle stages

- families in which violence or abuse is occurring, including physical, sexual and emotional abuse
- families adjusting to physical illness.

It may be useful for clinical psychologists to incorporate these type of distinctions into the way they organize the classification of referrals. In the audit form presented in Figure 5.9 in Chapter 5 (p. 182), cases are classified as focal problem or multi-problem referrals.

ETHICAL PROBLEMS WITH ICD 10 AND DSM IV TR

At an ethical level, diagnoses pathologize youngsters who are relatively powerless to resist this process. That is, diagnoses focus on weaknesses rather than strengths and are couched in a pathologizing pejorative discourse. The process of traditional diagnosis may lead youngsters, their families and the community to view diagnosed children as defective. If labelling leads to stigmatization, then it may only be justifiable to the extent that the diagnoses given, lead to treatment which ameliorates the problems described by the label. Incidentally, the same argument holds for labelling families as dysfunctional. A counterargument to this overall objection to labelling is that it is not the label which leads to stigmatization but the behavioural difficulties which the youngster exhibits (Cantwell & Rutter, 1994; Taylor & Rutter, 2002). My own view is that, probably, the problems and the label combine to lead to stigmatization but that the benefits of some form of labelling probably outweigh the costs. However, labelling should be as benign as possible. The massive over-emphasis on pathology with little regard for personal strengths and resources shown by the DSM and ICD system is unjustifiable. It would be very empowering for children and families to receive feedback like the following:

- *Our assessment shows that this youngster has personal strengths and skills and is well supported by his family and school and so presents with less severe sleep and mood problems than would otherwise occur following a trauma. The official ICD 11 and DSM V diagnosis is **robust personal and family coping syndrome**.*

Instead, our current classification systems informs feedback that is pathologizing such as:

- *Our assessment shows that this youngster, following exposure to a trauma suffers from intrusive memories, attempts to avoid or suppress these, and episodes of anxiety. The official ICD 10 and DSM IV TR diagnosis is of **post-traumatic stress disorder**.*

Within the family therapy tradition, there is a practice of routinely focusing on strengths and solutions rather than weaknesses and problems, which might well be adopted by clinical psychologists (Carr, 2000b).

PRACTICAL PROBLEMS WITH ICD 10 AND DSM IV TR

At the pragmatic level, surveys show that clinicians find the DSM system unhelpful in routine clinical practice (Jampala, Sierles & Taylor, 1986). A diagnostic label, or even a full multi-axial list of labels, offers very limited guidance on how to proceed clinically. For example, if a child has a diagnosis of conduct disorder, it is difficult to develop a coherent treatment plan without a formulation that specifies the patterns of interaction in which the specific conduct difficulties are embedded and the protective factors, particularly the parenting resources, present in the case. In practice, many clinicians give DSM diagnoses as an administrative chore since in the US insurance companies often link payment to the presence of a DSM diagnosis. In parts of Europe, particularly in the public health services, funding may be linked to the completion of administrative forms on each patient seen, and these forms include a requirement to give an ICD diagnosis.

A FRAMEWORK FOR THE CLASSIFICATION OF PROBLEMS

The framework used in this book for classifying the main problems with which clinical psychologists have to deal when working with children, adolescents and families is presented in Table 3.7. Problems are organized developmentally by the stage of the child's life at which they usually emerge. Thus a distinction is made between those that typically occur first during the pre-school years, those that commonly emerge in middle childhood and those that are principally a concern in adolescence. Problems associated with two major sources of stress (abuse and developmental transitions such as bereavement or divorce) have been categorized separately.

Pre-school problems include difficulties associated with sleeping and toileting. Feeding difficulties (often included as a pre-school problem in other texts) are considered with neglect and non-organic failure to thrive. Specific and general learning difficulties, developmental delays and pervasive developmental disorders such as autism are also included as problems which first come to attention in the pre-school years.

Conduct problems and attention deficit hyperactivity problems, both of which involve externalizing behavioural difficulties are included in the list of problems which typically emerge in middle childhood. The internalizing behavioural difficulties which are included here are anxiety problems, somatic

Table 3.7 Broad problem areas in clinical child psychology

Problems in early childhood	Sleeping problems Toileting problems Learning disabilities Pervasive developmental disorders
Problems in middle childhood	Conduct problems Attention deficit hyperactivity disorder Anxiety problems Repetition problems Somatic complaints
Problems in adolescence	Drug abuse Mood regulation problems Eating disorders Schizophrenia
Problems associated with child abuse	Physical abuse problems Emotional abuse and neglect-related problems Sexual abuse-related problems
Problems associated with major developmental transitions	Substitutive childcare-related problems Separation and divorce adjustment problems Grief associated with bereavement and life-threatening illness

complaints and repetition problems such as obsessive compulsive disorder, tics and Tourette's syndrome.

In adolescence, the main externalizing problem included is drug abuse and the internalizing problems are depression, eating disorders such as anorexia and schizophrenia.

Under the general heading of problems associated with abuse, distinctions are made between those associated with physical abuse, sexual abuse and emotional abuse along with related problems such as neglect and non-organic failure to thrive. Under the heading of problems associated with developmental transitions, reactions to divorce, bereavement and placement in care are considered. Problems associated with abuse and major life transitions have been separated out from other types of problems because they may occur at any point in the child's development and because they place unique types of demands on clinical psychologists.

The framework for classifying problems set out in Table 3.7 is by no means exhaustive. Many problems have been excluded. However, it covers most of the problems seen in routine clinical practice and offers an overall framework within which problems as defined in DSM IV TR, ICD 10 and elsewhere may be incorporated.

EPIDEMIOLOGY

While the classification of childhood disorders addresses the question 'How many different sort of problems are there?', the central question for epidemiology is 'How many children in the population have these problems?' Epidemiology is also concerned with the identification of factors associated with the distribution of diagnoses within populations. Data on the overall prevalence of psychological difficulties in a number of countries are presented in Table 3.8. In all studies the Rutter B Teacher's Questionnaire, a well-validated instrument, was used to screen cases (Rutter, 1967). Children scoring above the cut-off score of 9 on this scale were defined as having psychological problems of sufficient severity to warrant psychiatric diagnosis. From the table it is clear that the prevalence of childhood psychological problems varies from a low of 4% to a high of 23% depending on geographical location. Higher rates are associated with urban rather than rural location and with Westernized rather than Oriental culture.

The following are some of the broad conclusions that can be drawn from Table 3.9, where data from Meltzer, Gatward, Goodman & Ford's (2000) study of over 10,000 UK children aged 5–15 are presented.

- Overall, 9.5% of children have psychological disorders of some sort.
- Rates of psychological disorders increase with age. The rate for five- to ten-year-olds is 8.2% and for 11- to 15-year-olds is 11.2%.
- Rates of psychological disorders are higher for boys. The rate for boys is 11.4% and for girls it is 7.6%.

Table 3.8 Prevalence of childhood psychological disorder as assessed by Rutter's Teacher's Questionnaire in a series of international studies

Author	Year	Country (region)	n	% Psychological disorder
Venables	1983	Mauritius	1063	23%
Rutter	1975	UK (London)	1689	19%
Minde	1975	Uganda	577	18%
Jeffers	1991	Ireland (Dublin)	2029	17%
Porteous	1991	Ireland (Cork)	733	15%
Matsuura	1993	Korea	1975	14%
O'Connor	1988	Ireland (Clare)	1361	11%
Rutter	1975	UK (Isle of Wight)	1279	11%
McGee	1984	New Zealand	951	9%
Matsuura	1993	China	2432	8%
Matsuura	1993	Japan	2638	4%

Note: Adapted from Carr (1993). Cases scoring 9 or more on the Rutter B scale were classified as deviant and all percentages are rounded up to whole numbers.

Table 3.9 Prevalence of psychological disorders as assessed by the DAWBA in boys and girls in the UK

			Age		
Problem area	*Diagnostic category*	*Gender*	*5–10 years* (n = 5830)	*11–15 years* (n = 4608)	*All* (n = 10,438)
Conduct	**Conduct disorders**	Boys	6.5	8.6	5.3
		Girls	2.7	3.8	
	Attention deficit disorders	Boys	2.6	2.3	1.4
		Girls	0.4	0.5	
Emotion	**Depression**	Boys	0.2	1.7	0.9
		Girls	0.3	1.9	
	Anxiety disorders	Boys	3.2	3.9	3.8
		Girls	3.1	5.3	
	Depression and anxiety disorders	Boys	3.3	5.1	4.3
		Girls	3.3	6.1	
Less common	**PDD, eating disorders, tic**	Boys	0.8	0.3	0.3
		Girls	0.2	0.0	
All disorders		Boys	10.4	12.8	11.4
		Girls	5.9	9.6	7.6
		Boys and Girls	8.2	11.2	9.5

Note. DAWBA, Development and Well-being Assessment. All rates are percentages and are based on Table 4.1, p. 33. in Meltzer et al. (2000).

- Conduct disorders are more prevalent than emotional disorders, which in turn are more prevalent than ADHD. Overall 5.3% have conduct problems, 4.3% have emotional problems, .9% have ADHD and less than .5% have less common problems (pervasive developmental disorders, eating disorders and tics).
- Conduct problems are twice as common in boys as girls and rates of conduct problems increase with age.
- ADHD is five times more common in boys than girls but rates do not increase with age.
- Overall rates of emotional disorders are similar in pre-adolescent boys and girls. Rates almost double in adolescence, but the increased rate is greater for girls.

THE EFFECTIVENESS OF PSYCHOLOGICAL THERAPY

A series of meta-analyses involving over 200 studies and 11,000 cases have concluded that, on average, a child receiving psychological treatment scores higher on measures of symptomatic improvement than approximately 75% of untreated controls, and that these gains are maintained at follow-up (Fonagy et al., 2002, Chapter 1; Weisz & Kazdin, 2003). This large effect associated with the psychological treatment of children is similar to that obtained in meta-analyses of adult psychotherapy outcome studies. However, not all cases are equally likely to respond to treatment. Some of the more important variables that influence the degree to which cases are likely to respond to treatment are presented in Table 3.10. This list is based on reviews of the child psychotherapy and the family therapy process and treatment outcome literature (Carr, 2000a, 2002a; Fonagy et al., 2002; Kazdin & Weisz, 2003; Sprenkle, 2002; Weisz & Weiss, 1993). From Table 3.10 the following conclusions of relevance to clinical practice may be drawn.

Child characteristics

Diagnosis, co-morbidity, severity, chronicity and the age and gender of the child all affect response to treatment. Cases where the principal diagnosis is a pervasive developmental disorder show less improvement than those characterized by internalizing and externalizing disorders. The presence of co-morbidity and severe problems is also associated with a poorer response to treatment. Cases with a later age of onset and briefer duration show greater improvement than chronic cases with early onset. Younger cases show greater improvement than older cases and girls show greater improvement than boys.

Table 3.10 Factors influencing the outcome of psychological treatment of children

Domain	Variable	Good treatment response	Poor treatment response
Child	Diagnosis	Internalizing and externalizing disorders	Pervasive developmental disorders
	Co-morbidity	Single diagnosis	Co-morbid diagnoses
	Severity	Mild problems	Severe problems
	Chronicity	Later age of onset and briefer duration	Chronic cases with early onset
	Age	Younger cases	Older cases
	Gender	Female	Male
Family	Parental adjustment	Good health and adjustment	Psychological or physical health problems
	Marital satisfaction	Marital satisfaction	Marital discord
	Family functioning	Flexible family functioning	Family disorganization
	Father absence	Father is involved	Father is not involved
	SES	High socioeconomic status	Low socioeconomic status
Professional network	Agency involvement	Single agency involvement	Multi-agency involvement
	Coercive referral	Regular referral	Coercive referral
	Solicited referral	Solicited referral	Regular referral
Treatment system	Therapeutic alliance	Positive alliance	Poor alliance
	Therapeutic model	Cognitive-behavioural better than systemic, humanistic and psychodynamic models	
	Therapeutic modality for internalizing behaviour problems	Individual, group and family modalities	
	Therapeutic modality for externalizing and severe debilitating problems	Extensive family involvement	Individual or group formats
	Therapy duration	10 sessions and booster sessions	Less than 10 sessions without follow-up
	Therapist commitment to the model	Therapist is committed to the model	Therapist is not committed to the model
	Treatment manuals	Flexible use of manualized treatments	Rigid use of treatment manuals or non-manualized therapies
Evaluation system	Outcome measure	Specific measures of goal attainment	General measures
	Outcome rater	Independent observers, therapists and parents	Children receiving treatment, their peers and their teachers

Note: Information in this table is based on data reviewed in Carr, 2000a, 2002a; Fonagy et al., 2002; Kazdin and Weisz, 2003; Sprenkle, 2002; Weisz and Weiss, 1993.

Family factors

Parental mental health, family dysfunction, marital discord and father absence all influence the degree to which cases respond to treatment. Cases in which parents have psychological or physical health problems or criminal involvement show less improvement than cases without these difficulties. Cases characterized by marital discord and severe family disorganization show less improvement than cases where these difficulties are absent. Cases where the father is not involved in the child's life or in the child's treatment show less improvement than cases where the father is involved and these cases like those where the family is from a lower socioeconomic group, are more likely to drop out of therapy.

Professional network and referral system

Cases where many agencies and professionals are involved show less improvement than cases where only one agency or professional is involved. This is because cases with severe problems tend to be involved with multiple agencies and because multiple agencies often have co-ordination problems. Cases referred from a coercive referral source such as a child protection agency or probation service are more likely to drop out of treatment. This is usually because treatment is construed as a punitive rather than a supportive experience. Cases which are referred for treatment rather than solicited through newspaper advertisements for a treatment study show less improvement. This is because solicited cases are more motivated to engage in treatment and often have less severe problems.

Treatment system

Cases where there is a positive therapeutic alliance characterized by warmth, empathy and positive regard show more improvement than cases where there is a poor alliance. Greater improvement occurs when the therapist is committed to the model. Interventions based on systemic, cognitive-behavioural and psychodynamic models are all associated with improvement. Overall, behavioural therapies are marginally more effective than other types of interventions. But many effective behaviour therapy programmes include extensive family involvement and a sensitivity to problems and strengths of family systems and their relationship to children's difficulties. For specific problems, specific techniques are associated with greater improvement. Individual, group and family modalities are effective formats for internalizing behaviour problems. For externalizing problems, pre-school problems, pervasive developmental disorders and psychoses, a treatment format that includes extensive family involvement is more effective than programmes which rely exclusively on individual or group formats. Most improvement is made rapidly in the first ten sessions and, while improvement continues beyond this, it is at a far slower rate. Occasional booster sessions prevent relapse particularly with externalizing behaviour problems. Greater improvement occurs when therapists flexibly use clearly articulated manualized treatments rather than rigidly adhering to treatment manuals or using non-manualized therapies.

Evaluation system

Greater improvement is detected by specific measures of goal attainment compared with general measures of improved functioning. Greater improvement is detected by independent observers, therapists and parents compared with children receiving treatment, their peers and their teachers.

SUMMARY

Currently, the DSM IV TR and ICD 10 multi-axial classification systems are used in the US and Europe respectively to facilitate clinical practice, communication and research. These systems have the advantages of being multi-axial, including diagnostic criteria and allowing for the coding of psychosocial stresses and adaptive functioning. However, both the DSM IV TR and ICD 10 have poor coverage, high levels of co-morbidity on axis I and in most instances only fair to low levels of reliability and validity. The problems of poor coverage, high co-morbidity and low reliability may be due to the dimensional distribution of most behaviour problems within the population. A further problem with both systems is the privileging of the individual rather than the family or network as the primary unit of analysis. The prevalence of psychological problems in international studies varies from 4% to 23% and rates are higher in Western urban centres. Prevalence rates vary with gender and age. Meta-analyses of treatment outcome studies show that after treatment about 75% of treated cases are better off than untreated controls and these gains are maintained at follow-up. A variety of client, therapist, treatment and professional network variables effect outcome.

EXERCISE 3.1

Work in groups of three.

*   Use the data in Table 3.9. to draw six graphs. Put age on the x axis and prevalence rate on the y axis. Use a solid line for males and a dotted line for females. Inspect the six graphs.
*   Write down some hypotheses to account for the difference in patterning

of prevalence rates of psychological problems for boys and girls at different ages as depicted in your graphs.

FURTHER READING

American Psychiatric Association (2000). *Diagnostic and Statistical Manual of the Mental Disorders (Fourth Edition-Text Revision, DSM-IV-TR)*. Washington, DC: APA.

Carr, A. (2000a). *What Works With Children and Adolescents? A Critical Review of Research on Psychological Interventions with Children, Adolescents and their Families*. London: Routledge

Carr, A. (2002). *Prevention: What Works? A Critical Review of Research on Psychological Prevention Programmes with Children, Adolescents and their Families*. London: Brunner-Routledge.

Fonagy, P., Target, M., Cottrell, D., Phillips, J., & Kuttz, Z., (2002). *What Works for Whom? A Critical Review of Treatments for Children and Adolescents*. New York: Guilford Press.

Kazdin A. & Weisz, J. (2003). *Evidence-Based Psychotherapies for Children and Adolescents*. New York: Guilford Press.

World Health Organization (1996). *Multi axial Classification of Child and Adolescent Psychiatric Disorders: ICD 10 Classification of Mental and Behavioural Disorders in Children and Adolescents*. Cambridge: Cambridge University Press.

Zero to Three (1994). *Diagnostic Classification: 0–3: Diagnostic Classification of Mental Health and Developmental Disorders of Infancy and Early Childhood*. Arlington, VA: National Centre for Clinical Infant Programs.

WEBSITES

DSM IV TR: http://www.appi.org/dsm.cfx
ICD 10: http://www.who.int/msa/mnh/ems/icd10/icd10.htm
SC:0–3: http://www.zerotothree.org/bookstore/index.cfm?pubID=2514

Table 3.11 Structured interviews and screening instruments for assessing psychological symptomatology in children

CAPA	Child and Adolescent Psychiatric Assessment	Dr Adrian Angold: http:// devepi.mc.duke.edu/CAPA.html Angold, A. & Costello, E. (2000). The Child and Adolescent Psychiatric Assessment (CAPA). *Journal of the American Academy of Child and Adolescent Psychiatry*, 39, 39–48
CAS	Child Assessment Schedule	Dr Kay Hodges, Eastern Michigan University, Department of Psychology, 537 Mark Jefferson, Ypsilanti, MI 48179, USA Hodges, K., Gordon. Y. & Lennon, M. (1990). Parent-child agreement on symptoms assessed via a clinical research interview for children: the Child Assessment (CAS). *Journal of Child Psychology and Psychiatry*, 31, 427–436
DICA	Diagnostic Interview for Children and Adolescents	Dr Wendy Reich: wendyr@twins.wustl.edu http:// www.psychpress.com.au/cat/shop/ productdetails.asp?ProductID=88 Reich, W. (2000). Diagnostic Interview for Children and Adolescents (DICA). *Journal of the American Academy of Child and Adolescent Psychiatry*, 39, 59–66
ISCA	Interview Schedule for Children and Adolescents	Dr Maria Kovacs, Western Psychiatric Institute and Clinic, University of Pittsburgh School of Medicine, 3811, O'Hara Street, Pittsburgh, PN, 15213, USA Sherrill. J. & Kovacs, M. (2000). Interview schedule for children and adolescents (ISCA). *Journal of the American Academy of Child and Adolescent Psychiatry*, 39, 67–75
KSADS	Schedule for Affective Disorders and Schizophrenia for School Age Children	Dr Paul Ambrosini: Paul.Ambrosini@drexel.edu Ambrosini, P. (2000). Historical development and present status of the Schedule for Affective Disorders and Schizophrenia for School-Age Children (K-SADS). *Journal of the American Academy of Child and Adolescent Psychiatry*, 39, 49–58

Continued

Table 3.11 continued

DISC	Diagnostic Interview Schedule for Children	Dr David Shaffer: http://www.c-disc.com/who.htm Shaffer, D., Fisher, P., Lucas, C., Dulcan, M. & Schwab-Stone, M. (2000). NIMH Diagnostic Interview Schedule for Children version IV (NIMH DISC-IV): Description, differences from previous versions, and reliability of some common diagnoses. *Journal of the American Academy of Child and Adolescent Psychiatry*, 39, 28–38
DAWBA	Development and Well-being Assessment	Dr Richard Goodman: http://www.dawba.com/ Goodman, R., Ford, T., Richards, H., Gatward, R. & Meltzer, H. (2000). The Development and Well-Being Assessment: Description and initial validation of an integrated assessment of child and adolescent psychopathology. *Journal of Child Psychology and Psychiatry*, 41, 645–55
PAPA	Preschool Age Psychiatric Assessment	Dr Helen Link Egger, Developmental Epidemiology Center, Duke University Health Systems, DUMC Box 3454, Durham, NC 27710. PAPA contact is Ed Potts epotts@psych.duhs.duke.edu Egger, H. & Angold, A. (2004). The Preschool Age Psychiatric Assessment (PAPA): A structured parent interview for diagnosing psychiatric disorders in preschool children. In R. Delcarmen-Wiggens & A Carter (Eds.). A. *Handbook of Infant and Toddler Mental Health Assessment* (pp. 223–246). New York: Oxford University Press
ASEBA	Achenbach System of Empirically Based Assessment	Dr Tom Achenbach: http://www.aseba.org/
SDQ	Strengths and Difficulties Questionnaire	Dr Richard Goodman: http://www.sdqinfo.com/

Chapter 4

The consultation process and intake interviews

The framework set out in Figure 4.1. outlines the stages of consultation from the initial receiving of a referral letter to the point where the case is closed. In the first stage, a plan for conducting the intake interview is made using the framework in Figure 4.2. The second stage is concerned with the processes of engagement, alliance building, assessment and formulation. In the third stage, the focus is on case management, the therapeutic contract, and the management of resistance. In the final stage, disengagement or re-contracting for further intervention occurs. In this chapter principles of good clinical practice for each of these stages of the consultation process will be given.

STAGES OF THE CONSULTATION PROCESS

In clinical child psychology, consultation is usefully conceptualized as a developmental and recursive process. At each developmental stage, key tasks must be completed before progression to the next stage. Failure to complete the tasks of a given stage before progressing to the next stage may jeopardize the consultation process. For example, attempting to conduct an assessment without first contracting for assessment may lead to co-operation difficulties if the child or parents find the assessment procedures arduous. Consultation is a recursive process insofar as it is possible to move from the final stage of one episode of consultation to the first stage of the next. What follows is a description of the stages of consultation and the tasks entailed by each.

STAGE 1: PLANNING

In the first stage of consultation the main tasks are to plan who to invite to the first session or series of sessions and what to ask them. If there is confusion about who to invite, a network analysis may be conducted. In planning

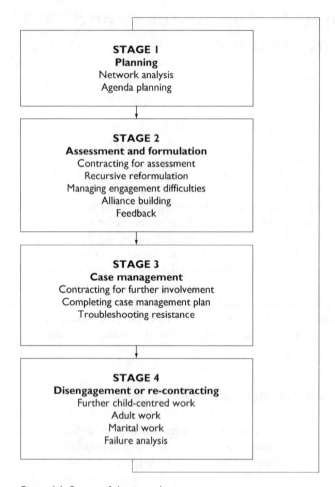

Figure 4.1 Stages of the consultation process

an agenda, a routine intake interview and a core test battery may be supplemented by questions and tests which take account of the specific features of the case.

Network analysis

To make a plan about who to invite to the sessions, the psychologist must find out from the referral letter or through telephone contact with the referrer who is involved with the problem and tentatively establish what roles they play with respect to it. With some cases this will be straightforward. For example, where parents are concerned about a child's enuresis it may be sufficient to invite the child and the parents. In other cases, where school, hospital staff or social services are most concerned about the case, the decision about who to invite to the first interview is less straightforward. In complex cases it is particularly important to analyse network roles accurately before deciding who to invite to the first session. Most network members fall into one or more of the following categories.

- the *referrer*: to whom correspondence about the case should be sent
- the *customer*: who is most concerned that the referral be made
- the *child* or children with the problem
- the legally responsible *guardians*: who are usually the parents but may be a social worker or other representative of the state
- the primary *caregivers*: who are usually the parents but may be foster parents, residential childcare staff or nursing staff
- the child's main *teacher*
- the *social control agents*, such as social workers or probation officers
- other *involved professionals*, including the family doctor, the paediatrician, the school nurse, the parent's psychiatrist, etc.

Certain key network members constitute the minimum sufficient network necessary for effective case management. These include the customer, the legal guardians, the caregivers and the referred child. Psychologists and members of their clinical teams cannot work effectively without engaging with these key network members. Ideally, all members of the minimum sufficient network should be invited to an intake meeting. If this is not possible, then individual meetings or telephone calls may be used to connect with these key members of the network. Where psychologists are working as part of multi-disciplinary teams, often the main customer for a psychological assessment is another team member. In such instances it is often useful to meet with the parents of the child and the referring team member briefly to clarify the reason for the referral and the implications of the psychologist's report for the type of service the child and his family will receive once the assessment is completed. Failure to convene such meetings often results in confusion or co-operation difficulties. Other common engagement difficulties have been described elsewhere (Carr, 2000b).

Often the assessment process is conducted over a number of sessions. To develop a thorough understanding of the presenting problems and related issues, a number of different types of assessment meetings may be conducted. These may include some or all of the following depending upon the case:

- child-centred assessment interview and testing session
- parental interviews
- nuclear family interviews

THE REFERRAL
- The referrer
- The customer
- The child and the reason for referral
- The legally responsible guardians
- The primary caregivers
- The child's main teacher
- The social control agents
- Other involved professionals

TYPES OF MEETINGS USED FOR ASSESSMENT
- Child-centred assessment
- Parental interview
- Nuclear family interview
- School interview
- Extended family interview
- Interview with other involved professionals
- Professional network meeting
- Team meeting
- Case conference

THE HISTORY OF PRESENTING PROBLEMS AND MAINTAINING FACTORS
- Main problems as identified by referrer, child's parents and other significant network members
- History of their development
- Previous successful and unsuccessful solutions
- Network members views on causes of problems and possible solutions
- Denial of the problem
- Lack of commitment to resolving the problem
- Inadvertent reinforcement
- Insecure attachment
- Coercive parent–child processes
- Over-involved parent–child processes
- Disengaged parent–child relationship
- Inconsistent discipline
- Confused communication
- Triangulation
- Chaotic family organization
- Father absence
- Marital discord

CHILD DEVELOPMENTAL HISTORY
The first five years
- Particular strengths shown in first five years
- Pregnancy and birth problems

- Major protective factors and strengths of family members
- The major transitions that the family has made through the family lifecycle
- Current stage of the lifecycle
- Supportive relationships for the child and caregivers within the network
- Stressful relationships for the child and caregivers within the network
- Family factions and patterns particularly multi-generational patterns

PARENT–CHILD RELATIONSHIPS
- Parents' style for meeting child's need for safety particularly with infants and toddlers and problems with neglect
- Parents' style for meeting child's needs for physical care, food, shelter, clothing and problems with neglect
- Parents' style for meeting the child's needs for emotional care, warmth, acceptance and love throughout childhood and adolescence (and problems with abuse or neglect)
- Parents' style for meeting the child's needs for control, clear limits and discipline particularly in middle childhood and adolescence (and problems with being too punitive and abusive or over-indulgent)
- Parents' style for meeting the child's needs for intellectual stimulation particularly in infancy and early childhood (and problems with neglect)
- Parents' style for meeting the child's needs for age-appropriate autonomy and responsibility particularly in adolescence (and problems with being too demanding or too lax and over-protective)

PARENT–PARENT RELATIONSHIPS
- People involved in parenting the child including biological parents, step-parents, foster parents, other family members
- Quality of marital relationship and degree of sharing of childcare if child lives with married or co-habiting parents
- Support network available to single parents
- Quality of co-operative parenting relationship if parents are separated and child lives with one parent but visits the other regularly

LIVING CONDITIONS AND FINANCIAL RESOURCES
- Location in community and proximity to schools, shops, extended family, etc. or problem with isolation
- Ratio of number of people to number of rooms and problems with crowding
- Quality of living quarters and problems with safety or hygiene
- Parental financial resources and need or entitlement to benefits

INVOLVEMENT WITH OTHER PROFESSIONALS AND AGENCIES
- List of other involved agencies
- Duration of involvement
- Reasons for involvement

- Physical health and any early childhood illnesses
- Feeding and eating patterns and problems
- Sleeping pattern, age when first slept through night and sleep problems
- Physical growth and any problems with height or weight being below 3rd centile
- Sensory and motor development and any delays in motor development
- Bowel and bladder control, age when toilet training was complete and any soiling or wetting problems
- Temperament and attachment and any attachment problems
- Language development and any language delays
- Cognitive development and any problems with sustaining attention and solving puzzles and games
- Social development and adjustment to pre-school and any attachment problems or peer problems
- Emotional regulation and problems with persistent crying
- Anger control and problems with tantrums

Middle childhood 6–12 years
- Particular strengths shown in middle childhood
- Physical health and illnesses during middle childhood
- Academic performance and cognitive development and any attainment problems
- Internalization of rules and moral development during middle childhood and any conduct problems
- Emotional regulation, anxiety and depression in middle childhood
- Making and maintaining friendships and peer problems during middle childhood

Adolescence 12–18 years
- Physical health and illnesses during adolescence
- Academic performance and cognitive development in adolescence and any problems with schoolwork
- Rule-following in adolescence and any conduct problems at home, school or in the community
- Adjustment within the peer group in adolescence and any problems with making and maintaining friendships or membership of deviant peer group
- Emotional regulation, anxiety and depression in adolescence
- Eating pattern in adolescence and any indication of anorexia or bulimia
- Experimentation with or abuse of drugs and alcohol
- Psychotic features in adolescence

FAMILY DEVELOPMENTAL HISTORY AND GENOGRAM
- Current household membership
- Extended family membership
- Other network members
- Identifying information such as names, ages, occupations and locations of important family and network members
- Major illnesses and psychosocial problems including hospitalizations, physical and psychological problems and criminality

SCHOOL CONTACT
- Current and past academic performance (including standardized test scores if available
- Current and past performance at sports, drama and other non-academic pursuits
- Current and past relationships with teachers
- Current and past relationships with peers
- Teacher's role in the network
- Teacher's beliefs about the problem and solution
- Teacher's prediction about how the case will work out
- Availability of remedial tuition
- Degree of parent–teacher co-operation
- Amount of child–teacher contact
- Expectations for good conduct
- Expectations for academic attainment
- Pupil involvement in school affairs
- Use of praise-based motivation

OBSERVATIONS OF CHILD AND CHILD'S VIEWPOINT
- Child's account of problem, coping strategies and defences
- Child's account of parents and teacher's views of problem
- Child's genogram and lifeline
- Child's perception of relationships with parents and teachers
- Child's cognitive and academic strengths and weaknesses
- Child's self-esteem, locus of control, self-efficacy and attributional style
- Child's capacity to make and maintain friendships and social problem-solving skills
- Child's account of situations requiring protective action (abuse or suicidal intent)
- The child's wishes for the future
- Child's account of situations requiring major changes in living arrangements (parental custody or foster care)
- Child's capacity to engage in individual, group, or family therapy and to respond to behavioural programmes

FORMULATION
- Pre-disposing factors
- Precipitating factors
- Maintaining factors
- Protective factors

POSSIBLE INTERVENTION OPTIONS
- Take no immediate action
- Reassess periodically
- Refer to another professional within the team for consultation
- Refer to another professional or residential facility outside the team
- Offer focal intervention to the child, parents, family or school
- Offer multi-systemic intervention alone or with other professionals or residential facility to the child, parents, family or school

Figure 4.2 A framework for planning the agenda for assessment interviews

- school interviews
- extended family interviews
- interviews with other involved professionals
- clinical team meetings
- professional network meetings
- statutory case conferences.

Following an intake interview, some combination of these various types of meeting will typically be planned to achieve certain assessment goals. It is important to distinguish between these different types of meeting and to keep records of which network members attended particular meetings, the reasons for their attendance, the information obtained; and the case management decisions made particularly in statutory cases. Record keeping and report writing will be discussed fully in Chapter 5. Written or verbal consent must be obtained from parents or guardians when other involved professionals or teachers are to be contacted as part of the assessment procedure. The child information form set out in Figure 4.3 includes requests for consent to contact the child's teacher, family doctor and other involved professionals. This form can be sent to literate parents to complete before the intake interview or it may be completed as part of routine intake interviewing procedures.

Agenda planning

Planning what questions to ask or what investigative procedures to use in a preliminary consultation session and subsequent assessment sessions will depend on the problem posed in the referring letter, the preliminary hypothesis that the clinician has about the case and the routine assessment procedures typically used by the psychologist in such cases.

If the referrer's concerns are vague, much time may be saved by phoning the referrer and requesting clarification. In short, by asking 'What question do you want answered?' or 'What problem do you want solved?' For example, during a clarification phone call a family doctor who initially asked for a psychological assessment for a nine-year-old boy (Ronny Boyle), indicated that there were three main problems: (1) encopresis; (2) school attainment problems; and (3) home-based behavioural difficulties. An assessment of all three was required along with recommendations for the school on the management of the scholastic difficulties and behavioural family therapy for the other two problems. Clinical psychologists have a responsibility to educate those that use their services about types of cases that may be referred to them and the types of assessment, treatment and case management services that they offer. Clarifying referral questions is one way of educating referrers about these issues.

INTAKE INFORMATION FORM

Please read the information in this box and complete this form before talking to your psychologist. You may ask any questions about this during your first meeting.

Voluntary attendance. Our clinic offers help to young people with problems of living and their families. Attendance at this clinic is voluntary. You may attend if you wish.

Both parents are invited. We find that it is most helpful if the young person with the problem and both parents attend the first appointment. Fathers have a particularly important contribution to make to our understanding of young people's problems and to their resolution.

First appointments. Your first appointment will last about 2 hours. During this meeting the young person and both parents may give their view of the problem, the things that you have tried to do in the past to solve it, and information about the young person's development. Sometimes, the young person is invited to complete some reading tests and tests of ability and to fill out some questionnaires.

Other appointments. At the end of the first appointment we will let you know if our service can offer you help with the problem of living that led you to visit us. We will offer you further appointments at times that are convenient to you at that point. If you cannot attend an appointment, please call us at least 2 days before the appointment so we can book in another person.

Confidentiality. In our clinic all staff work as part of team. The team includes experienced senior psychologists, psychologists in training who work under the supervision of senior psychologists, and professionals in other disciplines such as speech and language therapy, paediatrics, social work, occupational therapy, and psychiatry. Everything that you say to your psychologist is confidential to our team.

The only circumstances under which we are obliged to give information to other people about your case is where a member of your family is at risk of serious harm.

We will not give information about your case to others, such as the young person's school, without your consent.

Annonymized case reports. As a routine part of psychologists' training they are required to write case reports for examination at the university where they are training. All identifying details of your child and family will be omitted from such reports.

Psychological reports. If you would like a psychological report sent to the young person's school, to your family doctor or to some other professional, discuss this with your psychologist.

Please sign the next line to indicate that you consent to the conditions of service outlined in this box.

Signature of parent_____

Please complete this form. The information you give here will be used to help us understand your child's difficulties. If there are any questions that you cannot answer or do not wish to answer for private reasons, please leave the answer boxes blank. Thank You.

Please put your name and address and telephone number in the box opposite.	
What is your child's name?	
What is your child's age?	
What is your child's date of birth?	
What is your main concern about your child's behaviour and/or school work?	

Figure 4.3 Intake information form   (*Continued overleaf*)

Please name anyone outside the family who is particularly concerned about your child's behaviour or school work, such as a teacher, social worker or family doctor.			
Who is your family doctor?			
May I contact your family doctor?	Yes	No	Please sign, if you give your consent. I_____ give consent for _____ to contact my family doctor.
What is your child's present school, class and what is the name of your child's main teacher?			
May I contact your child's main teacher?	Yes	No	Please sign, if you give your consent. I_____ give consent for _____ to contact my child's teacher.
Can you please send me a recent end-of-term school report?	Yes	No	If you have not given it to me already, please enclose this when returning the questionnaire.
Was your child assessed by a psychologist, social worker or doctor before?	Yes	No	Please give brief details
If a report was prepared may I contact this person and ask them to send it to me?	Yes	No	Please sign, if you give your consent. I_____ give consent for_____ to contact _____
Has your child received treatment or remedial tuition for his or her problems?	Yes	No	Please give brief details
Has your child language problems?	Yes	No	Please give brief details
Has your child problems with reading or other schoolwork?	Yes	No	Please give brief details
Is your child very disobedient or disruptive at home?	Yes	No	Please give brief details
Is your child very disobedient or disruptive at school?	Yes	No	Please give brief details
Is your child sad, frightened, withdrawn or upset at home?	Yes	No	Please give brief details
Is your child sad, frightened, withdrawn or upset at school?	Yes	No	Please give brief details

Figure 4.3 Continued

			Please give brief details
Has your child sleeping or feeding problems?	Yes	No	
Has your child toileting problems?	Yes	No	Please give brief details
Has your child a medical condition, such as one of these listed, that caused particular stress? • Headaches • Stomach aches • Asthma • Head injury • Other	Yes	No	Please give brief details
Have any of the child's relatives (including yourself or the child's other parent) got language problems, reading problems, behaviour problems, mood problems or medical problems?	Yes	No	Please give brief details
Was the pregnancy with this child normal?	Yes	No	Please give brief details
Was the delivery normal?	Yes	No	Please give brief details
Has your child had any major illnesses and if so please give details?	Yes	No	Please give brief details
Has your child's hearing always been normal?	Yes	No	Please give brief details
Does your child wear glasses?	Yes	No	Please give brief details
In your opinion was the development of your child's ability to walk, run, jump and so forth normal?	Yes	No	Please give brief details
Is your child left-handed?	Yes	No	Please give brief details
In your opinion, was your child's language development normal?	Yes	No	Please give brief details
Has your child always been able to make friends?	Yes	No	Please give brief details
Please list all the pre-schools and schools your child has attended giving the dates of attendance		1. _____ 2. _____ 3. _____ 4. _____	

(Continued overleaf)

Is your child in the top third, the middle third or the bottom third of his class in terms of his or her overall marks?			Top third Middle third Bottom third		
Does your child like going to school?	Yes	No	Please give brief details		
Does your child resist or refuse to do homework?	Yes	No	Please give brief details		
Please list your children's names and ages in order and indicate if any of them have learning problems or behaviour problems			Name Age Learning or behavioural problem 1. _____ 2. _____ 3. _____ 4. _____ 5. _____ 6. _____ 7. _____		
Do you believe that any changes within your child's home or school such as the following are contributing to your child's current problems? • Changing school • Bullying at school • Moving house • Family member's illness • Parental unemployment • Birth of a sibling • Adoption of a child • Parental separation • Bereavement • Other major changes or conflicts at home or school	Yes	No	Please give brief details		

If you wish, please use this space to give your opinion about your child's difficulties and to provide any other relevant information.

Figure 4.3 Continued

Agendas for parent and family interviews

It is important to acknowledge that psychologists do not typically begin intake interviews with a completely open mind about the presenting problems. The referrer's question, along with the information provided by the referrer and in the intake information form (contained in Figure 4.3), will give rise to certain hunches or hypotheses. These are typically informed by experience with similar cases and a knowledge of the relevant literature. The more explicit these hypotheses are made, the better, since they will inform some of the lines of questioning followed in a preliminary interview or some of the tests used in a preliminary consultation session.

For all problems, it is important to include in preliminary hypotheses or formulations and related lines of questioning a consideration of pre-disposing, precipitating, maintaining and protective factors. Literature about such factors has been reviewed in Chapter 2. Pre-disposing, precipitating, maintaining and protective factors to consider in all cases are summarized in Figure 2.1 (p. 42). Specific factors to consider for particular problems are given in Chapters 5–24. Pre-disposing factors are those biological or psycho-logical features of the child or negative aspects of the early parent–child relationship or family situation that have rendered the child or members of the network vulnerable to developing either the problem behaviour or the behaviours which maintain it. Precipitating factors are those events that have led to the onset of the problem. These may take the form of acute life stresses, illness or injury, and transitions in the individual or family life cycle. Maintaining factors are those biological and psychological character-istics of the child or parents along with patterns of interaction within the family, the treatment system, or the wider social network which allow the problem to persist. Protective factors are those biological and psychological characteristics of the child or parents along with patterns of interaction within the family, the treatment system, or the wider social network which prevent problems from deteriorating and which have positive implications for response to treatment and prognosis.

In the case of Ronny Boyle, one hypothesis was that his reading difficulties arose from a genetic predisposition of the type which typically underpins specific reading difficulties and that it was maintained by a lack of adequate recognition and remediation. A second hypothesis was that conflictual parent–child and teacher–child relationships pre-disposed Ronny to developing tantrums and encopresis. For the encopresis, there may also have been a pre-disposing organic factor. For both of these problems it was assumed that specific life stresses precipitated their onset or exacerbation. With respect to maintaining factors, the hypothesis was that the parents and teacher were probably engaged in a pattern of interaction with Ronny that inadvert-ently reinforced all three problems. Also, academic failure and related self-esteem problems, it was guessed, might maintain the behaviour problems. A psychometric assessment of Ronny's abilities (of the type described in Chapter 8) and interviews with the parents and teachers largely supported these hypotheses.

History of the problem

The opening item on the agenda of the parent interview, once a contract for assessment has been established is usually the history of the presenting problems. This typically involves questions about the nature, frequency and intensity of the problems; previous successful and unsuccessful solutions to these problems and family members' views on the causes of these problems and possible solutions that they suspect may be fruitful to explore in future. In listening to replies to these inquires and requesting elaboration about the social context within which the problems have been occurring, particular attention should be paid to possible problem-maintaining interaction patterns associated with any of the following processes, all of which have been described in Chapter 2:

- denial of the problem
- lack of commitment to resolving the problem
- inadvertent reinforcement
- insecure attachment
- coercive parent–child processes
- over-involved parent–child processes
- disengaged parent–child relationship
- inconsistent discipline
- confused communication
- triangulation
- chaotic family organization
- father absence
- marital discord.

Child developmental history

For inquiring about the child's development, it is useful to routinely employ a fairly comprehensive framework based on the material covered in Chapter 1. In inquiring about the first five years, the following broad areas deserve consideration:

- particular strengths shown in the first five years
- pregnancy and birth problems
- physical health and any early childhood illnesses
- feeding and eating patterns and problems

- sleeping pattern: age when child first slept through the night, and sleep problems
- physical growth and any problems with height or weight being below the third centile
- sensory and motor development and any delays in motor development
- bowel and bladder control, age when toilet training was complete and any soiling or wetting problems
- temperament, attachment and any attachment problems
- language development and any language delays
- cognitive development and any problems with sustaining attention and solving puzzles and games
- social development and adjustment to pre-school and any attachment problems or peer problems
- emotional regulation and problems with persistent crying
- anger control and problems with tantrums.

With regard to the middle childhood period from six to twelve years, the following areas should be investigated in some detail when taking a developmental history:

- particular strengths shown in middle childhood
- physical health and illnesses during middle childhood
- academic performance and cognitive development and any attainment problems
- internalization of rules and moral development during middle childhood and any conduct problems
- emotional regulation, anxiety and depression in middle childhood
- making and maintaining friendships and peer problems during middle childhood.

Inquiries about development in adolescence should cover the following areas:

- physical health and illnesses during adolescence
- academic performance and cognitive development in adolescence and any problems with schoolwork
- rule-following in adolescence and any conduct problems at home, school or in the community
- adjustment within the peer group in adolescence and any problems with making and maintaining friendships or membership of deviant peer group
- emotional regulation, anxiety and depression in adolescence
- eating pattern in adolescence and any indication of anorexia or bulimia
- experimentation with or abuse of drugs and alcohol
- psychotic features in adolescence.

Family development

In addition to a child developmental history, it is important to include family development and interaction as part of the agenda for the intake interview. Information yielded by observations made during a family interview and interview material may be recorded in narrative form or as part of a geno-gram. Symbols for genogram construction are set out in Figure 4.4. Inquiries

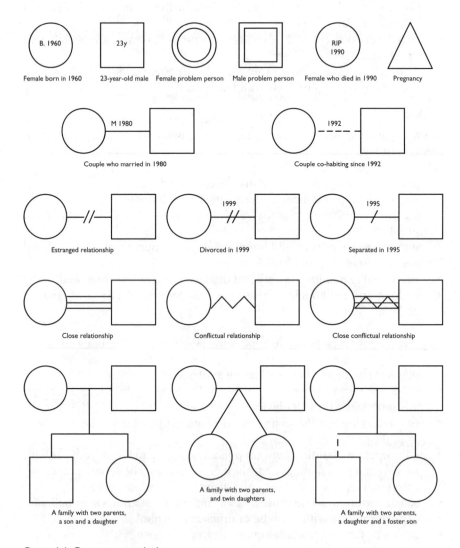

Figure 4.4 Genogram symbols

about family membership, structure and development should cover the following areas:

- current household membership
- extended family membership
- other network members
- identifying information, such as names, ages, occupations and locations of important family and network members
- major illnesses and psychosocial problems, including hospitalizations, physical and psychological problems and criminality
- major protective factors and strengths of family members
- the major transitions that the family has made through the family lifecycle
- current stage of the lifecycle
- supportive relationships for the child and caregivers within the network
- stressful relationships for the child and caregivers within the network
- family factions and triangulation patterns, particularly multi-generational patterns.

In observing and inquiring about parent–child relationships, the following points, which have been discussed in Chapters 1 and 2, when relevant, should form part of the intake agenda:

- parents' style for meeting child's need for safety particularly with infants and toddlers and problems with neglect
- parents' style for meeting child's needs for physical care, food, shelter, clothing and problems with neglect
- parents' style for meeting the child's needs for emotional care, warmth, acceptance and love throughout childhood and adolescence (and problems with abuse or neglect)
- parents' style for meeting the child's needs for control, clear limits and discipline, particularly in middle childhood and adolescence (and problems with being too punitive and abusive or over-indulgent)
- parents' style for meeting the child's needs for intellectual stimulation, particularly in infancy and early childhood (and problems with neglect)
- parents' style for meeting the child's needs for age-appropriate autonomy and responsibility particularly in adolescence (and problems with being too demanding or too lax and over-protective).

A consideration of the relationships between parents and their capacity to jointly meet the child's needs should also be part of the family assessment agenda. The following points deserve routine exploration:

- people involved in parenting the child including biological parents, step-parents, foster parents, other family members
- quality of marital relationship and degree of sharing of childcare, if the child lives with married or co-habiting parents

- support network available to single parents
- quality of co-operative parenting relationship if parents are separated and the child lives with one parent but visits the other regularly.

The physical and social context of the family is a further issue for inclusion on the family assessment agenda. Some important issues requiring routine assessment include the following:

- location of the family in the community and proximity to schools, shops, extended family, etc. or problems with isolation
- ratio of number of people to number of rooms and problems with crowding
- quality of living quarters and problems with safety or hygiene
- parental financial resources and need or entitlement to benefits.

When working with multi-problem families, in which there is multi-agency involvement, it is critical to clarify the following points as part of the broader ecological assessment of the family:

- list of other involved agencies
- duration of involvement
- reasons for involvement.

The developmental interviewing framework presented here and summarized in Figure 4.2. is based on the material covered in Chapters 1 and 2. The framework outlines the content areas that are important to cover when conducting a routine child and family assessment and may serve as a template for interviewing parents and other members of the child's network.

An example of a genogram for Ronny Boyle based on a family interview is presented in Figure 4.5. From this case example, it is apparent that Ronny is a middle child living with his mother, father and siblings. His father, like Ronny, has a history of literacy problems. Ronny's tantrums date back two years to the birth of his brother and his encopresis dates back a year to his older sister's departure to boarding school. This event was a major loss for Ronny because he has a close relationship with his sister. Ronny has a close conflict-ual relationship with his mother and a distant relationship with his father (a pattern which commonly maintains rather than resolves child behaviour problems) and these relationships between Ronny and his parents resemble the types of relationships that the parents had in their families of origin. Overall, the Boyles have experienced a considerable build-up of life stress in the four years prior to the referral. There have been two bereavements in father's family of origin, the birth of a difficult-temperament child and the older daughter's departure to boarding school. The stresses may have compromised the parents' capacity to manage Ronny's difficulties. This example illustrates the way genograms may offer a pictorial summary of

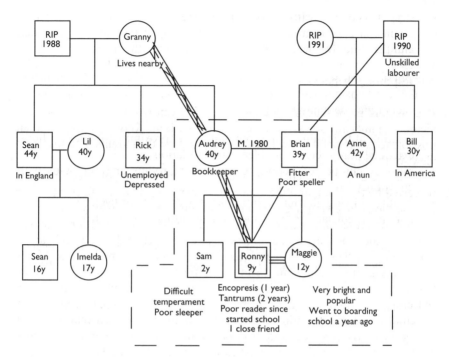

Figure 4.5 The Boyle genogram completed in 1994

significant individual developmental and family factors in complex cases. A fuller account of genogram construction is given in McGoldrick, Gerson & Shellenberger (1999) and Carr (2000b).

Agendas for child-centred interviews

In addition to parental or family interviews, it is good practice to routinely conduct a child-centred assessment. The following are key areas to include in child-centred assessments:

- child's account of problem, coping strategies and defences
- child's response to parents and teacher's views of problem
- child's genogram and lifeline
- child's perception of relationships with parents and teachers
- child's cognitive and academic strengths and weaknesses
- child's self-esteem, locus of control, self-efficacy and attributional style
- child's capacity to make and maintain friendships and social problem-solving skills
- child's account of situations requiring protective action (abuse or suicidal intent)

- child's account of situations requiring major changes in living arrangements (parental custody or foster care)
- child's wishes for the future
- child's capacity to engage in individual, group, or family therapy and to respond to behavioural programmes.

It is usually more fruitful to conduct a child-centred assessment once the views of significant adults in the child's network are known, since it is then possible to ask the child how he or she responds to the parents' and teachers' views of the problem.

With pre-adolescent children, the emotional climate of the family as perceived by the child, and the child's response to significant life events he or she mentions in giving a biographical account, may be assessed using the symbols presented in Figure 4.6. The child is introduced to the four faces that represent the emotions of happiness, sadness, anger and worry or fear. A genogram may then be drawn with the child and inquiries made about who is the family is most happy, most sad, most angry and most worried. A wavy line may then be drawn, with one end reflecting birth and the other end reflecting the present moment. It may be divided into one-year sections and the child asked about significant events that happened in each year. It is best to begin with the past year and work backwards, since recent events are more easily recalled. The child may be asked what type of feelings he or she experienced during the significant events and these may be recorded onto the lifeline.

In Figure 4.6, an example of Ronny Boyle's personal genogram and lifeline is given. From the genogram it is apparent that Ronny sees everyone in the family, except his sister who has left for boarding school, as experiencing negative emotions. He views himself and his mother as sad, his brother as worried and his father as angry. His lifeline shows that this was not always the case. His pre-school years were happy, except when he went to hospital following a fall. However, once he started school he became sad because no matter how hard he tried he could never read as well as the other children. He became convinced that he was stupid and it was this belief that made him sad. The birth of his brother who didn't sleep well and cried a lot, made his mother continually irritable and Ronny became very angry. Then when his older sister, Maggie, went to boarding school about a year before the assessment he became very sad. The lifeline is a succinct graphic representation of the child's developmental history and may be routinely used in conjunction with the genogram to obtain the child's view of the situation. In light of his lifeline and genogram, Ronny's wishes were for his sister to visit home more often, for him to succeed in school and for his parents to be happier.

Special areas to address in child-centred assessments are described in other chapters. Procedures for conducting psychometric assessments of abilities are described in Chapter 8. An approach to interviewing children where there

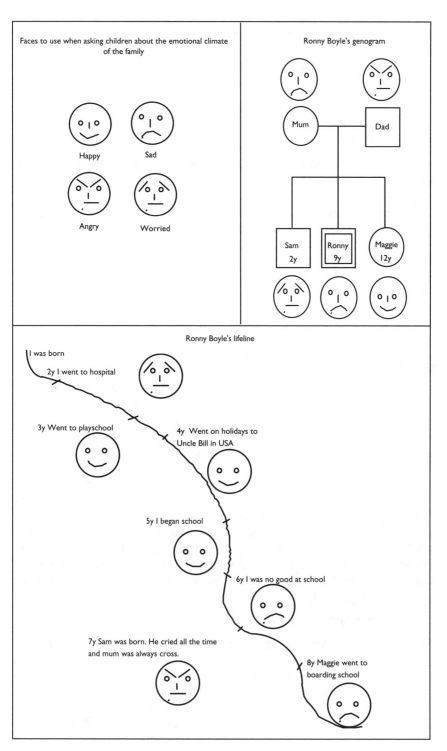

Figure 4.6 Child-centred assessment: example of a genogram, lifeline and indicators of emotional climate used in a child-centred assessment

may be a suicide risk is given in Chapter 16. Chapters 19, 20 and 21 contain suggestions on interviewing children in child protection cases. A guide to interviewing children about custody and access where parents have separated is given in Chapter 23.

Agendas for school contact

What follows is a list of items which may form the agenda for an interview with children's teachers or school staff:

- current and past academic performance (including standardized test scores or psychometric reports if available)
- current and past performance at sports, drama and other non-academic pursuits
- current and past relationships with teachers
- current and past relationships with peers
- teacher's role in the network
- teacher's beliefs about the problem and solution
- teacher's prediction about how the case will work out
- availability of remedial tuition
- degree of parent–teacher co-operation
- amount of child–teacher contact
- school's expectations for good conduct from the child
- school's expectations for academic attainment
- pupil's involvement in school affairs
- teacher's use of praise-based motivation.

This agenda is based on the relevant material covered in Chapters 1 and 2. In the case of Ronny Boyle, the teacher was highly sympathetic to Ronny and guessed that he might have a learning difficulty, but the school was under-resourced and so little had been done about Ronny's reading difficulties. The teacher was willing to work closely with the parents but had not done so because he felt they were antagonistic to the school. Fortunately, this was not the case and a paired reading programme (described in Chapter 8) was set up.

Psychometric assessment agendas

Some paper and pencil instruments that may be used as an adjunct to clinical interviews are listed in Table 4.1. These represent a *core battery* of psychosocial measures that I have found to be particularly useful in clinical practice. The parents may be asked to complete the Child Behaviour Check-list (Achenbach & Rescorla, 2000, 2001) or the Strengths and Difficulties Questionnaire scale (Goodman, 2001). The former gives a more detailed profile but the latter is a more rapid screening instrument. There are teacher

Table 4.1 Psychometric instruments that may be routinely used as an adjunct to clinical interviews in the assessment of child and family problems

Construct	Instrument	Publication	Comments
Child's behaviour problems	Achenbach System for Empirically Based Assessment ASEBA	Achenbach, T. M., & Rescorla, L. A. (2000). *Manual for ASEBA Preschool Forms & Profiles*. Burlington, VT: University of Vermont, Research Centre for Children, Youth, & Families. Achenbach, T. M., & Rescorla, L. A. (2001). *Manual for ASEBA School-Age Forms & Profiles*. Burlington, VT: University of Vermont, Research Centre for Children, Youth, & Families. http://www.aseba.org/	Each of the ASEBA instruments contains about 110 items and yields a total problem score, scores for internalizing and externalizing behaviour problems; scores for up to 8 empirically derived syndromes; and scores for DSM oriented scales. There are versions for children 1.5–5 and 6–18 years. Parent, teacher, self-report and clinician versions are available. Norms are US based
	Strengths and Difficulties Questionnaire SDQ	Goodman, R. (2001). Psychometric properties of the Strengths and Difficulties Questionnaire (SDQ). *Journal of the American Academy of Child and Adolescent Psychiatry*, 40, 1337–1345. http://www.sdqinfo.com/	Each of the SDQ instruments contains about 25 items and yields scores for conduct, emotional, hyperactive and peer problems and pro-social behaviour. The age span is 5–15. There are parent, teacher and self-report versions. Norms are UK based
	Health of the Nation Outcome Scales for Children and Adolescents HoNOSCA	Gowers, S.G., Harrington, R.C., & Whitton, A. (1998). *HoNOSCA Report on research and development.* London CRU. http://www.liv.ac.uk/honosca/Home.htm	HoNOSCA is a clinician rating scale which yields a total score and scores for 13 areas: anti-social behaviour, over-activity, self-injury, substance misuse, scholastic or language skills, physical illness or disability problems, hallucinations and delusions, somatic symptoms, emotional symptoms, peer relationships, self-care, family relationships, and school attendance. Ratings are made on 5-point scales and self-rated and parental-rated versions of the instrument are also available. The HoNOSCA was developed in the UK

(Continued)

Table 4.1 continued

Construct	Instrument	Publication	Comments
	Children's Global Assessment Scale (C-GAS)	Shaffer, D., Gould., M., Brasis, J., Ambrosini, P., Fisher, P., Bird, H., & Aluwahlia, S. (1983). A children's global assessment scale (C-GAS). Archives of General Psychiatry, 40, 1228–1231. http://depts.washington.edu/wimirc/Index.htm	This is a 100-point rating scale for assessing a child's general functioning
Parental mental health	General Health Questionnaire-28 (GHQ-28)	Goldberg, D. P. (1978). The General Health Questionnaire. Windsor, Berks: NFER-NELSON. http://www.nfer-nelson.co.uk/	This 28-item instrument yields an overall score and sub-scale scores for somatic complaints, anxiety, depression and social dysfunction. A cut-off score of 5 may be used to classify respondents as showing particularly severe mental health problems
Child and parent's self-esteem	Battle Culture Free Self-Esteem Inventories (BCFSEI-3)	Battle, J. (2002). Culture-Free Self-Esteem Inventories. Examiner's Manual (Third Edition). Austin, TX: Pro-ed. http://www.jamesbattle.com/cfsei.htm	This suite of inventories includes short (30-item) and long (60-item) versions of child and adult self-esteem inventories. In addition to yielding a general self-esteem score, the inventories give a range of domain specific scores
Locus of control	Nowicki Strickland locus of control scale	Nowicki, S. & Strickland, B. (1973). A locus of control scale for children. Journal of Consulting and Clinical Psychology, 40, 148–155	This 40-item scale measures locus of control (expectations that reinforcement is under personal control)
Perceived social support	Multidimensional Scale of Perceived Social Support (MSPSS)	Dahlem, N. W., Zimet, S. G. & Walker, R. (1991) The Multidimensional Scale of Perceived Social support: A Confirmation Study. Journal of Clinical Psychology, 47, 756–761	This 12-item scale for completion by adolescents and adults gives an overall score and sub-scale scores for perceived social support from family, friends and significant others. Items are rated on seven-point rating scales

Perceived family stress due to life events and changes	FILE: Family Inventory of Life Events and Changes	McCubbin, H., Patterson, J., & Wilson, L. (1982). Family Inventory of Life Events and changes: FILE. In D. Olson, H. Mc Cubbin, H. Barnes, A. Larsen, M. Muxen, & M. Wilson (Eds.) *Family Inventories*. (pp.69–88). University of Minnesota, St Paul, MN	This 71-item self-report life events schedule yields an overall score in life change units. The life change units are based on a US standardization study. Parent and adolescent versions of the scale are available
Perceived family functioning	Family Assessment Device (FAD)	Kabacoff, R. Miller, I., Bishop, D., Epstein, N. & Keitner, G. (1990). A psychometric study of the McMaster Family Assessment Device. *Journal of Family Psychology*, 3, 431–439	This 60-item self-report inventory for completion by adolescents and adults yields scores on the following sub-scales: problem solving; communication; roles; affective responsiveness; affective involvement; behaviour control; general functioning. The instrument is standardized and computer scoreable on a PC. A rating scale version for completion by clinicians is also available
	Global Assessment of Relational Functioning Scale (GARF)	GAP (1996). Global Assessment of Relational Functioning Scale (GARF): I. Background and rationale. *Family Process*, 35, 155–172	This is a 100-point rating scale included in the appendix of DSM IV TR to give an index of overall family functioning
Marital satisfaction	Kansas Marital Satisfaction Scale KMS	Schumm, W.R., Paff-Bergen, L.A., Hatch, R.C., Obiorah, F.C., Copeland, J.M., Meens, L.D., Bugaighis, M.A. (1986). Concurrent and discriminant validity of the Kansas Marital Satisfaction Scale. *Journal of Marriage & the Family*, 48, 381–387	This 3-item scale yields a single index of marital satisfaction. A seven-point response format is used for each of the three items
Parenting Satisfaction	Kansas Parent Satisfaction Scale (KMS)	James, D. E., Schumm, W.R., Kennedy, C. E., Grigsby, C. C., Shectman, K. L. Nichols, C. W. (1985). Characteristics of the Kansas Parental Satisfaction Scale among two samples of married parents. *Psychological Reports*, 57, 163–169	This 3-item scale yields a single index of the parents' satisfaction with the parent–child relationship. A seven-point response format is used for each of the three items

versions of both of these scales that may be sent to the school and for teenagers, there are also self-report versions. These may be mailed to prospective clients prior to the intake interview.

The third edition of the Battle Culture-Free Self-Esteem Inventory (Battle, 2002); the Nowicki Strickland (1973) Locus of Control Scale and the Family Assessment Device (Kabacoff, Miller, Bishop, Epstein & Keitner, 1990) may be completed by most children aged over eight during the child-centred assessment to give standardized assessments of self-esteem, self-regulatory beliefs and perceived family functioning.

After the intake interview, a package of self-report measures may be completed by one or both parents to assess various aspects of parental and family functioning including parental mental health (General Health Questionnaire 28; Goldberg, 1978); parental perception of family functioning (The Family Assessment Device; Kabacoff et al., 1990); parental perception of overall stresses faced by the family (Family Inventory of Life Events and Changes; McCubbin, Patterson & Wilson, 1982); parenting satisfaction (Kansas Parent Satisfaction Scale; James et al., 1985); marital satisfaction (Kansas Marital Satisfaction Scale; Schumm et al., 1986); and social support available to parents (Multidimensional Scale of Perceived Social Support; Dahlem, Zimet & Walker, 1991). In selecting each of these instruments, a compromise was reached among the following group of competing factors: the relevance of the instrument to a contextual approach to assessment, its psychometric properties, its brevity and its user-friendliness.

The Children's Global Assessment Scale (C-GAS; Schaffer et al., 1983), the Global Assessment of Relational Functioning Scale (GARF; GAP, 1996); and Health of the Nation Outcome Scales for Children and Adolescents (HoNOSCA; Gowers, Harrington & Whitton, 1998) have also been included in Table 4.1 because of their ease of use, their promising reliability and validity and their value in summarizing psychologists' overall impressions of the level of functioning of children and families.

For particular problems, in addition to this core battery of general measures, more specific instruments may be used. In Chapters 5–24, specialist instruments for use with specific clinical problems are listed. Corcoran and Fischer's (2000) compendium of brief, problem-focused assessment scales is a useful source for assessment instruments for specific problems.

STAGE 2: ASSESSMENT AND FORMULATION

The more important features of the assessment and formulation stage, which may span a number of sessions, are: establishing a contract for assessment, working through the assessment agenda and recursively refining the preliminary formulation in the light of the information obtained, dealing with engagement problems, building a therapeutic alliance and giving feedback.

Contracting for assessment

At a cognitive level, contracting for assessment involves the psychologist and clients clarifying expectations and reaching an agreement to work together. The first task is to explain what assessment involves and to offer the parents, the child and each relevant member of the network a chance to accept or reject the opportunity to complete the assessment. For most parents, this will involve outlining the way in which the interviews and testing procedures will be conducted. The concept of a family interview with adjunctive individual interviews and testing sessions is unusual for many parents. Most parents need to be told about the time commitment required. An assessment will usually require between one and three sessions. It is important to highlight the voluntary nature of the assessment. It is also important to clarify the limits of confidentiality. Normally, the contents of sessions are confidential unless there is evidence that a family member is a serious threat to themselves or to others. For example, where there is evidence of suicidal intent or child abuse, confidentiality may be breached.

With children and teenagers, misconceptions need to be dispelled. For example, some children think that they will be involuntarily admitted to hospital and others believe that they will be put in a detention centre. In some instances, children may not wish to complete the assessment but their parents may be insistent. In others, parents may not wish to complete the assessment but a referring physician or social worker may forcefully recommend attendance. In such situations, the therapist may facilitate the negotiation of some compromise between parties. The contracting for assessment is complete when family members have been adequately informed about the process and have agreed to complete the assessment.

Recursive re-formulation

The assessment phase of the overall consultation process involves conducting the interviews or administering tests to check out the accuracy of the formulations and hypotheses made during the planning phase and modifying the formulations or hypotheses in the light of the information gained in the interview or testing sessions. In practice, the first round of interviewing and testing may not only lead to a modification of the preliminary formulation but may raise further hypotheses that need to be checked out with further interviews or tests. This recursive process, which characterizes the assessment and formulation stage, is diagrammed in Figure 4.7. The process comes to an end when a formulation has been constructed that fits with: significant aspects of the child's problems, with network member's experiences of the child's problems and with available knowledge about similar problems described in the literature. This formulation should point to one or more options for case management. Options for case management will be dealt with below.

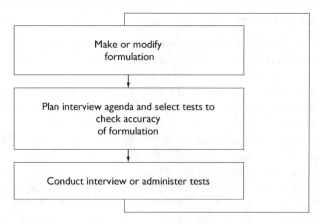

Figure 4.7 Process of recursive re-formulation

Engagement difficulties

The process of contracting for assessment does not always run smoothly. Engagement problems are to be expected. Non-attendance and inaccurate referral information are two of the more important obstacles to establishing a contract for assessment. When none of the people invited to the intake interview attends, phone the person that you have identified as the customer immediately and clarify why the family has not shown up. Non-attendance, in our experience, may be due either to practical difficulties or to a failure to identify the true customer for consultation. Non-attendance due to an inaccurate analysis of the problem system is best dealt with by arranging a meeting with the referrer to clarify who the customer for consultation is. Non-attendance due to practical problems occurs most frequently with chaotic families invited to attend a public clinic. In these instances, intake interviews may best be conducted in the clients' homes. Sometimes the information contained in the referral letter, or indeed through a referral phone call, is wildly inaccurate and clients indicate that the child-centred referral problem was only a red flag to mark a profound adult-centred or marital life difficulty. It is good practice to acknowledge the validity of clients by using a small child-focused problem as a way of checking out the therapist's trustworthiness before mentioning more profound difficulties with which they want assistance. Re-contracting for personal or marital work is usually deferred until after the child-focused problems have been dealt with. A fuller description of engagement difficulties is given elsewhere (Carr, 2000a).

Alliance building

In addition to providing information, the process of assessment also serves as a way for the psychologist, the child, the parents and members of the network to build a working alliance. Building a strong working alliance with the child and key members of the child's family and network is essential for valid assessment and effective therapy. *All other features of the consultation process should be subordinate to the working alliance*, since without it clients drop out of assessment and therapy or fail to make progress. The only exception to this rule is where the safety of the child or family member is at risk, when protection takes priority over alliance building. Research on common factors that contribute to a positive therapeutic outcome and ethical principles of good practice point to a number of guidelines which psychologists should employ in developing a working alliance (Carr, 2000a, 2002a; Fonagy et al., 2002; Kazdin & Weisz, 2003; Lambert, 2003; Sprenkle, 2002):

- When communicating with the child, parents and network members, the psychologist's communication style should be characterized by warmth, empathy and genuineness.
- The psychologist should form a collaborative partnership with the child, the parents and other members of the child's network.
- Assessment should be conducted from the vantage point of respectful curiosity.
- An invitational approach should be adopted in which children and family members are invited to participate in assessment and case management procedures.
- The inevitability of transference and countertransference reactions within the therapeutic relationship should be acknowledged.

Warmth, empathy and genuineness

Warmth, empathy and genuineness have repeatedly been shown to be significant contributors to therapeutic progress since Carl Rogers first highlighted their importance (Beutler, Machado & Neufeldt, 1994). When communicating with the child, parents and network members, the psychologist's warmth, empathy and genuineness should allow members of the network to experience the psychologist as understanding (but not necessarily condoning) their actions and their viewpoint. Warmth, empathy and genuineness allow clients to have the experience of being accepted and understood. There is no place for blaming within the therapeutic relationship. While parents may create a context within which children's problems develop, usually this occurs inadvertently. Where it occurs intentionally, typically wider social or historical factors have created a context within which the parents' intention to harm a child has evolved. Blaming is a concept useful in the judicial system where seeking justice is the primary goal. Within psychological practice, where understanding and promoting problem formulation and problem resolution are the main goals, warmth, empathy and genuineness are the most important features of the relationship. This guideline is relevant to work with all families including those where abuse, neglect and domestic violence have occurred. This is because understanding the position of a person who has abused another does not necessarily entail condoning the abuse.

Collaborative partnership

The psychologist should attempt to form a collaborative partnership with the child, the parents and other members of the child's network so that responsibility for the tasks of assessment and case management may be shared. This feature of the therapeutic alliance has been highlighted by cognitive therapists (Friedberg & McClure, 2002). Psychologists and families with whom they work are both experts, but in different areas. Family members are experts on the specific features of their own family and details of their unique problems. Psychologists are experts on general scientific and clinical information relevant to child and family development and the broad class of problems of which the client's is a specific instance. In managing the task of empowering parents and children to find solutions to their problems, psychologists bring expert knowledge about the psychology of such problems in general to bear on the clients' specific problem. This expertise comes from scientific literature, clinical training, clinical experience and personal psychotherapeutic work. However, the children and families whom psychologists help are experts on the details of their own problems and the way in which these are managed within their own families.

Respectful curiosity

Systemic therapists have argued that the danger of undermining the complexity of clients and their problems may be avoided if the psychologist adopts a position of respectful curiosity (Cecchin, 1987). With respectful curiosity, it is assumed that there are always multiple ways of constructing or understanding problems and the constellation of maintaining factors within which they are embedded. So the psychologist continually strives to uncover new information about the problem and potential solutions and invites the family to consider what the implications would be if the difficulties were viewed from multiple different perspectives. Ultimately, the aim of the consultation process is not to find the *true* formulation of a problem but to construct the *most useful* formulation of a problem, which both fits with the facts of the situation, and which opens up many feasible options for problem resolution. An attitude of respectful curiosity helps us avoid sterile diagnostic labelling or forcing clients to occupy theoretical procrustean beds.

An invitational approach

With an invitational approach, all attempts to influence children and their parents are presented as invitations to action. Coercive directiveness or inappropriate non-directiveness are avoided. This position has been most clearly articulated by clinical psychologists from the constructivist tradition (Kelly, 1955). The invitational approach allows family members to have the experience of choosing to participate in activities which constitute the consultation process and to avoid the experience of being neglected through excessive non-directiveness or coerced through excessive directiveness. This experience of choice associated with an invitational approach increases the probability that family members will co-operate with arduous tasks such as keeping diaries or completing a cognitive assessment. In treatment, an invitational approach offers children and parents a sense of control and ownership when they choose to accept the invitation to be coached in the development of new skills or offered new ways of construing their problems and possible solutions to these.

Transference and countertransference

Transference and countertransference reactions are an inevitable feature of the therapeutic alliance, and the acceptance of this may help psychologists manage co-operation difficulties which often occur in the course of the consultation process (Carr, 1997). Clients and therapists inadvertently bring to the working alliance attitudes, expectations, emotional responses and interactional routines from early significant care-giving and care-receiving relationships. These transference and countertransference reactions, if unrecognized, may compromise therapeutic progress. However, if recognized and accurately understood, they may contribute significantly to resolving the presenting problems (Malan, 1995).

Often children, parents or network members do not follow through on tasks that they have agreed to complete, fail to turn up to appointments or insist on prolonging the consultation process apparently unnecessarily. This occurs despite their avowed wish to solve the presenting problems! Clients' co-operation difficulties and resistance require careful analysis, and methods for doing this will be described in a later section. At this point it is sufficient to mention that in some instances clients have difficulty co-operating with therapy because of transference. That is, they transfer onto the psychologist relationship expectations that they had as infants of parents whom they experienced as either extremely nurturing or extremely neglectful. Karpman's triangle (1968), which is set out in Figure 4.8, is a useful framework for understanding transference reactions. Clients may treat the psychologist as a nurturent parent who will rescue them from psychological pain caused by some named or unnamed persecutor, without requiring them to take

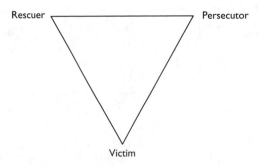

Figure 4.8 Karpman's triangle

responsibility for solving the presenting problems. For example, a demoralized parent may look to the psychologist to rescue her from what she perceives to be a persecuting child who is aggressive and has poor sleeping habits. Alternatively, clients may treat the psychologist as a neglectful parent who wants to punish them and so they refuse to fulfil the consultation contract. For example, a father may drop out of therapy if he views the psychologist as persecuting him by undermining his values or authority within the family. In some instances, clients alternate between these extreme transference positions. When parents develop these transference reactions, it is important to recognize them and discuss once again with clients their goals, and the responsibilities of the psychologist and family members within the assessment or treatment contract. In other instances, it may be appropriate to interpret transference by pointing out the parallels between clients current relationships with the psychologist and their past relationship with their parent. However, such interpretations can only be offered in instances where a strong therapeutic alliance has developed and where clients are psychologically minded.

Most psychologists experience some disappointment or frustration when clients do not follow through on tasks that they have agreed to complete, when they fail to turn up to appointments or where they insist on prolonging the consultation process without making progress towards treatment goals. These negative emotions are experienced whether the co-operation problems are due to transference or other factors. In those instances where a psychologist's negative reactions to co-operation problems are out of proportion to the clients' actual behaviour, the psychologist is probably experiencing countertransference. That is, he or she is transferring relationship expectations based on early life experience onto current relationships with clients. Karpman's triangle (set out in Figure 4.8) offers a valuable framework for interpreting such reactions. Inside many clinical psychologists there is a *rescuer* who derives self-esteem from saving the client/*victim* from some *persecuting* person or force. Thus, in situations where the child is perceived as the victim and the parent fails to bring the child for an appointment, a counter-transference reaction, which I have termed *rescuing the child*, may be experienced. With multi-problem families, in which all family members are viewed as victims, there may be a preliminary countertransference reaction of *rescuing the family* (from a persecuting social system). If the family does not co-operate with therapy, or insists on prolonging therapy without making progress, the countertransference reaction of rescuing the family may be replaced by one of *persecuting the family*. When this countertransference reaction occurs repeatedly, burnout develops (Carr, 1997).

The origin of the urge to rescue experienced by many clinical psychologists is complex and unique to each of us. A consistent theme, however, among helping professionals is the need to rescue others as a symbolic way of rescuing some archaic vulnerable aspect of the self. This aspect of the self often owes its genesis to the experience of some unmet childhood need. Indeed, the value of personal therapy as part of psychologists' continuing professional development is that it allows us to gain insight into these intrapsychic dynamics and work through them so that we are freer to take a neutral and curious stance when dealing with our clients' resistances.

Countertransference reactions may also be sparked off by particular personal characteristics of clients or the types of problems with which they present. Some therapists may find that they are particularly attracted to rescuing the women and children in families and to persecuting the males. Others may find that this pattern of countertransference only occurs in families where a bereavement has occurred, or where delinquency is the presenting problem. Families where child abuse has occurred typically elicit strong countertransference reactions to both clients and other professionals and these are discussed in Chapter 21 (Carr, 1997).

Formulation and feedback

The assessment is complete when the presenting problem and related difficulties are clarified; related pre-disposing, precipitating, maintaining and protective factors have been identified; a formulation has been constructed; possible goals have been identified; options for case management or treatment have been identified and these have been discussed with the family.

A formulation is a mini-theory that explains why the presenting problems developed, why they persist, what protective factors either prevent them from becoming worse or may be enlisted to solve the presenting problems. To construct a formulation, first a problem list is drawn up, which includes all the significant problems that have been identified during the assessment, such as encopresis, attainment problems, conduct difficulties and so forth. Second, salient points from all of the assessment interviews and testing sessions are abstracted, labelled and listed. These salient points are those which may have a role in causing the child's problems, such as stressful life events or problematic parent–child relationships. Third, salient points are then categorized as those which may play a role in maintaining one or more of the problems; those which precipitated either the onset of the problems or made the problems sufficiently severe to warrant referral; and those background factors which pre-disposed the child to developing his or her current difficulties. These pre-disposing factors, precipitating factors and maintaining factors may then be linked into the most useful and coherent mini-theory possible. In addition protective factors that may have implications for treatment and the prognosis of the case should be listed.

Abstracting, classifying and combining salient points into coherent formulations is a demanding process, which requires both clinical acumen and a good knowledge of the literature. Frameworks for identifying salient points and categorizing them, for a variety of specific problems are presented throughout the text and all are variations on the framework presented in Figure 2.1 (pp. 42–43). For example, in Chapter 10 a framework is given for identifying pre-disposing, precipitating and maintaining factors in cases where conduct problems are the central concern.

The importance of formulation cannot be over-emphasized. The process of constructing a formulation is the process of linking academic knowledge of theory and research to clinical practice. If the working alliance is the engine that drives the therapeutic process, formulation is the map that provides guidance on what direction to take.

With the Boyle family, it appeared that Ronny was pre-disposed to developing reading problems (his reading quotient of 80 was significantly below his full-scale IQ of 125) for genetic reasons and the difficulties were maintained by lack of remedial tuition at school. The multiple family bereavements, birth of a difficult-temperament child and transition of the oldest daughter to boarding school in the four-year period prior to referral placed a high level of stress on the whole family and so pre-disposed all members to have difficulty in resolving new difficulties. Against a back-drop of these pre-disposing factors, it appears that the change in family relationships that accompanied the birth of Ronny's younger brother, Sam, precipitated the onset of his tantrums and conduct difficulties. He probably felt displaced from his role as the youngest and only male child. A year later, the loss of social support which occurred when Ronny's eldest sister moved to boarding school precipitated the onset of the encopresis. The conduct and toileting difficulties appeared to be maintained by entrenched behaviour patterns and belief systems. Ronny was regularly involved in failure experiences in school and coercive interactions with his mother, to which his father was peripheral. Underpinning these interaction patterns was Ronny's belief system, characterized by low self-esteem and low-self efficacy; his mother's increasingly negative beliefs about him and his father's minimization of these difficulties.

However, a large number of protective factors were also present in the

Boyle case. Ronny was a bright child, of easy temperament, with good planning skills and a sense of humour who was capable of making and maintaining friendships. He had experienced no early losses, originally had a secure attachment to his mother, and was placed in a school where, although under-resourced, he had a teacher who was sympathetic to his reading problems. Furthermore, the family as a whole had a good social support network.

Once a formulation such as this has been constructed, feedback is given to the family about the formulation and options for the future management of the case are considered. The level of detail used in giving feedback needs to be matched to the family's cognitive ability to comprehend it and their emotional readiness to accept it. As part of the alliance-building process it is usually easiest for families if the protective factors are listed first, and then the section of the formulation explaining the aetiology of the problem is given. This process of presenting protective factors first generates a sense of hope. It is also important to empathize with each person's position when outlining the way in which the problem appears to have evolved. Usually, family members are well intentioned but, under stress and without adequate information, they inadvertently contribute to problem development or maintenance. In the process of feeding back some or all of the formulation to family members, in order to maintain a good working alliance it is useful to regularly check that the family has understood and accepted the formulation so far. Once the family has understood and accepted the formulation, broad options for case management may be outlined. It is futile to discuss case management options if the parents or legal guardians deny the problem or refuse to accept even part of the formulation.

Case management options

These may be derived from the formulation by speculating about what features of problem-maintaining behaviour patterns and belief systems would have to change for the problem to be resolved. The literature on effective treatments in similar cases should be considered. Most case management options fall into the following categories:

- take no immediate action
- psychoeducation and periodic reassessment
- refer to another professional within the psychologist's multi-disciplinary team for consultation, for example, audiology, speech therapy, social work or physiotherapy
- refer to another professional or residential facility outside the multi-disciplinary team
- offer focal and circumscribed psychological intervention to the child, parents, family or school

- offer multi-systemic intervention alone or in conjunction with other professionals or residential facility to the child, parents, family or school.

In some cases, the process of assessment and formulation leads to problem resolution and no further action is required. Two patterns of assessment-based problem resolution are common. In the first, the problem is re-framed so that the family no longer sees it as a problem. For example, the problem is redefined as a normal reaction, a developmental phase or an unfortunate but transient incident. In the second, the process of assessment releases family members' natural problem-solving skills and they resolve the problem themselves. For example, many parents, once they discuss their anxiety about handling their child in a productive way during a family assessment interview, feel released to do so.

In cases of specific or general physical, linguistic, academic or intellectual disabilities, psychoeducation and periodic reassessment may be a central recommendation. Psychoeducation may involve the provision of oral and written information about the condition and about support groups and legal educational or remedial entitlements. Reassessment may be advised on an annual basis or at critical points in the lifecycle where major placement or resourcing decisions have to be made such as school entry, changing schools or leaving school.

In cases of sensory, physical, linguistic or intellectual disabilities, multi-disciplinary assessment is vital. Referrals to paediatric medicine, physiotherapy, speech and language therapy, occupational therapy, social work, audiology should all be considered. It is crucial to consider a referral to paediatric medicine if there is a suspicion that psychological symptoms may reflect an underlying organic condition such as thyrotoxicosis (which may present as an anxiety-like disorder) or seizure disorder (which may present as day-dreaming). Likewise, a referral to child psychiatry should be considered in cases where psychotic or hypomanic features are central to the presentation, where a hospital admission may be required in cases of self-harm or where detoxification following substance abuse is required. In cases where child abuse has occurred or is suspected, national policy and local guidelines concerning interagency co-operation and reporting such cases to the statutory authorities should be followed. A fuller discussion of these issues is contained in Chapters 19, 20 and 21.

A number of general intervention strategies are discussed later in this chapter. Detailed guidelines on specific focal or multi-systemic interventions for children and members of their networks for particular problems are given in Chapters 6 to 24.

STAGE 3: CASE MANAGEMENT

When parents and their children have completed the assessment stage, have accepted the formulation, and are aware of the broad possibilities for case management, it is appropriate to progress to the stage of case management. The central tasks of this stage are contracting for further involvement to achieve specific goals, participating in the completion of the agreed case management plan and troubleshooting resistance. If, at this stage, it is apparent that other family problems, such as parental depression or marital discord require attention, referrals for this work may be made and it may be conducted concurrently with the programme that focuses explicitly on the child's problems. Alternatively, addressing these difficulties may be postponed until after the child-focused difficulties have been resolved.

Contracting for case management and goal setting

The contracting process involves inviting parents and children to make a commitment to pursue a specific case management plan to reach specific goals. This plan may include one or more of the case management options discussed in the previous section. Where part of the plan includes either focal or multi-systemic intervention, goal setting is particularly important. Clear, realistic, visualized goals that are fully accepted by all family members and that are perceived to be moderately challenging are crucial for effective therapy (Carr, 1997). Goal setting takes time and patience. Different family members may have different priorities when it comes to goal setting and negotiation about this is essential. This negotiation must take account of the costs and benefits of each goal for each family member.

In this context it is important to give parents and children clear information about research on the costs and benefits of psychological interventions and the overall results of outcome studies (Carr, 2000a, 2002a; Fonagy et al., 2002; Kazdin & Weisz, 2003; Sprenkle, 2002). Broadly speaking, most effective psychological interventions which have been developed for children and adolescents are effective in only 66–75% of cases and about 10% of cases deteriorate as a result of interventions. The more protective factors that are present in a given case, the more likely it is that therapy will be effective. If therapy is going to be effective most of the gains for most types of child and family therapy are made in the first six to ten sessions. Relapses are inevitable for many types of problems and periodic booster sessions may be necessary to help children and families handle relapse situations. With chronic problems and disabilities, further episodes of intervention are typically offered at life-stage transitions.

It is usually a more efficient use of time to agree on goals first, before discussing the details of how they might be achieved. The contracting session is complete when all involved members of the child's network necessary for implementing the case management plan agree to be involved in an episode of consultation to achieve specific goals. In these cost-conscious times, in public services or managed care services, therapeutic episodes should be time limited to between six and ten sessions, since most therapeutic change appears to happen within this time frame.

At this point, or indeed earlier in the consultation process, children or parents may point out that they have been through unsuccessful treatment programmes in the past, and that it appears that the psychological assessment or treatment programme being offered is similar to that which failed before. History of previous treatment, will have been assessed using the assessment protocol outlined in Figure 4.2 (pp. 108–9), so you will be familiar with the material the family wishes to discuss if it is raised at this point in the consultation process. However, it may be useful for concerned family members to be invited to give their views on previous unsuccessful treatment programmes. It may also be appropriate to invite family members to ventilate the feelings of fear, anger or demoralization that have led them to question the value of embarking on yet another treatment programme. Against this backdrop, the similarities and differences between those unsuccessful programmes and the services that are being offered may be outlined. In many instances there will be many similarities, as most psychosocial interventions involve meeting regularly and talking about problems and their solution using some type of psychosocial or biomedical model as a problem-solving framework. There are some important differences between the approach to consultation described here and other routine treatments that focus on one system (e.g. the child as an individual) or one type of intervention (e.g. support). The multi-systemic contextual approach to the practice of clinical psychology described here assumes that children's problems are complex and deserve thorough assessment. This assessment may be multi-disciplinary and will take into account the team's observations of the child but also those of the parents, teachers and other involved professionals. All of the information is integrated into a formulation, which is a map of how the problem evolved and is maintained. Treatment plans are based on this map and on evidence about the types of treatments that have been shown to work in scientific studies of similar sorts of problems. Where treatment programmes that have failed in the past are recommended as part of the consultation approach described here, it may be that in the past they were tried for too short a time, inappropriately applied or used alone rather than as part of a multi-systemic package. For example, the use of a reward system in isolation for a week to treat encopresis will usually be ineffective. However, a reward system used over a period of months may be one component of an overall effective treatment programme. Similarly, long-term, non-directive family therapy will usually be ineffective in the treatment of conduct problems but brief behavioural family therapy may be highly effective. Families may find it useful to explore these comparisons between previously ineffective treatment experiences and those being offered before committing themselves to a treatment plan.

Completing case management plans

Typical case management programmes include one or more of the following elements:

- a family-based approach
- psychoeducation
- monitoring problems
- communication training
- problem-solving training
- providing support and coaching parents in providing support
- coaching in using reward systems
- coaching in behavioural control
- coaching in tension reduction
- coaching children in cognitive coping strategies
- home–school liaison
- troubleshooting resistance
- co-ordinating multi-disciplinary and school input.

Family-based treatment approach

A family-based approach to children's psychological problems aims to help family members communicate clearly and openly about the problem and related issues, to decrease the emotional intensity of parent–child interactions related to the problem, to encourage joint parental problem solving with respect to the child's difficulties, to optimize parental support of the child and to optimize parents' use of healthcare resources and support groups. Where fathers are unavailable during office hours, it is worthwhile making special arrangements to schedule at least a couple of family sessions which are convenient for the father, since the participation of fathers in family-based therapy is associated with a positive outcome (Carr, 2000b). Where parents are separated or divorced, it is particularly important to arrange some sessions with the non-custodial parent, since it is important that both parents adopt the same approach in understanding and managing the child's difficulties.

Psychoeducation

In psychoeducational sessions parents, children and their siblings are given both general information about the problem and a specific formulation of the child's particular difficulties. Simplicity and realistic optimism are central to good psychoeducation. It is important not to overwhelm parents and children with information, so a good rule of thumb is to think about a case in complex terms but explain it to clients in as simple terms as possible. Put succinctly:

- *Think complex–talk simple.*

Good clinical practice involves matching the amount of information given about the formulation and case management plan to the client's readiness to understand and accept it. A second important rule of thumb is to engender a realistic level of hope when giving feedback by focusing on strengths and protective factors first, and referring to aetiological factors later. Put succinctly:

- *Create hope–name strengths.*

In psychoeducation, information on clinical features, pre-disposing, pre-cipitating, maintaining and protective factors may be given along with the probable impact of the problem in the short- and long-term on cognition, emotions, behaviour, family adjustment, school adjustment and health. Fact sheets about common psychological problems are available in Rose and York (2004). Details of the treatment programme should be given both orally and in written form, if appropriate, in a way that is compressible to the parents and the child. It is important to highlight the child and family's protective factors and strengths that increase the probability that the child will respond positively to treatment. This should be balanced with a statement of the sacrifices that the child and family will have to make to participate in the treatment programme. Common sacrifices include, attending a series of consultation sessions, discussing difficult issues openly, completing home-work assignments, being prepared for progress to be hampered by setbacks, learning to live with ongoing residual difficulties, accepting that episodes of therapy are time limited and accepting that, at best, the chances are only two out of three that therapy will be helpful. Psychoeducation should empower parents and children. It should allow them to reach a position where they can give a clear account of the problems and the correct way to manage it. Psycho-education may be offered in individual sessions, family sessions or group sessions. For some problems, such as diabetes, interactive instructional soft-ware programs are available that permit children to learn about their illness at their own pace. These have the advantage of being highly motivating for children and exciting to use. However, such programs should always be sup-plemented with individual consultations to answer the child's specific ques-tions. Family psychoeducation sessions allow the family to develop a shared understanding of the illness. Group psychoeducation offers a forum where children and parents can meet others in the same position and this has the benefit of providing additional support for family members. A wide variety of parent and child information books, work-books, games and activities is available and may also be used for psychoeducational purposes. At the end of many of the chapters in this text, such resources are listed. However, it is vital that whatever information is given to parents or children is consistent with the approach that you are taking in your formulation and treatment programme.

Separating the problem from the person, re-framing and re-labelling are three specific psychoeducational techniques that are used throughout the process of consultation.

In *separating the problem from the person*, the child's difficulties are defined as distinct from the child's identity and the child is described as being aligned with the parents and other network members in requiring a solution to the problem. Thus the child and parents may be described as a team who are working together to find a way to deal with a fiery temper, a difficult temperament, ADHD, anxiety, depression, encopresis, diabetes, addiction or whatever the problem happens to be. With young children, the problem may be externalized and personified and the child and family's task defined as defeating the personification of the problem. For example, encopresis may be personified as *sneaky-poo*, obsessive-compulsive disorder may be personified as *Mr Too-tidy* and so on. The parent's role become supporting the child in running sneaky-poo or Mr Too-tidy out of the child's life. This strategy has been pioneered by White and Epston (1990) and a particularly detailed treatment programme for using this technique in the management of obsessive-compulsive disorder is given in Chapter 13. The process of separating the problem from the person and then externalizing the problem counters the destructive tendency to label the child as the problem.

With *re-framing*, clients are offered a new framework within which to conceptualize a sequence of events, and this new way of conceptualizing makes it more likely that the problem will be resolved rather than maintained (Carr, 2000b). For example, where a mother and child become involved in heated arguments about the child's reluctance to apologize for hitting his sister, the mother may frame this as evidence that the child is intrinsically delinquent and say that this is the reason that she usually leaves these situations in frustration while her child is still screaming at her. This situation may be re-framed by pointing out that the child looks to the parent to learn self-control and it is difficult to learn self-control if uncontrolled behaviour like screaming is used to obtain relief. That is, the relief provided by the mother withdrawing from the situation before the child has stopped screaming and apologized to his sister. From this example, it may be seen that, here, re-framing is part of a psychoeducational input on managing aggressive behaviour, which provides a rationale for the mother using a reward system for increasing positive behaviour (like apologizing) or a behavioural control system for decreasing negative behaviour (such as screaming). With re-framing, the problem is contextualized and described as part of an interactional process rather than as an intrinsic characteristic of the child.

Re-labelling is way of altering parents and children's negative or pessimistic attributions and cognitive biases. With re-labelling, the psychologist routinely offers positive or optimistic labels for ambiguous behaviour as a substitute for negative or pessimistic labels. So where a parent says 'He was standing there *lazy and stupid* doing nothing, so I *told* him to get on with it', the psychologist may re-label this by saying 'When he was there *thinking through what to do next,* you *encouraged* him to start his homework'. Where a parent says 'She needs to be at home when she is this *ill*', the sentiment may be re-framed as 'While she is *recovering*, she needs to spend some time at home'. With re-labelling, children and families are offered optimistic ways of construing events, which open up possibilities for collaboration and problem solving as an alternative to pessimistic constructions of the problem, which engender polarization and problem maintenance (Carr, 2000b).

Monitoring problems

For most difficulties, it is useful to train children and/or parents to regularly record information about the main presenting problems, the circumstances surrounding their occurrence and the degree to which children and other family members complete therapeutic homework tasks or adhere to treatment regimes (Herbert, 2002). Intensity ratings, frequency counts, durations and other features of problems or symptoms may be recorded regularly. Intrapsychic and interpersonal events that happen before, during and after problems may also be noted. When inviting parents and children to use a monitoring system, the chances of them co-operating is better if a simple system is used to start out with. Later, more complex versions of it may be developed. Suggestions for monitoring particular types of problems and examples of monitoring charts are given throughout Chapters 6 to 24.

Information from monitoring charts should be reviewed regularly and family members may be invited to speculate on the reasons for changes in problems and related events. Where monitoring charts show that specific stimuli are associated with problems, ways of eliminating these stimuli may be examined. For example, in the case of asthma, the level of dust in a child's environment may be reduced. If eliminating problem-eliciting stimuli is not possible, ways of helping youngsters cope with these stimuli may be explored. For example, youngsters may be trained to cope with low levels of the stimulus first before being exposed to high levels of the stimulus. This is the rationale for systematic desensitization to anxiety-provoking situations, discussed in Chapter 12. Alternatively, youngsters may be trained to interpret the stimulus in a way that leads to positive rather than negative affect. This is the principle underlying the CTR cognitive coping strategy outlined below (p. 151) and in Chapter 12. Where clear patterns of parent–child interaction are associated with problems, family members may be invited to brainstorm ways of altering these interpersonal sequences. To do this, they may require training in communication and problem-solving skills.

Communication skills

Where parents and children have difficulties communicating clearly with each other about how best to manage the presenting problems, communication training may be appropriate. A common problem is that parents have difficulty listening to their children and children have difficulties clearly articulating their views to their parents. A second common communication problem is the difficulty parents have in listening to each other's views about how best to manage the child's difficulties in a non-judgemental way. In some instances parents and children have never learned communication skills. In others, good communication skills have been acquired but intoxication or intense emotions such as anger, anxiety or depression prevent parents and children from using these skills. Training in using communication skills is appropriate in the former situation but in the latter the key problem to be solved is how to arrange episodes of communication which will be uninfluenced by intoxication or negative mood states. Communication skills may be artificially sub-divided into those used for listening and those used for telling somebody something. These skills are listed in Table 4.2. Parents and children need, first, to be given an intellectual understanding of these skills. Then the psychologist should model the skills for the clients. Clients should at this point be invited to try using the skills to discuss a neutral topic in the

Table 4.2 Guidelines for listening and communication skills

Specific guidelines	General guidelines
Listening skills • Listen without interruption • Summarize key points • Check that you have understood accurately • Reply	• Make a time and place for clear communication • Remove distractions and turn off the TV • Discuss one problem at a time • Try to listen with the intention of accurately remembering what was said • Try to listen without judging what is being said
Communication skills • Decide on specific key points • Organize them logically • Say them clearly • Check you have been understood • Allow space for a reply	• Avoid negative mind-reading • State your points without attacking the other person • Avoid blaming, sulking or abusing • Avoid interruptions • Take turns fairly • Be brief • Make congruent I statements

session. Let the episode of communication run for five or ten minutes, and take notes of various difficulties that occur. Then give feedback and, in the light of this, ask clients to complete the episode again. Typical mistakes include interrupting before the other person has finished, failing to summarize what the other person said accurately, attributing negative malicious intentions to the other person when they have not communicated that they hold such intentions, failing to check that the message was accurately sent, failing to check that the message has been accurately received, blaming and sulking. Once clients can use the skills to exchange views on a neutral topic, they may then be used to exchange views on emotionally loaded issues in the session first and later at home. Communication homework assignments should be highly specific, to prevent clients from lapsing into poor communication habits. Thus, specific members of a family should be invited to find out the other person's views on a specific topic. A time and place free of distractions should be agreed and a time limit of no more than twenty minutes set for initial communication assignments and forty minutes when skills are better developed.

Problem-solving skills

When it is apparent that parents or children need to take a more systematic approach to resolving problems, problem-solving skills training is appropriate. Joint problem-solving training for parents is useful where parents have difficulty co-operatively developing plans for solving children's difficulties. Joint problem-solving training for adolescents and parents may be useful where parents and teenagers are having difficulty negotiating about the youngster's increasing autonomy. Individual problem-solving training for youngsters may be helpful when children have specific peer group or academic problems that they repeatedly fail to solve, such as joining in peer activities without aggression or managing homework assignments set by their teachers. As with communication difficulties, clients may have difficulties solving problems because they lack the skills or because intoxication, negative mood states or other factors interfere with the use of well-developed skills. Where such factors are present, therapy should focus on removing these obstacles to effective problem solving. In problem-solving training, the sequence of stages described for communication training should be followed with a progression from explanation of the skills listed in Table 4.3, to modelling, to rehearsal in the session with the focus on a neutral topic. Feedback should be given during rehearsal until the skills are well developed. Then clients may be invited to use the skills to solve emotionally laden problems. When families are observed trying to solve emotionally laden problems, often the first pitfall they slide into is that of problem definition. Many clients need to be coached in how to translate a big vague problem into a few small, specific problems. A second pitfall involves trying to solve more than one

Table 4.3 Guidelines for problem-solving skills

Specific guidelines	General guidelines
• Define the problem	• Make a time and place for clear
• Brainstorm options	communication
• Explore pros and cons	• Remove distractions and turn off the TV
• Agree on a joint action plan	• Discuss one problem at a time
• Implement the plan	• Divide one big problem into a few small
• Review progress	problems
• Revise the original plan	• Tackle problems one at a time
	• Avoid vague problem definitions
	• Define problems briefly
	• Show that the problem (not the person) makes you feel bad
	• Acknowledge your share of the responsibility in causing the problem
	• Do not explore pros and cons until you have finished brainstorming
	• Celebrate success

problem at a time. A third area of difficulty is helping clients to hold off on evaluating the pros and cons of any one solution until as many solutions as possible have been listed. This is important, since premature evaluating can stifle the production of creative solutions. Often, families need to be coached out of bad communication habits in problem-solving training such as negative mind-reading, where they attribute negative thoughts or feelings to others, blaming, sulking and abusing others. Where families with chronic problems successfully resolve a difficulty, a vital part of the coaching process is to help them celebrate this victory.

Providing support

In many instances, children, adolescents and parents referred for consultation lack social support. This deficit can be addressed by providing a forum where clients may confide their views and feelings about their problem situation. Children and adolescents may be seen individually or in groups and given space to talk about their problems or to use symbolic play or artistic media such as painting, drawing, poetry writing and so forth to articulate their views and feelings about their situation. Parents may be provided with sessions separately from the children, either individually, as couples or in groups, to ventilate their intense emotions and concerns about their children's difficulties. Regardless of the forum used, the responsibility of the psychologist is to:

• help clients find a medium through which they can express their thoughts and feelings

- create a climate in which the clients experience empathy, warmth and genuineness from those providing the support.

In some instances, it may be possible to refer clients to self-help support groups where others with similar problems meet and provide mutual support. Some such groups provide information, ongoing weekly support, and in some instances arrange summer camps for children.

For children, particularly those who have become embroiled in coercive problem-maintaining interaction patterns, an important intervention is to train parents in providing their children with support.

Parents may be coached in joint sessions with their children in how to do this. The guidelines for supportive play set out in Table 4.4 are first explained. Next, the psychologist models inviting the child to select a play activity and engaging in child-led play, while positively commenting on the child's activity, praising the child regularly and avoiding commands and teaching. Then the parent is invited to copy the psychologist's activity and feedback is given to parents on what they are doing well and what they need to do more of. Finally, the parent and child are invited to complete a twenty-minute daily episode of child-led play to increase the amount of support the child experiences from the parent.

Table 4.4 Guidelines for supportive play

Specific guidelines	*General guidelines*
• Set a specific time for 20 minutes supportive play per day • Ask the child to decide what he or she wants to do • Agree on an activity • Participate wholeheartedly • Run a commentary on what the child is doing or saying, to show your child that you are paying attention to what they find interesting • Make congruent 'I like it when you . . .' statements, to show your child you feel good about being there • Praise your child repeatedly • Laugh and make physical contact through hugs or rough and tumble • Finish the episode by summarizing what you did together and how much you enjoyed it	• Set out to use the episode to build a positive relationship with your child • Try to use the episode to give your child the message that they are in control of what happens and that you like being with them • Try to foresee rule-breaking and prevent it from happening or ignore it • Avoid using commands, instructions or teaching • Notice how much you enjoy being with your child

Reward systems

Where the goal of treatment is to help children learn new habits such as going to bed on time, taking medication, playing co-operatively with a sibling or coping with anxiety-providing situations, reward systems may be used (Herbert, 2002). Guidelines for using rewards systems are presented in Table 4.5. Reward systems may be introduced to parents and children in conjoint family sessions or in parent training sessions from which the child is absent. Whatever format is used, it is critical that the target behaviour is clearly defined, is monitored regularly and is rewarded promptly, using a symbolic system of points, tokens, stars or smiling faces that is age appropriate and acceptable to the child. Examples of smiling face and points charts are given in Chapter 10. The symbolic reward system must be backed by tangible rewards or prizes, which are highly valued, so that the child may buy these with points or tokens after they have accumulated a sufficient number. When points systems are ineffective, it may be that some adult in the child's environment, such as a non-custodial parent in the case of children from separated families, is not committed to implementing the system. In other instances, the target behaviours may be ambiguous or the number of points

Table 4.5 Guidelines for reward systems

Specific guidelines	General guideline
• Define the target behaviour clearly • Decide when and where the monitoring will occur • Make up a smiling-face chart or points chart • Explain to the child that they can win points or smiling faces by carrying out the target behaviour • Ask the child to list a set of prizes that they would like to be able to buy with their points or smiling faces • Agree on how many points or faces are necessary to buy each prize • Follow through on the plan and review it for effectiveness	• Present the reward system to your child as a way of helping him or her learn grown-up habits • All parental figures in the child's network should understand and agree to using the system • Use a chart that is age appropriate. Smiling faces or stars are good for children and points may be used for adolescents • The sooner points are given after completing the target behaviour, the quicker the child will learn • Highly valued prizes lead to faster learning • Try to fine-tune the system so that successes are maximized • If prizes are not being won, make the target behaviour smaller and clearer or the cost of prizes lower and make sure that all parent figures understand and are committed to using the system • If the system is not working, do not criticize the child • Always keep the number of target behaviours below five

required to win a prize too high. Troubleshooting these difficulties is a routine part of coaching families in using reward systems.

Behavioural control skills

Where parents have difficulties helping children to avoid engaging in aggressive and destructive behaviour, training in behaviour control skills is appropriate (Herbert, 2002). Guidelines for a behavioural control programme are set out in Table 4.6. This type of programme may be explained to parents alone or in the presence of their children in conjoint family sessions. The format preferred by the parent should be used. The programme should be framed as a way for helping the child to develop self-control skills. Specific negative or aggressive behaviours are defined as targets for which time-out from reinforcement is given. When these behaviours occur, the parent gives a command to the child to stop and this may be followed-up by two warnings. If children comply they are praised. If not, they are brought to time-out without any display of anger or any reasoned explanation being given at that time. The time for reasoned explanation is at the outset of the programme or when it is being reviewed, not following misbehaviour. During time-out, the child sits on a chair in the corner of the kitchen, the hall or their bedroom away from

Table 4.6 Guidelines for behaviour control programmes

Specific guidelines	General guidelines
Behaviour control programme • Agree on a few clear rules • Set clear consequences • Follow through • Reward good behaviour • Use time-out or loss of privileges for rule-breaking • Monitor change visibly **Time-out** • Give two warnings • Bring the child to time-out without negative emotion • After five minutes engage the child in a positive activity and praise him for temper control • If rule-breaking continues, return child to time-out until thirty seconds of quietness occurs • Engage in positive activity with child and praise for temper control	• Set out with the expectation that you can teach your child one good habit at a time • Build in episodes of unconditional special time into behavioural control programme • Frame the programme as learning self-control • Involve the child in filling in, designing and using the monitoring chart or system • Monitor increases in positive behaviour as well as decreases in negative behaviour • Do not hold grudges after episodes of negative behaviour • Avoid negative mind-reading • Avoid blaming, sulking or abusing • Ask for spouse support when you feel bad about the programme • Celebrate success

family activities and interesting or reinforcing events or toys. Following a period of two to five minutes (depending on the child's age), the child is invited to rejoin family activities and is engaged in a stimulating and rewarding exchange with the parent. If children misbehave or protest aggressively while in time-out, they remain there until they have been compliant and quiet for thirty seconds before rejoining family activities and engaging in a stimulating interaction with the parent. Running a behavioural control programme for the first two weeks is very stressful for most families. The normal pattern is for the time-out period to increase in length gradually and then eventually to begin to diminish. During this escalation period, when the child is testing out the parents' resolve and is having a last binge of self-indulgence before learning self-control, it is important to help families maintain the unconditionally supportive aspect of family life. There are two important interventions that may be useful here. First, spouses may be invited to set aside special time where the focus is on mutual marital support. Second, parents may plan episodes of supportive play with the children. The important feature of spouse support is that the couple set aside time to spend together without the children to talk to each other about issues unrelated to the children. In single-parent families, parents may be helped to explore ways for obtaining support from their network of friends and members of the extended family.

Tension reduction skills

Training in tension reduction skills may be included in treatment programmes where physiological arousal associated with anxiety, anger or other emotions is a central problem. Progressive muscle relaxation exercise, breathing exercises, visualization skills and auto-hypnosis are described in Chapter 12. With adolescents it may be appropriate to offer training in these tension reduction skills directly to the youngster. With children, parents may be coached in helping youngsters to work though these tension reduction routines.

Cognitive coping strategies

The types of internal or external stimuli to which children and parents attend prior to and during episodes of the presenting problem, the way in which they evaluate these stimuli and the behavioural and interpersonal patterns that they develop as a result of making these interpretations may all contribute to the maintenance of the presenting problems. Children and parents may be helped to cope with problematic situations more effectively by learning specific coping strategies, such as distraction, where the aim is to avoid attending to distressing stimuli or reinterpretation of problematic situations in ways that are less distressing. The CTR method for training children to interpret situations in less distressing ways is described in Chapter 12. Children are invited to Challenge threatening or depressing thoughts by asking themselves what the other possible interpretations of the situation are; to Test-out what evidence there is for the threatening or depressing outcome and the other more benign possible outcomes; and to Reward themselves for testing out the less dysfunctional interpretation of the situation.

Home–school liaison

Where factors within the school environment maintain children's difficulties or where children show school-based problems, liaison with the school is vital. The most effective way to conduct school liaison is to meet with the child's teacher and parents, outline the formulation of the problem in a tentative way, check that this is accepted by the teacher and parents and then explore options for action or suggest a particular way in which the school and parents may jointly contribute to the resolution of the child's problems. A home–school reporting system for use with hyperactive children is described in Chapter 11 and the way in which the school may be involved in the management of school refusal is described in Chapter 12.

Troubleshooting resistance

It is one of the extraordinary paradoxes of clinical psychology that clients go to considerable lengths to seek professional advice on how to manage their difficulties and often do not follow through on such advice or other responsibilities entailed by the treatment contract. This type of behaviour has traditionally been referred to as non-compliance or resistance. Accepting the inevitability of resistance and developing skills for managing it is central to the effective practice of clinical psychology (Anderson & Stewart, 1983).

Clients show resistance in a wide variety of ways. Resistance may take the form of not completing tasks between sessions, not attending sessions or refusing to terminate the therapy process. It may also involve not co-operating during therapy sessions. For clients to make progress with the resolution of their difficulties the therapist must have some systematic way of dealing with resistance (Carr, 2000b). First, describe the discrepancy between what clients agreed to do and what they actually did. Second, ask about the difference between situations where they managed to follow through on an agreed course of action and those where they did not. Third, ask what they believed blocked them from making progress. Fourth, ask if these blocks can be overcome. Fifth, ask about strategies for getting around the blocks. Sixth, ask about the pros and cons of these courses of action. Seventh, frame a therapeutic dilemma which outlines the costs of maintaining the status quo and the costs of circumventing the blocks.

When resistance is questioned, factors that underpin it are uncovered. In some instances unforeseen events – acts of God – hinder progress. In others, the problem is that the clients lack the skills and abilities that underpin resistance. Where a poor therapy contract has been formed, resistance is usually due to a lack of commitment to the therapeutic process. Specific convictions which form part of clients' individual, family or culturally based belief systems may also contribute to resistance, where the clients' values prevent them from following through on therapeutic tasks. The wish to avoid emotional pain is a further factor that commonly underpins resistance. Finally, transference may also contribute to resistance. This issue has been discussed in a previous section.

Questioning resistance is helpful only if a good therapeutic alliance has been built. Clients who feel that they are being blamed for not making progress will usually respond by pleading helplessness, blaming the therapist or someone else for the resistance, or distracting the focus of therapy away from the problem of resistance into less painful areas. Blaming, distraction or pleading helplessness often elicit countertransference reactions on the therapist's part, which compound rather than resolve the therapeutic impasse. The most common of these is persecuting the family, which has already been mentioned in the section on transference and countertransference.

Co-ordinating multi-disciplinary input

Complex case management plans require a designated key worker, a clear system for monitoring and recording the progress of the plan, and a system where members of the professional network and the family network regularly review progress and deal with co-ordination difficulties. In writing this text, I have addressed most of the practice issues to psychologists who will be designated key workers or case managers. Where psychologists adopt this role, a paper-based or computer-based system for keeping track of multi-systemic intervention programmes is vital if such plans are not to flounder. A front sheet should be placed in the file or on the database that specifies the following points:

- the name of each sub-component of the programme (e.g. social skills training, family therapy, speech therapy)
- a very brief statement of the goal for each component (e.g. develop friendship skills, improve home-based conduct problems)
- the names of the professional responsible for implementing the sub-components
- the number of sessions and dates of these (if that is feasible)
- the review dates for the overall multi-systemic programme
- the case manager or key worker responsible for convening review meetings.

With complex cases, review meetings for the network of involved professionals are particularly important since they provide a forum within which all involved professionals may share information and strive to retain a shared view of the case formulation, goals and management plan. Without a shared view, the opportunities for synergistic service delivery may be lost.

When convening a review meeting, particularly where difficulties have developed in the co-ordination and delivery of the agreed multi-systemic programme, set clear goals. Such goals typically include clarifying or refining the formulation and agreeing on roles and responsibilities. Open review meetings with introductions, if any team members have not met, and set the agenda and the rules for participation clearly. Make sure that everyone gets a fair hearing by helping the reticent to elaborate their positions and the talkative to condense their contributions. Summarize periodically, to help members maintain focus. Above all, retain neutrality by siding with no one and curiously inquiring about each person's position. Use time-out, if necessary, to integrate contributions, refine the formulation and elaborate options for action. Once the meeting accepts the refined formulation, request a commitment to develop or refine the action plan. Then work towards that by examining options and agreeing on which team members are responsible for particular parts of the programme. Minute all agreements and agree on further review dates.

When contributing to a review meeting, prepare points on your involvement in the case, your hypotheses and plans. Use slack time at the beginning of the meeting or during the tea break to build good working alliances with team members. Always introduce yourself before making your first contribution if you are new to the team. Outline your involvement first and hypotheses and plans later. Make your points briefly and summarize your points at the end of each major contribution. When you disagree, focus on clarifying the issue not on attacking the person with whom you disagree. Keep notes on who attended the meeting, on the formulation, and the plan agreed. If you have unresolved ambivalent feelings after the meeting, discuss these in supervision. A fuller account of convening and contributing to network meetings is given elsewhere (Carr, 1995).

STAGE 4: DISENGAGING OR RE-CONTRACTING

The process of disengagement begins once improvement is noticed. The interval between sessions is increased at this point. The degree to which goals have been met is reviewed when the session contract is complete or before this, if improvement is obvious. If goals have been achieved, the family's beliefs about the permanence of this change is established. Then the therapist helps the family construct an understanding of the change process by reviewing with them the problem, the formulation, their progress through the treatment programme and the concurrent improvement in the problem. Relapse management is also discussed (Marlatt & Gordon, 1985). Family members are helped to forecast the types of stressful situations in which relapses may occur, their probable negative reactions to relapses and the ways in which they can use the lessons learned in therapy to cope with these relapses in a productive way. Disengagement is constructed as an episodic event rather than as the end of a relationship. This is particularly important when working with families where members have chronic problems. In some instances, the end of one therapeutic contract will lead immediately to the beginning of a further contract. This subsequent contract may focus on the original child-centred problems, marital difficulties, or individual work for the adults in the family. Referral to other therapists or agencies for this further work may be appropriate. If goals are not reached, it is in the clients' best interests to avoid doing more of the same (Segal, 1991). Rather, therapeutic failures should be analysed in a systematic way. The understanding that emerges from this is useful both for the clients and for the therapist. From the clients' perspective, they avoid becoming trapped in a consultation process that maintains rather than resolves the problem. From the therapists' viewpoint it provides a mechanism for coping with burnout that occurs when multiple therapeutic failures occur.

Failures may occur for a number of reasons (Carr, 2000b). First, they may occur because of the engagement difficulties. The correct members of the child's network may not have been engaged. For example, where fathers are not engaged in the therapy process, dropout is more likely. The construction of a formulation of the presenting problem which does not open up possibilities for change or which does not fit with the family's belief systems is a second possible reason for failure. A third reason why failure occurs may be that the case management plan was not appropriately designed, the therapeutic alliance was poorly built, or the psychologist had difficulties in offering the family invitations to complete the therapeutic tasks. Problems with handling families' reservations about change, and the resistance that this may give rise to, is a fourth and further source of failure. Disengaging without empowering the family to handle relapses is a fifth possible factor contributing to therapeutic failure. A sixth factor is countertransference. Where countertransference reactions seriously compromise therapist neutrality and the capacity to join in an empathic way with each member of the problem-system, therapeutic failure may occur. Finally, failure may occur because the goals set did not take account of the constraints within which family members were operating. These constraints include biological factors such as illness, psychological factors such as intellectual disability, economic factors such as poverty, social factors such as general life stress, and broader sociocultural factors such as minority-group membership. Factors that influence therapy outcome identified in meta-analyses of the treatment outcome literature are summarized in Table 3.10 (p. 99), and a consideration of these may be useful in the analysis of treatment failures.

The analysis of treatment failure is an important way to develop therapeutic skill.

In some cases, psychologists may find it necessary to seek supervision for managing loss experiences associated with disengaging from both successful and unsuccessful cases. Where therapy has been unsuccessful, disengagement may lead to a sense of loss of professional expertise. Loss of an important source of professional affirmation and friendship are often experienced when therapists disengage from successful cases.

SUMMARY

The consultation process may be conceptualized as a developmental and recursive process involving the stages of planning, assessment and formulation, case management and disengagement or re-contracting. In the planning stage, network analysis provides guidance on who to invite to the intake interview. The minimum sufficient network necessary for an assessment to be completed includes the customer, the legal guardians, the caregivers and the referred child. In planning an agenda, a routine intake interview and a core test battery may be supplemented by questions and tests that take account of the specific features of the case. The routine interview and test battery should cover the child's individual physical, cognitive and psycho-social developmental history and an assessment of the family's development and functioning with particular reference to parent–child relationships; inter-parental relationships and the wider social network within which the family is embedded. Assessment of unique features of the case should be based on a preliminary formulation that contains hypotheses about pre-disposing, precipitating, maintaining and protective factors associated with the presenting problems. To develop a thorough understanding of the presenting problems and related issues, a number of different types of assessment meetings may be necessary. These may include some or all the following, depending on the case: child-centred assessment interviews and testing sessions, parental interviews, nuclear family interviews, school interviews, extended family interviews with other involved professionals, clinical team meetings, professional network meetings and statutory case conferences.

Establishing a contract for assessment, working through the assessment agenda and recursively refining the preliminary formulation in the light of the information obtained, dealing with engagement problems, building a therapeutic alliance and giving feedback are the more important features of the assessment and formulation stage, which may span a number of sessions. All other features of the consultation process should be subordinate to the working alliance, since without it clients drop out of the consultation process. The working alliance with the child, parents and network members should be a collaborative partnership characterized by warmth, empathy and genuineness, respectful curiosity and an invitational approach. The inevitability of transference and countertransference reactions within the therapeutic relationship should be acknowledged. Towards the end of the assessment phase a formulation is constructed. A formulation is a mini-theory that explains why the presenting problems developed, why they persist, what protective factors either prevent them from becoming worse or which may be enlisted to solve the presenting problems. The formulation is fed back to the family as a basis for a therapeutic contract. The level of detail used in giving this feedback needs to be matched to the family's cognitive ability to comprehend it and their emotional readiness to accept it. As part of the alliance-building process it is usually best if the protective factors are listed first and linked to possible case management options. Most case management options fall into the following categories: no immediate action, provide psychoeducation and reassess periodically, refer to another professional within the team, refer to another professional or residential facility outside the team, offer a focal psychological intervention and offer a multi-systemic intervention.

A therapeutic contract, based on the formulation begins with goal setting. Clear, realistic, visualized goals that are fully accepted by all family members and that are perceived to be moderately challenging are crucial for effective therapy. The costs and benefits of goals to involved members of the network must be considered as part of the contracting process. Case management and treatment plans for the problems of children and adolescents should be premised on a family-based approach. Such plans may include psychoeducation, monitoring problems, communication and problem-solving training and arranging the provision of support for children and parents. Treatment may also involve coaching in using reward systems and teaching children behavioural control skills. Coaching in tension reduction and cognitive coping strategies for children may be appropriate in other instances. In cases where the school or other professionals and agencies are involved, the co-ordination of multi-disciplinary and school input may be required. Complex case management plans require a designated key worker, a clear system for monitoring and recording the progress of the plan and a system whereby members of the professional network and the family network regularly review progress and deal with co-ordination difficulties. To work within such a system, skills for both managing and contributing to network meetings are required. Inevitably, co-operation difficulties occur during therapy and case management. These may be due to a lack of skills on the clients part or to complex factors that impinge on clients' motivation to resolve their difficulties. A systematic method for analysing resistance and resolving it is required to complete case management plans. Disengagement is considered when the end of the therapeutic contract is reached. If goals have not been achieved, this should be acknowledged and referral to another agency considered. Where goals have been reached, relapse management and the options for future booster sessions considered. In cases where further child problems or adult problems have emerged, a new contract for work on these issues may be offered.

EXERCISE 4.1

Work in teams of two to four members. Decide who to invite and what to ask in a first interview with the following case. In conducting a network analysis, first draw a genogram. In deciding what to ask, construct a preliminary formulation containing hypotheses about pre-disposing precipitating, maintaining and protective factors.

> Dear Team
>
> *Re: Paul O'Brien (aged ten)*
>
> Paul has been giving his mother a lot of grief recently since he came out of hospital. He was admitted to Church Street about two months ago following an accident in which he broke an arm and a leg after falling off the scaffolding in a building site in Howth. He is back at school and on a walking stick. He can't manage crutches because of his broken arm. The main problems seem to be defiance and disobedience. He is also occasionally tearful at school and has been sent home once or twice because the teachers felt he was not fit for school.
>
> He is one of three children. His parents were both previously married and he lives with his natural sister, Olive, and his stepfather's son, Jim. They have been together for about four years and most of the upheaval following the separations and all that seems to have passed.
>
> They all get on fine, but Paul's problems are a major worry for his mother, largely because they are getting worse rather than improving as time goes by. Please assess and advise.

EXERCISE 4.2

Work in pairs. Familiarize yourself with the material presented in Tables 4.2 to 4.6. For each of the skills (communication, problem solving, supportive play, reward systems, behavioural control), role-play explaining the skill to your partner as if he or she were the parent of a referred child. Ask your partner for feedback on how you might improve your presentation. Reverse roles and repeat the exercise.

FURTHER READING AND RESOURCES

Carr, A. (2006). *Family Therapy: Concepts, Process and Practice* (Second Edition). Chichester, UK: Wiley.

Corcoran, K. & Fischer, J. (2000). *Measures for Clinical Practice: A Sourcebook: Volume 1: Couples, Families, and Children* (Third Edition). New York: Free Press. (*Contains full reproductions of many useful brief assessment instruments such as those listed in Table 4.1 along with norms, scoring instructions and basic psychometric information.*)

O'Reilly, G. (2005). *A Teenager's Guide to Life*. Dublin, Ireland: Pscyhology Department, University College Dublin.

WEBSITES

Harcourt Assessment-Psychological Corporation (tests): http://www.harcourt-uk.com/

NFER Nelson (tests): http://www.nfer-nelson.co.uk/

Psychological assessment resources (tests): http://www.parinc.com/

Smallwood (self-help): http://www.smallwood.co.uk/

Speechmark (self-help): http://www.speechmark.net/

Western Psychological Services (tests): http://www.wpspublish.com/

Factsheets on common psychological problems given in this book and containing links to websites for parent and professional support and interest groups can be downloaded from the website for Rose, G. & York, A. (2004). *Mental Health and Growing Up. Fact sheets for Parents, Teachers and Young People* (Third edition). London: Gaskell: http://www.rcpsych.ac.uk

Chapter 5

Report writing

Psychologists have a duty to their clients to maintain confidentiality, and so all reports about clients should be managed with this as a central guiding principle. In all circumstances where psychologists wish to exchange information with other members of the client's professional or social network, the client's consent should be sought. Confidentiality may be broken only in circumstances where to maintain confidentiality would place the client or some other person in danger (British Psychological Society, 1995). Such circumstances are discussed in Chapter 16, which deals with self-harm, and Chapters 19, 20 and 21, where child abuse is addressed.

Report writing is central to the practice of clinical child psychology. The limitations of our memories require us to keep detailed accounts of complex information about our clients. An accurate account of information gained in interviews, testing sessions and meetings with other professionals is the basis on which a formulation is constructed and a treatment plan developed. Records also help us to keep track of progress with case management plans. At the end of an episode of consultation, a summary of the episode provides information that may be useful to ourselves or our colleagues in helping clients should they return for a further episode of consultation in the future.

During the process of assessment and case management, other members of the professional network, such as colleagues from our team, family doctors, referring agents, teachers and other involved professionals, may require verbal or written reports. Clients and members of the family system may also benefit from having written communication about aspects of the consultation process. In some cases it may be necessary to write specialized reports for courts or as assignments for clinical psychology training programmes. On an annual basis it may be necessary to write a service report. This chapter gives guidelines for writing the following types of report:

- progress notes
- comprehensive assessment reports
- end-of-episode case summaries

- verbal reports to clients and colleagues
- correspondence to clients and colleagues
- court reports
- case study reports
- annual service reports and clinical audit.

A guideline, which applies to all forms of reports, is to always write in such a way that you would be prepared to give your case files or service reports to clients and their families to read. This guideline helps us to inhibit the tendency to lapse too deeply into the pejorative deficit-discourse that unfortunately holds considerable sway in the mental health field (Gergen, 1994).

PROGRESS NOTES

When making progress notes about clinical cases, five categories of information should always be recorded:

- Time
- Attendance
- Review
- Agenda
- Plan

The first letters of these category names form the acronym TARAP. The issues covered by each category are expanded below.

Time

This category includes the date, day, time and duration of the session. It may also be useful to include the number of the session, particularly if working within a time-limited contract for assessment or intervention. Often, in clinical psychology, time-limited contracts of six, ten or twenty sessions are used.

Attendance

The people who attended the session and those who were invited and did not attend may be noted in this category. In the case of total non-attendance (or DNAs, as they are often called) it is important to record what steps were taken to inquire about reasons for non-attendance, especially where there are risks of self-harm or child abuse.

Review

A review of significant events that may have occurred since the previous session are recorded here. Changes in the presenting problem and factors related to its resolution or maintenance should be reviewed. Inquiries should also routinely be made about completion of assessment tasks such as self-monitoring and treatment tasks, such as practising particular parent–child interaction skills. In the case of an initial session, changes that have occurred since the referral was made may be noted.

Agenda

Information about the main *content* issues and the main *processes* that occurred may be recorded in this category. In assessment sessions common content issues are child and family development, problem formation and resolution or psychometric testing procedures and results. Process issues may include the quality of the working alliance and the impact of this on the validity of the information obtained. A good working alliance is essential for a valid assessment to be conducted. Themes covered in the sessions may be noted along with significant therapeutic processes.

Plan

Future action for clients, network members and the psychologist may be noted in this category. Assessment or treatment tasks that clients have been invited to complete may be noted here. Network members invited to the next session or referral of family members to other professionals for consultation also deserve mention at this point in the progress notes. Assessment procedures or particular therapy-related themes which may be included on the agenda for the next session may also be noted in this category along with hypotheses requiring further exploration.

The TARAP format for making progress notes is appropriate for assessment and treatment sessions with clients and members of their family networks. It is also useful to adhere to this format in recording information from case conferences and team meetings. Examples of assessment and treatment progress notes are presented in Figures 5.1 and 5.2, respectively.

COMPREHENSIVE ASSESSMENT REPORT

In Chapter 4 it was mentioned that distinctions may be made between the assessment and case management stages of the consultation process. The comprehensive assessment report is typically written at the end of the assessment

Time. 14.12.95. Thursday, 12.00 noon, 90 minutes. Second family assessment interview.

Attendance. Joe (father), Molly (step-mother) and Trevor were invited. Only Molly attended.

Review. None of the monitoring tasks was completed. All family members have the flu. Molly has been very depressed and Trevor (aged 15) continues to stay out till 2.00 a.m. and to hit his step-mother if she objects to him coming home late.

Agenda. Detailed exploration of the violent episodes was the central agenda of the session and the provision of support for Molly, who was very demoralized. Improving attendance was also examined. The episodes occur on days when Joe and Trevor fight before Trevor goes out with his mates. Where he goes and whether he takes drugs or if drink are involved is unknown, but Molly thinks he is *'doing Speed'*. He has never hit her in Joe's presence and only strikes out if she criticizes him for disobedience. He is always apologetic the next day. Molly is at her wits end and says she cannot take any more. She agreed she needs Joe's help to manage this. She phoned Joe in the session. He agreed to an appointment on Tuesday to further assess the pattern of interaction around the violence.

Plan. Meet with Molly and Joe on Thursday next at 12.00 noon. Molly was asked to write down the sequence of events that occurs each night there is no violence and each night there is.

Boris O'Toole
Clinical Psychologist in Training

Figure 5.1 Example of progress notes from an assessment session

Time. 12.2.96. Monday, 12.00 noon, 60 minutes. Second treatment session.

Attendance. Joe (father), Molly (step-mother), Trevor (15 years old), Tina (9-year-old step-sister) and Kate (10-year-old step-sister) were invited. All attended.

Review. Joe and Molly completed the task of listing three main house rules (Curfew of 10.00 p.m. on week nights and 11.00 p.m. at week-ends; no hitting; jobs including dustbins, garden and shopping will be rewarded).

Trevor completed the task of listing what he wants (curfew of 1.00 a.m. all week and 2.00 a.m. at week-ends; no hassle from Molly; permission and funds to visit mother in UK regularly).

Agenda. Negotiation of curfew times was the central agenda of the session. The grief and anger associated with his parents' separation; his difficulty in accepting Molly as an authority in the home; his wish to visit his mother in the UK were discussed.

Plan. Negotiation between Trevor and Molly and Joe about curfew time to occur for two periods of 20 minutes in next 10 days. Trevor to write a letter to Maeve (his mother) expressing wish to visit. Next appointment 22.2.96 at 12.00 noon.

Boris O'Toole
Clinical Psychologist in Training

Figure 5.2 Example of progress notes from a treatment session

stage and as the basis from which to conduct case management. This type of report represents a summary and integration of information obtained throughout the assessment process, which may have spanned a number of sessions and include a review of reports from other professionals. The comprehensive assessment report is written primarily for the psychologist and members of the psychologist's team. All other reports and correspondence are based on this document. It should usually include sections on the issues listed below.

Child demographic information

The child's name, date of birth and address should be given, along with names addresses and contact numbers for parents, legal guardians and foster-parents where relevant.

Referral information

This section includes the referring agent's name, address and contact number, the central problems that led to the referral or the principal referral question. It is also useful to include here details of significant members of the child's professional network, such as the name address and contact numbers of the child's school and family doctor. It is also useful to include the name of the person who instigated the referral.

Sources

The sources of information on which the report is based should be listed. These sources include all assessment sessions with dates and a note of who attended the sessions. If previous reports by psychologists, school teachers, physicians, social workers or other professionals were used these, too, should be noted. Where a child presents with school problems, ideally two or three recent school reports should be consulted to assess change in the child's behaviour over time.

History of the presenting problem

This section should include an account of how the problem developed and previous attempts to solve the presenting problem. The role of other involved professionals may be mentioned here. If medical, psychiatric or social work reports are available salient points from these may be summarized in this section.

The child's developmental history

Reference should be made to significant events or abnormalities in physical, cognitive and psychosocial development. Otherwise it is sufficient to note that development was within normal limits.

The family history and a genogram

Family membership, family members' characteristics, parent–child relationships, parental co-operation, family stresses and supports, significant family relationship patterns and significant achievements or difficulties in managing family transitions over the lifecycle should all be mentioned in this section.

Current cognitive abilities

Reference may be made here to the results of psychometric assessments of the child's abilities, to academic progress as outlined in at least two recent school reports and to reports from speech therapy or other sources relevant to the child's cognitive development. In presenting psychometric test results include the following information:

- the tests used
- the number and duration of testing sessions
- the impact of co-operation, physical factors (noise, cold, crowding, etc.), extraneous psychosocial factors (e.g. exhaustion or fear of childcare proceedings) and medication on the validity of the results
- an interpretation of the results specifying the child's overall ability level, the presence of specific or general learning difficulties and attainment levels for reading, language and other areas if these were assessed.

Where test results are broadly within the normal range, keep this section brief. Where the full pattern of test results is critical to the formulation and management of the case, a complete table of test results may be appended to the report and a detailed analysis of results may be given in this section. A fuller account of cognitive assessment, learning difficulties and guidelines for writing reports in such cases is given in Chapter 8.

Current psychosocial adjustment

Reference may be made here to the outcome of individual sessions with the child and to parents' and teachers' reports of the child's current behaviour at home and at school. Scores on standardized instruments such as the Child Behaviour Checklist or the Teacher Report Form may be given in this section, along with the results of objective or projective personality tests.

Formulation

A brief restatement of the central problems should be given here, along with an explanation of how they developed based on salient points drawn from previous sections of the report. Reference should be made to pre-disposing, precipitating and maintaining factors. In addition, protective factors and family strengths that have a bearing on the prognosis should be mentioned. In some situations it may be useful to give a differential diagnosis and a diagnosis before a formulation is offered.

Recommended case management plan

A prioritized list of options for case management may be listed here. Taking no further action, periodic reassessment, referral to another team member for consultation, referral elsewhere for consultation, focal intervention or multi-systemic intervention should all be considered. Where a multi-systemic intervention programme is central to the management plan, details of the components of the programme and the professionals responsible should be indicated. A key worker responsible for reviewing progress at designated times should be specified.

Signature

Most agencies have a policy about signing reports. Unless there are ethical reasons for not doing so, follow this policy, particularly if you are still in training. If there is no policy in your agency and you are in training, write your name and degrees on one line and underneath 'Clinical Psychologist in Training' (in Ireland and the UK) or 'Clinical Psychologist Intern' (in Canada and the US). In addition, your supervisor's name, degrees and appointment are also written on the report, which is co-signed.

Comprehensive assessment reports are usually written up by the key worker for the case. An example of such a report is presented in Figure 5.3.

Under some circumstances it may be useful to use computer-aided systems for report writing. I have typically found that editing such reports on a word processor eliminates any time-saving advantage they may have. However, details of two such systems are included in the Further Reading and Websites sections at the end of this chapter.

END-OF-EPISODE CASE SUMMARY

In Chapter 4 it was noted that psychological consultation is a developmental and recursive process involving the stages of planning, assessment, case management and re-contracting or disengagement. When clients conclude the re-contracting or disengagement stage, an end-of-episode case summary may be written. This report summarizes progress made as a result of implementing the case management plan. An end-of-episode case summary should contain the following sections:

- the formulation
- the implementation of the case management plan
- the outcome.

The formulation outlined in the comprehensive assessment report may be restated in the first section of the end-of-episode case summary. In the second section, a summary of the case management plan that was implemented should be given. It is also useful to note here any co-operation or co-ordination difficulties that occurred and how various resistances within the client's network were managed. In cases which did not respond to treatment, a hypothesis about the reasons for treatment failure should be given. Any new

PSYCHOLOGICAL REPORT

Child demographic information.
Trevor Sullivan (DOB 1.12.1980). 222 Windgate Road, Howth, Dublin 13. Phone: 83258888
The following people live at the above address
Father: Joe Sullivan
Step-mother: Molly Rourke
Step-sisters: Kate and Tina Rourke
Trevor's mother Maeve Sullivan lives at 36, The Rise, Luton, UK. Phone: 0044-1356-334412

Referral information.
Trevor was referred by Dr Gilhooley, 33 Sutton Cross, Sutton, Dublin 13. Phone: 832572723.
The referral was marked urgent and dated 3.12.1995. The principal concern, expressed by his father, Joe, was Trevor coming home at 2.00 a.m., three hours after he was due.
Trevor is a pupil at the Bracken Park High School, Shieldrake Road, Sutton. The year head is Mr Burke. Phone 832565654.
Joe gave written consent for the school to be contacted for an academic report and a behaviour checklist to be completed.

Sources.
This assessment report is based on five assessment interviews.
7.12.95. 12.00 a.m., 90 minutes. Trevor, Joe and Molly attended as requested.
7.12.95. 4.30 p.m., 30 minutes. Phone interview with Maeve.
14.12.95. 12.00 a.m., 90 minutes. Molly attended alone. Other family members were invited but could not come due to illness.
21.12.95. 12.00 a.m., 60 minutes, Trevor, Joe, Molly, Tina and Kate attended as requested
11.1.96. 10.00 a.m., 120 minutes, Trevor attended alone for psychometrics (WISC IV and WIAT II) and a child-centred interview as requested.
Two school reports (December 1994 and July 1995) were provided by Bracken Park and Mr Burke completed a behaviour checklist (Achenbach's Teacher Report Form). I also spoke with him on the phone on 7.12.95.
Joe completed the intake form and the Child Behaviour Checklist.

History of the presenting problem.
The problem began during the summer shortly after Trevor's mother Maeve moved to the UK with her new partner, Roy McFadden. He became very withdrawn at home and gradually began to stay out later at night. He also stopped talking to Molly, his step-mother for about a month in September and early October. Joe, Trevor's father, has tried to talk Trevor round, with little success. He has also tried ignoring the problem, which also has had little impact. Molly has tried confronting Trevor, but this has led to her being hit by Trevor, so she has backed off now.

Developmental history.
Trevor's physical, cognitive and psychosocial development have broadly been within normal limits. He was hospitalized briefly at the age of 5 when he broke his arm after falling off a bicycle. He was always an only child and adjusted well to this status. Trevor could make and maintain friendships satisfactorily. His transitions into school and from primary to secondary school all occurred without incident. In the year prior to his parents' separation he became quite withdrawn, but once the separation occurred and regular access was arranged this withdrawal, which was largely evident at home, ceased.

Genogram.

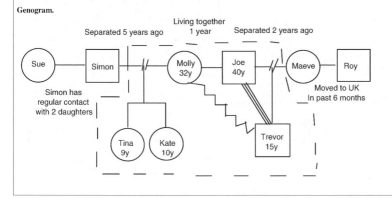

Figure 5.3 Example of a comprehensive assessment report   Continued

Family history.
The family composition is shown in the genogram. Trevor is the only child of Joe and Maeve, who separated two years ago following a period of gradual distancing. During the year or two prior to the separation, Joe was intensely involved with his work and Maeve had an affair with Roy. For about eighteen months following the separation (January 1994 to June 1995) Maeve and Roy lived near Joe, who retained custody of Trevor by agreement. Regular access occurred and this was satisfactory. During this period Joe met Molly and she and her two daughters moved in with Joe and Trevor. This new arrangement worked fairly well until last June when Maeve and Roy moved to the UK, because Roy's company transferred him to Luton. There has been little contact between Maeve and Trevor. However, she sent him a birthday card and some cash for his recent birthday. Trevor has been deeply hurt by his mother's move to the UK, and his sadness and anger about this find expression in his defiance of Joe and Molly's rules about 11.00 p.m. curfew; his aggression towards Molly; and his refusal to respond to Maeve's attempts to set up access visits. Joe, Maeve and Molly have not yet found a way to co-operatively support Trevor during this difficult period and also to set limits on his defiant and aggressive behaviour. However, relationships between Joe, Maeve and Molly are sufficiently flexible to indicate that co-operation about these issues is a possibility.

Tina and Kate have formed non-conflictual relationships with Trevor and Joe and have regular access visits with their father. However, the two girls have moved schools to St Frances in September and are not settling in well. Both have had episodes in the past 3 months of school refusal.

While Joe's physical and mental health have been fine over the past year, he has been exhausted in the past couple of months because he has been working double shifts on a regular basis. Molly, has a longstanding recurrent mood disorder and she has been particularly low in the past two months. Two particular stresses that have exacerbated her low mood in the past couple of months are the violent exchanges with Trevor and Tina and Kate's school problems.

Maeve is working long hours and has been unable to arrange a 3-day visit to Ireland to meet with Trevor, who, incidentally, has said he will not talk to her if she visits.

Cognitive abilities.
In a single two-hour session the WISC IV and the reading subtests of the WIAT II were administered to Trevor, who was 15 years and 0 months at the time of the assessment. He co-operated well with the assessment procedures so the obtained results may be interpreted as a valid estimate of his abilities. On the WISC IV, his full-scale IQ of 115 fell within the high average range of general intellectual abilities (110–119). His scores on the four main factors of the WISC IV also fell within the high average range and his subtest scatter on the WISC IV was unremarkable. On the WIAT II his reading comprehension and spelling scores were 118 and 117, respectively. These were consistent with his overall ability level. An examination of two recent school reports showed that Trevor has consistently been in the top third of his class for most academic subjects and has a particular aptitude for languages.

Psychosocial adjustment.
On the Child Behaviour Checklist, which was jointly completed by Joe and Molly, and on the self-report equivalent of this checklist (the Youth Self-Report Form), Trevor scored in the clinical range (above a T-score of 63) on both the internalizing and externalizing scales. However, on the Teacher Report Form, his scores on these scales were within the normal range. These results indicate that at home Trevor, his step-mother and father agree that he is showing clinically significant levels of conduct problems (aggression and defiance) and emotional problems (withdrawal and low mood). However, at school these conduct and emotional problems are not evident. This conclusion is consistent with the results of an individual interview with Trevor, who said that at school he can escape from 'the hassles of home'. In an individual interview Trevor also described how he interpreted his mother's move to England as a personal rejection, for which he finds it difficult to forgive her.

Formulation.
Trevor is a 15-year-old boy who, in the past six months, has been refusing to come in at night on time and who has been physically aggressive to his step-mother, Molly, when confronted about this defiance. Trevor has also shown low mood and withdrawal at home. These problems were precipitated by his mother's departure to the UK in June. The problems are an expression of his sadness and anger at his mother's departure. Pre-disposing factors include his parents' separation two years ago and the formation of the blended family in which he now resides. The problems are maintained by certain difficulties that have prevented Joe, Maeve and Molly from reaching a co-operative plan about how best to manage Trevor. These difficulties include Joe's recent exhaustion associated with working double shifts; Molly's recurrent mood problems, which are currently worse because of her daughters' problems in settling into school and the fact that Trevor has hit her on a number of occasions; and Maeve's work commitment which prevent her from visiting Trevor. The problems are also maintained by Trevor's interpretation of his mother's move to the UK as rejection and by his inability to deal with his feelings of grief and anger in a socially appropriate way. Looking at protective factors, Trevor's adjustment prior to this episode was within normal limits. Also Joe, Maeve and Molly are committed to solving this difficulty and making the new family arrangement work. Trevor has shown signs of remorse for his violence to Molly. And both Joe and Molly support Trevor's need to maintain a relationship with his mother in the UK. Also, despite the family-based difficulties, Trevor's school performance is within normal limits.

Recommended Case Management Plan
The family will be offered a series of six sessions. The suggested aims of this family work will be negotiating house rules and a system for implementing these that is acceptable to Joe, Molly and Trevor; helping Trevor, Molly and Joe develop a way to avoid future violent episodes; and helping Maeve, Trevor, Joe, and Molly find a way for Trevor and his mother to have regular contact. It may be necessary to invite Maeve to at least one session. In addition, Trevor will be offered a place in our adolescent group (which will be starting in March) to focus on anger management and examine his interpretation of his mother's move to the UK. The key worker for the case is Boris O'Toole. Progress review will occur in team meetings on 29.3.96 and 3.5.96.

Boris O'Toole, BA, MSc   Richard Kimbell, PhD, Reg Psychol AFPsSI, C Psychol AFBPsS
Clinical Psychologist in Training   Consultant Clinical Psychologist

Figure 5.3 Continued

information that came to light and led to the original formulation being substantially revised should be noted. The final section of an end-of-episode summary should note the degree to which specific treatment goals were met, along with other positive or negative changes. Follow-up plans for booster sessions or relapse management should also be noted. Where re-contracting for further work occurs, details of this should be recorded. An example of an end-of-episode case summary report is given in Figure 5.4.

VERBAL REPORTS

During the consultation process it may be necessary to give verbal reports to clients and colleagues in feedback sessions, team meetings and case conferences. In preparing verbal reports, first identify the audience to whom your report will be addressed. Is it a client, a social worker, a paediatrician, a

---

END-OF-EPISODE CASE SUMMARY

Trevor Sullivan (DOB 1.12.1980) 222 Windgate Road, Howth, Dublin 13. Phone: 83258888

Formulation.
Trevor is a 15-year-old boy who, in the six months prior to referral, was refusing to come in at night on time and who had been physically aggressive to his step-mother, Molly, when confronted about this defiance. Trevor had also shown low mood and withdrawal at home. These problems were precipitated by his mother's departure to the UK in June 1995. The problems seemed to be an expression of his sadness and anger at his mother's departure. Pre-disposing factors included his parents' separation two years prior to referral and the formation of the blended family in which he now resides. The problems were maintained by certain difficulties that prevented Joe, Maeve and Molly from reaching a co-operative plan about how best to manage Trevor. These difficulties included Joe's exhaustion associated with working double shifts; Molly's recurrent mood problems, which at referral were worse because of her daughters' problems in settling into school and the fact that Trevor had hit her on a number of occasions; and Maeve's work commitments which prevented her from visiting Trevor. The problems were also maintained by Trevor's interpretation of his mother's move to the UK as rejection and by his inability to deal with his feelings of grief and anger in a socially appropriate way. There were also protective factors in this case. Trevor's adjustment prior to this episode was within normal limits. Joe, Maeve and Molly were committed to solving this difficulty and making the new family arrangement work. Trevor had shown signs of remorse for his violence to Molly. And both Joe and Molly support Trevor's need to maintain a relationship with his mother in the UK. Also, despite the family-based difficulties, Trevor's school performance was within normal limits.

Case Management.
The family was offered a series of six sessions to work on negotiating house rules and a system for implementing these; helping Trevor, Molly and Joe develop a way to avoid future violent episodes; and helping Maeve, Trevor, Joe, and Molly find a way for Trevor and his mother to have regular contact. Five sessions were held focusing on these three issues. In the third of these, Maeve flew over from Luton to Dublin. This was a turning point in the case. Access arrangements were agreed and since then Trevor has flown to the UK on a bargain flight on two occasions using money he earns from doing household chores including painting the windows and rebuilding the patio. The violent episodes have not recurred. On those nights when he goes out, Trevor usually comes home on time.

Trevor attended the adolescent group for 8 sessions. He used the group to ventilate his feelings about his mother leaving Ireland and adjusting to his current living arrangements. Part of this involved taking responsibility for hitting Molly, for which he expressed remorse.

Outcome.
While the problems that led to Trevor's referral have been resolved, Molly continues to suffer from a recurrent mood disorder and Joe is finding this difficult to live with. At the end of this episode of treatment Joe and Molly asked to be referred for marital therapy and this has been arranged.

Boris O'Toole, BA, MSc	Richard Kimbell, PhD, Reg Psychol AFPsSI, C Psychol AFBPsS
Clinical Psychologist in Training	Consultant Clinical Psychologist

Figure 5.4 Example of an end-of-episode case summary

psychiatrist, a speech therapist or a mixed group of professionals? Then, clarify what sort of question to which you believe they require an answer. Do they want to know if your assessment indicates a child has a learning problem, or is at risk for abuse, or has responded to treatment? From your progress notes or the comprehensive assessment report, abstract the points that you are confidently able to make to answer the question. If you are unable to answer the question on the basis of the available information, arrange interviews or testing sessions to obtain such information if this is feasible and within the remit of your professional role.

Then prepare the list of points you wish to make in the meeting to answer the inquiries you know or guess are of central concern to your audience. Frame the points in language and at a level of technical sophistication that will be optimally intelligible to the audience. So, for example, it may be useful to give detailed psychometric information in a verbal report to a neuropsychologist but of little use to give such information to an orthopaedic surgeon or occupational therapist. In some instances, you will be unable to offer valid information to other professionals. For example, in some cases, risk of child abuse is difficult to confidently assess and in others, intelligence is difficult to assess because of co-operation problems. In such instances it is important to report that you are unable to answer the questions posed.

When making a verbal report to any audience state:

•   the question you aimed to answer
•   the source of your information and your confidence in its reliability and validity
•   the key pieces of information that answer the question (and no more).

If you are presenting information in a team meeting or case conference and do not know all of the participants, it is important to identify yourself as a clinical psychologist (or a clinical psychologist in training working under the supervision of a senior staff member).

If information presented by other professionals in a team meeting or case conference is inconsistent with your findings, think through the possible reasons for the discrepancy between the two sets of information before offering your opinion on this to the team or conference. Discrepancies between professional reports are common. The important issue to resolve is why the discrepancy occurred, not which view is correct and which is incorrect. Discrepancies may be due to the time and place where the assessment was conducted, the assessment or treatment methods used, the informants, the level of co-operation between the client and the professional and a wide range of other factors. Further guidelines for participating in team meetings are presented in Chapter 4 in the section on completing case management plans.

CORRESPONDENCE WITH PROFESSIONALS

All correspondence should be written with the concerns of the recipient of the letter in mind. Before writing a letter, clarify what question the recipient would like answered. Common questions are:

- Has the client been placed on the waiting list or has he or she been assessed?
- Why is this child behaving in an unusual way and what can be done about it?
- Have you been able to help this child and family manage the problem?
- Should we be co-ordinating our input to this case?

Decide what precise pieces of information the recipient would like abstracted from your case file to answer their question. Judge in what level of detail and what degree of technical sophistication they would like such information. Account should be taken of their knowledge of developmental psychology, psychometrics, family therapy and so forth. If any action will be required on their part, in response to your letter, decide exactly what it is that you are suggesting they do to help the client.

Routinely in most public service agencies, letters are written to referrers following the receipt of a referral to indicate that the referral has been placed on a waiting list. Letters are also written following a period of assessment to indicate the way the case has been formulated and the recommended case management plan. Finally, letters are also written at the end of an episode of contact to inform the referrer of the outcome of any intervention programme.

Having talked with more than 1000 professional recipients of psychologists' reports on both sides of the Atlantic over the past twenty-five years, one reasonably valid conclusion may be drawn: clinical psychologists' reports are too long and often the key information required by the referrer is buried under a mountain of unnecessary detail.

When a referral is received, it is sufficient to return a single-sentence letter indicating that the case will be placed on a waiting list and seen within a specified time frame. Following a preliminary interview or series of assessment sessions, it is sufficient to write a brief letter specifying the referral question, the assessment methods used, the formulation and the case management plan. A common mistake here is to send referrers (particularly family doctors) unwanted comprehensive assessment reports. It may be useful to conclude letters summarizing preliminary assessments by noting that a comprehensive report is available on request. An example of a letter to a family doctor summarizing a preliminary assessment is presented in Figure 5.5. In closing letters to referrers, it is sufficient to restate the initial question, the formulation, the case management plan, the degree to which it was

Dear Dr Gilhooley

Re: Trevor Sullivan, 222 Windgate Road, Howth.

Many thanks for referring this 15-year-old to me. I have seen Trevor, his father Joe, his step-mother Molly and his two step-sisters on three occasions for assessment interviews and spoken to his mother, Maeve (who lives in Luton), on the phone.

You mentioned that the father's main concern was with Trevor's refusal to come in at a reasonable hour at the week-ends. It also appears that the boy regularly hits his step-mother, Molly, if she confronts him about transgressions of house rules (including coming in late) in his father's absence. Trevor has also shown low mood and withdrawal at home but not at school.

These problems were precipitated by his mother's departure to the UK in June. The problems are an expression of his sadness and anger at his mother's departure. Predisposing factors include his parents' separation two years ago and the formation of the blended family in which he now resides. The problems are maintained by certain difficulties that have prevented Joe, Maeve and Molly from reaching a co-operative plan about how best to manage Trevor. These difficulties include Joe's recent exhaustion associated with working double shifts; Molly's recurrent mood problems which are currently worse because of her daughters' problems in settling into school, and the fact that Trevor has hit her on a number of occasions; and Maeve's work commitment which prevent her from visiting Trevor. The problems are also maintained by Trevor's interpretation of his mother's move to the UK as rejection and by his inability to deal with his feelings of grief and anger in a socially appropriate way.

Looking at protective factors, Trevor's adjustment prior to this episode was within normal limits. Also Joe, Maeve and Molly are committed to solving this difficulty and making the new family arrangement work. Trevor has shown signs of remorse for his violence to Molly. And both Joe and Molly support Trevor's need to maintain a relationship with his mother in the UK. Also, despite the family-based difficulties, Trevor's school performance is within normal limits.

Today, all parties in the family agreed to attend for a series of six sessions with a view to negotiating house rules, managing the violence and arranging a way for Trevor and his mother to have some contact. In addition, Trevor has agreed to attend our adolescent group which will be starting in March.

I shall write again when Trevor and the family have completed this programme.

Yours sincerely

Boris O'Toole, BA, MSc   Richard Kimbell, PhD, Reg Psychol AFPsSI, C Psychol AFBPsS
Clinical Psychologist in Training   Consultant Clinical Psychologist

Figure 5.5 Example of a letter to a referring agent

implemented and the outcome. The text from an end-of-episode case summary may be used as basis for writing a closing note to a referrer.

Asking other professionals to follow a particular course of action in a letter is more likely to lead to confusion than to co-ordinated action. It is better practice to outline your formulation in a letter and invite other professionals to join you in a meeting to discuss joint action than to ask them to implement a programme you have already designed.

CORRESPONDENCE WITH CLIENTS

Letters may be used to help clients remember what was said during consultation and to highlight key aspects of sessions. Case formulations, test results, instructions for completing specific tasks may all be given in written form. Letters also provide a medium for involving absent members of the family in the therapeutic process. For example, if a father or sibling is unable to attend a session, a letter may be sent summarizing the session and asking for the absent member's viewpoint. Letters may be used creatively as a medium for re-framing problems. For example, if parents view a child as intrinsically bad, and evidence comes to light during some aspect of consultation that the child's misbehaviour is situational, a letter may be written to the parent asking for their view on the fact that in certain situations the child's behaviour seems to be within normal limits. Detailed examples of all of these ways of using correspondence with clients are given in Carr (1995).

When writing a letter to a client, first clarify what you want to achieve by writing the letter. Do you want to inform the client or invite them to behave differently? Ideally, what impact would you like the letter to have on the client? Second, guess what is on the client's mind and how the client will be likely to respond to the information or invitation that you offer. In some instances clients will receive information positively and respond to invitations to change their behaviour quite flexibly. In other situations, clients' ability level, their fear or anger that they are being negatively labelled by the psychologist or their belief that the invitation in the letter to view the problem differently or behave differently will lead to some negative outcome may prevent them from understanding information or following through on invitations contained in letters. The third step in writing letters to clients is to decide how information or invitations should be framed so that they have the desired impact. Where clients have limited abilities, use simple language. Where there is a danger that clients may feel blamed for failing to solve the problem, acknowledge client strengths and commitment to change. Where clients fear that looking at the problem differently or behaving differently will lead to negative outcomes, highlight the benefits of accepting the invitation but also the dangers of accepting the invitation without due consideration and deliberation. An example of a letter to a client is contained in Figure 5.6.

Dear Martha:

We met today to discuss Brian's temper tantrums. I think that you have been very patient in putting up with them for so long. This patience will stand to you if you decide to try the two things we agreed today. These were:
1. To spend 20 minutes a day playing with Brian in the kitchen with the TV turned off.
2. To give 2 warnings if he refuses to follow the rules for bed time or meal time. If he does not obey on the third time, he is to be put in time-out for 3 minutes or until he stops screaming for 30 seconds.
I told you that things will get worse before they get better with Brian. So you may want to put off starting with these two new things until you are sure you are ready.
I will see you next Tuesday at 10.00 am in the clinic.

Yours sincerely,

Boris O'Toole, BA, MSc   Richard Kimbell, PhD, Reg Psychol AFPsSI, C Psychol AFBPsS
Clinical Psychologist in Training   Consultant Clinical Psychologist

Figure 5.6 Example of a letter to a client

COURT REPORTS

On occasion, psychologists are asked to write reports on the psychological adjustment of children for use in court. Such requests may come from a wide variety of sources including parents, legal guardians (where children are in the care of the State), solicitors or lawyers (acting on behalf of children, their parents or guardians), courts (where an independent opinion is required or following a subpoena) and insurance companies (where claims following accidents are being made).

Most court reports written by clinical psychologists working in child and family mental health fall into four categories:

- road traffic accidents
- child protection
- juvenile justice
- parental custody and access disputes.

With road traffic accidents, the central concern typically is the degree to which the child's cognitive and emotional well-being has been impaired as a result of the accident and the possible prognosis. In such instances, head injury (Chapter 8), impact of other physical injuries (Chapter 14), and post-traumatic stress reactions (Chapter 12) are routinely assessed along with other relevant areas such as bereavement (Chapter 24) when a fatality has occurred during the accident.

In child protection cases the principal concerns are usually the validity of the evidence for the occurrence of child abuse, the credibility of the child's statement, the impact of the abuse on the child and the future needs of the child, with particular reference to the changes that would have to be made in order for the child's family to offer adequate protection against further abuse. Physical child abuse, neglect and sexual abuse are covered in Chapters 19, 20 and 21. In Chapter 22, the transition from the family to residential child care is considered and this may be of relevance in child abuse cases which lead to out-of-family placements.

Requests for court reports in the juvenile justice area usually involve youngsters who have conduct problems (including drug abuse) which are significant enough to bring them to the attention of the police. Assessment of factors contributing to youngsters' anti-social behaviour is typically requested, along with recommendations for treatment and case management. Conduct problems and drug abuse are dealt with in Chapters 10 and 15.

The principal concern in parental custody and access disputes is how the child's needs for contact with both parents may best be met following parental separation or divorce. Psychological factors relevant to divorce are considered in Chapter 23.

Court reports should open with a statement of the clinical psychologist's qualifications and credentials to establish the psychologist's credibility in the eyes of the court. Professional qualifications, professional status with respect to national registration or chartering procedures, primary employer and other agencies or universities with which the psychologist is affiliated should all be mentioned. In addition, the amount of experience with similar cases should be stated, particularly if evidence on a rare condition or a psychologically complex issue is being given. Here is an example of how to write an opening paragraph of a court report:

> This report is written by Dr Finn MacCool. I hold a doctorate in clinical psychology from Tara University and Masters and Bachelors degrees in psychology from the University of Howth. I am a Registered Psychologist with the Psychological Society of Ireland and a Chartered Clinical Psychologist with the British Psychological Society. I have been employed as a Clinical Psychologist with the Fianna's Health Board since 1990. I also work as a Senior Tutor with the Clinical Psychology Training programme at Tara University. Over the past 5 years, I have conducted consultations with more than 50 cases of childhood sexual abuse. I have also trained colleagues within psychology and other disciplines in the assessment and management of cases where child protection is a central concern.

Following this type of introductory paragraph, the format for a comprehensive psychological assessment may be followed with some minor modifications. Where there are conflicting opinions within the family and professional network about how to manage the case, particular attention should be paid in the section on the source of the referral and the referral question to specifying how the results of the psychological report may help to resolve these differences of opinion. For example:

> X believes A and Y believes B. These opinions have been formed without access to the results of a psychological assessment. One function of the psychological assessment reported below was to throw light on the relative validity of each of these positions.

Following the section on formulation, in child protection, custody and access, and juvenile justices cases, the main options for case management and the pros and cons of each should be given. Finally, in a section headed 'Recommendations', a concise recommended action plan should be given, which reflects your opinion about which of the options discussed in the previous section is best to follow.

In cases where the central question is the immediate and long-term impact of injuries sustained in a road traffic accident, following the formulation, a section on prognosis should be included. It is important to outline the short- and long-term impact of the injuries on the child's physical, cognitive, academic, social and emotional functioning. Reference should be made to both clinical experience and research on the outcome for similar cases.

Presenting evidence in court is a complex process and requires considerable skill. A useful training resource is the Expert Testimony: Developing Witness Skills pack available from the British Psychological Society (1996). Useful examples of court reports are given in Black et al. (1998) and Munsinger & Karlson (1996).

CASE STUDY REPORTS

In many clinical psychology training programmes, conceptual clinical skills are assessed by case study. Case studies are an opportunity for candidates to demonstrate that they can bring their knowledge of relevant psychological literature to bear on the way in which they conceptualize and manage clinical problems. The precise requirements for writing a case study report vary from one clinical psychology training programme to another. The guidelines presented here are those used in our doctoral programme in clinical psychology at University College Dublin.

Case studies should be based on clients with whom the candidate has had clinical involvement as the key worker or as a co-worker with another clinician. The scientist–practitioner model should be used. That is, scientific knowledge and systematic investigative and intervention methods must be brought to bear on a specific clinical problem in an interpersonally sensitive way. A knowledge of the relevant literature must be demonstrated. A case study should highlight the candidate's ability to formulate and test clinical hypotheses. The ability to synthesize salient points from a range of investigative procedures into a comprehensive formulation should be clearly shown. A case study should indicate that the candidate can develop (and in some instances implement) case management plans which follow logically from the formulation. Interpersonal sensitivity and an awareness of process and ethical issues should also be demonstrated in case study reports.

A case study may focus on describing how assessment procedures were used to resolve a diagnostic issue and arrive at a coherent integrative formulation. In other instances, case studies may show how assessment and formulation led to the development and implementation of a case management or treatment plan. Where candidates had primary responsibility for implementing one aspect of this plan, particular attention may be paid to that in the case report. Where clients with similar problems have received group treatment, an entire group may serve as the focus for the case study. In such instances, a generic formulation of the problem addressed by the group treatment programme may be presented.

A case study should follow the outline structure presented in Box 5.1 and contain no more than 4000 words (excluding appendices and references). Copies of reports, correspondence, and test forms may be included in appendices. Client's names and other identifying information should be deleted from these documents to preserve confidentiality. Consent for writing case studies should be obtained at the outset of the assessment and treatment contract. This issue is covered in the intake form in Figure 4.3 (pp. 111–114). Where the case study format given in Box 5.1 is clearly unsuitable, candidates may order and organize case material and relevant information from the

Box 5.1 Framework for writing a case study

---

1. Demographic information about the case and the referral process
- Demographic information
- Referral agent, instigator of the referral and reason for referral
- History of the presenting problem
- Relevant background individual and family psychosocial and medical history
- Previous and current assessment and treatment

2. Review of relevant literature
- Classification, epidemiology, clinical features, course, assessment, treatment and controversial issues
- Reference to ICD and DSM and other relevant classification systems
- Reference to major clinical texts and recent relevant literature (particularly review papers, book chapters, assessment manuals, treatment manuals and handbooks)

3. Preliminary hypotheses and preliminary formulation of problem
- Hypotheses and proposed plan for testing hypotheses
- Preliminary formulation of the problem from a theoretical perspective

4. Assessment
- Procedures used, e.g. interviews, psychometric tests, observation sessions
- Rationale for choice
- Child's developmental history with particular reference to salient features
- Family's developmental history and genogram with particular reference to salient features
- Current cognitive functioning (including a table of test results if cognitive tests were conducted)
- Current psychosocial adjustment (including results of behaviour checklists and personality tests)

5. Formulation
- Implications of data from assessment for preliminary formulation and hypotheses
- Integration of assessment data into a comprehensive formulation highlighting pre-disposing, precipitating, maintaining and protective factors

6. Case management
- Consider options for action in the light of formulation (taking no further action; periodic reassessment; referral to another team member for consultation; referral elsewhere for consultation; focal intervention; or multi-systemic intervention)
- Choice of option and reason for choice in light of formulation
- Description of programme plan and goals of programme
- Review of progress in the light of goals
- Evaluation of outcome specifying assessment instruments used (graph changes in problems or symptoms if appropriate; at a minimum pre- and post-treatment measures may be used. Single case designs may be used if appropriate)

7. Process issues
- Impact of clinician–client relationship factors on the consultation process
- Impact of interprofessional and interagency relationships on the consultation process

8. Ethical issues
Ethical issues and the way they were managed should be addressed. Common issues include:
- The ability of children to give informed consent
- Confidentiality of child reports
- Child protection where there is a suspicion of abuse
- Conflict of interests of parents, children, teachers and other professionals

9. Summary and conclusions
- Reason for referral
- Summary of assessment and formulation
- Summary of treatment
- Recommendation or future management

10. References and appendices
- No more than 10 references, most of which should be to key review articles, book chapters, manuals, and handbooks, should be included as references and these should be in the format used in Journal of Consulting and Clinical Psychology, or the Irish Journal of Psychology which follow the BPS or APA referencing styles
- All relevant test result forms; checklists; reports from other professionals; correspondence; client drawings, etc. should be included as appendices with identifying information deleted

literature in a way which is most coherent. Although psychologists in clinical training usually choose to write-up cases where the work proceeded smoothly in accordance with a treatment manual, the client improved and was satisfied with services received, it may be more useful to write-up work that is more representative of routine practice. Indeed, the purpose of the case study is to demonstrate learning, reflection and professional development, and it is often in difficult work with clients where things do not go smoothly, where clients are challenging or do not improve, that we learn most. Such case studies may provide excellent opportunities for reflection and development.

The relationships between progress notes, assessment reports, end-of-episode case summaries, verbal reports, correspondence and special reports associated with specific cases is diagrammed in Figure 5.7. Assessment reports and case summaries are based on a synthesis of salient points from progress notes. Verbal reports, correspondence and special reports are abstracted from assessment reports and case summaries.

SERVICE REPORTS AND CLINICAL AUDIT

On an annual basis it is useful for clinical psychology service departments to produce reports which describe their performance over the preceding twelve-month period. Such reports are useful for service planning and for keeping managers, service purchasers and funders abreast of departmental performance. Most psychology departments provide the following categories of service:

• clinical services to clients

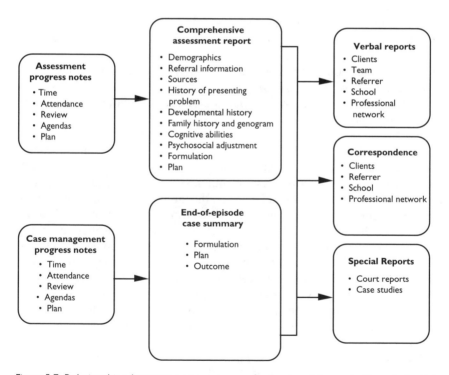

Figure 5.7 Relationships between various types of reports arising out of psychological consultations

- consultation and education to other professionals and agencies
- research, including surveys of population needs, waiting-list analyses and programme evaluation.

Sections on each of these areas of service provision should be included in an annual report, usually in the order in which they have been listed above. The section on research should contain a list of projects and authors. For each project, the following summary information may be provided:

- the aims of the research
- the methods used
- the time taken to complete the project
- the principal findings
- recommendations for service development.

Full copies of important research projects may be included as appendices to an annual report, if appropriate.

In the consultation and educational services section of an annual report, the following information may be given:

- a list of staff providing such services
- professionals or agencies receiving consultation or educational services or programmes
- the areas of education or consultation covered in the programmes
- the amount of time involved
- survey data or qualitative feedback on satisfaction with the consultation or educational process.

In an annual report, the section on clinical services to clients is usually presented first, since it is usually of greatest interest to service funders and providers alike. The section usually contains a description of the types of services offered, the staff who offer these, the target population for whom the service is intended and the avenues of referral. It is then followed by an account of the number and type of cases that received consultation, with a breakdown of the way they were referred, their demographic and clinical characteristics, the amount of input made to cases, the response of cases to the assessment and treatment process, the clients' satisfaction with treatment and the referring agents' satisfaction with the service provided. This information is obtained through clinical audit. The forms in Figures 5.8, 5.9 and 5.10 may be used to conduct such an audit and provide information areas mentioned above.

Some comments on the three forms will clarify how they may be used. For each case, the form in Figure 5.8 is completed at the end of an episode of consultation by the key worker. Most of the items are self-explanatory,

Information	Variable		Computer code
Names_____ _____ _____ Address_____ _____ _____ Phone	**Case identification** details and case number		1. Case identity
Referrer_____ Address_____ _____ _____ _____ Phone	**Referral source** Self Family doctor School Hospital Social services Other	1 2 3 4 5 6	2. Referrer
Main problems 1._____ 2._____ 3.	**Case type** Focal problem Complex multi-problem Complex child abuse	1 2 3	3. Case type
Main DSM or ICD Diagnosis	**Diagnosis** ICD or DSM		4. Diagnosis
Child's age	**Age** Pre-school (0–4) Pre-adolescent (5–11) Young adolescent (12–16) Older adolescent (16–18)	1 2 3 4	5. Age
Child's gender	**Gender** Male Female	1 0	6. Gender
Father's occupation_____ _____ Mother's occupation_____ _____	**Socioeconomic status** Higher prof/manager Lower prof/manager Non-manual (other) Skilled manual Semi-skilled Unskilled Unemployed	1 2 3 4 5 6 7	7. SES
Assessment completed and formulation agreed	**Assessment** Yes No (dropped out)	1 0	8. Assessment
Therapy contract goals 1._____ 2._____ 3._____	**Therapy** Therapy not offered (assessment only) Dropout Minimal goal attainment Partial goal attainment Full goal attainment	0 1 2 3 4	9. Therapy
Number of hours input including individual and family sessions, network consultation, telephone contact, etc.	**Staff input in hours**		10. Hours

Figure 5.8 Clinic audit form

although Item 3, where case type is coded, deserves explanation. A distinction may be made between cases where the presenting problems are relatively circumscribed (for example, learning difficulties and behavioural problems in a nine-year-old boy from an intact family that is otherwise functioning

You recently attended our service. We are writing to ask for your help. We want to improve the service we offer to children and families. So we would value your opinion on the service you received. Please fill out this form. Then return it to us in the enclosed stamped addressed envelope. Thank you.

Please **circle your answer** to each of the following questions

1. Have the problems that led to you coming to our service improved?	No they are worse 1	No they are the same 2	Yes there is some improvement 3	Yes there is a lot of Improvement 4
2. With respect to these problems, to what extent has our service met your needs and those of other family members?	None of our needs have been met 1	Only a few of our needs have been met 2	Most of our needs have been met 3	Almost all of our needs have been met 4
3. In an overall general sense, how satisfied are you with the service you received?	Quite dissatisfied 1	Mildly satisfied 2	Mostly satisfied 3	Very satisfied 4
4. If you wanted help again, would you come back to our service?	No definitely not 1	No I don't think so 2	Yes I think so 3	Yes definitely 4
5. When you were coming to the clinic, did you want to come?	No definitely not 1	No I don't think so 2	Yes I think so 3	Yes definitely 4
6. What is your role in the family?	Mother	Father	Child	Other

What was **most helpful** about the service?

What was **least helpful** about the service?

Thank you for returning this form in the enclosed SAE

Figure 5.9 Client audit form

You recently referred _____ to our service. As part of our routine clinical audit system, we would like your opinion on the service you received from our centre with respect to this family. Please fill out this form and return it to us in the enclosed stamped addressed envelope. Thank you.

Please **circle your answer** to each of the following questions

1. Have the problems that led to the referral of this family improved?	No they are worse 1	No they are the same 2	Yes there is some improvement 3	Yes there is a lot of Improvement 4
2. To what extent has our service met the child and family's needs?	None of their needs have been met 1	Only a few of their needs have been met 2	Most of their needs have been met 3	Almost all of their needs have been met 4
3. In an overall general sense, how satisfied are you with the service we provided for the child and family and yourself as the referrer?	Quite dissatisfied 1	Mildly satisfied 2	Mostly satisfied 3	Very satisfied 4
4. If you wanted to refer this or similar children and families for help in the future would you refer to our service?	No definitely not 1	No I don't think so 2	Yes I think so 3	Yes definitely 4
5. Have you had to provide the child and family with less of **YOUR TIME**, since referring the case to our centre?	No definitely not 1	No I don't think so 2	Yes I think so 3	Yes definitely 4
6. Has the **RISK** of abuse or self-injury been reduced since the referral (if it is a self-harm or child protection case)?	Not applicable 0	No definitely not 1	Possibly 2	Yes definitely 3
7. Has the **MANAGEMENT** of the case become **SIMPLER** since the referral (if this is a complex multiproblem case with many agencies involved)?	Not applicable 0	No definitely not 1	Possibly 2	Yes definitely 3
8. Who was most concerned that the referral be made originally?	Myself 1	The family 2	The school 3	Social services 4

What was the **most helpful** aspect of their service?

What was the **least helpful** aspect of their service?

Thank you for returning this form in the enclosed SAE

Figure 5.10 Referrer audit form

fairly well), and complex multi-problem cases (for example, runaway and fire-setting behaviour in a twelve-year-old girl who has been living with her depressed mother and step-father and whose step-sister is in foster care). Some complex multi-problem cases may be classified as involving child abuse or neglect. It is useful to classify these separately because most services identify service provision in the child protection area as a priority.

Items 8 and 9 of the Clinic Audit Form collect data on whether assessment and therapy phases of the consultation process were completed and the degree to which goals were attained. Thus, they furnish information on outcome from the therapist's perspective. Information on improvement in the presenting problem from the client's and referrer's perspective are furnished by the first item both on the Client Audit Form and on the Referrer's Audit Form.

Scores on items 2, 3 and 4 of the Client Audit Form may be summed to produce an index of the client's satisfaction with the service offered. The three items have been adapted from Larsen et al.'s (1979) Client Satisfaction Scale. (The three items formed the briefest reliable and valid scale from a psychometric analysis of eighty-one items.) Scores on items 2, 3 and 4 of the Referrer Audit Form may be summed to give an index of referrer satisfaction.

Items 5 and 6 of the Client Audit Form give information on the client's motivation to attend for consultation and their role in the family.

The lessening of a referrer's perception of a case as 'extremely complex to manage' or as 'posing a risk of child abuse or violence' have been identified as important indices of the usefulness of consultation to statutory social workers (Manor, 1991). For this reason, items 6 and 7 have been included in the Referrer Audit Form. Item 5, which assesses the degree to which systemic consultation reduces the amount of time the referrer has to devote to the case, was identified by family doctors as a valuable index of the usefulness of a consultation service for children and families (Carr, McDonnell & Owen, 1994).

Both the Client and Referrer Audit Forms give an opportunity for the respondent to comment on the most and least helpful aspects of the service. These qualitative data may suggest particular ways in which aspects of the consultation process or service delivery system may be improved. Illustrative comments may be drawn from the qualitative data and included in the body of a service report to flesh out and concretize the implication of the quantitative data.

The three forms have been developed in the light of the available literature on audit in the child and family mental health field and of our own experience with audit in a busy child and family clinic (Berger, Hill, Sein, Thompson & Verduyn 1993; Carr et al., 1994). Of course, the forms will probably require some local modifications if you want to use them within your service. However, if you do modify them, it is worth keeping in mind the criteria that were used during their development. First, the forms collect essential information only. Many available audit systems are wonderfully comprehensive (e.g. Berger et al., 1993). However, our experience is that, after an initial rush of enthusiasm, staff forget to complete large, comprehensive audit forms and clients do not return them. Second, the forms are designed so that the information from them may easily be entered into a computer database. The information on the Clinic Audit Form may be converted to ten computer code numbers in the right-hand column. Information from the Client Audit Forms may be computer coded as six numbers: one for each item. Information from the Referrer Audit Form may be entered into a computer database as eight number codes. The third feature of the system is that it is compact. Each form is only a single side of a single page. The fourth, important, characteristic of the system is that it is as simple and unambiguous as possible. The final attribute of the system deserving mention is its user-friendliness for staff, referrers and clients.

All three audit forms may be used with every case. However, this may be time consuming and expensive. A good compromise is to complete a clinic audit form on every case and to invite a subsample of referrers and clients to complete audit forms. A useful framework for conceptualizing the study of outcomes in clinical practice is presented in Berger (1996).

SUMMARY

Progress notes about clinical cases allow us to remember the complex information which is gathered during the assessment process. Five categories of information may be recorded at the end of each assessment session: Time, Attendance, Review, Agenda, Plan. These may be remembered because the combined first letters of the category names form the acronym TARAP.

With any case, at the end of the assessment stage the contents of the assessment progress notes may be drawn together into a comprehensive assessment report which summarizes details of the referral; the sources of information on which the report is based; salient points concerning the history of the problem, the child and the family; the child's current cognitive and psychosocial status; a formulation of the main problems and a case management plan. Throughout the case management process, progress notes may be recorded following the TARAP system. At the end of an episode, a case summary may be written containing the formulation, a summary of how the plan was implemented and the outcome to which it led.

During the consultation process, and when closing a case at the end of an episode, it may be necessary to keep clients and colleagues informed of progress through verbal or written reports. In preparing such reports or letters, first identify the audience to whom your report will be addressed. Clarify the sort of question to which they require an answer. Compose the list of points you wish to make to answer these inquiries. Frame the points in language and at a level of technical sophistication that will be optimally intelligible to the audience. Where you wish to engage in a programme of joint action with another professional, it is better practice to outline your formulation in a letter and invite your colleague to join you in a meeting to discuss joint action, than to ask them to implement a programme you have already designed.

Court reports written by clinical psychologists working in child and family mental health fall into four categories: assessment of the sequelae of road traffic accidents, child protection assessments, juvenile justice case assessments and assessments of children's needs in parental custody and access disputes. These reports should begin with a statement of the psychologist's credentials and experience. They should then follow the format of comprehensive assessment reports with some modification to the final paragraphs. In the case of children's adjustment following a road traffic accident, court reports should conclude with a prognostic statement based on clinical experience and research evidence from similar cases. In the other types of cases listed above, a consideration of the pros and cons of the main case management options should be given followed by recommendations for action.

In many clinical psychology training programmes, case study reports are used to assess conceptual clinical skills. In many instances such reports are required to be premised on the scientist–practitioner model. That is, scientific knowledge and systematic assessment and treatment methods are brought to bear on specific clinical problems in an interpersonally sensitive way. This chapter has outlined a framework for such reports. While this framework broadly follows the format of a comprehensive assessment report followed by an end-of-episode summary report, it incorporates a brief literature summary, an explicit preliminary formulation and a section in which process and ethical issues are considered. The framework also requires the inclusion of references and appendices.

To aid service development and provide service funders with accurate information on performance, clinical psychologists may produce annual service reports. An annual clinical psychology service report may include sections on the main areas of service provision, such as clinical services, consultation and education services and research. The results of a clinical audit which incorporates standard data on each case and feedback from clients and referrers may be incorporated into sections on clinical service provision.

EXERCISE 5.1

1   Divide the class into two groups. One group take the role of the assessment team and the other take the role of the Sullivan–Rourke family (Molly, Joe, Trevor, Tina and Kate) described in Figures 5.1, 5.2, 5.3, 5.4 and 5.5.

2   All members of both teams are invited to read the material in Figures 5.1–5.5.
3   The family team are invited to take ten minutes to enter into the roles of the Rourke–Sullivans by imagining and discussing what happened between the second (14.12.95) and third (21.12.95) assessment sessions.
4   The assessment team are invited to develop an assessment agenda to follow for the third assessment session and elect a member to conduct a twenty-minute interview with the group role-playing the family. This elected person should then conduct the assessment interview and the remaining members of the group should each independently write a progress note in the TARAP format.
5   All class members should de-role at this point. Members of the assessment team should read out the TARAP format progress notes. Each member of the class may note the similarities and differences between the notes made.

EXERCISE 5.2

Use the TARAP progress note system, the comprehensive assessment report system and the end-of-episode case summary system with one of your current cases.

FURTHER READING

Black, D., Harris-Hendricks, J. & Wolkind, S. (1998). *Child Psychiatry and the Law* (Third Edition). Gaskell and Royal College of Psychiatrists: London. (*Contains examples of court reports.*)
British Psychological Society (BPsS) (1996). Expert testimony: developing witness skills. BPsS. 48 Princess Road East, Leicester LE1 7DR. Tel: 0044-(0)116-254-9568. http://www.bps.org.uk (*Contains video training tapes, tutors manual, self-help guide and student support materials.*)
McGoldrick, M., Gerson, R. & Schellenberger, S. (1999). *Genograms: Assessment and Intervention.* New York, Norton.

WEBSITES

Genogram programmes are available at: http://www.genogram.org/ and http://genogram.freeservers.com/index.html
Report writing software is available at: http://www.parinc.com/

Problems of infancy and early childhood

Chapter 6

Sleep problems

This chapter describes the stages of sleep before considering the classification and clinical features of sleep disorders. The evidence-based assessment and management of various sleep problems are discussed (Douglas, 1989, 2005; Ferber & Kryger, 1995; Goodlin-Jones & Anders, 2004; Horne, 1992; Mindell & Owens, 2003; Ramchandani, Wiggs, Webb & Stores, 2000; Stein & Barnes, 2002; Stores, 2001; Stores & Wiggs, (2001).

When children have sleep problems, particularly settling and night-waking problems, and parents have tried over a period of months or years to solve the problem with little success, further family difficulties occur that may compound the sleep problems. These difficulties include exhaustion, parental depression, marital discord, deterioration in parent–child relationships, and a reduction in the number and quality of socially supportive interactions.

A wide variety of solutions have been tried in most families referred to clinical psychologists with children's sleep problems as the central concern. These may include sedation, night feeding, ignoring night-time crying, having the child sleep alone, having the child sleep with the parents, having a fixed bedtime, having a variable bedtime, prayer, faith healing and so on. An abundance of conflicting advice from a variety of professional and non-professional sources will have been offered. When parents arrive in the psychologist's office they are invariably at their wits end. It is therefore critical that the psychologist's approach to helping parents and their children solve such problems is both well informed on the one hand and sympathetic and supportive on the other.

STAGES OF SLEEP

Polysomnography (PSG) provides information about physiological changes that occur in electrical brain activity (electro-encephalogram; EEG), muscle tension (electromyogram; EMG), eye movements (electro-oculogram; EOG), and respiration during sleep. PSG records are rated using Rechtschaffen and Kales (1968) sleep stage criteria. With these criteria a distinction may be made between two sleep states: rapid eye movement (REM) sleep and non-rapid eye movement sleep (NREM). During REM sleep the EEG pattern approximates that of wakefulness. In addition, the eyes, while closed, move rapidly and continuously, low muscle-tone occurs and, if awakened, vivid dream experiences are reported. Four stages of NREM sleep are distinguished: stages 1 and 2 are associated with light sleep and stages 3 and 4 with deep sleep from which it is difficult to be awakened. Because of the low frequency of the EEG wave patterns that characterize stages 3 and 4, deep sleep is also known as slow-wave sleep (SWS). PSG studies show that throughout the night there is a cyclical alternation between NREM and REM sleep. The patterning of stages and NREM–REM cycles is referred to as sleep architecture. The architecture of sleep changes over the course of the lifespan (Roffwarg, Muzio & Dement, 1966). NREM–REM cycles lengthen from fifty minutes in infants to about ninety minutes in adults. Up until the age of three months, infants enter REM sleep directly from wakefulness. After three months, sleep typically begins with stage 1 NREM sleep. REM accounts for 90% of sleep in neonates and 50% of sleep in first year of life; this declines to about 20% in adulthood.

There is some consensus that the function of SWS may be restorative (Horne, 1992). Growth hormone output occurs during SWS. Children with chronic sleep disturbance due to asthma or a breathing-related sleep disorder in which there are periods during which they do not breath (such as obstructive sleep apnoea) have retarded growth, as do emotionally deprived children, who engage in little SWS. Controversy continues about the function of REM sleep. It may be that it plays some role in facilitating the maturation and fine-tuning of the central nervous system. It has also been argued that REM sleep may play a role in the consolidation of memories acquired during daytime activity.

The amount of time children spend asleep decreases with age. A graph of typical sleep requirements of children at various ages is presented in Figure 6.1. New-borns sleep an average of 16.5 hours per day, one-year-olds on average sleep for 13.75 hours per day, five-year-olds sleep for about 11 hours per night and by 10 years of age the average sleep duration for children is 9.75 hours (Ferber, 1985). However, there is considerable variability among children in the duration of sleep, although this too decreases with age. On average, two-year-olds wake about three times each night. However, the majority (about 75%) have self-soothing skills and are able to return to sleep without parental intervention (Minde et al., 1993). Breast-fed children tend to wake more frequently during the night than artificially fed children and Wright, McLeod & Cooper (1983) found that, on average, bottle-fed children slept through the night at eleven weeks in contrast to breast-fed children, who slept through at thirteen weeks.

Although there is considerable controversy about infants sleeping in their parents' beds, a UK-based survey showed that among children with

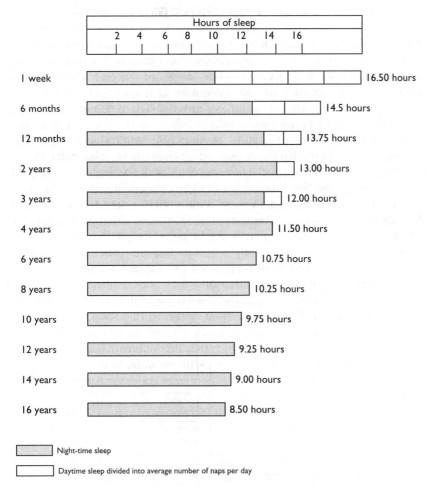

Figure 6.1 Typical sleep requirements in childhood

Note: Adapted from Ferber (1985).

night-waking problems it is quite common; 35% of infants who had night-waking difficulties slept with their parents compared with 7% of controls (Richman, 1981). There is no right or wrong answer when it comes to parents making a decision about children sleeping in their beds. In many primitive societies all family members sleep together until children are quite old, since this allows the parents to protect the children from predators and to keep the child warm. Children sleeping in their parents' bed only becomes a problem deserving clinical intervention when its impact on the parents and children becomes excessively negative.

CLASSIFICATION AND EPIDEMIOLOGY

Within DSM IV TR a distinction is made between primary sleep disorders on the one hand and those which occur secondary to another psychological condition, a medical condition or substance use on the other (APA, 2000a). The primary sleep disorders classified in DSM IV TR are set out in Figure 6.2. Within this classification system a distinction is made between the dyssomnias and the parasomnias. With the dyssomnias, the central problem is the amount, timing or quality of sleep. Behavioural and physiological abnormalities occurring during sleep characterize the parasomnias. Chapter 5 of ICD 10, which classifies psychological problems, uses a slightly different system and this is presented in Figure 6.3 (WHO, 1996). The major distinction between dyssomnias and parasomnias is not so clearly made. Also, narcolepsy and breathing-related sleep disorders are included in Chapter 6 of ICD 10 as primarily physiological rather than psychological disorders. Diagnostic criteria for the dyssomnias and parasomnias adapted from DSM IV TR and ICD 10 are presented in Tables 6.1 and 6.2.

Two other systems in which sleep disorders are classified and described deserve mention: the Revised International Classification of Sleep Disorders (ICSD-R; American Sleep Disorders Association, 1997) and the Diagnostic

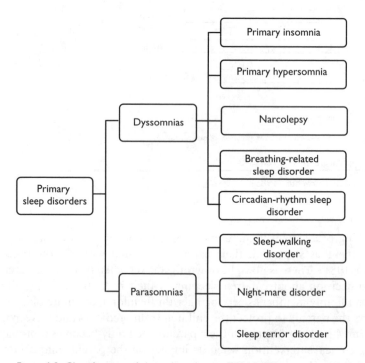

Figure 6.2 Classification of sleep disorders in DSM IV TR

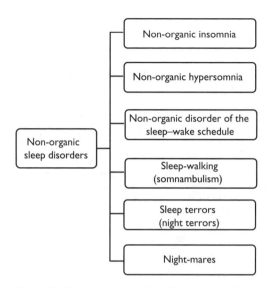

Figure 6.3 Classification of sleep disorders in ICD 10

Classification of Mental Health and Developmental Disorders in Infancy and Early Childhood (DC: 0–3; Zero to three, 1994). In the ICSD-R, over eighty different sleep disorders are classified as: (1) dyssomnias; (2) parasomnias; and (3) sleep disorders associated with mental, neurological or other medical disorders. For clinical assessment, the ICSD-R gives a three-axis system for coding sleep disorders: (1) abnormalities identified through specific sleep investigations; (2) co-morbid physical disorders; and (3) co-morbid psychological disorders. The ICSD-R was developed for adults and is currently of limited relevance to children, but the next revision is expected to take greater account of issues relevant to children and adolescents. In the DC: 0–3, distinctions are made between disorders of initiating sleep (settling problems), maintaining sleep (night waking), excessive somnolence, irregular sleep–wake schedules and disorders associated with sleep-stage or arousal (e.g. night terrors). Diagnostic criteria are not given. However, Goodlin-Jones and Anders (2004) have developed diagnostic criteria for young children with sleep onset and night-waking problems (Table 6.3). The empirically derived Sleep Problems Syndrome Scale from Achenbach and Rescorla's (2000) Child Behaviour Checklist (CBCL) for children aged 1.5–5 years is also included in this table for comparative purposes. The syndrome scale assess general sleep-onset and night-waking problems. Thus the CBCL is a reliable way to screen for general sleep problems in infants and toddlers, and this may be followed up with more detailed assessment of specific sleep disorders.

International epidemiological data from studies in industrialized countries suggest that a quarter to a third of pre-schoolers have sleep problems, the

Table 6.1 Diagnostic criteria for dyssomnias from DSM IV TR and ICD 10

	DSM IV TR	ICD 10
Insomnia	A. The predominant complaint is difficulty initiating or maintaining sleep, or non-restorative sleep for at least a month	A. Difficulty falling asleep, maintaining sleep or poor quality of sleep
	B. The sleep disturbance or associated daytime fatigue causes clinically significant distress	B. Episodes occur three times a week for at least a month
	C. The sleep disturbance does not occur exclusively during another sleep disorder such as narcolepsy or a parasomnia	C. A preoccupation with the sleeplessness and excessive concern over its consequences
	D. The sleep disturbance does not occur exclusively during another psychological disorder such as depression or anxiety	D. Sleep disturbance causes marked distress and impaired functioning
	E. The disorder is not due to the effects of substance or drug or a general medical condition	
Hypersomnia	A. The predominant complaint is excessive sleepiness for at least a month as evidenced by either prolonged sleep episodes or daily daytime sleep episodes (which are developmentally inappropriate)	A. Excessive daytime sleepiness or sleep attacks not accounted for by an inadequate amount of sleep or prolonged transition to wakefulness
	B. The excessive sleepiness cannot be accounted for by another sleep disorder	B. Sleep disturbance occurring daily for at least a month or for recurrent periods of shorter duration causing marked distress or impaired functioning
	C. The symptoms are not due to another psychological disorder	C. Absence of auxiliary symptoms of narcolepsy (cataplexy, hypnogogic or hypnopompic hallucinations and sleep paralysis) or evidence of sleep apnoea
	E. The disorder is not due to the effects of a substance or drug or a general medical condition	D. Not due to a medical condition
Narcolepsy	A. Irresistible attacks of refreshing sleep that occur daily over at least 3 months	Not included in Chapter 5 of ICD 10
	B. The presence of at least one of the following:	
	1. Cataplexy (brief episodes of sudden bilateral loss of muscle tone often in association with intense emotion)	

	2. Recurrent intrusions of elements of REM sleep into the transition from sleep to wakefulness as manifested by hypnopompic or hypnogogic hallucinations or sleep paralysis at the extremities of sleep episodes C. The disorder is not due to the effects of a substance or drug or a general medical condition	
Breathing-related sleep disorders	A. Sleep disruption leading to excessive sleepiness or insomnia due to a sleep-related breathing condition (obstructive or central sleep apnoea syndrome or central alveolar hypoventilation syndrome) B. The disorder is not due to another psychological disorder or the effects of a substance or drug or a general medical condition	Not included in Chapter 5 of ICD 10
Circadian rhythm sleep disorder	A. A persistent or recurrent pattern of sleep disruption leading to excessive sleepiness or insomnia that is due to a mismatch between the persons circadian rhythm and the sleep–wake schedule required by the person's environment B. The sleep disturbance causes clinically significant distress C. The symptoms cannot be accounted for by another sleep disorder or psychological disorder D. The disorder is not due to the effects of a substance or drug or a general medical condition	A. The person's sleep–wake pattern is out of synchrony with the sleep–wake schedule that is normal for a particular society and shared by most people in that cultural environment B. Insomnia during the major sleep period and hypersomnia during the waking period are experienced nearly every day for a month or recurrently for shorter periods C. Symptoms cause marked distress or impaired functioning

Note: Adapted from DSM IV TR (APA, 2000a) and ICD 10 (WHO, 1992, 1996).

Table 6.2 Diagnostic criteria for parasomnias from DSM IV TR and ICD 10

Night-mares	A. Repeated awakenings from the major sleep period, usually during the second half, with detailed recall of extended and extremely frightening dreams, usually involving threats to survival, security or self-esteem	A. Awakening from sleep with detailed and vivid recall of intensely frightening dreams, usually involving threats to survival, security, or self-esteem; the awakening may occur at any time during the sleep period but typically during the second half
	B. On awakening from the frightening dreams the person usually becomes oriented and alert (in contrast to the disorientation that follows sleep terrors and some forms of epilepsy)	B. The individual rapidly becomes oriented and alert upon awakening from the dream
	C. The symptoms cause clinically significant distress	C. Symptoms cause marked distress or impaired functioning
	D. The symptoms do not occur exclusively during another psychological disorder (e.g. PTSD) and are not due to the effects of a substance or drug or a general medical condition	
Sleep terrors	A. Recurrent episodes of abrupt awakening accompanied by a panicky scream during the first third of the major sleep episode	A. Recurrent episodes of awakening from sleep with a panicky scream and displaying intense anxiety, body motility, and autonomic hyperactivity such as tachycardia, rapid breathing, dilated pupils, and sweating
	B. Intense fear and autonomic arousal manifested by tachycardia, rapid breathing and sweating	
	C. Unresponsiveness to reassurance during the episode	B. Episodes last up to 10 minutes and occur during the first third of nocturnal sleep
	D. No dream recall and amnesia for the episode	C. Unresponsiveness to reassurance and disorientation and perseverative movements during the episode
	E. Episodes cause clinically significant distress	
	F. The symptoms are not due to the effects of a substance or drug or a general medical condition	D. Minimal recall of the event limited to one or two fragmentary images
		E. No evidence of a physical disorder such as a brain tumour or epilepsy
Sleep-walking	A. Recurrent episodes of rising from bed during the first third of the major sleep period and walking about	A. Recurrent episodes of rising from bed, usually during the first third of nocturnal sleep, and walking about

B. While sleep-walking the person is expressionless, unresponsive and resistant to waking

C. Amnesia for the episode on awakening

D. No impairment of cognitive functioning within minutes of awakening

E. Episodes cause clinically significant distress

F. The symptoms are not due to the effects of a substance or drug or a general medical condition

B. Blank staring face and unresponsive during an episode

C. No recollection for the episode upon awakening

D. Within several minutes of waking from the episode, no cognitive or behavioural impairment

E. No evidence of an organic mental disorder or a physical disorder such as epilepsy

Note: Adapted from DSM IV TR (APA, 2000a) and ICD 10 (WHO, 1992, 1996).

most common of which are settling and night waking (Goodlin-Jones & Anders, 2004). Accurate data on the prevalence of hypersomnia, narcolepsy, breathing-related sleep disorders and night-mares are unavailable. Night terrors have a prevalence of 1–6% and sleep-walking disorder has a prevalence of 1–5% in children (APA, 2000a).

CLINICAL FEATURES AND AETIOLOGICAL FACTORS

Clinical features of children's sleep problems along with a consideration of relevant aetiological factors will be outlined below (Goodlin-Jones & Anders, 2004; Horne, 1992; Mindell & Owens, 2003; Schaefer, 1995; Stein & Barnes, 2002; Stores, 2001). Settling and night-waking problems are the most commonly referred and so will be considered first. Some cases of night waking are due to nightmares and these will be considered second. Sleep terrors, sleep-walking and other parasomnias will be dealt with next. Finally, conditions which are associated with excessive daytime sleepiness (other than night waking) will be discussed.

Settling and night-waking problems

Difficulties in going to sleep and persistent night waking (which fall under the DSM or ICD diagnosis of insomnia) are by far the most common sleep problems in pre-school children. The DSM and ICD definitions of insomnia have limitations when applied to infants and young children since childhood insomnia does not often lead the child to experience clinically significant distress. However, most parents experience clinically significant distress in their attempts to cope with the child's difficulty in initiating and maintaining

Table 6.3 Goodlin-Jones and Anders classification and diagnostic criteria for sleep-onset and night-waking disorders and ASEBA Sleep Problems Syndrome scale

Sleep-onset problems	Night waking	ASEBA Sleep Problems Scale CBCL 1.5–5 years
For infants 12–24 months: 1. Takes more than 30 minutes to fall asleep 2. Parent remains in child's room until sleep onset 3. More than three parent–child reunions involving protests, bids or struggles occur	For infants 12–24 months, more than three wakings per night totalling more than 30 minutes	Doesn't want to sleep alone Trouble sleeping Night-mares Resists bed Sleeps little Talks or cries in sleep Wakes often
	For toddler 24–36 months, two or more wakings per night totalling more than 20 minutes	
	For children over 36 months, two or more wakings per night totalling more than 10 minutes	
For toddlers over 24 months: 1. Takes more than 20 minutes to fall asleep 2. Parent remains in child's room until sleep onset 3. More than two parent–child reunions involving protests, bids or struggles occur	For wakings, the child must have been asleep for more than 10 minutes and must signal the caregiver by crying or calling	
An episode is diagnosed if two of three criteria are met:	A night-waking *disorder* is diagnosed if there are five to seven episodes per week for more than a month	
A settling *disorder* is diagnosed if there are five to seven episodes per week for at least a month	A night-waking *disturbance* is diagnosed if there are two to four episodes per week for more than a month	
A settling *disturbance* is diagnosed if there are two to four episodes per week for at least a month	A night-waking *perturbation* is diagnosed if there is one episode per week for more than a month	
A settling *perturbation* is diagnosed if there is one episode per week for at least a month		

Note: Adapted from Goodlin-Jones and Anders (2004) and Achenbach and Rescorla (2000).

sleep. The proportion of children showing such problems reduces with age (Horne, 1992).

Two distinct constellations of factors are associated with night waking: one largely constitutional or biological and the other psychosocial or interactional (Minde et al., 1993). Constitutional factors include peri-natal complications, colic, allergies, asthma, milk intolerance, over-sensitivity or under-sensitivity to external stimuli and difficult temperament. This constellation of factors probably represents a biologically based problem with arousal regulation. Where infants who have arousal regulation difficulties try to settle or return to sleep after awakening they are unable to soothe themselves because their arousal level will not alter in response to their self-soothing attempts. Alternatively, they may find that awareness of internal or external stimuli maintains their arousal level.

Psychosocial factors associated with settling difficulties and night waking include mother–child attachment difficulties and maternal anxiety or depression. Where there is a secure mother–infant attachment, the mother will allow the infant sufficient time alone when settling or during night-waking episodes to employ self-soothing skills to return to sleep. In cases where an anxious mother–infant attachment has developed, the mother does not leave the infant alone long enough before sleep or during a night-waking episode to develop self-soothing skills.

In any given case, some combination of arousal regulation biological factors and attachment-related psychosocial factors may pre-dispose the infant to developing problems with settling or night waking and maintain the sleep problem when it occurs. Night feeding may further compound settling and night-waking difficulties. Night feeding can lead to less daytime feeding, to more wet nappies and related discomfort and to waking at night.

Many children have settling and night-waking problems from birth. Others develop them following some precipitating event or set of circumstances. Such precipitating factors may be biological or psychosocial. Biological factors include serious illness or injury. Stressful life events, particularly separation from the primary caregiver (usually the mother) or the occurrence of an event that threatens the child or the family, such as a house burglary, are the most common psychosocial factors contributing to the development of settling and waking difficulties in children who have already developed a robust sleep routine. These precipitating factors may lead to physical discomfort and/or anxiety and heightened arousal which the child is unable to regulate. So the child has difficulty falling asleep or returning to sleep after being awakened by physical discomfort or night-mares.

Night-mares

Night-mares are vivid, frightening dreams which occur during REM sleep (Mooney & Sobocinski, 1995). Typically, the child awakes abruptly in a state of anxiety from a vividly recalled frightening dream. Occasionally, sleep paralysis may occur. That is the lack of muscle tone and motor inhibition that characterizes REM sleep may persist into the waking state. Night-mares may occur as an isolated problem as with DSM IV TR's night-mare disorder defined in Table 6.1. However, in clinical practice they usually occur as part of a more global anxiety response to a perceived threat to the child's safety, security or self-esteem or to the safety of the family. Thus they may occur as one aspect of separation anxiety, post-traumatic stress disorder or generalized anxiety disorder. These and other anxiety problems are discussed in Chapter 12.

Night-mares, like other aspects of anxiety may be maintained by both child and family factors. The adoption of a threat-oriented cognitive set where the child is hypervigilant and interprets both internal and external cues as threatening may maintain the occurrence of night-mares. Parent–child interactions characterized by high levels of anxiety where the child is inadvertently reinforced for adopting a threat-oriented cognitive set may also maintain anxiety. Night-mares may also be maintained by non-supportive parent–child patterns of interaction within which children are unable to ventilate their fears. Such non-supportive patterns of interaction may range from situations where there is parent–child conflict to those where neglect and physical or sexual abuse are occurring. Child abuse and neglect are discussed more fully in Chapters 19, 20 and 21.

Night terrors, sleep-walking and other parasomnias

Night terrors and sleep-walking occur during SWS. They are developmental conditions for which there is often a positive family history and most children mature out of them by adolescence (Guilleminault, 1987). These parasomnias are probably all part of the same nosological continuum and are quite distinct from night-mares, which are anxiety related and occur during REM sleep.

Night terrors are often mistaken for night-mares. However, there are distinct differences. With night terrors, usually the child sits up in bed and screams loudly or bolts out of bed and moves frantically, as if trying to escape. The child looks terrified, is hyperaroused and is unresponsive to comforting. With night-mares, the child rarely screams and usually responds to reassurance. On awaking from a night terror, there is no detailed recall of a vivid dream, whereas this is a characteristic feature of a night-mare. Night terrors typically occur during the first third of the sleep period whereas night-mares typically occur during the second half of the night.

In sleep-walking episodes, which typically last about 20 minutes, the child usually leaves the bed, may get dressed and walks unresponsively about the house and is resistant to awakening. The main danger with sleep-walking is that the child will be inadvertently injured during the episode.

Head-banging, rocking, tooth-grinding (bruxism) and sleep-talking all occur in NREM sleep stages 1 and 2. While all of these parasomnias may lead to anxiety for the parent or child, injury resulting from head-banging and tooth-grinding is the main clinical concern associated with this group of conditions.

In some forms of epilepsy, attacks occur during sleep and these may involve movements and vocalizations that can be mistaken by parents for parasomnias or night-mares (Stores, 2001). Typically complex partial seizures of this sort are frequent and very brief, lasting less than a minute and so are clearly distinguishable from night-mares, in which no movement occurs and parasomnias in which movement lasts for longer periods.

Daytime sleepiness

Excessive daytime sleepiness in infants and children may occur because of disruption of night-time sleep caused by settling difficulties or persistent night waking discussed above (Horne, 1992; Stores, 2001). Breathing-related sleep disorders, in which the child is frequently aroused throughout the night because of respiration difficulties is a second common cause of daytime sleepiness in both children and adolescents. The breathing difficulties may be due to central alveolar hypoventilation or sleep apnoea. With central alveolar hypoventilation, respiratory hypoventilation worsens during sleep but there are no apnoea spells. With sleep apnoea, the child has episodes of 10 seconds or more during which breathing ceases. Usually episodes of loud snoring also occur.

A distinction is made between central and obstructive sleep apnoea with the latter usually being due to hyperplastic tonsils and adenoids and the former to a lack of diaphragmatic effort. Obstructive sleep apnoea is associated with obesity, rhinitis, hayfever and chronic upper airway infections. While children with sleep apnoea show excessive daytime sleepiness, they also display a broad range of personal difficulties related to the condition. These include irritability, hyperactivity, a reversion to nocturnal enuresis and poor school performance. In children, adenotosillectomy may lead to a marked improvement in breathing during sleep, reduced daytime sleepiness and improved psychosocial and educational adjustment (Stradling, Thomas, Warley, Williams & Freeland, 1990). In infants, some cases of sudden infant death syndrome (SIDS), have been related to central sleep apnoea (Stores, 2001).

In teenagers, daytime sleepiness may result from sleep apnoea, a circadian rhythm disorder or narcolepsy. With a circadian rhythm disorder, a mismatch has developed between the teenager's circadian rhythm and the sleep–waking schedule demands of the environment. Usually this mismatch results from going to sleep late and rising late.

Narcolepsy, a lifelong hereditary condition with onset in adolescence, is characterized by frequent brief sleep attacks, brief attacks of cataplexy in which there is a loss of muscle tone, sleep paralysis and hypnopompic or hypnogogic hallucinations. These occur as the child is entering sleep or waking. Often teenagers suffering from narcolepsy fear that they are going insane because of the bizzareness of these hallucinations. The cataplexy, sleep paralysis and hallucinations all represent the intrusion of REM phenomena into waking life.

Klein–Levin syndrome, which occurs typically at puberty, is characterized by recurrent outbreaks, of about two weeks duration, of hypersomnia, hyperphagia, aggression and sexual disinhibition (Stores, 2001). Often there is a prodromal phase characterized by fever, vomiting, photophobia and irritability. The condition usually resolves in late adolescence.

PRE-DISPOSING FACTORS

PERSONAL PRE-DISPOSING FACTORS

Biological factors
- Peri-natal complications
- Allergies
- Asthma
- Food intolerance
- Colic

Psychological factors
- Sensitivity to external stimuli
- Difficult temperament

CONTEXTUAL PRE-DISPOSING FACTORS

Parent–child factors in early life
- Attachment problems

Exposure to family problems in early life
- Maternal anxiety or depression

PERSONAL MAINTAINING FACTORS

Biological factors
- CNS immaturity (for night terrors and sleep problems)
- Airway obstruction due to infection, rhinitis, hayfever, or enlarged tonsils (for breathing related sleep disorders)

Psychological factors
- Poor self-soothing skills (for reducing arousal in settling or night-waking problems)
- Worrying about threats to safety, security

PERSONAL PROTECTIVE FACTORS

Biological factors
- Good physical health

Psychological factors
- Easy temperament
- High self-esteem
- Internal locus of control
- High self-efficacy
- Optimistic attributional style
- Good self-soothing skills

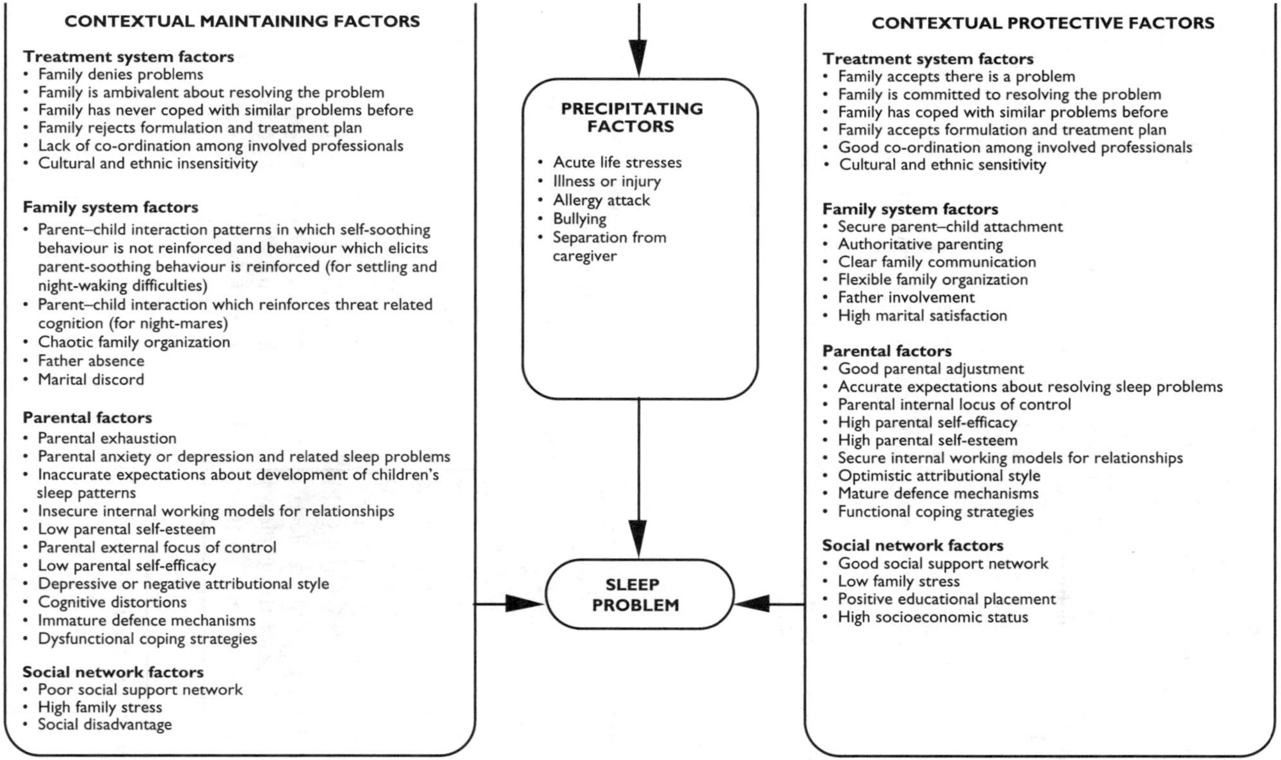

CONTEXTUAL MAINTAINING FACTORS

Treatment system factors
- Family denies problems
- Family is ambivalent about resolving the problem
- Family has never coped with similar problems before
- Family rejects formulation and treatment plan
- Lack of co-ordination among involved professionals
- Cultural and ethnic insensitivity

Family system factors
- Parent–child interaction patterns in which self-soothing behaviour is not reinforced and behaviour which elicits parent-soothing behaviour is reinforced (for settling and night-waking difficulties)
- Parent–child interaction which reinforces threat related cognition (for night-mares)
- Chaotic family organization
- Father absence
- Marital discord

Parental factors
- Parental exhaustion
- Parental anxiety or depression and related sleep problems
- Inaccurate expectations about development of children's sleep patterns
- Insecure internal working models for relationships
- Low parental self-esteem
- Low parental external focus of control
- Depressive or negative attributional style
- Cognitive distortions
- Immature defence mechanisms
- Dysfunctional coping strategies

Social network factors
- Poor social support network
- High family stress
- Social disadvantage

PRECIPITATING FACTORS

- Acute life stresses
- Illness or injury
- Allergy attack
- Bullying
- Separation from caregiver

SLEEP PROBLEM

CONTEXTUAL PROTECTIVE FACTORS

Treatment system factors
- Family accepts there is a problem
- Family is committed to resolving the problem
- Family has coped with similar problems before
- Family accepts formulation and treatment plan
- Good co-ordination among involved professionals
- Cultural and ethnic sensitivity

Family system factors
- Secure parent–child attachment
- Authoritative parenting
- Clear family communication
- Flexible family organization
- Father involvement
- High marital satisfaction

Parental factors
- Good parental adjustment
- Accurate expectations about resolving sleep problems
- Parental internal locus of control
- High parental self-efficacy
- High parental self-esteem
- Secure internal working models for relationships
- Optimistic attributional style
- Mature defence mechanisms
- Functional coping strategies

Social network factors
- Good social support network
- Low family stress
- Positive educational placement
- High socioeconomic status

Figure 6.4 Factors to consider in childhood sleep problems

ASSESSMENT OF CHILDREN WITH SLEEP PROBLEMS

In assessing children with sleep problems, it is important to inquire both about details of the child's sleeping routines and about the psychosocial context within which these problematic sleep routines occur, including a consideration of pre-disposing, precipitating, maintaining factors. Figure 6.4 provides a framework for assessing contextual factors of particular relevance to the aetiology of sleep problems in infants and children. This framework is intended as a supplement to routine assessment procedures described in Chapter 4.

Sleep routines

Inquiries about sleep routines and problems should focus on:

- bedtime routines
- night-waking routines
- daytime sleeping routines.

Bedtime routines

When asking about bedtime routines it is important to identify factors that may promote the development of good sleep habits and those that may maintain a disturbed sleeping pattern. Find out when the child is last fed and changed before bedtime, since both hunger and a wet, uncomfortable nappy may prevent the child from settling. Ask about who puts the child to bed, where and at what time this occurs. If this occurs following a set routine, good sleep habits are being fostered. If the time, place and people involved in bedtime routines change erratically, this may be contributing to settling difficulties. Inquire about how parents or carers respond while the child is waiting to go to sleep and how long this process takes. Ask if the child is permitted to use self-soothing skills or if the parent rocks or feeds the child to help soothe the child to sleep. Children who are allowed to master self-soothing skills tend to develop good settling habits. Where parents do not permit children to develop these skills, settling problems may occur. Long sleep-onset periods exhaust parents and are very stressful.

Night-waking routines

Inquiries about night-waking patterns should clarify first if night-mares, night terrors, sleep-walking, sleep-talking, rocking, head-banging, bruxism, breathing difficulties or other parasomnias precipitate episodes of night waking. Inquiries about when waking occurs, how often it occurs, for how long the child remains awake and how the return to sleep is managed should also be made. As with assessing bedtime routines, ask if the child is permitted to use self-soothing skills to return to sleep or if the parent rocks or feeds the child to help soothe the child to sleep.

Daytime sleeping routines

Daytime sleeping and activity patterns should also be assessed since daytime naps or inactivity may prevent night-time sleeping. Where a child's daytime sleep greatly exceeds the norms presented in Figure 6.1, this hypothesis should be further investigated. In assessing daytime sleeping routines, the amount of daytime sleeping and circumstances surrounding daytime naps should be explored. In particular, inquiries should be made about the number of naps per day, the times at which they occur, the duration of each nap, whether they were initiated and ended by the child or the parent and any factors that alter the child's typical pattern.

Sleep diaries

Information from assessment interviews may be supplemented with sleep diary records (Douglas & Richman, 1985; Stores, 2001). The sleep diary contained in Figure 6.5 may be photocopied and enlarged to A3 size for parents to complete. It is useful for parents to keep a sleep diary throughout the course of both assessment and treatment, since sleep diaries allow improvement or deterioration in sleep problems to be continuously monitored.

Special assessment procedures

Psychometric instruments that may be a useful supplement to information provided by interview and sleep diaries are listed in Table 6.4. Video and audiotape recordings may usefully be used in the preliminary assessment of breathing-related sleep disorders. Actiometres, which are small wrist-watch-like devices, may be used to assess movement during sleep and distinguish fairly accurately periods of sleep and wakefulness (Stores, 2001). Where sleep apnoea or night-time seizures are suspected, or where other assessment procedures yield confusing results, children should be referred for PSG assessment.

Pre-disposing factors

Pre-disposing biological factors deserving particular attention during assessment include peri-natal difficulties, allergies, asthma, food intolerance, colic, hypersensitivity to external stimuli and difficult temperament. All of these factors may make it difficult for children to use self-soothing routines to

	Monday	Tuesday	Wednesday	Thursday	Friday	Saturday	Sunday
Time the child was put to bed							
Length of time it took to fall asleep							
What the child did while waiting to fall asleep							
What the parents did while the child was waiting to fall asleep							
Number of wakings in the night							
Length of each night-waking							
What the child did while trying to return to sleep							
What the parents did while the child was trying to return to sleep							
Time the child awoke in the morning							
Time child spent in parent's bed at night							
Number of daytime naps							
Duration of daytime naps							
Events preceding daytime naps							
Events following daytime naps							

Figure 6.5 Sleep diary

Note: Photocopy this page and enlarge to A3 size so it can be used as a diary.

Table 6.4 Psychometric instruments that may be used in the assessment of children's sleeping and eating problems

Construct	Instrument	Publication	Comments
Sleep-related behaviours	Paediatric Sleep Questionnaire	Chervin, R., Hedger, K., Dillon, J., & Pituch, K. (2000). Pediatric Sleep Questionnaire (PSQ): validity and reliability of scales for sleep-disordered breathing, snoring, sleepiness and behavioural problems. Sleep Medicine, 1, 21–32.	This extensive questionnaire covers al aspects of sleep-related problems and behaviour; personal and family sleep, medical and psychiatric history. It is available at http://www.rch.org.au/clinicalguide/pages/sleep_handouts.html
	The Sleep Disturbance Scale for Children	Bruni, O., Ottaviano, S., Guidetti, V., Romoli M., Innocenzi, M., Cortesi, F. & Giannotti, F. (1996). The Sleep Disturbance Scale for Children (SDSC). Construction and validation of an instrument to evaluate sleep disturbances in childhood and adolescence. Journal of Sleep Research, 5, 251–61.	This 27-item scale evaluates most common sleep disturbances in children
	Sleep Questionnaire	Simmonds, J. & Parraga, H. (1982). Prevalence of sleep disorder and sleep behaviours in children and adolescents. Journal of the American Academy of Child Psychiatry, 21, 383–388.	This scale evaluates most common sleep disturbances in children. The questionnaire includes 25 items for which five-point response scales are provided and 29 items for which yes/no response categories are given
	Children's Sleep Habits Questionnaire	Owens, J., Spirito, A. & McGuinn, M. (2000). The Children's Sleep Habits Questionnaire (CSHQ): psychometric properties of a survey instrument for school-aged children. Sleep, 23, 1043–51.	This scale evaluates most common sleep disturbances in children

Continued

Table 6.4 Continued

Construct	Instrument	Publication	Comments
Daytime sleepiness	Epworth Sleepiness Scale	Johns, M. (1991). A new method for measuring daytime sleepiness: The Epworth Sleepiness Scale. *Sleep*, 14, 540–545.	For each of 8 items respondents indicate on a scale from 0 to 3 the likelihood that they would fall asleep
Night-time coping	Night-time Coping Inventory	Mooney, K. (1985). Children's night-time fears: Ratings of content and coping behaviours. *Cognitive Therapy and Research*, 9, 309–319.	Twenty coping strategies to deal with night-time fears are rated on 5-point scales. Strategies fall into six categories: self-control; social support; clinging to inanimate objects; control over inanimate objects; control over inanimate environment; control over others

regulate their arousal levels. Attachment problems and parental anxiety or depression may compromise the parents' capacity to create a social context within which the child develops a view of the world as a safe and secure place where self-soothing skills may be developed.

Precipitating factors

While some sleep problems are present from birth, for others there are clearly identifiable precipitating factors which deserve careful assessment. Biological factors which may precipitate the onset of sleep problems include illnesses, injuries or the development of allergies. Stressful life events, such as entering school, being abused and separations from caregivers are typical psychosocial factors that may precipitate sleep problems.

Maintaining factors

Specific repetitive patterns of interaction between children and parents typically maintain some sleep problems. With many settling difficulties and night waking, the pattern usually involves the parents permitting the child to have extended daytime naps and not permitting the child to have opportunities for self-soothing during the settling period or following night waking. For the child, there is a repeated pattern of engaging the parent in soothing behaviour rather than persisting with self-soothing behaviour. For settling and night-waking problems associated with night-mares, parent–child interactions that intensify rather than alleviate the anxiety which finds expression in the night-mare may maintain the sleep problems. The child's anxiety may be maintained by continual exposure to situations which pose a threat to the child's safety, security or self-esteem, such as ongoing bullying or abuse. In other situations, the anxiety may occur as part of a reaction to an acute trauma. That is, as part of a post-traumatic stress disorder. Where children are not offered a supportive context within which to process anxiety associated with such trauma, and are encouraged to repress or avoid experiencing the intrusive emotions and images of the trauma, these factors may maintain the occurrence of night-mares. Co-morbid conditions may maintain sleep problems through biological or psychosocial mechanisms. Such co-morbid conditions include autism, ADHD, depression, anxiety, cerebral palsy, neuromuscular disease and visual impairment. With sleep apnoea, airway obstruction may maintain the breathing-related sleep problem. Night terrors, sleep-walking and other parasomnias are probably maintained by nervous system immaturity.

Where children have sleep problems, particularly settling and night-waking problems, and parents have tried over a period of months or years to solve the problem with little success, further family difficulties occur that may compound the sleep problems. Parents become sleep-deprived and exhausted. Their capacity to maintain a co-operative and satisfying marital relationship may deteriorate. Major arguments may occur in the middle of the night as parents disagree on how best to manage the child's sleep difficulties. The deterioration in the marital relationship and exhaustion may in turn lead to curtailment of the couple's social life and a reduction in the amount and quality of social support available to each partner. This absence of support in turn may further diminish their capacity to manage the child's sleep difficulties. As sleep difficulties persist, the quality of parent–child relationships may also deteriorate. This may be compounded by factors related to other children in the family. Where there are other children in the family who have not had sleep difficulties, parents may construe the child with sleep difficulties as wholly problematic and in contrast construe the sibling without sleep problems as wholly good. Where all children in the family have had sleep problems, parents' tolerance and capacity for positive parent–child relationships may become extremely eroded by the ongoing sleep deprivation and exhaustion. Where there are no siblings, parents may become particularly resentful that their once satisfying marriage has become conflict-ridden as a result of the child's sleep difficulties. They may also come to doubt their adequacy as parents in the light of their repeated failure to solve the child's sleep difficulties. That is, their parenting self-efficacy beliefs may diminish. Where mothers are pregnant with their second child and their first continues to have sleep difficulties, a sense of despair may occur as the parents anticipate managing the persisting sleep difficulties of the first-born child and the additional demands of the new-born sibling. As with all family problems, external stresses, such as those associated with parental work situations, may further erode the energy that parents have available to deal with the sleep difficulties.

Protective factors and family resources

The probability that a sleep management programme will be effective is influenced by a variety of protective factors associated with the child and the family. It is important that these be assessed and included in the later formulation, since it is protective factors that usually serve as the foundation for therapeutic change. Easy temperament and a wish to solve the sleep problem are two important protective factors associated with the child as an individual. Parental commitment to resolving the problem, strong parental self-efficacy beliefs, secure parent–child attachment, marital satisfaction, the availability of social support and low extra-familial stress are important contextual protective factors.

Most parents will have tried a wide variety of solutions to their children's sleep problems before consulting a clinical psychologist. It is important to obtain a clear detailed account of each solution that was tried, because often valid sleep management practices have been used by parents but not for long enough or under unfavourable circumstances. For example, parents who used systematic ignoring of night-time crying for two nights while on holiday in a caravan when their child has an ear infection made little impact on the child's night-waking problem. However, the same strategy applied for a longer duration at home while the child was healthy helped the child develop self-soothing skills that permitted a return to sleep following night waking. If it is suggested that methods that have led to failure be tried again without previous failures with such methods being first discussed and reasons for the failure being clarified, then parents may become disillusioned with the consultation provided by the clinician.

Formulation

Salient features from the assessment should be drawn together into a formulation that begins with a statement of the central features of the sleep problems and then links these to pre-disposing, precipitating and maintaining factors. Protective factors and family resources that have implications for resolving the problem should also be mentioned. The case example in Box 6.1 is written in the format of a formulation. This formulation suggests certain treatment goals and may provide the basis for developing a treatment or case

Box 6.1 Case example of a child with a sleep problem

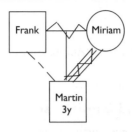

Martin is a three-year-old boy who has problems with both settling down to sleep at night and returning to sleep following night waking. He currently takes about thirty minutes to settle at night (at some time between 6 and 8 o'clock) and usually does so while being held by his mother and being bottle-fed on soya milk because he is allergic to cows milk. He wakes every night on one or two occasions (often at about 1 a.m. and 4 a.m.) and returns to sleep in the parents' bed, where he typically spends the second half of the night, only after being changed and bottle-fed.

He was pre-disposed to developing these sleeping problems because he had both milk intolerance and asthma. In addition he has a difficult temperament with marked irregularity in developing routines and intense arousal to minor stimuli. His asthma has led to a number of quite serious attacks, for which he was hospitalized.

The sleep difficulties are maintained by the lack of opportunity Martin has for developing self-soothing skills that do not involve feeding. The pre-sleep feeds and being held by the mother prevent the developing of self-soothing skills. A further factor maintaining the night-waking is the large feeds, which lead to later discomfort when he wets his nappy. Lengthy daytime naps are a third factor maintaining both the settling and night waking difficulties.

The daytime naps, pre-sleep feeding, holding and the inclusion of Martin in the parents' bed in the second part of the night occur because of a combination of parental exhaustion and anxiety. Both parents have become exhausted by three years of broken sleep. Since the asthma attacks, the parents, particularly Miriam (the mother), have also developed anxiety about his well-being. The anxiety about the child's health and exhaustion has placed a strain on the marital relationship and the management of the child is now largely Miriam's responsibility, with Frank making little input and offering little support. Often, Frank sleeps alone because he finds that he cannot meet the demands of a pressured work situation if his sleep is broken by Martin's night waking.

Protective factors in this case include the parents' commitment to jointly resolving the problem, their excellent relationship with Martin and their capacity to work co-operatively with the clinical team.

management plan. Goals might include the reduction in the length of time it takes for Martin to settle and helping Martin to develop self-soothing skills so that he can return to sleep unaided when he awakes at night. A reduction in the duration and frequency of daytime naps and the provision of opportunities to develop self-soothing skills are possible methods suggested by the formulation for achieving these goals. Finally, the formulation highlights the fact that if the management programme is to succeed it must take account of the parental exhaustion, anxiety and marital tension which have evolved around the child's sleeping difficulties.

MANAGEMENT OF SLEEP PROBLEMS

For settling and night waking, which are the most common sleep problems, the structured approach described below conducted over about five sessions has been shown to be highly effective (Ramchandani et al., 2000). The development of a working alliance and a shared understanding of the problem occurs during the assessment and formulation process. The working relationship ideally should be one where the parents experience the clinician as collaborating with them in helping the child to develop settling and self-soothing skills. Contracting for a sleep management programme and goal setting is particularly important because the process of following through on most sleep management programmes is so demanding. This is especially the case for parents who are already exhausted, anxious, unsupported, engaged in marital conflict or stressed by extra-familial pressures. Parents should be offered a time-limited contract for a specific number of sessions to achieve particular goals. For example, six sessions over 12 weeks to reduce settling time to 10 minutes and to help the child to develop self-soothing skills so that he can return to sleep unaided when he awakes at night. It is also important to warn parents that the process can be demanding and so the timing of the programme should not coincide with the occurrence of other family stresses, such as Christmas or an excessively busy work period for either parent. Where appropriate, parents should be encouraged to mobilize social support from each other, friends or the extended family. For example, parents may be invited to set aside one evening a week when they go out for a drink or a meal as a couple and take turns of 15 minutes listening actively to their partner and avoiding evaluating or arguing with the content of what the partner says. Where sleep management programmes fail, it is usually because other family stresses, lack of social support, inter-parental co-operation difficulties, parental depression or other parental and family problems have prevented parents from following through on agreed sleep management programme plans (Douglas, 1989, 2005).

A unique sleep management programme is required for each child. Such programmes are developed in light of the formulation and typically include some of the following strategies, which are based on the behavioural principles of shaping, fading, discrimination training, extinction and reinforcement and on cognitive principles of script and schema development (Douglas & Richman, 1985):

- gradual reduction or elimination of daytime sleeping

- gradual reduction or elimination of pre-sleep feeds or drinks
- the development of pleasant bedtime routines
- gradual or sudden movement of bedtime routines from a time when the child is highly likely to sleep to an earlier time
- gradual or sudden provision of opportunities to use self-soothing skills while the child is first going to sleep
- gradual or sudden provision of opportunities to use self-soothing skills following night waking
- coaching children in self-soothing relaxation skills
- reward training and extinction.

For some of these strategies the choice is between an abrupt or sudden change and a gradual change. Because infants typically respond to sudden changes in routines with persistent crying, and because this is particularly stressful for both the child and the parents, where possible gradual change procedures are preferable. Also, most parents will have received advice to use sudden change procedures and found these to be ineffective and distressing, so will be reluctant to try them again. For example, most parents will have been advised to let their children cry until the child falls asleep. Many parents manage this approach for three or four consecutive nights but eventually lift the child to prevent the crying, which has become intolerable for them. This invariably leads to the child's crying persisting for more than five or six nights after this. The duration of the crying also extends so many parents revert to lifting, rocking or soothing the child and give up attempts to help the child develop self-soothing skills.

Reducing daytime sleeping

Reduction of daytime sleeping may be achieved by helping children to cut down on the number of daytime naps they take or the duration of daytime naps. Napping may be replaced by activities that the child finds enjoyable. Naps may be shortened by waking the child after a set time has elapsed. Parents find this process demanding because often the child's daytime naps afford the exhausted parent an opportunity to doze or spend some time doing something other than caring for the infant.

Eliminating pre-sleep feeds

Where children have large feeds before settling, the time lapse between these feeds and sleeping may be gradually extended and the time of the last nappy change brought gradually closer to bedtime so that the chances of the child awakening because of the discomfort of a wet nappy are minimized. In cases of night waking where children return to sleep following feeding, the frequency and extent of these may be gradually reduced.

Developing bedtime routines

Pleasant bedtime routines including washing, changing, comforting, cuddling a special doll or teddy bear, story telling and singing may be developed and standardized so that the child can learn exactly what to expect at bedtime. Through this type of discrimination training the child develops a bedtime script. Where part of the sleep problem is children's reluctance to go to bed early, these routines may first be conducted at a time when the child is most likely to sleep and then they may gradually be moved to an earlier time in the evening.

Gradual provision of self-soothing opportunities

The gradual provision of opportunities for the child to use self-soothing to settle or return to sleep involves developing a hierarchy of situations from the child falling asleep in the parents arms to the child falling asleep alone with the parent out of view and then allowing the child to master each step in the hierarchy. Here is one example of such a hierarchy adapted from Jo Douglas' (1989) work:

1 Place cushions on the lap so the child is falling asleep with less physical comfort.
2 Reduce the tightness of the embrace and encourage the child to sleep more horizontally on the lap or the couch.
3 Place the child in bed to fall asleep after a brief cuddle on the lap but lean over the bed and comfort the child with gentle holding and stroking.
4 Encourage falling asleep in bed but reduce holding and stroking.
5 Sit beside the bed and touch the child gently while falling asleep.
6 Sit beside the bed but do not touch the child.
7 Move the chair two feet from the bed and avert gaze while the child falls asleep.
8 Move to the other side of the room while the child falls asleep.
9 Move out of eyesight while the child falls asleep.
10 Stand outside the door while the child falls asleep.

Coaching in relaxation skills

After the age of three, children may be coached by the clinician or the parent in self-soothing relaxation skills. Simplified progressive muscle relaxation training and sleep inducing guided imagery may be used. With very young children aged three to four years, I have found a simple four-muscle-group version of relaxation training very effective with toddlers. The four exercises are:

• clench and relax the hands

- point the toes upwards and relax them
- hunch the shoulders and relax them
- tense the stomach muscles after inhaling and relax them on exhaling.

For guided imagery, any image that reduces arousal may be used. For example, imagining the sun going down and the wind dying or a bird flying into the distance have been found by many children to be arousal reducing. With young children, variations on sheep-counting tend to increase arousal because counting is not an automatic skill and so requires concentration and heightened arousal. Some children find they can learn to use recordings of particular pieces of music and recorded stories to reduce their arousal and soothe themselves to sleep.

Reward training and extinction

Using a smiling-face chart like that presented in Figure 6.6 or small prizes from a prize-box may be used to reinforce appropriate sleep-related behaviour, such as preparing for bed at a set time, drinking the last drink of the day an hour before bedtime, avoiding calling parents to the bedroom after they have said their final good night and using self-soothing skills following night waking rather than entering the parents' bed. Rewarding these behaviours increases the likelihood they will recur and the child will develop appropriate sleep habits. Inappropriate sleep-related behaviours may be extinguished by ignoring them. Thus, objecting to beginning the bedtime routine or calling for the parent to come to the room following the last good night may all be ignored and eventually these inappropriate habits will rarely recur. As with all sleep management techniques, it is important that the parents' intention to help the child develop self-soothing and sleep management skills is explained to the child and that the rationale for the procedure is outlined to the child in terms that he or she can understand. If the child understands that reward training and extinction are being used to help him or her 'become a big boy or girl', and are not viewed as punishments which define the child as 'a bad boy or girl', then the chances of co-operation and problem resolution are maximized.

The effectiveness of reward training may be improved by initially rewarding all approximations to appropriate sleep-related behaviour so as to gradually shape appropriate sleep behaviour. The effectiveness of extinction, where children enter the parents' bed, may be increased if parents in an unemotive way return the child to bed immediately they enter the parents' bedroom and ignore subsequent calling out.

For rewards to be maximally effective, they should be highly valued by the child and given as close to the behaviour they are rewarding as possible, unless doing so would disrupt the development of appropriate sleep behaviour. If a reward chart is being used, it should be discussed with the child in a

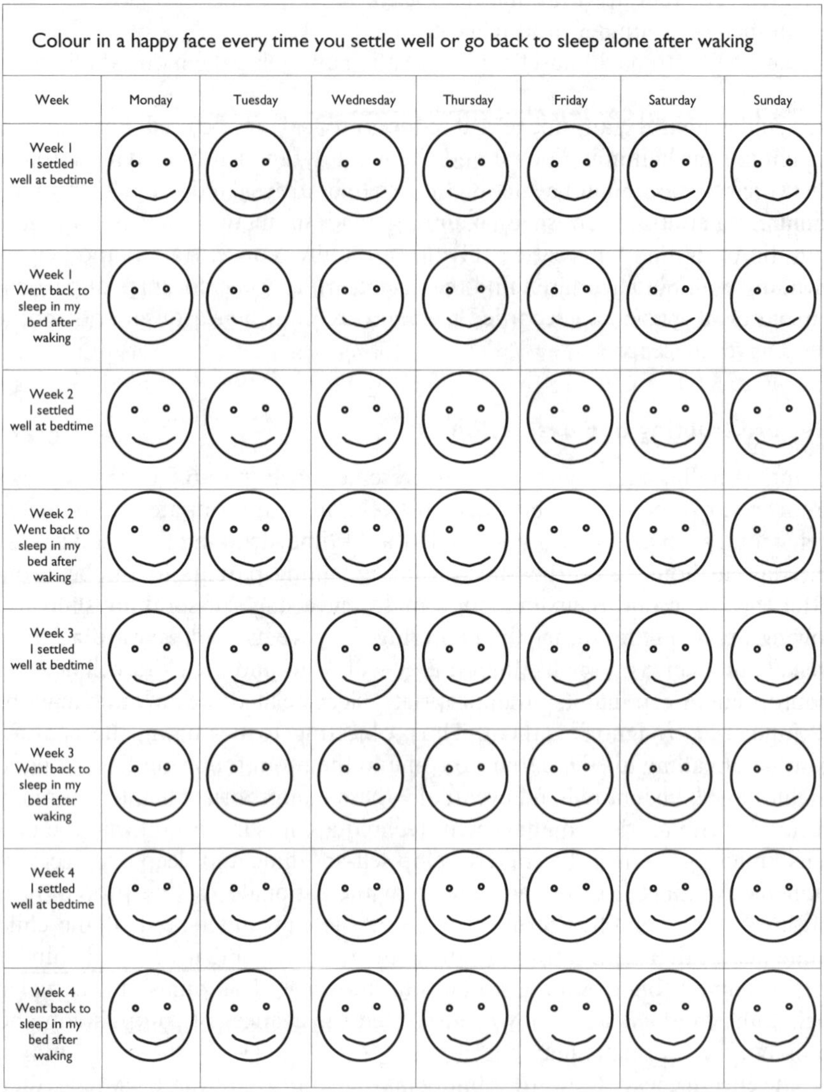

Week	Monday	Tuesday	Wednesday	Thursday	Friday	Saturday	Sunday
Week 1 I settled well at bedtime							
Week 1 Went back to sleep in my bed after waking							
Week 2 I settled well at bedtime							
Week 2 Went back to sleep in my bed after waking							
Week 3 I settled well at bedtime							
Week 3 Went back to sleep in my bed after waking							
Week 4 I settled well at bedtime							
Week 4 Went back to sleep in my bed after waking							

Colour in a happy face every time you settle well or go back to sleep alone after waking

Figure 6.6 Child's smiling-face chart for sleep problems

way that allows the child to see that colouring in a face or getting a sticker to put on the chart is a highly desirable event. If a prize bag is being used, the little prizes in the bag should be small treats, toys or food that the child likes a lot and prefers to other alternatives. Bedtime routines may be rewarded before the child goes to sleep (provided the rewards do not involve eating tooth-rotting sweets or candy!). Appropriate behaviour following night waking is probably best rewarded the next morning, since to reward at night might interfere with a return to sleep.

Treatment of circadian rhythm disorder

In circadian rhythm disorder there is a mismatch between the circadian rhythm and the sleep–waking schedule demands of the environment. Usually this mismatch results from going to sleep late and rising late. The mismatch may be overcome by moving bedtime forward three hours each day and avoiding daytime naps until the required bedtime is reached (Horne, 1992). Thus a child who will not sleep until 9.00 p.m., and the parents would like bedtime to be 6.00 p.m. would be set a schedule to go to sleep at 12.00 midnight, 3.00 a.m., 6.00 a.m., 9.00 a.m., 12.00 a.m., 3.00 p.m., 6.00 p.m. over a seven-day period. This is an exhausting process and requires considerable planning.

Treatment of night-time fears and night-mares

Reassurance that the bedroom is a safe place and that night-mares are only dreams is the appropriate way to manage mild bedtime fears. However, when children develop night-time fears significant enough to lead to a referral to a clinical psychologist, it is unlikely that such simple reassurance will be of much value in helping the child develop a less troubled sleep pattern. Typically, the night-time fears and night-mares occur as part of a broader reaction to a life situation that involves threats to the child's safety, security or self-esteem. Such threats may include moving house, changing school, parental separation, parental hospitalization, birth of a sibling, car accidents, burglary, bullying and physical or sexual abuse. Bedtime fears and night-mares may reflect the child's attempt to process and gain control over incomprehensible or threatening features of their current life situation (Mooney & Sobocinski, 1995).

In such situations, non-abusing parents may be coached in listening to their children's fears, facilitating their expression and empathizing with them. Parents may also be coached in teaching their children relaxation skills to reduce arousal. This facilitative approach may be modelled by the therapist first and later the parents may be given feedback on their attempts to facilitate their child's expression of fears and develop relaxation and arousal reduction skills. This type of therapy, which draws on both cognitive behaviour therapy and attachment theory, allows the child to process the negative affect, to develop a coherent cognitive model of what may be an overwhelmingly confusing situation, to overcome avoidance routines in which both parent and child avoid talking about the anxiety-provoking life situation and to strengthen their view of the facilitative parent as a secure base (Mooney & Sobocinski, 1995). With night-mares this approach may be supplemented with either systematic desensitization or flooding, in which the child, through a process of guided imagery, is gradually or abruptly exposed to the feared images from the night-mares and helped to cope with them. A variety of coping strategies may be employed, including using relaxation skills or mastery-oriented self-statements and imagery.

Where sleep paralysis occurs following night-mares, children may be shown how to terminate such paralysis by engaging in sustained voluntary eye movements. Physical contact from the parent may also terminate this very frightening state.

Managing food intolerance

Physical discomfort associated with cows milk intolerance was identified as an important factor causing sleep difficulties in about 10% of referrals to a paediatric sleep clinic and these cases showed normalization of sleep patterns after five weeks when milk products were removed from the children's diets (Kahn et al., 1989). Soya milk or goats milk may be used as alternatives to cow's mild in such cases.

Treatment of parasomnias

For all the parasomnias, but particularly night terrors and sleep-walking, it is important to reassure parents and children that parasomnias do not reflect psychological maladjustment but rather CNS immaturity, which most children grow out of by the end of adolescence. Practical methods for preventing inadvertent self-injury may be explored for those parasomnias where risks of injury are present. Sleep terrors and sleep-walking can be controlled in some instances by administering benzodiazepines at bedtime to reduce stage 4 activity (Stores, 2001).

Treatment of night terrors

For night terrors, the management approach of choice is waking treatment (Lask, 1995). On five successive nights parents observe their child sleeping and note the time at which the night terror episodes occur. If the episodes tend to occur at a relatively fixed time, parents are advised to wake their child ten to fifteen minutes before the night terror is expected and to keep the child awake for fifteen minutes. This procedure should be followed for five to seven consecutive nights. If terrors do not occur at a fixed time parents are advised to watch for signs of autonomic arousal preceding night terror episodes and to immediately wake their child if such signs occur. In such cases, this procedure should be followed for five to seven consecutive nights. Lask (1995) found that 80% of a series of over fifty cases recovered within a week with this management approach. Waking treatment probably prevents the occurrence of night terrors by interrupting faulty slow-wave sleep patterns. In Lask's treatment protocol, this waking method was supplemented with family support and education about sleep.

Management of disorders of excessive daytime sleepiness

The differential diagnosis of obstructive sleep apnoea which leads to excessive daytime sleepiness and narcolepsy is best made in a sleep laboratory, where those episodes during which the child stops breathing may clearly be identified or their presence outruled. Where it is clear that episodes of sleep apnoea are not present and that the child is getting a good night's sleep, it is probable that narcolepsy is present, particularly if sleep paralysis, hypnogogic hallucinations and cataplexy are present. Parent education about this lifelong disorder, sleep hygiene counselling and pharmacological management are the main components of a comprehensive treatment approach to narcolepsy (Guilleminault & Pelayo, 2000). With respect to education it should be made clear that narcolepsy is not a reflection of laziness or emotional disturbance but a neurological condition of unknown aetiology. With respect to sleep hygiene, children should be allowed two fifteen-minute daytime naps. Teenagers should be advised to avoid alcohol, street drugs and not to drive. Regular sleeping hours and regular exercise are also advised. From a pharmacological perspective, the ideal treatment is a stimulant to combat daytime sleepiness and a tricyclic agent to counteract cataplexy. Commonly used stimulants include pemolin sodium, methylphenidate and dexamfetamine. Imipramine is the most commonly used tricyclic.

Where the results of a sleep laboratory assessment show that obstructive sleep apnoea is present, the treatment of choice is adenotosillectomy (Palasti & Potsic, 1995). Where children have neuromuscular disorders, an uvulopalatopharyngoplasty may be indicated. Here the uvula, the tonsils and a portion of the soft palate are removed. Artificial airways such as nasopharyngeal tubes and nasal continuous positive airway pressure are alternatives. However, these are usually not well tolerated by children and so are not long-term solutions. If these procedures fail then a tracheotomy is the final treatment option.

SUMMARY

Sleep is not a unitary state but includes fifty to ninety-minute cycles of slow-wave sleep, which is guessed to be restorative, and rapid eye movement sleep, which may be important for cognitive development and efficiency. With age, overall sleep requirements decrease and sleep architecture changes. Cycles lengthen towards ninety minutes and the amount of REM sleep in each cycle decreases.

A distinction can be made between dyssomnias and parasomnias which are the two main types of sleep problem. Dyssomnias include those problems characterized by abnormalities in the amount, timing or quality of sleep. Settling and night waking are the most common dyssomnias in pre-school children. Behavioural and physiological abnormalities occurring during sleep characterize the parasomnias. Night-mares, night terrors and sleep-walking are among the more common parasomnias. While up to 25% of pre-schoolers display dyssomnias, probably less than 10% display parasomnias.

In assessing children with sleep problems, it is important to inquire both about details of the child's sleeping routines and about the psychosocial context within which these problematic sleep routines occur. Salient features from the assessment should be drawn together into a formulation, which begins with a statement of the central features of the sleep problems and then links these to pre-disposing, precipitating and maintaining factors. Protective factors and family resources that have implications for resolving the problem should also be mentioned.

A unique sleep management programme, developed in the light of the formulation, should be drawn up in each case. Where psychosocial factors are central to the maintenance of the problems, the plan should be based on the following principles: gradual reduction or elimination of daytime sleeping, gradual reduction or elimination of pre-sleep feeds or drinks, the development of pleasant bedtime routines, gradual or sudden movement of bedtime routines from a time when the child is highly likely to sleep to an earlier time, gradual or sudden provision of opportunities to use self-soothing skills while the child is first going to sleep, gradual or sudden provision of opportunities to use self-soothing skills following night waking, coaching children in self-soothing relaxation skills, reward training and extinction. Circadian rhythm disorder may be managed by moving bedtime forward three hours each day.

For the management of night-mares, parents may be coached in listening to their children's fears, facilitating their expression and empathizing with them. Parents may also be coached in teaching their children relaxation skills to reduce arousal associated with night-time fears. Exposure-based therapies such as systematic desensitization and flooding may complement such family-based approaches to the treatment of night-mares. Where sleep problems are associated with food intolerance, substitute foods such as soya milk or goats milk may be used as alternatives to cows milk. For all the parasomnias it is important to reassure parents and children that parasomnias do not reflect psychological maladjustment but rather CNS immaturity, which most children grow out of by the end of adolescence. Practical methods for preventing inadvertent self-injury may be explored for those parasomnias where risks of injury are present. Sleep terrors and sleep-walking can be controlled in some instances by administering benzodiazepines at bedtime to reduce stage 4 activity, although the management approach of choice is waking treatment. Parent education, sleep hygiene counselling and pharmacological management are the main components of a comprehensive treatment approach to narcolepsy. For sleep apnoea, the treatment of choice is adenotosillectomy.

EXERCISE 6.1

Construct a preliminary formulation and treatment plan for this case.

> Joe and Fay Roberts are at their wits' end. Their two-year-old, Rudy, has settling and night-waking problems. She naps about four or five times per day. She will not settle when put down and cries or screams until her mother or father lifts her. Eventually she nods off when being fed. She continues to be breast-fed regularly on demand. At night she wakes two or three times, often with a wet nappy (diaper). She will return to sleep only if fed. She often sleeps the second half of the night in the parents' bed, which is not a problem for Joe or Fay. However, the sleep-loss both are experiencing is leading to exhaustion for both of them. Joe recently changed jobs and has on some occasions slept in the spare room because he finds he cannot meet the demands of his job after repeated night wakings. Fay, who had intended to return to work when Rudy was about a year old, now says she could not imagine ever having sufficient energy or confidence to go back to work. The couple rarely go out with their friends and see little of the extended family. Most of the week-end is devoted to housework or sleeping.

FURTHER READING

Ferber, R. & Kryger, M. (1995). *Principles and Practice of Sleep Medicine in the Child.* Philadelphia, PA: Saunders.

Mindell, J. & Owens, J. (2003). *A Clinical Guide to Paediatric Sleep: Diagnosis and Management of Sleep Problems.* Philadelphia: Lippincott Williams & Wilkins.

Schaefer, C. (1995). *Clinical Handbook of Sleep Disorders in Children.* Northvale, NJ: Jason Aronson.

Stores G & Wiggs, L. (2001). *Sleep Disturbance in Children and Adolescence with Disorders of Development; Its Significance and Management.* London: MacKeith Press.

Stores, G. (2001). *A Clinical Guide to Sleep Disorders in Children and Adolescents.* Oxford: Oxford University Press.

READING FOR PARENTS

Daymond, K. (2001). *The ParentTalk Guide to Sleep*. London: Hodder and Stoughton.

Douglas, J. & Richman, N. (1984). *My Child Won't Sleep*. Harmondsworth, UK: Penguin.

Durand, V. (1998). *Sleep Better: A Guide to Improving Sleep for Children with Special Needs*. Baltimore, MD: Paul H Brookes.

Ferber, R. (1985). *Solve Your Child's Sleep Problems*. London: Dorling Kindersley.

Lansky, V. (1991). *Getting Your Child to Sleep . . . and Back to Sleep*. Deephaven: The Book Peddlers.

Quine, L. (1997). *Solving Children's Sleep Problems: A Step by Step Guide for Parents*. Huntingdon: Beckett Karlson.

Weissbluth, M. (1987). *Sleepwell*. London: Unwin.

WEBSITES

Factsheets on the sleep problems covered in this book can be downloaded from the website for Rose, G. & York, A. (2004). *Mental Health and Growing Up. Fact sheets for Parents, Teachers and Young People* (Third edition). London: Gaskell: http://www.rcpsych.ac.uk/info/mhgu/

Chapter 7

Toileting problems

The development of bladder and bowel control occurs in a stage-wise manner in most children during the first five years of life (Buchanan, 1992; Clayden, Taylor, Loader, Bortzkowski & Edwards, 2002; Houts, 2003; Murphy & Carr, 2000a; Walker, 2003). In the first months of life the child is incontinent. Gradually the child develops bowel control at night. This is followed by the development of bowel control during the day. Next, the child learns to control the bladder during the day and finally most children by the age of five learn to control their bladder at night. Most children follow this sequence, although there is some variation within the population. Girls develop bowel and bladder control more quickly than boys. By four years of age most children have developed bowel control and by five most children have developed bladder control so these ages are used as the cut-off ages for diagnosing encopresis and enuresis, respectively.

Enuresis and encopresis – or wetting and soiling – are the main toileting problems which come to the attention of clinical psychologists. A case example of enuresis is presented in Box 7.1; Box 7.2 gives a case example of encopresis. Children are typically referred for treatment with toileting or elimination problems if they fail to achieve bladder and bowel control by the age of four or five years. These problems are of concern to clinical psychologists, principally because they have a negative impact on children's social and educational development. Children with elimination problems may be excluded from school, ostracized by their peers and they may develop conflictual relationships with their parents. This in turn can lead to the development of academic attainment problems, low self-esteem, and secondary emotional or conduct problems.

This chapter, after considering the classification, epidemiology and clinical features of elimination problems, considers a variety of theoretical explanations concerning their aetiology, along with relevant empirical evidence. The assessment of enuresis and encopresis will then be outlined and an approach to the treatment of these problems will be given.

Box 7.1 A case example of enuresis

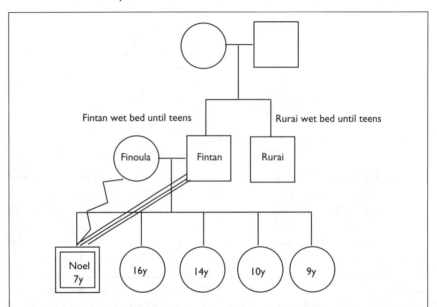

Noel, aged seven, was referred because he had never developed nocturnal bladder control, with one exception. When on holiday with his aunt in Cork in the summer before the referral was made, he did not wet the bed once. The wet beds which followed this incident led to considerable conflict between Noel and his mother, Finoula, who interpreted the relapse as an act of deliberate aggression against her. The parents, Finoula and Fintan, since Noel was about four years of age, had alternated between taking a lenient understanding approach and a critical punitive approach. They had difficulty agreeing on how best to manage the problems and it often led to acrimonious rows, with Fintan arguing for the lenient approach and Finoula advocating a more punitive management style. By the time the referral was made, relationships between Noel and his parents had deteriorated to an all-time low.

Besides the enuresis, Noel's developmental history was essentially normal. His academic performance was excellent and he had no psychosocial adjustment problems, other than those that arose between himself and his parents as a consequence of his enuresis. He took great care to wash thoroughly each morning and so did not have an odour of urine which might give his peers reason to mock or bully him at school.

Noel was the youngest and only boy in a family with five children. His four sisters have no continence problems and are well adjusted. There is a family history of bedwetting on the father's side. Noel's father, Fintan, and his uncle, Rurai, wet their beds until they were in their teens.

Box 7.2 A case of encopresis

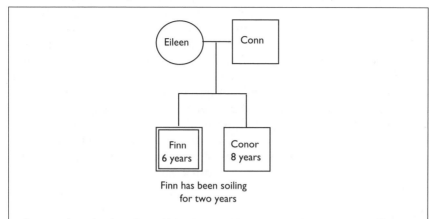

Finn has been soiling
for two years

Finn, aged six, developed good bowel control by the age of four but began soiling at six. The soiling occurred at night and occasionally in school. It was the embarrassment and secondary peer problems that were evolving in response to his soiling in school that led to the referral.

Finn had suffered alternately from gastroenteritis and constipation during the three months prior to the onset of the encopresis. He had developed an anal fissure which became infected. Subsequently he avoided the bathroom because of an intense and growing fear that the fissure would recur. He developed chronic constipation, for which he was given laxatives. This led to overflow incontinence and strengthening of his fear and avoidance of the toilet.

Finn was one of two children, his brother being two years his senior. Both boys fitted in well at school before the encopresis occurred. The parents were both professionals, and had excellent relationships with the boys. But they were in despair because they felt helpless when faced with Finn's problem.

DIAGNOSIS, CLINICAL FEATURES AND CLASSIFICATION

Elimination problems constitute a heterogeneous group of disorders and any classification system must take account of a number of important distinctions. First, both wetting and soiling may occur exclusively during the day, exclusively during the night or at any time. Second, with primary enuresis and encopresis, incontinence has been present from birth, but with secondary enuresis or encopresis, there has been a period of bowel or bladder control which at some point broke down. Third, with secondary enuresis and encopresis, a distinction may be made between cases where the wetting or soiling is intentional and those where it is unintentional. Fourth, with encopresis, at a symptomatic level, soiling may occur either with or without constipation and overflow incontinence. Fifth, elimination problems may occur as monosymptomatic presentations or as cases characterized by both faecal and urinary incontinence. Sixth, elimination problems may occur as an uncomplicated one or two symptom presentation or as part of a wider set of adjustment problems primarily related to a chaotic, stressful or abusive psychosocial environment; or as one aspect of a developmental disability or medical condition.

Table 7.1 shows that ICD 10 (WHO, 1992, 1996) and DSM IV TR (APA, 2000a) have taken many of these features into account in describing elimination disorders, but that few have been taken into account in sub-classification. In ICD 10, a distinction is made between enuresis and encopresis, but no attempt is made to further sub-classify elimination problems with different features. In DSM IV TR encopresis is sub-classified into a type characterized by constipation and overflow incontinence and a type where this feature is absent. With enuresis, three sub-types are recognized depending on the time of day when wetting typically occurs: diurnal, nocturnal and both.

EPIDEMIOLOGY

The epidemiology of enuresis and encopresis has been well summarized in DSM IV TR (APA, 2000a). Encopresis is not diagnosed until four years of age. At five years of age the prevalence of encopresis is about 1%. Enuresis is not diagnosed until five years of age. The prevalence of enuresis among five year olds is 7% for males and 3% for females. At ten years of age the prevalence is 3% for males and 2% for females. At age eighteen, 1% of males have enuresis and fewer females suffer from the condition. This gradual reduction in the prevalence of elimination disorders with increasing age is illustrated in Figure 7.1. Secondary elimination problems most commonly occur between five and eight years. The male:female ratio for elimination disorders is about 2:1.

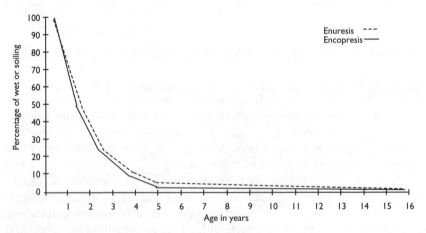

Figure 7.1 Prevalence of wetting and soiling from birth to adolescence

Note: Based on Buchanan (1992) and Houts et al. (1994).

Table 7.1 Diagnostic criteria for elimination disorders in DSM IV TR and ICD 10

	DSM IV TR	*ICD 10*
Enuresis	A. A repeated voiding of urine into bed or clothes (whether involuntary or intentional) B. The behaviours clinically significant as manifested by either a frequency of twice a week for at least 3 consecutive months or the presence of clinically significant distress or impairment in social, academic (occupational) or other important areas of functioning C. Chronological age of at least 5 years (or equivalent developmental level) D. The behaviour is not due exclusively to the direct physiological effect of a substance (e.g a diuretic) or a general medical condition such as spina bifida Specify type: Nocturnal only. Diurnal only. Nocturnal and diurnal	A disorder characterized by the involuntary voiding of urine, by day and/or by night, which is abnormal in relation to the individual's mental age and which is not a consequence of a lack of bladder control due to any neurological disorder, to epileptic attacks, or to any structural abnormality of the urinary tact The enuresis may have been present from birth or it may have arisen following a period of acquired bladder control The later onset variety usually begins at the age of 5 to 7 years The enuresis may constitute a monosymptomatic condition or it may be associated with a more widespread emotional or behavioural disorder Emotional problems may arise as a secondary consequence of the distress or stigma that results from enuresis, the enuresis may form part of some other psychiatric disorder or both the enuresis and the emotional/behavioural disturbance may arise in parallel from related aetiological factors There is no straightforward way of deciding between these alternatives
Encopresis	A. Repeated passage of faeces into inappropriate places (e.g. clothing or floor) whether involuntary or intentional B. A least one such event per month for at least 3 months C. Chronological age is at least 4 years (or equivalent developmental level	Repeated voluntary or involuntary passage of faeces, usually of normal or near normal consistency in places not appropriate for that purpose in the individual's own sociocultural setting There are three main aetiological patterns: • First, the condition may represent a lack of adequate toilet training, with the history being one of continuous failure ever to acquire adequate bowel control

Continued

Table 7.1 Continued

DSM IV TR	ICD 10
D. The behaviour is not due exclusively to the direct physiological effect of a substance (e.g a laxative) or a general medical condition except through the mechanism of constipation Specify type: With constipation and overflow incontinence. Without constipation and overflow incontinence	• Second, it may reflect a psychologically determined disorder in which there has been normal physiological control over defecation but, for some reason a reluctance, resistance or failure to conform to social norms in defecation in acceptable places • Third, it may stem from physiological retention, involving impaction of faeces, with secondary overflow. Such retention may arise from parent–child battles over bowel training or from withholding faeces because of painful defecation as a consequence of an anal fissure or gastrointestinal problem In some instances the encopresis may be accompanied by smearing of faeces over the body or over the external environment and there may be anal fingering and masturbation. In such instances it usually forms part of a wider emotional or behavioural disorder

Note: Adapted from DSM IV TR (APA, 2000a) and ICD 10 (WHO, 1992, 1996).

For treated cases, motivation and adherence to behavioural treatment programme regimes are the best predictors of positive outcome (Buchanan, 1992; Kaplan & Busner, 1993). The number of first-degree relatives with bedwetting problems is the single most accurate predictor of a poor prognosis for enuretics (Barclay & Houts, 1995). With encopresis, a poor prognosis has been found in cases characterized by highly coercive or intrusive parent–child interaction (Kelly, 1996).

AETIOLOGICAL THEORIES

Aetiological theories of elimination problems fall into six categories: biological, developmental, psychopathological, psychodynamic, behavioural and family systems. The principal features of these theories and their treatment implications are sketched in Table 7.2.

Table 7.2 Aetiological theories of elimination disorders

Theory	Theoretical principles	Principles of treatment
Biological	Elimination problems are due to genetic factors or to urinary or anorectal structural or functional abnormalities	Medication or surgery to rectify abnormalities or training in how to cope with them
Developmental	Elimination disorders are part of a specific or general developmental delay	Reassurance and behavioural training
Psychopathological	Elimination disorders are part of broader set of psychological problems Psychopathology may cause elimination disorders Psychopathology may arise from elimination disorders Behaviour problems and elimination problems may both be an expression of underlying psychopathology	Psychological treatment for both the elimination problem and the psychopathology
Psychoanalytic	Elimination problems are an expression of unconscious conflicts associated with neglectful or coercive parental toilet training during the anal stage of development	Psychodynamic play therapy to help resolve conflicts underpinning elimination problems
Behavioural	Lack of positive reinforcement for appropriate toileting or the association of toileting with pain or other aversive experiences prevents the development or maintenance of appropriate toileting habits	Behavioural programme to learn appropriate toileting habits
Family systems	Primary elimination problems may be due to living in a chaotic family environment. Secondary elimination problems may arise from acute stressful life events and family lifecycle transitions. Elimination problems may be maintained by coercive, intrusive, or triangulating interaction patterns with parents or caregivers	Family therapy to alter interaction patterns that maintain the elimination problems

Biological theories

Biological explanations of enuresis and encopresis point to the importance of genetic and constitutional factors in the aetiology of elimination problems. Findings concerning the role of biological factors in the aetiology of enuresis and biological treatments of enuresis have been reviewed by Clayden et al. (2002), Walker (2003) and Barclay and Houts (1995). Approximately 70% of children with enuresis have a first-degree relative who has a history of bedwetting, suggesting the importance of genetic factors in enuresis. Compared with other variables assessing psychological adjustment or physical health, the single major predictor of the outcome for children with enuresis is the number of first-degree relatives having similar problems. Enuresis has also been found to be associated with urinary tract infections, urinary tract abnormalities, a low functional bladder volume and constipation. While antibiotic treatment may relieve urinary tract infections, they have little impact on enuresis. Surgery to rectify urinary tract abnormalities is ineffective in alleviating enuresis. Treatment of constipation, however, may lead to a resolution of enuresis and this is probably most effective in those cases where the faecal mass has reduced functional bladder capacity. Nocturnal enuresis is associated with an abnormal vasopressin circadian rhythm. However, treatment of enuresis with vasopressin (also known as DDAVP, desamino-D-arginine) is effective in only a minority of cases and there is a high relapse rate (Kaplan & Busner, 1993). The observation that the antidepressant, imipramine, leads to immediate cessation of nocturnal enuresis and its withdrawal leads to an immediate relapse in most cases has led to speculation about abnormalities of the neuroamine system contributing to the aetiology of enuresis. Anticholinergic drugs such as belladonna, propantheline, oxybutynin chloride and terodeiline delay the desire to void and increase functional bladder capacity. They have little effect on nocturnal enuresis but are effective in reducing daytime wetting. However, all of the anticholinergic drugs have unpleasant side effects such as dry mouth, blurred vision, dizziness, headache and nausea.

The role of biological factors in the aetiology of encopresis has been reviewed by Clayden et al. (2002), Walker (2003) and Buchanan (1992). Abnormalities in anorectal sensory and motor function, the presence of a megacolon, Hirschsprung's disease, spina bifida and cerebral palsy may all lead to encopresis. Where there are abnormalities of anorectal sensory functioning, the child is unaware of the need for defecation and so fails to develop adequate control of the sphincter to prevent soiling, whereas with poor anorectal motor functioning the child is aware of the need to control the sphincter but is unable to. In some instances this may be due to internal sphincter hypertrophy. In Hirschsprung's disease, inadequate innervation of the intestines (which is diagnosed by biopsy) prevents the motility of faeces through the intestines. This leads to chronic constipation and in some cases overflow incontinence. About 10% of referrals with chronic constipation have Hirschsprung's disease. In spina bifida, there are typically severe abnormalities of the sensory and motor nerves to the legs, bowel and bladder. In cerebral palsy, impairment of the motor nerves of the central nervous system may prevent the development of adequate bladder and bowel control in some cases.

Developmental theories

Developmental hypotheses about the aetiology of elimination disorders view enuresis and encopresis as part of a delay in reaching normal developmental milestones. Relevant research in this area has been reviewed by Clayden et al. (2002), Walker (2003) and Buchanan (1992). Elimination problems are more common among children with both specific developmental delays characterized by a failure to reach motor, speech and social milestones on time and minor neurological abnormalities. They are also more common among children with general developmental delays characterized by low IQ and a diagnosis of intellectual disability. Encopresis is more common among children with low birth weight. There may also be a critical period for learning bladder-control skills. Enuresis is more likely to develop in youngsters who do not begin toilet training until after eighteen months.

Psychopathological hypotheses

Psychopathological hypotheses about the links between psychological adjustment and elimination problems fall into three categories. The first hypothesis is that an underlying psychopathology leads to the development of elimination problems. The second hypothesis is that the elimination problems (and the response of others to these difficulties) place stress on the child and this leads to the development of psychological problems. The third hypothesis is that some underlying psychopathology gives rise to a range of behavioural difficulties of which elimination problems are one subset (Shaffer, 1994). Research relevant to these three hypotheses has been reviewed by Shaffer (1994) and Buchanan (1992). A co-morbid psychological diagnosis is present in only a minority of children with enuresis and encopresis. However, clinically significant psychological problems are approximately four times more common among enuretics than children with normal bladder control and no specific diagnostic category is associated uniquely with elimination problems; rather, a range of internalizing and externalizing difficulties is shown. Co-morbidity is more common among girls, youngsters with secondary enuresis, and in cases of diurnal enuresis. It has consistently been found that successful symptomatic treatment of elimination problems leads to improvement in other behavioural and psychological problems. Thus for a majority of children with elimination disorders, it is probably the case that the elimination problems are partially or completely responsible for the other observed psychological difficulties.

Psychodynamic theories

In psychodynamic theories, wetting and soiling are explained as expressions of unconscious intrapsychic conflicts which have their roots in non-optimal parent–child relationships during the anal period of psychosexual development. Specifically, the parent may have been overly lax and negligent or overly coercive and controlling during the stage of development when toilet training is a central concern (e.g. Anthony, 1957). Negligence on the parents' part, according to this theory, may lead to suppressed aggression, which finds expression in elimination problems. Coercive control on the parents' part may lead to anxiety about soiling and subsequent constipation with overflow soiling. Individual psychotherapy, play therapy or art therapy, which aims to permit the child to express and resolve the conflicted feelings that underpin the elimination problems, are the principal treatments to have arisen from the psychodynamic tradition. Outcome studies of such therapy have shown that it is rarely effective in helping youngsters develop bowel and bladder control (Kaplan & Busner, 1993). However, case reports suggest that psychodynamically oriented play and art therapy may be useful to help youngsters increase their self-esteem and self-efficacy beliefs where these have diminished due to the negative response of family, peers and teachers to the elimination problems (Kelly, 1996).

Behavioural theories

Behavioural theories have highlighted the role of inappropriate reinforcement schedules in the development of primary enuresis and encopresis and avoidance conditioning in the aetiology of secondary encopresis (e.g. Fielding & Doleys, 1988). With primary enuresis and encopresis, bladder filling or rectal distension and sphincter relaxation have not become discriminative stimuli for appropriate toileting habits. Furthermore, when appropriate toileting behaviours have occurred they have not been adequately reinforced. With secondary encopresis, pain or other aversive events may have led to avoidance of the toilet and the consequent development of constipation and overflow incontinence. In addition, parental attention following soiling or wetting may inadvertently reinforce such elimination problems. There is also the possibility that unsuccessful attempts to resolve elimination problems and the negative physical and psychosocial consequences of enuresis and encopresis may lead to the development of learned helplessness and low self-efficacy beliefs (Sluckin, 1981). According to behavioural explanations of enuresis and encopresis, treatment should focus on sensitizing children to bodily sensations that precede urination and defecation so that these become effective discriminative stimuli. Where avoidance behaviours have developed desensitization to toileting situations should be arranged. Finally, successive approximations to appropriate toileting behaviour should be reinforced so that normal toileting habits are learned. Treatment for both enuresis and encopresis based on these principles have been shown in many outcome studies to be remarkably effective and are described in detail below (Buchanan, 1992; Clayden et al., 2002; Houts, 2003; Murphy & Carr, 2000a; Walker, 2003).

Family systems theories

Family systems theories of elimination problems have focused on the roles of patterns of family interaction in the maintenance of elimination problems (Kelly, 1996; White, 1984). When elimination problems develop, children may become triangulated into stressful patterns of interaction with their parents or caregivers. Within such patterns, one parent interacts with the child in an over-protective intrusive manner, while the other adopts a critical and distant position with respect to the child. Parental disagreements about how to mange the elimination problems are not openly addressed but are detoured through the child. For the child to recover, the family must be helped to replace these problem-maintaining behaviour patterns with alternative ways of managing the elimination difficulties that involves greater parental co-operation. There is some evidence that family therapy may be as effective as behavioural treatments for encopresis (Richman, 1983).

A number of acute and chronic family stresses have been found to be associated with enuresis and encopresis (Buchanan, 1992; Clayden et al., 2002; Houts, 2003; Murphy & Carr, 2000a; Walker, 2003). Stressful life events such as birth of a sibling, parental separation, disruptions of parental care, placement in institutional care, head injury, physical or sexual abuse and exposure to a natural disaster may all precipitate the onset of secondary enuresis and, in some instances, encopresis. Enuresis and encopresis are more common among children exposed to chronic stresses associated with a chaotic family environment such as marital discord, parental adjustment problems (including criminality, chronic illness and chronic psychological problems), financial difficulties and crowding. Taken together, these findings suggest that a chaotic family environment may pre-dispose youngsters to have elimination problems, probably because the routines required for developing bowel and bladder control skills are not provided. These results also suggest that exposure to an acute family stress may disrupt well-established toileting habits.

ASSESSMENT

In assessing elimination problems it is important to first clarify the following issues:

- whether the elimination problems include enuresis only, encopresis only, or both
- whether the problems are diurnal or nocturnal or both
- whether the incontinence is primary and has been present since birth or secondary and has developed following a period of continence
- whether secondary incontinence is intentional or unintentional
- whether encopresis occurs with or without constipation and overflow incontinence
- whether the incontinence is a feature of a wider set of adjustment problems associated with chaotic, stressful or abusive environment
- whether the incontinence is a feature of a developmental disability or medical condition.

It is good practice to arrange for a thorough paediatric medical examination to check abnormalities of the urethra, urinary tract infections, constipation, gastrointestinal illness, megacolon, Hirschsprung's disease and so forth. Over the course of the first few sessions, the pattern of soiling and wetting may be tracked by inviting parents to monitor toileting using the chart presented in Figure 7.2. This chart can be helpful later for goal setting. Data collected during assessment may be used as a baseline against which to evaluate progress in treatment. Diet, fluids, exercise and laxative use may be monitored during assessment using the chart set out in Figure 7.3. This chart may also be used during treatment to monitor adherence to healthy eating and exercising routines. The questionnaires that assess parental attitudes (included in Table 7.3) may also be used as part of the intake assessment in cases of enuresis. Parents who have particularly negative attitudes, as assessed by these questionnaires are more likely to drop out of treatment, so focusing on modifying parental attitudes may be particularly important in those cases.

Along with the areas addressed in a routine preliminary evaluation (described in Chapter 4) the features set out in Figures 7.4 and 7.5 should be covered in a preliminary interview with cases where elimination problems are the central concern.

Pre-disposing factors for enuresis

From Figure 7.4 it may be seen that genetic vulnerability, urinary tract abnormalities, low functional bladder volume and the possibility of abnormal vasopressin circadian rhythms can all be considered when identifying possible biological pre-disposing factors in cases of enuresis. Psychosocial

	Monday	Tuesday	Wednesday	Thursday	Friday	Saturday	Sunday
Dry and clean at 8.00 a.m.							
Comment on • Size of accident (1–10) • Antecedents • Use of alarm • Consequences							
Dry and clean at 12.00 noon							
Comment on • Size of accident (1–10) • Antecedents • Use of alarm • Consequences							
Dry and clean at 4.00 p.m.							
Comment on • Size of accident (1–10) • Antecedents • Use of alarm • Consequences							
Dry and clean at 8.00 p.m.							
Comment on • Size of accident (1–10) • Antecedents • Use of alarm • Consequences							
Dry and clean at 12.00 midnight							
Comment on • Size of accident (1–10) • Antecedents • Use of alarm • Consequences							
Dry and clean at 4.00 a.m.							
Comment on • Size of accident (1–10) • Antecedents • Use of alarm • Consequences							

Figure 7.2 Parent recording chart for monitoring changes in soiling and/or wetting

pre-disposing factors include the presence of a developmental delay, failure to start toilet training before the critical age of eighteen months and residing in a chaotic family environment.

Precipitating factors for enuresis

While primary enuresis is present from birth, secondary enuresis may be precipitated by biological factors such as a urinary tract infection,

	Monday	Tuesday	Wednesday	Thursday	Friday	Saturday	Sunday
Breakfast Foods Fluids							
Morning Laxatives							
Morning Snack							
Morning Exercise							
Lunch Foods Fluids							
Lunch time Laxatives							
Afternoon Snack							
Afternoon Exercise							
Evening meal Foods Fluids							
Evening time Laxatives							
Evening Snack Pre-bed fluids							
Evening Exercise							

Figure 7.3 Parent recording chart for monitoring diet, fluids, exercise and laxative use

gastrointestinal illness or constipation. Psychosocial precipitating factors include coercive or intrusive toilet training and stressful life events, including sexual abuse, although this may lead to enuresis indirectly by precipitating a urinary tract infection.

Maintaining factors for enuresis

Enuresis may be maintained by children's learned helplessness and low self-efficacy beliefs that the situation cannot be changed by them. It may also be maintained in some instances by negative affectivity. Specifically, anger associated with coercive parent–child interaction or anxiety associated with intrusive interaction relating to urination. Biological factors may also be involved in the maintenance of enuresis and these include urinary tract infections and abnormalities, low functional bladder volume and abnormal vasopressin circadian rhythms.

Table 7.3 Psychometric instruments that may be used as an adjunct to clinical interviews in the assessment of enuresis

Instrument	Publication	Comments
Parental Tolerance Scale	Morgan, R. & Young, G. (1975). Parental attitudes and the conditioning treatment of childhood enuresis. *Behaviour Research and Therapy*, 13, 197–199	This 20-item scale inquiring about beliefs and attitudes concerning enuresis gives an overall index of the degree to which the parent is tolerant or intolerant of the child's enuresis. High intolerance scores are predictive of treatment drop-out
Parental Nuisance Value Scale	Morgan, R. & Young, G. (1975). Parental attitudes and the conditioning treatment of childhood enuresis. *Behaviour Research and Therapy*, 13, 197–199	Parents indicate which of 25 childhood problems are a greater nuisance than enuresis. Where parents view enuresis a greater nuisance than most other childhood problems, there is a greater likelihood of treatment drop-out

Protective factors for enuresis

The probability that an enuresis treatment programme will be effective is influenced by a variety of protective factors associated with the child and the family. It is important that these be assessed and included in the later formulation, since it is protective factors that usually serve as the foundation for therapeutic change. A wish to resolve the toileting problem, an ability to co-operate with the treatment team, positive child and parent adjustment, and good overall marital and family functioning are the main protective factors to consider in cases of enuresis.

Pre-disposing factors in encopresis

Figure 7.5 shows that for encopresis genetic vulnerability, a congenital megarectum, anorectal abnormalities including limited sensations for rectal filling and Hirschsprung's disease are the principal biological pre-disposing factors deserving consideration in a clinical assessment. Important psychosocial pre-disposing factors include the presence of a developmental delay and residing in a chaotic family environment.

Precipitating factors in encopresis

While primary encopresis may be present from birth, secondary encopresis may be precipitated by biological factors such as dietary changes which give

PRE-DISPOSING FACTORS

PERSONAL PRE-DISPOSING FACTORS

Biological factors
- Genetic vulnerabilities
- Urinary tract abnormalities
- Low functional bladder volume
- Abnormal vasopressin circadian rhythms

Psychological factors
- Developmental delay with intellectual or physical disability

CONTEXTUAL PRE-DISPOSING FACTORS

Parent–child factors in early life
- Late to start toilet training

Exposure to family problems in early life
- Family disorganization

PERSONAL MAINTAINING FACTORS

Biological factors
- Urinary tract abnormalities
- Urinary tract infections
- Low functional bladder volume
- Abnormal vasopressin circadian rhythms

Psychological factors
- Aggression towards parents for coercive approach to enuresis
- Anxiety about enuresis due to parents, coercive or intrusive approach to enuresis

PERSONAL PROTECTIVE FACTORS

Biological factors
- Good physical health

Psychological factors
- High IQ
- Easy temperament
- High self-esteem
- Internal locus of control
- High self-efficacy
- Optimistic attributional style
- Mature defence mechanisms
- Functional coping strategies

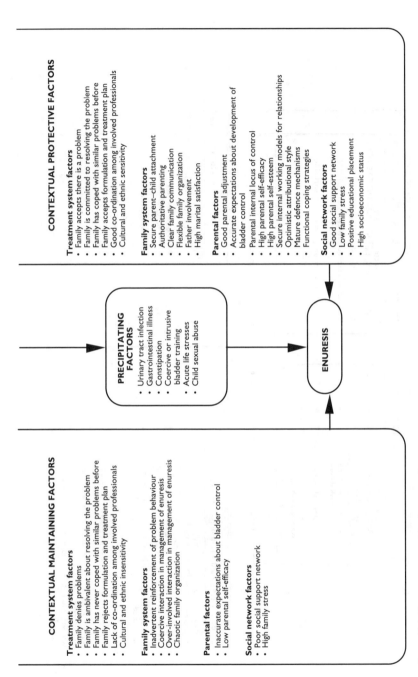

CONTEXTUAL MAINTAINING FACTORS

Treatment system factors
- Family denies problems
- Family is ambivalent about resolving the problem
- Family has never coped with similar problems before
- Family rejects formulation and treatment plan
- Lack of co-ordination among involved professionals
- Cultural and ethnic insensitivity

Family system factors
- Inadvertent reinforcement of problem behaviour
- Coercive interaction in management of enuresis
- Over-involved interaction in management of enuresis
- Chaotic family organization

Parental factors
- Inaccurate expectations about bladder control
- Low parental self-efficacy

Social network factors
- Poor social support network
- High family stress

PRECIPITATING FACTORS
- Urinary tract infection
- Gastrointestinal illness
- Constipation
- Coercive or intrusive bladder training
- Acute life stresses
- Child sexual abuse

ENURESIS

CONTEXTUAL PROTECTIVE FACTORS

Treatment system factors
- Family accepts there is a problem
- Family is committed to resolving the problem
- Family has coped with similar problems before
- Family accepts formulation and treatment plan
- Good co-ordination among involved professionals
- Cultural and ethnic sensitivity

Family system factors
- Secure parent–child attachment
- Authoritative parenting
- Clear family communication
- Flexible family organization
- Father involvement
- High marital satisfaction

Parental factors
- Good parental adjustment
- Accurate expectations about development of bladder control
- Parental internal locus of control
- High parental self-efficacy
- High parental self-esteem
- Secure internal working models for relationships
- Optimistic attributional style
- Mature defence mechanisms
- Functional coping strategies

Social network factors
- Good social support network
- Low family stress
- Positive educational placement
- High socioeconomic status

Figure 7.4 Factors to consider in enuresis

PRE-DISPOSING FACTORS

PERSONAL PRE-DISPOSING FACTORS

Biological factors
- Genetic vulnerabilities
- Congenital megarectum
- Anorectal abnormalities
- Poor sensation of rectal filling
- Hirschprung's disease

Psychological factors
- Developmental delay with intellectual or physical disability

CONTEXTUAL PRE-DISPOSING FACTORS

Parent–child factors in early life
- Parents did not teach bowel control

Exposure to family problems in early life
- Family disorganization

PERSONAL MAINTAINING FACTORS

Biological factors
- Megacolon
- Internal sphincter hypertrophy
- Poor sensation of desire to defecate leading to further constipation and overflow soiling
- Overflow soiling due to laxative use when severely constipated

Psychological factors
- Avoidance of defecation due to fear of anal-fissure-related pain
- Aggression towards parents for coercive approach to encopresis
- Low self-efficacy beliefs and learned helplessness due to failure to resolve encopresis and stigma associated with it

PERSONAL PROTECTIVE FACTORS

Biological factors
- Good physical health

Psychological factors
- High IQ
- Easy temperament
- High self-esteem
- Internal locus of control
- High self-efficacy
- Optimistic attributional style
- Mature defence mechanisms
- Functional coping strategies

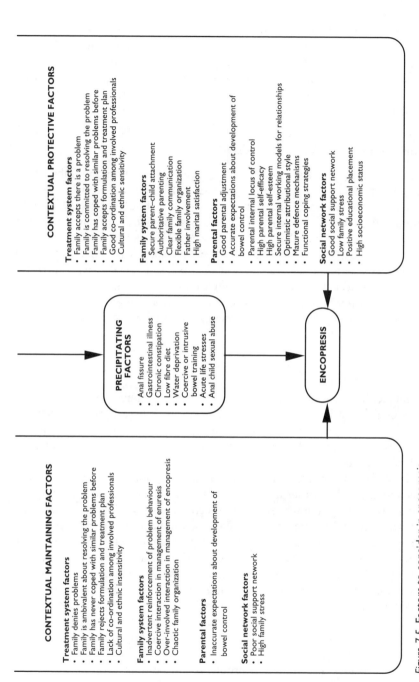

CONTEXTUAL MAINTAINING FACTORS

Treatment system factors
- Family denies problems
- Family is ambivalent about resolving the problem
- Family has never coped with similar problems before
- Family rejects formulation and treatment plan
- Lack of co-ordination among involved professionals
- Cultural and ethnic insensitivity

Family system factors
- Inadvertent reinforcement of problem behaviour
- Coercive interaction in management of enuresis
- Over-involved interaction in management of encopresis
- Chaotic family organization

Parental factors
- Inaccurate expectations about development of bowel control

Social network factors
- Poor social support network
- High family stress

PRECIPITATING FACTORS
- Anal fissure
- Gastrointestinal illness
- Chronic constipation
- Low fibre diet
- Water deprivation
- Coercive or intrusive bowel training
- Acute life stresses
- Anal child sexual abuse

ENCOPRESIS

CONTEXTUAL PROTECTIVE FACTORS

Treatment system factors
- Family accepts there is a problem
- Family is committed to resolving the problem
- Family has coped with similar problems before
- Family accepts formulation and treatment plan
- Good co-ordination among involved professionals
- Cultural and ethnic sensitivity

Family system factors
- Secure parent–child attachment
- Authoritative parenting
- Clear family communication
- Flexible family organization
- Father involvement
- High marital satisfaction

Parental factors
- Good parental adjustment
- Accurate expectations about development of bowel control
- Parental internal locus of control
- High parental self-efficacy
- High parental self-esteem
- Secure internal working models for relationships
- Optimistic attributional style
- Mature defence mechanisms
- Functional coping strategies

Social network factors
- Good social support network
- Low family stress
- Positive educational placement
- High socioeconomic status

Figure 7.5 Factors to consider in encopresis

rise to chronic constipation. Such changes include water deprivation and a low level of fibre. Gastrointestinal illness or an anal fissure may also precipitate overflow incontinence by a process of avoidance conditioning. Psychosocial precipitating factors include coercive or intrusive toilet training and stressful life events, including anal sexual abuse, although this may lead to encopresis indirectly by causing an anal fissure, which in turn leads to avoidance of defecation, constipation and overflow incontinence.

Maintaining factors in encopresis

Encopresis may be maintained by avoidance of defecation and subsequent chronic constipation, poor sensation of rectal filling and overflow soiling possibly associated with occasional laxative use. Encopresis may also be maintained by children's learned helplessness and low self-efficacy beliefs about their ability to resolve their encopresis. The soiling may also be maintained, in some instances, by negative affectivity, specifically anger associated with coercive parent–child interaction or anxiety associated with intrusive interaction relating to defecation. Biological factors such as the presence of a megacolon or internal sphincter hypertrophy may also maintain encopresis.

Protective factors deserving assessment in cases of encopresis are similar to those listed above for enuresis.

Formulation

Salient features from the evaluation interviews and home-monitoring exercises may be integrated into a formulation. Where it is clear that the presentation is monosymptomatic, the discrete programmes for enuresis and encopresis described below are appropriate. In cases where the elimination problem is part of a wider set of adjustment difficulties and problems in the child's social network, treatment should address both the elimination problems and the child's other difficulties. For example, if a child presents with enuresis secondary to a urinary tract infection, and overflow encopresis secondary to an anal fissure, and both of these problems are in turn secondary to chronic sexual abuse, a management programme which addresses the child protection issues (such as that described in Chapter 21) and a medical and psychological treatment programme for the elimination problems may be the most appropriate intervention. If a child with encopresis is being bullied at school and this bullying occurs in the school toilets, school-based intervention to deal with the bullying may be required and additional treatment of the encopresis may be necessary, particularly if constipation has developed.

In most instances, elimination problems can be treated on an outpatient basis. However, where there have been repeated treatment failures, where there are serious medical complications, where an enema under sedation is required and where the parents lack the psychological resources to implement a home-based programme, hospitalization may be necessary.

Creating a facilitative family environment

To maximize the chances of learning bladder- or bowel-control habits, parents must work with the psychologist to create a facilitative environment within which the child can be treated. This is an environment in which parents send the child the message that: (1) they love and respect the child; (2) they see the enuresis or encopresis as a problem which is non-intentional and experienced by the child as uncontrollable; (3) they believe the child has great courage for coping with the elimination problems and has the ability to learn bladder or bowel control by jointly working with the parent and psychologist.

Parents may be coached to follow a number of simple guidelines which help create a facilitative environment. These include spending one period of twenty minutes a day engaged in supportive play following the guidelines set out in Table 4.4 in Chapter 4 (p. 148); reducing other demands and stresses on the child; avoiding criticism, scolding or punishment for lack of bladder or bowel control, or the demands that the enuresis or encopresis programme places on parents and other family members; offering praise and encouragement for progress no matter how small the gains are; helping the child to keep a regular predictable routine for eating, sleeping and exercising; and ensuring that the technical aspects of the programme (such as the urine alarm, laxatives, star charts and other specific elements described below) are all managed as directed by the psychologist.

Where one parent has become embroiled in a battle with the child over bowel or bladder control, it may be easier for all involved if this parent agrees to distance him- or herself from managing the problem and allow the less involved parent to take a more active role. In practice, this often means inviting the child's mother to distance herself from the management of the elimination problem and inviting the child's father to take a more central role (Carr, 1995).

For parents to be able to offer this type of facilitative environment for their child, they must be helped to understand the aetiology of the children's elimination problems and the factors that maintain them, and to give up the idea that elimination problems are an expression of laziness, defiance, attention seeking or an underlying pervasive psychological disorder. Some specific guidelines for educating parents about enuresis and encopresis are given below. In educating parents about the development of bowel and bladder control it is vital to point out that relapses are inevitable; this pre-empts relapse-related demoralization.

For children to be able to respond to this type of facilitating environment, they must be empowered to view the elimination problem as separate from their identity. White (1984) uses the process of externalization to help children do this. He personifies the problem of encopresis by naming it 'sneaky-poo' and then works collaboratively with the child and the parents to help the child master this adversary. This process of externalization is particularly useful for helping children who have developed low self-esteem to reconstruct a view of themselves as good and worthwhile, and the elimination problem as an external stress (a nuisance) with which they must cope with the help of their parents and the psychologist.

Specific treatment programmes that are particularly effective for the management of enuresis and encopresis and which have been well researched will be described below. The likelihood of these programmes being effective is enhanced if they are offered within the context of a facultative environment and as part of a broader multi-systemic package of interventions, in cases where the elimination problem is but one of a wider set of adjustment difficulties. Where children are referred with elimination problems that have failed to respond to the treatments described below, in some instances treatment failure may have arisen from inadequate comprehensive assessment and failure to create a facilitative environment within which to conduct treatment. It is important to highlight this crucial contextual difference, when inviting parents and children to embark, once again, on a programme which they view as having been ineffective.

Treatment of enuresis

Where physical factors, such as urinary tract infections, are implicated in the aetiology of a case of enuresis, these should be treated before psychological intervention is attempted. From a psychological perspective, both nocturnal and diurnal enuresis may be most effectively treated with programmes that have an enuresis alarm as their central component (Houts, 2003). The nocturnal enuresis alarm is a device that includes a pad or mat, which goes under the child's sheet, and a battery-powered alarm bell or buzzer. If the child wets the bed the dampness of the sheet closes a circuit of wires in the pad and the alarm sounds. This leads the child to wake during urination. By a process of conditioning, after a number of trials, the child comes to associate the desire to void the bladder with the process of awakening. For diurnal enuresis, a mini-pad is placed in the underwear and a small vibrating alarm is discretely placed under the clothing in contact with the skin. If the child begins to urinate, the circuit in the pad is closed and the vibrating alarm alerts the child to the necessity to use the bathroom. By a process of conditioning, the desire to urinate comes to be associated with the wish to visit the bathroom.

Treatment with a routine enuresis alarm leads to improvement in 60–90% of cases (Houts, 2003). Treatment failures are due to using an alarm that is not loud enough to awake the child fully, not supervising children urinating in the bathroom following waking and not persisting with the programme for long enough. Usually, between twelve and sixteen weeks treatment is required. The average relapse rate for treatment with an enuresis alarm is about 40%. About 68% of these relapsers can be successfully re-treated. Demoralization following relapse may prevent parents from re-treating their children using the enuresis alarm following treatment. A variety of strategies have been incorporated into pad and bell programmes to decrease the relapse rate to around 20% (Azrin & Besalel, 1979; Azrin, Sneed & Fox, 1974; Houts, 2003). These have included:

- psychoeducation
- rehearsal of toileting
- cleanliness training and reward systems
- retention control training
- over-learning
- dry bed training.

Psychoeducation

The central feature of psychoeducation is that the parents and child must be helped to view the enuresis as a developmental delay: a failure to learn a set of habits due to a delay in the development of the neural pathways that govern bladder control. Where the child presents with secondary enuresis, the idea that physical and psychological stresses can lead to setbacks in normal development that are outside of the child's control may be offered as an explanation for the child's condition. This way of viewing the development of bladder control also offers a rationale for explaining relapses to parents. Pointing out that relapses are inevitable is important, since it pre-empts relapse-related demoralization.

Rehearsal

With rehearsal of toileting, an hour before retiring the child lies on the bed, counts to fifty, walks to the toilet, attempts to urinate and returns to bed. This routine is conducted on the first night of treatment and throughout treatment after each episode of wetting, once the sheets have been changed. It helps the child to develop the habit of visiting the bathroom and urinating.

Cleanliness training and reward systems

Cleanliness training aims to increase the probability that children will avoid bedwetting by reinforcing bladder control and requiring children to take responsibility for managing the consequences of wetting their beds. With cleanliness training, children are required to change their sheets and pyjamas following each episode of wetting. With reward systems, a reward chart, such as that presented in Figure 7.6, is used and children colour in smiling faces for every dry night.

Retention control training

Retention control training aims to help children increase functional bladder capacity while awake, and this in turn is expected to reduce the probability of

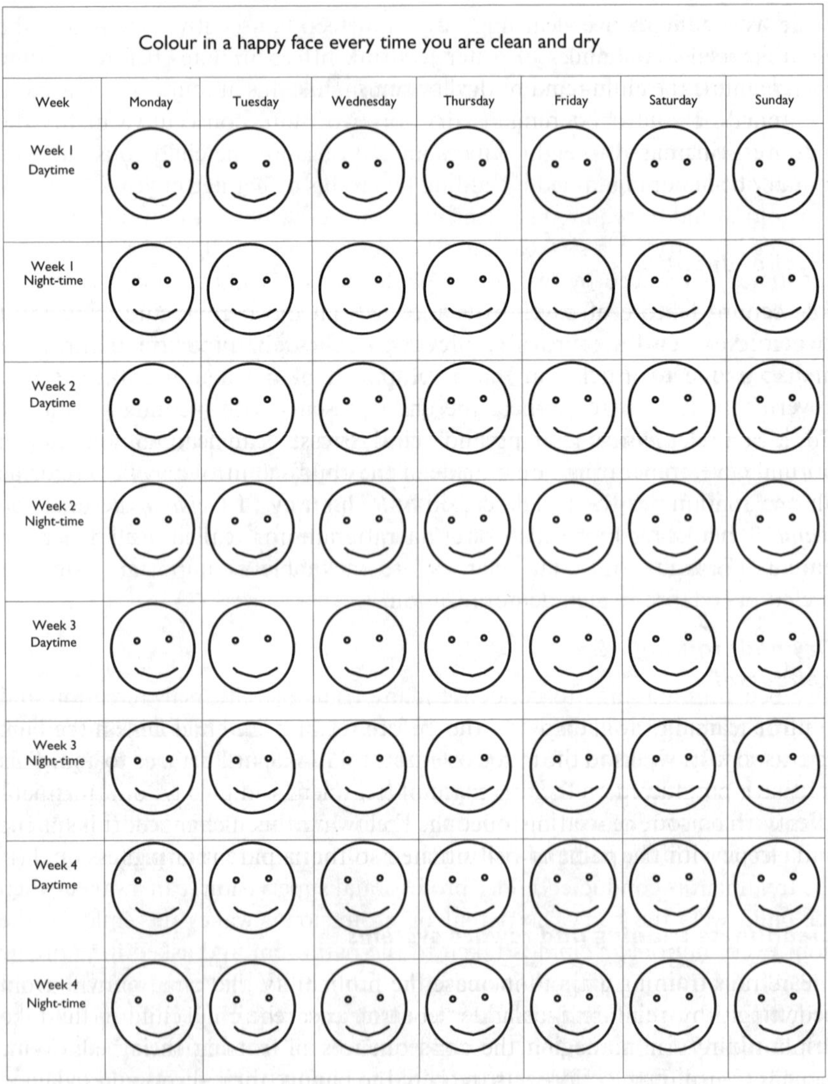

Colour in a happy face every time you are clean and dry							
Week	Monday	Tuesday	Wednesday	Thursday	Friday	Saturday	Sunday
Week 1 Daytime	☺	☺	☺	☺	☺	☺	☺
Week 1 Night-time	☺	☺	☺	☺	☺	☺	☺
Week 2 Daytime	☺	☺	☺	☺	☺	☺	☺
Week 2 Night-time	☺	☺	☺	☺	☺	☺	☺
Week 3 Daytime	☺	☺	☺	☺	☺	☺	☺
Week 3 Night-time	☺	☺	☺	☺	☺	☺	☺
Week 4 Daytime	☺	☺	☺	☺	☺	☺	☺
Week 4 Night-time	☺	☺	☺	☺	☺	☺	☺

Figure 7.6 Child's star chart for enuresis and encopresis

bedwetting. With retention control training, at a preset time each day children are given fluid to drink and asked to tell the parent when they wish to urinate. At this point they are asked to delay urination for three minutes and the next time for six minutes and so on until they can delay for forty-five minutes. For a successful delay the child is given a reward.

Over-learning

Over-learning aims to help children increase functional bladder capacity while asleep. With over-learning, after fourteen consecutive dry nights the child is given four ounces of water to drink fifteen minutes before bedtime each night. If the child remains dry for two nights, this amount is increased to six ounces. If the child remains dry for two more consecutive nights the amount is increased to eight ounces and so on until the child consumes the number of ounces obtained by adding two to his or her age in years. So a six-year-old would be required to drink eight ounces, which is the average normal bladder capacity for a six-year-old. If a wet bed occurs, the amount of water consumed is reduced by two ounces, and then the child gradually increases the amount taken each night by two ounces once two consecutive dry night are achieved. This over-learning procedure stops when fourteen consecutive dry nights are recorded.

Education, cleanliness training and using reward systems, retention control training and over-learning have all been incorporated in a very effective urine alarm programme, which is described in *Bedwetting: A Guide for Parents and Children* (Houts & Liebert, 1984). This programme is called 'Full Spectrum Home Training'.

Dry bed training

Dry bed training aims to condense many trials of rehearsal, retention and control training, awakening to the enuresis alarm and cleanliness training into a very brief period of time (Azrin et al., 1974). With dry bed training, an intensive programme of training occurs on the first night. This begins with twenty trials of rehearsal of toileting. Following this, the child drinks fluids and sleeps with the pad and bell situated so that a parent or professional (if the treatment is conducted under professional supervision) can awaken when the child wets the bed. The parent or professional wakes the child on the hour every hour. The child is taken to the bathroom and asked if he or she can refrain from urinating for one more hour. If so, the child refrains from urinating; if not the child urinates. In either case, the child is given fluids to drink and returns to bed. If the child can refrain from urinating, he or she returns to bed. If the child wets the bed, the parent or professional awakened by the alarm supervises the child changing sheets and pyjamas, and twenty trials of rehearsal of toileting before returning to sleep. Following this night of intensive training, on subsequent nights the child is only woken once per night and no additional fluids are given. On the second night the parents wake the child after two hours and ask him or her to urinate. On the third night this waking occurs at 2.5 hours. Each night the waking time is advanced by thirty minutes if, and only if, the bed is dry. If the child wets twice in one week the schedule is restarted.

Typically, treatment for nocturnal enuresis spans twelve weeks for children who wet once per night and up to sixteen weeks for those who wet more than once per night (Houts, 2003). Parents, either alone or with their children, usually attend a series of ten training and monitoring sessions, with sessions being spaced further apart as treatment progresses. However, in a proportion of cases less intensive contact may lead to good results, provided adequate support materials are provided. Hunt and Adams (1989) showed that parents given well-designed home treatment manuals and a demonstration video pack required less than 2.5 hours of professional input and their children made gains comparable to those of more intensive behavioural programmes.

Treatment of encopresis

Reviews of treatment outcome studies show that joint paediatric and psycho-logical treatment programmes can lead to recovery for up to 77% of children (Buchanan, 1992; Walker, 2003). Treatment should be tailored to target significant pre-disposing or maintaining factors identified in the formulation. The main components of effective treatment programmes are:

- psychoeducation
- clearing the faecal mass
- bowel retraining.

Psychoeducation

With psychoeducation, parents and children must be helped to view the encopresis as a developmental delay or an understandable physical problem. This process is more complex for encopresis than for enuresis since a variety of mechanisms contribute to the problem. First, children may soil if there has been a developmental delay in the maturation of the neural pathways that govern bowel control. These neural pathways can be likened to telephone-lines for explanatory purposes and it may be explained that some children soil because they are not getting the message that they need to defecate. Such neural problems may occur as a result of a specific medical condition, a specific developmental delay or as part of a more general developmental delay. Second, if a child has a large rectum, it can hold many stools and when this occurs the rectum grows larger and develops strong walls. The strong walls do not relax easily. This leads to the gradual development of a hard faecal mass. For explanatory purposes, this may be likened to a traffic-jam. Third, if laxatives are given to treat such chronic constipation, some loosening of the edges of the faecal mass may occur, and this may seep out through the anus unnoticed because the anus may have become insensitive to sensations arising from soft stools, due to the prolonged presence of the large faecal mass; this is overflow incontinence. Fourth, when eventually some large hard faeces are passed, considerable pain may be experienced and in the worst cases an anal fissure develops. This leads to avoidance of defecation, since defecation precipitates immediate and intense pain. Often this avoidance of defecation is experienced as involuntary. Thus, children who are frightened to defecate but have sufficient courage to attempt to do so find that such attempts are futile because the twinges of pain lead to the sphincter contracting. Involuntary inhibition of defecation may also occur secondary to a gastrointestinal illness. Fifth, the stress of chronic constipation, anal discomfort and soiling may lead children and their parents to be bad tempered, to misunderstand each other and to argue about toileting and other issues. The anxiety and anger associated with such conflicts may lead to some loosening of stools and this may seep out around the edge of the faecal mass resulting in further soiling. Sixth, the situation may be made worse if the child eats a low-fibre diet and does not exercise regularly. Often, these dietary and exercise problems occur after the child has developed chronic constipation. Constipated children rarely feel like eating high-fibre food or engaging in vigorous exercise.

Not all of these mechanisms operate in all cases of encopresis. However, offering this type of explanation to parents and children and identifying those processes that are operating in their particular case, may help parents develop sufficient understanding to offer a facilitative environment for the treatment of encopresis. Clayden and Agnarsson's *Information Booklet for Children and Parents* (which is reproduced in Buchanan, 1992) offers a simple account of the processes that contribute to encopresis described above.

In the light of this type of explanation of encopresis, the parent and child may be informed that the most effective treatment is to remove the faecal mass (if one is present) and to use a set of routines to train the child's bowel to work regularly and effectively.

Clearing the faecal mass

The following procedures to clear a faecal mass have been found to be effective as part of a comprehensive management programme (Buchanan, 1992). First, stool softeners may be used (e.g. docusate three times per day). Stool softeners allow the stool to absorb water and gradually become eroded. Second, if the stool is soft but still retained, picosulphate (laxoberal or picolax) may be taken orally to flush out the lower bowel. Picosulphate leads to excess fluid flushing through the intestines and this may sweep the retained stool (softened by the stool softener) ahead of it. Third, regular senna (senokot or senna tablet) may be given daily in a single dose. Senna is a powerful and effective laxative. This may be augmented with lactulose or methyl cellulose to prevent the stools from drying out. Often, children with a tendency towards chronic constipation require regular senna for up to year to prevent a redevelopment of the faecal mass. Fourth, if the faecal mass begins to build up again, picosulphate may be taken at week-ends. The precaution of taking this step at week-ends is necessary since picosulphate may lead to accelerated stools, which are difficult to control and may lead to soiling at school if a toilet is not easily accessible. Finally, if the stool softener (docusate) and picosulphate are insufficient to dissolve and evacuate the faecal mass, an enema with or without sedation may be considered. The use of these various medications and procedures for break down of the faecal mass, is typically managed by a paediatrician or in some instances by the family doctor.

Bowel retraining

Once the faecal mass has been removed (in those cases where one was present) a bowel retraining programme may be followed. Routines for the following four areas should be included in such a programme:

- laxative use
- toileting
- accident management
- diet and exercise.

For all four areas, reward systems using adaptations of the chart presented in Figure 7.6 may be used.

With laxative use, the parents and child, in conjunction with the psychologist and other relevant team members such as paediatrician or family doctor, agree on a regular schedule for laxative use. With children prone to chronic constipation this is essential. The child may colour in a face on the reward chart each time the laxative is successfully taken and this may be accompanied by praise for taking the laxative and also for remembering that it was time to take the laxative if the child indicated that it was the appropriate time for medication.

With toileting, regular times for visiting the toilet and attempting to defecate need to be established. For example, there may be agreement that the child will attend the toilet after each morning and evening meal. A plan for parental supervision of this schedule should be agreed. Where children have developed a fear of visiting the toilet or defecation due to previous painful experiences associated with toileting (such as an anal fissure), a desensitization programme may be necessary, in which the child is trained to relax in the presence of increasingly anxiety-provoking stimuli, such as being outside the bathroom door, being in the bathroom, sitting on the toilet and straining to defecate and so forth. The principles of systematic desensitization are discussed in Chapter 12. Parents may be trained to supervise the implementation of such desensitization programmes.

For both regular toileting and for completing steps in a desensitization programme, a reward chart coupled with praise and encouragement may be used to reinforce appropriate toileting behaviour or successive approximations to proper toilet usage. It is important to reinforce effort (such as visiting the toilet) as well as performance (defecation). So, in cases where desensitization is unnecessary, the child may be given one reward on the chart for visiting the toilet and sitting there for five minutes. Two rewards on the chart may be given for defecation. In cases where desensitization is necessary, a reward on the chart should be given for each step or successive approximation to appropriate toilet use, no matter how small. The reinforcement value of reward charts may be increased by tailoring their design to the children's wishes and interests. For example, youngsters interested in football could be given stickers of football players from their favourite team to stick on the chart, rather than colouring in a smiling face. With young children, advent calendars which contain a series of numbered doors behind which a piece of chocolate is hidden may be used. Parents should be helped to avoid using coercion and punishment since they increase the probability of relapse. Parents should be encouraged to use praise liberally with their children for all approximations to proper toilet usage.

With very young children who are very frightened for sitting on a potty, defecation in a nappy or diaper may initially be rewarded as the first approximation to defecation in a potty. The rationale for beginning shaping by first reinforcing defecation needs to be carefully explained to parents who have inadvertently been reinforcing faecal retention by praising their children for having clean nappies or diapers and punishing them for soiling. With young children, special devices such as musical pots or musical toilet seats may be used to offer immediate reinforcement when a stool is passed. With older children, sitting on the toilet may be made intrinsically reinforcing by providing them with interesting activities such as reading stories, listening to music, or playing hand-held electronic games while sitting on the toilet.

For school-aged children particularly, a routine for accident management needs to be developed. Youngsters should be helped to make a discrete 'clean-up kit' to put in their school bag. This may include clean underwear, tissues, wet-wipes and a plastic bag for storing the soiled underwear.

Where children have constipation problems, a high-fibre diet and six to eight glasses of water per day are essential. Fruit, vegetables and high-fibre breakfast cereals should all be a regular part of the child's diet and each meal should contain a portion of food with a high-fibre content. Foods that slow the movement of the bowels, such as milk and milk-based products, should be taken in moderation. Sweets should be avoided before meals since they reduce appetite and make it difficult for children to eat the high-fibre food essential for good bowel motility. A dietician may be consulted where advice on the development of a high-fibre diet for a specific case, which does not respond to this simple approach, is required. Regular daily exercise increases bowel motility and a schedule of such regular activity should be drawn up in cases where children have developed a sedentary lifestyle. Reward charts may be used to motivate children to adhere to particular dietary and exercise routines.

Biofeedback

In some cases, children may be unable to learn to recognize when they are about to defecate. In such instances biofeedback may be useful adjunct to the programme described here (Olness, McFarland & Piper, 1980).

There is wide variability in the duration of effective treatment for children with encopresis. A good rule of thumb is that an initial series of three or four paediatric appointments are necessary to assess the child's physical health and arrange clearance of the faecal mass. It is useful if the psychologist becomes involved with the parents and child as early as possible and the ideal is for them to be given an initial joint consultation with the paediatrician and psychologist. During this period, the psychologist's main role is to educate the parents and child and build a good working alliance. After initial assessment, between six and ten follow-up appointments with the psychologist focusing on the bowel retraining programme described above is usually required. These appointments may span up to eighteen months, with initial appointments occurring weekly and later appointments occurring less frequently.

SUMMARY

Elimination problems constitute a heterogeneous group of disorders that result from a failure to develop bowel and bladder control in the first five years of life. Enuresis and encopresis may be primary or secondary, occur alone or together, occur diurnally or nocturnally or both, be intentional or unintentional and occur as a monosymptomatic presentation or as part of a wider set of adjustment problems. Under 3% of ten-year-olds have elimination problems and their prevalence reduces markedly over adolescence. Hypotheses derived from biological, developmental, psychopathological, psychodynamic, behavioural and family systems theories have inspired most of the research on elimination disorders. Both biological and psychosocial pre-disposing factors have been identified for the elimination disorders and these include structural and functional urethral and anorectal abnormalities, developmental delays and a chaotic family environment. Biological and psychosocial precipitating factors have also been identified, with urinary tract infections or chronic constipation falling into the former category and life stresses including sexual abuse falling into the latter category. Both biological and psychological factors may maintain elimination problems. With enuresis, chief among these are urinary tract infections, failure to become conditioned to recognize bladder filling as a discriminative stimulus for toileting and negative parent–child interactions. A multi-disciplinary programme that aims to resolve physical problems and arrange appropriate family work and home-based conditioning is the treatment of choice for enuresis. Secondary encopresis, which is by far the most common, is typically maintained by a vicious cycle of toilet avoidance, chronic constipation and overflow incontinence along with low self-efficacy and negative parent–child interactions. A multi-disciplinary programme which aims to resolve the constipation and arrange appropriate family work and home-based conditioning is the treatment of choice for encopresis.

EXERCISE 7.1

Terry, aged seven, has been referred for consultation because of soiling and wetting problems. He wets his bed a few nights per week and soils his pants during the day. The soiling mainly occurs at week-ends. Both problems are increasing tensions within the family. Terry is the eldest of five children and lives with his mother and step-father in a rented apartment. His mother has a history of depression and has been treated with antidepressants by the family doctor on a number of occasions.

- Draw up a preliminary formulation or hypothesis.
- How would you assess this case?
- What difficulties would you expect to encounter during assessment and treatment?
- How would you manage these?

FURTHER READING

Buchanan, A. (1992). *Children Who Soil. Assessment and Treatment*. Chichester: Wiley.
Herbert, M. (1996). *Toilet Training, Bedwetting and Soiling*. Leicester: British Psychological Society.

FURTHER READING FOR PARENTS AND CHILDREN

Azrin, N. & Besalel, V. (1979). *A Parent's Guide to Bedwetting Control*. New York: Simon & Schuster.

Clayden, G. & Agnarsson, V. (1992). *Constipation in Childhood: Information Booklet for Children and Parents*. In Appendix A of: Buchanan, A. (1992). *Children Who Soil. Assessment and Treatment*. Chichester: Wiley.

Houts, A. & Liebert, R. (1985). *Bedwetting: A Guide for Parents and Children*. Springfield, II: Charles C Thomas.

Galvin, M. & Ferrero, S. (1991). *Clouds and Clocks: A Story for Children Who Soil*. Washington, DC: Magination Press.

WEBSITES

Education and Resources for Improving Childhood Continence (ERIC): http://www.eric.org.uk/

Factsheets on wetting and soiling can be downloaded from the website for Rose, G. & York, A. (2004). *Mental Health and Growing Up. Fact sheets for Parents, Teachers and Young People* (Third edition). London: Gaskell: http://www.rcpsych.ac.uk

Chapter 8

Intellectual, learning and communication disabilities

This chapter considers intellectual, learning and communication disabilities. The ways in which problems in these areas are classified in DSM IV TR (APAa, 2000) and ICD 10 (WHO, 1992, 1996) are set out in Figures 8.1 and 8.2. Both systems distinguish between general intellectual disabilities (or mental retardation) on the one hand and all other learning and communication problems on the other. Indeed, in both systems, intellectual disability (or mental retardation) is coded on a separate axis. Both systems also distinguish between specific communication disorders and other specific learning disorders associated with the development of academic and motor skills. Finally, both systems distinguish between learning problems that have been present from birth and acquired learning problems, of which those associated with head injury are probably the most important in clinical practice with children and adolescents. Finer distinctions made within the ICD and DSM systems for the sub-typing of learning and communication problems will be discussed in subsequent sections of this chapter.

The chapter is organized as follows. Accounts of clinical features, epidemiology, outcome, aetiology and *specific* approaches to assessment and intervention will be given for each of the following four clusters of problems:

- intellectual disabilities
- specific developmental language delays
- specific learning disabilities
- acquired learning difficulties that may follow from traumatic brain injury.

The chapter will close with a discussion of *general* principles that apply to the use of psychometric tests in clinical practice and a consideration of prevention.

In deciding on the level of detail to include in this chapter, account has been taken of the way in which many professional training programmes in clinical psychology are structured in Ireland and the UK. In addition to a course on child and adolescent clinical psychology, for which books like this are the major text, students usually complete additional courses on

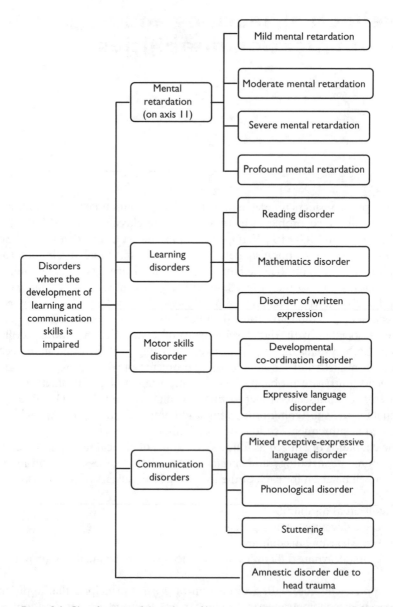

Figure 8.1 Classification of disorders of learning and communication in DSM IV TR

intellectual disability (O'Reilly et al., 2005), psychological testing (Sattler, 2001a,b; Sattler & Dumont, 2004) and neuropsychology (Reynolds & Ray, 1997). The information presented in this chapter is intended as a very brief supplement to these other courses.

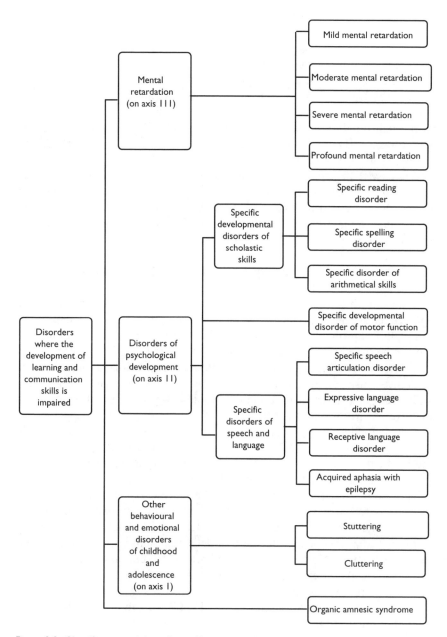

Figure 8.2 Classification of disorders of learning and communication in ICD 10

INTELLECTUAL DISABILITY

A case of intellectual disability (ID), of the type often seen in child and family psychology clinics, is presented in Box 8.1. In this chapter the term 'intellectual disability' will be used to refer to what is called 'mental retardation' in parts of the USA, 'learning difficulties' in the UK, and 'mental handicap' in parts of Ireland and elsewhere. A thorough discussion of the evolution of the term 'intellectual disability' is given in Parmenter (2001). Table 8.1 presents definitions of ID from three widely used classification systems: ICD 10 (WHO, 1996), DSM IV TR (APA, 2000a) and AAMR 10 (Luckasson et al., 2002). AAMR 10 is the tenth revision of the American Association for Mental Retardation's manual – *Mental retardation: definition, classification and systems of support* (Luckasson et al., 2002). Also included in the table in the column summarizing the ICD 10 definition of ID is reference to the disability model described in the World Health Organization's International Classification of Functioning, Disability and Health (ICF; WHO, 2001).

Deficits in both intellectual functioning and adaptive behaviour are central to the definitions of ID in all the three systems in Table 8.1. In addition to these deficits, the criterion that the diagnosis of ID be made before the age of eighteen is specified in the DSM and AAMR, but not ICD definition, although it is probably implicit in the ICD system. There is also an acceptance in the three systems that functional deficits are indicated by scores of 70 or below on reliable and valid appropriately standardized psychometric assessment instruments. A list of widely used intelligence tests for people of different ages is given in Table 8.2. Table 8.3 gives a list of widely used adaptive behaviour scales.

Explicit models of key factors that affect functioning in people with ID have been offered by the World Health Organization in the ICF (WHO, 2001) and by the AAMR 10. In the ICF model, levels of functioning and disability are conceptualized as being determined by health status (disease of disorders), bodily functions and structures (impairments), activity limitations, restrictions to participation in community life, and environmental barriers and hindrances. Within the AAMR 10 model, a person's level of functioning is conceptualized as being affected by intellectual abilities; adaptive behaviour; participation, interactions and social roles in the community; health; and the wider social context. The impact of these five factors on functioning is mediated by the availability of supports.

The following ranges are used in DSM IV TR for sub-classification of ID by level of intellectual functioning:

- mild: IQ level 50–55 to 70 (approximately)
- moderate: IQ level 35–40 to 50–55
- severe: IQ level 20–25 to 35–40
- profound: IQ level below 20–25.

Box 8.1 A case of intellectual disability

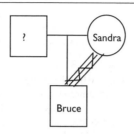

?   Sandra

Bruce

Bruce, aged seven, was referred by his teacher because of concerns about his lack of academic progress and conduct problems. Bruce was the only child in a single-parent family, that had moved to the district three years previously. His unemployed mother, Sandra, was known to Social Services and there had been an ongoing concern that Bruce may have been at risk for neglect. Records from Sandra's previous health district indicated that, while in secondary school, she had been psychologically assessed and found to be functioning in the IQ range of 50–70, associated with mild intellectual disability. Sandra and Bruce lived in a council apartment where the preliminary assessment was conducted. The family's living arrangements were chaotic, with no routines for eating, sleeping, management of finances, punctual school attendance, baby-sitting or hygiene. Sandra found coping with Bruce extremely challenging, although the mother and child had a strong mutual attachment.

A psychometric evaluation of Bruce showed that on the WISC-IV he had a Full Scale IQ of 68 with an unremarkable sub-test profile. On the Wide Range Achievement Test-1 I I, he obtained reading, spelling and arithmetic scores which fell below the second percentile and were, therefore consistent with his overall level of ability. On both the Child Behaviour Checklist and the Teacher Report Form, Bruce's scores on the Externalizing Scale fell above the 98th percentile, confirming the presence of clinically significant conduct problems both at home and at school. On the Adaptive Behaviour Scale (School Edition), independent functioning and communication were the two principal areas in which adaptive behaviour deficits were detected.

Taken together, these results indicated that Bruce had a mild intellectual disability characterized by difficulties in the areas of academic attainment, independent functioning, communication and controlling aggression and destructiveness.

Bruce was living within an isolated single-parent family, and while his mother provided emotional care, she needed a substantial amount of support to be able to provide Bruce with the supervision, structure and intellectual stimulation required for him to function optimally. Arrangements were made for Sandra to receive behavioural parent training to manage Bruce's aggression at home and to develop play routines so that she could meet Bruce's need for intellectual stimulation. In addition, a home-help was organized to offer support with household management. At school, a curriculum more closely suited to Bruce's ability level was selected.

Ongoing interagency liaison with Social Services was arranged, since Social Services continued to monitor the family for child protection risk.

Table 8.1 Diagnostic criteria for intellectual disability

ICD 10/ICF	DSM IV TR	A AMR 10
For a definite diagnosis of mental retardation there should be a: (A) reduced level of intellectual functioning resulting in (B) diminished ability to adapt to the daily demands of the normal social environment. The assessment of intellectual level should be based on clinical observation, standardized ratings of adaptive behaviour and psychometric test performance. **Mild mental retardation** • An IQ of between 50 and 69 • A mental age of 9 to 12 years in adults. Children may have some learning difficulties in school • Many adults will be able to work, maintain good social relationships and contribute to society **Moderate mental retardation** • An IQ of between 35 and 49 • A mental age of 6 to 9 years in adults. Most children will show marked developmental delays but most can learn to develop some degree of independence in self-care and acquire adequate communication and academic skills	Mental retardation: A. Significantly subaverage mental functioning shown by an IQ of approximately 70 or below on an individually administered IQ test (for infants, a clinical judgement of significantly subaverage intellectual functioning) B. Concurrent deficits or impairments in present adaptive functioning (i.e. the person's effectiveness in meeting the standards expected for his age or her age by his or her cultural group) in at least two of the following areas: • communication • self-care • home living • social–inter-personal skills • use of community resources • self-direction • functional academic skills • work • leisure • health and safety C. The onset is before 18 years of age Code as: Mild: IQ level 50–55 to 70 (approx) Moderate: IQ level 35–40 to 50–55	Mental retardation is a disability characterized by significant limitations both in: (A) intellectual functioning and in (B) adaptive behaviour as expressed in conceptual, social, and practical adaptive skills (C) this disability originates before age 18 For a diagnosis there must be: • A standardized intelligence test score 2 standard deviations below the mean • A standardized rating of adaptive behaviour in one or more domains (conceptual social or practical) 2 standard deviations below the mean Five assumptions are entailed by this definition: 1. Limitations in present functioning must be considered within the context of community environments typical of the individual's age peers and culture 2. Valid assessment considers cultural and linguistic diversity as well as differences in communication, sensory, motor and behavioural factors 3. Within an individual, limitations often co-exist with strengths 4. An important purpose of describing limitations is to develop a profile of needed supports

- Adults will need varying degrees of support to live in the community

Severe mental retardation

- An IQ of between 20 and 34
- A mental age of 3 to 6 years
- Likely to result in continuous need for support

Profound mental retardation

- An IQ of below 20
- A mental age less than 3 in adults
- Severe limitation in self-care, continence, communication and mobility

Model of intellectual disability

In ICF functioning and level of disability are determined by:

- Health status (disease of disorder)
- Bodily functions and structures (impairments)
- Activities (limitations)
- Participation (restrictions)
- Environmental factors (barriers and hindrances)
- Personal factors (demographic profile)

Diagnosis coded on Axis III for children
Diagnosis coded on Axis I for adults

Severe: IQ level 20–25 to 35–40
Profound: IQ level below 20–25.

Diagnosis coded on Axis II

5. With appropriate personalized supports over a sustained period, the life functioning of the person with mental retardation generally will improve

Model of intellectual disability

The definition is based on a model in which level of individual functioning is defined by status on 5 factors:

- intellectual abilities
- adaptive behaviour
- participation, interactions and social roles
- health
- social context

The impact of these five factors on functioning is mediated by supports

Note: Adapted from DSM IV TR (APA, 2000a), ICD 10 (WHO, 1996), ICF (WHO, 2001) and AAMR 10 (Luckasson et al., 2002).

In the DSM, but not the ICD system, category boundaries have bandwidths of five points to take account of test measurement error. In the AAMR 10 system, it is possible to classify cases in a variety of ways depending on the function of classification. For service development and interprofessional communication, it may be appropriate to classify by level of disability (mild, moderate, severe or profound). For research purposes, it may be appropriate

Table 8.2 Psychometric instruments for the assessment of intelligence and general cognitive abilities

Age range where instrument is particularly useful	Instrument	Comments
Infancy	Bailey, N. (1993). *Bailey's Scales II*. San Antonio, TX: Psychological Corporation	• It yields scores on mental and motor development scales and includes an infant behaviour record • Contains over 100 items and requires about an hour to administer • Standardized in the US on children age 1–42 months
	Huntley, M. (1996). *Griffiths Mental Development Scales from Birth to Two Years*. UK. Association for Research on Infant and Child Development Griffiths, R. (1970). *Griffiths Mental Development Scales*. High Wycombe, Bucks: Test Agency	• Yields a general quotient and six sub-scale scores: locomotor; personal–social; hearing and speech; eye and hand co-ordination; performance; and practical reasoning • Contains over 100 items and takes about an hour to administer • Standardized in the UK on children aged 1 month to 8 years
Toddlers under 5	McCarthy, D. (1972). *McCarthy Scales of Children's Abilities*. San Antonio: Psychological Corporation	• Yields scores on a general scale and five sub-scales (verbal; perceptual-performance; quantitative; memory and motor) • Contains 18 tests and takes about an hour to administer • Standardized in the US on children 2.5–8.5 years
	Kaufman, A. & Kaufman, N. (2004). *Kaufman Assessment Battery for Children. Second Edition (KABC-II)*. Circle Pines, MN: American Guidance Service	• Yields scores for components of both the Luria neuropsychological model and the Cattell–Horn–Carroll model • On the Luria model gives an index of overall intelligence and non-verbal intelligence as well as four scale scores (sequential processing; simultaneous processing; planning ability; learning ability)

	Wechsler, D. (2003). *Wechsler Preschool and Primary Scale of Intelligence-III (WPPSI-III)*. San Antonio, TX: Psychological Corporation	• On the Cattell–Horn–Carroll model gives an overall fluid crystallized index and a non-verbal index as well as five sub-scale scores (visual procession, short-term memory, fluid reasoning, long-term storage and retrieval and crystallized ability) • Contains many sub-tests and takes an hour to administer • Standardized in the US on children aged 2.5–18 years
	Wechsler, D. (2004). *Wechsler Preschool and Primary Scale of Intelligence-III UK (WPPSI-III)*. San Antonio, TX: Psychological Corporation	• Validated in the US and UK • For children aged between 2:6 and 3:11, 4 core sub-tests and 1 supplemental sub-test taking 25–35 minutes to administer yield a full scale IQ, verbal IQ, and performance IQ • For children aged between 4:0 and 7:3, 7 core sub-tests and 5 supplemental sub-tests taking 40–50 minutes to administer yield a full scale IQ, verbal IQ, performance IQ and a Processing Speed Quotient
Under 5s (but also over 5s and adolescents)	Elliott, C. (1996). *British Ability Scales. Second Edition. (BAS II)*. Windsor: NFER Nelson	• Yields index of intelligence, reading, spelling, arithmetic and various cognitive skills • Contains 21 sub-tests and brief or long versions may be administered • Standardized in the UK on children aged 2–18 years
	Roid, G. (2003) *Stanford-Binet Intelligence Scales, Fifth Edition (SB-V)*. Itasca, IL Riverside Publishing. http://www.riverpub.com/products/clinical/sbis/home.html	• Yields a full scale IQ, verbal and non-verbal IQ and scores on five factors – Fluid Reasoning, Knowledge, Quantitative Reasoning, Visual–Spatial Processing, and Working Memory • Contains 10 sub-tests • Normed on a stratified random sample of 4800 individuals that matches the 2000 US Census

Continued

Table 8.2 Continued

Age range where instrument is particularly useful	Instrument	Comments
Children over 6 and adolescents	Wechsler, D. (1991). *Wechsler Intelligence Scale for Children. Third Edition (WISC-III).* San Antonio, TX: Psychological Corporation Wechsler, D. (1992). *Wechsler Intelligence Scale for Children. Third Edition UK (WISC-III^uk).* San Antonio, TX: Psychological Corporation	• Validated in US and UK • Yields a full scale IQ and verbal and performance IQs • Also yields four factor scores (verbal comprehension; perceptual organization; freedom from distractibility and processing speed) • Contains 13 sub-tests and takes about an hour to administer
	Wechsler, D. (2003). *Wechsler Intelligence Scale for Children. Fourth Edition (WISC-IV).* San Antonio, TX: Psychological Corporation Wechsler, D. (2004). *Wechsler Intelligence Scale for Children. Fourth Edition UK (WISC-IV^uk).* San Antonio, TX: Psychological Corporation	• Validated in the US and UK • Designed to incorporate advances in theoretical ideas on intelligence, the WISC-IV contains 11 core sub-tests and 5 supplemental sub-tests • Yields a full scale IQ, a verbal comprehension index, a perceptual reasoning index, a working memory index, and a processing speed index
Adolescents and adults	Wechsler, D. (1999). *Wechsler Adult Intelligence Scale – Third Edition (WAIS-III).* San Antonio, TX: Psychological Corporation Wechsler, D. (1999). *Wechsler Adult Intelligence Scale – Third Edition (WAIS-III^uk).* San Antonio, TX: Psychological Corporation	• Validated in the US and UK • Yields a full scale IQ and verbal and performance IQs • Contains 12 sub-tests and takes about an hour to administer
	Weschler, D. (1999). *Wechsler Abbreviated Scale of Intelligence. (WASI).* San Antonio, TX: Psychological Corporation	• Validated in the US • Normed for people 6–89 years • Yields a full scale IQ and verbal and performance IQs • Contains 4 sub-tests: Vocabulary, Similarities, Block Design, and Matrix Reasoning: • 4-sub-test from takes 30 min to administer and 2-sub-test form can be administered in 15 min.

Table 8.3 Psychometric instruments for the assessment of adaptive behaviour

Instrument	Comments
Lambert, N., Nihira, K. & Leyland, H. (1993). *Adaptive Behaviour Scale-School Version Second Edition*. Washington, DC: AAMR Nihira, K., Leyland, H. & Lambert, N. (1993). *Adaptive Behaviour Scale-Residential and Community Version Second Edition*. Austin, TX: Pro-ed	• Yields scores in multiple adaptive behaviour domains (e.g. independent functioning, physical development, economic activity) and problem behaviour domains (e.g. violent or destructive behaviour) • Standardized in the US on large population of 3- to 69-year-olds • Contains over 100 items and takes 30 minutes for a parent or caretaker to complete
Sparrow, S., Balla, D. & Cicchetti, D. (1984). *Vineland Adaptive Behaviour Scales*. Pine Circles, MN: American Guidance Service	• Yields scores in four domains: communication; daily living skills; socialization; and motor skills. The expanded version also includes a maladaptive behaviour domain • Standardized in the US on a population of 3000 0- to 19-year-olds • There are three versions: survey form; expanded form and classroom edition • The expanded form contains over 500 items and takes an hour for a parent or caretaker to complete. The other two forms contain between 200 and 300 items and take about 30 minutes to complete
Bruininks, R., Woodcock, R., Weatherman, R. & Hill, B. (1996). *Scales of Independent Behaviour – Revised*. Ithaca, IL: Riverside	• Yields scores on multiple adaptive behaviour sub-scales grouped into four domains (motor; social interaction and communication; personal living and community living) and 8 maladaptive behaviour sub-scales grouped into three domains (internalized behaviour problems; externalized behaviour problems and social maladaptive behaviour) • Standardized in the US on children and adults • Contains over 300 items and takes an hour for a parent or caretaker to complete. There is a 32-item short form, which can be completed in 10 minutes. There is also an early development form • The scale is a component of the Woodcock Johnson Psychoeducational Battery
Adams, G. (1999). *Comprehensive Test of Adaptive Behaviour – Revised*. Seattle, WA: Educational Achievement Systems. http://www.edresearch.com	• Yields scores for self-help skills, home living skills, independent living, social skills, sensory and motor skills, language and academic skills • Normed on large USA sample of children and adults • Contains 495 male and 523 female items and yields scores on adaptive behaviour and problematic behaviour and can be completed using data from teachers and parents or carers

Continued

Table 8.3 Continued

Instrument	Comments
Harrison, P. & Oakland, T. (2000). *ABAS. Adaptive Behaviour Assessment System.* San Antonio, TX: Psychological Corporation	• Yields scores for 10 DSM IV specified areas of adaptive behaviour: communication, functional academics, health and safety, self-care, social, community use, home living, leisure, self-direction and work • Normed on large USA sample of children and adults • Scores are linked to WISC III and WAIS III

to classify cases by aetiology. For placement within residential care facilities, it may be appropriate to classify by level of adaptive behaviour. For service funding, it may be appropriate to classify by level of support required (intermittent, limited, extensive or pervasive).

Epidemiology

Using a criterion of an IQ below 70 and impaired adaptive behaviour, the overall prevalence of ID is between 1 and 3% (Fryers, 2000; Volkmar & Dykens, 2002). About 85% of people with ID fall into the mild range, 10% into the moderate range, 3–4% into the severe range and 1–2% into the profound range. These figures are based on epidemiological community surveys. Typically administrative prevalence rates are lower than those from such surveys. For example the national administrative prevalence of ID in Ireland in the year 2000 was 0.7% and of these cases 41% had mild disabilities, 36% moderate, 15% severe and 4% profound (Mulvaney, 2000). Clearly, many cases of mild ID went undetected in Ireland in 2000. Autism and other pervasive developmental disorders, psychoses, disruptive behaviour disorders, especially attention deficit hyperactivity disorder (ADHD), challenging behaviour, epilepsy, and sensory and motor impairments are all far more common among people with intellectual disabilities (Carr & O'Reilly, 2005). The best prognosis occurs for people with mild disabilities and good adaptive behavioural skills who have few co-morbid difficulties and come from stable families and contexts within which there is a good deal of support (Dosen & Day, 2001; Kaski, 2000; Volkmar & Dykens, 2002).

Clinical features

Children with mild, moderate, severe and profound intellectual disabilities have different profiles of clinical features in terms of IQ and adaptive behaviour.

Mild ID

These children have IQs below about 70 and above 50–55, and comparable levels of adaptive behaviour deficits. They are slower to develop communication and adaptive behavioural skills during their pre-school years than children of normal ability. However, by five years of age they can interact socially with a degree of competence. They show little significant sensorimotor impairment. However, during their primary school years they show significant difficulties in acquiring academic skills, such as those required for reading, writing and arithmetic. It is often because of these difficulties that they are referred for psychological assessment. Unlike children with specific learning disabilities, such as dyslexia, children with mild intellectual disabilities have pervasive rather than circumscribed academic difficulties and their overall IQ falls below 70. In contrast, children with specific learning disabilities have IQs above 70 and circumscribed academic difficulties. With sufficient educational supports most children and adolescents with mild intellectual disabilities can develop some academic and vocational skills.

Moderate ID

These children have IQs above 35–40 and below 50–55 and comparable levels of adaptive behaviour deficits. They show a significant developmental delay in the acquisition of gross motor, fine sensorimotor, communication and adaptive behavioural skills during the pre-school years, which often leads to a referral for psychological assessment. During their childhood years some develop skills to interact socially with adults and peers with a degree of competence, while others have great difficulty developing such skills throughout their lives. During their primary school years they show significant difficulties in acquiring basic academic skills. With sufficient educational supports and an appropriate curriculum, some children and adolescents with moderate intellectual disabilities can develop some academic and vocational skills.

Severe ID

These children have IQs above 20–25 and below 35–40. They also have comparable levels of adaptive behaviour deficits. They show a pronounced developmental delay in the acquisition of gross motor, fine sensorimotor, communication and adaptive behaviour skills during the pre-school years. This often leads to a referral for psychological assessment prior to three years of age. During their primary school years some develop skills to interact socially with adults and peers, whereas others have great difficulty developing such skills throughout their lives. During their primary school years the focus is appropriately on acquiring adaptive behavioural skills rather than academic skills. With sufficient educational supports and an appropriate curriculum, some adolescents with severe intellectual disabilities can develop a small reading vocabulary, which is useful for interpreting public signs or notices.

Profound ID

These children have IQs below 20–25. They show a very marked developmental delay in the acquisition of gross motor, fine sensorimotor, communication and adaptive behavioural skills. This usually leads to a referral for psychological assessment prior to three years of age. Because of restricted mobility, incontinence and difficulty acquiring communication skills, as children, adolescents and adults, people with profound disabilities usually require intensive supports to maximize their quality of life. A highly structured environment with an individualized relationship with a caregiver is an appropriate level of support for people with severe ID.

Aetiology

Historically, in what has come to be termed the 'two group' approach, children with intellectual disabilities were classified into those whose ID was due to known organic causes, such as Down syndrome, and those where it was assumed that social disadvantage was the primary aetiological factor (Kaski, 2000; Volkmar & Dykens, 2002). Within this system, the 'organic' group tended to have more severe intellectual disabilities than the 'environmental' group. The former were typically classified as having moderate, severe or profound intellectual disabilities, and the latter as having mild disabilities. However, for many cases a range of biomedical and psychosocial risk factors that occur during the pre-natal, peri-natal and post-natal period may be identified (Friedman & Chase-Lansdale, 2002; Kaski, 2000, Luckasson et al., 2002; Volkmar & Dykens, 2002).

Biological aetiological factors

ID may be caused by genetically determined syndromes with behavioural phenotypes of which Down syndrome and fragile X syndrome are by far the most common. Metabolic disorders such as phenylketonuria and congenital hypothyroidism may contribute to the development of intellectual disability. Fortunately, both of these can be treated: hypothyroidism with thyroxine and PKU with a diet low in phenylalanine. Increasing maternal age (over thirty years) and maternal illness, particularly HIV infection, hepatitis, rubella, diabetes, cytomegalovirus (which causes inflammation of brain tissue), toxoplasmosis (which destroys brain tissue) and bacterial meningitis are risk factors for ID, as is maternal exposure to potential toxins such as lead or radiation. During the peri-natal period, prematurity, low birth weight, birth injury, and neo-natal disorders are all significant risk factors for delayed cognitive development. Important neo-natal disorders include seizures, infections, respiratory distress or anoxia indicated by low Apgar scores, or brain haemorrhage. The infant's post-natal medical status is typically expressed as an Apgar score. Apgar scores range from 0 to 10, with scores below 4 reflecting sufficient difficulties to warrant intensive care. The score is based on an evaluation of the infant's skin colour (with blue suggesting anoxia), respiration, heart rate, muscle tone, and response to stimulation. After birth, ID may be caused by many factors including traumatic brain injury, malnutrition, seizure disorders and by degenerative disorders (Goodman, 2002). Identifying specific aetiological biomedical factors is important for good clinical practice. In some instances, such as PKU or hypothyroidism, ID may be prevented. In cases where ID is associated with a particular syndrome or behavioural phenotype, then information on the course and outcome for the condition may be used in planning supports. Genetic counselling may be given to families in instances where there is evidence for the role of genetic factors in the aetiology of ID. Also, families may benefit from membership of support groups formed specifically for parents of children with particular syndromes.

Psychosocial aetiological factors

Poverty; maternal malnutrition; lack of access to pre-natal and birth care; disorganized parental behaviour; parental drug, alcohol and nicotine use; domestic violence; child abuse and neglect; inadequate child education and parental support and institutional upbringing are important psychosocial social risk factors for intellectual disability (Friedman & Chase-Lansdale, 2002). Pre-, peri- and post-natal family supports, therapy, parent training and child stimulation may modify the impact of these risk factors (Lange & Carr, 2002; O'Sullivan & Carr, 2002).

Assessment and differential diagnosis

The process of assessment and diagnosis of ID is usually carried out by a multi-disciplinary team, which may include members of the following professions: paediatrics; nursing; clinical, educational or school psychology; speech and language therapy; teaching; psychiatry; neurology; social work; occupational therapy and physiotherapy. The composition of the assessment team, the way clinical and administrative responsibilities are shared within teams and the way people are referred for assessment will vary, depending on local practices; health, education and social service systems and overall policies and legislation, all of which vary from one jurisdiction to another. For clinical psychologists in training, it is important when working on a disability placement or internship to find out how local guidelines are used to implement national policies. For qualified professionals it is vital to keep abreast of changes in policy, practices and funding systems for people with disabilities.

In some instances, the risk of ID will be detected through post-natal screening procedures and it may be possible to prevent the development of ID. For example, in Ireland, the UK and many other countries, a test for PKU is routinely conducted shortly after the child is born, since, as has been previously mentioned, early detection of this disorder permits the prevention of ID through dietary intervention. In clinical practice the range of disorders to include in the differential diagnosis depends on the degree of ID, the presence and extent of co-morbid physical and mental health problems, the age of the client, and the observational skills and communication skills of the client's primary carers. Children with specific syndromes that have distinctive clinical features such as Down syndrome, children with low birth weight, distress at birth, sensory or motor disabilities or severe ID will be detected early, usually by a paediatrics service through observation and monitoring of attainment of sensorimotor milestones. As part of the differential diagnostic process, psychologists may need to make distinctions between ID, language delay and specific learning disabilities. They may also need to decide in specific cases if co-morbid disorders are present, notably autism, ADHD and epilepsy.

ID versus language delay

Once there is evidence of a developmental delay, to determine whether it is a specific language delay or a general delay in cognitive development, formal psychological assessment of intellectual abilities, adaptive behaviour and language development may be conducted and repeated at six-monthly or annual intervals, coupled with direct observation of the child and interviews with parents. Where test scores, clinical observations and data from parental interviews consistently indicate an IQ below 70 and deficits in adaptive behaviour, then a diagnosis of ID may be made. Where children have sensory and motor deficits, psychometric instruments listed in Table 8.4 may be used. With developmental language delay or motor delay, the child shows delayed development in a circumscribed area but age-appropriate development in other areas. This may be indicated by a major discrepancy of one or two standard deviations between scores on a standardized language test such as the *Reynell Developmental Language Scales. III*, listed in Table 8.6, and scores which fall in the normal range on a non-verbal test of general intelligence such as the *Leiter International Performance Scale – Revised*, listed in Table 8.4. The diagnostic criteria for developmental language delay are given in Table 8.5.

ID versus specific learning disabilities

School-aged children or adolescents with mild or moderate intellectual disabilities that have gone undiagnosed during the pre-school years, are typically

Table 8.4 Instruments for assessing children with motor and sensory impairments

Disability	Assessment instruments	Comments
Motor disability	Verbal subtests of WPPSI-III; WISC-III; WISC-IV; WAIS-III & SB-V	• Gives verbal IQ or estimate of Full Scale IQ
	Dunn, L. & Dunn, L. (1981). *Peabody Picture Vocabulary Test-Revised.* Circle Pines: MN: American Guidance Service	• Yields measure of receptive language
Hearing disability	Performance subtests of WPPSI-III; WISC-III; WISC-IV; WAIS-III & SB-V	• Gives non-verbal IQ or estimate of Full Scale IQ
	Roid, G. & Miller, L. (1997). *Leiter International Performance Scale-Revised.* Odessa, FL: Psychological Assessment Resources	• Give a measure of non-verbal ability • Standardized on over 2000 US normal and clinical children aged 2–20 • Requires 40 minutes for administration
Visual disability	Verbal subtests of WPPSI-III; WISC-III; WAIS-III & SB-V	• Gives verbal IQ or estimate of Full Scale IQ
	Davis, C. (1980). *Perkins-Binet Tests of Intelligence for the Blind.* Watertown, MA: Perkins School for the Blind.	• Gives Full Scale IQ
	Newland, T. (1971). *Blind Learning Aptitude Test.* Champaign, IL: University of Illinois Press	• Gives index of overall ability

referred to psychologists for assessment of scholastic attainment often coupled with either behaviour problems or day-dreaming. The principal differential diagnosis in such school-age children is between a specific learning disability and a general ID. Diagnostic criteria for specific learning disabilities are given in Table 8.7. Children with specific learning disabilities obtain full scale IQ scores above 70 and scores on standardized achievement tests, such as those listed in Table 8.6, that fall below the level expected, given their overall IQ. In the manual for the WIAT II (listed in Table 8.6), tabular systems are given for deciding whether achievement test scores are significantly below the level expected for the child's IQ on a Wechsler intelligence test. Where a person's scores on tests of both intelligence and achievement fall below 70, and the person shows other adaptive behaviour deficits, then a diagnosis of ID may be made.

Table 8.5 Diagnostic criteria for developmental language delay

	DSM IV TR	ICD 10
Mixed receptive-expressive language disorder	A. The scores obtained from a battery of standardized individually administered measures of both receptive and expressive language development are substantially below those obtained from standardized measures of non-verbal intellectual capacity. Symptoms include those for expressive language disorder as well as difficulty understanding words, sentences, or specific types of words such as spatial terms B. The difficulties with receptive and expressive language significantly interfere with academic or occupational achievement or with social communication C. Criteria are not met for a pervasive developmental disorder D. If mental retardation, a speech-motor or sensory deficit or environmental deprivation is present, the language difficulties are in excess of those usually associated with these problems	A specific developmental disorder in which the child's understanding of language is below the appropriate level for his or her mental age. In almost all cases, expressive language is markedly disturbed and abnormalities in word-sound production are common Failure to respond to familiar names by the first birthday; inability to name a few objects by 18 months or failure to follow simple, routine instructions by the age of 2 years should be taken as significant signs of delay. Later difficulties include inability to understand grammatical structures (negatives, questions or comparatives) and lack of understanding if more subtle aspects of language (such as tone of voice)
Expressive language disorder	A. The scores obtained from a battery of standardized individually administered measures of expressive language development are substantially below those obtained from standardized measures of both non-verbal intellectual capacity and receptive language development. The disturbance may be manifest by symptoms that include having a markedly limited vocabulary, making errors in tense, or having difficulty recalling words or producing sentences with developmentally appropriate length or complexity B. The difficulties with expressive language significantly interfere with academic or occupational achievement or with social communication	A specific developmental disorder in which the child's ability to use expressive spoken language is markedly below the appropriate level for his or her mental age, but in which language comprehension is within normal limits. There may or may not be abnormalities in articulation The absence of single words (or word approximations) by 2 years and the failure to generate simple two-word phrases by 3 years should be taken as significant signs of delay. Later difficulties include restricted vocabulary development; overuse of a small set of general words; difficulties in selecting appropriate words; word substitutions; short utterances; immature sentence structure; syntactical errors,

C. Criteria are not met for a mixed receptive-expressive language disorder or a pervasive developmental disorder	especially omissions of word endings or prefixes; misuse or failure to use prepositions, pronouns, articles, and verb and noun inflections. Incorrect over-generalizations of rules may occur as may lack of sentence fluency and difficulties in sequencing when recounting past events. There may also be delays or abnormalities in word-sound production
D. If mental retardation, a speech-motor or sensory deficit or environmental deprivation is present, the language difficulties are in excess of those usually associated with these problems	

Note: Adapted from DSM IV TR (APA, 2000a) and ICD 10 (WH0, 1992, 1996).

ID and autistic spectrum disorders (ASD)

With pre-school children, particularly those who show moderate, severe or profound levels of ID, the possibility of co-morbid ASD should be born in mind. Children with ID and co-morbid ASD show both delayed development as indicated by full scale IQs below 70 and varying degrees and patterning of qualitative impairments in reciprocal social interaction and communication as well as restricted, stereotyped behaviour patterns. The diagnostic criteria for autism and the assessment of ASD are considered in Chapter 9.

ID and attention deficit hyperactivity disorder (ADHD)

As has been mentioned, often when school-aged children with undetected learning disabilities are referred for assessment, in addition to scholastic problems, behavioural difficulties are also a concern. Behavioural difficulties may be assessed using the parent and teacher versions for Strengths and Difficulties Questionnaire (SDQ; see Figure 4.7) or the Child Behaviour Checklist (CBCL) and Teacher Report Form (TRF). These instruments will indicate the extent of the behaviour problems and the degree to which these are coupled with attention problems suggestive of ADHD. Diagnostic criteria for ADHD are given in Chapter 11.

ID and epilepsy

As has already been mentioned, when school-aged children with undetected learning disabilities are referred for assessment, in addition to scholastic problems, day-dreaming can also be a concern. In some instances, children with intellectual disabilities lose concentration and do not focus on their schoolwork. However, frequently what appears to be day-dreaming are petite mal epileptic 'absences'. If children report 'losing time' or not being aware of what is happening during these episodes, a referral for neurological assess-ment and an EEG are required to determine if a diagnosis of a seizure

Table 8.6 Tests for assessing language and attainment problems

Instrument	Comments
Edwards, S., Fletcher, M., Garman, A. Hughes, A., Letts, C. & I. Sinka (1997). *Reynell Developmental Language Scales. III.* Windsor: NFER-Nelson	• Measures children's expressive language and verbal comprehension • The Comprehension Scale comprises 62 items organized into 10 sections: single words, relating two-named objects, agents and actions, clausal constituents, attributes, noun phrases, locative relations, verbs and thematic role assignment, vocabulary and complex grammar and inferencing • The Expressive Scale compromises 62 items organized into 6 main sections: simple words, verbs and phrases, inflections – plurals and third person and past tense, clausal elements, auxiliaries – negatives and questions and tags, complex structures – initiation and correction of errors and utterance completion • UK norms available for children aged 15 months to 7 years
Weschler, D. (2001). *Wechsler Individual Achievement Tests II (WIAT-II).* San Antonio, TX: Psychological Corporation Wechsler, D. (2005). *Wechsler Individual Achievement Test – II UK (WIAT-II^{uk}).* San Antonio, TX: Psychological Corporation	• For reading, yields measures of word reading, reading comprehension and pseudoword decoding • For written language, yields scores for spelling and written expression • For oral language, yields measures of listening comprehension and oral expression • For mathematics, yields scores for mathematical reasoning and numerical operations • Standardized in the US and UK on children aged 4 and up and adults
Wilkinson, G. (1993). *Wide Range Achievement Test – 3 (WRAT-3).* Wide Range Inc, 15 Ashley Place, Suite 1a, Wilmington Delaware 19804–1314. Phone 302–652–4990	• For pre-school and primary school children and adults aged 5 years to 75 years • Contains three subtests and takes about 30 minutes to administer • Yields word recognition spelling and arithmetic quotients • Standardized in the US

disorder is appropriate. More than a quarter of people with intellectual disabilities also have epilepsy, which can be controlled in most cases with anti-convulsant medication. Distress associated with the reactions of the child, parents and teachers to seizures may be greatly reduced if a definitive diagnosis is given, clear psychoeducation about epilepsy offered and an appropriate medication regime put in place. Epilepsy is discussed in Chapter 14.

Table 8.7 Diagnostic criteria for specific learning disabilities

	DSM IV TR	ICD 10
Reading disorder	A. Reading achievement as measured by individually administered standardized tests of reading accuracy or comprehension is substantially below that expected given the person's chronological age, measured intelligence and age-appropriate education. B. The disturbance significantly interferes with academic achievement or activities of daily living that require reading skills. C. If a sensory deficit is present, the reading difficulties are in excess of those usually associated with it.	The child's reading performance should be significantly below the level expected on the basis of age, general intelligence, and school placement and not due to visual acuity problems. Performance is best assessed by means of an individually administered, standardized test of reading accuracy and comprehension. In early stages of learning there may be difficulties in reciting the alphabet, naming letters or rhyming. Later there may be difficulties in oral reading such as omissions, substitutions, distortions, or additions. Slow reading speed, frequent loss of place, and reversals may also occur. Comprehension problems such as inability to recall facts read and inability to draw conclusions from material read may also occur. In later childhood and adulthood spelling difficulties may predominate with phonological errors being the most common.
Mathematics disorder	A. Mathematical ability as measured by individually administered standardized tests is substantially below that expected given the person's chronological age, measured intelligence and age-appropriate education. B. The disturbance significantly interferes with academic achievement or activities of daily living that require mathematical ability. C. If a sensory deficit is present, the difficulties in mathematical ability are in excess of those usually associated with it.	The child's arithmetical performance should be significantly below the level expected on the basis of his or her age, general intelligence, and school placement, and is best assessed by means of an individually administered standardized test of arithmetic. Reading and spelling should be within the normal range. The difficulties in arithmetic should not be due to grossly inadequate teaching, or to the direct effects of defects of visual, hearing, or neurological function and should not have been acquired as a result

Continued

Table 8.7 Continued

DSM IV TR	ICD 10
	of any neurological, psychiatric or other disorder.
	The arithmetic difficulties that occur are various but may include failure to understand the concepts underlying particular arithmetic operations; lack of understanding of mathematical terms or signs; failure to recognize numerical symbols; difficulty in carrying out standard numerical manipulations; difficulties in understanding which numbers are relevant to the arithmetic problem being considered; difficulty in properly aligning numbers or in inserting decimal points or symbols during calculations; poor spatial organization of arithmetic calculations; and inability to learn multiplication tables.
	There may be impairment of visuo-spatial skills.

Note: Adapted from DSM IV TR (APA, 2000a) and ICD 10 (WHO, 1992, 1996).

Assessment of support needs

In addition to the differential diagnosis of ID, support needs should be assessed. In the AAMR 10, supports fall into nine areas: (1) human development; (2) teaching and education; (3) home living; (4) community living; (5) employment; (6) health and safety; (7) behavioural; (8) social; and (9) protection and advocacy (Luckasson et al., 2002). The nature and intensity of supports required in each of these areas depends on the discrepancy between the requirements and demands of a child's social environment on the one hand and their intellectual capabilities, adaptive skills and risk and protective factors on the other. The desired outcomes from using supports include enhanced independence, relationships, and contributions to society; school and community participation and personal well-being. The intensity of supports any person with an ID needs will vary across situations and stages of the lifecycle. Distinctions are made in AAMR 10 between intermittent, limited, extensive or pervasive levels of support. A child requiring intermittent supports needs the support at specific times on an 'as-needed' basis, such as during lifecycle transitions or crises. A child requiring limited supports needs the support consistently rather than intermittently, but for a time-limited period. A child requiring extensive supports needs regular, long-term support in at least some living environments. This includes daily supports at home, school or work. A child requiring pervasive supports needs constant, high-intensity support across all living environments, and these supports are potentially life sustaining, for example, long-term residential care. The AAMR 10 manual recommends that individualized support plans be written for all children with intellectual disabilities to specify how support activities will address support requirements, and to prioritize the interests and preferences of children and families. Plans should include a system for monitoring goal attainment, should favour supports in the client's natural social network and should specify the agencies and people responsible for finding and implementing the plan. In Ireland and the UK, such individualized support plans will include individual educational plans (IEPs) and requirements for family support.

Intervention: four common problem areas

Typically, clinical psychologists who work with families containing a child with an ID are required to offer assessment and intervention services to deal with the following broad problem areas:

- psychoeducation
- organization of appropriate supports and periodic review
- offering life skills training for the child
- providing consultancy to manage challenging behaviour
- counselling during lifecycle transitions and supporting families in dealing with the grief process.

What follows is a brief account of the main practice-related issues in each of these areas. Typically clinical psychologists working in this area offer their services as part of a multi-disciplinary team.

Psychoeducation

The aim of psychoeducation in cases of ID is to help parents and other family members understand their child's diagnosis and its implications for the child's development. It is very difficult for most parents to acknowledge and appreciate the implications of the diagnosis of ID, since the diagnosis violates their expectations associated with having a completely healthy child. Most parents experience shock and denial (two elements of the grief process described below). Psychologists on multi-disciplinary teams have a responsibility to help team members give parents and family members a clear, unified and unambiguous message about the diagnosis, since this is what the parents require to work through their denial and get on with the process of accepting their child's disability and dealing with it in a realistic way. Parents should be given information on the normative status of their child's cognitive abilities and adaptive skills and supports necessary for the child to live a normal life. The way in which such supports may be accessed should also be clarified. The main pitfall in psychoeducation is to give parents ambiguous information that allows them to maintain the erroneous belief that their child has no disability or a transient condition that will resolve with maturation.

Organization of appropriate supports and period review

Following the first comprehensive assessment and feedback of diagnostic information, as part of a multi-disciplinary service, clinical psychologists may have a role in organizing and arranging the delivery of appropriate supports for children with intellectual disabilities and their families. The appropriateness of these supports in meeting the changing needs of the child and the burden of care shouldered by the family require periodic review and revision. For good practice in this area, the child and family's support needs must be clearly stated in concrete terms. The precise action plans for arranging supports must be agreed with the family and the professional network, the precise roles and responsibilities of members of the professional network in providing supports must be agreed, the way in which the provision of supports will be resourced financially must be agreed and the timetable of periodic review dates must be drawn up (Coyle, 2005). Central to this type of system is the concept of a key worker who holds administrative responsibility for insuring the child's support plan is implemented. Even the most robust system of this type will flounder without an organizational structure which requires key workers to take responsibility for co-ordinating the implementation of support plans. The terminology used to describe these individualized support plans vary from country to country. However, the principles of good practice remain the same. Also the precise role of the clinical psychologist in relation to other professionals, including educational and school psychologists, will vary depending on local and national policy.

Life skills training

The principles of applied behavioural analysis and behaviour modification may be used for designing skills development programmes and training parents and school staff to implement these to help the child develop life skills (O'Reilly et al, 2005; Sigafoos, O'Reilly & Green, 2005; Wehmeyer & Lee, 2005).

Challenging behaviour

When self-injurious, aggressive and destructive behaviour occur, assessing the contextual factors that maintain these problems and developing programmes to help children with intellectual disabilities and members of their networks resolve these difficulties is an important part of the psychologist's role. Interventions to reduce the frequency of challenging behaviours should be based on a thorough functional analysis of the immediate antecedents and consequences of such behaviours which may maintain them. A wider ecological assessment is also required to identify both personal attributes and relatively enduring features of the physical and social environment which may predispose children and their carers to become involved in mutually reinforcing patterns of behaviour that maintain aggressive and self-injurious behaviour (Emerson, 2001; Kennedy & Carr, 2002; Oliver, 1995).

Two common behavioural patterns that may maintain self-injurious behaviour (but which may equally apply to aggressive behaviour) have been described in detail by Oliver (1995). In the first pattern, a period of social isolation leads the child to a state of heightened need for social contact and challenging behaviour occurs. In response to this, the carer provides social contact until the child's need for contact is satiated. When the child's need for contact ceases, it is more likely that the child will engage in challenging behaviour again, since this has been positively reinforced by the carer's attention. It is also more likely that the carer will provide social contact in response to challenging behaviour, since giving attention leads the adult ultimately to experience relief (associated with negative reinforcement) when the challenging behaviour ceases.

In the second pattern, the carer places demands on the child and, in response, the child engages in challenging behaviour, which leads the adult to cease placing demands on the child. When the episode ceases, the child is more likely in future to engage in challenging behaviour when demands are placed on him or her, because in the past this has led to a cessation of demands (negative reinforcement). The adult is more likely to stop making demands in response to challenging behaviour because this has led to a cessation of the child's challenging behaviour (negative reinforcement). This pattern is discussed more fully in Chapter 10.

Environmental pre-disposing factors for challenging behaviour include: disruptions of the sleep–waking cycle, disruptions of daily routines, life transitions, living in authoritarian social environments entailing many demands, living in social environments where there is limited contact with carers or teachers due to high staff–student ratios, living in social environments where carers provide few routines and little structure for the child, living in environments where carers are not sensitive to fluctuations in the child's moment-to-moment needs and frustration tolerance.

Personal pre-disposing factors for challenging behaviour include: a greater degree of ID, fewer adaptive behaviours, more limited expressive language, co-morbid autism, co-morbid sensory and motor disabilities and the presence of particular syndromes such as Lesch–Nyhan, Smith–Magenis and de la Tourette's syndrome. Many of these pre-disposing factors, limit the availability of alternative responses of equivalent efficiency through which the child can alleviate the need to make social contact with carers or reduce the demands made by carers.

A functional analysis will identify proximal and distal antecedents and consequences of challenging behaviour. The analysis will suggest potential interventions, and these may fall into three broad categories: (1) changing proximal or distal antecedents to pre-empt the occurrence of the challenging behaviour; (2) changing the immediate consequences of challenging behaviour to prevent its reinforcement; and (3) functional equivalence training, which provides the child with a more adaptive response that is as efficient as the challenging behaviour for meeting the child's need that was met by the challenging behaviour.

Family grief counselling at lifecycle transitions

Parents, siblings and other family members may require counselling at critical lifecycle transitions, such as the diagnosis of ID, the transition to school, leaving school, entering supported employment, leaving home, the onset of parental decline and parental death.

Initially, when parents are informed that their child has an ID, a grief process is set in motion which includes the sub-processes of shock; denial; emotional turmoil involving disappointment, anger and guilt; and acceptance. The way the news of handicap is broken affects parents' satisfaction with the consultation service received. The following factors are particularly important: the approachableness of the clinician and the degree to which the clinician understands the parents' concerns, the sympathy of the clinician, the directness and clarity of communication (Quine & Rutter, 1994). This issue has been mentioned above in the section on psychoeducation; grief processes are discussed more fully in Chapter 24.

Throughout the lifecycle, at each transition the family is reminded of the loss of the able-bodied child that was initially expected and the grief process recurs, albeit in a progressively attenuated form (Blancher & Kraemer, 2005; Goldberg, Magrill, Hale, Damaskinidou & Tham, 1995). Lifecycle transitions are particularly strong triggers for family grief processes, since they entail unique features when compared with lifecycle transitions associated with able-bodied children. For example, the transition to school may entail a higher level of concern because of fears that the disability may prevent the child from forming peer relationships and fitting in. The leaving home transition may occur later in life, if at all. The impending death of the parents may be a particular source of anxiety, since a major concern may be who will care for the disabled child when the parent has died. An important function of the clinical psychologist is to help families both mourn their disappointments but also celebrate the achievements of their children with intellectual disabilities. This may involve offering family counselling or therapy, or offering support and supervision to key workers providing this service.

SPECIFIC LANGUAGE DELAY

A distinction may be made between secondary language delay (due to ID, autism, hearing loss or some such condition) and specific language delay. Specific language delays can be sub-classified as expressive, which are the most common, and mixed receptive-expressive, which are the most debilitating (Bishop, 2002; Rapin, 1996; Whitehurst & Fischel, 1994). This distinction is the central organizing principle in the classification of language disorders in DSM IV TR (APA, 2000a) and ICD 10 (WHO, 1992, 1996). A case example of a child with a receptive-expressive language delay is presented in Box 8.2. Diagnostic criteria for specific language delays from DSM IV TR and ICD 10 are presented in Table 8.5 (pp. 274–275). Children with receptive delays only are very rare. In addition to these distinctions, it is useful to describe language difficulties in terms of phonology, semantics, syntax, pragmatics and fluency.

Phonology

Phonological difficulties are manifested as inaccurate articulation of specific sounds, typically consonants rather than vowels. The following consonants tend to pose the most difficulties: *r, l, f, v*, and *s*. For example, omissions such as *ee* for *sleep*; substitution such as *berry* for *very* and cluster reduction such as *ream* for *cream*. Where these phonological problems reflect a pre-schooler's difficulty in the motor skills required for correct articulation, the prognosis for both language development and reading skills is good, and such children are indistinguishable from their peers by middle childhood. Phonological disorder and specific speech articulation disorder are the terms used to describe this condition in the DSM and the ICD respectively.

Where phonological difficulties reflect a lack of phonological awareness, such as an inability to use rhyme and alliteration the prognosis for the development of reading skills is poor. However, this relationship between problems with phonological awareness and ability to use rhyme and alliteration also holds for children who have no phonological expressive language difficulties. This issue is discussed more fully in the section on dyslexia (see pp. 290–291).

Box 8.2 A case of developmental language delay

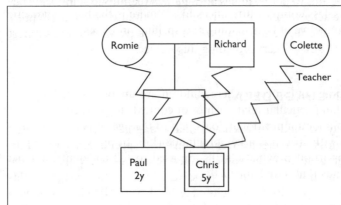

Chris was referred at age five because his parents and school teacher were concerned about his conduct problems and communication abilities. He was frequently disobedient, seemed to selectively misunderstand instructions and commands given to him by his parents and teachers and only used a limited range of words in speaking with others. His mother was finding that managing his difficulties and the demands of her two-year-old, Paul, was very stressful. A psychological assessment showed that on both the Child Behaviour Checklist and the Teacher Report Form, Chris's scores on the externalizing scales fell above the 98th percentile and well within the clinical range. On both the Leiter scale and the performance scale of the WPPSI-III, Chris's performance was within the normal range but on the Reynell, receptive and expressive language quotients below the 3rd percentile were obtained. Together, these results indicated that Chris had a specific mixed receptive-expressive language disorder with secondary conduct problems. These probably arose from difficulties in comprehending and internalizing rules for appropriate conduct at home and at school. A home- and school-based behavioural management programme and involvement of a speech and language therapist in the multi-disciplinary management of the case followed from this preliminary psychological assessment.

Semantics

With semantic difficulties, the child has a restricted vocabulary and so under-stands the meaning of a limited number of words and can only use a limited number of words to verbally communicate with others.

Syntax

Problems with syntax or grammar include restricted length of utterance and restricted diversity of utterance types. By two years of age, most children should be using multi-word utterances. Children with specific language delays characterized by syntactical difficulties are unable to use such multi-word utterances at this stage. Later on, they are slow to use multi-clausal sentences such as 'Where is the ball, that I was playing with yesterday?' They will be confined to using less complex utterances like 'Where is the ball?' Syntactic difficulties are predictive of later reading and spelling problems.

Pragmatics

Problems with pragmatics occur where children are unable to use language and gestures within particular relationships or contexts to get their needs met or achieve certain communicational goals. Up to the age of two years, integrating gestures with speech is a key pragmatic skill. In pre-schoolers up to the age of 5, important pragmatic skills are used to tell coherent extended stories about events that have happened.

Fluency

Stuttering and cluttering are distinctive fluency problems, with the latter involving a rapid rate of speech and consequent breakdown in fluency and the former involving repetitions, prolongations and pauses that disrupt the rhythmic flow of speech.

Epidemiology

Up to 17% of two-year-olds; 8% of three-year-olds; and 3% of five-year-olds have expressive language delay. The male–female ratio is between 3 and 5:1. The majority of children with specific language delay recover by five years of age and have few later adjustment problems (Whitehurst & Fischel, 1994).

Between 2 and 3% of six- to seven-year-olds have phonological disorders but most outgrow these problems and only 0.5% of seventeen-year-olds present with this problem, which is more prevalent in boys than girls. The vast majority of children with phonological problems in the pre-school years have no later academic or adjustment problems (Whitehurst & Fischel, 1994).

The prevalence of stuttering among children is about 1% and it is three times more common among boys than girls. Up to 60% of cases recover spontaneously before the age of sixteen years (APA, 2000a).

Co-morbid conduct problems are common among children with specific language delays, particularly children with severe receptive-expressive disorders. Baker and Cantwell (1982) found that conduct problems occurred in up to 95% of cases of specific receptive-expressive language disorder; 45% of cases of expressive language disorder and 29% of case of articulation disorder.

Specific reading retardation is common among children whose specific language disorder persists beyond the pre-school years. Bishop and Adams (1990) found that specific reading retardation occurred in only 3–7% of children with specific language delay whose language problem resolved by five-and-a-half years of age. However, 35–46% of cases with persistent specific language disorders developed specific reading retardation at school.

Aetiology

Available longitudinal evidence supports the view that there is a hierarchy of vulnerability in the components of language that are effected in cases of specific language delay and children who change symptoms over time during recovery move up this hierarchy (Whitehurst & Fischel, 1994). The hierarchy, moving from the most to the least vulnerable component, is as follows:

1   expressive phonology
2   expressive syntax and morphology
3   expressive semantics
4   receptive language.

Thus a child with expressive semantic problems with maturation when these semantic problems resolve, will develop expressive syntax and morphology problems rather than receptive language problems. This hierarchy of vulnerability has led to the view that some aetiological factors must be common to all language disorders. However, there is no doubt that some factors are specific to particular disorders.

All language delays are more common in boys than girls, so some gender-related biological factors are probably involved in the aetiology of all language problems. A delay in the development of speeded fine motor skills (but not general clumsiness) has been found to characterize most specific language delays. Both the language delay and the motor delay may reflect an underlying neurological immaturity, which finds expression in slow information processing and limited information-processing capacity (Bishop, 1992).

Genetic factors play a significant role in most secondary language delays and in specific receptive-expressive language disorders but probably not in early specific expressive language delay (Whitehurst & Fischel, 1994).

Otitis media (middle ear infection) in twelve- to eighteen-month period has been shown to precede rapidly resolving specific expressive language delay at two years, and expressive language delay at two years is associated with problems in oral motor development (Whitehurst & Fischel, 1994).

It is unlikely that psychosocial factors play a major aetiological role in most cases of specific developmental language delay. However, they may play a role in maintaining language problems (Whitehurst & Fischel, 1994). Low socioeconomic status, large family size and problematic parent–child interaction patterns involving conduct problems characterize many cases of language disorder, and the more severe the disorder, the worse the conduct problem. Evidence suggests that a variety of mechanisms may link these psychosocial factors to language problems. First, language problems may lead to frustration in the areas of communicating with others or achieving valued goals; this frustration finds expression in misconduct. Second, children with language problems may have difficulty controlling their conduct with inner speech. Third, parents with poor parenting skills and multiple stresses (such as large family size and low socioeconomic status) may become trapped in coercive cycles of interaction with their children (such as those described in Chapter 10). These coercive interaction patterns may then prevent the children from developing language skills through engaging in positive verbal exchanges with their parents. A final possibility is that conduct problems and language problems may both be expressions of an underlying neurological immaturity.

Assessment and intervention

Psychological assessment of language problems should ideally be conducted by a multi-disciplinary team (American Academy of Child and Adolescent Psychiatry, 1998a,b,c). A full paediatric assessment of the child should be conducted to detect the presence of problems such as otitis media and to rule out the presence of neurological and medical conditions such as Duchenne muscular dystrophy. An audiological examination should be conducted to outrule hearing impairment.

In addition to routine interviewing, observation and completion of behaviour checklists and adaptive behaviour scales, assessment should involve the administration of standardized receptive and expressive language tests, along with a measure of non-verbal intelligence. A number of psychometric instruments that are useful in the assessment of communication problems are listed in Table 8.6. Where measures of non-verbal intelligence, receptive and expressive language and adaptive behaviour all fall two standard deviations below the mean (or a standard score of 70), then the language problem is secondary to ID. Where the non-verbal intelligence score is within the normal range, and receptive or expressive language quotients fall 1.5 to two standard deviations below average, a diagnosis of specific language disorder may be made and reference should be made to diagnostic criteria presented in Table 8.5.

Specific language delay may be distinguished from the following three syndromes (Bishop, 2002):

- autism
- Landau–Kleffner syndrome
- elective mutism.

Specific language delay may be distinguished from autism by a number of features. Autistic children show more echolalia, pronominal reversal, stereotyped utterances, lack of gesture, undue sensitivity to noise and lack of imaginative play. A full account of autism is given in Chapter 9.

Specific language delays that are present from birth are distinguished in ICD 10 from acquired aphasia with epilepsy (Landau–Kleffner syndrome). In this syndrome, a child with normal cognitive and linguistic skills loses expressive and receptive language skills while retaining normal intelligence. Concurrently there are EEG bilateral temporal lobe abnormalities and seizures consistent with a diagnosis of epilepsy. The onset of the Landau–Kleffner syndrome occurs between three and seven. About a third of cases recover and two-thirds retain a severe mixed receptive-expressive language disorder. The cause of the disorder is unknown but it is presumed to be due to an inflammatory encephalitic process.

Specific language delays and Landau–Kleffner syndrome should be distinguished from elective or selective mutism. This is a condition in which the child's speech and language abilities remain intact but are not used in particular circumstances for psychosocial reasons. Typically, children with this condition speak to family members and close friends privately in the home but not to teachers or to people in public. The parents may be asked to tape-record a private conversation with the child and this provides sufficient information to make the differential diagnosis. A family-based approach to the management of this condition is described in Chapter 12.

In cases of specific expressive language disorder, there is little evidence to suggest that pre-school interventions add much to recovery rates, which occur due to maturation (Bishop, 2002; Whitehurst & Fischel, 1994). Parents may be given this information and advised not to try to coerce the child to talk and to accept that intervention may be offered if no improvement has occurred by the time the child has reached five years of age. However, behavioural parent training may be offered to help parents manage co-morbid conduct problems. This type of treatment is described in Chapter 10.

In cases of specific receptive-expressive language disorders and secondary language disorders, referral for an individualized speech therapy programme, involvement of parents in implementing aspects of the programme in the home and placement of the child in a therapeutic school environment (ideally in a mainstream school) are the principal types of treatment that, singly or in combination, have been shown to have positive short-term effects (Whitehurst & Fischel, 1994). Typically, these speech and language programmes need to be conducted in conjunction with home- and school-based behavioural management programmes, such as those mentioned in Chapter 10, focusing on the child's conduct problems.

Two recent innovations in speech and language therapy, Hannen and FastForward, deserve mention. With the Hannen approach, parent–child interactions are videotaped and these are used as a basis for instruction with parents (Girolametto, Weitzman & Pearce, 1996). With the FastForward programme, children engage in computer-based language skill training embedded in attractive computer games (Tallal, Miller & Bedi, 1996). Preliminary evidence for the effectiveness of both approaches is promising.

SPECIFIC LEARNING DISABILITIES

The DSM IV TR (APA, 2000a) and ICD 10 (WHO, 1992, 1996) classification systems distinguish specific learning disabilities from both ID (or mental retardation), specific language delays and acquired learning problems associated with traumatic brain injury. Both systems then offer a sub-classification of specific scholastic disabilities through reference to the specific skill in which the deficits are shown, e.g. reading, spelling and arithmetic. These classification systems have been presented in Figures 8.1 and 8.2.

Epidemiology

In a major UK epidemiological study of over 1200 nine- to ten-year-olds, Lewis, Hitch & Walker (1994) found that 3.9% had specific reading difficulties or dyslexia, 1.3% had specific arithmetic difficulties and an additional 2.3% had both arithmetic and reading difficulties. The male:female ratio for specific reading difficulties was 3:1, but with specific arithmetic difficulties and combined specific reading and arithmetic difficulties the male:female ratio was approximately 1:1. Cases were defined as having specific academic difficulties if their Full Scale IQ was above 90 and their attainment quotient was below 85. Meltzer et al. (2000), in a UK national epidemiological study of children aged between five and fifteen, found that overall 5% of children has specific reading or spelling difficulties. The rate of these specific learning difficulties were 17% for children with ADHD, 13% for children with conduct disorder, 11% for children with emotional disorders and 4% for children without other psychological disorders.

A deficit in phonological processing is a core characteristic of children with dyslexia (Maughan, 1995; Snowling, 1996, 2002; Vellutino, Fletcher, Snowling & Scanlon, 2004). Word identification problems are due to deficiencies in phonological awareness, alphabetic mapping and phonological decoding. These deficiencies lead to problems in forming connective bonds between the spoken and written word. Current research shows that reading difficulties are not due to problems in the visual system leading to letter reversals and difficulties with word recognition, as was previously thought (Vellutino et al., 2004). While the basic phonological deficit central to dyslexia commonly persists into adulthood, a proportion of dyslexic children continue to show improvements in reading skills in adulthood, provided they are supported by their families, given additional tuition in school and practice reading regularly with manageable and motivating materials. In later life, good adjustment is associated with selecting a job that fits with personal strengths and does not require a major literacy component. The development of a positive self-image and the reduction in associated anti-social behaviour was also associated with this positive environment.

Clinical features of specific reading disability

Of the three specific learning disorders, specific reading disorder or dyslexia is probably the most important from a clinical perspective. This is because of the significance of literacy as a social skill and because of the clear link between reading problems and conduct problems. Also, far more is known about reading problems than about other specific learning difficulties. For these reasons, the main focus in this section will be on specific reading retardation or dyslexia. A typical case example of dyslexia is presented in Figure 8.3. The figure includes a full psychometric report along with guidelines for parents on helping their child with reading and spelling. This detailed sample report is given because specific reading disability is such a common co-morbid problem for youngsters referred for psychological consultation. (The level of detail given in the report may not always be necessary, and account should be taken of the requirements and skills of parents, teachers and others to whom the report is to be sent.)

Diagnostic criteria for specific reading disorders are presented in Table 8.7 along with the criteria for specific mathematics disorder for comparative purposes. The most noteworthy feature of these criteria is that specific learning disabilities are diagnosed principally on the basis of psychoeducational assessment. Children must return attainment scores on standardized tests that fall significantly below their age and intelligence level for a diagnosis to be made.

A variety of approaches to the sub-typing of reading disabilities have been taken. Rutter and Yule (1975), in the Isle of Wight studies, distinguished between specific reading retardation and general reading backwardness. Specific reading retardation was defined as the co-occurrence of normal intelligence with specific severe retardation in reading skills. This was found to be associated with early specific language disability, to be three times more common in boys and for there to be a high genetic risk of the disorder in families where male parents also suffered from specific reading difficulties. A strong association between conduct disorder and specific reading retardation was also found. In contrast, general reading backwardness was defined as reading problems co-occurring with a low IQ. It was found to be equally common in boys and girls and to be associated with mild neurological difficulties, visuo-motor skills deficits and social disadvantage.

Morris (1988), in a wide-ranging review of attempts to sub-classify children with specific reading disabilities, pointed out that sub-classification systems must take account of the fact that children with specific reading difficulties may also show specific spelling and arithmetic difficulties, they may have co-morbid specific language difficulties and they may differ in the degree to which they show deficits in phonological awareness on the one hand and visual discrimination and visual sequential memory deficits on the other. Attempts to tailor remedial reading programmes for sub-types of specific reading disability to capitalize on children's strengths have not been overwhelmingly successful.

Aetiology

The aetiology of specific reading retardation or dyslexia may be understood within the context of theories about the development of reading skills. Traditionally, two theories about the development of reading skills have been proposed. *Phonic theory* argues that, in order to read, children must first learn the sounds associated with letters, and then use these phonic building blocks to read and spell whole words (Perfetti, 1985). The argument is that children build up the word *cat* from the three sounds associated with the letters *c*, *a* and *t*. In contrast, *whole language theory* argues that children learn to recognize whole words rather than piecing together individual letter or sounds. According to whole language theory, the sound of unfamiliar words are learned by guessing from the meaning of the context within which they occur and obtaining feedback from a teacher (Goodman, 1976). So the child may assume that the word *cat* sounds like cat because it occurs under the picture of a cat or in a sentence that says '*the dog chased the cat*'.

Phonological theory gave rise to the phonic method of teaching reading, which requires the child to learn corresponding sounds for each letter. The whole language theory spawned a variety of contextual teaching methods, for example the *look and say* method, in which the child is taught to recognize whole words in context. Neither theory has received wholesale support from experimental studies of reading or studies of children with reading disabilities (Snowling, 1996). However, it does appear that children use both phonic-decoding strategies and whole-language contextual strategies, depending on their developmental level of reading skill, their familiarity with the material and the costs and benefits of accurate performance.

The theory of reading that has received widest support argues that children's perception of rhyme and alliteration is the most important precursor of reading skills (Snowling, 1996). This position entails the view that children may take a word like *cat* and break it into an onset: *c*, and a rhyme: *at*. They can use this skill to help them read unfamiliar words like *mat*, *sat* or *pat*. This involves an awareness of the similar sounds (phonological similarity) of the rhyming words and also an awareness of the similar appearance (orthographic similarity) of the words that rhyme. A large body of evidence shows that children who develop the skills of recognizing phonological and orthographic similarities at an early age become good readers and that those who do not develop reading problems.

Dr Alan Carr
BA, MA, PhD, Reg Psychol FPsSI, C. Psychol, AFBPsS.
Registered Psychologist
Chartered Clinical Psychologist

Clanwilliam Institute, Clanwilliam Terrace, Dublin 2
(01) 6762881

CONFIDENTIAL AND WITHOUT PREJUDICE

PSYCHOLOGICAL REPORT ON: Roy Murphy, Windgate Road, Howth, Dublin 13.

DATE OF ASSESSMENT: 27.3.2004

DATE OF BIRTH: 22.12.1993

AGE: 10 years 3 months.

PREPARED FOR: Mr & Mrs Murphy, Windgate Road, Howth, Dublin 13.

Dear Mr & Mrs Murphy:
Thank you for asking me to conduct a psychological assessment with Roy and for completing the Child Information Questionnaire. Thank you also for sending me copies of two recent school reports and for arranging for Mr Potts to complete the Teacher Report Form. The principal concerns appear to be Roy's poor school work, his difficulty in completing homework in a reasonable time, and his conduct problems at school.

SCHOOLING
Roy is a pupil at the National School in Howth where at present he is in fourth class and his class teacher is Mr Potts. Roy reports having a good working relationship with his class teacher.

From Roy's two recent school reports (1.2.03 & 6.2.04) and the Teacher Report Form completed by Mr Potts, it is apparent that Roy's teachers believe that his attendance and punctuality are acceptable, as is his oral language and performance in PE.

However, his written work, spelling and maths are below the level expected given his oral language ability.

He shows little effort to learn, little interest in school work and has difficulty concentrating, organizing and completing school work assignments, and learning new material. His academic attainments place him in the lower third of his class.

He also has difficulty following school rules and this leads to disruptive behaviour.

He appears to be easily hurt when corrected and complains of feeling worthless. He worries, complains of headaches and stomach cramps.

Despite his current academic and behavioural problems, Roy is not receiving remedial tuition.

Roy requires glasses for reading and often does not wear them.

He previously was a pupil at St Anthony's National School in Fairview between September 1998 and June 2002.

DEVELOPMENT
From the information you gave me my impression is that Roy's development has been broadly within normal limits.

There are two noteworthy features in his medical history. There were perinatal difficulties with the umbilical chord. Roy also has had asthma for a number of years.

Roy currently has no major developmental sensory, motor or social difficulties.

At home he complains of disliking school and homework and finds it difficult to complete his homework in a reasonable time.

In the past 2 years Roy has been exposed to a high level of life stress. He has moved house and changed school from an all boys school in Fairview to a mixed school in Howth. Two of his grandparents have died and his father had a heart attack.

Fortunately, Roy comes from a resourceful family, and so has been helped in a supportive way to manage this stress and deal with the challenges of the past two years.

Figure 8.3   A report on a case of specific reading disorder (or dyslexia)

From the behaviour checklists completed by his teacher and parents it may be concluded that his behaviour, while sometimes challenging is, broadly, within normal limits and reflects no major psychological disturbance.

TESTS ADMINISTERED
In a single two-hour session the following tests were administered:
- The Wechsler Intelligence Scale for Children (Fourth Edition) (WISC-IV)
- The Wechsler Individual Achievement Tests (Second Edition) (WIAT-II)

Roy co-operated well with all the testing procedures, so the obtained results may be interpreted as a valid estimate of his abilities.

INTERPRETATION OF THE TEST RESULTS
A comprehensive table of test results is appended to this report. What follows is my interpretation of these results.

Roy's full scale IQ of 101 falls at the 53rd percentile which means that out of 100 children of his age he would be more intelligent than 53 of them. This score is in the average range of general intellectual abilities (90-109).
The possible ranges are

130 +	Exceptional
120-129	High
110-119	High average
90-109	Average
80-89	Low average
70-79	Low
69 and below	Exceptionally low

On the WISC-IV, overall intellectual ability is broken down into four distinct areas:
- Verbal comprehension (which covers the skills used for language use and verbal reasoning)
- Perceptual reasoning (which includes skills such as those used by children when they solve problems involving patterns and designs or architects when they design a house)
- Working memory (which refers to the capacity to concentrate, remember and manipulate sequences of symbols that have been heard but not seen)
- Processing speed (which refers to the capacity to concentrate on and rapidly manipulate sequences of symbols that have been seen but not heard)

Compared to the other three areas, Roy obtained a particularly high score (115) for verbal comprehension which fell within the high average range (110-119).

His scores for perceptual reasoning (92) and processing speed (102) fell within the normal range (90-109).

His score for working memory fell within the low average range (80-89). His score on this dimension was 89 and it fell at the 23rd percentile. Thus, he would have less well-developed working memory than 23 of his peers. This is unfortunate, since a well-developed working memory is one of the core abilities required for developing reading skills.

On the WIAT-II attainments in our areas were assessed:
- Oral language (including listening comprehension and oral expression)
- Reading (including word reading, reading comprehension and pseudoword decoding)
- Written language (including spelling and written expression)
- Mathematics (including mathematical reasoning and numerical operations).

Roy's oral language score (81) fell at the 10th percentile. Thus compared to 100 boys of his won age, his language skills would be better developed than only 10 of them. Roy's composite language score and both his listening comprehension and oral expression scores fell within the low average range (80-89).

Roy's reading score (75) fell at the 5th percentile. Thus compared to 100 boys of his own age, his reading skills would be better developed than only 5 of them. Roy's composite reading score and his word reading, reading comprehension and pseudoword decoding scores fell within the low range (70-79).

Roy's written language score (82) fell at the 12th percentile. Thus compared to 100 boys of his own age, his written language skills would be better developed than only 12 of them. Roy's composite written language score and both his spelling and written expression scores fell within the low average range (80-89).

Roy's mathematics score (96) fell at the 39th percentile. Thus compared to 100 boys of his own age his mathematical skills would be better developed than only 39 of them. Roy's composite mathematics score and both his mathematical reasoning and numerical operations scores fell within the normal range (90-109).

ANALYSIS OF ATTAINMENT AND STUDY SKILLS PROBLEMS AND STRENGHTS
Most of Roy's reading errors were with large or irregular words and involved refusals and substitutions. With substitutions there was a tendency to phonetically decode the first few letters of each word and then guess at the remainder. In other cases Roy substituted words that were semantically plausible.

Many of the spelling errors involved spelling irregular words phonetically. Roy needs to learn rules for spelling irregular words.

Roy read at a moderate speed, but mispronounced many words and often was unclear about the meaning of the passage.

Continued

In a free writing assignment Roy wrote in legible, but untidy, printed script. The ideas were logically and coherently organized, but his spelling difficulties peppered the whole assignment and he worked slowly. This is consistent with the reports of his teachers that he has difficulty finishing work assignments and his parents report that he has difficulty completing homework.

With arithmetic, he showed a clear understanding of addition, subtraction, multiplication and division. However, he was unable to complete problems involving long division, long multiplication, decimals, fractions or minutes and hours.

With individual instruction, Roy showed that he was capable of understanding and completing academic assignments in a clinical setting. He also showed a capacity to learn new literacy and numeracy skills with individual instruction, provided the material was presented at a pace that matched his abilities.

However, he reported that he finds independent study and homework very difficult because he cannot sustain concentration for long periods and also because, for him, remembering material that he has read is difficult.

He finds group instruction problematic because he has difficulty keeping up with the pace at which the material is presented.

CONCLUSIONS

Roy is a 10 year old child of normal intelligence with well developed verbal comprehension skills but who has a specific learning difficulty. The core problem is poorly developed working memory. That is, Roy's capacity to remember and process sequences of auditorally presented symbols is very poorly developed. These learning difficulties account for his problems with spelling and reading. His motivation, mood and conduct difficulties are secondary to his specific learning difficulty. These may have been exacerbated by the considerable life stress to which he has been exposed over the past two years.

Roy' ability profile (normal intelligence with a specific learning difficulty) is typical of youngsters, who like him appear to be reasonably intelligent in conversation, but who fail to develop skills necessary for written academic work. It is also common for youngsters with this profile to become demoralized, because when they put in the same amount of effort as their peers, at school they make far less progress. They begin to avoid work and this often leads to conflict with their teachers and parents who become frustrated with their lack of motivation and progress.

PROGNOSIS

The prognosis for Roy, if he is provided with remedial support, is good because of three important positive factors present in this case. First, Roy has sufficiently well developed verbal comprehension skills to be able to understand and benefit from remedial support. Second, Roy comes from a stable and supportive family. Third, Roy is attending a highly supportive school in which care has been taken to provide accurate and up-to-date information on his current status and which has not excluded him despite his academic and conduct problems. However, it is important to stress that Roy will not grow out of his specific learning difficulty. Rather, with remedial support he will learn to compensate for it.

RECOMMENDATIONS

1. Roy's teachers need to be made aware of his specific learning disability.

2. Arrangements should be made for Roy to receive regular remedial tuition on an individual or small group basis. The school may wish to use this report as a basis for making an application for additional resources. If state funding for remedial support cannot be arranged, private tuition may be arranged through the Association for Children and Adults with Learning Difficulties.

3. A clear routine for homework needs to be established and maintained. (Notes on this are enclosed with this report.)

4. Paired reading should be carried out at home on a regular basis. (Notes on this are enclosed with this report.)

5. Simultaneous oral spelling (SOS) should be used routinely at home as the method for learning new spellings. (Notes on this are enclosed with this report.)

6. Roy may need to be re-assessed on an annual basis if difficulties continue but especially before the Junior and Leaving Cert. examinations. Re-assessment may indicate that an application for special consideration to be given to Roy in these exams is advisable.

If you have any further questions please contact me.

Dr Alan Carr,
BA, MA, PhD, Reg Psychol FPsSI, C. Psychol, AFBPsS.
Registered Psychologist & Chartered Clinical Psychologist

Figure 8.3 Continued

Scale	Score	Percentile rank	Interpretation Under 69: exceptionally low 70–79: low 80–89: low average 90–109: average 110–119: high average 120–129: high Above 130: exceptional
Full scale IQ **from WISC IV**	101	53	Full scale IQ was within the normal range (90–109)
Verbal comprehension Index from WISC IV	115	84	Verbal comprehension was within the high average range (110–119)
Perceptual Reasoning Index from WISC IV	92	30	Perceptual reasoning was within the normal range (90–109)
Working memory from WISC IV	89	23	Working memory was within the normal range (90–109)
Processing Speed from WISC IV	102	55	Processing speed was within the low average range (90–109)
Oral Language from WIAT II	81	10	Oral language was within the low average range (80–89)
Reading from WIAT II	75	5	Reading was within the low range (70–79)
Written language from WIAT II	82	12	Written language was within the low average range (80–89)
Mathematics from WIAT II	96	39	Mathematics was within the normal range (90–109)

Summary of psychological test results for Roy Murphy DOB 22.12.93. Age 10 y. 3 m.

Continued

GUIDELINES FOR PARENTS
OF CHILDREN WITH SPECIFIC LEARNING DIFFICULTIES

BE REALISTIC WITH YOUR CHILD

Be honest with your child. Don't say that there is nothing wrong. No one knows better than your child that something is wrong. Your child has a specific learning difficulty. Your child's problems with literacy and or numeracy skills are not due to laziness, disobedience or illness. They are due to a specific learning difficulty.

The core problem is that your child's apparatus for manipulating sequences of symbols (such as the sounds and shapes of letters) is not working properly. Compared to other children, it is harder for your child to recognize, remember and use sequences of symbols. This is unfortunate since most schoolwork such as reading, spelling and arithmetic involves using symbols. Children with specific learning difficulties learn symbolic material more slowly than other children. They also use different strategies just as people with colour blindness learn how to distinguish colours using special strategies.

BE REALISTIC WITH YOURSELF

Your child's difficulties are not your fault, so don't blame yourself. Specific reading difficulties are not caused by parents treating their child the wrong way. If you have become embroiled in arguments with your child about homework, reading and spelling, this is understandable. You want your child to learn and do well and you may have been frustrated by the lack of progress.

Right now there are very specific things that you can do.
- Take a positive approach to your child
- Help your child develop a homework routine
- Read with your child every day
- Help your child with spellings every day

Here are some guidelines to follow to help you do these things.

TAKE A POSITIVE APPROACH

Take a positive approach with your child when discussing learning. Let your child know that your are on his or her side. Here are some things said by parents that children told me made all the difference to them:
- *You can learn even though you have a learning difficulty. I know you can because you are bright*
- *We'll get a routine for your homework that helps you learn and leaves time for play*
- *We'll read together every day, for fun*
- *We'll do some spellings every day but not too many*
- *Remember I 'm in this with you and I believe you can do well*

HOME WORK ROUTINES

Set a fixed time and place for homework each day. Set a time when your child is not tired. Provide your child with a quiet, well lit, warm place for doing homework. Provide dictionaries, encyclopaedias or atlases as well as pens, pencils, markers and paper if necessary.

At the outset of the homework session clarify what has to be done. Many children with specific learning difficulties have problems writing down homework off the board quickly. If this is occurring, discuss it with the teacher who will want to help resolve the problem.

Ask your child to allot a set amount of time for each topic. Some children can make work plans like this and follow through independently. If your child is like this, praise him or her. If not help your child set up a work plan. If sticking to it is a problem, use a points system where points are earned for completing each section of the plan on time. Points may be accumulated and used to get a prize at the end of the session. Design the system so as to maximize the chances of success by breaking big tasks into small manageable tasks. If using this type of system does not reduce your child's homework time to a reasonable length, discuss the possibility of reducing your child's homework load with the teacher.

Provide help as required when your child is doing homework. If your child wants to know how to pronounce or spell a word, provide the information requested. Avoid giving a reading or spelling lesson since this will disrupt the development of independent homework skills. Set aside separate times for joint reading and spelling lessons. Guidelines for these are set out on the next page.

LISTENING TO YOUR CHILD READ. PAIRED READING

Set aside a 10 - 15 minute period each day when you can read with your child. Choose a place free from distractions. Then follow the steps for paired reading set out below.

1. Ask your child to choose a book to read.

2. Sit side by side, so both of you can see the text.

3. Begin by reading the text together and adjust your speed and rhythm so you are both reading in time together.

4. When your child is ready to read alone, he or she should tap you on the arm. This is the signal for you to be silent and let your child read alone.

5. When your child gets a word wrong or can't read a word don't let him or her struggle for more than 5 seconds. Just tell your child what the word is. Let your child read it correctly and praise him or her for it. Don't analyse the word phonetically and try to teach your child how to spell it.

6. Don't read for more than 15 minutes. Talk with your child about the story you have read. Ask questions posed by the story. Answer any questions your child may have.

7. Be as patient as you can. Speak to your child in a quiet calm voice. Make your directions short and simple.

This method is called paired reading. Children who do paired reading with their parents show reading improvements at 3 times the speed of children who don't do paired reading. This conclusion was drawn from research on hundreds of children in the UK with reading problems. Paired reading allows children to read interesting material, to control the amount of help they get from parents, to be praised for success and to get as little criticism as possible. Paired reading allows parents to enjoy their children's success without the drudgery of labouring over their mistakes. Above all paired reading allows a child with a specific reading disability to experience fluent reading. This experience of fluent reading will motivate your child to put in the hand work necessary to learn how to read fluently.

HELPING YOUR CHILD LEARN SPELLINGS. SIMULTANEOUS ORAL SPELLING

Set aside a 10 minute period each day for helping your child with spelling. Spelling lists should be short and contain no more than 5 words. The same spelling list should be used for 3 nights in a row. This means that no more than 10 new words can be learned in a week. Follow the routine described for each word.

1. Write the target word out or make it with plastic letters. Tell your child how to say the word and what it means.

2. Ask your child to copy the target word and simultaneously to say the name of each letter as it is being written.

3. Ask your child to check that each letter he or she has written is the same as each letter in the target word.

4. When your child has copied a word correctly three times using steps 2 and 3, ask your child to look at the target word for a few seconds, cover up the target word, and write it from memory while simultaneously saying the name of each letter as it is being written.

5. Ask your child to check that each letter he or she has written is the same as each letter in the target word. When your child has copied a word correctly three times from memory, move on to learning the next word in the spelling list.

6. Make sure your child practises each word following this routine for 3 consecutive daily sessions.

This way of learning spelling is called the SOS method: **S**imultaneous **O**ral **S**pelling. Dr Lynette Bradley at Oxford University has shown that this method is almost twice as effective as other common methods of learning spelling, such as simple writing or simple repetition. SOS is a multi-sensory learning method. When your child uses the SOS method he or she is using all sensory channels to learn how to spell a new word. Your child is using visual, auditory and motor/movement channels to take in the spelling pattern of the new target word. Your child is also using his or her intelligence to check that they have not jumbled the order of letters by mistake. The SOS method also involves over-learning. Each word is practised for 3 days in a row. This helps your child remember each new word he or she learns. The method is slow. Only 10 new words can be learned per week. However, it is effective for children with specific learning difficulties.

Assessment

With specific reading difficulties and other specific learning problems, it is essential that there be close liaison between the clinical psychologist, the child's teacher, the parents, the child and other pertinent professionals (especially educational and school psychologists if they are involved). Routine interviews with parents and teachers should be conducted, copies of past school attainment reports should be obtained and behaviour checklists, such as those in the ASEBA or SDQ (listed in Table 4.1), should be completed by both parents and teachers. Routine screening for visual or hearing impairment should also be conducted. General principles for psychometric assessment of children's abilities are discussed in a later section of this chapter. Here, psychometric methods for assessing specific reading difficulties will be dealt with.

To diagnose specific learning disabilities, assess attainments with standardized tests such as the WIAT-II or WRAT-3 (listed in Table 8.6) and intelligence with tests such as the WISC-IV or BAS-II (listed in Table 8.2). The attainment–ability score discrepancy method or observed–predicted attainment score discrepancy method may be used to evaluate the presence of a specific learning difficulty. With the attainment–ability score discrepancy method, if any attainment score falls 1.5 standard deviations (about 22 points) below the Full Scale IQ score, then a specific learning difficulty in that area may be diagnosed. The observed and predicted attainment score method can be used if there is a table in the manual of the attainment or ability test that gives expected attainment scores associated with IQ level. From such tables, predicted attainment levels may be determined. The statistical significance of discrepancies between predicted and observed attainment levels may be evaluated with reference to tables of such discrepancies given in the manual. For both procedures, there is an assumption that the child had co-operated well with testing procedures and has had adequate opportunity to develop reading skills.

A further issue for assessment, once the presence of a specific learning difficulty has been established, is the pattern of specific cognitive deficits that underpins it and the pattern of specific strengths that may be tapped in a remedial reading programme. This pattern of cognitive strengths and weaknesses may be determined by inspecting the score scatter of the ability test. In Figure 8.3, an example of this type of analysis is given with respect to the WISC-IV. In Table 8.8 an approach to WISC-IV interpretation is given.

The Aston Index (Aubrey, Eaves, Hicks & Newton, 1982) contains subtests that specifically assess visual sequential memory, auditory sequential memory, sound blending and sound discrimination. It is common practice for remedial reading programmes to take account of the child's pattern of cognitive strengths and weaknesses, profiled using the results of the Aston, the WISC or BAS tests despite the fact that there is no evidence to show that this

Table 8.8 A procedure for interpreting the WISC-IV

Step	Procedures
1. Interpret Full Scale IQ (FSIQ)	• Assign the FSIQ score to an ability level (e.g. high average) and give a percentile rank • If the FSIQ is below 70, consider general intellectual disability as a hypothesis deserving further testing • If the FSIQ is above 70 and there are attainment problems, consider specific learning disability, motivational or situational problems in school, or sensory difficulties as hypotheses deserving further testing
2. Interpret the scatter of the four indices	• Assign verbal comprehension (VCI), perceptual reasoning (PRI), working memory (WMI), and processing speed (PSI) index scores to ability levels and give them percentile ranks • Differences between index scores of about 10 points should be interpreted • If there are no significant differences between the four index scores and if the FSIQ is below 70, consider general intellectual disability as a hypothesis deserving further testing • If there are attainment problems, a FSIQ above 70 and significant differences between index scores, consider specific learning disability, ADHD, traumatic brain injury, high functioning autism, Asperger's syndrome, sensory or motor disabilities, or situational influences on test behaviour or school performance as hypotheses deserving further testing
3. Interpret low PSI profile	• If PSI is more than 5 points lower than the other three indices, consider and test the following hypotheses: motor disability, head injury, or specific learning disability with written expression being the key area affected
4. Interpret low WMI profile	• If WMI is lower than the other three indices, consider and test the following hypotheses: specific learning disability with reading being the key area affected
5. Interpret low VCI profile	• If VCI is lower than the other three indices, consider and test the following hypotheses: specific language delay
6. Interpret low PRI profile	• If PRI is lower than the other three indices, consider and test the following hypotheses: specific learning disability with mathematics being the key area affected
7. Interpret high PRI profile	• If PRI is higher than the other three indices, consider and test the following hypotheses: autism

Continued

Table 8.8 continued

Step	Procedures
8. Interpret low PSI and WMI profile	• If PSI and WMI are both lower than the other two indices, consider and test the following hypothesis: ADHD
9. Interpret strengths from index and sub-test scatter	• Where indices are about 10 or more points above FSIQ interpret this as indicating strengths in that area
	• Where sub-test scores are 3 or more points above the mean sub-test score for the profile, interpret these as areas of strength

Note: Based on information in the WISC-IV manual and at http://www.psychcorp.com.au/ WISC-IV%20report%203.pdf and Sattler and Dumont (2004).

approach is any more effective than using a programme built on paired reading, phonics and simultaneous oral spelling (Snowling, 2002).

Where a very brief screening test is required prior to a full assessment, Fawcett and Nicholson (1996, 1997) have developed the Dyslexia Screening Test and the Dyslexia Early Screening Test, which detect the presence of cognitive deficits associated with specific learning difficulties.

Intervention

It is essential that remediation programmes for children with specific reading difficulties be based on a thorough assessment of the child's abilities and the potential resources within the family, the school and the wider professional network for remediating the child's reading difficulties. All programmes for children with specific reading disability should be highly *structured* with material increasing in difficulty as the child progresses. Material should be presented in a *sequence* and there should be a *cumulative* acquisition of reading and spelling skills (Reid, 2003).

Remediation tutorial programmes that include both training in reading passages of text and the use of exercises to improve phonic awareness (such as rhymes and alliteration) have better outcomes in terms of teaching decoding and spelling skills compared with methods that focus on the use of contextual cues and meaning-based strategies (Snowling, 1996).

Paired reading

Parental involvement in brief periods of daily paired reading is a highly effective preventative and treatment strategy for children with reading difficulties (Hewison, 1988; Topping, 1986). With this strategy, parents are trained to sit with their children and simultaneously read with them until the child is ready to read independently. During this phase, the child's errors are corrected by the parent modelling correct pronunciation of the appropriate word. Once children are ready to read independently, they use a non-verbal signal to indicate that parents should be silent and listen to them reading unaided. When children encounter errors they use a non-verbal signal to instruct parents to model the correct pronunciation of the difficult word for them. They then proceed with independent reading. The paired reading process, is a packaged set of routines to help parents provide what Vygotsky (1934/1962) referred to as scaffolding to facilitate the development of the child's emergent reading skills.

Simultaneous oral spelling

Multi-sensory approaches to spelling have been found to be effective for children with specific reading difficulties and of these, simultaneous oral spelling is particularly useful (Thompson, 1990). To learn a specific word, the child is first given a model word to copy. The child copies the model and concurrently says each letter aloud as it is copied so that visual, auditory and kinaesthetic modalities are used simultaneously to learn the spelling. After each trial, the child is required to check, letter by letter, what he or she has written against the model word. After three consecutive correct trials the procedure is repeated, but the model word is covered once it has been inspected and is written from memory. This procedure is followed with small groups of words, which are practised for three consecutive days, after which most children find the spellings have been learned. This multi-sensory approach may be used by children in conjunction with their parents, in working through a typical primary school spelling curriculum. However, in my clinical experience it works best when small groups of spellings are targeted each week and children are allowed to work at a pace that leads to the greatest rate of success. It may be coupled with a reward chart to maintain motivation. Notes for parents on paired reading and simultaneous oral spelling are contained in Figure 8.3.

Study skills

Adolescents with specific reading difficulties can, to some degree, offset the handicap entailed by their reading difficulties by developing good study skills. These include time management, active reading and mapping. With time management the three main skills are making a calendar of time slots, chunking work material, prioritizing chunks and slotting them into the calendar at appropriate times and troubleshooting when difficulties occur while implementing the study plan. In making a calendar of time slots, youngsters should be encouraged to take account of whether they work best in the morning or the evening, their span of concentration (which for most teenagers is about fifty minutes), and their work and leisure commitments. In chunking and prioritizing work, account should be taken of how much material may reasonably be covered in a fifty-minute slot, which topics can be studied for multiple consecutive periods and which are best studied for a single period sandwiched in between other topics. When troubleshooting difficulties, the overall goal of the study plan should always be given priority and the need for regular reinforcement and leisure activities, which the adolescent should construe as being his or her own reward for completing part of the study plan. Inevitably, parts of the plan will go awry. Improvising, rescheduling and avoiding catastrophizing, are key troubleshooting skills. Challenging cata-strophic thoughts is discussed in Chapter 12, where anxiety disorders are considered.

Active reading involves following a routine to actively extract meaning from texts and remember extracted points as coherent knowledge structures. The first step is to scan the text, noting the headings, and reading the over-view and summary if these are provided. In light of this scanning process, the second step is to list the main questions that may be answered by a detailed reading of the chapter. The third step is to read each section with a question in mind and at the end of the section write down the answer to the question that has arisen from reading the section. When this process has been completed for all sections, the fourth step is to re-read the questions and answers that have been composed a couple of times. Then with the answers covered, the questions should be asked once more and the answers recited from memory. The next step involves reviewing the accuracy of these answers. The final stage is try to draw out a visuo-spatial representation of the material, and post this *cognitive map* on the wall of the study for frequent inspection:

- step 1: scan
- step 2: question
- step 3: read and write answers
- step 4: re-read questions and answers
- step 5: recite answers to questions
- step 6: review accuracy of answers
- step 7: map new knowledge and post it on the wall.

Psychometric reports for specific learning difficulties

The general principles set out in Chapter 5 apply to writing reports to parents and members of the professional network about specific learning difficulties. However, it is often necessary to offer quite detailed and complex feedback to non-specialists and so writing psychometric reports requires additional skills. An example of a routine psychometric report for a child with a specific learning difficulty is presented in Figure 8.3. Also included in this figure are some guidelines for parents on helping their children with literacy skills.

HEAD INJURY

Many children who sustain head injuries develop transient or chronic learning difficulties. Commonly these learning difficulties are associated with
behavioural problems. An example of such a case is presented in Box 8.3.

Box 8.3 A case of traumatic brain injury

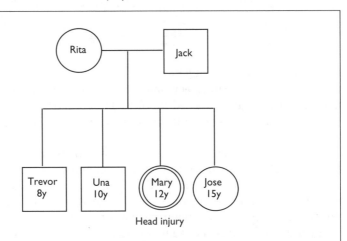

Head injury

Mary, aged twelve, was referred for routine psychological assessment a month
after involvement in a road traffic accident in which she sustained a closed head
injury. Her GCS at admission was 6 and at 24 hours was 9. She regained full
consciousness within 24 hours. A CAT scan confirmed the presence of bilateral
insults to the temporal and frontal lobes. Her EEG was within normal limits and
their was no evidence of seizure activity.

The central referral question concerned her prognosis in terms of attainment
problems and behavioural adjustment, which had been within normal limits prior to
the accident.

Her developmental history, as given by her mother was unremarkable, with her
development on sensorimotor, language, cognitive and social parameters falling
broadly within the normal range. An inspection of her school reports showed that
she was in the top 10% of her mixed-ability class. Samples of her school work and
this information suggested that her pre-morbid functioning was probably in the high
average range of general intellectual abilities.

The Child Behaviour Checklist was completed by her mother during the fourth
week following the trauma. Her scores on the anxiety/depression and attention
problem sub-scales fell within the clinical range.

She co-operated well with psychological assessment procedures; exhibited no
impairment of hearing or sight and was on no medication; so the results of the
psychological assessment were interpreted as a valid description of her level of
functioning a month following the trauma.

The WISC-IV and the WIAT-II were administered, along with the Wide Range
Assessment of Memory and Learning. She returned a full scale IQ that fell at the
lower end of the normal range. Her verbal skills, which were in the high average
range, were significantly less impaired than her working memory and processing

speed, which fell in the low average range. Both her verbal and visual memory showed significant impairment. She returned language and reading quotients that fell within the normal range and written language and mathematics quotients that fell within the low average range.

Her parents and teachers were informed of her psychological status and it was mentioned that gradual recovery over a 12-month period could be expected. Biannual reassessments for two years were arranged. Family work focusing on helping the parents and siblings to support Mary during her recovery was arranged. Meetings were held with her parents and teachers to plan her re-introduction into school.

Learning difficulties arising from traumatic brain injury typically involve problems in remembering new information or recalling previously learned information and are classified in DSM IV TR (APA, 2000a) and ICD 10 (WHO, 1992, 1996) as amnestic or amnesic disorders. Diagnostic criteria are presented in Table 8.9.

The main role of the clinical psychologist in these cases is to clearly document the child's competencies and disabilities and track these over time, while offering support and guidance to the child, parents and teachers during the recovery process. This functional approach to acquired learning difficulties is not concerned with predicting particular brain lesions from patterns of psychometric test findings in conjunction with other clinical data, or in tracking or predicting co-variation in brain–behaviour relationships over time; such skills require advanced training in neuropsychology (Reynolds & Ray, 1997). Where detailed evaluation of brain–behaviour linkages are required, a referral to a specialist neuropsychologist should be made.

Epidemiology

A number of conclusions may be drawn from literature on the epidemiology of traumatic brain injury (Goodman, 2002; Middleton, 2001; Snow & Hooper, 1994). The incidence of traumatic brain injury is twice as common among adolescents as pre-adolescents, and twice as common among boys as girls. For children under fourteen the incidence is approximately 200/100 000 per annum. For adolescents (fourteen to nineteen years old), the incidence is 550/100 000. Children with emotional, behavioural and learning difficulties from low socioeconomic status groups are at greater risk for traumatic brain injury, and children who have sustained a head injury are more likely to sustain a second injury. Road traffic accidents and falls are the principal causes of head injuries.

While head injury leads to cognitive and social adjustment problems, improvement in these areas occurs over time (Middleton, 2001; Snow & Hooper, 1994). Most of the limited amount of longitudinal data come from studies of non-penetrative head injuries. Different recovery patterns are

Table 8.9 Diagnostic criteria for learning disorders caused by head injury

DSM IV TR Amnestic disorder due to head trauma	ICD 10 Organic amnesic syndrome
A. The development of memory impairment as manifested by impairment in the ability to learn new information or the inability to recall previously learned information	A syndrome of prominent impairment of recent and remote memory. For a definitive diagnosis it is necessary to establish:
B. The memory disturbance causes significant impairment in social or occupational functioning and represents a significant decline from a previous level of functioning	A. Presence of a memory impairment manifest in a defect of recent memory (impaired learning new material); anterograde and retrograde amnesia, and a reduced ability to recall past experiences in reverse order of their occurrence
C. The memory disturbance does not occur exclusively during the course of a delirium or dementia	
D. There is evidence from the history, physical examination, or laboratory findings that the disturbance is the direct physiological consequence of a general medical condition (including physical trauma)	B. History or objective evidence of an insult to, or a disease of, the brain (especially with bilateral involvement of the diencephalic and medial temporal structures)
Code as transient or chronic if impairment is less or more than one month respectively	C. Absence of a defect in immediate recall of disturbances of attention and consciousness and of global intellectual impairment
	Confabulations, lack of insight and emotional changes are additional, although not necessary, pointers to the diagnosis

Note: Adapted from DSM IV TR (APA, 2000a) and ICD 10 (WHO, 1992, 1996).

shown by cases with mild and severe traumatic head injury. In most studies, severe head injury is defined as a score of 8 or less on the Glasgow Coma Scale (Teasdale & Jennett, 1974); the occurrence of post-traumatic amnesia for more than seven days, as assessed objectively by an instrument such as the Children's Orientation and Amnesia Test (Ewing-Cobbs, Levin, Fletcher, Miner & Eisenberg, 1990) and evidence of a mass lesion from a CT or MRI scan. These indices are described in more detail below.

Post-traumatic seizures are more common in cases of severe head injury. In comparison with mild cases, children with severe head injury tend to show greater deficits in most areas of cognitive functioning including memory, attention, visuo-spatial abilities and verbal abilities. But in comparison with mild cases, severe cases also show greater recovery of cognitive functioning, most of which occurs within twelve months of the injury. However, children with head injury continue to show gradual recovery of cognitive functioning for up to five years following injury, and possibly for longer. Recovery of cognitive functioning is associated with a gradual improvement in academic functioning. In comparison with mild cases, severe cases show pronounced difficulties in adaptive behaviour and psychological adjustment and available evidence shows that these problems persist for one to two years following injury, although they may persist for longer. In DSM IV TR these are referred to as *personality changes due to a general medical condition*. Labile, disinhibited, aggressive, apathetic, or paranoid are the principal types of personality changes specified. In ICD 10 these adjustment problems are referred to as *personality* and *behavioural disorders due to brain damage*. The applicability of these diagnostic categories to children and adolescents has not been researched.

The outcome in cases of head injury is related to pre-morbid adjustment, severity of the head injury, intracranial pressure, rate of recovery of specific functions, presence of seizures and psychosocial adversity (Goodman, 2002; Middleton, 2001; Snow & Hooper, 1994). Better pre-morbid adjustment is associated with a better outcome. The prognosis is best for cases of mild head injury, and the more rapidly a function re-emerges following injury the better the prognosis for that function. The presence of high intracranial pressure, seizures and psychosocial adversity increases the risk of long-term psychological adjustment difficulties. Outcome is unrelated to the gender of the child.

Neurological development and traumatic brain injury

The psychological sequelae of head injury are usefully considered within the context of available evidence on the two-stage development of the CNS (Rutter & Rutter, 1993). In the first phase of development there is a proliferation of nerve cells, which migrate to their final destination within the brain or spinal chord. Concurrently there is an elaboration of connections between neurons, which is marked by an increase in the number of synapses and of neurotransmitters to permit the transmission of signals across these synapses or neural junctions. By the end of infancy this process gives way to the second phase, when half of the nerve cells selectively die off so that only specific networks of connections between nerve cells are preserved. This subtractive second phase is best thought of as a fine-tuning process, during which specific neural networks become associated with specific functions. This fine-tuning process is to some degree dependent on sensory input, hence the importance of early infant sensory and intellectual stimulation. Such stimulation in part determines the nature and complexity of preserved neural networks and has implications for which nerve cells die off. The second stage is not complete until mid-adolescence.

This model of brain development allows coherent explanations to be offered for clinically observed patterns of recovery from brain damage at different ages. Three distinct patterns have been clinically identified, although carefully controlled longitudinal studies have not yet been conducted to verify these clinical observations. Each pattern is associated with different stages of the lifecycle. The acquisition of specific skills may appear normal when unilateral or bilateral brain damage occurs pre-natally or during infancy. However, overall intelligence may be somewhat impaired. From the toddler period through to mid-adolescence, recovery from bilateral brain damage may be as poor as in adults but recovery of specific skills following unilateral damage may be more pronounced than for adults. After mid-adolescence, lasting skills deficits result from both unilateral and bilateral brain damage. We may hypothesize that the lack of specific skills deficits associated with brain damage in infancy may be due to the capacity of the CNS for reorganization during this period. However, once the subtractive second phase begins in toddlerhood, only some degree of reorganization (associated with unilateral damage) becomes possible.

Assessment

When a child is referred for psychological consultation following traumatic head injury, some basic referral questions may be answered by most clinical psychologists without specialist neuropsychological training. For example, those that inquire about the general prognosis in terms of academic attainment, functional limitations and behavioural problems, and those that require the development of programmes for the management of the sequelae of traumatic brain injury. In routine clinical psychology practice, the framework presented in Figure 8.4 may be used as a guide to assessing factors that may have implications for prognosis and treatment (Fletcher, 1988).

In the practice of specialist neuropsychology, more complex models which include a greater range of variables are required as a basis for answering highly specific question about current and probable future brain–behaviour relationships (Reynolds & Ray, 1997). Where answers to such specific questions are required, referral to a specialist neuropsychologist should be made. What follows are some comments on the assessment of a number of the variables listed in Figure 8.4 (those variables included in Figure 8.4 that have already been discussed in Chapter 4 will not be considered in detail here).

Biological indices of functioning immediately following traumatic brain injury

Usually a full medical assessment will have been carried out immediately following injury. Interpreting this medical information is an important first

PRE-DISPOSING FACTORS

PERSONAL PRE-DISPOSING FACTORS

Biological factors
- Genetic vulnerabilities
- Pre- and peri-natal complications
- Early insults, injuries and illnesses

Psychological factors
- Low intelligence
- Difficult temperament
- Low self-esteem
- External locus of control

CONTEXTUAL PRE-DISPOSING FACTORS

Parent–child factors in early life
- Attachment problems
- Lack of intellectual stimulation
- Authoritarian parenting
- Permissive parenting
- Neglectful parenting
- Inconsistent parental discipline

Exposure to family problems in early life
- Parental psychological problems
- Parental alcohol and substance abuse
- Parental criminality
- Marital discord or violence
- Family disorganization
- Deviant siblings

Stresses in early life
- Bereavements
- Separations
- Child abuse
- Social disadvantage
- Institutional upbringing

PERSONAL PROTECTIVE FACTORS

Biological factors
- Good physical health

Psychological factors
- High IQ
- Easy temperament
- High self-esteem
- Internal locus of control
- High self-efficacy
- Optimistic attributional style
- Mature defence mechanisms
- Functional coping strategies

PERSONAL MAINTAINING FACTORS

Biological factors
- Dysregulation of physiological systems impaired by brain damage

Psychological factors
- Low self-efficacy
- Dysfunctional attributional style
- Negative cognitive distortions
- Immature defence mechanisms
- Dysfunctional coping strategies

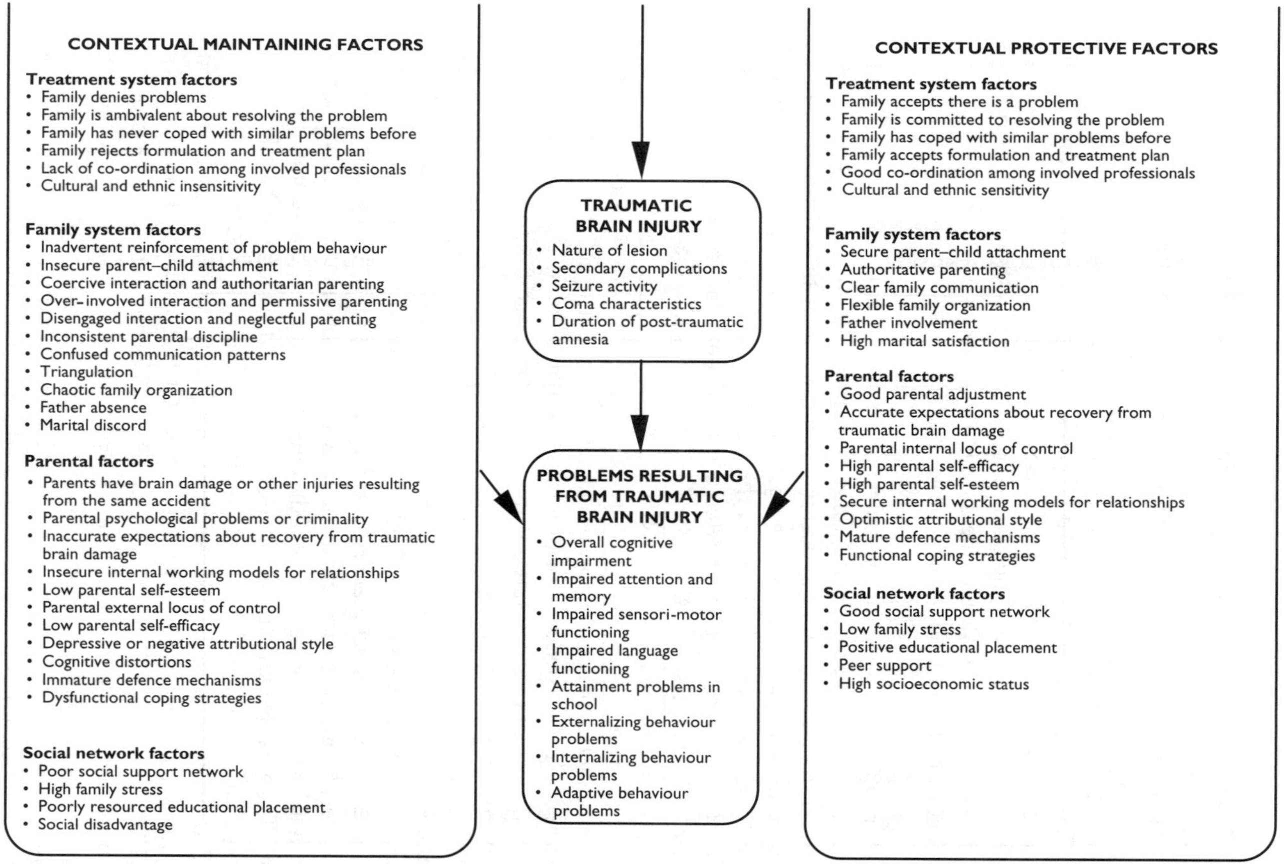

CONTEXTUAL MAINTAINING FACTORS

Treatment system factors
- Family denies problems
- Family is ambivalent about resolving the problem
- Family has never coped with similar problems before
- Family rejects formulation and treatment plan
- Lack of co-ordination among involved professionals
- Cultural and ethnic insensitivity

Family system factors
- Inadvertent reinforcement of problem behaviour
- Insecure parent–child attachment
- Coercive interaction and authoritarian parenting
- Over-involved interaction and permissive parenting
- Disengaged interaction and neglectful parenting
- Inconsistent parental discipline
- Confused communication patterns
- Triangulation
- Chaotic family organization
- Father absence
- Marital discord

Parental factors
- Parents have brain damage or other injuries resulting from the same accident
- Parental psychological problems or criminality
- Inaccurate expectations about recovery from traumatic brain damage
- Insecure internal working models for relationships
- Low parental self-esteem
- Parental external locus of control
- Low parental self-efficacy
- Depressive or negative attributional style
- Cognitive distortions
- Immature defence mechanisms
- Dysfunctional coping strategies

Social network factors
- Poor social support network
- High family stress
- Poorly resourced educational placement
- Social disadvantage

TRAUMATIC BRAIN INJURY
- Nature of lesion
- Secondary complications
- Seizure activity
- Coma characteristics
- Duration of post-traumatic amnesia

PROBLEMS RESULTING FROM TRAUMATIC BRAIN INJURY
- Overall cognitive impairment
- Impaired attention and memory
- Impaired sensori-motor functioning
- Impaired language functioning
- Attainment problems in school
- Externalizing behaviour problems
- Internalizing behaviour problems
- Adaptive behaviour problems

CONTEXTUAL PROTECTIVE FACTORS

Treatment system factors
- Family accepts there is a problem
- Family is committed to resolving the problem
- Family has coped with similar problems before
- Family accepts formulation and treatment plan
- Good co-ordination among involved professionals
- Cultural and ethnic sensitivity

Family system factors
- Secure parent–child attachment
- Authoritative parenting
- Clear family communication
- Flexible family organization
- Father involvement
- High marital satisfaction

Parental factors
- Good parental adjustment
- Accurate expectations about recovery from traumatic brain damage
- Parental internal locus of control
- High parental self-efficacy
- High parental self-esteem
- Secure internal working models for relationships
- Optimistic attributional style
- Mature defence mechanisms
- Functional coping strategies

Social network factors
- Good social support network
- Low family stress
- Positive educational placement
- Peer support
- High socioeconomic status

Figure 8.4 A framework for assessment of adjustment problems in cases of traumatic brain injury

step in the process of psychological assessment. Information should be abstracted from the medical notes on the following items:

- Nature of the lesion and supporting results from skull X-rays, CT and MRI scans.
- Secondary complications, such as raised intracranial pressure, hypoxia, ischemia, cerebral oedema, haemorrhage, cerebral atrophy or enlargement of ventricles.
- Seizure activity and supporting EEG results along with information about the patient's anti-convulsant medication.
- Coma characteristics, including the initial and 24-hour ratings on the Glasgow Coma Scale and the duration of coma.
- The duration of traumatic amnesia.

Over 90% of cases of paediatric traumatic brain damage are non-penetrative closed head injuries (Snow & Hooper, 1994). That is, the skull is not fractured, or if fracturing occurs it is linear rather than depressed. Such injuries, in contrast to penetrative injuries, tend to be associated with diffuse rather than focal lesions. However, the results of skull X-rays, CT scans and MRI scans may be used to draw conclusions about the location and extent of the structural lesions. A neuroanatomical atlas may be consulted to aid interpretation of such reports (Menkes, 1990).

Secondary neuronal damage may occur due to hypoxia associated with poorly oxygenated blood supply or ischaemia where obstructed blood flow has occurred. Cerebral oedema (or brain swelling) or haemorrhaging may lead to increased intracranial pressure and further brain damage. Cerebral atrophy and enlargement of ventricles may also occur secondary to traumatic brain injury.

Immediate or delayed seizure activity may occur following traumatic brain injury, with such activity being more common in cases of severe injury. However, it is worth keeping in mind that seizure activity in some cases may precede, or indeed, precipitate events leading to traumatic brain injury. Where EEG results indicate that seizure activity or post-traumatic epilepsy is present, it is important to determine if the child is taking anti-convulsant medication. The possible sedative effects of such medication should be taken into account when conducting and interpreting psychological tests.

Patients who sustain head injuries are typically rated on admission and 24 hours later on the Glasgow Coma Scale (GCS; Teasdale & Jennett, 1974). The Glasgow Coma Scale rates the quality of the child's motor response to a verbal command or physical stimulus, verbal response to a question and the presence or absence of eye-opening responses to speech or touch on ordinal scales and sums the results to give a score, which can range from 3 (indicating a profound coma) to 15 (reflecting an alert state). Ratings of 8 or less indicate a profound coma and, in many studies, a rating of 8 or less is taken to indicate the presence of severe traumatic brain injury.

The duration of post-traumatic anterograde amnesia (PTA) is typically timed from the point at which the person regains consciousness following coma and is characterized by an inability to remember new information. The period ends when the person's capacity to recall some recent events is restored, but some retrograde amnesia (loss of memory prior to the injury) may remain. The Children's Orientation and Amnesia Test (COAT; Ewing-Cobbs et al., 1990) is a useful method for rating recovery from amnesia.

Problems resulting from traumatic brain injury

Following traumatic brain injury, problems with cognitive functioning, academic attainment and behavioural adjustment may occur. The youngster's status in each of these domains may be assessed using appropriate psychometric instruments. Cognitive functioning should be assessed with a battery of tests, which cover memory and attention; non-verbal, sensorimotor abilities; and verbal and language abilities. A battery including tests such as the WISC-IV, the WIAT-II and the Wide Range Assessment of Memory and Learning (Sheslow & Adams, 2004), may be used for this. Details of the WISC-IV have been presented in Table 8.2 and the WIAT-II is mentioned in Table 8.6. The Wide Range Assessment of Memory and Learning, which was standardized in the US on a representative sample of over 2000 children aged between five and seventeen offers a comprehensive assessment of memory functioning. Behavioural problems may be assessed using the ASEBA or SDQ checklists (listed in Table 4.1) and competencies may be assessed using a broad social functioning scale such as the Vineland Adaptive Behaviour Scale (listed in Table 8.3).

Pre-disposing, maintaining and protective factors

Routine interviewing and assessment procedures (described in Chapter 4) may be used to assess pre-disposing, maintaining and protective factors, all of which have implications for the child's recovery. The child's pre-morbid adjustment, parental coping resources and social disadvantage should be explored in some detail in the family interview. The resources available to the school, particularly the possibility of some individual or small-group tuition, along with the capacity of the school to work closely with the psychologist and other members of the assessment team in implementing programmes to help the child manage the sequelae of traumatic brain injury are important areas to probe in school-based interviews.

Intervention

Routine intervention with the child, family and school in cases of traumatic brain injury should include:

- psychoeducation where prognostic information is provided
- periodic reassessment where recovery is regularly tracked
- parent and child counselling on the management of memory problems, seizure activity, and the emotional and behavioural sequelae of traumatic brain injury.

General prognostic information may be offered on the basis of the review of longitudinal outcome studies summarized earlier in this chapter. For more specific prognostic information, a specialist neuropsychological consultation should be arranged.

On the basis of a functional analysis of specific situations at home and at school, in which children show particularly disruptive forgetting, seizure activity, emotional distress or behavioural problems, individualized programmes may be developed. These programmes may be developed on the basis of the principles set out in the neuropsycholgical rehabilitation literature (e.g. Anderson, Northam, Hendy & Wrennall, 2001; Yeates, Ris & Taylor, 1999) and general clinical intervention literature such as that presented in other chapters of this book.

Programmes targeting memory problems may centre on helping the child to develop strategies to get through each day without missing-out important aspects of daily routines, rather than on improving memory functioning. Developing systematic routines, arranging the environment so that it is very predictable and using lists and alarm timers may be tested as possible environmental interventions. Coaching youngsters to organize material that has to be learned into a coherent visual or linguistic map, helping them to use multi-sensory learning methods where auditory, visual and kinaesthetic channels are used simultaneously to learn new information and encouraging over-learning are skills-based strategies for improving memory that may be tested with individual cases.

Programmes to alter seizure activity may include interruption of pre-seizure behavioural chains, desensitization to seizure-producing stimuli and the removal of the positive and negative reinforcing social consequences which follow from seizure activities.

Programmes targeting emotional problems such as anxiety and depression, and conduct problems such as aggression and impulsivity, may be developed for children with traumatic brain damage in the same way as those for children who have these problems but who have not suffered from brain damage. Such interventions are discussed in Chapters 10, 11, 12 and 17. Central organizing themes in working with children and families where traumatic brain injury has occurred are parental guilt for not preventing the accident and grief associated with the loss of the health child. A fuller discussion of grief processes is given in Chapter 24.

For language problems, referral to a speech therapist may be made and, in the case of motor impairments, referral to a physiotherapist is appropriate. Multi-disciplinary co-ordination of various components of an overall treatment programme is essential where a number of professionals are contributing to rehabilitation.

PSYCHOMETRIC TESTS AND CLINICAL PRACTICE

Psychometric tests are central to clinical practice in cases of learning and communication problems. This part of the chapter deals with three issues. First, some guidelines for evaluating new tests will be given; second, there will be a discussion of some aspects of the most popular ability tests; finally, guidelines for practice in cases where psychometric assessment forms part of the overall evaluation process will be outlined.

Evaluating new tests

Psychometric tests are useful tools for assessing learning and communication problems. The production and marketing of these tests is also big business and practising clinicians are regularly flooded with advertisements for new instruments that make claims they often do not live up to. Professional associations such as the British Psychological Society and the American Psychological Association periodically publish standards that may be used by individual clinicians as evaluating tests. Such standards require regular revision because of the growth of increasingly sophisticated test-construction technology.

However, in selecting new tests four issues should be taken into consideration:

- norms
- reliability
- validity
- user-friendliness.

Norms

Ideally, a test should be standardized on the population from which your clinical cases will be referred. The normative sample should be large and representative of the population containing your referrals. This will usually mean that the population is the same nationality and falls within the same age bracket as the cases you intend to assess using the test. Often, however, this ideal cannot be achieved. For example, here in Ireland, we routinely use ability and intelligence tests standardized on UK and US populations of children. Tests that are standardized on small, unrepresentative samples of children who do not closely resemble the population from which your referrals are drawn should not be used, since valid conclusions may not be drawn from clients' scores on them.

Reliability

Reliability refers to the stability and consistency of test or scale scores across items, raters and testing occasions. Ideally, tests should be highly reliable with internal consistency reliability co-efficients and test–retest reliability co-efficients of .9 or greater. Internal consistency co-efficients, of which Crohnbach's alpha is the most common, indicate the degree to which all of the items in the test reliably contribute to the overall test score. Test–retest reliability co-efficients indicate the stability of test scores over time. In the case of rating scales, inter-rater reliability of greater than .9 is also desirable. This indicates that when two people rate the same case using the rating scale, they make similar ratings. Tests and rating scales that have reliability co-efficients below .7 are not clinically useful.

Validity

A valid test is one which measures that construct which it purports to measure. Ideally, there should be data to show that a test has concurrent criterion validity, predictive criterion validity and construct validity. For concurrent and predictive criterion validity, a series of studies should be cited in the test manual to show that the test scores correlate highly with the status of cases on meaningful criteria at the same point in time and some time after the test has been administered. For example, the results of a new intelligence test should correlate with results of other intelligence tests given at the same time or some time (say a year) after the first period of testing. For construct validity, studies should be cited in the test manual which show that the test has relationships with other constructs entailed by well-validated theories. For example, high scores on an adaptive behaviour scale dimension would be expected to correlated negatively with scores on the Child Behaviour Checklist. In cases where a test is expected to measure a number of factors (such as verbal and non-verbal intelligence) the construct validity of the test is supported by studies which show that the factors the test is intended to measure are consistent with the results of a factor analysis.

User friendliness

A user-friendly test has convenience features that make it attractive to clients and clinicians. Tests that engage clients' interest, sustain their motivation and do not distress or bore them are user friendly. Tests that are easy to administer, quick to score and have features that minimize the chances of clerical errors are user friendly for clinicians. It is also helpful if tests form part of a suite of tests that are similarly scored and normed. The Wechsler intelligence and achievement tests are a good example of this. Finally, it is useful if tests include a facility for computer administration, scoring or report writing. For example, Dougherty (1996) has developed a software package for writing standard reports based on a number of commonly used attainment and achievement tests. Standard reports may be imported into a word processing package and customized for each client. Only computerized reports that permit such customization are desirable for good practice.

The WISC and other IQ tests

David Wechsler has developed the most widely used set of intelligence tests and related tests of ability in the English-speaking world. Details of recent versions of these are given in Tables 8.2 and 8.6. The bulk of children referred to child and adolescent psychologists with learning problems as a primary or secondary difficulty are between the ages of six and seventeen. For this reason, the Wechsler test specifically for this age group will now be considered in detail. The test is the Wechsler Intelligence Scale for Children, which is now in its Fourth Edition (WISC-IV). Previous versions of the WISC have been widely used in the US, the UK, Ireland and elsewhere. For toddlers too young to compete the WISC there is the Wechsler Preschool and Primary Scale of Intelligence (now in its third revision: WPPSI-III). This is suitable for children aged three to seven years. With older teenagers and adults aged sixteen and over, the Wechsler Adult Intelligence Scale (now in its third revision: WAIS-III) may be used. The Wechsler Abbreviated Scale of Intelligence (WASI) is a four-sub-test scale for use with people aged between six and eighty-nine years. There is also a suite of Wechsler individual ability tests to assess language, literacy and numeracy skills. These are the Wechsler Individual Attainment Tests (now in their second revision: WIAT-II); details of these are given in Table 8.6.

Comparison of WISC scores with other Wechsler tests

Comparisons of full scale IQ (FSIQ) scores on past versions of the WISC, WPPSI, WAIS and WASI show that significant discrepancies occur (Sattler, 1992, 2001a; Sattler & Dumont, 2004). This must be borne in mind when conducting follow-up assessments of children who were previously assessed with other revisions of a similar Wechsler test (e.g. following-up a child with the WISC-IV who was previously assessed with the WISC-III) and also when following-up children previously assessed with other tests (e.g. following up a child with the WISC-IV who was previously assessed with the WPPSI-R). These discrepancies across different revisions and versions of the test are documented in Jerry Sattler's books (1992, 2001a; Sattler & Dumont, 2004). The full scale IQ of the WISC-IV has been found to be about 3 points lower than that of the WISC-III, the WAIS-III and the WASI, but less than a point different from the WPPSI-III.

Practice effects and short forms of the WISC-III

Where repeated testing is conducted over time, it is important to take account of gains made due to practice effects. Over a three-week period on Wechsler tests, gains of up to 8 points may occurs in FSIQ; 2 points in verbal IQ and 8 points in perceptual IQ. These gains are also documented in Jerry Sattler's books (1992, 2001a; Sattler & Dumont, 2004). Short forms of Wechsler tests may be used for preliminary screening, for assessing children with sensory or motor impairments who are unable to complete the full test, for assessing overall ability when this issues is a peripheral part of the overall assessment or for research purposes. Vocabulary and block design is the most reliable and valid two-sub-test short form of most Wechsler tests, which include both a verbal and a performance sub-test. Results of short forms may be converted to IQs using the tables provided in Jerry Sattler's books (1992, 2001a; Sattler & Dumont, 2004). A less sophisticated approach is to divide the sum of the scaled scores by the number of sub-tests administered and multiply by total number of sub-tests in the full version of the test. However, this approach yields a crude estimate and does not take account of varying sub-test reliability.

Alternatives to Wechsler's tests

Important alternatives to Wechsler's approach to test development include the Stanford–Binet (now in its fifth edition) and the British Ability Scales (now in its second edition) details of which are given in Table 8.2. Both of these tests have a wide age range and may be used with children from pre-school years right up to late teenage years, and the Stanford–Binet may be used with adults. The British Ability Scales is widely used in the UK.

Guidelines for using tests in clinical practice

Use a core battery approach

Ability tests may be used to check out hypotheses or as a vehicle for establishing a relationship with the child and generating hypotheses about their difficulties. For hypotheses generating, clinicians should have a core battery of tests with which they become very familiar. For hypothesis testing, clinicians should carefully select specific tests which are added onto the core battery to assess specific functions or deficits.

Take account of sensorimotor and medication factors

Before testing, check the child's sensory or motor functioning and medication usage with the referring agent. If the child has sensory or motor deficits, specific tests will need to be chosen for the assessment session. Medication may affect the child's alertness. All of these factors may have implications for the duration of the assessment or the number of sessions required for its completion.

Explain procedures

Explain the administration of the tests to both the parents and the children. Testing may be described as a way of finding out what the child's strengths are and how he or she can take advantage of these strengths in learning new skills at school and at home. For younger children, explain that the tests are a series of puzzles or games that most children like to try out. Explain to parents and children how long the testing will take, when they will receive the results and what use will be made of the results. With young children, give explanations in terms they can understand: 'This will be like a full morning in play-school. We will have a break for juice and biscuits just like you have at play-school.'

Start with an ice-breaker

In setting up the testing situation, meeting the child in the waiting room, bringing him or her to your office, engaging in pre-testing interaction and completing the tests, try to visualize it from the child's viewpoint and make arrangements that will maximize the child's motivation and performance within the boundaries set by the standard procedures in the manual. Have an *ice-breaker* activity prepared for the child to absorb his or her attention as soon as they enter the testing situation. The more attractive this is the better. However, it should be an activity from which the child will find it easy to disengage when you are ready to begin formal testing. Drawing a self-portrait or a house, tree and person with big felt-tipped pens is a useful ice-breaker.

Make a smooth transition to testing

Make a smooth transition from the ice-breaker to the first sub-test to be administered. To the child, the more this transition seems like a direct continuation in a sequence of enjoyable activities, the better. Arrange the manual, stopwatch and all testing materials and recording forms so that they are easily accessible to you but not the child. Arrange the seating and desk or table so that the specific material you wish the child to manipulate is easily accessible to the child. Let the child know that the testing situation involves spending a small period of time on a lot of tasks, rather than a long period of time on a single task.

Manage family members sensitively

If parents remain with children during testing, place their chairs outside the child's visual field and ask parents to help their children to concentrate and develop a good working relationship with you by remaining silent. Giving the parent a Child Behaviour Checklist or Strengths and Difficulties Question-naire and other paper and pencil instruments to complete may offer them a way to remain present to support their child without compromising the valid-ity of the testing procedures. Parents may wish to remain with their children throughout testing procedures when they are very young, when they have particular types of disabilities, or when the parent and child have separation anxiety. It is important to always respect the parent's wish to remain with the child during assessment procedures, except in certain child-protection assessment situations. This issue is discussed in the chapter on child sexual abuse. If other children are present during testing (for example where testing is conducted in the child's home), give them an absorbing task to do, such as drawing or writing a story.

Manage children's adjustment to the session sensitively

Reward children with smiles and praise for motivation, effort and co-operation, not for giving the correct response. Where children say *I don't know* instantly to all items, encourage them to guess. If they give wild guesses, encourage them to think through their answers before replying. If anxiety, anger, excitability, boredom or sadness begin to interfere with a child's motiv-ation and performance, decide whether to distract the child from these experiences by helping him or her to focus concentration on the testing situ-ation, or whether to take a break from the testing procedures. Often, child-ren's off-task comments and behaviour give important clinical information about the child's problems. It may give information about how long they can concentrate for, what sorts of material or situations interfere with their on-task behaviour; what types of life themes pre-occupy them; and how they respond to being given space to ventilate their feelings or efforts to refocus their attention.

Modify standard procedures if necessary

If children have problems completing all tests in a single session, spread tests across a number of sessions. Follow the instructions in the manual unless the child's characteristics (e.g. sensory impairment, motor impairments, behavioural difficulties, difficulties related to medication) or characteristics of the situation (e.g. limited amount of time available, distracting or noisy clinical environment) make modifications necessary. Make a note of all modifications to standard procedures and take these into account when drawing conclusions. Make a note of the level of co-operation shown by the child in completing the testing and the degree to which this detracts from the reliability and validity of the obtained results. Record all answers and times (for timed responses) accurately.

Score tests accurately

Score tests according to the manual. Double-check computations; double-check conversions from raw scores to normed scores; tabulate results. Wherever possible, express results as percentiles, since these are easy for parents and other professionals to interpret.

Give feedback to parents

At the conclusion of a testing session, praise the child for sustained effort. Then try to put yourself (metaphorically) in the parents' shoes. Parents will have had concerns about the tests, their child's abilities and so forth and will want, in many instances, to know exactly what the results were. At least four options are open here. The first is to let parents know how well the child co-operated with the testing procedure and assure the parent that the result of the tests will be valid because of the level of motivation and co-operation shown. Then invite parents to a subsequent appointment where the results will be given when the scoring is complete and has been considered in the light of data from other sources such as other members of a multi-disciplinary team and the school. The second option is to ask the parents to wait in the clinic while scoring and interpretation is completed and then convene a feedback meeting. The third option is to let the parent know that further testing is required and arrange further appointments. The final option is to let the parents know that valid results could not be obtained and to make arrangements for further case management that take account of this.

Work co-operatively with schools

Once parents have understood the implications of psychometric results and related clinical findings, a plan for communicating these results to the child's teachers and discussing how an appropriate programme of remedial education may be developed, resourced and implemented needs to be worked out. A useful framework for joint working with families and schools has been described by Dowling and Osborne (1994).

Prevention

Early intervention programmes for children with ID, either alone or accompanied by physical disability, have been shown to have an impact on later adjustment, although the extent and durability of this effect remains a matter for debate. Such programmes focus on skills training for the child in conjunction with parent support and training (Lange & Carr, 2002; O'Sullivan & Carr, 2002). Controversy remains about the value of early intervention programmes for speech and language disorders, particularly in the case of expressive language disorders and articulation problems (Snowling, 2002). With specific reading retardation and other specific learning disabilities, there is agreement that the earlier these problems are recognized and remedial tuition started, the better, although there are few data to support this position (Maughan, 1995; Topping, 1986). With head injury, teaching children safety skills such as wearing helmets when riding bicycles is central to prevention, and programmes to teach such skills can be effective (Weiss, 1992).

SUMMARY

This chapter considered general and specific learning disabilities, communication problems and the learning difficulties that occur following traumatic brain injury. Between 1 and 3% of the population may be classified as having intellectual disabilities. Discrete genetic and organic factors are implicated in the aetiology of moderate and severe disability, whereas polygenetic influences and psychosocial adversity underpin mild ID. Intervention programmes include psychoeducation, organization of appropriate supports and periodic review, offering life skills training for the child; providing consultancy to manage challenging behaviour, counselling during family lifecycle transitions and supporting families in dealing with the grief process.

Specific language delays may be sub-classified as expressive, which are the most common, and mixed receptive-expressive delays, which are the most debilitating. Language delays may involve difficulties with phonology, semantics, syntax, pragmatics and fluency. There is a hierarchy of vulnerability in the components of language that are effected in cases of specific language delay; expressive phonology is the most vulnerable component, through expressive syntax and morphology, expressive semantics, to receptive language, which is the least vulnerable component. Specific language delays are most common among children under five and they are far more common among boys. They are associated with co-morbid conduct problems and later reading difficulties. Genetic factors play a central role in the aetiology of many language delays. Otitis media may play a role in expressive language disorders and psychosocial disadvantage may also play an aetiological role in some cases. In differential diagnosis, specific language delay should be distinguished from the following three syndromes, autism, Landau–Kleffner syndrome and elective mutism. Multi-disciplinary assessment and referral for individualized speech therapy are central to the management of specific language delays.

Up to 5% of children suffer from specific learning disabilities and, of these, specific reading disability is the most common. Genetic factors probably play an important role in the aetiology of these disorders, although psycho-social factors may maintain the secondary conduct and emotional problems that typically develop in youngsters with such disabilities. Psychometric evaluation followed by home–school liaison and remedial tuition is the management approach of choice.

Learning difficulties arising from traumatic brain injury typically involve problems in remembering new information or recalling previously learned information and are classified in DSM IV TR and ICD 10 as amnesic disorders. Following traumatic brain injury, children may show cognitive, attainment and behavioural difficulties. The severity of these difficulties is influenced by biological factors associated with the injury, pre-disposing personal and contextual factors associated with premorbid functioning, personal and contextual maintaining factors and personal and contextual protective factors. Important biological factors for later adjustment include the nature of the lesion, secondary complications, seizure activity, coma duration and the duration of traumatic amnesia. Intervention in cases of traumatic brain injury should include psychoeducation where prognostic information is provided; periodic reassessment where recovery is regularly tracked and counselling on the management of memory problems, seizure activity and the emotional and behavioural sequelae of traumatic brain injury.

In selecting psychometric tests for use in the assessment of learning and communication problems, the availability of appropriate norms and the adequacy of their reliability, validity and user friendliness should be taken into account. Routinely using a core test battery, with supplementary tests added as required, is a particularly manageable way to deal with cohorts of cases requiring psychometric assessment of learning and communication problems. In assessing any case, the impact of sensorimotor problems and medication factors should be taken into account. Testing procedures should be explained at the outset and a sensitive approach to parents and children taken in managing their adjustment to the testing situation. Standard testing procedures should only be modified if this is absolutely necessary to accommodate to the child's unique disabilities. Tests should be accurately scored and feedback given sensitively. Co-operative work with parents and schools may follow.

Early intervention programmes for children with ID either alone or accompanied by physical disability, have been shown to have an impact on later adjustment and these programmes focus on skills training for the child in conjunction with parent support and training.

EXERCISE 8.1

If Bruce and Sandra mentioned, in Box 8.1, were referred to you when Bruce was eleven following an incident where he hit and injured his mother, how would you go about conducting an assessment of the situation?

EXERCISE 8.2

Work in groups of five. Three people take the roles of Roy Murphy and his parents mentioned in Figure 8.3. The other two people take the role of a clinical team. The team's task is to explain the test results to Mr and Mrs Murphy and Roy and then coach them in how to do paired reading and simultaneous oral spelling.

EXERCISE 8.3

With respect to the case described in Box 8.2, work in triads taking the roles of psychologist, mother and father. The psychologist must give the parents the information arising from the assessment. The parents enter this interview with the view that Chris is naughty, just like his cousin. The mother thinks that this is because the father is too lenient. The father blames Chris's mis-behaviour on his TV-watching habits. The teacher has hinted that the boy has an ID.

EXERCISE 8.4

With respect to the case described in Box 8.3, what feedback would you give Mary and her parents.

FURTHER READING

Dowling, E. & Osborne, E. (1994). *The Family and The School. A Joint Systems approach to Problems with Children* (Second Edition). London: Routledge.

Flanagan, D. & Kaufman, A. (2004). *Essentials of WISC-IV Assessment*. New York: Wiley.

Luckasson, R., Borthwick-Duffy, S., Buntinx, W., Coulter, D., Craig, E., Reeve, A., Schalock, R., Snell, M., Spitalnik, D., Spreat, S., & Tasse, M. (2002) *Mental Retardation: Definition, Classification, and Systems of Supports* (10th Edition). Washington, DC: American Association on Mental Retardation.

Reid, G. (2003). *Dyslexia: A Practitioner's Handbook* (Third Edition). Chichester: Wiley.

Reynolds, C. & Ray, I. (1997). *Handbook of Clinical Child Neuropsychology* (Second Edition). New York: Plenum.

Sattler, J. (2001). *Assessment of Children. Behavioural and Clinical Applications* (Fourth Edition). San Diego, CA: Sattler. http://www.sattlerpublisher.com/

Sattler, J. & Dumont, R. (2004). *Assessment of Children with the WISC IV and WPPSI III Supplement*. SanDiego: Sattler. http://www.sattlerpublisher.com/

Wall, K. (2003). *Special Needs and Early Years Practice. A Practitioner's Guide*. London: Paul Chapman.

WEBSITES

American Association of Mental Retardation: http://www.aamr.org/

American Speech–Language–Hearing Association: http://www.asha.org

Brain Injury Association: http://www.biausa.org

British Dyslexia Association: http://www.bda-dyslexia.org.uk/

British Institute for Learning Disabilities: http://www.bild.org.uk

Dyslexia Institute: http://www.dyslexia-inst.org.uk

Headway – for Brain Injury Association: http://www.headway.org.uk/

International Dyslexia Association: http://www.interdys.org/

Internet Resources for Speech & Language: http://library.hcs.ucl.ac.uk/Links/SLT.htm

Speech and Language specialists – Fast Forward: http://www.scientificlearning.com/

Speech and Language specialists – Hannen: http://hanen.velocet.ca/

Factsheets on the specific and general learning disabilities given in this book can be downloaded from the website for Rose, G. & York, A. (2004). *Mental Health and Growing Up. Fact sheets for Parents, Teachers and Young People* (Third edition). London: Gaskell: http://www.rcpsych.ac.uk

Chapter 9

Autism and pervasive developmental disorders

Autism (Kanner, 1943) and other pervasive developmental disorders (or autistic spectrum disorders as they are also termed) entail substantial social, communicative and behavioural problems (Lord & Bailey, 2002; Volkmar, Lord, Bailey, Schultz & Klin, 2004). The early and accurate identification, evaluation and management of children with these problems is essential. Working in partnership with parents and teachers is central to good practice in this area (Lord & National Research Council, 2001). As youngsters move towards adulthood, promoting skills for independent living, insofar as that is possible within the constraints entailed by the disability, becomes the primary goal. The outcome for children with autism is poor. From 61 to 73% are unable to live independently and only 5–17% reach a stage where they can live a normal social and vocational life (Gillberg & Coleman, 2000). Children with a non-verbal IQ in the normal range and some functional language skills by the age of five have the best prognosis. However, under-estimating the potential of children with pervasive developmental disorders to develop life skills is the major pitfall to be avoided. Catherine Maurice's account of how she used behavioural methods to help two of her own children achieve a high level of functioning should offer hope to parents and professionals who treat children with this disorder (Maurice, 1993). A case of autism is presented in Box 9.1. This chapter, after considering the classification, epidemiology and clinical features of autism and other pervasive developmental disorders, considers a variety of theoretical explanations concerning their aetiology, along with relevant empirical evidence. The assessment of autism and an approach to its management is then given.

CLASSIFICATION AND EPIDEMIOLOGY

Children who show extremely marked abnormalities in their capacity for reciprocal social interaction, in communication and language development, in the development of symbolic play and in addition display restricted, repetitive patterns of activities and interests from infancy are classified within ICD

Box 9.1 A case of autism: Tom and the light box

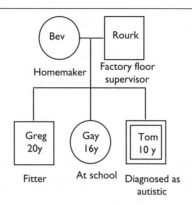

Tom was seen for consultation in a special educational setting at age ten. The immediate concern was his persistent flicking of light switches, which was causing much disruption throughout the school and was a particular problem because on a number of occasions fuses had blown as a result of the switch flicking. Also Tom responded to all attempts to control this behaviour with extreme aggression. In a preliminary consultation he made no eye contact and showed no emotional response to the interview situation. He showed little emotional attachment to his teacher who accompanied him and who had known him for about three years. Within the school he had no friends and no interest in making friends. He had no sense of humour and was unable to share a joke with his classmates. His sentences were very short and he spoke mainly in response to questions. He was unable to recount a story at length about events that had happened in the preceding week, such as a visit of a juggler to the school. He described the action of turning on and off light switches using a neologism. He would say *Want switchlik*. Often this statement would be accompanied by stereotyped flicking movements of the fingers in front of the eyes. His cherished possessions were a collection of four model cars, each of which had doors or bonnets that opened and clicked shut. Tom appeared to get most pleasure from opening and closing the doors and bonnets but showed little interest in using the cars for make-believe car chases or other such games involving imagination and symbolic play. At dinner time in the school he would become very upset and angry if required to sit anywhere other than in his usual place and refused food unless it was served in an orange bowl. His Full Scale IQ was in the low average range but there was a marked difference between his verbal IQ and his performance IQ in favour of the latter. Tom's parents had a good relationship with the school staff and worked very co-operatively with them in implementing behavioural programmes developed within the school at home. These programmes focused on helping Tom develop various communication and life skills. Tom's diagnosis had been made at about three years of age. For his first years of life, Tom's parents noticed his lack of communication with them but assumed that he would grow out of this, a position supported by a number of health professionals who were consulted at the time. Tom's mother went through a period of self-blame where she was convinced that some failure on her part to correctly care for her child had led to his difficulties. A multi-disciplinary assessment at the age of five led to the diagnosis of autism and placement in a school for children with learning difficulties The switch flicking problem was dealt with by building Tom a battery-powered light box with a regular wall switch on top and a torch bulb on the side which lit up when the switch was flicked. Tom liked this a lot and eventually transferred his passion for switch flicking from the classroom switch to the light box.

10 (WHO, 1992, 1996) and DSM IV TR (APA, 2000a) as having pervasive developmental disorders. Autism, first described by Leo Kanner in 1943, is the most common of these disorders with a current prevalence rate of 10 per 10,000 (Fombonne, 2003). The prevalence of autism reported in epidemiological studies has increased in recent years, although it is difficult to determine whether this reflects an increase of the disorder within the populations studied, methodological features of investigations or changes in clinical and administrative diagnostic practices in health and educational services (Volkmar, Klin & Cohen, 2004a). The male:female ratio for autism is 3 or 4:1. There is a strong association between intellectual disability and sex ratio. The highest male:female ratios have been found in children with IQs in the normal range and the lowest ratios occur where children have profound intellectual disabilities (Volkmar et al., 2004a). While the syndrome of autism will be the central focus for this chapter, a number of other less common pervasive developmental disorders listed in both ICD 10 (Figure 9.1) and DSM IV TR (Figure 9.2) deserve some elaboration (Volkmar et al., 1997a).

Asperger's (1944) syndrome, like autism, is characterized by abnormalities in reciprocal interactions and restricted, repetitive patterns of activities and interests (Frith, 2004). However, it differs from autism insofar as no delay in language development or intellectual development occurs. Often, people with Asperger's syndrome have outstanding memories for facts and figures. The prevalence of Asperger's syndrome is about 2.5 per 10,000 (Fombonne, 2003). Currently there is little empirical evidence to show that children diagnosed with Asperger's syndrome differ on clinical, experimental or neurobiological variables from those with IQs within the normal range and a diagnosis of autism (Macintosh & Dissanayake, 2004). In view of this, many argue that the two disorders are best conceptualized as belonging to an autistic spectrum, although this is still an area of controversy (Frith, 2004; Wing, 1996).

Rett's syndrome, like autism, is also characterized by abnormalities in social and language development and accompanied by repetitive behaviour patterns (Kerr, 2002; Van Acker, 1997). However, it is not evident from birth. Rather, the onset of the disorder occurs between five and thirty months and is accompanied by a deceleration in head growth. Among the most noticeable features are the loss of purposeful hand movements and the development of stereotyped hand-washing movements. Severe or profound intellectual disability accompanies Rett's disorder and epilepsy occurs in most cases before adolescence. The syndrome has only been observed in girls. The prevalence of Rett's syndrome is 1 per 10,000 females (Kerr, 2002).

Childhood disintegrative disorder (or Heller's syndrome) entails the social, communicative and behavioural features of autism but follows a period of normal development of at least two years (Volkmar et al., 1997b). The prevalence of childhood disintegrative disorder is about 1 per 50,000 (Volkmar et al., 2004b).

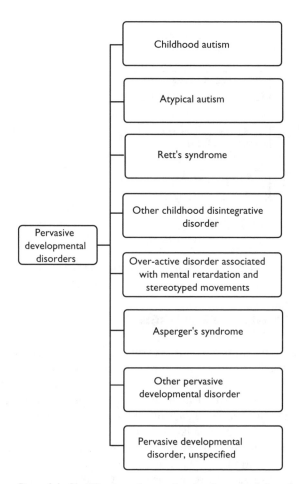

Figure 9.1 Classification of pervasive developmental disorders in ICD 10

In DSM IV TR, the diagnosis of 'Pervasive developmental disorder – not otherwise specified' (PDDNOS) is given where the onset of autistic features occurs after three years of age or where not all symptoms are present. In the ICD 10, the term 'atypical autism' is used for such cases. The epidemiology of this condition is unknown. However, it is probably more common than autism and Asperger's syndrome because the overall prevalence of all autism spectrum disorders in children under seven is about 60 per 10,000 (Johnstone & MRC Autism Review Group, 2001) and the combined prevalence for autism and Asperger's is under 13 per 10,000.

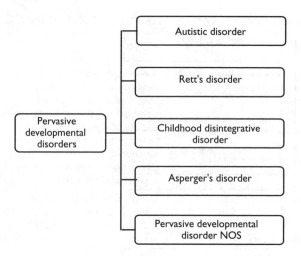

Figure 9.2 Classification of pervasive developmental disorders in DSM IV TR

DIAGNOSIS AND CLINICAL FEATURES

A triad of deficits typify most autistic children (Volkmar et al., 2004a). These are often called Wing's triad, after the eminent researcher Lorna Wing. These deficits occur in social development, language and behaviour, particularly imaginative or make-believe play. Abnormalities in social behaviour that first appear in infancy include the absence of eye-to-eye signalling, the absence of the use of social or emotional gestures, a lack of reciprocity in social relationships, attachment problems such as an inability to use parents as a secure base, little interest in peer relationships, lack of empathy and little interest in sharing positive emotions such as pride or pleasure with others. Language development in autistic children is usually delayed and the language of autistic children is characterized by a variety of pragmatic abnormalities, including pronominal reversal, echolalia, neologisms and speech idiosyncrasies. With pronominal reversal, the child uses the pronoun *you* in place of the pronoun *I*. With echolalia the child repeats the exact words that someone has said to them with the same intonation. Autistic children rarely engage in extended conversations focusing on social or affective topics, and display little creativity in language use. The behaviour of autistic children is characterized by stereotyped repetitive patterns and confined in its range by the restricted interests that most autistic children display. There is also a strong desire to maintain routines and sameness and a resistance to change. Imaginative or make-believe play is virtually absent. Diagnostic criteria for autism and Asperger's syndrome from DSM IV TR and ICD 10 are presented in Table 9.1.

Table 9.1 Diagnostic criteria for autism and Asperger's syndrome in DSM IV TR and ICD 10

Disorder	DSM IV TR	ICD 10
Autism	A. At least six of the following with at least two items from 1 and one each from 2 and 3:	A pervasive developmental disorder defined by the presence of abnormal and/or impaired development that is manifest before the age of 3 years, and by the characteristic type of abnormal functioning in three areas of social interaction, communication and restricted repetitive behaviour
	1. Qualitative impairment in social interaction as manifested by at least two of the following: (a) marked impairments in the use of multiple non-verbal behaviours such as eye-to-eye gaze, facial expression, body postures, and gestures to regulate social interaction (b) failure to develop peer relationships appropriate to developmental level (c) a lack of spontaneous seeking to share enjoyment, interests, or achievements with other people (d) lack of social or emotional reciprocity	Usually there is no prior period of unequivocally normal development but, if there is, abnormality become apparent before the age of 3 years. There are always qualitative impairments in reciprocal social interaction. These take the form of an inadequate appreciation of socio-emotional cues, as shown by a lack of responses to other people's emotions and/or a lack of modulation of behaviour according to social context; poor use of social signals and a weak integration of social, emotional, and communicative behaviours; and, especially, a lack of socio-emotional reciprocity
	2. Qualitative impairments in communication as manifested by at least one of the following: (a) delay in, or total lack of, the development of spoken language (b) in individuals with adequate speech, marked impairment in the ability to initiate or sustain a conversation with others (c) stereotyped and repetitive use of language or idiosyncratic language (d) lack of varied, spontaneous make-believe play or social imitative play appropriate to developmental level	Similarly qualitative impairments in communication are universal. These take the form of a lack of social usage of whatever language skills are present; impairment of make-believe and social imitative play; poor synchrony and lack of reciprocity in conversational interchange; poor flexibility in language expression and a relative lack of creativity and fantasy in thought processes; lack of emotional response to other people's verbal and non-verbal overtures; impaired use of variations in cadence or emphasis to reflect communicative modulation; and a similar lack of accompanying gesture to provide emphasis or aid meaning in spoken communication
	3. Restricted repetitive and stereotyped patterns of behaviour, interests, and activities as manifested by at least one of the following: (a) encompassing preoccupation with one or more stereotyped and restricted patterns of interest that is abnormal either in intensity or focus (b) apparently inflexible adherence to specific, non-functional routines or rituals	

Continued

Table 9.1 Continued

Disorder	DSM IV TR	ICD 10
	(c) stereotyped and repetitive motor mannerisms (d) persistent preoccupation with parts of objects B. Delays or abnormal functioning in at least one of the following areas, with onset prior to age 3 years: (1) social interaction, (2) language as used in social communication, or (3) symbolic or imaginative play C. The disturbance is not better accounted for by Rett's Disorder or Childhood Disintegrative Disorder.	The condition is also characterized by restricted, repetitive and stereotyped patterns of behaviour, interests and activities. These take the form of a tendency to impose rigidity and routine on a wide range of aspects of day-to-day functioning; this usually applies to novel activities as well as to familiar habits and play patterns In early childhood there may be attachment to unusual, typically non-soft objects. The children may insist on the performance of particular routines or rituals of a non-functional character; there may be stereotyped preoccupations with interests such as dates, routes or timetables; often there are motor stereotypies; a specific interest in non-functional elements of objects (such as their smell or feel) is common; and there may be resistance to changes in routine or details of the personal environment
Asperger's syndrome	A. Qualitative impairment in social interaction as manifested by at least two of the following: 1. marked impairments in the use of multiple non-verbal behaviours such as eye-to-eye gaze, facial expression, body postures, and gestures to regulate social interaction 2. failure to develop peer relationships appropriate to developmental level 3. a lack of spontaneous seeking to share enjoyment, interests, or achievements with other people 4. lack of social or emotional reciprocity B. Restricted repetitive and stereotyped patterns of behaviour, interests, and activities as manifested by at least one of the following: 1. encompassing preoccupation	A disorder characterized by the same kind of qualitative abnormalities of reciprocal social interaction that typify autism, together with a restricted stereotyped, repetitive repertoire of interests and activities The disorder differs from autism primarily in that there is no general delay or retardation in language or in cognitive development Most individuals are of normal intelligence but it is common for them to be markedly clumsy There is a strong tendency for the abnormalities to persist into adolescence and adult life and it seems they represent individual characteristics that are not greatly

with one or more stereotyped and restricted patterns of interest that is abnormal either in intensity or focus

2. apparently inflexible adherence to specific, non-functional routines or rituals
3. stereotyped and repetitive motor mannerisms
4. persistent preoccupation with parts of objects

C. The disturbance causes clinically significant impairment in social, occupational, or other important areas of functioning

D. There is no significant general delay in language (e.g. single words used by 2 years and communicative phrases by 3 years)

E. There is no clinically significant delay in cognitive development or in the development of age-appropriate self-help skills, adaptive behaviour (other than social interaction) and curiosity about the environment in childhood

F. Criteria are not met for another specific pervasive developmental disorder or schizophrenia

affected by environmental influences

Psychotic episodes occasionally occur in adult life

Note: Adapted from DSM IV TR (APA, 2000a) and ICD 10 (WHO, 1992, 1996).

In addition to these social, linguistic and behavioural deficits, children with autism may have a variety of associated features, particularly in the affective, cognitive and physical domains deserving clinical inquiry. Some of these are listed in Table 9.2. The affective and emotional expressions of autistic children are typically inappropriate to the social context within which they occur. For example, many autistic children like Tom in the case example presented in Box 9.1 are unable to appreciate a joke. Intense tantrums and negative emotional displays may occur as an expression of resistance to change. In addition, many autistic children have fears and phobias.

In the cognitive domain, it is noteworthy that about 75% of children with autism have IQs below 70 and the characteristic profile is for the non-verbal or performance IQ score to be greater than the verbal IQ. An IQ above 50, especially a verbal IQ above 50, is a particularly significant protective factor associated with a better prognosis. Age-appropriate language development at five years is also a good prognostic sign. Some youngsters with autism have islets of ability. For example, they may be able to play many tunes by ear or

Table 9.2 Clinical characteristics and associated features of autism

Domain	Feature
Interpersonal adjustment	• Inability to empathize with others • Lack of understanding of rules governing social interaction • Lack of reciprocity in social interaction • Impaired ability to form loving relationships
Language	• Developmental language delay • Lack of social conversation • Lack of creative use of language in conversation • Pronominal reversal • Echolalia • Neologisms • Idiosyncratic use of language
Behaviour	• Absence of imaginative play • Stereotyped behaviour patterns, routines and rituals • Resistance to change
Affect	• Inappropriate emotional expression • Occasionally intense negative emotional response to change • Fears and phobias are common in younger cases
Cognition	• Over 75% have an IQ below 70 • Visuo-spatial IQ greater than verbal IQ • Islets of ability • Difficulties with social problem solving
Physical condition	• Up to 33% of cases develop epilepsy in late adolescence. • Enuresis and encopresis are common in younger cases • A minority show self-injurious behaviour (head-banging or biting)

remember a catalogue of facts. However, the most noticeable cognitive deficit in autism is an inability to solve social or interpersonal problems. About a third of children with autism initially develop language skills but lose these towards the end of the second year.

In the domain of physical development, up to a third of autistic children develop epilepsy in late adolescence. Many have elimination problems, including encopresis and enuresis. Some also develop physical complications due to self-injurious behaviour, such as head-banging or biting. Children with autism have larger heads than normal during childhood, an abnormality that is not present at birth and one that resolves with age.

THEORETICAL FRAMEWORKS

Theories of autism fall into three broad categories: psychogenic, biogenic and cognitive. Psychogenic theories argue that psychosocial processes are central in the aetiology of autism, whereas biogenic theories look to biological factors as the basis for the condition. Cognitive theories are concerned not with identifying the primary causes of autism but with explaining the patterning of symptoms in terms of specific underlying cognitive deficits. A summary of some of the more important theories in each of these categories is presented in Table 9.3.

Table 9.3 Theories of autism

Theory type	Sub-type and source	Principles
Psychodynamic theory	Bettleheim (1967)	Autistic withdrawal occurs as a response to inadequate parenting. Echolalia and insistence on sameness are an expression of hostility associated with unmet needs Long-term non-directive psychotherapy offers a substitute for the inadequate parent–child relationship and leads to a reduction in withdrawal and expressions of hostility
Biological theories	Gillberg & Coleman (2000)	Autism and ASD are a group of neurodevelopmental disabilities or syndromes which reflect injury to a final common pathway. This may be caused by many different disease processes involving genetic factors, intrauterine insults, or peri-natal factors or some combination of these
Broad-band cognitive theories	Weak central coherence Happé & Frith (1996)	People with autism do not have the irresistible urge to make sense of the global features of a situation and process information piece-meal rather than in context. They take a bottom-up rather than top-down approach to managing informational input
	Executive dysfunction Ozonoff (1997)	Executive function deficits account for communicative and behavioural features and possibly for some of the social features of autism.

Continued

Table 9.3 continued

Theory type	Sub-type and source	Principles
		Executive functions include the abilities to disengage for the external context; to inhibit unwanted responses; to plan actions; to maintain a cognitive set and stay on task; to monitor performance and use feedback to take corrective action; and to flexibly shift cognitive set
Narrow-band cognitive theories	Theory of mind deficit Baron Cohen et al. (2000)	The social and communicative features of autism are due to an inability to form cognitive representations of other's mental states
	Information-processing deficit Hermelin & O'Connor (1970)	Autistic children have encoding, sequencing and abstraction deficits which account for delayed language development
	Joint attention deficit Mundy & Neale (2001)	A deficit in the capacity to jointly attend to events with others and to preferentially orient towards social rather than inanimate events impairs the development of language, social communication and theory of mind in children with autism
	Imitation deficit Rogers & Bennett (2000)	A deficit in the capacity to imitate others impairs the development of intersubjectivity and executive functioning and accounts for language and social deficits in autism
	Emotion perception deficit Hobson (1993)	Autistic children's inappropriate affect is due to an abnormality in the way they process information about facial expressions of emotion
	Evaluative appraisal autobiographical memory deficit Jordan & Powell (1995)	In autism there is an episodic autobiographical memory deficit which is due to an inability to evaluatively appraise the significance of events related to the self. Children with autism, therefore, have problems recalling events as having happened to themselves

Psychogenic theories

Early theories about the aetiology of autism attributed the social, linguistic and behavioural features to emotional difficulties that derived from exposure to inadequate parenting. For example, Bettelheim (1967) argued that autistic withdrawal was the child's response to cold, unemotional, inadequate parenting. Some of the annoying features of autism, such as echolalia, insistence on sameness and stereotyped rituals were viewed as expressions of hostility towards parents who were thought to be perceived by the child as failing to fulfil his or her needs. Long-term non-directive psychodynamic psychotherapy, which focused on helping children deal with the central emotional difficulty, was identified as the treatment of choice. The aim of the therapy was to provide a substitute parent–child relationship that would meet the child's needs for warmth and acceptance. In some instances, psychotherapy for parents to help them resolve the emotional difficulties that underpinned their inadequate parenting, was also recommended. These theories evolved within the psychodynamic tradition at a time when psychodynamic studies of children separated from their parents during the war or through hospitalization highlighted the value of parental emotional warmth and availability or a psychotherapeutic substitute for this in helping children to cope with separation.

Psychogenic theories, which point to the quality of parenting and patterns of family interaction as the primary cause of autism, have not been supported by carefully controlled studies which reveal no such abnormalities in the families of autistic children (e.g. Koegel, Schreibman, O'Neill & Burke, 1983). Controlled studies of treatments based on the psychogenic model, such as psychodynamic play therapy, and more recent offshoots of this such as holding therapy and gentle teaching are unavailable (Finnegan & Carr, 2002). Despite this lack of evidence for the psychogenic theories of autism, the position is still popularized in publications such as Skynner and Cleese's (1983) pop psychology book *Families and How to Survive Them*. This is unfortunate, since the idea that parents are responsible for their children's disability places additional stress on the parents of children with autism, something that they could well do without.

Most recent research points to the neurobiological aetiology of autism and to the centrality of cognitive rather than emotional factors as underpinning the main clinical features (Volkmar et al., 2004a). Furthermore, behavioural studies point to the importance of directive behavioural methods rather than non-directive psychotherapeutic methods in the treatment of autistic children (Finnegan & Carr, 2002). While therapeutic input to parents of children with autism is warranted, it should aim at supporting parents and training them to implement carefully designed behavioural programmes rather than correcting some underlying intrapsychic or interpersonal deficit (Lord & National Research Council, 2001).

Biological theories

Biological theories of autism have attempted to account for the condition through reference to genetic factors, intrauterine environmental factors, peri-natal complications, neuroanatomical factors, neurochemical factors, physio-logical factors or some combination of these (Gillberg & Coleman, 2000). Evidence from twin and family studies show that genetic factors contribute to the development of autism and that the mode of transmission is quite com-plex and probably involves multiple genes. In a small proportion of cases (5–10%) autism may be due to single gene disorders or chromosomal abnormalities (Johnstone & MRC Autism Review Group, 2001) including Fragile X anomaly and tuberose sclerosis. Tuberose sclerosis is a neurocuta-neous disorder characterized by skin lesions and neurological features; both epilepsy and learning difficulties also occur in many cases. Past reports of an association between autism and phenylketonuria have not been replicated (Volkmar et al., 2004a). The risk of parents having a second child with autism is between 3 and 7%.

A higher incidence of pre- and peri-natal problems has been found in children with autism including advanced maternal age, birth order (first- or fourth-born or later), use of medication, alcohol and drug abuse, prematur-ity, post-maturity, early or mid-trimster bleeding and obstetric complications. However, the current consensus is that there is insufficient evidence to sup-port a contributory link between these factors and autism (Johnstone & MRC Autism Review Group, 2001). Past reports of an association between autism and congenital rubella have not been replicated (Volkmar et al., 2004a). The hypothesis that ingestion of mercury or lead can lead to autism has not been supported (Johnstone & MRC Autism Review Group, 2001).

Considerable controversy has surrounded the hypothesis that the process of immunization with the measles, mumps and rubella (MMR) vaccine may lead to autism. Currently the weight of evidence suggests no causal link between MMR and autism (Johnstone & MRC Autism Review Group, 2001; Volkmar et al., 2004a).

The hypothesis that gastrointestinal difficulties, specifically altered intes-tinal permeability, can result in nervous system dysfunctions that underpin autism has led to the development of treatments involving casein- and gluten-free diets. Insufficient evidence is available at present to judge the validity of this hypothesis (Johnstone & MRC Autism Review Group, 2001).

The precise biological characteristics that are genetically transmitted or that develop as a result of congenital infection or obstetric complication and which underpin the clinical features of autism are still unclear despite extensive research investigating the neuroanatomical, neurochemical and psychophysiological characteristics of people with autism (Bailey, Phillips & Rutter, 1996; Gillberg & Coleman, 2000). However, four recent findings sug-gest important areas for future research (Johnstone & MRC Autism Review

Group, 2001; Volkmar et al., 2004a). First, the brain size of people with autism is greater than that of normal, and this difference is greatest in toddlers whose brain size may be up to 10% greater than normal controls. This enlargement is not present at birth, is not associated with higher IQ and diminishes with age. Second, brain centres for processing emotions (amygdala) and face perception (fusiform face area) are less active in people with autism than in normal controls, and degree of social disability is correlated with level of activation in the face perception area. Third, in a significant minority of children with autism (about 30%) there is a dysregulation of the serotonin system. Finally, about a third of people with autism have epilepsy, the onset of which is most common in early childhood or late adolescence.

Cognitive theories

Cognitive theories of autism posit central cognitive deficits, which may account for some or all of the clinical features and symptoms that characterize the condition. These theories may be classified as narrow-band or broad-band, depending on the magnitude of the cognitive dysfunction that is suggested to underpin the symptoms of autism (Bailey et al., 1996). Two theories identify broader cognitive deficits as central to autism and there is some evidence to support both positions. Central coherence theory posits a difficulty with managing information input as the underlying difficulty in autism, whereas executive function theory specifies that the main deficit is in problem-solving output. Happé & Frith (1996) have argued that an underlying problem in autism is the lack of a strong drive for central coherence. Thus, people with autism do not have the irresistible urge to make sense of the global features of a situation that most people experience. Thus they process information piece-meal rather than in context. They take a bottom-up rather than top-down approach to managing informational input.

Ozonoff (1997) argues that executive dysfunction is central to autism. Executive functions include the abilities to disengage for the external context, to inhibit unwanted responses, to plan actions, to maintain a cognitive set and stay on task, to monitor performance and use feedback to take corrective action and to flexibly shift cognitive set.

In contrast to these broad-band theories, there are six main narrow-band theories that implicate deficits in social cognition as central to autism and there is some evidence to support all six positions (Bailey et al., 1996; Volkmar et al., 2004a). Baron-Cohen has shown that people with autism lack *a theory of mind* or are *mind blind* and consequently are unable to form cognitive representations of mental states, an ability that typically emerges at about two years and subserves imaginal play (Baron-Cohen, Tager-Flusberg & Cohen, 2000). This theory accounts for the observations that children with autism show deficits in social behaviour that involve representing others' mental states, such as keeping secrets or pro-declarative pointing (to draw another's attention to an object) whereas deficits do not occur in social behaviours involving rote learning (such as using a standard introduction) or manipulation of objects such as pro-imperative pointing (to get a required object from another). This theory has led to the development of an important intervention programme, the goal of which is to teach autistic children to mind-read (Howlin, Baron-Cohen & Hadwin, 1999). This programme is effective, but the skills have not been shown to generalize beyond the training situation.

Hermelin and O'Connor (1970) found that autistic children had difficulties with encoding, sequencing and abstraction and that these differences contributed to their delayed language development.

Mundy and Neale (2001) argue that a deficit in the capacity to jointly attend to events with others and to preferentially orient towards social rather than inanimate stimuli impairs the development of language, social communication and theory of mind in children with autism.

Rogers and Benneto (2000) proposed that a deficit in the capacity to imitate others impairs the development of intersubjectivity and executive functioning and that this accounts for language and social deficits in autism.

Hobson (1993) has shown that autistic children process information about the facial expressions of emotions differently from normal children, and so do not respond appropriately to emotional displays of others.

Jordan and Powell (1995) have argued that, in autism, there is an episodic autobiographical memory deficit that is due to an inability to evaluatively appraise the significance of events related to the self. Children with autism have difficulty experiencing events as happening to them, so they have problems recalling events as having happened to themselves. They argue that teaching children with autism should focus on helping them develop evaluative appraisal skills, to attach personal significance to events and to develop episodic autobiographical memory. That is, to operate as if they had an experiencing self.

It seems quite probable that some combination of all of these cognitive deficits account for the clinical features of autism. Future research will aim to clarify this and also the relationship between these cognitive deficits and the neurobiological correlates of autism.

ASSESSMENT

Many of the issues covered in the assessment and management of youngsters with intellectual disabilities apply to autism and readers may wish to refer to Chapter 8, in which intellectual disability is discussed.

Multi-disciplinary assessment

Assessment of autism should ideally be conducted by a multi-disciplinary and multi-agency team over an extended period of time in partnership with parents (American Academy of Child and Adolescent Psychiatry, 1999a; Charman & Baird, 2002; Jordan, 2005; Lord & Bailey, 2002; Lord & National Research Council, 2001). Clinical psychology, educational psychology, paediatric medicine, speech and language therapy, special education, occupational therapy, community nursing and child psychiatry are among some of the disciplines that may be involved in such teams. Both health and education agencies may collaborate in service delivery to families with children who have pervasive developmental disorders or autism spectrum disorders.

Pacing the assessment

The process of diagnosis for parents is challenging, since it involves making sense of their child's unusual behaviour, giving up the idea that this behaviour is something transitory their child will grow out of, grieving the loss of the 'normal child' the parents wished for and beginning to accept that developing a functional long-term relationship with health and educational services will offer their child the best chance for living a full life. Thus, assessment and diagnosis is best conceptualized as a major family transition, a process that takes time. It is therefore appropriate to spread the interviews and assessments over a number of weeks and adopt a collaborative position during the diagnostic process. This position involves letting the parents know, early in the process, the diagnostic criteria for autism spectrum disorders and other possibilities in the differential diagnosis and then, after each investigation, discussing with the parents the degree to which the new information fits with the diagnostic criteria. In this way, towards the end of the diagnostic process, parents 'discover' for themselves that their child has an autistic spectrum disorder. This process should be paced in a way that fosters a good working relationship with parents, so that the transition from diagnosis to treatment planning is smooth. If the assessment and diagnostic process occurs too rapidly, parents may reject the diagnosis and/or enter into unproductive conflict with health and educational professionals about the diagnosis or treatment plan. It is reasonable to spread an assessment over six or eight weeks. It is usually inappropriate to conduct the assessment in a single session.

Parental interviews

A developmental and family history and routine child and family evaluation following the guidelines set out in Chapter 4 should be completed with the parents. Parental reports of autistic-like behaviour in the areas of social interaction, communication and restricted activity may be obtained by routine clinical interview. However, this should be supplemented with a standardized interview such as the ADI-R or the DISCO listed in Table 9.4. In addition to these autism-specific instruments, it may be valuable to ask parents to complete one of the adaptive behaviour scales listed in Table 8.3 (p. 267) to throw light on the level of social functioning of the child and the areas of strength and weakness.

Table 9.4 Psychometric instruments that may be used as an adjunct to clinical interviews in the assessment of autism

Construct	Instrument	Publication	Comments
Autistic behaviour	Autism Behaviour Checklist (ABC)	Krug, D., Arick, J. Almond, P. (1980). Behaviour checklist for identifying severely handicapped children with high levels of autistic behaviour. *Journal of Child Psychology and Psychiatry*, 21, 221–229	This 57-item instrument provides scores on five dimensions: sensory; relating; body and object use; language; social and self-help. Scores on these may be summed to give an overall intensity score. It may be used with school-aged children
	Social Communication Questionnaire (SCQ)	Rutter, M., Bailey, A., Lord, C. & Berument, S. (2003). *Social Communication Questionnaire*. Los Angeles, CA: Western Psychological Services	This 40-item questionnaire derived from the ADI-R is a useful screening instrument
	Autism Diagnostic Observation Schedule (ADOS)	Lord, C., Rutter, M. & DiLavore, P (1997). *Autism Diagnostic Observation Schedule-Generic (ADOS-G)*. New York: The Psychological Corporation	Ratings are made on the basis of a 20-minute interview with the child who must have expressive language of at least the three-year level
	Autism Diagnostic Interview-Revised (ADI-R)	LeCouteur, A., Lord, C. & Rutter, M. (2003). *Autistic Diagnostic Interview-Revised (ADI-R)*. Los Angeles, CA: Western Psychological Services	A DSM IV or ICD 10 diagnosis may be given on the basis of a 90-minute interview with a parent or carer

Diagnostic interview for social and communication disorders (DISCO)	Wing, L., Leekham, S.R., Libby, S.J., Gould, J. & Larcombe, M. (2002). The diagnostic interview for social and communication disorders: background, inter-rater reliability and clinical use. *Journal of Child Psychology and Psychiatry*, 43, 307–25	This very detailed interview schedule yields the full range of ASD diagnoses
The Childhood Autism Rating Scale (CARS) for Diagnostic Screening and classification of autism	Schopler, E. Richler, R., Renner, B. (1986). *The Childhood Autism Rating Scale (CARS) for Diagnostic Screening and Classification of Autism.* New York: Irvington. (Order CARS from Western Psychological Services 12031 Wilshire Boulevard, Los Angeles, California 90025–1251. Phone 1–800–648–8857. Order a CARS training video from Health Sciences Consortium 201 Silver Cedar Court, Chapel Hill, NC, 27514–1517. Phone 919–942–8731)	Pre-school-aged children may be rated on the 15 scales that make up this instrument. These are: relationships with people; imitation; affect; use of body; relation to non-human objects; adaptation to environmental change; visual responsiveness; auditory responsiveness; near receptor responsiveness; anxiety reaction, verbal communication; non-verbal communication; activity level; intellectual functioning; general impressions. Ratings are made after observation and routine psychometric ability testing
Gilliam Autism Rating Scale (GARS)	Gilliam, J. (1991). *Gilliam Autism Rating Scale.* Odessa, FL. Psychological Assessment Resources. http://www.parinc.com	This rating scale for completion by teachers or parents provides scores on stereotyped behaviours; communication; social interaction; and developmental disturbances

Continued

Table 9.4 continued

Construct	Instrument	Publication	Comments
Educational skills	Psycho-Educational Profile Revised (PEP-R)	Schopler, E., Reichler, R., Bashford, A., Lashing, M. & Marcus, L. (1990). *Psychoeducational Profile Revised (PEP-R)*. Austin, TX: Pro-ed. (Order from PRO-ED, 8700 Shoal Creek Blvd., Austin, TX 78758. Phone 512–451–3246)	This set of ability scales for pre-school and school-age children yields scores on imitation, perception motor, eye–hand integration, cognitive-perform-ance, and cognitive-verbal skills
	Adolescent and Adult Psycho-Educational Profile (AAPEP)	Mesibov, G. Schopler, E. & Caison, W. (1989). *Adolescent and Adult Psycho-Educational Profile (AAPEP)*. Austin, TX: Pro-ed	This assessment package includes home and school-based checklists and a set of performance tasks which are administered as tests and scored from direct observation
	Autism Screening Instrument for Educational Planning (ASIEP)	Krug, D., Arick & Almond, P. (1996). *Autism Screening Instrument For Educational Planning. Second Edition. Odessa, FL*. Psychological Assessment Resources, (PAR, PO Box 998, Odessa Florida, 33556. Phone 1–800–331–8378)	This kit includes an autism behaviour checklist; a method for rating a sample of vocal behaviour; a method for rating social interaction; a method for making an educational assessment; and a method for assessing prognosis of learning

Teacher interviews

Where children are attending school, appropriate standardized rating scales from the list given in Table 9.4 (such as the Gilliam Autism Rating Scale) and the school edition of the Adaptive Behaviour Scale (which is listed in Table 8.3) may be given to teachers to complete to supplement interview information.

Psychometric assessment of abilities and language

With the child, tests of intelligence and language should be administered. A list of intelligence tests appropriate to children of different ages is given in Table 8.2 (pp. 264–266). It is important to use an instrument that includes measures of non-verbal abilities such as the revised Leiter International Performance Scale listed in Table 8.4 (p. 273) when assessing children suspected of having autism, since often they perform particularly well on non-verbal tests. Some language tests that may be used in the assessment of autism are listed in Table 8.6 (p. 276). If there is a speech and language therapist on the assessment team, it may be appropriate for such a professional to conduct the language assessment. Psychoeducational profiles of strengths and weaknesses which may be useful for planning treatment and education programmes should be obtained using instruments such as the revised Psychoeducational Profile or other such instruments listed in Table 9.4. For diagnostic purposes, information from the psychometric assessment and observation of the child during this process may be systematized using the Childhood Autism Rating Scale listed in Table 9.4.

Specialist assessments

In addition to parent and teacher interviews and psychometric assessment of the child, a number of specialist evaluations that are outside the remit of the clinical psychologist may be required in the evaluation of children suspected of having autism. A thorough audiological evaluation may be necessary in cases where children show very limited response to sound. If possible, a home observation session should be conducted to observe the child's behaviour in his or her natural surroundings. A full paediatric physical examination should routinely be conducted as part of the multi-disciplinary assessment of a child suspected of having autism. If seizure activity is suspected, an EEG should be completed to check for the presence of epilepsy.

Differential diagnosis

Information from involved professionals may be pooled with three aims in mind. First, the degree to which the child meets the diagnostic criteria for autism or Asperger's syndrome listed in Table 9.1 or another autistic spectrum disorder must be determined. Second, the confidence with which alternative diagnoses may be ruled out must be assessed. Third, define the child's areas of strength and weakness, and outline the implications of this profile for planning treatment and education. Autism may be distinguished from other pervasive developmental disorders in the ways described in the earlier section on diagnosis. The following conditions should also be included in the differential diagnosis of autism (Lord & Bailey, 2002):

- severe hearing impairment
- intellectual disability
- developmental language disorders
- elective mutism

- reactive attachment disorder
- childhood schizophrenia.

Children with severe hearing impairment may be screened out on the basis of the results of the audiological examination. These deaf children who do not have autism can usually make eye contact and engage in sign-based reciprocal social interaction. Children with intellectual difficulties, but who do not have autism, do not show deficits in reciprocal social interaction and their language development is typically consistent with their overall level of intellectual ability. Children with developmental language problems do not show the non-verbal communication problems that typify children with autism nor do they show the restricted repetitive behaviour patterns characteristic of autistic children (Bishop, 2002; Rapin, 1996). In contrast to the pervasive problems associated with autism, normal interpersonal interactions, language development and behaviour within the context of the home characterize children who are electively mute, although at school or in places other than the home they typically do not speak. The similarities between some children who have suffered severe psychosocial deprivation and developed reactive attachment disorder and those with autism may be quite marked. For example, severe psychosocial deprivation may lead to language delay, unusual interpersonal behaviour and stereotyped behaviour patterns. However, such children tend to make appropriate use of what language they have to engage in reciprocal social interaction and their behaviour and communication tends to normalize gradually when placed in a normal social environment. Finally, children with childhood schizophrenia typically have a history of relatively normal development prior to the onset of the condition. They also do not show the language comprehension difficulties typical of autism.

Profiling

In profiling strengths and weaknesses of youngsters with autism and other pervasive developmental disorders it may be useful to categorize them under the following headings (which are not mutually exclusive) for the purposes of treatment planning:

- problem-solving abilities both verbal and non-verbal, academic and life-skills development
- communication skills and language development
- challenging behaviours, such as aggression or self-injury
- family's coping resources.

These broad categories for profiling strengths and weaknesses map onto the four main classes of goals of comprehensive treatment programme, which are to enhance communicative skills, foster the development of problem-solving skills, decrease challenging behaviours and help parents to cope with the pervasive developmental disorder (Rutter, 1985c).

TREATMENT

There is no cure for autism (Cohen & Volkmar, 1997). At best, youngsters with this condition may be helped to develop skills to partially compensate for their communicative, cognitive and behavioural deficits and parents may be helped to cope with their children more effectively so that youngsters and their families can lead as normal a life as possible (Finnegan & Carr, 2002; Lord & National Research Council, 2001; Simpson, 2005). Comprehensive programmes that exemplify best practice involve the following components:

- psychoeducation, in which parents are given information about their child's diagnosis, prognosis and available services
- advice and support in arranging educational placement
- family-based approach to long-term management
- structured teaching as a central method for designing learning activities
- behaviour modification as a central approach for teaching skills and dealing with challenging behaviour
- self-care and educational skills training
- communication skills training and speech and language therapy
- management of challenging behaviour (including pharmacological and psychological approaches)
- respite care.

Psychoeducation

The first step in treatment is explaining the diagnosis and making the disorder coherent to parents. The following points may be useful in explaining autism. Autism is a disorder that is caused by biological factors that are poorly understood. It is a chronic lifelong neurodevelopmental disability, not a time-limited emotional reaction to a stressful family situation. Children with autism cannot guess what others are thinking or feeling and so cannot predict the behaviour of others. They also have a strong wish to maintain predictable routines and to live in an orderly world. In addition, many are very sensitive to sound, light or touch. These core difficulties make it hard for them to share attention with others and jointly watch an event. They make it difficult for autistic children to show warmth towards others, to empathize with others, to communicate effectively, to hold conversations that involve turn-taking and respecting the other person's viewpoint and to flexibly adapt to changing circumstances. The desire for predictability may lead to the development of rigid routines and habits that involve repetition. This desire for predictability may also lead to little creativity. People with autism also have difficulty developing a conscience, since this involves imagining the effect that their actions have on others. The difficulty that people with autism have in imagining what others think means that they may find other people (who they view as unpredictable) very threatening, particularly if they disrupt their routines. This may lead to aggression towards others who attempt to change their routines. Often this aggression is expressed in an extreme way since the child with autism has little awareness of the impact the expression of aggression has on others. Repetitive self-harm, since it is highly predictable, may be experienced as desirable or pleasurable. Reacting aggressively to normal levels of visual, auditory and touch stimuli, or withdrawal, rocking or other self-soothing routines may be used to cope with heightened sensitivity to sensory stimulation.

In the long term, with structured teaching and skills training, youngsters with autism can learn to communicate with others, care for themselves, avoid challenging behaviour and manage productive work routines, provided a highly structured approach to teaching is taken which takes account of their need for a highly predictable environment. The degree of independence they gain as adults is dependent on the level of structured teaching they receive as children.

Educational placement

A central issue in the treatment of youngsters with autism is whether they should be placed in special schools exclusively for children with autism or whether they should be placed in mainstream schools attended by children without disabilities and provided with additional support (Harris & Handleman, 1997; Wall, 2004). No comparative data are available on which approach is most effective, so policy and practice decisions on this issue are influenced by ethical and pragmatic considerations. Ethically, there is widespread agreement that children with disabilities such as autism should be provided with every opportunity to live as normal a life as possible and, for this reason, autistic children should be educated in mainstream schools with additional support provided. However, pragmatically, it is often difficult to arrange for sufficient support within mainstream schools to be provided to allow a child with autism to received an adequate education within that context. It is often easier to centralize the special educational resources required for children with autism. Of course, national policy, the views of autism advocacy groups, and the way in which funding from statutory and voluntary sources are allocated all determine the availability of mainstream or centralized special educational placements.

For pre-school and school-aged children with autistic spectrum disorders, optimal programmes have certain key features (Lord & National Research Council, 2001). These include early entry into the programme (at two or three years); participation in the programme for at least 25 hours per week, twelve months per year; engagement in repeated, brief structured learning activities using an evidence-based teaching approach; the use of teaching methods that capitalize on children's strengths to overcome their weaknesses; adequate staff training to be able to deliver an evidence-based teaching programme; a curriculum that is developmentally appropriate and covers an appropriate mix of communication, social, play and academic skills training; access for pupils to a supervised comfortable low-stimulation environment as required when over-stimulated; low pupil:staff ratio (2:1 maximum); an evidence-based approach to managing challenging behaviour; inclusion of parents in setting educational goals and working with school staff to help their children achieve these; regular assessment of goal attainment and modification of the teaching programme in light of re-assessment; and the statement of children's educational goals in observable measurable terms.

Family-based approach to management

The emphasis in effective programmes is on a collaborative working relationship with parents (Lord & National Research Council, 2001; Marcus, Kunce & Schopler, 1997; Simpson, 2005; Wall, 2004). Parents must be centrally involved in developing individual educational and therapeutic programme plans and collaboratively involved in their delivery. It is also acknowledged that parents require support from professionals and the parents of other children with autism to help them work through the grief process associated with adjusting to having a child with this disability. A fuller discussion of this issue is contained in Chapter 8 in relation to intellectual disability, and grief processes are discussed in detail in Chapter 24. The best results have been obtained where parents are involved in intensive structured educative programmes such as the TEACCH (Treatment and Education of Autistic and related Communication handicapped CHildren) programme, developed by Schopler, or in intensive behavioural training programmes, such as those developed by Lovaas and based on the principles of applied behavioural analysis (Finnegan & Carr, 2002). In both instances, professionals train and support parents to provide an environment for their child which promotes skills development.

Early Bird – a programme developed by the National Autistic Society for helping parents of autistic children – is widely used in the UK (Shields, 2001). It includes eight weekly psychoeducational training sessions and a manual for parents, which gives reliable information on autism. These group-based sessions also provide parents with support. In the Early Bird programme, a couple of home visits are conducted in which video feedback is used to help parents develop appropriate communication and child management skills. Parents learn to use the Picture Exchange Communication System (PECS), a pictorially based way of communicating with autistic children (Bondy &

Frost, 1994); the TEACCH structured learning programme developed by Schopler (Schopler, 1997; Schreibman & Koegel, 1996; Koegel & Koegel, 1996); and how to use HANEN routines for promoting early parent-child interaction and facilitating language development (Sussman, 1999). Details of the Early Bird, PECS, TEACCH and HANEN programme materials are available at their websites (listed at the end of this chapter).

Structured teaching

Schopler and the group that developed the TEACCH system place structured learning at the heart of their very comprehensive approach to autism (Schopler, 1997). The TEACCH approach aims to make the world intelligible to the autistic child by acknowledging deficits (such as communication problems and difficulties in social cognition) and structuring learning activities so that they capitalize on the strengths of children with autism. Children with autism have excellent visual processing abilities, good rote memory abilities and many have unique special interests. Thus, learning activities should be structured so that the child can visualize what is expected to achieve success. Activities should depend on memory for sequences of tasks and the content of the tasks should capitalize on any special interests that the child has shown. So, for example, photographs of stages of task completion should be used rather than extensive verbal instructions, where language development is delayed. If the child is interested in toy cars, then these may be used to teach counting or language.

Schopler's group uses a system where two clinicians work with each case: one is designated the child therapist and the other is the parent consultant (Schopler, 1997). At each clinical contact, the child therapist works directly with the child, developing a written programme of home teaching activities for the parent to carry out each week. Concurrently, the parent consultant works with the parent, reviewing and planning future child management strategies for developing productive routines and managing challenging behaviour. Parents are invited to observe the programmes developed by the child therapist and practise these with the child at home for about twenty minutes per day. Typical programmes involve four or five activities, selected to match the child's profile of strengths and weaknesses. Schopler and his group have catalogued the types of activities that may be included in such programmes in a series of publications and videotapes, which are available at the TEACCH website. Parents are advised to develop highly structured work routines with their children. The same time and place for work should be used each day and the environment should be free of distractions. Materials for tasks to be completed should be placed on the left and, when the work is finished, the materials should be stored in a tray on the right marked *finished*. Parents are shown how to model all activities for their children and then to instruct them and give feedback in simple language. This highly structured approach capitalized on the affinity that children with autism have for sameness and their resistance to changes of routine.

Behavioural treatment

Behaviourally based treatment programmes have been shown to lead to significant skills gains and reductions in challenging behaviours in controlled studies (Finnegan & Carr, 2002; Lovaas, 1987; Lovaas, & Smith, 2003; McEachin, Smith & Lovaas, 1993). Within these programmes, on the basis of a broad developmental analysis of skills and deficits and a fine-grained behavioural analysis of skill use, or lack thereof, in particular situations, a set of highly specific treatment goals are established and behavioural methods for achieving these specified. Common treatment goals include reducing ritualistic and aggressive or self-injurious behaviour and enhancing communication, interaction, play, cognitive skills and self-care skills. Parents and school staff, or other involved front-line professionals such as nurses or childcare workers, are trained to implement these programmes. Some examples of typical problems and behavioural treatment strategies for the domains of communication, skills development and challenging behaviour are presented in Table 9.5.

The behavioural programme for which best evidence of efficacy is available is Ivar Lovaas' Young Autism Programme (Lovaas & Smith, 2003). Details of Lovaas' programme are available at his website (listed at the end of this chapter). Within the programme, pre-school children aged two to five years receive about forty hours of one-to-one therapist-delivered behavioural intervention per week in addition to parent-delivered intervention in their home environment. Broad goals are broken down into small behavioural targets and discrete trial training is used to help children develop skills. Here, in a one-to-one situation, therapists give short, simple instructions, carefully prompt (and later fade-out prompts) for the target skill being taught, give immediate reinforcement for appropriate responses or approximations to these. There are six stages to the programme:

- In the first stage a teaching relationship is established. This is very challenging for therapists, parents and supervisors since attempts to directly instruct autistic children usually lead to avoidance or escape behaviour often involving aggression or self-injury. The therapist selects a simple target behaviour, such as sitting on a chair or putting a brick in a bucket and reinforces all approximations to this, while not reinforcing avoidant or escape behaviour.
- In the second stage, which may last up to four months, foundational skills are taught, including receptive language skills such as coming to the therapist on request, imitating gross motor action such as clapping or waving, imitating fine motor actions such as facial expressions, matching

Table 9.5 Examples of behavioural treatment strategies for managing problems presented by children with autism

Domain	Problem	Treatment strategy
Skills development	Impaired understanding	Simplified communication, selection of materials at appropriate developmental level, break down large task into small steps
	Lack of initiative	Structured learning with child-selected materials and tasks that maximize probability of success to maximize motivation
	Lack of persistence	Immediate intermittent natural reinforcement for successful performance and unsuccessful attempts
	Lack of generalization	Train the skill in multiple contexts and use prompts to remind the child that the skill has been learned
Language and communication	Lack of language skills	Direct instruction in language use Instruction in sign language
	Failure to use language socially	Modelling and coaching Differential reinforcement Focus on communication rather than speech
	Lack of conversational reciprocity	Coaching in reciprocal conversation
	Social isolation	Planned periods of interaction
Challenging behaviour	Aggressive or self-injurious response to identifiable environmental changes	Remove precipitating stimuli or desensitize child to these Coach the child in self-control skills and re-inforce the use of these to manage challenging behaviour
	Apparently unprovoked aggressive or self-injurious behaviour initiated to get something or to avoid something	Coach in skills necessary to get desired reinforcer or avoid negative stimulus (if this is appropriate) Desensitize child to avoided stimulus and re-inforce the child for approaching it Use time-out or restraint as an adjunct to all of the above

and sorting objects into categories, and basic self-care skills such as dressing. Generalization is facilitated by arranging for the child to complete skills in therapeutic and home environments with prompts and reinforcements given by parents and other members of the child's social network.

- In the third stage, which may last more than six months, the focus is on expressive communication skills and advanced self-care skills, including toileting. With expressive communication, children are taught to make speech sounds first, then to form words and finally to make sentences. Where children do not develop expressive language, written or pictorial communication may be used.

- In the fourth stage, which may last a year, children gradually enter normal pre-school classes, beginning with as little as ten minutes per day pre-school. In one-to-one out-of-class sessions, children are taught play and pretend skills and age-appropriate peer activities, such as singing songs, saying rhymes and playing games. These skills help them adjust to the normal pre-school situation. Children enter normal pre-schools rather than special pre-schools because they contain children who can act as good role models and teachers with relatively high expectations. These two factors facilitate development.
- In the fifth stage, which may last more than a year, children learn to use advanced language skills, advanced interaction skills (including understanding other people's perspectives), and life skills such as helping with chores. The pre-school teacher plays an increasing role in prompting and shaping new skills.
- In the sixth stage children make the transition from pre-school to normal primary school, if they have developed sufficient skills to do so. Teachers rather than therapists take an increasing role in instructing children. However, if children do not make progress, they repeat the first year of primary school. Some children go on to complete normal primary school and some are placed in special educational placements.

The programme is staff intensive and four levels of staff are involved: student therapists, senior therapists, case supervisors and programme directors. All staff, including student therapists, are highly trained in the principles and practice of social learning theory and applied behaviour analysis. Interventions teams containing about five student therapists, a senior therapist, a supervisor and director are assigned to each child. Each student therapist works more than five hours per week with a child and attends a one-hour meeting with the family, senior therapist, supervisor and director. After six months, student therapists who have developed adequate clinical skills may become senior therapists. After 1500 hours of practice and demonstrating a high level of clinical skill, senior therapists may become supervisors. Programme directors usually have a doctorate in clinical psychology. Parents play a central role in the programme. They are involved in preliminary assessment, work five hours a week with the therapist in the first stage of treatment and help implement skills training generalization routines throughout the programme. They are also involved in organizing the transition into pre-school and school and work collaboratively with programme staff in this regard.

Skills training

Children with autism may have a variety of difficulties in learning self-care and academic skills (Bregman & Gerdtz, 1997). In all instances, the curriculum materials should be matched to the child's developmental stage. Where low IQ or limited language usage prevents or impairs the child's understanding, simplified verbal or pictorial communication methods may be used. Large tasks should be broken down into smaller more manageable tasks that make success more likely. Where children show a lack of initiative, they should be encouraged to choose the learning materials in which they are most interested, and the tasks should be structured so as to maximize success. So if the child is learning a new skill, trials of learning the new unfamiliar skill should be interspersed with trials of executing related skills that have already been mastered. Where children show a lack of resistance in learning a new skill, reinforcement should be arranged so that it is delivered intermittently, on a variable interval or ratio schedule. However, when it is delivered, the child should receive it immediately and naturally occurring reinforcers rather than contrived reinforcers (such as sweets or candy) should be used. Generalization of skills learned in one context to multiple contexts is a major problem in the education of children with autism. Ideally, children should be encouraged and prompted to exercise newly learned skills in many different environments and reinforced for doing so since this maximizes the chances of generalization occurring.

Communication training

In the domain of language and communication, the speech and language curriculum should be geared to the developmental level of the child. If there are some language skills, these may be built on, but where all linguistic skills are absent then sign language may first be taught since this may promote the later development of speech (Schuler, Prizant & Wetherby, 1997). Alternatively, the Picture Exchange Communication System (PECS) may be used to help children communicate their needs pictorially (Bondy & Frost, 1994). Coaching involving modelling, encouragement, reinforcement and feedback for both effort and successive approximations within a moderately structured setting for brief periods of up to thirty minutes per day may be used. Where children have speech and language skills but do not use them within a social context, modelling and reinforcement of all communicative attempts within a naturalistic setting may be used to increase social speech and communication (Prizant, Schuler, Wetherby & Rydell, 1997). Initially, the emphasis should be on communication rather than speech. Where children do not initiate and sustain reciprocal social interactions with others, periods of interaction with teachers, parents and peers need to be planned, attempts at social interaction should be prompted and all efforts or approximations to conversation reinforced.

The refinement of communication skills such as the appropriate use of intonation, non-verbal gestures, and the correction of echolalia, pronominal reversal and speech idiosyncrasies may also be achieved through behavioural training using the coaching methods described above. Video modelling and video feedback may be useful aids in this process. However, this is a long and arduous process because of the way the child with autism views the self and others. Children with autism cannot understand social signals such as smiles, or other non-verbal gestures. They must learn about social rules and then learn to apply them. This is much like an adult learning a second language, which is necessarily a slow process. It was noted earlier that Jordan and Powell (1995) argue that, in autism, there is an episodic autobiographical memory deficit. This is due to an inability to evaluatively appraise the significance of events related to the self. Children with autism, therefore, have difficulty experiencing events as happening to them, so they have problems recalling events as having happened to themselves and communicating these to others in reciprocal social interactions. On this basis, Jordan and Powell argue that teaching children with autism should focus on helping them develop evaluative appraisal skills so that they attach personal significance to events and so develop episodic autobiographical memory. The development of such a memory, by prompting and coaching in recalling and recounting significant events that have happened to them each day, may provide a basis for greater reciprocal interaction.

The Child's Talk project is an evidence-based ASD communication programme, from the UK, in which parents receive psychoeducation and training in specific parent–child communication skills (Aldred, Green & Adams, 2004). Parents are trained to enhance parent–child joint attention to facilitate the development of children's capacity for social referencing. Parents are shown how to replace intrusive parental demands with sensitivity and responsivity to children's ongoing actions by providing an accurate and supportive commentary on their children's behaviour. Parents are trained in how to show children the way language can be used to achieve pragmatic goals, by translating their children's non-verbal communications into simple words. Parents are also shown how to consolidate their children's understanding by using repetitive and predictable language scripts in specific contexts to communicate specific meanings and intentions. The programme also includes coaching parents in using teasing, pauses and openings to encourage variations and expansions of their children's language and play and to expand children's language repertoires. Parents and pre-school children in the Child's Talk programme attend monthly sessions for six months and then less frequent sessions for a further six months. Video feedback is used to coach parents in communication training skills. They are invited to schedule daily thirty-minute sessions to use these skills to coach their children in the development of communication skills.

Challenging behaviour

The management of challenging behaviour in cases where children have intellectual disabilities is discussed in Chapter 8 and it was noted there that the first step in the management of aggression or self-injury is to conduct a thorough functional analysis (Kennedy & Carr, 2002). In conducting such an analysis in cases of autism, a number of additional points need to be taken into account. First, children with autism perceive many situations that might be non-threatening to others as particularly threatening or distressing. These situations include disruption of their routines or insistence that they transfer their attention from one activity to another. Second, children with autism cannot guess what others are thinking and predict how they will behave, so most of the time children with autism find the behaviours of others unpredictable, confusing and potentially distressing. Third, children with autism are unable to clearly predict or understand the impact that intense displays of aggression or self-injury have on others. Fourth, children with autism have difficulty regulating and controlling their own emotions including the display of aggression. Fifth, repetitive self-injury (such as head-banging), probably because it is predictable in its effects, may be intrinsically reinforcing for some children with autism. Sixth, over-sensitivity to stimuli may lead autistic children to react aggressively to what for other children would be normal levels of visual, auditory or touch stimulation.

In all cases where challenging behaviour is occurring, a thorough functional analysis should first be conducted. Where challenging behaviours typically occur in response to identifiable environmental stimuli, in some instances such stimuli may simply be removed. However, in many instances this is not possible because the stimulus is a necessary part of the child's environment, such as transition from one task to another, or from home to school. In these instances if the child is frightened of the stimulus, they may be desensitized to it. If they feel unable to cope with it, they may be coached in coping behaviours, such as predicting the occurrence of the stimulus, relaxing themselves or distracting themselves when the stimulus is present and then they may be reinforced for coping with the stimulus.

While some episodes of challenging behaviour are clearly a response to a discriminative stimulus, others enable the child to *get something or get out of something*. Where challenging behaviours are used to help the child gain something (such as attention) some functionally equivalent but less destructive skill may be taught to the child as a way of obtaining the desired reinforcer. Where the challenging behaviour is a way of avoiding a feared situation, the child may be desensitized to it and reinforced for coping with the feared stimulus when it occurs. Alternatively, the child may be helped to develop less destructive ways of avoiding the feared situation, if this is appropriate.

Psychopharmacological treatment

Medication is used in the treatment of children with autism (Fisman, 2002; Lord & Bailey, 2002; Volkmar et al., 2004a). In the past haloperidol was widely used to treat challenging behaviour. However, the extrapyramidal side effects and long-term risk of tardive dyskinesia are major drawbacks of haloperidol, which has now been superseded by newer neuroleptics, notably respirodone and olanzapine. A low dose of respirodone has been shown to be effective for reducing aggression in children with autism. For obsessional, repetitive, stereotyped behaviour, there is some evidence in selected cases for the effectiveness of specific serotonin re-uptake inhibitors (SSRIs). Psychos-timulant medication, notably methylphenidate, has been shown to reduce hyperactivity in children with autism, although it may exacerbate stereotyped behaviour. Anti-convulsants are widely used to control epilepsy in autism. For mood stabilization in children with autism, anti-convulsants (such as carbamezapine or sodium valporate) are commonly used in clinical practice. There is little evidence for the efficacy of secretin or vitamins in the treatment of autism, although proponents of such treatments have made unfounded claims for their effectiveness.

Respite care

Where the demands of caring for a child with autism periodically outstrip the family's coping resources, respite care may be arranged.

SUMMARY

Autism, Asperger's syndrome, PDDNOS, Rett's disorder and Heller's syndrome are the principal pervasive developmental disabilities. They entail substantial social, communicative, cognitive and behavioural problems. The majority of children with these disorders are unable to lead independent lives as adults. While autism and Asperger's syndrome are present from birth, Rett's and Heller's syndromes emerge during the pre-school years after a period of relatively normal development. The prevalence rate for autism, the most common of the pervasive developmental disorders, is 10 per 10,000, and autism is more common in boys. While psychogenic aetiological theories of autism were popular in the past, the available evidence now suggests that autism is a neurodevelopmental disability rather than an emotional reaction to a stressful family environment. A number of cognitive deficits have been implicated in the development of autistic symptomatology. Currently there is no cure for autism. Diagnostic and compensatory treatment programmes are the principal type of intervention offered by clinical psychologists as members of multi-disciplinary and multi-agency teams. The early and accurate identification, evaluation and management of children with these problems is essential. Clinicians work in partnership with parents to enhance children's communicative skills, foster the development of problem-solving skills and decrease challenging behaviours.

EXERCISE 9.1

Work in pairs. Read the case study in Box 9.1, the diagnostic criteria in Table 9.1 and the clinical features in Table 9.2. On the basis of the information given in Box 9.1, list the clinical features that Tom showed and the behaviours he exhibited which fit with the diagnostic criteria for autism. Then decide what specific further information you would require to be sure of your diagnosis.

FURTHER READING

Cohen, D., & Volkmar, F. (1997). *Handbook of Autism and Pervasive Developmental Disorders* (Second Edition). New York: Wiley.

Howlin, P. & Rutter, M. (1987). *Treatment of Autistic Children*. New York: Wiley.

Schloper, E., Lansing, M., & Reichler, R. (1979). *Individualised Assessment And Treatment For Autistic And Developmentally Disabled Children. Teaching Strategies for Parents and Professionals Volume 11*. Austin, TX: Pro-ed.

Schloper, E., Lansing, M., & Waters, L. (1980). *Individualised Assessment And Treatment For Autistic And Developmentally Disabled Children. Teaching Strategies for Parents and Professionals Volume 111*. Austin, TX: Pro-ed.

Volkmar, F., Cook, E., Pomeroy, J., Realmuto, G. & Tanguay, P. (1999). Practice parameters for the assessment and treatment of children and adults with autism and other pervasive developmental disorders. American Academy of Child and Adolescent Psychiatry working group on quality issues.. *Journal of the American Academy of Child and Adolescent Psychiatry*, 38 (12 Supplement), 32S–54S.

Wall, K. (2004). *Autism and Early Years Practice. A Guide for Early Years Professionals, Teachers and Parents*. London: Paul Chapman. (*This is an outstanding resource for UK practitioners, containing sound advice on practice and lists of websites and resources.*)

FURTHER READING FOR FAMILIES OF AUTISTIC CHILDREN

Attwood, T. (1998). *Asperger's Syndrome*. London: Jessica Kingsley.

Gillberg, C. (2002). *A Guide to Asperger Syndrome*. Cambridge: Cambridge University Press.

Grandin, T. & Scariano, M. (1986). *Emergence, Labelled Autistic*. London: Costello. (*Biographical account of autism.*)

Harris, S. (1994). *Siblings of Children with Autism. A Guide for Families*. Bethesda, MD: Woodbine House.

Howlin, P. (1998). *Children with Autism and Asperger's Syndrome. A Guide for Practitioner's and Carers.* Chichester: Wiley.

Jordon, R. & Powell, S. (1995). *Understanding and Teaching Children with Autism.* New York: Wiley.

Maurice, C. (1993). *Let me Hear Your Voice.* New York: Knopf. (*A mother's story of children's recovery following behavioural treatment.*)

National Autistic Society (1993). *Approaches to Autism* (Second Edition). London: National Autistic Society.

Vermeulen, P. (2000). *I am Special. Introducing Children and Young People to the Autistic Spectrum Disorder.* London: Jessica Kingsley.

Williams, D. (1992). *Nobody Nowhere.* London: Doubleday. (*Biographical account of autism.*)

Wing, L. (1996). *The Autistic Spectrum: A Guide for Parents and Professionals.* Constable: London.

WEBSITES

Autism Society of America: http://www.autism-society.org/

Center for the study of Autism: http: //www.autism.org

Hanen Centre for early language intervention: http://hanen.velocet.ca/

Lovaas Institute for Early Intervention – Applied Behaviour Analysis for autism: http://www.lovaas.com/

National Autism Society, UK: http://www.nas.org.uk/

Picture Exchange Communication System: http://www.pecs.com/

TEACCH structured learning for autism: http://www. teacch. com

Temple Grandin's first-person account website: http://www.templegrandin.com/ and http://www.templegrandin-autismvideos.com

Factsheets on autism and Asperger's syndrome can be downloaded from the website for Rose, G. & York, A. (2004). *Mental Health and Growing Up. Fact sheets for Parents, Teachers and Young People* (Third edition). London: Gaskell: http://www.rcpsych.ac.uk

Section III

Problems of middle childhood

Chapter 10

Conduct problems

Conduct problems constitute a third to a half of all clinic referrals (Burke, Loeber & Birmaher, 2002; Farrington, 1995; Kazdin, 1995; Loeber, Burke, Lahey, Winters & Zera, 2000). One of the most common referrals in child and family psychology is a boy in middle childhood who presents with conduct problems, specific learning difficulties and related family and school problems. Conduct problems are the single most costly disorder of childhood and adolescence for three reasons. First, they are remarkably unresponsive to treatment. Positive outcome rates for routine treatments range from 20 to 40%. Second, about 60% of children with conduct problems have a poor prognosis. A summary of some of the adult outcomes for children with conduct disorder is presented in Table 10.1. From this figure it is apparent that

Table 10.1 Outcome for adults identified as conduct disordered during childhood or adolescence compared with control groups

Criminality	More criminal behaviour, arrests, convictions, imprisonment and rates of driving while intoxicated
Mental health	Higher rates of psychiatric hospitalization and higher rates of all psychological symptoms, anti-social personality disorder, drug abuse and alcohol abuse
Physical health	Higher rates of hospitalization and mortality
Educational attainment	Higher rates of school drop-out and lower attainment levels
Occupational adjustment	Higher unemployment, lower occupational status if employed, more frequent job changes
Marital adjustment	Higher rates of separation, divorce and remarriage
Social adjustment Intergenerational transmission	Less contact with relatives, friends, neighbours and church More children with conduct problems

Note: Based on comparisons of referred cases of conduct disorder with clinical or normal controls or on comparisons of delinquent and non-delinquent youngsters cited in Burke et al. (2002); Farrington (1995); Loeber et al. (2000) and Kazdin (1995).

children with conduct disorder turn to adult criminality and develop anti-social personality disorders, alcohol-related problems and a variety of psychological difficulties. They also have more problems with health, educational attainment, occupational adjustment, marital stability and social integration. The third reason for the high cost of conduct problems is the fact that they are intergenerationally transmitted. Adults with a history of conduct disorder rear children with a particularly high prevalence of conduct difficulties.

A typical case example of a youngster with a conduct problem is presented in Box 10.1. After considering the classification, epidemiology and clinical features of conduct problems, this chapter considers a variety of theoretical explanations concerning their aetiology, along with relevant empirical evidence. The assessment of conduct problems and approaches to their treatment in middle childhood and adolescence is then given. The chapter concludes with some ideas on how to prevent conduct problems in populations at risk.

Box 10.1. Case example of conduct disorder. Bill, the boy on the roof

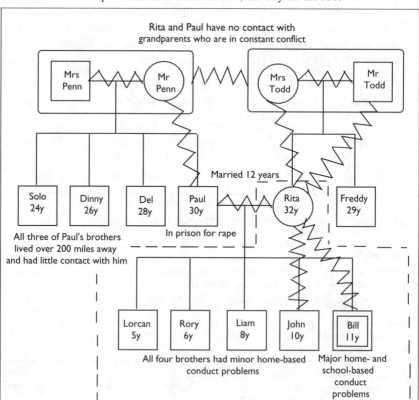

Referral. Bill, aged eleven, was referred by his social worker for treatment following an incident in which he had assaulted neighbours by climbing up onto the roof of his house and throwing rocks and stones at them. He also had a number of other problems, according to the school headteacher, including academic under-achievement, difficulty in maintaining friendships at school and repeated school absence. He smoked, occasionally drank alcohol, and stole money and goods from neighbours. His problems were long standing but had intensified in the six months preceding the referral. At that time his father, Paul, was imprisoned for raping a young girl in the small rural village where the family lived.

Family history. From the genogram it may be seen that Bill was one of five boys who lived with his mother at the time of the referral. The family lived in relatively chaotic circumstances. Prior to Paul's imprisonment, the children's defiance and rule breaking, particularly Bill's, was kept in check by their fear of physical punishment from their father. Since his incarceration, there were few house rules and these were implemented inconsistently, so all of the children showed conduct problems but Bill's were by far the worst. Rita had developed intense coercive patterns of interaction with Bill and John (the second eldest). In addition to the parenting difficulties, there were also no routines to ensure bills were paid, food was bought, washing was done, homework completed or regular meal and sleeping times were observed. Rita supported the family with welfare payments and money earned illegally from farm-work. Despite the family chaos, she was very attached to her children and would sometimes take them to work with her rather than send them to school because she liked their company.

At the preliminary interview, Rita said that 'her nerves were in tatters'. She was attending a psychiatrist intermittently for pharmacological treatment of depression. She had a long-standing history of conduct and mood regulation problems, beginning early in adolescence. In particular she had conflictual relationships with her mother and father, which were characterized by coercive cycles of interaction. In school she had had academic difficulties and peer relationship problems.

Paul, the father, also had long-standing difficulties. His conduct problems began in middle childhood. He was the eldest of four brothers, all of whom developed conduct problems, but his were by far the most severe. He had a history of becoming involved in aggressive exchanges that often escalated to violence. He and his mother had become involved in coercive patterns of interaction from his earliest years. He developed similar coercive patterns of interaction at school with his teachers, at work with various gangers and also in his relationship with Rita. He had a distant and detached relationship with his father.

Rita had been ostracized by her own family when she married Paul, who they saw as an unsuitable partner for her, since he had a number of previous convictions for theft and assault. Paul's family never accepted Rita because they thought she had '. . . ideas above her station'. Rita's and Paul's parents were in regular conflict, and each family blamed the other for the chaotic situation in which Paul and Rita had found themselves. Rita was also ostracized by the village community in which she lived. The community blamed her for driving her husband to commit rape.

Developmental history. From Bill's developmental history, it was clear that he was a difficult-temperament child who did not develop sleeping and feeding routines easily and responded intensely and negatively to new situations. His language development had been delayed and he had showed academic difficulties since his first years in school. On the positive side, Bill had a strong sense of family loyalty to his brothers and parents and did not want to see the family split up.

Psychometric assessment. On Child Behaviour Checklists, all five of the boys obtained externalizing behaviour problem scores in the clinical range, but Bill's were by far the most extreme. On Teacher Report Forms, of the five boys, only Bill obtained an externalizing behaviour problem score in the clinical range. A psychometric evaluation of Bill's abilities with the WISC-IV and the WRAT-3 showed that he was of normal intelligence, but his attainments in reading, spelling and arithmetic fell below the 10th percentile. From his WISC-IV sub-test profile, which included particularly low scores on Digit Span and Coding sub-tests, it was concluded that the discrepancy between attainment and abilities was accounted for by a specific learning disability.

School report. The headteacher at the school which Bill and his brothers attended confirmed that Bill had academic, conduct and attainment problems, but was committed to educating the boys and managing their conduct and attendance problems in a constructive way. The headteacher, Mr Dempsey, had a reputation (of which he was very proud) for being particularly skilled in managing children with problems.

Formulation. Bill was an eleven-year-old boy with a persistent and broad pattern of conduct problems both within and outside the home. He also had a specific learning disability and peer relationships problems. Factors which predisposed Bill to the development of these problems include a difficult temperament, a developmental language delay, exposure to paternal criminality, maternal depression and a chaotic family environment. The father's incarceration six months prior to the referral led to an intensification of Bill's conduct problems. The conduct problems were maintained at the time of the referral by engagement in coercive patterns of interaction with his mother and teachers, rejection of Bill by peers at school, and isolation of his family by the extended family and the community. Protective factors in the case included the mother's wish to retain custody of the children rather than have them taken into foster care, the children's sense of family loyalty and the school's commitment to retaining and dealing with the boys rather than excluding them for truancy and misconduct.

Treatment. The treatment plan in this case involved a multi-systemic intervention programme. The mother was trained in behavioural parenting skills. A series of meetings between the teacher, the mother and the social worker were convened to develop and implement a plan that insured regular school attendance. Occasional relief foster care was arranged for Bill and John (the second eldest) to reduce the stress on Rita. Social skills training was provided for Bill to help him deal with peer relationship problems.

CLASSIFICATION

Any system for classifying conduct problems must take account of the extraordinary variability that occurs in populations of youngsters with such difficulties (Burke et al., 2002; Hill, 2002; Kazdin, 1995; Loeber et al., 2000). Available research suggests that variability in conduct problems occur along the following axes:

- severity, from mild and infrequent to severe and frequent
- chronicity, from recent to long standing
- pervasiveness, from home-based to home-, school- and community-based

- age of onset of problems, from childhood onset to adolescent onset
- peer influences on conduct problems, from peer-group-based socialized conduct problems to solitary conduct difficulties
- the level of deceit involved, from overt aggression to covert stealing and lying
- the presence or absence of attention problems
- the presence or absence of hyperactivity problems
- the presence or absence of depression and other negative mood states
- the presence or absence of specific learning difficulties
- the degree of family disorganization.

As can be seen from Figures 10.1 and 10.2 different strategies have been used in DSM IV TR and ICD 10 to take account of variability along these axes. However, certain distinctions are present in both systems. First, a distinction is made between transient adjustment disorders involving circumscribed conduct problems on the one hand and more pervasive long-standing conduct problems on the other. This is a useful clinical distinction to make and in this chapter our main concern will be with long-standing pervasive disruptive externalizing behaviour problems. However, it is worth noting that in clinical practice the distinction between adjustment reactions and disorders is not always clear cut. The results of multi-variate studies suggest that adjustment disorders with a disturbance of conduct and disruptive behaviour disorders fall along a continuum of externalizing behaviour problems (Achenbach & Rescorla, 2000, 2001). A second distinction is that made between oppositional defiant disorder and conduct disorder with the former reflecting a less pervasive disturbance than the latter. Also, oppositional defiant disorder is often a developmental precursor of conduct disorder. The ICD system allows for peer influence on conduct problems to be accounted for by distinguishing between socialized and unsocialized conduct problems. In the DSM system a distinction is made between childhood-onset and adolescent-onset sub-types of conduct disorder. Conduct disorder with either co-morbid ADHD or depression are defined as distinct sub-types of the condition in the ICD

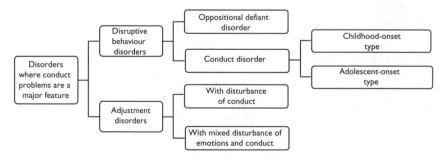

Figure 10.1 Classification of disruptive behaviour disorders in DSM IV TR

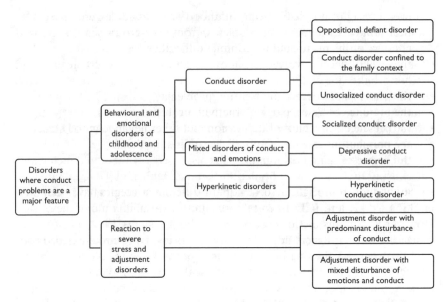

Figure 10.2 Classification of disruptive behaviour disorders in ICD 10

system, i.e. hyperkinetic conduct disorder and depressive conduct disorder. Within the DSM system, in contrast, co-morbid first axis diagnoses would be given in such cases. Neither the DSM IV TR nor the ICD 10 system make a distinction between the overt aggression versus covert deceit sub-types of conduct problems. Co-morbid learning problems and family difficulties are dealt with in both systems through multi-axial coding. In DSM IV TR, specific learning difficulties are coded as co-morbid diagnoses on axis 1, and level of family disorganization is coded on axis IV with other psychosocial and environmental problems. In ICD 10, specific learning difficulties are coded on axis II as specific delays in development and family disorganization is coded on axis V with other abnormal psychosocial situations (both these multi-axial systems are outlined in Table 3.1, p. 81).

EPIDEMIOLOGY

Overall prevalence rates for conduct disorders and oppositional defiant disorders vary from 4 to 14%, depending on the criteria used and the population studied (Carr, 1993; Cohen et al., 1993; Meltzer et al., 2000). Table 3.9 (p. 97) shows that, in a UK national epidemiological survey, the prevalence for conduct disorders was 5.3% (Meltzer et al., 2000). Oppositional defiant disorder is more common than conduct disorder; conduct disorders are more common than emotional disorders. They are more prevalent in boys than girls, with male:female ratios varying from 4:1 to 2:1. Rates of conduct disorder are higher for adolescents than children. These disorders are more common in low socioeconomic groups. In Western countries, over the past seventy years the prevalence of conduct disorder has increased five fold (Robins, 1999).

Co-morbidity for conduct problems and other problems, such as ADHD, emotional disorders, developmental language delay, and specific learning disabilities is quite common, particularly in clinic populations. Table 3.4 (p. 86) shows that the co-morbidity rate for conduct disorder and ADHD in community populations is 23.3%; Table 3.5 (p. 87) shows that the co-morbidity rate for aggression and attention problems based on the Child Behaviour Checklist (CBCL) in clinic populations is much higher, at 47%. In Table 3.4 (p. 86) it may be seen that co-morbidity rates for conduct disorder and emotional disorders in community populations is 16.9% for major depression and 14.8% for anxiety disorders. Table 3.5 (p. 87) shows that the co-morbidity rate for aggression and anxious/depressed problems based on the Child Behaviour Checklist in clinic populations is 41%.

DIAGNOSIS AND CLINICAL FEATURES

The DSM IV TR and ICD 10 diagnostic criteria and corresponding ASEBA CBCL sub-scales for oppositional defiant disorder and conduct disorder are given in Tables 10.2 and 10.3. For oppositional defiant disorder, the aggressive sub-scale from the CBCL profile for eighteen-month- to five-year-olds is given in Table 10.2, since, in clinical practice, often young children are referred with this problem and there is some evidence that oppositional defiant disorder may be a developmental precursor of conduct disorder (Burke et al., 2002; Hill, 2002; Loeber et al., 2000). For conduct disorder, the aggressive and rule-breaking sub-scales of the CBCL profile for six- to eighteen-year-olds have been included in Table 10.3, since, in clinical practice, conduct disorder is more common among older referrals. High scores on both the aggressive and rule-breaking behaviour sub-scale of the CBCL suggests the presence of socialized conduct problems, in which deviant peer-group relationships play a part, whereas elevations on the aggressive behaviour sub-scale only suggest the presence of an unsocialized conduct problem.

Table 10.4 presents the clinical features of oppositional defiant disorder and conduct disorder. The disorders are similar insofar as, in each, the main behavioural feature is a persistent pattern of anti-social behaviour characterized by defiance of authority and aggression. However, in oppositional defiant disorder the behavioural pattern is circumscribed and usually confined to the home, whereas with conduct disorder a more pervasive pattern of anti-social behaviour is present. This pattern extends to the school and community and involves deceitfulness, cruelty and other problems such as drug abuse.

Table 10.2 Diagnostic criteria for oppositional defiant disorder in DSM IV TR, ICD 10 and items from Achenbach's Aggressive Behaviour syndrome scale of the ASEBA system for 1.5- to 5-year-olds

DSM IV TR	ICD 10	ASEBA Aggressive Behaviour syndrome scale for 1.5- to 5-year-olds
A. A pattern of negativistic, hostile and defiant behaviour lasting at least six months, during which four or more of the following are present: 1. Often loses temper 2. Often argues with adults 3. Often actively defies or refuses to comply with adults' requests or rules 4. Often deliberately annoys people 5. Often blames others for his or her mistakes or misbehaviour 6. Is often touchy or easily annoyed by others 7. Is often angry or resentful 8. Is often spiteful or vindictive B. The disturbance in behaviour causes clinically significant impairment in social, academic or occupational functioning C. The behaviours do not occur exclusively during the course of a psychotic or a mood disorder D. Criteria are not met for conduct disorder or anti-social personality disorder	The essential feature of this disorder is a pattern of persistently negativistic, hostile, defiant, provocative and disruptive behaviour which is clearly outside the normal range of behaviour for a child of the same age in the same sociocultural context and which does not include the more serious violations of the rights of others associated with conduct disorder Children with this disorder tend frequently and actively to defy adult requests or rules and deliberately to annoy other people. Usually they tend to be angry, resentful, and easily annoyed by other people, whom they blame for their own mistakes and difficulties. They generally have a low frustration tolerance and readily lose their temper. Typically their defiance has a provocative quality, so that they initiate confrontations and generally exhibit excessive levels of rudeness, uncooperativeness and resistance to authority Frequently this behaviour is most evident in interactions with adults or peers whom the child knows well, and signs of the disorder may not be present during clinical interview The key distinction from other types of conduct disorder is the absence of behaviour that violates the law and the basic rights of others such as theft, cruelty, bullying, assault and destructiveness	**Self-regulation deficits** Selfish (P&T) Stubborn (P&T) Can't stand waiting (P&T) Easily frustrated (P&T) Angry moods (P&T) Screams (P&T) Accident prone (P&T) Unresponsive to punishment (P&T) Lacks guilt (P&T) **Aggression** Disturbs others (T) Mean to others (T) Teases others (T) Not liked by others (T) Attacks others (P&T) Hits others (P&T) Fights (P&T) Cruel to animals (T) **Destruction** Destroy own things (T) Destroys others' things (P&T) **Defiance** Uncooperative (P&T) Demands attention (P&T) Demanding (P&T) Defiant (P&T) Disobedient (P&T) Temper tantrums (P&T) Items marked (P) are on the parent report Child Behaviour Checklist Items marked (T) are on the Teacher and Caregiver Report form

Note: Adapted from DSM IV TR (APA, 2000a), ICD 10 (WH0, 1992, 1996) and ASEBA (Achenbach & Rescorla, 2000).

Table 10.3 Diagnostic criteria for conduct disorder in DSM IV TR, ICD 10 and items from Achenbach's Aggressive Behaviour and Rule Breaking syndrome scales of the ASEBA system for 6- to 18-year-olds

DSM IV TR	*ICD 10*	*ASEBA 6–18 year olds*
A. A repetitive and persistent pattern of behaviour in which the basic rights of others or major age-appropriate societal norms or rules are violated as manifested by the presence of three or more of the following criteria in the past 12 months with at least one criterion present in the past 6 months	Conduct disorders (CD) are characterized by a repetitive and persistent pattern of dissocial, aggressive or defiant conduct. Such behaviour, when at its most extreme for the individual should amount to major violations of age-appropriate social expectations, and is therefore more severe than ordinary childish mischief or adolescent rebelliousness.	**AGGRESSIVE BEHAVIOUR SYNDROME** **Self-regulation deficits** Stubborn (P&T&C) Easily frustrated (T) Speaks loudly (P&T&C) Screams (P&T&C) Sudden changes in mood (P&T&C) Explosive (T) Explosive (T) Sulks (P&T)
Aggression to people and animals 1. Often bullies threatens or intimidates others 2. Often initiates physical fights 3. Has used a weapon that can cause serious physical harm to others 4. Has been physically cruel to people 5. Has been physically cruel to animals 6. Has stolen while confronting a victim 7. Has forced someone into sexual activity	Examples of the behaviours on which the diagnosis is based include the following: excessive levels of fighting or bullying; cruelty to animals or other people; severe destructiveness to property; firesetting; stealing; repeated lying; truancy from school and running away from home; unusually frequent and severe temper tantrums; defiant provocative behaviour; and persistent and severe disobedience. Any one of these categories, if marked, is sufficient for the diagnosis, but isolated dissocial acts are not	**Aggression** Suspicious of others (P&T&C) Mean to others (P&T&C) Teases others (P&T&C) Threatens others (P&T&C) Attacks others (P&T&C) Gets in fights (P&T&C) **Destruction** Destroys own things (P&T&C) Destroys others' things (P&T&C) **Defiance** Demands attention (P&T&C) Argues a lot (P&T&C) Disobedient at school (P&T&C) Disobedient at home (P) Defiant (T) Loses temper (P&T&C)
Destruction of property 8. Has deliberately engaged in firesetting 9. Has deliberately destroyed others' property **Deceitfulness or theft** 10. Has broken into someone's house, building or car 11. Often lies to obtain goods or favours or avoid obligations 12. Has stolen items without confronting the victim	Exclusion criteria include serious underlying conditions such as schizophrenia, hyperkinetic disorder or depression	**RULE-BREAKING SYNDROME** **Rule breaking without guilt** Breaks rules (P&T&C) Shows no guilt (P&T&C)

Continued

Table 10.3 continued

DSM IV TR	ICD 10	ASEBA 6–18 year olds

Serious violation of rules
13. Often stays out late at night despite parental prohibitions (before 13 years of age)
14. Has run away from home overnight at least twice while living in parental home or once without returning for a lengthy period
15. Is often truant from school before the age of 13
 	
B. The disturbance in behaviour causes clinically significant impairment in social, academic or occupational functioning
 	
C. In those over 18 years, the criteria for anti-social personality disorder are not met
   Specify childhood-onset (prior to 10 years) or adolescent onset
   Specify severity (mild, moderate or severe)
	The diagnosis is not made unless the duration of the behaviour is 6 months or longer
	
	Specify: CD confined to family context where the symptoms are confined to the home
	
	Unsocialized CD where there is a pervasive abnormality in peer relationships
	
	Socialized CD where the individual is well integrated into a peer group
		Deviant peers
		Prefers older friends (P&T&C)
		Has bad friends (P&T&C)
		
		Overt conduct problems
		Tardy to school or class (T)
		Swears (P&T&C)
		Sets fires (P&C)
		Vandalism (P&T&C)
		Runs away from home (P&C)
		Truants from school (P&T&C)
		
		Covert conduct problems
		Lies and cheats (P&T&C)
		Steals from home (P&C)
		Steals outside home (P&T&C)
		
		Drug abuse
		Uses tobacco (P&T&C)
		Drinks alcohol (P&C)
		Uses drugs (P&T&C)
		
		Coercive sex
		Sex problems (P)
		Thinks about sex too much (P&T&C)
		Items marked (P) are on the Parent Report CBCL
		Items marked (T) are on the Teacher Report form
		Items marked (C) are on the Youth Self-Report form

Note: Adapted from DSM IV TR (APA, 2000a), ICD 10 (WHO, 1992, 1996) and ASEBA (Achenbach & Rescorla, 2001).

With respect to cognition, in both disorders there appears to be a limited internalization of social rules and norms. In both oppositional defiant disorder and conduct disorder there is a hostile attributional bias, where the youngster interprets ambiguous social situations as threatening and responds with aggressive retaliative behaviour.

With respect to affect, in both oppositional defiant disorder and conduct disorder, anger and irritability are the predominant mood states.

Table 10.4 Clinical features of disorders of conduct

	Oppositional defiant disorder	Conduct disorder
Cognition	• Limited internalization of social rules or norms • Interprets ambiguous social situations as threatening and responds with anti-social behaviour	• Limited internalization of social rules or norms • Interprets ambiguous social situations as threatening and responds with anti-social behaviour
Affect	• Anger and irritability	• Anger and irritability
Behaviour	• Persistent pattern of defiance towards adults in authority • Aggression • Temper tantrums	• Persistent broad pattern of anti-social behaviour • Defiance • Aggression • Destructiveness • Deceitfulness and theft • Cruelty • Truancy • Running away • Coercive sex • Pre-adolescent drug use
Physical condition		• Physical problems associated with risk-taking behaviour such as fighting, drug abuse or casual unsafe sex
Interpersonal adjustment	• Problematic relationships with parents	• Problematic relationships with parents, teachers and peers

With respect to physical health, youngsters with conduct disorders may have a variety of problems which result from risk-taking behaviour. For example, they may have injuries from involvement in fighting or dangerous driving. They may have addictions, infection or medical complications associated with illicit drug use or casual sexual relationships.

In both conditions there may be problematic relationships with significant members of the child's network. With oppositional defiant disorder the main relationship difficulties occur with parents and centre on the child's defiance. In conduct disorders, negative relationships with parents and teachers typically revolve around the youngster's defiant behaviour, and with peers the problems typically centre on aggression and bullying, which is guided by the hostile attributional bias with which conduct disordered youngsters construe many of their peer relationships. With conduct disorders there may also be problematic relationships with members of the wider community if theft or vandalism has occurred. Multi-agency involvement with juvenile justice or social work agencies are common. Also, because conduct disorder is associated with family disorganization, parental criminality and parental psychological adjustment difficulties, professionals from adult mental health and justice systems may be involved.

AETIOLOGICAL THEORIES OF CONDUCT DISORDER

Since the distinction between oppositional defiant disorder and conduct disorder is a relatively recent development, most theories in this area have been developed with specific reference to conduct disorder, but have obvious implications for oppositional defiant disorder, which is probably a developmental precursor of conduct disorder in many cases. Some of the more influential theories about the aetiology of conduct disorder are listed in Table 10.5 along with the implications of these theories for treatment. Let us consider each of these in turn.

Table 10.5 Psychological theories and treatments for conduct disorder

	Theory	Theoretical principles	Principles of treatment
Biological theories	**Genetic theory**	• A disposition to aggression is inherited	NA
	Neurotransmitter and hormonal theory	• A disposition to aggression is due to a dysregulation of neurotransmitter (serotonin and noradrenalin) and hormonal (testosterone and cortisol) systems	• Psychopharmacological treatment of aggression
	Arousal theory	• Children with conduct disorders have an impaired capacity for learning pro-social behaviour or for learning to avoid anti-social behaviour • Their genetically inherited low arousal levels make them less responsive to positive and negative reinforcement than normal children	• Highly structured and intensive behavioural treatment where immediate and intense consequences for rule-following and rule-breaking behaviour occurs
	Difficult temperament theory	• Difficult temperament is a risk factor for conduct problems because it leads to poor self-regulation and elicits punishment from caregivers	• Self-regulation skills training for youngsters and parenting skills training for caregivers

	Neuro-psychological deficit theory	• Neuropsychologically based deficits in language, verbal reasoning and executive functioning underpin self-regulation difficulties that contribute to conduct problems • They also lead to under-achievement, which leads to frustration and this contributes to aggressive behaviour	• Remedial interventions that facilitate the development of language and academic skills
Psychodynamic theories	Super-ego deficit theory	• Anti-social behaviour occurs because of either over-indulgent or punitive/negligent parenting • With over-indulgent parenting, the child internalizes lax standards • With punitive or negligent parenting, the child internalizes the parents aggressive or negligent style for dealing with relationships	• Residential group-based milieu therapy where staff consistently and compassionately enforce rules of conduct which reflect societal standards
	Attachment theory	• Children who are separated from their primary caretakers for extended periods of time during their first months of life fail to develop secure attachments • In later life they do not have internal working models to guide moral social interaction	• Treatment should provide a secure-attachment relationship which will lead to the development of appropriate internal working models for relationships
Cognitive theories	Social information-processing theory	• Children with conduct disorders attribute hostile intentions to others and respond with retaliatory aggression • The reactions of peers confirms the hostile attributional bias	• Group-based social problem-solving skills training
	Social skills deficit theory	• Children with conduct disorders lack the skills to generate alternative solutions to social problems and implement these • They use aggression to solve social problems	• Social skills training

Continued

Table 10.5 continued

	Theory	Theoretical principles	Principles of treatment
Social learning theories	**Modelling theory**	• Aggression is learned through a process of imitation or modelling the behaviour displayed by the parents or older siblings	• Family-based treatment to help parents model appropriate behaviour for their children or the provision of alternative models of appropriate behaviour in a residential or foster-care setting
	Coercive family process theory	• Children with conduct disorders learn their anti-social behaviours from involvement in coercive patterns of interaction with their parents • Social and economic stressors contribute to the parents' use of a coercive parenting style	• Family-based therapy to help parents and children break coercive patterns of interaction and to empower parents to manage life stresses which compromise their parenting effectiveness
Systems theories	**Structural family systems theory**	Conduct problems occur in disorganized families which lack: • communication and problem-solving skills • clear rules, roles, routines • clear boundaries and hierarchies • flexibility for managing lifecycle transitions such as children's entry into adulthood	• Family-based therapy to help families become more organized
	Sociological theory	• Within a socially disadvantaged delinquent sub-culture, theft and other anti-social behaviours are illegitimate means to achieve material goals valued by mainstream culture	• Treatment must provide delinquents and their peer groups with legitimate means to achieve societal goals through training and employment schemes
	Multi-systemic ecological theory	Conduct disorders are maintained by: • individual factors (such as hostile attributional bias, poor social skills, difficulties learning pro-social behaviour from	Multi-systemic treatment packages should include: • individual and group cognitive and social skills training to enhance pro-social

experience, academic learning difficulties)
- family factors (particularly parent–child attachment and discipline problems, marital discord and disorganization)
- school factors (such as poor attainment)
- community factors (such as involvement with deviant peers and drug abuse)

peer relationships and reduce involvement in deviant peer groups
- family therapy or treatment foster care to improve parent–child attachment and discipline and reduce family disorganization
- school-based interventions to deal with under-achievement

Biological theories

Biological theories have focused on the roles of genetic factors, difficult temperament, neurotransmitters and hormonal factors, arousal levels, and neuropsychological deficits in the aetiology of conduct problems (Raine, 2002).

Genetic theories

Many lines of research focus on genetic and constitutional aspects of children with conduct disorder, and these are guided by the hypothesis that biological factors underpin anti-social behaviour. The predominance of males among youngsters with conduct disorders, and the finding of heritability co-efficients between .2 and .8, with most being between .4, and .7, point to a role for genetically transmitted constitutional factors in the aetiology of conduct disorders (Simonoff, 2001). It may be that genetic factors associated with difficult temperament, dysregulation of certain neurotransmitter systems, lower level of autonomic arousal or certain neuropsychological deficits contribute to the development of anti-social behaviour. Early reports of a causal link between XYY syndrome and conduct problems have not been supported by later research. The association between XYY syndrome and conduct problems appears to be due the high rates of parental separation and maternal psychological problems that characterize the families of XYY children (Bolton & Holland, 1994).

Difficult temperament theory

According to this position, children with a difficult temperament are at risk for developing conduct disorders (Chess & Thomas, 1995). Difficult temperament and associated self-regulation deficits may make it challenging for these children to internalize and conform to social rules. Also, children with difficult temperaments may elicit punitive responses from their care-givers and so, through a process of modelling, develop a punitive or aggressive style for interacting with others. Available evidence shows that difficult temperament, which is partially inherited, is a risk factor for conduct disorders, but the link is not as strong as originally suspected (Hill, 2002). Interventions that aim to enhance youngsters' self-regulation skills, and non-punitive parenting practices derive from this theory. Evidence from treatment outcome studies shows that such interventions are effective in treating conduct disorders (Behan & Carr, 2000; Brosnan & Carr, 2000; Fonagy & Kurtz, 2002; Kazdin, 2003; Lochman, Barry & Pardini 2003; Richardson & Joughin, 2002).

Neurotransmitter and hormonal theories

These theories point to the role of one or more neurotransmitters or hormones as risk factors in the development of conduct disorders and to the role of psychopharmacological interventions for the management of aggressive behaviour (Lynn & King, 2002). Current hypotheses in this domain posit a link between conduct disorder or aggression and diminished noradrenaline, serotonin and cortisol levels and excess levels of testosterone. The evidence in this area, which is predominantly correlational, is not uniformly consistent so firm conclusions about the validity of these types of theories may not be drawn at this point (Earls & Mezzacappa, 2002; Hill, 2002).

Arousal theory

Children with conduct disorders have lower arousal levels than normal children, according to this theory, and so are fearless, stimulation seeking and less responsive to rewards and punishments (Raine, 1993, 2002). They have an impaired capacity for responding to the positive reinforcement that often follows pro-social behaviour or for avoiding punishments associated with anti-social behaviour. Thus they fail to learn pro-social behaviour or to avoid anti-social behaviour. In a series of studies, Raine (2002) has shown that low arousal (as indexed by heart rate and other psychophsiological measures) characterizes youngsters with conduct disorder. It is assumed that this abnormally low arousal level is inherited, and the results of twin studies partially support this (Kazdin, 1995). Treatment based on this hypothesis involves highly structured and intensive learning situations to facilitate internalizing social rules. The positive and negative reinforcers used must be highly valued and delivered immediately following responses. All rule infractions must lead to immediate withdrawal of desired stimuli. Rule following should be immediately and intensely rewarded on a variable interval schedule, since this leads to learning that is maximally resistant to extinction. These treatment implications of arousal theory have been incorporated into the design of residential token economies for delinquent adolescents, behavioural parent training programmes, school-based behavioural programmes and treatment foster care (Behan & Carr, 2000; Brosnan & Carr, 2000; Fonagy & Kurtz, 2002; Richardson & Joughin, 2002).

Neuropsychological deficit theory

Neuropsychologically based deficits in language development, verbal reasoning and executive functioning due to peri-natal complications, according to this position, underpin self-regulation difficulties that contribute to conduct problems (Moffit, 1993). They may also cause under-achievement, which leads to frustration and this contributes to aggressive behaviour. This position is supported by evidence that documents an association between conduct disorder and the following risk factors: maternal smoking, maternal malnutrition, peri-natal complications, structural abnormalities in the prefrontal cortex, specific language delays, verbal reasoning deficits, reading difficulties, self-regulation skill deficits and executive function deficits (Hill, 2002, Raine, 2002). Remedial interventions that facilitate the development of language and academic skills are the principal types of treatment deriving from this theory. Available evidence suggests that such interventions are most effective when incorporated into multi-systemic intervention programmes (Brosnan & Carr, 2000; Fonagy & Kurtz, 2002; Henggeler & Lee, 2003; Henggeler & Sheidow, 2003).

Psychodynamic theories

Classical psychoanalytic theory points to super-ego deficits and attachment theory highlights the role of insecure attachment in the development of conduct problems.

Super-ego deficit theory

Aichorn (1935) argued that anti-social behaviour occurs because of impoverished super-ego functioning. The problems with super-ego functioning were thought to arise either from over-indulgent parenting on the one hand or from punitive and neglectful parenting on the other. With over-indulgent parenting, the child internalizes lax standards and so feels no guilt when breaking rules or behaving immorally. In such cases, any apparently moral behaviour is a manipulative attempt to gratify some desire. With punitive or neglectful parenting, the child splits the experience of the parent into the *good caring parent* and the *bad punitive/neglectful parent* and internalizes both of these aspects of the parent quite separately with little integration. In dealing with parents, peers and authority figures, the child may be guided by either the internalization of the good parent or the internalization of the bad parent. Typically, at any point in time such youngsters can clearly identify those members of their network who fall into the good and bad categories. They behave morally towards those for whom they experience a positive transference and view as good, and immorally to those towards whom they have a negative transference and view as bad. Residential group-based milieu therapy where staff consistently and compassionately enforce rules of conduct that reflect societal standards is the principal treatment to evolve from this theoretical perspective. Within such a treatment programme, children gradually internalize societal rules, integrate the *good* and *bad* parental introjects, and develop a more adequate super-ego.

While there is little evidence for the effectiveness of psychoanalytically based treatment for conduct disorders (Kazdin, 1995), it has provided important insights into the impact of working with such youngsters on the dynamics within multi-disciplinary teams. For example, in my clinical experience, conduct-disordered youngsters who have internalized good and bad parental representations into the super-ego, typically project good parental qualities onto one faction of the multi-disciplinary team (typically the least powerful) and bad parental qualities onto the other team members (typically the most powerful). These projections elicit strong countertransference reactions in team members, with those receiving good projections experiencing positive feeling towards the youngster and those receiving bad projections experiencing negative feelings towards the youngster. Inevitably this leads to team conflict, which can be destructive to team functioning if not interpreted, understood and worked through.

Attachment theory

Bowlby (1944) pointed out that children who were separated from their primary caretakers for extended periods of time during their first months of life failed to develop secure attachments and so, in later life, did not have internal working models for secure trusting relationships. He referred to such children as displaying affectionless psychopathy. Since moral behaviour is premised on functional internal working models of how to conduct oneself in trusting relationships, such children behave immorally. Treatment according to this position should aim to provide the child with a secure-attachment relationship or corrective emotional experience that will lead to the development of appropriate internal working models. These, in turn, will provide a basis for moral action.

While the provision of a secure attachment experience within the context of outpatient weekly individual therapy is an ineffective treatment for children with conduct disorder, a secure attachment relationship is a central treatment component in some effective interventions, such as treatment foster care (Chamberlain & Smith, 2003). Here, the foster parents provide the child with a secure-attachment experience and couple this with good behavioural management. Recent research on the link between insecure attachment and conduct disorders has partially supported Bowlby's original observations (Hill, 2002).

Cognitive theories

Problems with social information-processing and social skills deficits are the principal factors highlighted in cognitive theories of conduct problems.

Social information-processing theories

Research on social information processing in youngsters with conduct disorders has shown that in ambiguous social situations their cognition is characterized by a hostile attributional bias (Crick & Dodge, 1994). Children with conduct disorders attribute hostile intentions to others in social situations where the intentions of others are ambiguous. The aggressive behaviour of children with conduct disorders in such situations is, therefore, intended to be retaliatory. The aggression is viewed as unjustified by those against whom it is directed and this leads to impaired peer relationships. The reactions of peers to such apparently unjustified aggression provides confirmation for the aggressive child that their peers have hostile intentions which justifies further retaliatory aggression.

Social skills deficit theory

A second line of research highlights the social skills deficits of children with conduct disorders (Spivack & Shure, 1982). These children lack the skills to generate alternative solutions to social problems such as dealing with an apparently hostile peer. They also lack the skills to implement solutions to social problems such as these. Within this cognitive-behavioural tradition group-based social skills programmes have been developed which aim to train youngsters in the following skills:

- correcting hostile attributional bias
- accurately assessing problematic social situations
- generating a range of solutions to such problem situations
- anticipating the immediate and long-term impact of these solutions
- implementing the most appropriate solution
- learning from feedback.

A growing body of data shows that group-based social problem-solving skills training is an effective component of broad, multi-systemic intervention packages for delinquent adolescents (Henggeler, Schoenwald, Bordin, Rowland & Cunningham, 1998; Kazdin, 2003).

Social learning theories

Modelling and coercive family processes have been identified by social learning theory as central to the development and maintenance of conduct problems.

Modelling theory

Bandura and Walters (1959) have taken the position that aggression, characteristic of children with conduct disorders, is learned through a process of imitation or modelling. In some instances it may be the behaviour displayed by the parents that the child imitates. Fathers of aggressive boys typically are aggressive. Mothers of such children are typically rejecting and discourage the expression of their children's dependency needs. It is this aggression and neglectful hostility that aggressive children are imitating. This position is supported by a large body of evidence, particularly that which points to the intrafamilial transmission of aggressive behaviour (Hill, 2002; Kazdin, 1995). According to modelling theory, treatment should aim to help parents model appropriate behaviour for their children, or provide alternative models of appropriate behaviour in a residential or treatment foster-care setting (Chamberlain & Smith, 2003).

Coercive family process theory

This position which is most clearly articulated by Patterson and his group (Patterson, Reed & Dishion, 1992) begins with the view that children with conduct disorders learn their anti-social behaviours from involvement in coercive patterns of interaction with their parents and these behaviours are then exhibited in school and community contexts. Marital discord, parental psychopathology, a variety of social and economic stressors and social isolation all contribute to the parents' use of a coercive parenting style. This style has three main features. First, parents have few positive interactions with their children. Second, they punish children frequently, inconsistently and ineffectively. Third, the parents of children with conduct problems negatively reinforce anti-social behaviour by confronting or punishing the child briefly and then withdrawing the confrontation or punishment when the child escalates the anti-social behaviour, so that the child learns that escalation leads to parental withdrawal. By middle childhood, children exposed to this parenting style have developed an aggressive relational style which leads to rejection by non-deviant peers. Such children, who often have co-morbid specific learning difficulties, typically develop conflictual relationships with teachers and consequent attainment problems. In adolescence, rejection by non-deviant peers and academic failure make socializing with a deviant delinquent peer group an attractive option. Patterson's group have shown that this developmental trajectory is common among youngsters who first present with oppositional defiant disorder. The delinquency of adolescence is a staging post on the route to adult anti-social personality disorder, criminality, drug abuse and conflictual, violent and unstable marital and parental roles for more than half of all youngsters with conduct disorder (Farrington, 1995). Therapy for families with pre-adolescent children based on this model aims to:

- help parents and children break coercive patterns of interaction
- help parents develop skills for disciplining children
- help parents and children develop positive patterns of interaction
- help parents manage personal psychopathology, marital discord and life stresses, which compromise their parenting effectiveness.

Behavioural parent training and treatment foster care are the principal formats within which such treatment is offered and there is considerable evidence for the effectiveness of both approaches (Behan & Carr, 2000; Brosnan & Carr, 2000; Fonagy & Kurtz, 2002; Richardson & Joughin, 2002).

Systems theories

Systems theories highlight the role of characteristics of family systems, broader social network systems and societal systems in the aetiology and maintenance of conduct problems.

Structural family systems theory

Within the family therapy tradition, the structural, functional and strategic schools have been most influential in offering a framework for understanding how conduct disorders are maintained by patterns of family interaction and how they may be resolved by intervening in these patterns (Colapinto, 1991; Madanes, 1991; Sexton & Alexander, 2003). At a structural level, families with youngsters who have conduct problems are more disorganized than other families. Rules, roles and routines are unclear. Communication is indirect, lacking in empathy and confusing. There is also an absence of systematic family problem-solving skills. The members are more emotionally disengaged from each other in comparison with other families. In addition, families with youngsters who display conduct problems have difficulties maintaining clear, unambiguous intergenerational hierarchies and negotiating lifecycle transitions.

With respect to ambiguous hierarchies, conduct problems are maintained if a youngster becomes involved in conflicting overt and covert hierarchies with the parents. The overt hierarchy in most families involves a spoken acceptance that both parents share a strong coalition around which there is a boundary that separates the parents hierarchically from the child, so that the child is to some degree subservient to the wishes of both parents. Where children have conduct problems, in addition to this overt hierarchy, there is typically a covert hierarchy in which the child and one parent share a strong cross-generational coalition around which there is a covert boundary that separates them hierarchically from the other parent. This covert hierarchy is not spoken about or denied. Usually it is the mother and child who share the covert coalition and the father that is hierarchically inferior to this dyad. Haley (1967) refers to this family structure as the pathological triangle. Not surprisingly, parents in these families often have marital difficulties.

With respect to lifecycle transitions, many families in our culture evolve through a series of predictable stages of the lifecycle, which have been outlined in Table 1.1 (p. 5). Haley (1980) has argued that some families with youngsters who have conduct problems become stuck at the stage of being a family with adolescents living at home and have difficulty making the transition to being a family in the empty nest stage of development. These families often display the structure described as the pathological triangle. The delinquent behaviour may serve the function of preventing the family from splitting up (Sexton & Alexander, 2003).

Family therapy based on structural and strategic systems theory aims to help families become more coherently organized by meeting with various family members together and in sub-groups to:

- develop explicit rules, roles and routines
- develop clear and direct communication styles
- develop systematic family problem-solving skills
- clarify hierarchies so that there are clear intergenerational boundaries
- help family members negotiate lifecycle transitions such as leaving home.

There is some evidence that family therapy based on these structural and functional principles is a more effective treatment for pre-adolescents and young adolescents with conduct problems than either non-directive family therapy or individual therapy (Brosnan & Carr, 2000; Fonagy & Kurtz, 2002; Sexton & Alexander, 2003).

Sociological theories

A variety of sociological theories have posited a causal link between deviant anti-social behaviour typical of conduct disorders and aspects of the wider sociocultural context within which such behaviour occurs. Anomie theory is a commonly cited exemplar of this body of theories (Cloward & Ohlin, 1960). According to anomie theory, theft and other related anti-social behaviour, such as mugging and lying, are illegitimate means used by members of a socially disadvantaged delinquent sub-culture to achieve material goals valued by mainstream culture. Anomie is the state of lawlessness and normlessness that characterizes such sub-cultures. The consistent finding of a link between social disadvantage and delinquency, and between conduct disorder and deviant peer group involvement supports this theory (Hill, 2002). Treatment premised on this theory must provide delinquents and their peer groups with legitimate means to achieve societal goals. Remedial academic programmes, vocational training programmes and treatment foster care are the main treatment approaches implicated by this theory. There is some evidence for the efficacy of multi-systemic programmes that incorporate these elements with family therapy and for treatment foster care (Brosnan & Carr, 2000; Chamberlain & Smith, 2003; Fonagy & Kurtz, 2002; Henggeler et al., 1998).

Multi-systemic ecological theory

This position entails the view that multiple systems (including the individual, the family, the school and the community) are involved in the genesis and maintenance of conduct problems and consequently effective treatment must target multiple systems rather than any single system (Henggeler et al., 1998). Bronfenbrenner's (1986) model of ecologically nested systems is the foundation for this theory. Conduct disorders, it is argued, are maintained by multiple factors in these multiple ecologically nested systems. Important individual factors include difficult temperament, early separation experiences, hostile attributional bias, poor social skills, difficulties learning pro-social behaviour from experience and academic learning difficulties. Family factors include family disorganization, ambiguous family hierarchies, parent–child attachment difficulties, parenting and discipline problems, marital discord and difficulty negotiating family lifecycle transitions. School factors include patterns of interaction that maintain school-based discipline problems, attainment difficulties and lack of educational resources. Community factors include involvement with deviant peers, drug abuse and involvement in poorly co-ordinated multi-agency networks.

Treatment based on this model must be individually tailored and based on a multi-system ecological assessment. Treatment packages should include:

- individual and group cognitive and social skills training
- family therapy to reduce family disorganization
- school-based interventions to deal with interactional patterns that maintain school-based conduct problems and under-achievement
- peer-group-based interventions to enhance pro-social peer relationships and reduce involvement in deviant peer groups.

There is some evidence that this approach is effective (Brosnan & Carr, 2000; Fonagy & Kurtz, 2002; Henggeler & Lee, 2003; Henggeler & Sheidow, 2003).

ASSESSMENT

Assessment of conduct problems and related clinical features may be conducted using the diagnostic criteria and guidelines set out in Tables 10.2, 10.3, 10.4. In addition to the routine assessment procedures and instruments described in Chapter 4, the instruments listed in Table 10.6 may be used. However, they add little to the SDQ or ASEBA suite of instruments, which are recommended for routine use with all cases. The framework presented in Figure 10.3 can be used as a guide to the assessment of pre-disposing, precipitating, maintaining and protective factors. An enormous body of empirical work has led to the identification of risk factors that pre-dispose youngsters to develop conduct problems and to personal and contextual factors that maintain these problems once they occur (Burke et al., 2002; Farrington, 1995; Hill, 2002; Kazdin, 1995; Loeber et al., 2000; Patterson, et al., 1992; Rutter, Giller & Hagell, 1998). The basis for our knowledge about precipitating factors and protective factors is less extensive (Fergusson & Lynskey, 1996). The information presented in Figure 10.3 and the discussion below is based on the extensive reviews of studies of risk and protective factors associated with the conduct problems cited above.

Table 10.6 Psychometric instruments that may be used as an adjunct to clinical interviews in the assessment of conduct

Instrument	Publication	Comments
Revised Behaviour Problem Checklist (RBPC)	Quay, H. & Peterson, D. (1996). Revised Behaviour Problem Checklist. Odessa, FL: Psychological Assessment Resources	This 89-item scale completed by parents or teachers yields scores on 6 empirically derived factors: conduct disorder, socialized aggression, attention problems, anxiety withdrawal, psychotic behaviour and motor excess. Norms are available for children and adolescents aged 5–18
Eyberg Child Behaviour Inventories (ECBI)	Eyberg, S. & Pincus, D. (1999). *ECBI: Eyberg Child Behaviour Inventory and SESBI-R Sutter-Eyeberg Student Behaviour Inventory – Revised Professional Manual.* Odessa, FL: Psychological Assessment Resources	These 36-item rating scales yields a single score on a conduct problems dimension. Items are rated as present or absent and intensity ratings on a 7-point scale are also given. Norms are available for pre-school and school-aged children of 2–16 years

Pre-disposing factors

Figure 10.3 shows that pre-disposing risk factors for conduct disorder may be classified as those uniquely associated with the child and those associated with the social context within which the child lives.

Personal pre-disposing factors

Both biological and psychological factors may pre-dispose youngsters to developing conduct disorders. At a biological level, genetic factors may play a role in the aetiology of some cases of conduct disorder. The precise avenue through which genetic factors influence the development of conduct disorders is unclear. It may be that the genetic pre-disposition involves the physiological substrate governing arousal level or temperament. It may also be that dysreguation of neurotransmitters, such as serotonin and noradrenaline, or hormones, such as testosterone and cortisol, are involved in this physiological substrate.

Youngsters with difficult temperaments and co-morbid ADHD are at particular risk for developing conduct disorder. This may be because their difficulty in regulating negative emotional states, such as anger and irritability; their difficulty in regulating their activity level makes it more probable that they will experience affective or impulsive states that find expression in behaviour that violates social rules. Alternatively, difficulties in regulating affective states or impulses may make it difficult for them to internalize social rules. A further alternative is that some combination of both of these processes link temperament and ADHD to the development of conduct problems.

Once conduct problems develop, the age of onset, type, frequency, seriousness and pervasiveness of the problems have prognostic implications. Youngsters who first show conduct problems in early childhood and who frequently engage in many different types of serious misconduct such as aggression, destructiveness and deceitfulness in a wide variety of social contexts including the home, the school and the community have a particularly poor prognosis. This is probably because severe conduct problems with an early onset develop within disorganized family contexts that both engender them initially and then maintain them. Home-based conduct problems when they become entrenched and severe spread to the school and peer group. Non-deviant peers tend to reject youngsters with conduct problems and label them as bullies, forcing them into deviant peer groups, which maintain conduct problems and encourage community-based delinquency. Many schools are not sufficiently well resourced to manage severe conduct problems and so deal with youngsters with conduct problems in ways that reinforce them. Low IQ and learning difficulties are also pre-disposing factors for conduct disorder. These issues of school-based attainment and conduct problems will be taken up below in the section on contextual maintaining factors.

PRE-DISPOSING FACTORS

PERSONAL PRE-DISPOSING FACTORS

Biological factors
- Genetic vulnerabilities
- Low-arousal levels

Psychological factors
- Low intelligence
- Difficult temperament
- Low self-esteem
- External locus of control
- Co-morbid ADHD or learning difficulties
- Early onset of aggressive behaviour
- Many frequent serious anti-social acts in multiple settings

CONTEXTUAL PRE-DISPOSING FACTORS

Parent–child factors in early life
- Attachment problems
- Lack of intellectual stimulation
- Authoritarian parenting
- Permissive parenting
- Neglectful parenting
- Inconsistent parental discipline

Exposure to family problems in early life
- Parental psychological problems
- Parental alcohol and substance abuse
- Parental criminality
- Marital discord or violence
- Parent separation
- Family disorganization
- Deviant siblings
- Large family size and middleborn

Stresses in early life
- Bereavements
- Separations
- Child abuse
- Social disadvantage
- Institutional upbringing

PERSONAL MAINTAINING FACTORS

Biological factors
- Social learning difficulties due to low arousal

Psychological factors
- Poor internal working models for relationships
- Hostile attributional bias
- Low self-efficacy
- Immature defence mechanisms
- Dysfunctional coping strategies

PERSONAL PROTECTIVE FACTORS

Biological factors
- Good physical health

Psychological factors
- High IQ
- Easy temperament
- High self-esteem
- Internal locus of control
- High self-efficacy
- Optimistic attributional style
- Mature defence mechanisms
- Functional coping strategies

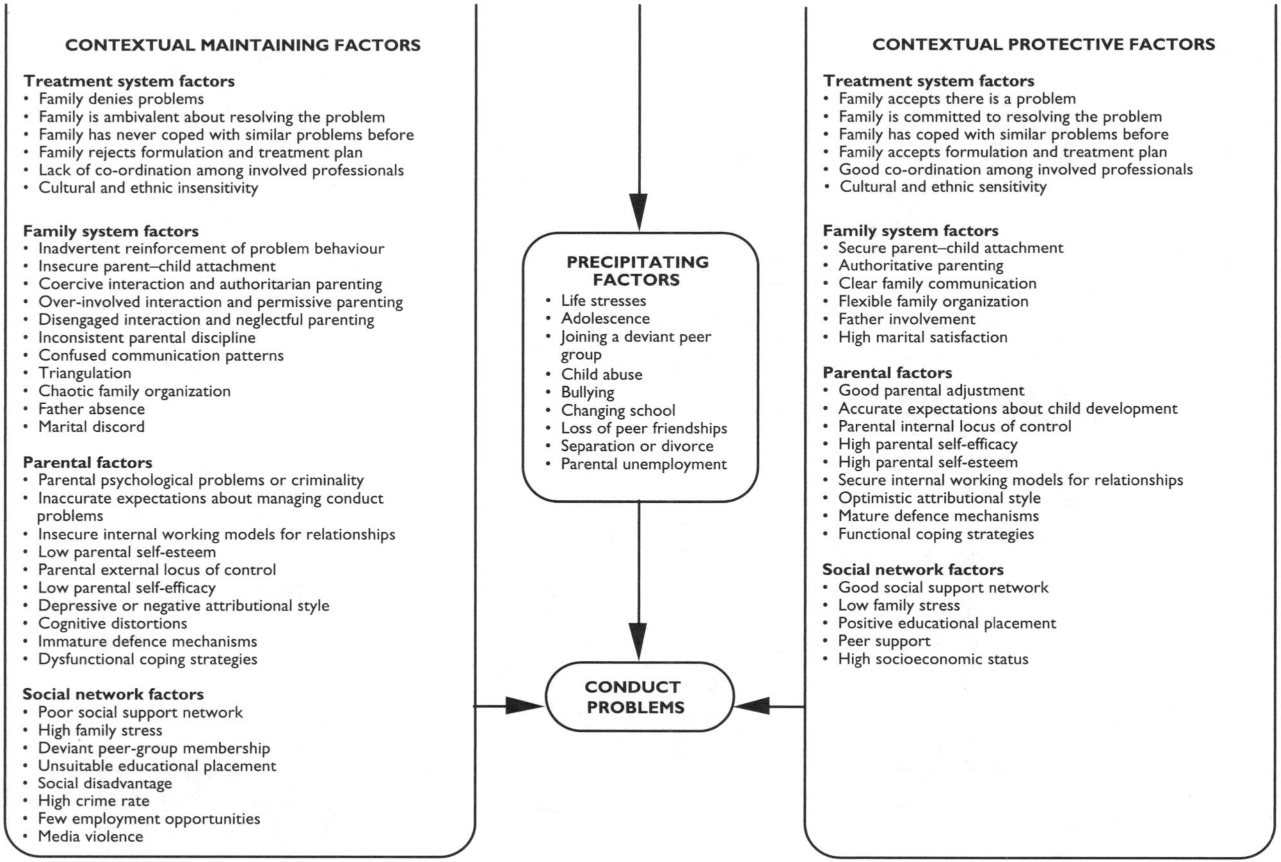

CONTEXTUAL MAINTAINING FACTORS

Treatment system factors
- Family denies problems
- Family is ambivalent about resolving the problem
- Family has never coped with similar problems before
- Family rejects formulation and treatment plan
- Lack of co-ordination among involved professionals
- Cultural and ethnic insensitivity

Family system factors
- Inadvertent reinforcement of problem behaviour
- Insecure parent–child attachment
- Coercive interaction and authoritarian parenting
- Over-involved interaction and permissive parenting
- Disengaged interaction and neglectful parenting
- Inconsistent parental discipline
- Confused communication patterns
- Triangulation
- Chaotic family organization
- Father absence
- Marital discord

Parental factors
- Parental psychological problems or criminality
- Inaccurate expectations about managing conduct problems
- Insecure internal working models for relationships
- Low parental self-esteem
- Parental external locus of control
- Low parental self-efficacy
- Depressive or negative attributional style
- Cognitive distortions
- Immature defence mechanisms
- Dysfunctional coping strategies

Social network factors
- Poor social support network
- High family stress
- Deviant peer-group membership
- Unsuitable educational placement
- Social disadvantage
- High crime rate
- Few employment opportunities
- Media violence

CONTEXTUAL PROTECTIVE FACTORS

Treatment system factors
- Family accepts there is a problem
- Family is committed to resolving the problem
- Family has coped with similar problems before
- Family accepts formulation and treatment plan
- Good co-ordination among involved professionals
- Cultural and ethnic sensitivity

Family system factors
- Secure parent–child attachment
- Authoritative parenting
- Clear family communication
- Flexible family organization
- Father involvement
- High marital satisfaction

Parental factors
- Good parental adjustment
- Accurate expectations about child development
- Parental internal locus of control
- High parental self-efficacy
- High parental self-esteem
- Secure internal working models for relationships
- Optimistic attributional style
- Mature defence mechanisms
- Functional coping strategies

Social network factors
- Good social support network
- Low family stress
- Positive educational placement
- Peer support
- High socioeconomic status

PRECIPITATING FACTORS
- Life stresses
- Adolescence
- Joining a deviant peer group
- Child abuse
- Bullying
- Changing school
- Loss of peer friendships
- Separation or divorce
- Parental unemployment

CONDUCT PROBLEMS

Figure 10.3 Factors to consider in childhood conduct problems

An external locus of control and low self-esteem may also pre-dispose youngsters to developing conduct problems. The belief that major sources of reinforcement are outside of one's control and negative self-evaluative beliefs may cause frustration, which finds expression in aggressive and destructive acts.

Contextual pre-disposing factors

With respect to pre-disposing family-based risk factors, conceptual distinctions may be made between those associated with the parent–child relationship, those associated with the overall family structure and style of functioning and those reflective of chronic early life stress.

Neglect, abuse, separations, lack of opportunities to develop secure attachments and harsh, lax or inconsistent discipline are among the more important aspects of the parent–child relationship that place youngsters at risk for developing conduct disorder. Separation and disruption of primary attachments through neglect or abuse may prevent children from developing internal working models for secure attachments. Without such internal working models, the development of pro-social relationships and behaviour is problematic. With abuse and harsh discipline, children may imitate their parent's behaviour by bullying other children or sexually assaulting them. Lax disciplinary procedures fail to provide children with a set of social norms to internalize and to guide pro-social behaviour. Inconsistent discipline allows children to learn that, on some occasions, it is possible to get away with anti-social behaviour, and by implication that they should test every situation to check if it is one of these instances where there will be no consequences for negative behaviour. Coercive family process, described earlier is an important facet of this.

Youngsters who come from families where parents are involved in criminal activity, have psychological problems or who abuse alcohol are at risk for developing conduct problems. Parents involved in crime may provide deviant role models for children to imitate and both psychological difficulties, and alcohol abuse may compromise parents' capacity to nurture and socialize their children. Risk factors related to the marital relationship range in severity from marital discord, through marital violence to parental separation. Marital problems contribute to the development of conduct problems in a number of ways. First, parents experiencing marital conflict or parents who are separated may have difficulty agreeing on rules of conduct and how these should be implemented. This may lead to inconsistent disciplinary practices. An important instance of this is Haley's (1967) pathological triangle, described earlier, in which a parent and child form a covert coalition that is hierarchically superior to the other parent's position within the family. Inconsistent discipline, especially when it occurs within the context of a pathological triangle, may lead to conduct difficulties in the ways described in the previous paragraph. Second, children exposed to marital violence may imitate this in their relationships with others and display violent behaviour towards family, peers and teachers. Third, parents experiencing marital discord may displace anger towards each other onto the child in the form of harsh discipline, physical or sexual abuse. This in turn may lead the child, through the process of imitation, to treat others in similar ways. Fourth, where children are exposed to parental conflict or violence, they experience a range of negative emotions including fear that their safety and security will be threatened, anger that their parents are jeopardizing their safety and security, sadness that they cannot live in a happy family, and conflict concerning their feelings of both anger towards and attachment to both parents. These negative emotions may find expression in anti-social conduct problems. Fifth, where parents are separated and living alone, they may find that the demands of socializing their child through consistent discipline, in addition to managing other domestic and occupational responsibilities alone, exceeds their personal resources. They may, as a result of emotional exhaustion, discipline inconsistently and become involved in coercive problem-maintaining patterns of interaction with their children.

Factors which characterize the overall organization of the family may predispose youngsters to developing conduct problems. Middleborn children with deviant older siblings in large poorly organized families are at particular risk for developing conduct disorder. Such youngsters are given no opportunity to be the sole focus of their parents' attachments and attempts to socialize them. They also have the unfortunate opportunity to imitate the deviant behaviour of their older siblings. Overall family disorganization with chaotic rules, roles and routines; unclear communication and limited emotional engagement between family members provide a poor context for learning pro-social behaviour and it is therefore not surprising that these, too, are risk factors for the development of conduct problems.

Social disadvantage, low socioeconomic status, poverty, crowding and social isolation are broader social factors that pre-dispose youngsters to developing conduct problems. These factors may increase the risk of conduct problems in a variety of ways.

First, low socioeconomic status and poverty put parents in a position where they have few resources upon which to draw in providing materially for the family's needs, and this in turn may increase the stress experienced by both parents and children. There may be insufficient money for food, clothing and housing of adequate size and comfort. The housing arrangements may be crowded. The temperature within the house or apartment may be poorly regulated. For children, the stress associated with this material discomfort may find expression in conduct problems. The availability of funds for babysitters when parents need a break from cramped quarters may be scarce. This factor becomes all the more significant if the nuclear family are socially isolated from the family of origin and has no network of socially supportive friends on whom it can depend for such help. Coping with all of these material stresses may compromise parents' capacity to nurture and discipline their children in a tolerant manner.

The meaning attributed to living in circumstances characterized by low socioeconomic status, poverty, crowding and social isolation is a second way that these factors may contribute to the development of conduct problems. The media in Western societies glorify wealth and the material benefits associated with it. The message given in the media is, if you want to be worthwhile and valued, then you should have wealth to purchase cars, clothes, holidays and a range of consumer goods. The implication is that to be poor is to be worthless. Both parents and children with low socioeconomic status and little money living in crowded accommodation isolated from social support may experience frustration when they receive the media's message about their worth. This frustration may find expression in violent anti-social conduct or in theft as a means to achieve the material goals glorified by the media.

A third way that social disadvantage may contribute to the development of conduct problems hinges on the psychological resources of the parents. Parents of low socioeconomic status may bring with them limited psychological resources for managing the difficult task of socializing children. For example, they may have limited education and poorly developed problem-solving skills. These limited psychological resources may be insufficient for the task of socializing children when coupled with other material resource problems such as poverty, crowding and isolation or other risk factors such as having a child with a difficult temperament who becomes involved in a delinquent sub-culture.

Precipitating factors

Conduct problems may have a clearly identified starting point associated with the occurrence of a particular precipitating event or they may have an insidious onset where a narrow pattern of normal defiance and disobedience mushrooms into a full-blown conduct disorder. This latter course is associated with an entrenched pattern of ineffective parenting, which usually occurs within the context of a highly disorganized family.

Illness or injury (particularly brain injury); major stressful life events; transitions within the family lifecycle, particularly the onset of adolescence; and changes in the child's social network are the four main classes of event that can precipitate the onset of a major conduct problem. Major stressful life events can include financial problems, sudden unemployment, major family illnesses, changes in family residence and changes in family composition, including both losses and additions. Bereavement or parental separation are examples of losses. Additions include births, adoptions or situations where a step-parent joins a family. There are many processes by which such stressful life events precipitate the onset of conduct problems. Two of these are of particular importance. The first centres on the child's perception of the stressful event as threatening and the second centres on the demands that such stresses place on the parents. Where youngsters construe the stressful event as a threat to safety or security, then conduct problems may occur as a retaliative or restorative action. For example, if a family moves to a new neighbourhood, this may be construed as a threat to the child's security, since important peer relationships may be lost. The child's running away may be an attempt to restore the security that has been lost by returning to the old peer group. If a separated mother develops a relationship with a new partner, the child may believe that the security of his relationship with the mother is being threatened and try to punish the new partner through extensive misconduct. Where parents find that the stressful event drains their psychological resources, then they may have insufficient energy to consistently deal with their children's misconduct and so may inadvertently become involved in coercive patterns of interaction which reinforce the youngster's conduct problems. For example, parents preoccupied by major financial problems or serious illness may have little energy for dealing consistently with misbehaviour.

The transition to adolescence may precipitate the development of conduct problems largely through entry into deviant peer groups and associated deviant recreational activities such as drug abuse or theft. With the increasing independence of adolescence, the youngster has a wider variety of peer group options from which to choose, some of which are involved in deviant anti-social activities. Where youngsters already have developed some conduct problems in childhood, and have been rejected by non-deviant peers, they may seek out a deviant peer group with which to identify and within which to perform anti-social activities such as theft or vandalism. Where youngsters who have few pre-adolescent conduct problems want to be accepted into a deviant peer group they may conform to the social pressure within the group to engage in anti-social activity.

Maintaining factors

Factors that maintain conduct disorders may be conceptually divided into those that fall within the personal and contextual domains.

Personal maintaining factors

Youngsters' conduct problems may persist because of social learning difficulties due to low arousal. That is, such youngsters may be particularly unresponsive to punishment on the one hand, and so have difficulty learning to avoid misconduct, while also being unresponsive to positive reinforcement on the other hand and so have difficulty developing pro-social behaviour.

Conduct problems may also be maintained by the absence of internal working models of secure attachment to guide moral interpersonal behaviour. This may be coupled with poor social problem-solving skills and a hostile attributional bias where the ambiguous social behaviour of others is interpreted as intentional aggression. These factors prevent youngsters from developing relationships with others based on trust, co-operation and commitment. The inability to form such relationships may maintain conduct problems by continually leading to the exclusion of youngsters from non-deviant peer groups and forcing them repeatedly into deviant social networks.

Immature defences such as displacement of anger or splitting and projection, where the youngster attributes positive qualities and intentions to certain parents, professionals, teachers or peers and negative qualities and intentions to others, may maintain conduct problems by engendering conflictual relationships with parents, peers, teachers and helping professionals.

Dysfunctional coping strategies, such as using drugs to regulate negative mood states, may maintain conduct problems, particularly if drug dependence develops. Youngsters who develop dependence may repeatedly steal to secure funds to buy the drugs required to prevent withdrawal symptoms from developing.

Contextual maintaining factors

Conduct problems may be maintained by a wide range of contextual factors. Within the youngster's family, problematic parent–child relationships, in which adequate support is not given to the child and where rules are either unclear or poorly enforced, may maintain conduct problems. Thus parent–child relationships characterized by insecure attachment, coercive interaction, inadvertent reinforcement of deviant behaviour, and harsh, lax, inconsistent or neglectful parenting may all maintain conduct problems. These types of problematic parent–child relationships are more likely to occur in family cultures characterized by confused communication, triangulation, and chaotic family organization. Such family cultures may be associated with problems within the parental system. Thus they may occur in families where there is marital discord or interparental violence or where the youngster's father lives outside the home and plays a marginal role in the child's life.

The parents' personal difficulties may maintain their children's conduct problem by compromising their capacity to offer adequate support and supervision to their children. Thus parents with debilitating psychological problems, such as depression or borderline personality disorder; inaccurate knowledge about child development and management of misconduct; low parental self-efficacy; an external locus of control and low self-esteem may lack the personal resources to consistently discipline their children and consistently offer care and understanding to them. Where parents lack internal working models for secure attachments, mature defence mechanisms and functional coping strategies for dealing with stress, they may find the challenges of parenting excessive and engage in interactions with their children which maintain their conduct problems.

Within the wider social system, high levels of stress associated with social disadvantage and low levels of social support may tax parents' personal coping resources to the limit and leave them depleted when faced with the challenges of dealing with children's conduct problems. In this sense conduct problems may be maintained by high levels of stress and low levels of support within the wider social network.

Where youngsters are exposed to deviant models through deviant peer-group membership and a sub-culture that endorses crime through residence in a high-crime area, their conduct problems may be maintained by these factors. This is particularly pertinent to situations where there are few employment opportunities or educational placements which can accommodate the youngsters' educational needs.

A number of educational factors, including the child's ability and achievement profile and the organization of the school learning environment, may maintain conduct problems. In some cases, youngsters with conduct problems truant from school and pay little attention to their studies and so develop achievement problems. In others, they have limited general abilities or specific learning difficulties and so cannot benefit from routine teaching practices. In either case, poor attainment may lead to frustration and disenchantment with academic work and this finds expression in conduct problems, which in turn compromise academic performance and future employment prospects.

Schools that are not organized to cope with attainment problems and conduct problems may maintain these difficulties. Routinely excluding or expelling such children from school allows youngsters to learn that, if they engage in misconduct, then all expectations that they should conform to social rules will be withdrawn. Where schools do not have a policy of working co-operatively with parents to manage conduct difficulties, conflict may arise between teachers and parents that maintains the child's conduct problems in much the same way as that described in Haley's pathological triangle. Typically, the parent sides with the child against the school and the child's conduct problems are reinforced. The child learns that if he misbehaves, and teachers object to this, then his parents will defend him.

These problems are more likely to happen where there is a poor overall school environment. Such schools are poorly physically resourced and poorly staffed so that they do not have remedial (or pastoral) tutors to help youngsters with specific learning difficulties. There are a lack of consistent expectations for academic performance and good conduct. There may also be a lack of consistent expectations for pupils to participate in non-academic school events, such as sports, drama or the organization of the school. There is typically limited contact with teachers. When such contact occurs, there is lack of praise-based motivation from teachers and a lack of interest in pupils developing their own personal strengths.

When youngsters with conduct problems are referred for treatment and the parents and involved professionals fail to develop a good working alliance and co-operative interprofessional relationships, then these treatment system problems may maintain the youngsters' conduct problems. Thus conduct problems may be maintained by parents' denial of their existence or refusal to accept the formulation and treatment plan, or by a sense of confusion engendered by a lack of co-ordination among various involved professionals, such as social workers, teachers, juvenile justice workers and so forth. Treatment systems that are not sensitive to the cultural and ethnic beliefs and values of the youngster's family system may maintain conduct problems by inhibiting engagement or promoting drop-out from treatment and preventing the development of a good working alliance between the treamtent team, the youngster and his or her family. Where parents have not dealt with similar problems in the past, they may feel overwhelmed by the challenge they pose. Where parents have come from a deviant family culture, they may be ambivalent about participating in treatment, since it may be the school or some other agency that sees the child's behaviour as problems and not the parents. In these instances, parents difficulties in co-operating fully with treatment may maintain their children's conduct problems.

Protective factors

The personal and contextual protective factors that increase the probability that youngsters with conduct problems will have a good outcome and respond to treatment are listed in Figure 10.3 (pp. 386–387).

Personal protective factors

Abilities, including high intelligence and good problem-solving skills; an easy temperament; adaptive beliefs, particularly those associated with high self-esteem, self-efficacy and an internal locus of control; and physical health are all important personal protective factors. So too is an optimistic attributional style and the use of mature defences and functional coping strategies. These factors may work through a variety of mechanisms. For example, youngsters may be helped to harness their intelligence and problem-solving skills to learn to cope with adverse family, school and vocational situations; to develop an understanding of the long-range consequences of repetitive conduct problems and pro-social behaviour; and to develop the requisite social and vocational skills necessary for a non-deviant career. Positive self-evaluative beliefs and the perception of the self as controlling important aspects of the environment may both be employed in therapy as a springboard from which the youngster can make decisions about how to control his or her future to avoid future misconduct and crime. The capacity to make and maintain new friendships is an important coping strategy for resolving conduct problems if youngsters are involved with deviant peer groups, which they may have to leave if they are to develop a non-deviant lifestyle.

Contextual protective factors

Positive family relationships, good parental adjustment, low stress and a high level of social support within the wider social network, a positive educational placement and co-operative relationships between parents and involved professionals are among the more important contextual protective factors in cases of conduct disorder. Where children have positive relationships with their parents and experience secure attachment within these relationships, then they are more likely to respond to beneficial changes in the parents' disciplining style arising from treatment. This will be most likely in families where parents have a strong marital relationship and where there is clear communication and considerable flexibility. Parents may be better able to respond to family-based treatments such as parent training where they are in good psychological health, have high self-esteem, an internal locus of control and high parental self-efficacy. A non-deviant support network and role model are also probably protective for the child because they provide valued models for good behaviour and opportunities to engage in routines that are non-deviant. Previous experience within the family of resolving similar problems is a protective factor since it may enhance self-efficacy beliefs and it is also evidence that the family have problem-solving skills that may be used to address the presenting problems. A better response to treatment may be expected where parents accept that there is a problem, are committed to resolving it and accept the treatment team's formulation and plan. Treatment systems that are sensitive to the cultural and ethnic beliefs and values of the youngster's family are more likely to help families engage with, and remain in treatment, and foster the development of a good working alliance. Good interprofessional and interagency communication and co-ordination may also lead to a more positive response to treatment.

FORMULATION

Formulation in cases where conduct problems are the main reason for referral are invariably complex, since typically youngsters with conduct problems come from complex multi-problem families. An example of a formulation for a relatively straightforward case is given in Box 10.1 (p. 362). The key to good formulation in cases of conduct disorder is to identify specific conduct problems or target behaviours requiring treatment, and then link these to ongoing interaction patterns in the home, school and community that maintain them. Against this back-drop, identify background pre-disposing factors and any recent events that precipitated the referral or a recent exacerbation of the youngster's anti-social behaviour. Once this explanation of the problems has been developed, all protective factors that might contribute to problem resolution may be listed.

Management of cases involving a youngster with conduct problems is typically complex because the families have often been the recipients of multiple previous interventions and are involved with multiple agencies. Professionals from the fields of child mental health, education, and juvenile justice may be involved with the child and siblings. Professionals from adult mental health and probation may be involved with the parents. Child protection and social welfare agencies may also be involved. It is therefore particularly important to follow guidelines for good practice set out in Chapter 4 in establishing an assessment contract with the family, the referring agency and other involved agencies if necessary.

With multi-problem families where there is multi-agency involvement, assessment is typically conducted over a number of sessions and involves meetings or telephone contact with the referring agent, the legal guardians of the child (if the child is not in the custody of the parents), the parents, other family members who have regular contact with the referred child, the involved school staff and other involved professionals. Home-based observation, observation of the child's behaviour at school and observation of interaction in a group setting in a clinic or residential assessment centre may all provide information on the types of conduct difficulties displayed by the youngster and the patterns of interaction in which they are embedded.

TREATMENT

Treatment contracts offered to families where children have conduct problems should be based on clear and comprehensive case formulations and aimed at specific treatment goals. The treatment literature underlines the extraordinarily poor outcome for cases of conduct disorder. Most traditional individual and group-based psychotherapeutic treatments have little sustained positive impact (Kazdin, 1997). However, recent research supports the effectiveness of family-oriented interventions along a continuum of care, which extends from behavioural parent training through family therapy and multi-systemic therapy to treatment foster care (American Academy of Child and Adolescent Psychiatry, 1997a; Behan & Carr, 2000; Brosnan & Carr, 2000; Lochman et al., 2005). Families of young children with less severe conduct problems may benefit from group-based behavioural parent training conducted on a weekly basis over three to six months. Families of older children and young adolescents with moderate conduct problems may require the more intensive intervention entailed by non-group-based parent training, family therapy and multi-systemic therapy. Here, treatment is delivered to a single family rather than on a group basis and may involve more than one contact per week over a period of up to two years, with treatment components focusing on enhancing parenting skills, improving parents' self-regulation skills, improving family communication and problem solving, improving school performance and enhancing the youngster's social problem-solving skills. Older adolescents with chronic pervasive conduct problems may require treatment foster care, which is a particularly intensive approach to treatment. This involves placement of the youngster with behaviourally skilled and professionally supervised foster parents for a period of up to nine months. Concurrently and afterwards, a multi-systmeic therapy package is offered to the youngster and his natural family with the aim of the adolescent returning home once his conduct problems have become manageable. For cases receiving multi-systemic therapy and treatment foster care, small case loads not exceeding five to ten cases per keyworker and 24-hour on-call availability for crisis intervention is an important feature of effective programmes. The team support required for the key worker in treatment foster care is specified in Chapter 22.

For all cases of oppositional defiant disorder and conduct disorder, a chronic-care rather than an acute-care model is the most appropriate to adopt. An intensive initial episode of therapy involving frequent contact and a high level of support should be followed by long-term but less intensive contact, except during lifecycle transitions and stressful crises. The following components are contained in effective treatment packages, although not all components will be necessary in all cases:

- psychoeducation
- monitoring anti-social and pro-social behavioural targets
- behavioural parent training with a focus on reward training and time-out
- family-based communication and problem-solving training
- home–school liaison meetings and remedial tuition
- child-based social problem-solving skills training
- parent counselling for managing personal or marital difficulties
- treatment foster care placement where families are extremely disorganized
- interprofessional and interagency co-ordination meetings.

In selecting specific components for inclusion in a treatment package or a specific case, interventions should target the systems in which the problems occur and are maintained. For oppositional defiant disorder that is limited to the family context, the treatment package may be based around behavioural parent training. With chronic adolescent conduct problems that occur in family, school and community settings, a multi-systemic intervention package may be required, which includes family communication and problem-solving training for implementing contingency management programmes as the central component.

In all treatment programmes, psychoeducation should be included so parents acquire a problem-solving framework within which to make sense of their children's problems and the patterns of interaction within which they are embedded. Training in monitoring target behaviours is essential in all programmes also.

Where children present with school-based conduct problems or co-morbid learning problems, home–school liaison meetings are essential, and remedial tuition is appropriate where there are attainment difficulties.

It is important to include child-based social problem-solving skills training, particularly where youngsters have difficulties making and maintaining friendships.

Where parents experience high levels of life stress, limited social support and few personal coping resources, then parent counselling or therapy for managing these difficulties may be necessary. Without such input, parents may become overwhelmed and fail to consistently implement behavioural management programmes with their children. Where parents become repeatedly overwhelmed by life stresses, coupled with the challenges of implementing behaviour programmes with their children, then treatment foster care may be appropriate. Initially, the child with the conduct disorder is placed with trained foster parents who implement a behavioural programme to reduce conduct problems, while concurrently the natural parents receive behavioural parent training. The child returns for increasingly longer visits to the natural family, who use the parenting training and support from the foster parents to implement behavioural programmes to modify the child's conduct problems and improve the quality of parent–child relationships.

In all cases where other professionals or agencies are involved, interprofessional or interagency co-ordination meetings are essential to insure that involved network members follow a co-ordinated plan.

What follows is a brief description of each of the possible components of a multi-systemic intervention programme for children and adolescents with conduct problems.

Psychoeducation

Conveying the idea that aggressive, destructive or defiant behaviour is not a reflection of an intrinsic negative characteristic of the child is central to psychoeducation in cases of conduct problems. Typically, by the time children have been referred for treatment, their parents have come to attribute all of their conduct problems to internal, global, stable negative factors.

Through psychoeducation, parents are helped to move from viewing the child's conduct problems as proof that he is *intrinsically bad* to a position where they view the youngster as *a good child with bad habits* that are triggered by certain stimuli and reinforced by certain consequences. When parents bring their child to treatment, typically they are exasperated and want the psychologist to take the child into individual treatment and *fix* him. Through psychoeducation, the parent is helped to see that the child's conduct problems are maintained by patterns of interaction within the family and wider social network and therefore family and network members must be involved in the treatment process. Parents may be helped to shift towards this more useful way of viewing their children's misconduct by observing and monitoring the impact of antecedents and consequences on their child's behaviour either in the clinic or at home. Within the clinic, one parent may be invited to engage the child in supportive play following the guidelines set out in Table 4.4 (p. 148). The other parent may be invited to observe this and note the impact of attention praise and laughter on increasing the frequency of positive behaviours and the impact of ignoring negative behaviours on decreasing their frequency. Alternatively, the session may be videotaped and reviewed by both parents with the therapist. In either case, the parent is asked to note how a specific target behaviour (such as hitting or playing appropriately) is controlled by antecedents (such as invitations or commands) and specific consequences (such as praise, attention, criticism or being ignored). Within the home, parents may be invited to keep a three-column diary of antecedents and consequences of specific positive and negative behaviours. These may be reviewed to show the relationships between specific behaviours and related contingencies. A sample three-column diary page is presented in Figure 10.4.

Explanations of Patterson's (1982) coercive cycle of interaction, where the child's escalating aggression is reinforced by causing the scolding parent to withdraw should also be given along with the rationale for time-out, the use of rewards systems and the use of supportive play. It is important to emphasize that time-out typically leads to an escalation of aggression initially before improvement occurs whereas with reward systems and supportive play there is a slow gradual and steady improvement in positive behaviour. Reward systems, behavioural control training using time-out and relationship enhancement using supportive play are all described in Chapter 4 and summaries of key features of these techniques are given in Tables 4.4, 4.5 and 4.6 (pp. 148–50).

From clients' perspectives it is more useful if psychoeducation is woven into the fabric of the entire treatment programme rather than offered in a single one-off session. Thus, in every session when monitoring charts and homework assignments are reviewed, this opportunity may be used to define the child's conduct problems as bad habits that may be changed through the use of behavioural parenting programmes, rather than intrinsic characteristics of the child.

Day and time	What happened **before** the target	**Target** behaviour	What happened **after** the target

Figure 10.4 Three-column chart for monitoring antecedents and consequences of positive and negative target behaviours

Monitoring

With conduct problems, during assessment a three-column chart such as that presented in Figure 10.4 may be used to identify antecedents and consequences of specific target behaviours during a specific time interval, such as between 6 and 7 p.m. each day. With such charts it is important to begin by monitoring no more than three negative behaviours and no more than three positive behaviours, since to try to do more than this may be confusing or tiring for the parents. Most parents need training in spotting instances of the target behaviour (such as hitting or helping) and in accurately describing the antecedents and consequences.

With pre-adolescent children, reward charts such as that presented in Figure 10.5 and time-out charts such as that presented in Figure 10.6 may be used as part of behavioural parent training. With teenagers, parents and children may keep a tally of points earned per day using a point system such as that presented in Figures 10.7 and 10.8. The home–school daily report card presented in Figure 10.9 may be used to help teachers and parents monitor progress on certain target behaviours throughout the school day.

With conduct problems, the process of monitoring progress using diaries or charts is important because it shows that the child's behaviour is partly controlled by antecedents and consequences. Monitoring may suggest ways that conduct problems may be reduced by altering antecedents or consequences. Monitoring of points earned through a reward system or time spent in time-out helps parents who often feel overwhelmed by their children's difficulties to see that they are making progress, and for young children gaining points, stars or smiling faces on a reward chart may be intrinsically reinforcing.

Behavioural parent training

With young children who have oppositional defiant disorders, training parents to use behavioural techniques for disciplining children and maintaining positive relationships with them is a core component of effective treatment. In such programmes, parents are helped, through psychoeducation, to view children's problems as being controlled by antecedent triggers on the one hand and positive and negative consequences on the other. They learn to identify and monitor positive and negative target behaviours. The also learn to pinpoint proximal and distal antecedents and positive and negative consequences using in-session observational training and monitoring charts such as those presented in Figure 10.4. Parents are coached in methods for developing solutions which involve using the principles of social learning theory to increase pro-social target behaviours and decrease aggression or other negative target behaviours. These solutions focus mainly on altering antecedents and consequences.

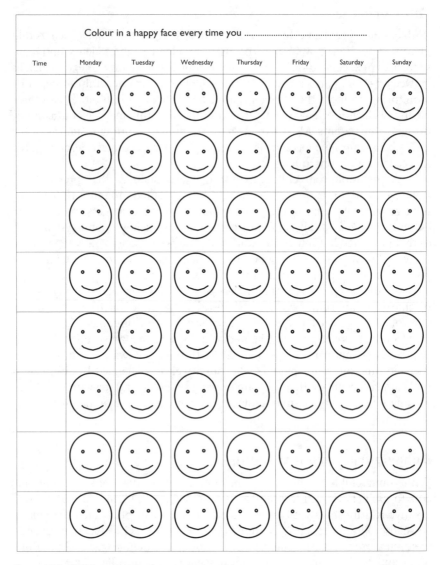

Figure 10.5 Child's star chart for conduct problems

Reducing anti-social behaviour

Solutions for decreasing anti-social behaviour by altering antecedents include: eliminating or reducing the conditions that precede aggressive behaviour, reducing children's exposure to situations in which they observe aggressive behaviour and reducing children's exposure to situations which

Date	Time going in	Number of minutes in time-out	Situation that led to time-out	Pleasant activity that happened afterwards

Figure 10.6 Time-out monitoring chart

they find aversive, uncomfortable or tiring, since such situations reduce their capacity to control aggression. In practice, such solutions often involve helping parents to plan regular routines for managing daily transitional events such as rising in the morning or going to bed at night, preparing to leave for school or returning home after school, initiating or ending leisure activities and games, starting and finishing meals and so forth. The more predictable these routines become, the less likely they are to trigger episodes

For these target behaviours you can earn points	Points that can be earned
Up by 7.30 a.m.	I
Washed, dressed and finished breakfast by 8.15 a.m.	I
Made bed and standing at door with school-bag ready to go by 8.30 a.m.	I
Attend each class and have teacher sign school card	I per class (max. 8)
Good report for each class	I per class (max. 8)
Finish homework	I
Daily jobs (e.g. taking out dustbins or washing dishes)	I per job (max. 4)
Bed on time (9.30 p.m.)	I
Responding to requests to help or criticism without moodiness or pushing limits	2
Offering to help with a job that a parent thinks deserves points	2
Going to time-out instead of becoming aggressive	2
Apologizing after rule-breaking	2
Showing consideration for parents (as judged by parents)	2
Showing consideration for siblings (as judged by parents)	2
Cash-in points for privileges and accept fines without arguing	2

Figure 10.7 Points chart for an adolescent

of aggression or other conduct problems. Within therapy sessions or as homework, parents and children may develop lists of steps for problematic routines, write these out and place the list of steps in a prominent place in the home until the routine becomes a regular part of family life. Parents may also be coached to teach their children to use internal speech (self-instructions) to both talk themselves through these predictable routines and to regulate negative mood states that may occur when routines are disrupted. For example, if a child becomes frustrated when unable to find a school-bag while completing a getting-ready-for-school routine, the parent may prompt the child to use

You can buy these privileges with points	Points	You must pay a fine for breaking these rules	Points
Can watch TV for 1 hour	10	Not up by 7.30 a.m.	1
Can listen to music in bedroom for an hour	5	Not washed, dressed and finished breakfast by 8.15 a.m.	1
Can use computer for 1 hour	5	Not made bed and standing at door with school-bag ready to go by 8.30 a.m.	1
Can stay up an extra 30 minutes in bedroom with light on	5	Not attend each class and not have teacher sign school card	1 per class
Can stay up an extra 30 minutes in living room	10	Bad report for each class	1 per class
Can have a snack treat after supper	20	Not finish homework within specified time	1
Can make a phone call for 5 minutes	10	Not do daily jobs (e.g. taking out dustbins or washing dishes)	1 per job
Can have a friend over for 2 hours	25	Not in bed on time (9.30 p.m.)	10
Can visit a friend for 2 hours	30	Respond to requests to help or criticism with moodiness, sulking, pushing limits or arguments	5
Can go out with friend to specified destination for one afternoon until 6.00 p.m.	35	Swearing, rudeness, ignoring parental requests	10 per event
Can go out with friend to specified destination for one evening until 11.00 p.m.	40	Physical aggression to objects (banging doors, throwing things)	20 per event
Can stay over at friend's house for night	60	Physical aggression to people	30–100
		Using others things without permission	30–100
		Lying or suspicion of lying (as judged by parent)	30–100
		Stealing or suspicion of stealing at home, school or community (as judged by parent)	30–100
		Missing class or not arriving home on time or being out unsupervised without permission	30–100

Figure 10.8 Adolescents' privileges and fines

Name_____Date_____

For his or her performance today, please rate this child in each of the areas listed below using this 5-point scale

1 Very poor	2 Poor	3 Fair	4 Good	5 Excellent

	Class 1	Class 2	Class 3	Class 4	Class 5	Class 6	Class 7	Class 8
Paying attention								
Completing classwork								
Following rules								
Other								
Teacher's initials								

Figure 10.9 Daily report card

self-instructions to calm down and conduct a systematic search for the school-bag rather than have a tantrum.

Solutions to reduce anti-social behaviour by altering consequences include helping parents to ignore minor displays of anti-social behaviour and using time-out or deprivation of privileges as a response to aggression or anti-social behaviour. Parents may also be helped to teach their children to use internal speech (self-instructions) to regulate their anti-social behaviour. Time-out has been described in Chapter 4 and guidelines for using it as part of a behaviour control programme are presented in Table 4.6 (p. 150). With time-out specific negative or aggressive behaviours are defined as targets for which time-out from reinforcement is given. When these behaviours occur, the parent gives a command to the child to stop and this may be followed up by two warnings. If children comply they are praised. If not they are brought to time-out without any display of anger or any reasoned explanation being given at that time. During time-out, the child sits on chair in the corner of the kitchen or in their bedroom away from interesting or reinforcing events or toys. Following a period of two to five minutes (depending on the child's age), the child is invited to rejoin family activities and is engaged in a stimulating and rewarding exchange with the parent. If children misbehave or protest aggressively while in time-out, they remain there until they have been compliant and quiet for thirty seconds before rejoining family activities and engaging in a stimulating interaction with the parent. With time-out, parents need to be told that initially the child will show an escalation of aggression and will offer considerable resistance to being asked to stay in time-out. However, this resistance will reach a peak and then begin to decrease quite rapidly. This predicted pattern may be monitored using the chart presented in Figure 10.6.

Increasing pro-social behaviour

Solutions to increase pro-social behaviour by altering antecedents include: increasing the conditions that precede pro-social behaviour, increasing children's exposure to situations in which they observe pro-social altruistic behaviour and increasing children's exposure to situations which they find emotionally satisfying, such as episodes of supportive play with parents as described in Table 4.4 (p. 148).

Solutions to increase pro-social behaviour by altering consequences include the use of reward systems such as those described in Chapter 4 and Table 4.5 (p. 149). With pre-adolescents, reward charts for children like that set out in Figure 10.5 may be used as part of such programmes. When the child accumulates a certain number of smiling faces these may be exchanged for a tangible and valued reward such as a trip to the park or an extra bedtime story. With teenagers, a points system may be used. Here points may be acquired by carrying out specific behaviours and points may be lost for rule-breaking. On a daily or weekly basis, points may be exchanged for an agreed list of privileges. An example of such a point system is set out in Figures 10.7 and 10.8. This system is a simplified version of that used by Chamberlain (1994) in her treatment foster-care programme.

Children's pro-social behaviour may also be increased through training parents in shaping. Here they are shown how to routinely give immediate praise for approximations to desired pro-social behaviour.

Parents may also be coached in modelling and reinforcing their children for using pro-social behaviours to achieve goals they typically achieve through aggression and destructiveness. Where such behaviours are complex, parents may be coached in breaking down large sequences of pro-social behaviour into small parts and rewarding children for completing each of the small steps.

Designing behavioural parent training programmes

In a typical behaviour control programme, for a specific set of positive and negative target behaviours, a clear set of rules and consequence is agreed. The importance of the parents following through on the consequences and of keeping a record of the frequency of positive and negative target behaviours is highlighted. Good behaviours are typically rewarded through praise and points recorded on a chart. These may be cashed in for rewards agreed between the parents and the child. Conduct problems and rule violations result in time-out or loss of privileges.

This type of behaviour control programme is more acceptable to children if it is framed as a game for learning self-control or learning how to be *grown up* and if the child is involved in designing and using the reward chart. Parents should be encouraged not to hold grudges after episodes of negative behaviour and time-out and also to avoid negative mind-reading, blaming, sulking or abusing the child physically or verbally during the programme. Implementing a programme like this can be very stressful for parents since the child's behaviour often deteriorates before it improves. Parents need to be made aware of this and encouraged to ask their spouses, friends or members of their extended family for support when they feel the strain of implementing the programme. Finally, the whole family should be encouraged to celebrate success once the child begins to learn self-control.

To increase the chances of a contingency-based behavioural control programme being effective, it is useful to arrange for parents and pre-adolescent children to have regular episodes of supportive play following the guidelines described in Chapter 4 and Table 4.4 (p. 148). With adolescents, some joint activity in which the adolescent takes a leading rather than a following role may be arranged. In either case, the function of these parent–child interaction episodes is to provide a forum within which the child regularly receives unconditional positive regard and attention from the parent. Parents need to be coached in how to finish these episodes by summarizing what the parent and child did together and how much the parent enjoyed it. Help the parent to view the episode as an opportunity for giving the child the message that he or she is in control of what happens and that the parent likes being with them. Advise the parent to foresee rule-breaking and prevent it from happening. Finally, invite parents to notice how much they enjoy being with their children.

Throughout the programme, all adults within the child's social system (including parents, step-parents, grandparents, childminders, etc.) are encouraged to work co-operatively in the implementation of the programme, since these programmes tend to have little impact when one or more significant adults from the child's social system does not implement the programme as agreed. Parents may also be helped to negotiate with each other so that the demands of disciplining and coaching the children is shared in a way that is as satisfactory as possible for both parents.

The first two weeks running a behavioural control programme are very stressful for most families. The normal pattern is for the time-out period to increase in length gradually and then eventually to begin to diminish. During this escalation period, when the child is testing out the parents' resolve and having a last binge of self-indulgence before learning self-control, it is important to help parents to be mutually supportive. The important feature of spouse support is that the couple set aside time to spend together without the children to talk to each other about issues unrelated to the children. In single-parent families, parents may be helped to explore ways for obtaining support from their network of friends and members of the extended family.

Three formats for behavioural parent training

This type of therapy has been shown to be effective in three main formats:

- behavioural family therapy
- small-group (ten to twelve members) parent training
- large-group (twenty to thirty members) parent training.

In the behavioural family therapy format, the parents, the parents and child or all members of the child's household attend sessions in the clinic or in the child's home. This has the advantage that parenting skills may be practised in the session and immediate feedback given to parents on their use of parenting skills and to the child on their use of self-control skills. However, it is costly of therapist time. In small-group parent training, parents are given instructions and video demonstrations and take part in rehearsal and role-playing exercises. It is not uncommon for children to be offered concurrent social skills training or structured activities in a separate room while the parent training occurs. This format has been used largely in clinic settings. While the benefits of immediate coaching in an actual family situation are not available when this approach is used, both parents and children receive the social support offered by other members of their training groups. Cunningham and his team have shown that large-group training offered in community settings such as schools or village halls with monthly follow-up booster sessions may be even more effective than the clinic-based, small-group treatment format (Cunningham, Bremmer & Boyle, 1995).

Not all cases can benefit from parent training. Chaotic families of low socioeconomic status tend to derive less benefit and are more prone to dropping out of routine treatment, unless the programme is offered following Cunningham's large-group format. Mothers who are categorized as having an attachment profile reflective of unresolved loss or trauma on the adult attachment interview benefit less from parent training programmes than mothers with secure attachment patterns (Routh, Hill, Steele, Elliott &

Dewey, 1995). These mothers are typically disorganized and disoriented and show lapses in speech when describing loss or trauma.

Well-validated and empirically supported programmes include the Incredible Years Programme (Webster-Stratton & Reid, 2003), the Parenting Plus Programme (Sharry & Fitzpatrick, 2000), and parent–child interaction therapy (Brinkmeyer & Eyberg, 2003). The Incredible Years programme and the Parenting Plus programme both use video modelling to teach parenting skills. The programmes include many videotaped vignettes of how to address specific parenting challenges, which parents can view, discuss and attempt to emulate. Versions of these programmes have been developed for children of different ages. The Incredible Years programme also includes additional modules for teaching children social problem-solving skills; for teaching parents self-regulation, problem-solving and communication skills; and for teaching school teachers how to use behavioural principles in the classroom. With parent–child interaction therapy, which is appropriate for children under six years of age, the therapist coaches parents in both supportive play and using behavioural control techniques such as reward systems and time-out, in a play-room situation with a one-way mirror and 'bug in the ear' communication system. Initially, the therapist briefs the parent in how to use supportive play or behavioural control systems and then models these skills. The parent then tries to use the skills with their own child in the play-room, while the therapist watches through a one-way screen and prompts, shapes and reinforces the parent through the 'bug in the ear' communication system.

Parenting-wisely is an interactive computer-based behavioural parent training programme (Gordon & Rolland-Stanar, 2003). The programme was designed specifically for parents and families who find it challenging to engage in group-based parent training or family therapy. Following a preliminary assessment session, parents are shown how to use the interactive programme to train themselves in parenting skills. The programme contains a series of vignettes that depict common parenting challenges. After viewing each of these, parents select and view further vignettes presenting one of a series of possible responses to these challenges. Thus they have the opportunity to see both appropriate effective and ineffective parenting responses and to receive feedback on their choices. Once they have seen a correct response, they are then given a knowledge test, to check that they have learned the parenting skill. Feedback on this test is also given to shape and reinforce parenting skill acquisition. The efficacy of the programme has been empirically supported.

Family-based communication and problem-solving training

To deal with adolescent conduct problems in most industrialized cultures, parents (and in some instances step-parents, foster parents and grandparents) must share a strong alliance and conjointly agree on household rules, roles and routines that specify what is and is not acceptable conduct for the teenager. Consequences for violating rules or disregarding roles and routines must be absolutely clear. Once agreed, rewards and sanctions associated with rules, roles and routines must be implemented consistently by parents (and step-parents, foster parents or grandparents if they are involved in the teenager's day-to-day life). Unilateral parent training with minimal involvement of the child in therapy can be effective with some pre-adolescents, but with the increased power and autonomy that comes with adolescence, involvement of parents and teenagers in a least some joint sessions becomes quite important, since rules and consequences must be negotiated. Invariably, parents and teenagers with conduct problem are unskilled in the art of negotiation and so it is not surprising that effective treatment programmes include communication and problem-solving training as the core component for adolescents with conduct difficulties (Chamberlain, & Smith, 2003; Henggeler & Lee, 2003; Sexton & Alexander, 2003). The aim of such training is to help parents and teenagers communicate clearly with each other and negotiate a set of rules, roles and routines and consequences associated with adhering to or breaking rules. Rules should be clear, negotiated and just or fair as judged by the norms of the family's culture. Routines should be predictable and regular within the constraints of the family's culture. Roles, particularly those of parents and children, should be unambiguous and separated by clear intergenerational boundaries.

In multi-problem families where adolescents have pervasive conduct disorders, training in communication skills must precede problem-solving skills training and negotiation of rules and consequences. It is not uncommon for such families to have no system for turn-taking, speaking and listening. Rarely is the distinction made between talking about a problem so that all viewpoints are aired and negotiating a solution that is acceptable to all parties.

The aim of communication skills training is to equip parents and teenagers with the skills required to take turns at speaking clearly and presenting their viewpoint in an unambiguous way on the one hand and listening carefully so that they receive an accurate understanding of the other person's viewpoint on the other. Coaching family members in communication skills may follow the broad guidelines set out in Chapter 4 and Table 4.2 (p. 145). The roles of speaker and listener are clearly distinguished. The speaker is invited to present his or her viewpoint, uninterrupted, and when, finished, the listener summarizes what he or she has heard and checks the accuracy of his or her recollection with the speaker. These skills are taught using non-emotive material using modelling and coaching. Then family members are shown how to list problems related to the adolescent's rule-breaking and discuss them one at a time, beginning with those that are least emotionally charged, with each party being given a fair turn to state their position or to reply. When taking a speaking turn, family members should be coached in how to decide on specific key points that they want to make, organize them logically, say them clearly and unambiguously and check that they have been understood. In taking a turn at listening, family members should be coached to listen without interruption, summarize key points made by the other person and check that they have understood them accurately before replying. Where-ever possible, 'I statements' rather than 'you statements' should be made. For example, 'I want to be able to stay out until midnight and get a cab home on Saturday' is an 'I statement'. 'You always ruin my Saturday nights with your silly rules' is a 'you statement'. There should be an agreement between the therapist and the family that negative mind-reading, blaming, sulking, abusing and interrupting will be avoided and that the psychologist has the duty to signal when this agreement is being broken.

Problem-solving skills training may follow the guidelines set out in Chapter 4 and Table 4.3 (p. 147). Family members may be helped to define problems briefly in concrete terms and avoiding long-winded, vague definitions of the problem. They should be helped to sub-divide big problems into a number of smaller problems and to tackle these one at a time. Tackling problems involves brainstorming options, exploring the pros and cons of these, agreeing on a joint action plan, implementing the plan, reviewing progress and revising the original plan if progress is unsatisfactory. However, this highly task-focused approach to facilitating family problem-solving needs to be coupled with a sensitivity to emotional and relationship issues. Family members should be facilitated in their expression of sadness or anxiety associated with the problem and helped to acknowledge their share of the responsibility in causing the problem but their understandable wish to deny this responsibility. Premature attempts to explore pros and cons of various solutions motivated by anxiety should be postponed until brainstorming has run its course. Finally, families should be encouraged to celebrate successful episodes of problem solving.

Families can use their communication and problem-solving skills to develop and implement programmes such as that presented in Figures 10.7 and 10.8. It may also be necessary for parents and teenagers to negotiate about the adolescent's behaviour at school and the peer group. In the following two sections home–school liaison and therapy for peer problems are discussed.

Home–school liaison meetings and remedial tuition

Many adolescents with conduct problems, engage in destructive school-based behaviour and have co-morbid learning difficulties. School interventions should address both conduct and academic problems. School-based conduct problems may be managed by arranging a series of meetings involving a representative of the school, the parents and the adolescent. The goal of these meetings should be to identify target conduct problems to be altered by implementing a programme of rewards and sanctions run jointly by the parents and the school, in which acceptable target behaviour at school is rewarded and unacceptable target behaviour at school leads to loss of privileges at home. Figure 10.9 presents an example of a daily report card for use in home–school liaison programmes. A critical aspect of home–school liaison meetings is facilitating the building of a working relationship between the parents and the school representative, since often with multi-problem families containing a child with conduct problems, family–school relationships are antagonistic (Dowling & Osborne, 1994). The psychologist should continually provide both parents and teachers with opportunities to voice their shared wish to help the child develop good academic skills and control over their conduct problems. Where youngsters also have academic under-achievement problems, it is important for the psychologist and teachers to take the steps necessary to arrange remedial tuition and study skills training as described in Chapter 8.

Social problem-solving skills training

Adolescents with conduct problems, it was noted earlier, often are character-ized by a hostile attributional bias and poor social problem-solving skills. These problems underpin their difficulties in making and maintaining non-deviant peer relationships. Typically the main peer problems faced by young-sters with conduct problems is that they are isolated and have difficulty joining a peer group or they are a member of a deviant peer group and have difficulty leaving this and joining a non-deviant peer group. Individual or group-based social problem-solving skills training may be used to help youngsters who have peer problems develop the skills necessary to manage peer-group relationships more effectively (Finch et al, 1993; Kazdin, 2003; Shure, 1992). In this type of treatment, the therapist takes an active role as a coach or instructor and trains the youngster to handle social situations in a systematic way. Examples of various social situations provide a focus for training sessions. Common social situations dealt with in this type of therapy include joining a group of peers who are already playing a game or involved in a discussion; contributing to a group discussion in a non-aggressive way, giving compliments, asking a peer to engage in an activity, handling refusals, managing differences of opinion and dealing with authority. The examples may be offered by the therapist or elicited from youngsters in the group. For each example, the therapist helps the youngster through modelling, role-play, shaping and reinforcement to develop the following skills:

- accurately assessing problematic social situations
- generating a range of solutions to such problem situations
- anticipating the immediate and long-term impact of these solutions
- implementing the most appropriate solution
- learning from feedback
- use self-instructions to guide oneself through these steps.

Special attention should be given to perspective taking and empathizing with the viewpoints of others and managing anger by reinterpreting situations and using distraction, breathing and relaxation skills. Youngsters may be encouraged to view ambiguous social situations positively and problematic social situations as opportunities to use their newly learned skills and master problems rather than as threats to their self-esteem. Insofar as this occurs, this type of therapy allows youngsters to correct their hostile attributional biases. Between sessions, homework assignments may be given, in which youngsters try out their newly learned skills and then report back to the therapist and the group on their successes and failures.

Parent counselling

Adolescents with pervasive conduct problems typically come from multi-problem families in which parents have limited resources for coping with high levels of stress and low levels of social support. Often, these parents find it difficult to follow through on plans to implement rules, roles and routines worked out in therapy sessions. The parents' own psychological difficulties, marital problems and life stresses prevent them from sticking to their plans to provide consistent rewards or sanctions for rule-following or rule-breaking behaviour, particularly during the early stages of therapy. As a result of this, the youngster's conduct problems persist.

There are two main types of effective solution to this problem: parent counselling and treatment foster care. With treatment foster care the child is placed with a foster family trained in social learning theory based methods for socializing children with conduct problems (Chamberlain & Smith, 2003). As the conduct problems abate, and as the natural parents are concurrently trained to negotiate with their youngster and implement consistent rewards or sanctions for rule-following or rule-breaking behaviour, the youngster spends increasingly longer visits with the natural parents. Thus the burden of socializing the child is shared by the natural parents and the foster parents. Treatment foster care is discussed more fully in Chapter 22.

With parent counselling, the parents are provided with individual or marital counselling to help them better manage their personal and marital difficulties so that these factors will not compromise their capacity to follow through on implementing consistent rewards or sanctions for rule-following or rule-breaking behaviour.

The art of effective family work with multi-problem families where children present with conduct problems is to keep a substantial portion of the therapy focused on resolving the conduct problem by altering the pattern of interaction between the child and the parents that maintains the conduct difficulties and only deviate from this focus into wider family issues, when it is clear that the parents will be unable to maintain focus without these wider issues being addressed. Where parents have personal or marital difficulties and require individual or marital counselling or therapy, ideally separate sessions should be allocated to these problems, other members of the involved professional network may be designated to manage them or a referral to another agency may be made. Common problems include maternal depression, social isolation, financial difficulties, paternal alcohol and substance abuse and marital crises. A danger to be avoided in working with multi-problem families is losing focus and becoming embroiled in a series of crisis intervention sessions that address a range of family problems in a haphazard way.

Interprofessional and interagency co-ordination meetings

Adolescents with pervasive conduct problems that occur in family, school and community settings typically become involved with multiple agencies and professions in the fields of health, education, social services and law enforcement. In addition, other members of their families commonly have connections to multiple agencies and professionals. Co-ordinating multi-systemic intervention packages and co-operating with other involved agencies for these multi-problem youngsters, from multi-problem families with multi-agency involvement, is a major challenge. First, it is important to keep a list of all involved professionals and agencies and to keep these professionals informed of your involvement. Second, arranging periodic co-ordination meetings is vital so that involved professionals and family members share a joint view of the overall case management plan. Guidelines for managing and contributing to such review meetings are given in Chapter 4.

CONSULTING TO HIGH-SUPPORT UNITS

Despite the lack of evidence for the efficacy of imprisonment or out-of-home institutional placement of youngsters with severe conduct disorders, this practice still occurs (Dowden & Andrews, 1999). Clinical psychologists may be asked to consult to such 'high-support' units, usually during crises where adolescents have become violent. Structured risk-assessment procedures such as the Historical Clinical Risk Management 20-item checklist may be used in making judgements about risk of future violence in specific cases (Webster, Douglas, Eaves & Hart, 1997). While violent youngsters in such units may have primary conduct disorders, their violence may be due to other conditions, such as paranoid schizophrenia, which require careful evaluation (Bailey, 2002). Following thorough assessment of such incidents, involving interviews with staff and residents, and immediate crisis intervention, five main classes of interventions may be considered to reduce the frequency of future episodes within whole units. The first of these is training staff at the high-support unit to set clear behavioural rules and routines and a points system for rewarding or sanctioning compliance with rules, like those given in Figures 10.7 and 10.8. The second is the introduction of a unit-wide anger management initiative for youngsters, such as Anger Replacement Training (Goldstein & Glick, 1987). The third intervention is training staff to minimize potential precipitating triggers for violent outbursts within the unit. This may involve developing a culture of calm respectful conversation that minimizes opportunities for communication difficulties or humiliation of youngsters; regular routines for eating, sleeping, working and exercising; and a non-stressful physical environment which does not entail excessive heat, cold, noise, crowding, etc. The fourth intervention is to train staff in de-escalation routines for use where youngsters are in danger of becoming violent. These routines involve ceasing confrontation; encouraging youngsters to use distraction, breathing and relaxation routines to calm down; using communication and active listening skills to clarify misunderstanding and providing a safe, face-saving way for the youngster to re-enter the routine of the unit after a potentially violent crisis. The final intervention is to support staff in developing and implementing a policy for using physical restraint in situations where de-escalation fails (American Academy of Child and Adolescent Psychiatry, 2002). Staff training in safe but effective restraint skill is a central part of such policies. Restraint routines should specify the number of staff required; the specific permissible holds; the duration of these holds; the conditions under which seclusion, physical or chemical restraint may be used; the nature and frequency of monitoring of youngsters' well-being during restraint; written documentation of the use of physical restraint; and the timing and nature of psychiatric and psychological assessment of youngsters following episodes of restraint.

PREVENTION

Clinical psychologists have an important role to play in designing and implementing primary prevention programmes for families at risk for conduct difficulties. Ideally, such programmes would be community based, target at-risk families and involve an empirically validated parent training programme (Prinz & Dumas, 2004; Sanders Markie-Dadds, Turner & Ralph, 2004). In the case of particularly high-risk groups, such as the socially disadvantaged, intensive home-visiting support services and child-centred pre-school stimulation programmes of the sort discussed in the chapters on physical abuse and neglect (Chapters 19 and 20) may be appropriate (Lange & Carr, 2002).

SUMMARY

Conduct problems are the most common type of referral to child and family outpatient clinics. Children with conduct problems are a treatment priority because the outcome for more than half of these youngsters is very poor in terms of criminality and psychological adjustment. In the long term, the cost to society for unsuccessfully treated conduct problems is enormous. DSM IV TR and ICD 10 have adopted different approaches to the sub-classification of conduct problems but both make clear distinctions between conduct problems with different ages of onset, pervasiveness and severity. Up to 14% of youngsters have significant conduct problems and these difficulties are far more common among boys. Co-morbidity for conduct disorders and both ADHD and emotional problems such as anxiety and depression is very high particularly in clinic populations. The central clinical features are defiance, aggression and destructiveness; anger and irritability; pervasive relationship difficulties within the family, school and peer group; and difficulties with social cognition. Specifically, there is a failure to internalize social norms and a negative bias in interpreting ambiguous social situations. Biological theories have focused on the roles of genetic factors, hormonal factors and arousal levels in the aetiology of conduct problems. Classical psychoanalytic theory points to super-ego deficits and object relations theorists highlight the role of disrupted attachments in the development of conduct disorders. Problems with social information processing and social skills deficits are the principal factors highlighted in cognitive theories of conduct problems. Modelling and coercive family processes have been identified by social learning theory as central to the development and maintenance of conduct difficulties. Systems theories highlight the role of characteristics of family systems, broader social network systems and societal systems in the aetiology and maintenance of conduct problems. Treatment of conduct problems must be based on a comprehensive formulation of the child and families difficulties which takes account of pre-disposing, precipitating and maintaining factors within the child, the family and the wider social system. Such formulations should be based on thorough multi-systemic assessment. With oppositional defiant disorders in pre-adolescent children whose problems are confined to the home, behavioural parent training is the treatment of choice. With older children and adolescents who present with pervasive conduct problems, a multi-systemic intervention programme targeting specific problem-maintaining processes or potential problem-resolving processes within the child, the family and the school is the most effective approach to treatment. Clinical psychologists have important roles to play in consulting to high-support units for violent delinquent youngsters and in the development of prevention programmes for at-risk populations.

EXERCISE 10.1

Ken is an eight-year-old child who is referred because he has reading difficulties and conduct problems at school. He is also very difficult to handle at home and rarely does as he is told. He hits his mother regularly, breaks his toys and steals. His mother, Sally, is twenty-six and is at her wits' end. She thinks Mrs Johnson, the headteacher, doesn't understand Ken and is picking on him. Sally is a single parent, having left Ronnie, Ken's father, seven years ago following a number of violent episodes. Ronnie has moved away from the town where Ken and Sally live and has little contact with them. Sally has had a series of live-in boyfriends but none in the past year. She has no siblings and her father is dead. Her mother has a serious alcohol abuse problem and contacts her periodically looking for money. Sally has been hospitalized three times for depression and is currently on anti-depressants. Sally would like something done about the school situation and Mrs Johnson would like treatment for Ken, who she thinks is emotionally disturbed.

1   Draw up a preliminary formulation for this case, specifying probable pre-disposing, precipitating, maintaining and protective factors.
2   Draw up a plan for your assessment interviews with the mother, child and headteacher, and list any tests or checklists you would use in this case.
3   Role-play the first interviews.
4   Role-play helping Sally identify two positive and two negative behavioural targets and training her to use time-out for the negative targets and a reward chart for the positive targets.

FURTHER READING

Alexander, J., Barton, C., Gordon, D., Grotpeter, J., Hansson, K., Harrison, R., Mears, S., Mihalic, S., Parsons, B., Pugh, C., Schulman, S., Waldron, H., & Sexton,

T., (1998). *Blueprints for Violence Prevention, Book Three: Functional Family Therapy (FFT)*. Boulder, CO: Center for the Study and Prevention of Violence. Available at: http://www.colorado.edu/cspv/publications/blueprints.html

Alexander, J. & Parsons, B. (1982). *Functional Family Therapy*. Monterey, CA: Brooks Cole.

Barkley, R. (1997). *Defiant Children: A Clinician's Manual for Assessment and Parent Training* (Second Edition). New York: Guilford Press.

Cavell, T. (2000). *Working with Aggressive Children: A Practitioners Guide*. Washington, DC: APA.

Chamberlain, P. (1994). *Family Connections: A Treatment Foster Care Model For Adolescents With Delinquency*. Eugene, OR: Castalia.

Dowling, E. & Osborne, E. (1994). *The Family and The School. A Joint Systems approach to Problems with Children* (Second Edition). London: Routledge.

Forehand, R. & McMahon, R (1981). *Helping the Non-Compliant Child: A Clinician's Guide to Parent Training*. New York: Guilford.

Goldstein, A. & Glick, B. (1987). *Anger Replacement Training. A Comprehensive Intervention for Aggressive Youth*. Champaign, IL: Research Press.

Henggeler, S., Mihalic, S., Rone, L., Thomas, C., & Timmons-Mitchell, J. (1998). *Blueprints for Violence Prevention, Book Six: Multisystemic Therapy (MST)*. Boulder, CO: Center for the Study and Prevention of Violence. Available at: http://www.colorado.edu/cspv/publications/blueprints.html

Henggeler, S., Schoenwald, S., Bordin, C., Rowland, M., & Cunningham, P. (1998). *Multisystemic Treatment of Antisocial Behaviour in Children and Adolescents*. New York: Guilford.

Herbert, M. (1987). *Behavioural Treatment of Children With Problems*. London: Academic Press.

Larson, J. & Lochman, J. (2002). *Helping School Children Cope with Anger. A Cognitive Behavioural Intervention*. New York: Guilford.

Sanders, M. & Dadds, M. (1993). *Behavioural Family Intervention*. Needham Heights, MA: Allyn & Bacon.

Sexton, T. L. & Alexander, J. F. (1999). *Functional Family Therapy: Principles of Clinical Intervention, Assessment, and Implementation*. Henderson, NV: RCH Enterprises.

Shure, M. (1992). *I Can Problem Solve (CPS): An Interpersonal Cognitive Problem Solving Program*. Champaign, IL: Research Press.

FURTHER READING FOR PARENTS

Barkley, R. (1998). *Your Defiant Child: Eight Steps to Better Behaviour*. New York: Guilford.

Forehand, R. & Long, N. (1996). *Parenting the Strong-Willed Child: The Clinically Proven Five Week Programme for Parents of Two to Six Year Olds*. Chicago: Contemporary Books.

Fogatch, M. & Patterson, G. (1989). *Parents & Adolescent Living Together. Part 1. The Basics*. Eugene, OR: Castalia.

Fogatch, M. & Patterson, G. (1989). *Parents & Adolescent Living Together. Part 2. Family Problem Solving*. Eugene, OR: Castalia.

Webster-Stratton, C. (1992). *Incredible Years: Trouble-Shooting Guide for Parents of Children Aged 3–8*. Toronto, Canada: Umbrella Press.

Sharry, J. (2002). *Parent Power: Bringing Up Responsible Children and Teenagers*. Chichester, UK: Wiley.

WEBSITES

Functional family therapy. E-mail address: jfafft@psych.utah.edu
Incredible years: http://www.incredibleyears.com/
Multisystemic family therapy: http://www.msstservices.com/
Oregon Treatment Foster Care. E-mail address: pattic@oslc.org
Parenting Plus: http://.parentsplus.ie, email:admin@parentsplus.ie
Parenting Wisely: http://www.familyworksinc.com/

Factsheets on the conduct problems and good parenting given in this book can be downloaded from the website for Rose, G. & York, A. (2004). *Mental Health and Growing Up. Fact sheets for Parents, Teachers and Young People* (Third edition). London: Gaskell: http://www.rcpsych.ac.uk

Chapter 11

Attention and over-activity problems

Attention deficit hyperactivity disorder (ADHD), attention deficit disorder (ADD), hyperkinetic disorder HKD, hyperkinesis, minimal brain dysfunction, minimal brain damage (MBD), and disorder of attention, motor control and perception (DAMP) are some of the terms used for a syndrome characterized by persistent over-activity, impulsivity and difficulties in sustaining attention (American Academy of Child and Adolescent Psychiatry, 1997b; Barkley, 2003; Gillberg, 2003; Kutcher et al., 2004; Nolan & Carr, 2000; Schachar & Tannock, 2002; Taylor, Sergeant & Doepfner, 1998; Warner-Rogers, 2002). Children with such difficulties were first described in modern medical literature by George Still in 1902. Throughout this chapter, preference will be given to the term 'attention deficit hyperactivity disorder' (ADHD), since this is currently the most widely used term. A case example of a child with ADHD is presented in Box 11.1. ADHD is a particularly serious problem because youngsters with the core difficulties of inattention, over-activity and impulsivity can develop a wide range of secondary academic and relationship problems. Attentional difficulties may lead to poor attainment in school. Impulsivity and aggression may lead to difficulties making and maintaining appropriate peer relationships and developing a supportive peer group. Inattention, impulsivity and over-activity make it difficult for youngsters with these attributes to conform to parental expectations, and so children with ADHD often become embroiled in chronic conflictual relationships with their parents. In adolescence, impulsivity may lead to excessive risk taking with consequent complications such as drug abuse, road traffic accidents and dropping out of school. All of these risk-taking behaviours have knock-on effects and compromise later adjustment. As youngsters with ADHD become aware of their difficulties with regulating attention, activity and impulsivity, and the failure that these deficits lead to within the family, peer group and school, they may also develop low self-esteem and depression. In light of the primary problems and secondary difficulties that may evolve in cases of ADHD, it is not surprising that for some the prognosis is poor. For two-thirds of cases, the primary problems of inattention, impulsivity and hyperactivity persist into late adolescence and

Box 11.1 Case example of ADHD: Timmy, the motorboat

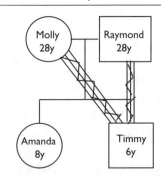

Referral. Timmy, aged six, was referred for assessment because his teachers found him unmanageable. He was unable to sit still in school and concentrate on his schoolwork. He left his chair frequently and ran around the classroom shouting. This was distracting for both his teachers and classmates. Even with individual tuition he could not apply himself to his schoolwork. He also had difficulties getting along with other children. They disliked him because he disrupted their games. He rarely waited for his turn and did not obey the rules. At home he was consistently disobedient and according to his father ran 'like a motorboat' from the time he got up until bedtime. He often climbed on furniture and routinely shouted rather than talked at an acceptable level.

Family History. Timmy came from a well-functioning family. The parents had a very stable and satisfying marriage and together ran a successful business. Their daughter, Amanda, was a well-adjusted and academically able eight year old. The parents were careful not to favour the daughter over her brother or to unduly punish Timmy for his constant disruption of his sister's activities. However, there was a growing tension between each of the parents and Timmy. While they were undoubtedly committed to him, they were also continually suppressing their growing irritation with his frenetic activity, disobedience, shouting and school problems. Within the wider family there were few resources that the parents could draw on to help them cope with Timmy. The grandparents, aunts and uncles lived in another county and so could not provide regular support for the parents. Furthermore, they were bewildered by Timmy's condition, found it very unpleasant and had gradually reduced their contact with Timmy's nuclear family since his birth.

Psychometric assessment and child interview. Psychometric evaluation showed that his overall IQ was within the normal range but Timmy was highly distractible and had literacy and numeracy skills that were significantly below his overall ability level. On both the Parent Report Child Behaviour Checklist and the Teacher Report Form Child Behaviour Checklist Timmy's scores were above the clinical cut-off for the attention problem sub-scale and the anxious/depressed sub-scale. Timmy, perceived himself to be a failure. He believed that he could not do anything right at home or at school and he was sad that the other children did not want to play with him. He believed that his teacher disliked him and doubted his parents' love for him.

Developmental history. There were a number of noteworthy features in Timmy's developmental history. He had suffered anoxia at birth and febrile convulsions in infancy. He had also had episodes of projectile vomiting. His high activity level and demandingness were present from birth. He also displayed a difficult temperament, showing little regularity in feeding or sleeping; intense negative emotions to new stimuli; and was slow to soothe following an intense experience of negative emotion.

Formulation. Timmy was a six-year-old boy with home- and school-based problems of hyperactivity, impulsivity and distractibility of sufficient severity to warrant a diagnosis of attention deficit hyperactivity disorder. Possible pre-disposing factors included anoxia at birth, subtle neurological damage due to febrile convulsions in infancy and a difficult temperament. In Timmy's case, ADHD had led to academic attainment difficulties; peer relationship problems and tension within the family. This wider constellation of difficulties underpinned Timmy's diminishing self-esteem, which in turn exacerbated his problems with attainment, peer relationships and family relationships. The absence of an extended family support system for the parents to help them deal with Timmy's difficulties was also a possible maintaining factor. Important protective factors in this case were the commitment of the parents to resolving the problem and supporting Timmy and the stability of Timmy's nuclear family.

Treatment. Treatment in this case involved both psychosocial and pharmacological intervention. The psychosocial intervention included parent and teacher education about ADHD; behavioural parent training; self-instructional training for the child; a classroom-based behavioural programme and provision of periodic relief care/holidays with specially trained foster parents. Timmy was also placed on methylphenidate.

for some of these the primary symptoms persist into adulthood. Roughly a third develop significant anti-social behaviour problems in adolescence, including conduct disorder and substance abuse, and for most of this sub-group, these problems persist into adulthood, leading to criminality. Occupational adjustment problems and suicide attempts occur in a small but significant minority of cases.

CLASSIFICATION AND CLINICAL FEATURES

In DSM IV TR (APA, 2000a), ICD 10 (WHO, 1992, 1996) and ASEBA (Achenbach & Rescorla, 2000, 2001) different terms are used for the syndrome of inattention, over-activity and impulsivity. Table 11.1 presents the DSM IV TR diagnostic criteria for ADHD, the ICD 10 criteria for hyperkinetic disorder and items from the ASEBA Attention Problems Syndrome scale. The most noteworthy feature of the syndromes described in the three systems is their similarity. Historically, a narrow definition of ADHD has been used in the UK, with great emphasis being placed on the stability of the over-activity problems across home and school contexts. In contrast, in the US, this cross-situation stability has not been a core diagnostic criterion (Hinshaw, 1994). Currently, the ICD criteria are stricter than those in the DSM. They stipulate that the *actual symptoms* of inattention, hyperactivity and impulsivity must be present in two or more settings, such as home and school, for a positive diagnosis to be made. In contrast, the more lenient

Table 11.1 Diagnostic criteria for attention and hyperactivity syndromes in DSM IV TR, ICD 10 and ASEBA

DSM IV TR *Attention deficit hyperactivity disorder*	ICD 10 *Hyperkinetic disorders*	ASEBA ATTENTION PROBLEMS SYNDROME
A. Either 1 or 2. 1. Six or more of the following symptoms of inattention have persisted for at least 6 months to a degree that is maladaptive and inconsistent with developmental level: **Inattention** a. Often fails to give close attention to details or makes careless mistakes in schoolwork, work or other activities b. Often has difficulty sustaining attention in tasks or play activities c. Often does not seem to listen when spoken to directly d. Often does not follow through on instructions and fails to finish schoolwork, chores or work duties e. Often has difficulty organizing tasks and activities f. Often avoids or dislikes tasks that require sustained mental effort g. Often loses things necessary for tasks or activities h. Is often easily distracted by extraneous stimuli i. Is often forgetful in daily activities 2. Six or more of the following symptoms of **hyperactivity-impulsivity** have persisted for at least 6 months to a degree that is maladaptive and inconsistent with developmental level:	The cardinal features are impaired attention and over-activity. Both are necessary for the diagnosis and should be evident in **more than one situation** (e.g. home or school) **Impaired attention** is manifested by prematurely breaking off from tasks and leaving activities unfinished. The children change frequently from one activity to another, seemingly losing interest in one task because they become diverted to another. These deficits in persistence and attention should be diagnosed only if they are excessive for the child's age and IQ **Over-activity** implies excessive restlessness, especially in situations requiring relative calm. It may, depending on the situation, involve the child running and jumping around, getting up from a seat when he or she was supposed to remain seated, excessive talkativeness and noisiness, or fidgeting and wriggling. The standard for judgement should be that the activity is excessive in the context of what is expected in the situation and by comparison with other children of the same age and IQ. This behavioural feature is most evident in structured, organized situations that require a high degree of behavioural self-control	**FOR 1.5- to 5-YEAR OLDS** **Inattention** Inattentive (T) Can't concentrate (P&T) Difficulty with directions (T) Fails to carry out tasks (T) **Over-activity** Can't sit still (P&T) Fidgets (T) Quickly shifts from one activity to another (P&T) Wanders away (P&T) Clumsy (P&T) **FOR 6- to 8-YEAR OLDS** **Inattention** Inattentive (P&T&C) Can't concentrate (P&T&C) Confused (P&T&C) Day-dreams (P&T&C) Stares blankly (P&T) Difficulty following directions in school (T) Fails to carry out tasks in school (T) Fails to finish tasks (P&T&C) Difficulty learning (T) Poor school work (P&T&C) Messy school work (T) Underachieving (T) **Over-activity** Can't sit still (P&T&C) Fidgets (T) Talks too much (T&C) Brags (T&C) Shows off (T&C) Whining (C) Makes odd noises (T) Apathetic in school (T) Irresponsible in school (T) Acts too young (P&T&C) **Impulsivity** Impulsive (P&TC)

Hyperactivity

a. Often fidgets with hands or feet or squirms in seat

b. Often leaves seat in classroom or in other situations in which remaining seated is expected

c. Often runs about or climbs excessively in situations in which it is inappropriate

d. Often has difficulty playing or engaging in leisure activities quietly

e. Is often on the go or acts as if driven by a motor

f. Often talks excessively

Impulsivity

g. Often blurts out answer before questions have been completed

h. Often has difficulty awaiting turn

B. Some of these symptoms were present before the age of 7 years

C. Some impairment from the symptoms is present in **two or more settings** (e.g. home and school)

D. Clinically significant impairment in social, academic or occupational functioning

E. Not due to another disorder

Specify:

Combined type if inattention and over-activity-impulsivity are present

Inattentive type if over-activity is absent;

Hyperactive-impulsive type if inattentiveness is absent

The characteristic behaviour problems should be of early onset (before the age of 6 years) and long duration

Associated features include disinhibition in social relationships, recklessness in situations involving some danger, impulsive flouting of social rules, learning disorders, and motor clumsiness

Specify:

Hyperkinetic disorder with disturbance of activity and attention when anti-social features of conduct disorder are absent

Hyperkinetic conduct disorder when criteria for both conduct disorder and hyperkinetic disorder are met

Talks out of turn (T)

Disturbs other children in school (T)

Disrupts discipline in school (T)

Items marked (P) are on the Parent Report CBCL

Items marked (T) are on the Teacher Report form

Items marked (C) are on the Youth Self-Report form

Note: Adapted from DSM IV TR (APA, 2000a) and ICD 10 (WHO, 1992, 1996) and ASEBA (Achenbach & Rescorla, 2000, 2001).

DSM criteria specify that only *impairment* in functioning arising from the symptoms, rather than the actual symptoms, must be present in two or more settings for a positive diagnosis.

Within ASEBA there are different item sets for 1.5- to five-year-olds and six- to eight-year-olds, reflecting developmental differences. For the 1.5- to five-year-olds, parent and teacher or caregiver report forms are available. For adolescents, there are parent, teacher and self-report forms. The various forms each contain a core set of items, which are common to all checklists, and in addition some items specific to either the home, school or self-report contexts. In Table 11.1 these have been grouped into those associated with inattention, over-activity and impulsivity to aid comparison with the DSM and ICD diagnostic criteria and to highlight the similarity of the three systems.

The clinical features of ADHD in the domains of cognition, affect, behaviour, physical health and interpersonal adjustment are presented in Table 11.2. With respect to cognition, short attention span, distractibility and an inability to foresee the consequences of action are the main features. Other important cognitive deficits include poor time estimation, poor planning skills, language delay, delayed internalization of speech, language impairment, learning difficulties, memory deficits and poor school performance. There is usually a poor internalization of the rules of social conduct and in some instances low self-esteem may be present. With respect to affect, excitability associated with lack of impulse control is the dominant emotional state. This may be coupled with depressed mood associated with low self-esteem in some cases. Also, anger associated with poor frustration tolerance may be a significant clinical feature. With ADHD it is the high rate of activity, common co-morbid aggressive anti-social behaviour, excessive risk taking, and under-developed adaptive behaviour associated with inattention that are the cardinal behavioural features. With respect to physical health in ADHD, youngsters may show immature bone growth and short stature. Neurological examination may reveal minor physical abnormalities and neurological soft signs. In some instances, food allergies may be present. Injuries or medical complications associated with anti-social or risk-taking behaviour, such as fighting and drug abuse, may also occur. Relationship difficulties with parents, teachers and peers are the principal interpersonal adjustment problems. Difficulties with turn-taking in games due to impulsivity make children with ADHD poor playmates. The failure of children with ADHD to internalize rules of social conduct at home and to meet parental expectations for appropriate social and academic behaviour leads to conflictual parent–child relationships. In school, youngsters with ADHD pose classroom management problems for teachers and these children invariably have problems benefiting from routine teaching and instructional methods. For these reasons, their relationships with teachers tend to be conflictual.

Table 11.2 Clinical features of ADHD

Domain	Features
Cognition	• Short attention span • Distractibility • Unable to foresee consequences of behaviour • Poor time estimation • Poor planning skills • Language delay, delayed internalization of speech and language impairment • Learning difficulties, memory deficits and poor school performance • Low self-esteem • Lack of conscience
Affect	• Poor self-regulation and lack of impulse control • Excitability • Low frustration tolerance and anger • Low mood
Behaviour	• High rate of activity • Delay in motor development and poor co-ordination • Low 'conditionability' • High level of risk-taking behaviour (e.g. sports and fast driving) • Underdeveloped adaptive behaviour
Physical condition	• Immature physical size and bone growth • Minor physical abnormalities • Neurological soft signs • Allergies • Increased respiratory infections and otitis media • Accident prone and high rate of injury
Interpersonal adjustment	• Problematic relationships with parents, teachers and peers

Historically, the following features have been used to sub-type ADHD:

• the pervasiveness of the problem
• presence or absence of both inattention and hyperactivity
• presence of co-morbid disorders.

The occurrence of the symptoms both within and outside the home, presence of both inattention and over-activity, and the presence of conduct disorder are all associated with a more serious condition, which is less responsive to treatment and which has a poorer outcome (McArdle, O'Brien & Kolvin, 1995). From Table 11.1 it may be seen that both the DSM and ICD distinguish between sub-types of ADHD depending on the patterning of symptomatology or the presence of co-morbid conditions. In DSM IV TR, the main distinctions are between cases where inattention and over-activity are present or absent, whereas co-morbid conduct problems is the basis for sub-typing in ICD 10.

The inattentive and over-active or combined sub-types of ADHD have distinct profiles (Barkley, 2003; Hinshaw, 1994). Children with the inattentive sub-type of ADHD, are described clinically as sluggish, apathetic, day-dreamers who are easily distracted and have difficulty completing assigned tasks within school because of learning difficulties. Within their family history there is a preponderance of learning disorders and emotional disorders, such as anxiety and depression. Those with the hyperactive-impulsive or combined sub-type of ADHD are characterized by extreme over-activity, oppositional and aggressive behaviours. Conduct problems are their most notable school-based difficulties and they have a high rate of school suspension and special educational placement. Within their family history they have a preponderance of anti-social problems such as drug abuse and criminality, and children with the hyperactive-impulsive profile are at risk for long-term anti-social behaviour problems and poor social adjustment. Children with the inattentive, hyperactive-impulsive and combined sub-types of ADHD have significant relationship difficulties with peers, school staff and family members and both respond to psychostimulant treatment, although the inattentive sub-type tends to respond to a lower dosage.

The primary distinction made in the ICD 10 system is between hyperkinetic conduct disorder, where a co-morbid conduct disorder is present, and cases where such co-morbidity is absent. Hinshaw (1994), in a review of differences between these two sub-groups, concluded that those children with co-morbid conduct disorder show greater academic problems and suffer more extreme relationship difficulties with peers, teachers and family members. While they show some response to psychostimulant treatment, they rarely respond to psychosocial individual and family interventions.

ADHD with co-morbid emotional disorders, such as anxiety or depression, is not sub-classified as a distinct condition within either ICD 10 or DSM IV TR. Children with such co-morbid profiles have been found to have a later onset for the disorder, fewer learning and cognitive problems and to be less responsive to stimulant medication than youngsters without co-morbid anxiety (Taylor, 1994).

Biederman et al. (1993) found distinctive CBCL profiles for ADHD children with and without other co-morbid problems. Those with ADHD obtained elevations only on the attentions problems sub-scale. Those with co-morbid conduct disorder showed elevations, in addition, on the delinquent (rule-breaking) behaviour and aggressive behaviour scales. Elevations on the anxious/depressed scale characterized cases with co-morbid anxiety disorders and elevations on thought problems and aggressive behaviour occurred in cases where there was a co-morbid mood disorder.

In Nordic countries, the diagnostic category of disorder of attention, motor control and perception (DAMP) is used by some clinicians to classify children with developmental delays or deficits in the areas of attention, gross and fine motor skills, perception and speech and language (Gillberg, 2003). DAMP is a modern attempt to operationalize the earlier term 'minimal brain dysfunction' (or damage). DAMP refers to ADHD with co-morbid developmental co-ordination disorder and specific language delay. The criteria for DAMP include both those for DSM ADHD and those for DSM developmental co-ordination disorder, which is characterized by a significant delay in the development of gross and fine motor skills and clumsiness. In severe DAMP significant speech and language delay may also be present. DAMP is, therefore, a broader category than DSM ADHD and far broader than ICD hyperkinetic disorder. The DAMP category is not in common use in Ireland, the UK, North America or Australia.

EPIDEMIOLOGY

Reviews of epidemiological studies of ADHD report overall prevalence rates varying from 1 to 20%, depending on the stringency of the diagnostic criteria applied, the data collection methods used and the demographic characteristics of the populations studied (Hinshaw, 1994; Schachar & Tannock, 2002; Swanson et al., 1998). Using stringent ICD 10 hyperkinetic disorder criteria demanding cross-situational stability of symptoms, a prevalence rate of 1% has been obtained in a UK national epidemiological study (Meltzer et al., 2000). Prevalence rates of 5–10% have been found in studies that use the more lenient DSM criteria and structured interviews. Prevalence rates of 10–20% have been found in studies where behaviour checklists were used.

The combined inattentive-hyperactive ADHD sub-type is by far the most common in clinical samples. In a study of a clinic sample of ADHD cases, Farraone, Biederman, Weber & Russell (1998) found that 60% of cases had the combined sub-type, compared with 30% who had the inattentive sub-type and 10% who had the hyperactive-impulsive sub-type.

The prevalence of ADHD varies with gender, age and geographical location (Schachar & Tannock, 2002). ADHD is more prevalent in boys than girls; in pre-adolescents than in late adolescents and among youngsters living in urban rather than rural communities.

Co-morbidity for conduct disorder and ADHD is quite prevalent in community populations. From Table 3.4 in Chapter 3 (p. 86) it may be seen that the co-morbidity rate for ADHD and conduct disorder based on standardized interviews (the DISC or the DICA) and DSM III diagnostic criteria is 23.3%. From Table 3.5 (p. 87) it may be seen that co-morbidity rates for the CBCL aggression syndrome and the CBCL attention problem syndrome (which are very similar to DSM conduct disorder and ADHD) is far higher in clinic populations (47%) than in community populations (28%).

Co-morbidity for emotional disorders and ADHD is quite prevalent in community populations. Table 3.4 shows that the co-morbidity rate for ADHD and major depression is 10.5% and for anxiety disorders is 11.8%. These co-morbidity rates are based on standardized interviews (the DISC or the DICA) and DSM III diagnostic criteria. From Table 3.5 it may be seen that co-morbidity rates for the CBCL attention problems syndrome and the CBCL anxious-depressed syndrome (which is similar to DSM anxiety disorders) is far higher in clinic populations (43%) than in community populations (28%).

Virtually all children with ADHD have attainment problems. However, co-morbid severe specific learning difficulties have been estimated to occur in 10–25% of cases (Hinshaw, 1994).

A significant proportion of youngsters with ADHD have co-morbid sleep disorders, tic disorders and developmental language delays (Barkley, 2003).

AETIOLOGICAL THEORIES

Many theories have been developed to account for ADHD (Tannock, 1998), some of which are summarized with their implications for treatment in Table 11.3. These theories fall into three main categories. First there are those that focus largely on the role of biological factors in the aetiology of ADHD. Second, there are intrapsychic theories, which attempt to explain the syndrome of inattention, over-activity and impulsivity through reference to a central underlying deficit. Third, there are those that deal with the role of psychosocial factors in the development and maintenance of the condition.

Biological theories

Hypotheses about the role of genetic factors, structural brain abnormalities, neurotransmitter dysregulation, hypoarousal and dietary factors have guided much research in the aetiology of ADHD.

Genetic hypotheses

Genetic hypotheses suggest that ADHD symptomatology or a pre-disposition to hyperactivity is inherited by children who develop the condition. In support of this hypothesis, twin, adoption and family studies all show that rates of ADHD are higher in the biological relatives of children with ADHD than those without the disorder (Barkley, 2003; Hinshaw, 1994; Schachar & Tannock, 2002; Tharper & Scourfield, 2002). Twin studies show that the heritability co-efficient for ADHD is at least .8 (which is higher than that for intelligence, typically estimated at .5 to .7); 20% of the variance in ADHD

Table 11.3 Theories of ADHD and treatment implications

	Theory	Theoretical principles	Principles of treatment
Biological theories	**Genetic hypothesis**	ADHD symptomatology, or temperamental over-activity which interacts with environmental factors to produce ADHD symptoms are inherited	Treatment should be based on a chronic care or coping model in which the child and family are offered episodes of brief intensive intervention within the context of a long-term relationship with the treatment service
	Organic deficit theory	ADHD is due to a structural or functional neurological deficit in the prefrontal cortex and related subcortical structures which subserve executive functioning	
	Neurotransmitter dysregulation hypothesis	ADHD is due to a dysregulation of dopaminergic system which subserves executive functioning and noradrenergic system, which inhibits over-activity in the prefrontal cortex and related subcortical structures	Psychostimulants may be used to rectify dysregulation of the dopamine system. Anti-depressants and noradrenergic agonists may be used to rectify dysregulation of the noradrenergic system
	Under-arousal hypothesis	Children with ADHD are psycho-physiologically less responsive to signal stimuli and this underpins their attentional problems, in that they require a great deal of stimulation to stay on task. Also their hyperactivity may reflect stimulus-seeking behaviour	Training in academic and social skills should include the use of vivid, arousing stimulus materials and contingency management should involve the use of highly salient reinforcers delivered immediately following appropriate responses
	Allergy hypothesis	ADHD is a cognitive and behavioural response to food intolerance	Specific foods to which the child is allergic should be identified and eliminated from the child's diet. Common foods for elimination include cows' milk, wheat flour, food dyes and citrus fruits

Continued

Table 11.3 continued

	Theory	Theoretical principles	Principles of treatment
Intrapsychic theories	**Inattention hypothesis**	A difficulty with sustaining attention underpins all of the features of ADHD including over-activity and impulsivity	In both academic and relational situations treatment should aim to help the child to compensate for specific psychological deficit (inattention, over-activity, impulsivity or rule-following problems)
	Over-activity hypothesis	A difficulty in regulating the rate of motor activity underpins all of the features of ADHD, including impulsivity and inattention	
	Impulsivity hypothesis	A difficulty in regulating the timing of responses to stimuli underpins all of the features of ADHD, including over-activity and inattention. The central difficulty in ADHD is an aversion to the experience of delay	
	Executive function hypothesis	ADHD arises from a core deficit in behavioural inhibition associated with, and reinforced by secondary deficits in (1) non-verbal working memory, (2) verbal working memory, (3) self-regulation of affect, arousal and motivation, and (4) verbal and behavioural creativity and fluency	
Systems theory		Conflictual parent–child relationships; conflictual marital relationships; wider family conflict; parental psychological problems and social disadvantage contribute to the development and maintenance of ADHD	Family interventions and school interventions which aim to alter conflictual patterns of interaction with family members, peers and school staff which maintain the academic and social adjustment difficulties

symptomatology may be accounted for by environmental factors. The nature and extent of the contribution made by genetic and environmental factors varies from case to case. Extreme levels of the temperamental characteristic of over-activity, which is normally distributed within the population and polygenetically determined, probably interacts with environmental factors (either intrauterine or psychosocial) to give rise to the clinical syndrome of ADHD. It may be that, in some cases, temperamentally over-active children sustain a pre-natal or early childhood neurological insult and go on to develop ADHD, whereas others with an over-active temperament develop the syndrome following participation in ongoing, non-optimal parent–child interactions. Molecular genetic studies have found an association between ADHD and the dopamine transporter gene (DAT1) and the dopamine D4 receptor gene (DRD4). The search for these genes was informed by evidence for dysregulation of the dopamine system in the prefrontal region of the brain, associated with executive function, in children with ADHD. For a very small sub-group of children with ADHD, the syndrome appears to be caused by a genetic condition resulting in a generalized resistance to thyroid hormone (Hauser et al., 1993).

Organic deficit hypothesis

The organic deficit hypothesis attributes ADHD to structural or functional brain abnormalities. In support of this hypothesis, sophisticated neuroimaging studies have shown that structural and functional abnormalities in the regions of the brain associated with executive function typify cases of ADHD (Barkley, 2003; Schachar & Tannock, 2002). Compared with normal children, those with ADHD have been found to have smaller and less symmetrical prefrontal and basal ganglia structures in the right cerebral hemisphere. These abnormalities may arise from genetic or adverse pre- or peri-natal factors. Pre- or peri-natal adversities more prevalent among youngsters with ADHD than normal children include maternal smoking and alcohol use during pregnancy, prematurity, low birth weight, birth complications, low fetal heart rate during delivery, small head circumference at birth, minor physical abnormalities, a high rate of diseases of infancy, lead poisoning and early head injury (Barkley, 2003). It is important to point out that these factors, which may contribute to the development of an organic deficit, are not unique to ADHD and occur also in youngsters with other disorders. Therefore they probably interact with other factors in contributing to the development of ADHD.

The genetic and organic deficit hypotheses underline the importance of a chronic care model in developing services for families of children with ADHD (Kazdin, 1997). Acute-care service models, which offer a single episode of time-limited intervention, according to the organic deficit model will probably be of little long-term value since the genetic disposition or organic deficit that under-pins the symptoms of inattention, over-activity and impulsivity will remain.

Neurotransmitter dysregulation hypothesis

The neurotransmitter dysregulation hypothesis attributes the symptoms of ADHD to abnormalities in neurotransmitter functioning in centres which subserve behavioural activation and executive functioning. There is growing evidence to show that a dysregulation of the dopamine and noradrenaline systems in the prefrontal cortex and basal ganglia occur in ADHD (Barkley, 2003; Schachar & Ickowitcz, 2000; Schachar & Tannock, 2002). The dopamine system sub-serves executive function. Stimulants such as methylphenidate, which affect the dopamine system, lead to a reduction in hyperactivity and inattention and an improvement in academic and social functioning, although positive effects dissipate when treatment ceases. This was first reported by Bradley in 1937. The noradrenergic system inhibits over-activity. Tricyclic anti-depressants and noradrenergic agonists such as clonidine, which affect the noradrenergic system, reduce hyperactivity but have little effect on attention problem in ADHD.

Hypoarousal hypotheses

The hypoarousal hypothesis explains hyperactivity and inattention as a failure to be sufficiently aroused by signal stimuli to attend to them and regulate activity levels. Hyperactivity may also, according to this hypothesis, reflect stimulus-seeking behaviour. Psychophysiological studies indicate that ADHD children show reduced psychophysiological responsiveness (as assessed by electroencephalograph (EEG), galvanic skin response (GSR) and heart rate) to novel stimuli with signal value (Barkley, 2003). However, similar unresponsiveness characterizes children with learning disorders and conduct disorders (Taylor, 1994). So hypoarousal is not a vulnerability unique to ADHD. The use of vivid stimuli in academic settings and highly salient and immediate reinforcers are implicated by the hypoarousal hypothesis. Reward systems and operant programmes conforming to these specifications have been found to have significant short-term effects (Pelham & Hinshaw, 1992).

Allergy hypotheses

The allergy hypothesis attributes the symptoms of ADHD to children's reaction to certain features of their daily diet. Originally Feingold (1975) argued that artificial food additives such as colorants accounted for a substantial proportion of ADHD symptomatology. However, controlled trials of additive-free diets did not support his position (Barkley, 1998b). Egger, Carter, Graham, Gumley and Soothill (1985) refined Feingold's original allergy theory and argued that particular children with ADHD may have unique allergy profiles and, if their diet is modified so as to exclude the precise substances to which they are allergic, then their activity and attention problems may improve. Carefully controlled dietary studies have supported Egger's theory (Egger et al., 1985).

Intrapsychic theories

Many intrapsychic theories have been developed to explain the patterning of symptomatology in ADHD. A small illustrative handful of these will be mentioned below. All attempt to show how the overall syndrome of inattention, over-activity and impulsivity may be accounted for by one or more underlying core deficits.

Inattention hypothesis

The inattention hypothesis argues that problems with sustaining attention on a single task and screening out other distracting stimuli is the core difficulty that under-pins the other symptoms of impulsivity and over-activity in ADHD (e.g. Douglas, 1983). That is, youngsters with ADHD at the outset of a task requiring attention will perform at a level equivalent to normal children but, over time, they will show more errors, which are directly attributable to the inability to sustain attention. This problem with sustaining attention leads them to change the focus of their attention frequently and this is manifested at a behavioural level as excessive impulsivity and over-activity. On certain laboratory tasks children with ADHD show a gradual deterioration in sustained attention. However, on other tasks they show immediate selective attention problems compared to normals and they also display over-activity while asleep (Barkley, 2003). These findings suggest that a deficit in sustained inattention alone cannot fully account for the ADHD syndrome.

Hyperactivity hypothesis

The hyperactivity hypothesis argues that a problem with inhibiting motor activity is the core deficit that under-pins the ADHD syndrome and can account for inattention and impulsivity (e.g. Quay, 1997; Schachar, 1991). A large body of evidence shows that hyperactivity is unique as a symptom to children with ADHD compared to children with other psychological problems, and that hyperactivity as a construct correlates with many academic indices of attentional problems (Barkley, 2003).

Impulsivity hypothesis

This hypothesis argues that a core problem in inhibiting cognitive and behavioural responses to specific stimuli leads to poor performance on tasks apparently requiring good attentional abilities and also to tasks requiring planning and careful regulation of behaviour. Thus the central problems in ADHD, according to this hypothesis, are with cognitive and behavioural impulsivity (Nigg, 2001). According to this theory, with academic tasks apparently requiring high levels of sustained attention, children with ADHD have problems using systematic cognitive problem-solving strategies because they are cognitively impulsive. Also, in both academic and social situations, children with ADHD engage in careless work practices in school and in socially inappropriate behaviour with peers, parents and teachers because they are behaviourally impulsive. There is some evidence to show that while children with ADHD may know and understand problem-solving skills and social skills, they fail to use them appropriately in academic and social situations (Barkley, 2003).

Executive function hypothesis

Russell Barkley (2003) argues that the symptoms of ADHD (impulsivity, over-activity and inattention) reflect a central deficit in the core executive function of behavioural inhibition that is neurodevelopmental (rather than social) in origin. Children with deficits in behavioural inhibition cannot delay immediate gratification so as to reap better rewards later. This core deficit in behavioural inhibition is associated with, and reinforced by secondary deficits in four other executive functions: (1) non-verbal working memory; (2) verbal working memory (or internalization of speech); (3) self-regulation of affect, arousal and motivation; and (4) verbal and behavioural creativity and fluency (or internalization of play). With poor verbal and non-verbal working memory, ADHD children cannot hold a picture of events in the mind, or obey a set of self-directed instructions and so delay gratification or sustain planned sequences of goal-directed behaviour. With poor self-regulation of affect, arousal and motivation, ADHD children have difficulty preventing strong emotional experiences and motives from interfering with planned goal-directed behaviour. With poor verbal and behavioural creativity and fluency, ADHD children have difficulty developing, rehearsing and implementing creative plans to achieve novel goals. The four secondary executive faction deficits, according to Barkley, reflect failures to internalize and privatize functions that, in early development, were external features of the child's interactions with caregivers. In normal development, the emergence of these four executive functions reflects a shift in the source of control of behaviour from external events to mental representations of events, from control by others to control by the self and from immediate to delayed gratification. This complex and elaborate executive function hypothesis has to some degree supplanted earlier simpler psychological theories and is partially supported by a growing body of empirical evidence (Barkley, 2003).

To compensate for deficits in attention, regulation of motor activity, impulsivity and executive function, various skills training programmes have been developed, largely within the cognitive-behavioural tradition. Self-instructional training for managing academic tasks and social skills training to manage relationship problems (particularly those involving peers) are the main types of skills taught within these programmes. Because of the negligible impact that such programmes had when conducted in isolation, they are now offered as one element of a multi-modal package involving stimulant medication, family intervention and school intervention (American Academy of Child and Adolescent Psychiatry, 1997b; Fonagy et al., 2002; Nolan & Carr, 2000; Schachar & Tannock, 2002; Taylor et al., 1998). Hinshaw (1994) has argued that it is probable that compensatory problem-solving and social-skills training programmes can have optimum effect when offered after a consistent home- and school-based contingency management programme has been established and stimulant treatment is in progress.

There is a growing consensus within the field that single-factor theories are unlikely to be able to explain the complex and heterogeneous population of youngsters who qualify for a diagnosis of ADHD (American Academy of Child and Adolescent Psychiatry, 1997b; Schachar & Tannock, 2002; Taylor et al., 1998). It is probable that a variety of biological and psychosocial factors interact in complex ways to give rise to the syndrome and that problems with a number of intrapsychic processes, particularly those involved in regulating both cognitive and motor responses, under-pin symptomatology. The symptomatology is probably partially maintained and exacerbated by problematic relationships within the family, the peer group and the school.

Systems theory

Systems theories have focused largely on the role of the family system or the wider social context in the aetiology and maintenance of ADHD. With respect to family problems, high stress and low support; parental psychological problems such as depression, aggression or alcohol abuse; exposure to marital discord; over-intrusive parenting and coercive parent–child interactions in childhood and adolescence have all been found to have associations with ADHD (Lange et al., 2005). With respect to the wider social system, the following factors have been found to be associated with ADHD: low socio-economic status, institutional upbringing, peer relationship problems and relationship problems with school staff (Barkley, 2003). A problem with much of the research on psychosocial factors in the aetiology and maintenance of ADHD is the fact that in many cases co-morbid conduct disorders are present and the risk factors that are identified, which bear a close resemblance to those identified for conduct disorders, may primarily be associated with the aetiology of conduct problems rather than ADHD. A second difficulty is untangling the causal chain and establishing which family and relationship difficulties precede the development of ADHD and are pre-disposing factors;

and distinguishing these from relationship difficulties that evolve in response to ADHD and possibly maintain or exacerbate the condition.

Behavioural parent training, family therapy and multi-systemic intervention programmes involving the child's wider social network have evolved from family systems theories of ADHD. These programmes focus on improving parenting skills and enhancing the child's relationships with members of the family and the wider network. Such programmes have been shown to have positive short-term effects on both symptomatology and social adjustment (Anastopoulos, Barkley & Shelton, 1996; Barkley, Guevremont Anastopoulas & Fletcher, 1992; Fonagy et al., 2002; Nolan & Carr, 2000).

ASSESSMENT

Assessment and management of children with syndromes involving inattention, hyperactivity and impulsivity should be offered within a chronic-care rather than an acute model. ADHD is a lifelong disorder for which children and families require ongoing treatment, usually in the form of episodes of intensive clinical contact at critical points in the child's lifecycle, interspersed with periods of less intensive monitoring and support. Episodes of intensive contact are required during the initial assessment and management period and at transitions from one educational setting to another or from school to work. In addition should evidence of the escalation of co-morbid conduct or emotional problems emerge, intensive intervention particularly for anti-social behaviour should be arranged, since children with ADHD with the poorest outcomes are those who develop co-morbid anti-social conduct problems. In addition to this episodic clinical input, youngsters with ADHD require ongoing appropriate remedial tuition.

The management of cases where inattention, over-activity and impulsivity are central concerns should begin with a thorough assessment. In addition to the routine areas for assessment set out in Chapter 4, the symptoms listed in Table 11.1 and the clinical features listed in Table 11.2 should be considered. The importance of obtaining reliable, valid and comparable accounts of the child's behaviour in home and school contexts cannot be over-emphasized. The ASEBA and SDQ checklists (listed in Table 4.1, p. 125) and the Conners' rating scales (listed in Table 11.4, p. 439) are particularly useful tools for this aspect of the assessment because they contain well-validated attention problems sub-scales and, in addition, furnish an assessment of co-morbid conduct and emotional problems which are often present. Children scoring above the clinical cut-off score on the attention problems sub-scales of these instruments and who meet the diagnostic criteria listed in Table 11.1 may be diagnosed as having ADHD.

A thorough psychometric assessment of intelligence, attainments and

Table 11.4 Psychometric instruments that my be used as an adjunct to clinical interviews in the assessment of ADHD

Construct	Instrument	Publication	Comments
ADHD symptomatology	Attention Deficit Hyperactivity Disorder Test	Gilliam, J. (1996). *Attention Deficit Hyperactivity Disorder Test.* Odessa, FL: PAR. http:// www.parinc.com	This 36-item test is based on DSM IV criteria and yields an overall score and sub-scale sores for hyperactivity, impulsivity and inattention. It was normed in 1994 on over 1200 cases of ADHD between ages 3 and 23 years
	Conners' Parent Rating Scale	Conners, C. (1997). *Connors Rating Scales. Revised Technical Manual.* North Tonawanda, New York. Multihealth Systems. http:// www.mhs.com	Connors' parent, teacher and self-report rating scales are available in short and long versions with a maximum item length of about 90 items for long versions and about 28 items for short versions. The long parent version yields scores for these factors: ADHD index, DSM IV symptom sub-scales, DSM IV inattentive, DSM IV hyperactive–impulsive, oppositonal, inattention, hyperactivity, anxious–shy, perfectionism, social problems, psychosomatic, Conner's' global index, restless–impulsive and emotional lability. There are normative data for children 3–17 years of age for parent and teacher versions and 12–17 years for the self-report version. All scales are hand and computer scoreable

Continued

Table 11.4 continued

Construct	Instrument	Publication	Comments
Situations in which ADHD symptoms occur	Home Situations Questionnaire (HSQ)	Barkley, R. (1997). *Defiant Children: A Clinician's manual for Parent Training (Second Edition).* New York: Guilford Press	On 16 items, parents indicate whether their child has behaviour problems in home and community situations and the severity of such problems if they exist. The HSQ gives a score for the number of situations in which problems occur and the overall severity of such problems
	School Situations Questionnaire (SSQ)	Barkley, R. (1997). *Defiant Children: A Clinician's manual for Parent Training (Second Edition).* New York: Guilford Press	On 12 items, parents indicate whether their child has behaviour problems in school situations and the severity of such problems if they exist. The SSQ gives a score for the number of situations in which problems occur and the overall severity of such problems

language, following the guidelines given in Chapter 8, is also essential in the assessment of children with ADHD, since most children with ADHD have learning problems and many have co-morbid developmental language delay and specific learning difficulties.

Ideally, psychological assessment of children with ADHD should be conducted as one element of a multi-disciplinary assessment. Where such multi-disciplinary assessments are being co-ordinated by a clinical psychologist, referral to paediatrics and speech and language therapy are particularly important. Referral for paediatric medical assessment should be routinely made to evaluate the impact of pre- and peri-natal factors, neurological status, minor physical anomalies and food allergies. Referral to speech and language therapy may be made to assess developmental language delay.

From the wealth of research generated on ADHD, and from clinical experience, pre-disposing, maintaining and protective factors for syndromes involving attentional problems, impulsivity and hyperactivity deserving consideration in the assessment of cases of ADHD have been summarized in

Figure 11.1. (American Academy of Child and Adolescent Psychiatry, 1997b; Barkley, 2003; Kutcher et al., 2004; Nolan & Carr, 2000; Schachar & Tannock, 2002; Taylor et al., 1998; Warner-Rogers, 2002). It is noteworthy that, unlike many other problems and conditions covered in this text, no precipitating factors have been reliably identified in the literature. Rather, it appears that ADHD usually evolves gradually over the first five years or is present from birth.

Pre-disposing factors

Both personal and contextual pre-disposing factors may be present in ADHD. Among the more important personal biological pre-disposing factors are: genetic vulnerability, pre-natal difficulties, maternal smoking during pregnancy, maternal alcohol use during pregnancy, low fetal heart rate during delivery, small head circumference at birth, minor physical abnormalities, anoxia at birth, low birth weight, a high rate of diseases of infancy, lead poisoning and early neurological insult. Difficult-temperament children are also pre-disposed to developing ADHD. Parental psychopathology, intrusive caregiver behaviour, exposure to marital discord and family disorganization, low socioeconomic status and an institutional upbringing are the principal contextual pre-disposing factors which may be considered in the assessment of ADHD. In many instances, clinical interviewing reveals that children with many personal biological pre-disposing factors develop mild ADHD, which is exacerbated through exposure to contextual psychosocial pre-disposing factors, most of which are chronic life stresses.

Maintaining factors

Both personal and contextual psychosocial factors may maintain ADHD. At a personal level, poorly developed internal speech and an associated developmental language delay may maintain inattention, over-activity and impulsivity. Co-morbid emotional and conduct disorders and specific learning difficulties may also maintain the symptoms of ADHD by diminishing the personal resources that the child has to consciously control attention, activity and impulsivity levels. Low task-related self-efficacy, immature defences and poor coping strategies may also maintain the condition. At a biological level, hypoarousal may maintain ADHD by making it difficult for youngsters to learn in situations where extremely salient stimuli and reinforcers are not available. Dysregulation of dopaminergic, adrenergic and noradrenergic neurotransmitter systems may also maintain ADHD.

At a contextual level, conflictual, coercive, negligent or intrusive relationships with parents may maintain ADHD, particularly if coupled with inconsistent parental discipline and inadvertent reinforcement of problem behaviours. ADHD is more likely to persist where children are triangulated in

PRE-DISPOSING FACTORS

PERSONAL PRE-DISPOSING FACTORS

Biological factors
- Genetic vulnerabilities
- Pre-natal difficulties
- Maternal smoking in pregnancy
- Maternal alcohol use in pregnancy
- Low fetal heart rate in labour
- Small head circumference at birth
- Minor physical abnormalities at birth
- Anoxia at birth
- Low birth weight
- Disease of infancy
- Lead poisoning
- Early neurological insult

Psychological factors
- Difficult temperament

CONTEXTUAL PRE-DISPOSING FACTORS

Parent–child factors in early life
- Intrusive parenting

Exposure to family problems in early life
- Parental psychological problems
- Marital discord or violence
- Family disorganization

Stresses in early life
- Social disadvantage
- Institutional upbringing

PERSONAL PROTECTIVE FACTORS

Biological factors
- Good physical health

Psychological factors
- High IQ
- Easy temperament
- High self-esteem
- Internal locus of control
- High self-efficacy
- Optimistic attributional style
- Mature defence mechanisms
- Functional coping strategies

PERSONAL MAINTAINING FACTORS

Biological factors
- Dysregulation of dopaminergic and noradrenergic systems
- Hypoarousal

Psychological factors
- Co-morbid developmental language delay and poorly developed internal speech to aid rule following
- Co-morbid specific learning disability
- Co-morbid conduct disorder
- Co-morbid emotional disorder
- Low self-efficacy
- Immature defence mechanisms
- Dysfunctional coping strategies

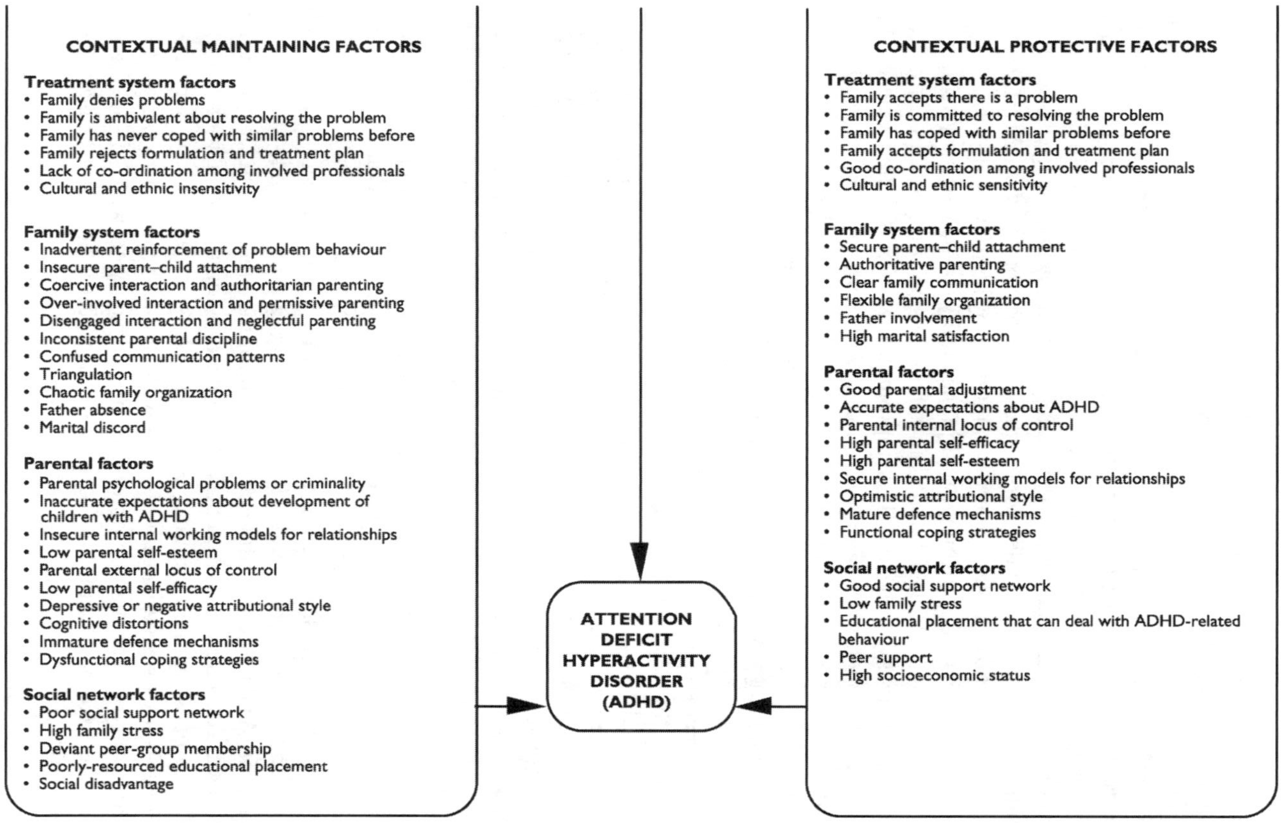

CONTEXTUAL MAINTAINING FACTORS

Treatment system factors
- Family denies problems
- Family is ambivalent about resolving the problem
- Family has never coped with similar problems before
- Family rejects formulation and treatment plan
- Lack of co-ordination among involved professionals
- Cultural and ethnic insensitivity

Family system factors
- Inadvertent reinforcement of problem behaviour
- Insecure parent–child attachment
- Coercive interaction and authoritarian parenting
- Over-involved interaction and permissive parenting
- Disengaged interaction and neglectful parenting
- Inconsistent parental discipline
- Confused communication patterns
- Triangulation
- Chaotic family organization
- Father absence
- Marital discord

Parental factors
- Parental psychological problems or criminality
- Inaccurate expectations about development of children with ADHD
- Insecure internal working models for relationships
- Low parental self-esteem
- Parental external locus of control
- Low parental self-efficacy
- Depressive or negative attributional style
- Cognitive distortions
- Immature defence mechanisms
- Dysfunctional coping strategies

Social network factors
- Poor social support network
- High family stress
- Deviant peer-group membership
- Poorly-resourced educational placement
- Social disadvantage

CONTEXTUAL PROTECTIVE FACTORS

Treatment system factors
- Family accepts there is a problem
- Family is committed to resolving the problem
- Family has coped with similar problems before
- Family accepts formulation and treatment plan
- Good co-ordination among involved professionals
- Cultural and ethnic sensitivity

Family system factors
- Secure parent–child attachment
- Authoritative parenting
- Clear family communication
- Flexible family organization
- Father involvement
- High marital satisfaction

Parental factors
- Good parental adjustment
- Accurate expectations about ADHD
- Parental internal locus of control
- High parental self-efficacy
- High parental self-esteem
- Secure internal working models for relationships
- Optimistic attributional style
- Mature defence mechanisms
- Functional coping strategies

Social network factors
- Good social support network
- Low family stress
- Educational placement that can deal with ADHD-related behaviour
- Peer support
- High socioeconomic status

ATTENTION DEFICIT HYPERACTIVITY DISORDER (ADHD)

Figure 11.1 Aetiological factors to consider in the assessment ADHD.

families characterized by chaotic organization, confused communication, marital discord and in which fathers play a peripheral role. Such patterns of parenting and family organization may be associated with parental psychological problems such as insecure internal working models for relationships, low self-esteem, low self-efficacy, external locus of control, dysfunctional attributional style, cognitive distortions, immature defences and poor coping strategies. Parents may also become involved in problem-maintaining interactions with their children if they have inaccurate knowledge about their child's condition and the developmental problems that go with ADHD.

ADHD symptomatology may be maintained by high levels of stress, limited support and social disadvantage within the family's wider social system, since these features may deplete parents' and children's personal resources for dealing constructively with ADHD symptomatology. For children whose educational placements are poorly resourced, with staff untrained to deal with ADHD and poor staff–student ratios, children may become involved in coercive patterns of interaction with teachers and peers that maintain ADHD symptomatology. When youngsters with ADHD are members of deviant peer groups, their conduct problems and impulsivity may be maintained by the deviant peer group through modelling deviant behaviour and reinforcing it.

Within the treatment system, a lack of co-ordination among involved professionals including teachers, psychologists, psychiatrists, paediatricians, speech therapists and so forth may maintain ADHD-related problems. Effective treatment for ADHD must be multi-modal and include pharmacological, psychological, pedagogical and other components. However, if children and parents view these components as competing rather than complementary solutions to ADHD, then the child's difficulties may get worse as a result of the family's interaction with an un-co-ordinated group of professionals. Where co-operation problems between families and treatment teams develop, and families deny the existence of the problem, the validity of the formulation or the appropriateness of the treatment programme, then the child's difficulties may persist. Treatment systems that are not sensitive to the cultural and ethnic beliefs and values of the youngster's family system may maintain ADHD-related difficulties by inhibiting engagement or promoting drop-out from treatment and preventing the development of a good working alliance between the treamtent team, the youngster and his or her family. Parents' lack of experience in dealing with similar problems in the past is a further factor that may compromise their capacity to work co-operatively with the treatment team and so may contribute to the maintenance of the child's problems.

Protective factors

The probability that a treatment programme for ADHD will be effective is influenced by a variety of personal and contextual protective factors. It is important that these be assessed and included in the later formulation, since it is protective factors that usually serve as the foundation for therapeutic change. Good health, a high IQ, an easy temperament, high self-esteem, an internal locus of control, high self-efficacy and an optimistic attributional style are all important personal protective factors. Other important personal protective factors include mature defence mechanisms and functional coping strategies, particularly good problem-solving skills and a capacity to make and maintain friendships.

Within the family, secure parent–child attachment and authoritative parenting are central protective factors, particularly if they occur within the context of a flexible family structure in which there is clear communication, high marital satisfaction and both parents share the day-to-day tasks of child care.

Good parental adjustment is also a protective factor. Where parents have an internal locus of control, high self-efficacy, high self-esteem, internal working models for secure attachments, an optimistic attributional style, mature defences and functional coping strategies, then they are better resourced to manage the symptoms of ADHD constructively. Of course, accurate knowledge about ADHD and the implications of ADHD for child development is also a protective factor.

Within the broader social network, high levels of support, low levels of stress and membership of a high socioeconomic group are all protective factors for children with ADHD. Where families are embedded in social networks that provide a high level of support and place few stressful demands on family members, then it is less likely that parents' and children's resources for dealing with ADHD will become depleted. A well-resourced educational placement may also be viewed as a protective factor. Educational placements where teachers have a clear understanding of ADHD and can provide instructional programmes tailored to the child's educational requirements protect the child from academic and vocational problems that arise in poorly resourced educational placements.

Within the treatment system, co-operative working relationships between the treatment team and the family and good co-ordination of multi-professional input are protective factors. Treatment systems that are sensitive to the cultural and ethnic beliefs and values of the youngster's family are more likely to help families engage with, and remain in, treatment and foster the development of a good working alliance. Families are more likely to benefit from treatment when they accept the formulation of the problem given by the treatment team and are committed to working with the team to resolve it. Where families have successfully faced similar problems before they are more likely to benefit from treatment and, in this sense, previous experience with similar problems is a protective factor.

FORMULATION

Salient points from assessment interviews with the parents, the child and school staff; and key results from behaviour checklists, psychometric evaluations, paediatric medical evaluation, speech and language assessment and other multi-disciplinary inputs should be integrated into a case formulation. The formulation should outline the principal clinical features shown by the child, the pre-disposing factors, the maintaining factors and the protective factors. An example of a formulation of a case of ADHD is given in the penultimate paragraph of the case study set out in Box 11.1. A management and treatment plan based on the formulation should be drawn up which attempts, in particular, to address maintaining factors.

TREATMENT

A multi-systemic treatment programme for children with ADHD includes the following elements (American Academy of Child and Adolescent Psychiatry, 1997b; Barkley, 1997, 1998a; Fonagy et al., 2002; Kutcher et al., 2004; MTA Cooperative Group, 1999; Pelham & Walker, 2005; Nolan & Carr, 2000; Schachar & Tannock, 2002; Taylor et al., 1998):

- psychoeducation
- psychostimulant medication
- family intervention to promote rule-following at home
- school intervention focusing on the management of school-based learning difficulties and conduct problems
- child-focused work to teach self-regulation skills
- dietary assessment and intervention.

Psychoeducation

Parents require clear authoritative information about the syndrome of inattention, hyperactivity and impulsivity. They need to be informed that the symptoms listed in Table 11.1 reflect the current consensus among clinicians and scientists working in this field. About 1 in 100 children suffer from the extreme type of this condition which is called attention deficit hyperactivity disorder (ADHD) in the US and hyperkinetic disorder in the UK.

The syndrome has had a variety of names over the years including hyperactivity, attention deficit disorder (ADD), minimal brain dysfunction and minimal brain damage (MBD).

There are many misconceptions about the aetiology and treatment of the syndrome of inattention, hyperactivity and impulsivity. ADHD probably arises from a genetic pre-disposition to having an over-active temperament interacting with pre-natal and peri-natal and early life factors of the type listed in Figure 11.1. While pre-existing family relationship problems do little to alleviate ADHD, they are probably not the primary cause. Because many parents blame themselves for the condition it is valuable to point out that in most cases the relationship problems that occur are a response to the syndrome rather than the cause of it.

It may also be pointed out that sympathetic management of the condition with stimulant medication, home- and school-based behavioural programmes, appropriate remedial tuition and counselling as required can help the young-ster cope with the syndrome without developing secondary emotional and conduct problems. In a small group of cases, food allergies may play a role and dietary management may be appropriate. Families that have the strength and determination to support their children in this way increase the chances of their child having a positive long-term outcome.

With respect to outcome, it should be mentioned that about a third of children learn to cope well with the syndrome and develop strategies for focusing attention and restraining their impulses to be over-active. This improvement is very gradual and occurs during adolescence. About a third, however, never achieve this type of control. These youngsters are usually those that develop secondary problems with aggression and anti-social behaviour. The remaining third show some improvement towards the end of adolescence, usually in the area of reduced levels of over-activity.

Parents and childen may be provided with reading materials written specifically for a lay audience on ADHD. A number of such texts are listed at the end of this chapter. Also information on websites listed at the end of the chapter may be given.

For families to be able to cope with ADHD throughout the child's development, membership of a support group for parents with children who have similar problems is advised. Provision of information on local support groups or establishing such groups where none exist is part of the clinical psychologist's psychoeducational remit.

Parents also require information on the rights of their child to appropriate educational resources and local guidance on how best to access these resources.

Parents may also be offered information on childproofing the home to make it safer for everyone to live in. Depending on the age of the child, this may include getting a stair gate and a fire guard; child-locks for cupboards, cabinets and drawers that contain knives, lighters and other dangerous items; arranging electrical items so as to minimize the chances of electrocution and so forth. With teenagers, the principal safety concern may be with managing the youngster's risk-taking activities, such as the wish to drive cars and motorbikes or engage in sports that entail high safety risks. The main advice that can be given is to listen carefully to the teenager's wishes but set clear limits that take account of the teenager's impulse control skills. These tend to develop much more slowly in youngsters with ADHD and so they cannot be permitted to engage in risky activities, like learning to drive, until they show clear evidence of a sufficient degree of impulse control.

Psychostimulant medication

Psychostimulant treatment should be offered as part of a multi-systemic intervention programme involving child-, family- and school-based psycho-social interventions. Psychostimulant treatment may be arranged in conjunction with a family physician, a paediatrician or child psychiatrist. However, it is important for the clinical psychologist liaising with a physician to follow guidelines for good practice, such as the NICE guidelines for treatment of ADHD with methylphenidate listed at the end of the chapter and those in other authoritative sources (American Academy of Child and Adolescent Psychiatry, 1997b; Fonagy et al., 2002; Schachar & Tannock, 2002; Taylor et al., 1998).

Stimulant treatment is contraindicated when children are under four years of age and where there is a history or high risk of cardiovascular disease, psychosis or tic disorders notably Tourette's syndrome. Stimulant treatment is less likely to be effective when children have a co-morbid anxiety disorder. Where parents or children have strong beliefs about the inappropriateness of using medication to manage children's attentional and impulsivity problems, adherence to a stimulant treatment regime will probably be poor even if the child shows a significant initial treatment response. Stimulant treatment may lead to secondary difficulties in families where a parent or sibling engages in drug abuse. In such cases, the drug abuser may use stimulants as a recreational drug. The financial costs of stimulant medication and the time and energy required by the parents, the school and the child to regularly adhere to the medication regime should be taken into account when considering stimulant treatment.

The main stimulants used are methylphenidate (Ritalin), dexamphetamine (Dexedrine), and pemoline (Cylert). Because the half-life of methylphenidate and dexamphetamine is about 3.5 hours, medication is usually prescribed as a split dose to be taken in the morning and at noon. A long-acting methylphenidate preparation (Concerta) and a slow-release preparation of amphetamines (Adderall) have been developed. These need only be taken once per day. Alternatively, pemoline, which is a longer-acting stimulant may be used.

Dosage is usually decided first on the basis of body weight and subsequently on symptomatic response to a trial of four to eight weeks. Details of dosages for psychostimulants and other medications used for ADHD are given in Spencer, Biederman and Wilens (2002).

Response to treatment may be monitored using the short, ten-item version of the Conners' Abbreviated Symptom Questionnaire (Conners, 1997). In monitoring treatment response, it is important to keep in mind that moderate dosages lead to maximum improvements in attention problems and high doses lead to maximum improvement in social and behavioural functioning. In clinical practice, the ideal is to find a dosage that optimizes both academic and social functioning.

Common side effects of psychostimulants include loss of appetite, sleep disruption, headaches and stomach aches. Although far less common, motor and vocal tics are the most worrying side effects of stimulant medication. Stimulants may speed the emergence of complex tics associated with Tourette's syndrome, which has a high co-morbidity with ADHD (see Chapter 13). A reduction in medication may control these various side effects. Height and weight should be plotted on growth charts during stimulant treatment, and if growth rate declines a six-week medication holiday should be taken.

Once medication is stopped, the benefits of psychostimulant treatment cease. In the long term, children probably do not develop a tolerance to psychostimulants. They also do not show a complete loss of personal responsibility for their behaviour and make external attributions (to psychostimulant medication) for all treatment gains.

The effects of stimulants are not specific to children with ADHD. Normal children and children with other diagnoses such as conduct disorder also show a reduction in activity level in response to psychostimulants. However, the best response has been found to be from children who show the most severe levels of over-activity and inattention and the absence of anxiety. Neurodevelopmental delays and family adversity are unrelated to treatment response.

About 75% of children with ADHD respond to psychostimulants generally, and about 60% respond to methylphenidate. For those who do not respond, there is some evidence that tricyclic anti-depressants or clonidine may be helpful in reducing ADHD symptoms (Fonagy et al., 2002).

Family intervention with children

Different types of family-intervention programme are required for pre-adolescent children and adolescents. For pre-adolescent children, the behavioural parent training programme described in Barkley's (1997) treatment manual has been found to be effective for approximately two-thirds of cases, compared with only a quarter of waiting-list controls (Anastopoulos & Farley, 2003). The programme consists of nine weekly sessions and so spans about two to three months.

The first session covers much of the material mentioned in the section on psychoeducation above. In the second session, a four-factor model of parent–child conflict is described and behaviour management principles are reviewed. The child's behaviour is explained as being influenced by: (1) intrinsic characteristics of the child such as temperament; (2) intrinsic characteristics of the parent; (3) overall family stresses; and (4) the immediate consequences of the child's behaviour. While the first three are important, the greatest influences on what children do in a given situation are their expectations of the consequences of their actions. Thus, the main things that the parents can do to help their child develop pro-social behaviour, according to this simple analysis, is to reward appropriate pro-social behaviour and make rewards unavailable for anti-social, inappropriate behaviour. This provides a rationale for the reinforcement skills learned in the next session.

It also follows from this analysis that the parents' behaviour is governed by the same four sets of factors. That is, the parents' response to the child is influenced by the parents' characteristics (particularly their expectations and stamina managing difficult behaviour), the child's characteristics (notably over-active temperamental style), family stresses (which may preoccupy parents and erode their patience for dealing with difficult child behaviour) and the consequences of the adults' behaviour. So, just as parents shape and influence the child's behaviour, so also the child shapes and influences the adults' behaviour by, for example, stopping screaming and hitting once the parents cease to place demands on the child for appropriate behaviour.

As a homework assignment, parents are invited to complete an inventory of their own characteristics, the child's characteristics and current family stresses.

In the third session parents are trained to positively attend to socially appropriate behaviour and to ignore inappropriate behaviour during episodes of special playtime. Special playtime is similar to supportive play as described in Table 4.4 (p. 148) and also in Chapter 10. During special playtime, which should occur for a regular period of fifteen to twenty minutes each day, the child selects an activity. The parent must avoid commands and questions when speaking with the child. All approximations to appropriate behaviour should be responded to with social reinforcement, that is, by the parent describing or acknowledging the child's action and praising or appreciating it. Inappropriate activities should simply be ignored. It is pointed out that as this style of interacting with the child evolves, the child will come to value parent–child interaction and so much briefer and less punitive strategies can later be used to discourage inappropriate behaviour.

In the fourth session, parents are trained to positively attend to socially appropriate behaviour and ignore inappropriate behaviour in situations where the child is playing independently. The main skill here is for parents to continually monitor the child's behaviour outside of special playtime, looking for instances of pro-social behaviour and offering social reinforcement wherever possible. Thus the quality of parent–child interaction within and outside of special playtime improves along with the probability that the child will engage in socially appropriate behaviour. There is also discussion of how to give commands effectively. Commands should only be given when the parent intends to follow through on them. They should be clear and simple, in a tone that conveys an expectation that they will be followed, and the parent should make eye contact with the child when giving the command. Qualifying information (such as 'You were very good this morning when you did what I asked . . .') should be omitted; it is a distraction for the child. It is also distracting if commands are phrased as questions rather than instructions. Other competing distractions (such as the TV) should be eliminated before commands are given. When a command has been given, it is important to ask the child to repeat the command to check that it has been heard and understood accurately. When training a child to follow commands, begin with instructions that he or she has shown some compliance with in the past, rather than those which have never been heeded. It is also better to select a time when the child is not exhausted, ill or otherwise distracted and can focus full concentration on responding to the command. All approximations to responding to a command appropriately should be socially reinforced. At the end of this session, parents are given a homework assignment of practising using positive reinforcement for independent play and compliance with commands given according to the guidelines given in the session.

In the fifth session, parents are trained in how to set up a reward system at home using points or tokens. These reward systems are similar to those described in Table 4.5 (p. 149) and also in Chapter 10. Parents are invited to draw up a list of daily, weekly and long-range treats, privileges and rewards that the child might like (a reinforcement menu) and a list of jobs or chores that must be done on a daily or weekly basis. Points that may be earned for completing jobs are noted beside each job on the list. Points required to buy an item off the reinforcement menu are put beside each item on the menu. With children eight years and under, plastic tokens from a board game or poker chips may be used as currency. With older children, ticks may be placed on a card or notebook that the child carries at all times. With children who have ADHD it is important that the tokens or points are delivered immediately following the execution of a pro-social target behaviour, that extra tokens are given when the child shows extra effort or better performance in completing a target task or behaviour and that the reward menu from which items can be bought with tokens contains highly valued items. For this reason, parents may wish to modify their reinforcement menus in consultation with their children after the session.

By this stage in the treatment programme, six to eight weeks will have elapsed, during which the quality of parent–child interaction will have improved significantly and be marked by many positive exchanges and a high rate of positive social reinforcement. Against this backdrop, in the sixth session parents are instructed in how to use response cost or the removal of tokens for punishing specifically targeted minor rule violations and non-compliance with commands. Thus, for non-compliance, children may lose the exact number of points that they would have gained if they had complied with a parental instruction.

The use of time-out from reinforcement for anti-social behaviour or aggression is also explained in detail. Time-out follows similar principles to those set out in Table 4.6 (p. 150) and discussed in Chapter 10. Parents are asked to select one or two particularly troublesome target anti-social behaviours to which time-out will be applied. Then the principles of the procedure are outlined. Time-out should be brief (the number of minutes of the child's age in years) and dispassionate and preceded by two warnings. During time-out, the child sits on a chair in a position away from the hub of family activity but easy to supervise, such as the corner of the kitchen. At the end of the specified brief period, provided tantrums or anti-social behaviour has ceased, the child should be given the command with which he or she did not comply that led to going into time-out. If the child complies, he or she receives no tokens but the parent should look for an opportunity as soon as possible to reinforce an appropriate behaviour. If the child does not comply following two warnings, he or she returns to the time-out chair and the cycle is repeated until compliance is achieved. As soon as possible after compliance, the child is rewarded for engaging in some other socially appropriate activity. Parents should be warned that, on the first few occasions time-out is used, the child's negative behaviour escalates before abating but, gradually, the duration of the child's response to time-out and the period in time-out reduces. Parents are instructed to use response cost, privilege removal, and physical restraint if the child leaves the chair.

In the seventh session the focus is on coaching parents in how to use time-out from reinforcement for a range of home-based rule violations including swearing, aggression and destructiveness.

In the eighth session parents are instructed in how to manage child behaviour problems when they occur in public places such as shops, restaurants and churches. Parents are coached in how to anticipate problems and develop plans to use social reinforcement, tokens, response cost and time-out in public settings.

In the final session the management of future problems, methods for working co-operatively with school staff, methods for dealing with co-morbid problems such as enuresis and encopresis (outlined in Chapter 7) are discussed. A booster session is normally offered a month or two after completion of the programme to troubleshoot any difficulties that the parents have in continuing to implement the parenting skills learned over the nine-session programme.

The programme described here is implemented in a flexible rather than a rigid manner. Parents are given handouts at the end of each session covering the main points made; these are available in Barkley's (1997) treatment manual. At the start of each session, homework is reviewed and difficulties with using the behavioural strategies are discussed and resolved. Throughout the programme parents are offered telephone back-up, which they are encouraged to use if they have particular difficulties with their children. Because of the flexibility of the programme, additional behaviour management strategies described in Chapter 10 for the management of oppositional defiant behaviour, may be incorporated into Barkley's behavioural parent programme for children with ADHD.

Family intervention with adolescents

While up to two-thirds of pre-adolescents with ADHD can benefit from family intervention, with adolescents various family-based interventions have been found to be effective in only about half this proportion of cases. Behavioural parent training, problem-solving and communication training, and structural family therapy have each been found to be effective in about a third of adolescents with ADHD (Anastopoulos et al., 1996). This is a sobering statistic, in view of the fact that these are probably the most effective available family intervention programmes for a wide range of other problems of childhood and adolescence.

With teenagers, the behavioural parent training programme described in the previous section requires some modification. For example, the reinforcement menu may include weekend rather than daily privileges and, for time-out and for rule-braking, parents are advised to prevent teenagers from going out and interacting with their peers for a brief specified period of time. However, problem-solving and communications training and structural family therapy both entail a treatment format that maximally involves the adolescent in treatment and may therefore be preferred on ethical grounds. Both may be conducted over about ten sessions spanning approximately three months, and there is no reason why elements of both approaches cannot be usefully combined into a course of treatment (Robin & Foster, 1989).

Problem-solving and communication training is a highly directive treatment programme with three core components: communication training, five-step behavioural problem-solving and cognitive restructuring. With communication training, active listening and sending clear messages are the main sets of skills in which family members are coached. Active listening involves not interrupting the speaker, summarizing key points made and checking that these have been accurately understood. Sending clear messages requires the speaker to make 'I statements' that reflect their views or wishes, to be clear and precise in making points, to avoid blaming and criticizing and to respect the need for equitable turn-taking so that listeners can check that they have understood the intended message. This is similar to the communication skills training described in Table 4.2 (p. 145) and discussed in Chapter 10.

In the five-step problem solving, teenagers and their parents are trained in how to pin-point commonly encountered adolescent problems, such as eating habits, cleaning bedrooms, completing chores, using the phone, spending money, choice of friends, dating, driving cars, doing homework, school achievement, time keeping, care of belongings and clothes, grooming and sibling quarrels. They are then coached in how to tackle one problem at a time in an unemotional way progressing through five steps. These are: (1) defining the problem; (2) suggesting solutions; (3) evaluating solutions and negotiating a consensus; (4) implementing the solution; and (5) verifying the outcome. This is similar to the problem-solving skills training described in Table 4.3 (p. 147) and discussed in Chapter 10.

Cognitive restructuring is an approach to modifying negative family beliefs and negative attributions that under-pin destructive interaction patterns. These beliefs may include the following themes:

- ruination: 'If I let him stay out late he will become a drug addict'
- approval: 'If my children don't agree with my rules, I am a bad parent'
- perfectionism: 'He should know how to do that schoolwork'
- obedience: 'He should be obedient always'
- self-blame: 'It's my fault that he turned out like this'
- fairness: 'Parents' rules should be fair according to my standards'
- autonomy: 'He's grown up and should be able to make his own decisions'

Problematic attributions include attributing negative intentions to others ('He's doing that just to annoy me') and attributing problems to relatively unchangeable personal traits or characteristics ('He did that because he's irresponsible/stupid/bad'). In cognitive restructuring, first the rigid polarized positions adopted by the parent and adolescent are described. Then, the negative beliefs and attributions that under-pin these are identified and family members are invited to re-evaluate or test these by checking out the other person's position or looking for evidence that contravenes the negative belief. They are then asked to re-frame the other person's action as being due to situational factors or benign intentions.

In structural family therapy (Minuchin, 1974), the over-riding structural goal of therapy is to help parents draw clear and appropriately permeable boundaries between themselves and the teenager, so that he or she can receive a clear, unified parental message about rules of conduct, and a clear and unified sense of support from the parents. This boundary-making may involve challenging cross-generational parent–child coalitions where, for example, rules made by one parent are undermined by another. It may involve challenging an enmeshed family structure where the adolescent is not permitted sufficient privacy and autonomy to individuate and is treated as a five year old rather than a fifteen year old. It may involve challenging a disengaged family structure where few rules are inconsistently applied with lax supervision.

Structural family therapy begins by identifying conflict-laden issues of primary concern and reviewing the way in which family members have tried to resolve these issues. Then, within the session, the family members are invited to re-enact problem-solving attempts and are coached in how to extend their natural problem-solving style further than the point at which they typically become stuck. In this coaching, the therapist may ask one member to withdraw from the discussion while the other two members try to solve the problem. For example, a teenager may be asked to remain silent while parents try to reach agreement on how to manage a discipline issue such as how late he or she should be allowed to stay out on Saturday. The therapist may side temporarily with one family member against another. For example, the therapist may side with the teenager (temporarily) and argue the case for more privacy and autonomy. Or the therapist may side with the parents (temporarily) and push for clearer rules and more supervision.

School intervention

The aim of school-based interventions is to provide the child with an appropriate level of teacher contact, an appropriate curriculum and a contingency management programme.

Where children with ADHD are included in regular classes, an additional teaching assistant for the teaching team working in the main classroom or additional out-of-class remedial tuition is required. This additional resourcing is required to help plan and deliver a modified teaching curriculum using structured behavioural methods to the child. The degree to which the routine class curriculum will require modification will depend on the precise nature of the learning difficulties and attainment problems identified in the psychological assessment. In primary school, most youngsters with ADHD require remedial tuition in reading and mathematics. In secondary school, tutoring in specific subjects may be necessary and study skills training is essential. Assessment of learning difficulties, remedial tuition and study skills training are discussed in Chapter 8.

An important part of the clinical psychologist's responsibilities is to liaise with appropriate colleagues in the educational system and indicate the need for additional resourcing, in a way that is helpful to both the child and the school. Administrative procedures for this type of liaison vary from country to country and district to district. Without appropriate resourcing and appropriate curriculum modification, it is often difficult to offer useful support and advice on behavioural management, since such advice usually involves substantial input from school staff, who are typically over-burdened with responsibilities. Indeed, when school-based behavioural programmes break down it is often because teachers had insufficient time to implement special programmes for the child with ADHD, due to the demands imposed on teachers by other members of the class.

A large body of research shows that children with ADHD may be motivated to develop appropriate academic skills and behaviour at school through the use of home–school reward systems and contingency management programmes (Wells, 2004). Specific target behaviours and academic goals are set jointly by the teacher, child, parent and psychologist, and a points system agreed. Points from this system may be used to buy items from a reinforcement menu at home or to achieve specific agreed privileges in school.

When setting academic targets, the materials should be pitched at the child's attainment level and broken into small units, with reinforcement given for completion of specific academic tasks (such as completion of a work sheet) rather than process behaviours (such as sitting still). Repetitive tasks should be avoided where possible. When setting behavioural targets for which the child can earn reinforcers, they should be highly specific and typically centre on following instructions to behave in a positive way rather than cease behaving in a negative way. A response–cost contingency should be used for rule violations, so that the child loses the number of points he would have gained for complying with the instruction.

Reinforcers (in the form of tokens for children under eight and ticks on a report card for older children) should be delivered immediately and frequently following the execution of target behaviours. When reinforcers are being given or response costs are being implemented, it is more effective to conduct this quietly, without drawing the attention of the class to the process, since the class's response may make both receiving and losing points equally reinforcing. There should be set times when the child can exchange tokens for items on the home or school reinforcement menu.

Once children show that they can respond to a continuous reward system such as this, written contingency contracts may be used, where the child agrees to carry out certain listed target behaviours and in return the teacher and parents agree to certain rewards if the targets are met and certain response costs where targets are not met.

With older children and teenagers, a daily report card system, such as that presented in Figure 10.9 (p. 406), may be used. Following each class, the teacher rates the child's performance on the four or five listed behaviours and initials the card. The points obtained may be used either at home or in school to purchase items from a reinforcement menu.

Child-focused interventions

Self-instructional training to improve academic skills (Meichenbaum, 1977) and a combination of self-awareness training and anger management training (Hinshaw, 1996) to enhance the use of social skills are well-validated, child-focused interventions that are optimally offered within a group context and as one element of a multi-systemic programme.

Self-instructional training aims to compensate for the internal speech deficiency present in ADHD. Initially, the therapist models the use of self-instructions by completing a task while saying self-instructions aloud. Children are next guided by therapist instructions in the completion of academic and social tasks, and later by self-instruction, which is faded to a whisper and then to internal speech (Meichenbaum, 1977). Tasks chosen for self-instructional training should initially be well within the child's competence and, once self-instructional skills have been developed, increasingly challenging tasks may be used. Self-instructions should include self-statements to clarify what the task demands are ('What do I have to do?'); to develop a plan ('I have to draw a picture'); to guide the child through the plan ('I'll hold the pencil and work slowly'); to cope with distraction ('I'll ignore that noise and stick to the job'); and to self-reinforce on-task behaviour ('Well done').

Youngsters with ADHD do not lack knowledge about social skills. Rather, they are unaware of their failure to use them and this leads to many relationship problems, particularly with peers. The match game can be used to help youngsters develop self-monitoring skills so that they can evaluate the degree to which their behaviour conforms to social norms (Hinshaw, 1996). In the match game, a target behaviour is chosen, for example co-operation with other group members. Then a recreational or academic group activity occurs, such as playing ball, telling stories, drawing or completing schoolwork. Throughout this period the therapist reinforces the target behaviour using tokens or points. After a period of an hour each child rates the degree to which he or she believes they performed the target behaviour throughout the hour on a five-point scale. The therapist also rates each child on a five-point scale. If a child's self-rating matches the therapist's rating then extra tokens are earned during the first few sessions of such a programme. Later in the programme the child must try to score above a particular level set by the therapist on the five-point rating scale and also match the therapist's rating of their behaviour in order to earn tokens in the match game. Most of the learning occurs at the end of each hour, when group members discuss the reason why discrepancies occurred between their ratings and the therapist's ratings of their behaviour. This type of discussion helps youngsters develop more accurate self-awareness concerning the degree to which they exhibit socially appropriate or inappropriate behaviour, a skill in which children with ADHD are deficient and which under-pins some of their relationship difficulties.

Controlling impulses, particularly aggressive impulses, may under-pin some of the peer-relationship difficulties shown by youngsters with ADHD. Hinshaw (1996) has shown that Novaco's anger management programme may be effective in reducing impulsive aggression among youngsters with ADHD (Feindler & Ecton, 1985; Novaco, 1975). In a group setting, youngsters are trained to recognize internal and external cues that precede episodes where impulsive anger is likely. They are then trained to identify coping strategies to avoid acting out the anger, such as breathing deeply or relaxing to reduce arousal, withdrawing from the situation, distracting themselves by counting to ten or thinking of something else, re-framing the provocation so that it is less provocative and using self-instructions to calm down. Once these skills have been learned, the therapist, by consent, arranges for each group member to be exposed to increasingly provocative situations. When one person is learning to use anger control skills, other group members are enlisted to taunt and provoke him. Successful anger control is reinforced by the therapist.

Dietary interventions

Egger et al. (1985) have shown that careful food allergy testing in specific cases may lead to the identification of a unique profile of substances, such as milk or wheat, to which children with ADHD are allergic. These foods may then be eliminated from the child's diet. Referral for paediatric and dietetic consultations are appropriate here.

Interventions for co-morbid problems

Where youngsters with ADHD have co-morbid problems, such as enuresis or depression, these may be assessed and managed concurrently following the guidelines for those problems presented elsewhere in this text.

SUMMARY

Attention deficit hyperactivity disorder is currently the most common term used for a syndrome characterized by persistent over-activity, impulsivity and difficulties in sustaining attention. About 1% of children have the extreme form of this syndrome, which is typically lifelong. Co-morbid developmental language delays, specific learning difficulties, elimination disorders, conduct disorders and emotional disorders are quite common. A poor outcome occurs for about a third of cases, who typically have secondary conduct and academic problems. Available evidence suggests that a marked genetic predisposition for an over-active temperament, which finds expression as a result of exposure to physical and psychosocial environmental risk factors during the pre- and peri-natal periods and early infancy, causes the syndrome. Adjustment problems shown by youngsters with ADHD are in part maintained by problematic relationships within the family, school and peer group. Multi-systemic treatment includes psychoeducation, psychostimulant treatment, family intervention, school intervention, self-regulation skills training and dietary control where food intolerance is present. In addition, assessment and treatment of co-morbid problems may be required.

EXERCISE 11.1

Work in groups of three to take the roles of psychologist and the parents in the case example presented in Box 11.1. The psychologist is invited to help the parents to set up a reinforcement menu and a list of target jobs or chores to be completed. Conduct this consultation as if it occurs halfway into a parent training programme and assume that a good relationship has developed.

EXERCISE 11.2

Four people take on the roles of the family members in the case example presented in Box 11.1. At least two others take the roles of a treatment team. Imagine Timmy is now 13. The family has returned for a further episode of treatment and has been working with you for two weeks. The main focus of concern is Timmy's refusal to come in on time at night. Help the family to use five-step problem solving to find a solution to this problem.

FURTHER READING

Barkley, R. (1997). *Defiant Children: A Clinician's manual for Parent Training* (Second Edition). New York: Guilford Press.

Barkley, R. (1998). *Attention Deficit Hyperactivity Disorder: A Handbook for Diagnosis and Treatment* (Second Edition). New York. Guilford.

Barkley, R. & Murphy, K. (1998). *Attention Deficit Hyperactivity Disorder: A Clinical Work* (Second Edition). New York: Guilford.

FURTHER READING FOR CLIENTS

Barkley, R. (2000). *Taking Charge of ADHD: The Complete Authoritative Guide for Parents* (Revised Edition). New York: Guilford.

Wender, P. (1987). *The Hyperactive Child Adolescent and Adult. Attention Deficit Disorder Through The Lifespan*. New York: Oxford University Press.

Quinn, P., Stern, J., & Russell, N. (1998). *The 'Putting on the Brakes' Activity Book for Young People with ADHD*. Washington, DC: Magination Press.

Quinn, P., Stern, J., & Russell, N. (2001). *Putting on the Brakes: Young People's Guide to Understanding Attention Deficit Hyperactivity Disorder*. Washington, DC: Magination Press.

Nadeau, K., Dixon, E., & Rose, J. (1998). *Learning to Slow Down and Pay Attention: A Book for Kids About ADD*. Washington, DC: Magination Press.

WEBSITES

ADDNet, the UK ADHD Website: http://www.btinternet.com/~black.ice/addnet/
ADHD website: http://www.mentalhealth.org.uk/page.cfm?pagecode=PMAMADWB
Attention Deficit Disorder Association, the US association: http://www.add.org/
New Zealand ADHD website: http://www.adhd.org.nz/
NICE Guidelines for treatment of ADHD with methylphenidate: http://www.nice.org.uk/pdf/Methylph-guidance13.pdf

Videos and manuals for parents and teachers produced by Russell Barclay include 'ADHD: What do we know?'; 'ADHD: What can we do?'; 'ADHD in the Classroom: Strategies for teachers'. They are available from: http://www.parinc.com

Factsheets on ADHD can be downloaded from the website for Rose, G. & York, A. (2004). *Mental Health and Growing Up. Fact sheets for Parents, Teachers and Young People* (Third edition). London: Gaskell: http://www.rcpsych.ac.uk

Chapter 12

Fear and anxiety problems

After considering normal fear, this chapter considers abnormal anxiety and its development, and the classification and epidemiology of anxiety disorders. There is then a discussion of the clinical features, aetiological theories, assessment, formulation and management of anxiety disorders in general. This is followed by detailed guidelines on the treatment of specific anxiety disorders, including separation anxiety, elective mutism, specific phobias, social phobia, generalized anxiety disorder, panic disorder and post-traumatic stress disorder.

Fear is the natural response to a stimulus that poses a threat to well-being, safety or security. This response includes cognitive, affective, physiological, behavioural and relational aspects (Morris & March, 2004; Ollendick & March, 2003; Silverman & Treffers, 2001). At a cognitive level, the stimulus or situation is construed as threatening or dangerous. At an affective level, there are feelings of apprehension, tension and uneasiness. At a physiological level, autonomic arousal occurs so as to prepare the person to neutralize the threat by fighting or fleeing from danger. With respect to behaviour, individuals may either aggressively approach and confront the danger, especially if they are trapped, or apprehensively avoid it. In the face of extreme threat, however, the person may become immobilized. The interpretation of situations as threatening and the patterning of aggressive or avoidant behaviour are both determined by, and have an impact on, the relational context within which they occur. For children, this context usually includes parents, siblings, school teachers and peers. From this analysis, it is apparent that fear is an adaptive response to danger. It is adaptive for the survival of the individual and, from an evolutionary perspective, it is adaptive for the survival of the species.

DEVELOPMENT OF FEARS AND ANXIETIES

From infancy through childhood into adolescence, the types of stimuli which elicit fear change, and these changes parallel developments in the individual's cognitive and social competencies and concerns (Ollendick, King & Yule, 1994; Öst & Treffers, 2001; Westenberg, Siebelink & Treffers, 2001). Stimuli which elicit fear at different stages of development are listed in Table 12.1. In the first six months, extreme stimulation such as loud sounds or loss of support elicit fear. However, with the development of object constancy and cause and effect schemas during the latter half of the first year, a normal concern about separation appears and the child fears strangers and separation from

Table 12.1 Fears at different ages

Age	Psychological and social competencies and concerns relevant to development of fears, phobias and anxiety	Principal sources of fear	Principal anxiety disorders
Early infancy 0–6 months	• Sensory abilities dominate infants' adaptation	• Intense sensory stimuli • Loss of support • Loud noises	
Late infancy 6–12 months	• Sensorimotor schemas • Cause and effect • Object constancy	• Strangers • Separation	
Toddler years 2–4 years	• Pre-operational thinking • Capacity to imagine but inability to distinguish fantasy from reality	• Imaginary creatures • Potential burglars • The dark	• Separation anxiety* • Selective mutism
Early childhood 5–7 years	• Concrete operational thinking • Capacity to think in concrete logical terms	• Natural disasters (fire flood thunder) • Injury • Animals • Media-based fears	• Animal phobia • Blood phobia
Middle childhood 8–11 years	• Esteem centres on academic and athletic performance in school	• Poor academic and athletic performance	• Test anxiety • School phobia
Adolescence 12–18 years	• Formal operational thought • Capacity to anticipate future dangers • Esteem is derived from peer relationships	• Peer rejection	• Social phobias • Agoraphobia • Panic disorder

Note: Based on Ollendick et al. (1994).
* Separation anxiety appears in early childhood but peaks in late childhood.

caretakers. In the toddler years, during the pre-operational period, the skills required for make-believe and imagination develop but those for distinguishing fantasy from reality are not yet acquired, and the child comes to fear imaginary or supernatural creatures. At this time mobility also increases and children come to fear animals and potential burglars. In early childhood, as their awareness of the natural world and of the world portrayed on the media develops, children come to fear natural disasters such as floods or thunder and lightening, and media-based fears such as epidemics of diseases. In middle childhood, failure in academic and athletic performance at school become a source of fear. With the onset of adolescence, the period of formal operational thinking, the capacity for abstract thought emerges. The youngster can project what will happen in the future and anticipate with considerable sophistication potential hazards, threats and dangers in many domains, particularly that of social relationships. Fears about peer rejection emerge at this stage.

A distinction may be made between normal adaptive fears, which are premised on an accurate appraisal of the potential threat posed by a stimulus or situation, and maladaptive fears, which are based on an inaccurate appraisal of the threat to well-being (Ollendick et al., 1994). Such maladaptive fear is usually referred to as anxiety. With phobic anxiety, the eliciting stimuli are confined to a clearly defined class of objects, events or situations. For example, a child with a dog phobia may appraise all dogs to be potentially dangerous because they may bite, and experience intense fear even when approached by a dog that has been shown to be tame and well trained. With generalized anxiety, the class of eliciting stimuli is less circumscribed and many aspects of the environment are interpreted as potentially threatening, even when there are no reasonable grounds for anticipating danger. Thus the person experiences a high ongoing level of anxiety. Spielberger (1973) has referred to phobic and generalized anxiety as state and trait anxiety, respectively. State anxiety is an acute transient experience which occurs in specific situations. Trait anxiety is a stable, enduring, chronic condition characterized by hyperarousal. Spielberger (1973) has developed a useful set of self-report questionnaires to measure state and trait anxiety in children (see Table 12.10, p. 498).

Table 12.1 shows that the emergence of maladaptive fears or anxieties, which involve the inaccurate appraisal of the potential threat posed by stimuli, follows a developmental course which parallels that of normal fears. Separation anxiety may present as a clinically significant problem at the transition to school, although it is noteworthy that separation anxiety disorder is most prevalent among children in middle childhood. Selective mutism, which is increasingly being conceptualized as an early variant of social phobia, also occurs first during the pre-school years (Freeman, Garcia, Miller, Dow & Leonard, 2004). The onset of animal phobias is most prevalent in early childhood. The onset of test anxiety and other types of performance anxiety peaks in middle childhood. Social anxiety, panic disorder and agoraphobia, which often occurs secondary to panic disorder, tend to first appear in adolescence, along with generalized anxiety.

From a clinical perspective, children are typically referred for treatment of an anxiety problem when it prevents them from completing developmentally appropriate tasks such as going to school or socializing with friends.

CLASSIFICATION

A system for classifying anxiety problems must take account of the developmental timing of their emergence, the classes of stimuli that elicit the anxiety, the pervasiveness and the topography of the anxiety response, and the role of clearly identifiable factors in the aetiology of the anxiety. Some attempt is made within both DSM IV TR (APA, 2000a) and ICD 10 (WHO, 1992, 1996) to take account of these various factors, as may be seen in Figures 12.1 and 12.2. Separation anxiety and selective mutism are clearly designated as childhood disorders in both systems. Furthermore, both systems distinguish between specific phobias, which are elicited by a designated class of stimuli, and generalized anxiety disorder, where many stimuli elicit the anxiety response. Among the phobias, distinctions are made between specific phobias, where the class of eliciting stimuli is narrow and the effects on the person's adjustment may be quite circumscribed on the one hand, and social phobia and agoraphobia where a broader class of stimuli are involved and the impact on the person's adjustment may be more pervasive on the other. Panic disorder, where discrete episodes of intense anxiety occur, is distinguished from other conditions, such as generalized anxiety disorder which have a different topography, with a moderate level of anxiety being experienced over a protracted time period. In both systems, post-traumatic stress disorder (PTSD), where a clear historical event may be pin-pointed as central to the aetiology of the condition, is distinguished from other anxiety disorders where such aetiological factors are not identifiable.

Obsessive-compulsive disorder (OCD) is classified with the anxiety disorders in both DSM IV TR and ICD 10. This decision may be due to the fact that eliciting stimuli give rise to obsessional anxiety which is avoided through the execution of compulsive rituals. On the grounds that OCD shares a genetic diathesis with tic disorders and, like tic disorders, involves repetitive actions which interfere with adjustment, I have elected to deal with both OCD and tic disorders elsewhere (in Chapter 13).

Both DSM IV TR and ICD 10 contain a number of less-clearly defined categories for anxiety disorders about which little is known, such as adjustment disorder characterized by anxiety.

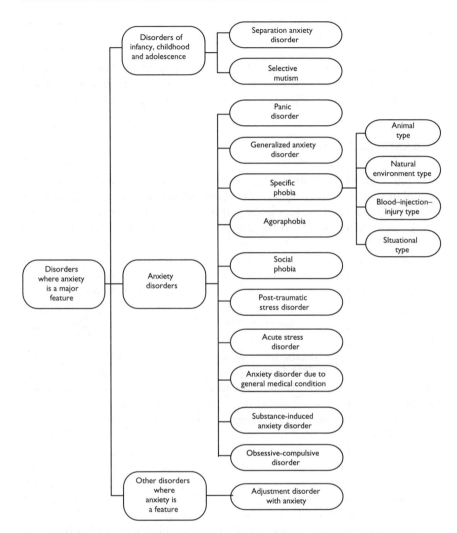

Figure 12.1 Classification of disorders where anxiety is a major feature in DSM IV TR

EPIDEMIOLOGY

Reviews of major epidemiological studies of childhood anxiety disorders allow the following conclusions to be drawn (Carr, 2004b; Freeman et al., 2004; Klein & Pine, 2002; Öst & Treffers, 2001; Verhulst, 2001): the overall prevalence for anxiety disorders in children and adolescents is approximately 6–10%, the approximate prevalence of separation anxiety is 3%, of selective mutism is less than 1%, of simple phobias is 3%, of social phobias is 1%, of

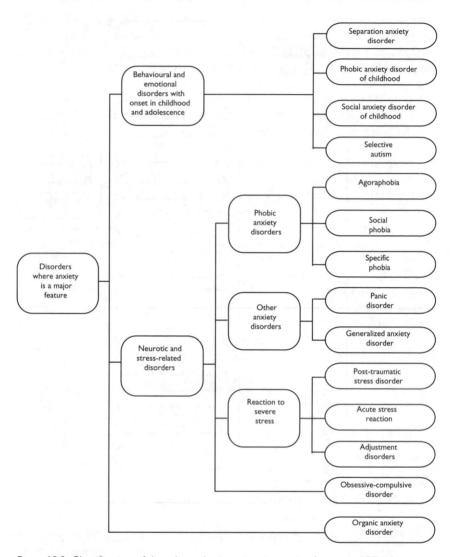

Figure 12.2 Classification of disorders where anxiety is a major feature in ICD 10

generalized anxiety disorders is 2% and of panic disorder is less than 1%. Community surveys show that 13–43% of girls and boys have experienced at least one traumatic event in their lifetime and, of these, 3–15% of girls and 1–6% of boys develop PTSD. Many children meet criteria for two or more anxiety disorders, so the prevalence rates for individual disorders sum to more than 10%.

Anxiety disorders are more prevalent in boys than girls. With respect to age trends, it has already been noted that separation anxiety, selective mutism and simple phobias are more common among pre-adolescents and generalized anxiety disorder, panic disorder and social phobia are more common among adolescents. Childhood anxiety disorders place children at risk for anxiety and mood disorders in adulthood.

Co-morbidity among anxiety disorders is quite high. In clinical samples, 50% of cases with one anxiety disorder also meet the diagnostic criteria for another anxiety disorder. In community samples, up to 39% of cases meet the criteria for two or more anxiety disorders.

From Table 3.4 (p. 86), it may be seen that co-morbidity rates for anxiety disorders with other disorders is also quite high in community populations. Co-morbidity with major depression is 16.2%, with conduct disorders is 14.8% and with attention deficit hyperactivity disorder is 11.8%.

Cases falling above the clinical cut-off score on the anxious/depressed syndrome scale of the Child Behaviour Checklist have clinically significant anxiety symptoms and epidemiological data concerning such children are therefore relevant here. Co-morbidity rates for such cases in community and clinic samples for other types of problem are presented in Table 3.5 (p. 87). For parent-reported symptomatology in clinic samples, it may be seen that the co-morbidity rate for the anxious/depressed syndrome with aggressive behaviour is 41%, with attention problems it is 43% and with somatic complaints it is 30%. For parent-reported symptomatology in community samples, it may be seen that the co-morbidity rates for the anxious/depressed syndrome with other types of problems is much lower. With aggressive behaviour, the co-morbidity rate is 26%, with attention problems it is 28% and with somatic complaints the rate is 15%. This pattern of higher co-morbidity rates in clinic compared with community samples is a ubiquitous finding and not unique to anxiety disorders.

DIAGNOSIS AND CLINICAL FEATURES

With separation anxiety, inappropriate fear is aroused by separation from an attachment figure. Although not the only cause of school refusal, it is one of the most common causes of this complaint. A typical case of separation anxiety and school refusal is presented in Box 12.1 and diagnostic criteria for separation anxiety from DSM IV TR (APA, 2000a) and ICD 10 (1992, 1996) are presented in Table 12.2. Separation anxiety with chronic school refusal is a serious condition since it has such a poor prognosis if left untreated. Some youngsters with this condition go on to develop panic disorder and agoraphobia (Silverman & Dick-Niederhauser, 2004).

With selective mutism the child speaks at home or with close friends and is mute at pre-school or school or with strangers. The condition typically begins in the pre-school years and is associated with social anxiety. A typical

Box 12.1 A case of separation anxiety and school refusal

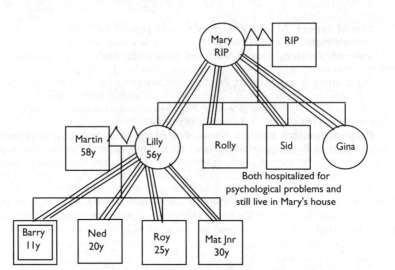

Both hospitalized for psychological problems and still live in Mary's house

Three brothers live at home and all had separation anxiety and school refusal in secondary school

Referral. Barry, aged eleven, was referred because he had not attended school for two months, following the Easter holidays in the year prior to his entry to secondary school. The family doctor could find no organic basis for the abdominal pain or headaches of which he periodically complained, particularly on the mornings when his mother asked him how his health was. Barry's friends visited him at week-ends and he went off cycling with them regularly. But on Monday mornings he was unable to get to school both because of the abdominal pains and also because of a sense of foreboding that something dangerous might happen to his mother. If forced to go to school he would become tearful or aggressive.

Family history. While, there was no serious threat to Barry's mother's health, Lilly, had a variety of complaints including rheumatism and epilepsy which compromised her sense of well-being. Her epilepsy was usually well controlled, but Lilly had experienced a number of grand mal fits in the six months prior to the referral. Barry was one of four children and all had histories of school refusal. Barry's three brothers aged 20, 25 and 30 all lived at home and had few friends or acquaintances. His eldest brother ran a computer software business from his bedroom. All of the boys had very close relationships with their mother and distant relationships with their father. The father, Martin, who was a healthy man, ran a corner shop and worked long hours. He left early in the morning and returned late at night. He was very concerned for the welfare of his son, Barry, and believed that his wife, Lilly, mollycoddled the boy. But he was reluctant to challenge her because he did not want to upset her. The parents had a history of marital discord and over the year prior to the referral had strongly disagreed about how to handle the boy's separation anxiety.

Two of Barry's uncles had psychological adjustment difficulties and both had been on medication, although, details of their problems were unavailable. These uncles had lived at home with their mother until her death and both of them and Lilly and her sister Gina had very close relationships with their mother, Mary, but distant relationships with their father. Lilly's parents had also quarrelled about how best to manage the children, with Mary being lenient and her husband being strict. Thus, the pattern of relationships in both Lilly's family of origin and Barry's family were very similar as can be seen from the genogram.

School report. At school, Barry was very popular, particularly because he generously shared candy and sweets from his father's shop with his peers. He had complained of bullying once or twice and on one occasion said the gym teacher victimized him.

Psychometric assessment. Psychometric assessment showed that Barry was of high average intelligence and his attainments in reading, spelling and arithmetic were consistent with his overall level of ability. His school reports were good and he was in the top third of his class with respect to ability.

Formulation. Pre-disposing factors in this case include a possible genetic vulnerability to psychological adjustment problem and the modelling experience of seeing his three brothers develop separation anxiety and subsequent school refusal. Barry's anticipation of the transition to secondary school in the autumn and his awareness of his mother's worsening health may have precipitated the onset of the separation anxiety. The anxiety and the school refusal were maintained by his mother's over-concern and the father's limited involvement in the management of the child's difficulties. It may also have been maintained by the availability of an active social life within the house (involving contact with his mother and three brothers) during school hours and outside school hours at the week-end. Protective factors included the good relationships that Barry had with both his teachers and peers at school and the willingness of the father to become involved in treatment.

Treatment. Treatment involved a series of family sessions and home–school liaison with the parents and school staff. Martin, the father eventually agreed to drive Barry to school regularly for a month and for a teacher to meet Barry in the car park and bring him into the classroom where he was to sit with two peers and work on a special project for 20 minutes before class started each day. Concurrently, weekly family sessions were held in which progress was assessed; a reward system for school attendance was set up; and the transition to secondary school was discussed. The mother, Lilly, also arranged for a series of consultations for her epilepsy, which became better controlled. Barry returned to school and moved to secondary school in the autumn. However, after Christmas, he relapsed and attempts to use a similar approach to treatment were unsuccessful. After missing a year of schooling he eventually was placed at a small tutorial centre where he remained until 16.

---

case of selective mutism is presented in Box 12.2 and diagnostic criteria from DSM IV TR and ICD 10 (in which the condition is termed elective mutism) are presented in Table 12.3.

Phobic anxiety is the intense fear which occurs when faced with an object, event or situation from a clearly definably class of stimuli which is out of proportion to the danger posed by the stimulus, and leads to persistent avoidance. In DSM IV TR, specific phobias are distinguished from social phobias and agoraphobia. Specific phobias are sub-divided in DSM IV TR into those associated with animals, injury (including injections), features of the natural environment (such as heights or thunder) and particular situations (such as elevators or flying). An example of a simple phobia is presented in Box 12.3

Table 12.2 Diagnostic criteria for separation anxiety disorder from DSM IV TR and ICD 10

DSM IV TR	ICD 10
A. Developmentally inappropriate and excessive anxiety concerning separation from home or those to whom the individual is attached as evidenced by three or more of the following: 1. Recurrent excessive distress when separation from home or major attachment figures occurs or is anticipated 2. Persistent and excessive worry about losing or about possible harm befalling a major attachment figure 3. Persistent and excessive worry that an untoward event will lead to separation from a major attachment figure (e.g. getting lost or being kidnapped) 4. Persistent reluctance or refusal to go to school or elsewhere because of fear of separation 5. Persistently and excessively fearful or reluctant to be alone or without major attachment figures at home or without significant adults in other settings 6. Persistent reluctance or refusal to go to sleep without being near a major attachment figure or to sleep away from home 7. Repeated night-mares about separation 8. Repeated complaints of physical symptoms (headaches, stomachaches, nausea and vomiting) when separation from major attachment figures occurs or is anticipated B. The disturbance last for at least 4 weeks C. It occurs before 18 years of age D. The disorder causes clinically significant distress or impairment of social or academic functioning E. The disorder does not occur exclusively during the course of a psychotic disorder and is not accounted for by panic disorder with agoraphobia	The diagnostic feature is a focused excessive anxiety concerning separation from those individuals to whom the child is attached that is not merely part of a generalized anxiety about multiple situations. The anxiety may take the form of: a. An unrealistic preoccupying worry about possible harm befalling major attachment figures or a fear that they will leave and not return b. An unrealistic preoccupying worry that some untoward event such as the child being lost, kidnapped or admitted to hospital will separate him or her from a major attachment figure c. Persistent reluctance or refusal to go to school because of fear about separation (rather than fear of events at school) d. Persistent reluctance or refusal to go to sleep without being near or next to a major attachment figure e. Persistent inappropriate fear of being alone f. Repeated night-mares about separation g. Repeated occurrence of physical symptoms (stomachaches or headaches) on occasions involving separation h. Excessive recurrent distress in anticipation of, during or after separation from a major attachment figure School refusal often represents separation anxiety but sometimes, especially in adolescence, it does not. The diagnosis rests on the demonstration that the common element giving rise to anxiety is separation from a major attachment figure

Note: Adapted from DSM IV TR (APA, 2000a) and ICD 10 (WHO, 1992, 1996).

and diagnostic criteria for both specific phobias and social phobias are presented in Table 12.4. With social phobias, the principal fear is of being evaluated by other unfamiliar people and behaving in an embarrassing way while under their scrutiny. Social phobia leads to a constricted social life.

Box 12.2 A case of selective mutism

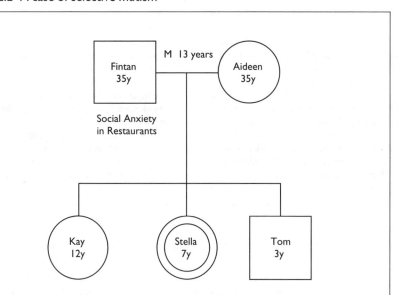

Referral. Stella Crow, a seven-year-old girl, referred by her general practitioner, had a four-year history of elective mutism, the onset of which coincided with the birth of her younger brother. Her refusal to speak was first noted at that time by the teachers at the playschool which she was attending. As a toddler, she got lost in a large shopping centre in a neighbouring town, and since then had displayed a strong fear of being left alone with strangers, a reluctance to venture far from the house alone and a marked reduction in the number of people with whom she was willing to talk. When we first met the Crows, Stella had been attending primary school for two years and had never spoken in that environment.

Family history. Stella lived with her parents, her older sister Kay (12 years) and her younger brother Tom (3 years). The parents were well adjusted, although Mr Crow has a history of mild social anxiety which prevented him from eating in restaurants on some occasions.

Past treatment. The school staff had initially waited for Stella to grow out of her mutism before taking a more active approach to the problem. After a year of little progress, the school staff, in conjunction with Mrs Crow, devised and implemented a programme during which Stella would read to her mother in the school classroom, while the teacher watched from a gradually reduced distance. Stella was making such good progress in reading aloud in the presence of the teacher that Mrs Crow silently left the classroom on one occasion, hoping that this would accelerate her programme. Unfortunately it precipitated a relapse. At the time of referral, some months after this incident, Stella's school, family and peer group had all accepted her elective mutism and developed ways of accommodating it. For example, her parents would taperecord her reading at home and bring this to school so that the school could provide Stella with reading material to match her ability. Her peers at school would communicate with her in sign language or by passing notes.

Formulation. Stella may have been pre-disposed to developing selective mutism because she had an inhibited temperament, probably inherited from her father. The onset of the condition was precipitated by the incident where she got lost while shopping. It was then exacerbated by the incident where, without Stella's consent, her mother left the classroom while Stella was reading to her mother and teacher. There were two maintaining factors. First, the mutism reduced social anxiety, and second, the parents, teachers and peers had accommodated to the mutism.

Treatment. A stimulus-fading programme was conducted on a daily basis over 8 weeks in which, through graded steps, Stella moved from reading to her mother sitting in close proximity in the school classroom to a situation where she read to her mother who stood just outside the doorway of the classroom. Concurrently, Stella's teacher and close friends, over the 8-week treatment programme, gradually moved from listening to her reading from outside the door to listening while sitting in close proximity to her. As Stella progressed through this programme and tolerated her mother's increasing distance and the greater proximity of her teacher and friends, she was rewarded with tokens for achieving each step. She exchanged these tokens for valued treats. After 8 weeks Stella spontaneously began to speak in class.

When youngsters experience generalized anxiety, they have an ongoing apprehension that misfortunes of various sorts will occur. Their anxiety is not focused on one particular object or situation. The child may also fear that he or she cannot stop worrying. An example of a case of generalized anxiety disorder is presented in Box 12.4 and diagnostic criteria are set out in Table 12.5.

With panic disorder there are recurrent unexpected panic attacks. These attacks are experienced as acute episodes of intense anxiety and are extremely distressing. Youngsters come to perceive normal fluctuations in autonomic arousal as anxiety provoking, since they may reflect the onset of a panic attack. Commonly, secondary agoraphobia develops. The youngster fears leaving the safety of the home in case a panic attack occurs in a public setting. A case example of panic attacks with agoraphobia is presented in Box 12.5 and diagnostic criteria for panic disorder and for agoraphobia are presented in Table 12.6.

Post-traumatic stress disorder (PTSD) occurs in many children following a catastrophic trauma which the child perceived to be potentially life-threatening for themselves or others. In PTSD, children have recurrent intrusive memories of the trauma that leads to intense anxiety. They try to avoid this by suppressing the memories and avoiding situations that remind them of the trauma. A case example of PTSD is presented in Box 12.6 and diagnostic criteria are set out in Table 12.7.

The clinical features of the six types of anxiety disorders described above are presented in Table 12.8. Clinical features in the domains of perception, cognition, affect, arousal, behaviour and interpersonal adjustment are given. With respect to perception, the six disorders differ in the classes of stimuli which elicit anxiety. With separation anxiety, the stimulus is separation from the caregiver. With selective mutism, the stimulus is threatening social situations. For phobias it is specific creatures (e.g. animals), events (e.g. injury),

Table 12.3 Diagnostic criteria for selective mutism from DSM IV TR and ICD 10

DSM IV TR *Selective mutism*	ICD 10 *Elective mutism*
A. Consistent failure to speak in specific social situations (in which there is an expectation for speaking, e.g. at school) despite speaking in other situations B. The disturbance interferes with educational or occupational achievement or with social communication C. The disturbance lasts for at least 1 month (not limited to the first month of school) D. Failure to speak is not due to lack of knowledge, or comfort with the spoken language required in the social situation E. The disturbance is not better accounted for by a communication disorder (e.g. stuttering) and does not occur exclusively during the course of a pervasive developmental disorder, schizophrenia or other psychotic disorder	The condition is characterized by a marked, emotionally determined selectivity in speaking, such that the child demonstrates his or her language competence in some situations but fails to speak in other (definable) situations. Most frequently the disorder is first manifest in early childhood. It occurs with the same frequency in the two sexes. It is usual for the mutism to be associated with marked personality features involving social anxiety, social withdrawal, social sensitivity and resistance or oppositional behaviour. Typically, the child speaks at home or with close friends and is mute at school or with strangers, but other patterns (including the converse) can occur. A substantial minority of children with selective mutism have a history of either some speech delay or articulation problems The diagnosis presupposes: (a) a normal or near-normal level of language comprehension; (b) a level of competence in language expression that is sufficient for social communication; and (c) demonstrable evidence that the individual can and does speak normally or almost normally in some situations The diagnosis excludes transient mutism as part of separation anxiety in young children, specific developmental disorders of speech and language, pervasive developmental disorders and schizophrenia

or situations (e.g. meeting new people) that elicits anxiety. With generalized anxiety disorder, the person interprets many aspects of the environment as potentially threatening. In panic disorder, somatic sensations of arousal such as tachycardia are perceived as threatening since they are expected to lead to a full-blown panic attack. With PTSD, internal and external cues that remind the person of the trauma that led to the disorder elicit anxiety.

Cognitions in all six anxiety disorders have the detection and/or avoidance

Box 12.3 A case of a specific phobia

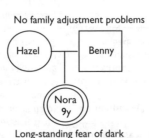

No family adjustment problems

Long-standing fear of dark

Nora, aged 9, was referred because of her fear of the dark. She wanted to go on a camping trip with the Brownies but was frightened because she would have to sleep in complete darkness. This was something she had never done. She always slept with the light on in her bedroom and with the door open and the landing light on. Her developmental history was unremarkable and she had never experienced a traumatic incident in the darkness. Her parents had tried to convince her to sleep with the light off, but she became so distressed on these occasions that they had stopped making such attempts and believed that she would eventually grow out of the darkness phobia. Nora was an only child and there was no family history of anxiety disorders or adjustment problems, nor was there a developmental history of a particularly traumatic incident. This uncomplicated simple phobia was treated with in vivo, parent-assisted systematic desensitization. Nora went camping and successfully slept in a dark tent for three nights.

of danger as the central organizing theme. In separation anxiety, children believe that they or their parents will be harmed if separation occurs. With selective mutism, the child believes that something threatening will happen if he or she speaks in school or other situations in which mutism occurs. With phobias, the child believes that contact with the feared object or creature, or entry into the feared situation, will result in harm, such as being bitten by a dog in the case of dog phobia or being negatively judged by strangers in the case of social phobia. With generalized anxiety, children catastrophize about many features of their environment. For example, they may fear that the house will burn down, their parents' car will crash, they will be punished for soiling their clothes, their friends will leave them and so forth. In panic disorder, the child believes that further panic attacks may be fatal and often secondary beliefs evolve that lead to agoraphobia. That is, youngsters believe that provided they stay in the safety of the home, the panic attacks are less likely to occur. With PTSD, there is a belief that provided the memories of the trauma are excluded from consciousness, the danger of re-experiencing the intense fear and danger associated with the trauma that led to PTSD can be avoided.

In all six of the anxiety disorders listed in Table 12.8, the beliefs about threat and danger are accompanied by an affective state, characterized by

Table 12.4 Diagnostic criteria for phobias from DSM IV TR and ICD 10

	DSM IV TR	ICD 10
Specific phobia	A. Marked and persistent fear that is excessive or unreasonable, cued by the presence or anticipation of a specific object or situation (e.g. flying, heights, animals, an injection, blood) B. Exposure to the phobic stimulus produces an immediate anxiety response which may take the form of a panic attack or, in children, may involve crying, tantrums, freezing or, clinging C. The person recognizes that the fear is excessive or unreasonable, although this feature may be absent in children D. The phobic situation is avoided or endured with intense anxiety or distress E. The avoidance or anxiety interferes significantly with personal, social or academic functioning F. If under 18 years of age, the duration is at least 6 months G. The anxiety and avoidance is not better accounted for by another disorder	Simple phobias are restricted to highly specific situations such as particular animals, heights, darkness, thunder, urinating or defecating in public toilets, the sight of blood and fear of exposure to specific diseases such as AIDS or VD All of the following must be fulfilled for a definite diagnosis: a. The psychological or autonomic symptoms must be primarily manifestations of anxiety and not secondary to other symptoms such as delusions or obsessional thoughts b. The anxiety must be restricted to the presence of a specific phobic object c. The phobic situation is avoided whenever possible
Social phobia	A. A marked or persistent fear of one or more social or performance situations in which the person is exposed to unfamiliar people or to possible scrutiny by others. The individual fears that he or she will act in a way that will be humiliating or embarrassing. In children the child must have the capacity for age-appropriate relationships with familiar people and the anxiety occurs in peer-group settings	Social phobias are centred around a fear of scrutiny by other people in comparatively small groups (as opposed to crowds), leading to avoidance of social situations. They may be discrete (i.e. restricted to eating in public, to public speaking, or to encounters with the opposite sex) or diffuse involving almost all social situations outside the family circle

Continued

Table 12.4 continued

	DSM IV TR	ICD 10
	B. Exposure to the feared social situation produces an immediate anxiety response, which may take the form of a panic attack or in children may involve crying, tantrums, freezing or shrinking from social situations with unfamiliar people	All of the following should be fulfilled for a definite diagnosis: a. The psychological or autonomic symptoms must be primarily manifestations of anxiety and not secondary to other symptoms such as delusions or obsessional thoughts
	C. The person recognizes that the fear is excessive or unreasonable, although this feature may be absent in children	b. The anxiety must be restricted to or predominate in particular social situations c. Avoidance of the phobic situations must be a prominent feature
	D. The feared social situations are avoided or endured with intense anxiety or distress	
	E. The avoidance or anxiety interferes significantly with personal, social or academic functioning	
	F. If under 18 years of age the duration is at least 6 months	
	G. The anxiety and avoidance is not better accounted for by another disorder	
	H. The fear is not related to a general medical or psychological condition such as Parkinson's disease or stuttering	

Note: Adapted from DSM IV TR (APA, 2000) and ICD 10 (WHO, 1992, 1996).

feelings of tension, restlessness and uneasiness. If the child is compelled to approach the feared stimuli, outbursts of anger may occur. For example, children with separation anxiety may have aggressive tantrums if forced to remain at school while their mothers leave. Similarly, selectively mute children may become oppositional if strongly urged to speak in school or other threatening situations. A similar display of anger may occur if children with water phobia are carried into a swimming pool by well-intentioned parents trying to teach them to swim. In PTSD, in addition to the affective experiences of uneasiness and tension, an affective experience of emotional blunting, arising from the child's attempt to exclude all affective material from consciousness may develop.

Box 12.4 A case of generalized anxiety disorder

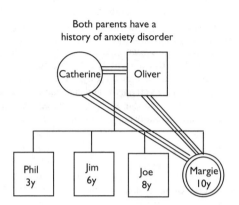

Both parents have a
history of anxiety disorder

Catherine Oliver

| Phil 3y | Jim 6y | Joe 8y | Margie 10y |

Referral. Margie, aged ten was referred because of excessive tearfulness in school, which had been gradually worsening over a number of months. The tearfulness was unpredictable. She would often cry when spoken to by the teacher or while playing with her friends during break time. In the referral letter her family doctor described her as *a worrier, like her mother.*

Presentation. In the intake interview Margie said that she worried about many routine daily activities and responsibilities. She worried about doing poorly at school, that she had made mistakes which would later be discovered, that her friends wouldn't like her, that her parents would be disappointed with the way she did her household jobs, that she would be either too early or too late for the school bus, that there would be no room for her on the bus and that she would forget her school books. She worried about her health and had frequent stomachaches. She also had wider-ranging fears about the safety of her family. She worried that the house would be struck by lightning, that the river would break its banks and flood the low-lying fens where she lived and that her house would be washed away. She had concerns about the future and worried that she would fail her exams; be unable to find a satisfactory job; fail to find a marital partner or marry an unsuitable person. She reported feeling continually restless and unable to relax.

Psychometric assessment. On the Child Behaviour Checklist and Teacher Report form Margie scored above the clinical cut-off for the Internalizing scale and showed elevations on all internalizing sub-scales. A psychometric assessment of her abilities showed that her IQ fell within the normal range and that her attainments in reading, spelling and arithmetic were consistent with her overall level of ability.

Family history. Margie was the eldest of four children and the only girl in the family. Both of her parents showed symptoms of anxiety in the intake interview and her mother had been treated with benzodiazepines for anxiety over a number of years. The parents regularly discussed their worries about their own health, safety and their own concerns about the uncertainty of the future. The father, Oliver, worked with an insurance company and frequently discussed accidents and burglaries that had befallen his clients. Margie regularly participated in these conversations, being the eldest child. The parents' chief concern was about Margie's tearfulness, which they viewed as unusual. Her worries and fears they saw as quite legitimate.

Margie had a couple of close friends with whom she played at the week-ends, but spent a lot of time in her parents' company.

Formulation. Pre-disposing factors in this case include a possible genetic vulnerability to anxiety and exposure to a family culture marked by a concern with safety and an over-sensitivity to danger. No clear-cut precipitating factor is apparent. Ongoing involvement in parental conversations about potential threats to the well-being of family members possibly maintained the condition, along with the attention and concern shown to Margie's tearfulness at school.

Treatment. Treatment in this case involved family work focusing on helping Margie and her parents reduce the amount of time they spent talking about danger and threats and increase the amount of time they spent engaged in activities and conversations focusing on Margie's strengths and capabilities. The parents were also helped to coach Margie in relaxation skills and mastery-oriented coping self-statements. Some reduction in anxiety and tearfulness occurred and Margie showed some improvement in her adjustment in school.

Table 12.5 Diagnostic criteria for generalized anxiety from DSM IV TR and ICD 10

DSM IV TR	ICD 10
A. Excessive anxiety and worry (apprehensive expectation), occurring more days than not for 6 months about a number of events or activities (such as school or work performance) B. The person finds it difficult to control the worry C. The anxiety or worry is associated with 3 of the following in adults or 1 of the following in children for more days than not in the past 6 months: 1. Restlessness or feeling keyed-up or on edge 2. Being easily fatigued 3. Difficulty concentrating or mind going blank 4. Irritability 5. Muscle tension 6. Sleep disturbance D. The focus of the anxiety or worry is not confined to features of an axis I disorder, such as gaining weight (anorexia nervosa) E. The anxiety or physical symptoms cause clinically significant distress or impairment in social, occupational, school and other important areas of functioning F. The disturbance is not due to the direct physiological effect of a substance	The essential feature is anxiety, which is generalized and persistent but not restricted to any particular environmental circumstance. The dominant symptoms are highly variable but complaints of continuous feelings of nervousness, trembling, muscular tension, sweating, light-headedness, palpitations, dizziness, and epigastric discomfort are common. Fears that the sufferer or a relative will shortly become ill or have an accident, are often expressed together with a variety of other thoughts and forebodings The sufferer must have the primary symptoms for most days for several weeks at a time, and usually for several months. These symptoms should usually involve elements of: a. apprehension (worry about future misfortune, feeling on edge, difficulty in concentrating) b. motor tension (restless fidgeting, tension headaches, trembling, inability to relax) c. autonomic over-activity (light-headedness, sweating, tachycardia, tachypnoea, epigastric discomfort, dizziness, dry mouth) In children frequent need for reassurance and recurrent somatic complaints may be prominent

Note: Adapted from DSM IV TR (APA, 2000a) and ICD 10 (WHO, 1992, 1996).

Box 12.5 A case of panic disorder with agoraphobia

Have illness/threat saturated family culture

Live in London and have little contact

Live locally and both have been hospitalized for psychological problems

At university Visits occasionally

Referral. Sandra, a fifteen-year-old girl, was referred because of anxiety about sitting exams. She lived with her grandparents, Ruth and Josh. She slept and ate well and appeared to be happy. However, she would not venture away from the house. A tutor from the local technical college at which she was enrolled had regularly brought schoolwork to her for about 9 months. The immanence of her O-level exams, which were due to be held at the college, precipitated the referral. She wanted to overcome her anxiety so that she could travel to college and sit her exams, which she had felt unable to complete the previous year due to anxiety.

History of the presenting problem. In a preliminary interview, conducted at her grandparents' house, she described a fear of leaving the safety of her own home and how this fear increased with distance from her house. The fear began during her mock O-level school exams a year previously. She had a panic attack and left the exam hall. She ran to her grandparents' house after this incident and subsequent attempts to return to school led to further panic attacks. Her family and the college staff, after some preliminary ineffective attempts to help her get out and about, gave up trying. On many occasions, when she found herself any distance from the house, she would begin to panic and run back quickly. This led to the symptoms of panic abating. One staff member at the college visited her and taught her some relaxation exercises. He suggested she use these to help her cope with attempts to leave the house, but she found them of little benefit. Eventually she settled for a house-bound life.

During the attacks she was afraid she would die. She couldn't catch her breath and felt dizzy. She also felt as if she were out of her body and as if the world was dream-like. The attack lasted no more than a few minutes. Subsequent attacks were similar to the first. On a couple of occasions, when she had sufficient courage to visit her friends, she had panic attacks. She described the fear of taking hot tea, which she might not be able to finish without scalding herself, should she experience a panic attack and need to run home quickly. She said she would not like to offend her friends by not finishing her tea. Sandra's principal fears were that she would have an attack and would not get home safely. She was therefore frightened of going on buses or in cars on the motorway. She was also frightened of queuing at the bank.

Family history. Sandra's parents were divorced. Her father, Des, was a police officer in London and had left her mother, Lynn, when Sandra was seven years old. Lynn lived near the grandparents, in a rural village about a three-hour drive from London. Lynn co-habited with Jeff whom she had met while hospitalized for depression. The mother had an extensive history of psychiatric treatment for anxiety disorders and depression. The grandparents and the mother were preoccupied with physical illness and psychological problems and regularly discussed threats to each other's well-being. There was also a view, based on Lynn's experiences, that psychological problems ran a chronic course and were unresponsive to psychological treatments. The grandparents and the mother had very close relationships with Sandra. Lynn was involved in regular conflicts with her mother over the suitability of Jeff as a partner for her. Sandra's brother, Paul, who attended university, visited her occasionally with his friends and she envied his lifestyle. He rarely joined in the conversations about illness at the grandparents' house. He was a drama enthusiast and Sandra would help him rehearse his lines when he visited. For Sandra, this was a welcome break from the regular conversation at her grandparent's house. Sandra had four or five friends who lived locally and two of these visited regularly.

Formulation. In this case, the principal pre-disposing factors were a genetic vulnerability to anxiety from the mother's side of the family and a family culture that focused on illness, fear, danger and anxiety. The exam situation was the principal precipitating factor. Multiple unsuccessful treatments and the experience of negative reinforcement afforded by escaping from threatening situations maintained the condition. Other maintaining factors included the father's lack of involvement in attempts to help Sandra recover, the grandparents' and mother's danger-saturated family culture and their beliefs that psychological problems had a chronic course and were unresponsive to treatment. However, two positive peer relationships and a desire for vocational progression were also present in this case and were important protective factors.

Treatment. Treatment in this instance began with family work involving the grandparents, the mother and on a couple of occasions the father to reduce the amount of illness- and anxiety-focused conversation to which Sandra was exposed and to challenge the beliefs that psychological problems were unresponsive to psychological treatments. This was followed with in vivo systematic desensitization coupled with a brief trial of Anafranil, but Sandra could not tolerate the side effects so the medication was discontinued. It was also arranged for her to sit exams at school in a private room. Following this, a work placement at a crèche and at an old folks home were arranged by the college staff. While Sandra made a good recovery, she suffered periodic relapses and re-referred herself for a number of further episodes of treatment over the following two years.

The patterning of arousal varies, depending on the frequency with which the youngster comes into contact with feared stimuli. With separation anxiety, hyperarousal occurs only when separation is threatened. With selective mutism, hyperarousal only occurs when the child is strongly urged to speak in school or threatening situations. With specific phobias, hyperarousal only occurs only in the presence of the feared object. With generalized anxiety disorder, there is a pattern of ongoing continual hyperarousal. With panic disorder and PTSD there is a moderate level of chronic hyperarousal punctuated by brief episodes of extreme hyperarousal. These occur in panic disorder

Table 12.6 Diagnostic criteria for panic disorder and agoraphobia from DSM IV TR and ICD 10

	DSM IV TR	ICD 10
Panic disorder	Recurrent unexpected panic attacks and at least one of the following: 1. Persistent concern about having additional attacks 2. Worry about the implications of the attack or its consequences (losing control, having a heart attack, going crazy) 3. A significant change in behaviour related to the attacks A panic attack is a discrete period of intense fear or discomfort in which at least four of the following symptoms developed and reached a peak within 10 minutes: 1. Palpitations or pounding heart 2. Sweating 3. Trembling or shaking 4. Sensations of shortness of breath or smothering 5. Feeling of choking 6. Chest pain or discomfort 7. Nausea or abdominal distress 8. Feeling dizzy, unsteady, light-headed or faint 9. Derealization (feelings of unreality) or depersonalization (detached from oneself) 10. Fear of losing control or going crazy 11. Fear of dying 12. Parasthesias (numbness or tingling sensations) 13. Chills or hot flushes	Several severe panic attacks within a period of about a month The dominant symptoms of a panic attack vary from person to person but sudden onset of palpitations, chest pain, choking sensations, dizziness, and feelings of unreality (depersonalization or derealization) are common. There is also, almost invariably, a secondary fear of dying, losing control, or going mad. Individual attacks usually only last for minutes. An individual in a panic attack often experiences a crescendo of fear and autonomic symptoms, which result in a hurried exit from wherever he or she may be. If this occurs in a specific situation such as on a bus or in a crowd, the patient may subsequently avoid that situation. Frequent and unpredictable panic attacks produce a fear of being alone or going into public places
Agoraphobia	A. Anxiety about being in places or situations from which escape might be difficult or in which help might not be available in the event of having a panic attack. Agoraphobic fears typically involve characteristic clusters of situations that include being outside the home alone; being in a crowd or standing in line; being on a bridge; or travelling in a bus, train, or automobile	Agoraphobia refers to an interrelated and overlapping cluster of phobias including a fear of leaving home; fear of entering shops, crowds, and public places or travelling alone in trains, buses or planes. Some sufferers become

Continued

Table 12.6 continued

DSM IV TR	ICD 10
B. The situations are avoided or endured with marked distress or anxiety about having a panic attack or require the presence of a companion C. The anxiety or avoidance behaviour is not better accounted for by another disorder Agoraphobia may occur with or without panic attacks	completely house-bound. Many are terrified by the thought of collapsing and being left helpless in public. The lack of an immediately available exit is one of the key features of many of these agoraphobic situations All of the following should be fulfilled for a definite diagnosis: a. The psychological or autonomic symptoms must be primarily manifestations of anxiety and not secondary to other symptoms such as delusions or obsessional thoughts b. The anxiety must be restricted to at least two of the following situations: crowds, public places, travelling away from home, travelling alone c. Avoidance of the phobic situation must be a prominent feature Agoraphobia may occur with or without panic attacks

Note: Adapted from DSM IV TR (APA, 2000a) and ICD 10 (WHO, 1992, 1996).

during panic attacks and in PTSD when memories of the traumatic event intrude into consciousness.

Avoidance behaviours characterize all anxiety disorders. With specific phobias, these may lead to only a moderate constriction in lifestyle. For example, a child may refuse to engage in sports or athletics, or to ride a bicycle, because of an injury phobia. However, with separation anxiety, selective mutism, generalized anxiety disorder, panic disorder and PTSD, the avoidance behaviour may lead the youngster to become house-bound. With PTSD, alcohol or drug abuse may occur. Alcohol and drugs are used to reduce negative affect and suppress traumatic memories. This type of self-medication is discussed more fully in Chapter 15.

Box 12.6 A case of PTSD

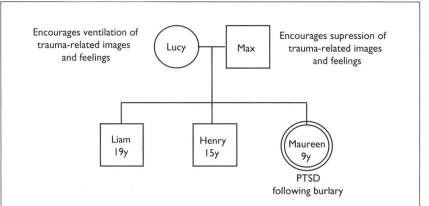

History of the presenting problem. Maureen, a nine-year-old was referred by the family doctor because of recurrent night-mares, a refusal to sleep in her own bed and withdrawn behaviour at school. These problems had developed following a burglary. The family were in the house when the burglary happened. The parents awoke and brought the three children into their room as quietly as possible. However, the burglar panicked when he heard this and ran up the stairs to the bedroom shouting violent threats. Maureen thought that the burglar was going to kill all members of the family. After an unsuccessful attempt to break down the bedroom door, the burglar left the house. When it was clear that the burglar had left the house, Maureen and the rest of the family went downstairs and saw that the ground floor of the house had been ransacked.

During assessment, Maureen said that she became anxious each evening as bedtime approached. She could only sleep with the light on. She had vivid night-mares about the robbery and in these her parents were killed. She could only return to sleep if her parents slept in her bed or she slept in theirs. During the day she had flashes of images of dark figures chasing her and also sudden pangs of fear. She found it hard to concentrate on her schoolwork or to join in games with her friends. She tried to deal with the flashes and pangs by putting them out of her mind or talking to her parents about them.

Maureen's two older brothers (aged fifteen and nineteen) and her parents, while shaken by the event, had similar but less pronounced symptoms. The family vacillated between reassuring Maureen that everything was all right now and urging her to forget the incident on the one hand and allowing her to ventilate her fears and ruminations on the other. Occasionally the parents, Lucy and Max argued about the best approach to managing the situation.

Formulation. No clear pre-disposing factors were identified in this case. The burglary precipitated the onset of Maureen's problems. The symptoms were maintained by Maureen's attempt to keep them out of her mind and her parents' partial support for using this coping strategy.

Treatment. Treatment in this case involved family work, which focused on helping the parents and two older brothers support Maureen while *exposed* to ongoing detailed vivid conversation about the burglary. Between sessions, arrangements were made for Maureen to sleep in her parents' bedroom for a number of months. She was also invited to record all her vivid trauma-related dreams and make pictures of them and bring them to the family sessions. To help

Maureen develop a sense of mastery, in the family sessions, family members re-told the dream stories but altered the endings so that Maureen vanquished the dark figures who chased her. A gradual reduction in night-mares, daytime intrusive images and emotions and avoidance behaviour occurred over a period of six months.

Table 12.7 Diagnostic criteria for PTSD from DSM IV TR and ICD 10

DSM IV TR	ICD 10
A. The person has been exposed to a traumatic event in which both of the following were present: 1. The person experienced, witnessed, or was confronted with an event that involved actual or threatened death or serious injury of self or others 2. The person's response involved intense fear, helplessness or horror or, in the case of children, disorganized behaviour B. The traumatic event is persistently re-experienced in one or more of the following ways: 1. Recurrent and intrusive distressing recollections of the event including thoughts, images, or in children repetitive play in which the themes of the trauma are re-enacted 2. Recurrent distressing dreams of the event or in children the dreams may have unrecognizable fearful content 3. Acting or feeling as if the traumatic event were recurring (including, hallucinations, illusions and dissociative flashbacks, or in children re-enactments) 4. Intense psychological distress to exposure to internal or external cues that symbolize the traumatic event 5. Physiological reactivity to exposure to internal or external cues that symbolize the traumatic event	This arises as a delayed and/or protracted response to a stressful event or situation of an exceptionally threatening or catastrophic nature, which is likely to cause pervasive distress to almost anyone (e.g. natural or man-made disaster, combat, serious accident, witnessing the violent death of others, being a victim of rape, torture, terrorism or another crime) Typical symptoms include episodes of repeated re-living of the trauma in intrusive memories (flashbacks) or dreams, occurring against the persisting background of a sense of numbness and emotional blunting, detachment from other people, unresponsiveness to surroundings, anhedonia, and avoidance of activities and situations reminiscent of the trauma. Commonly there is a fear and avoidance of cues that remind the sufferer of the original trauma. Rarely there may be dramatic acute bursts of fear, panic, or aggression triggered by stimuli arousing a sudden recollection and/or re-enactment of the trauma There is usually a state of autonomic hyperarousal with hypervigilance, enhanced startle reaction, and insomnia. Anxiety and depression are commonly associated with the above symptoms and signs and suicidal ideation is not infrequent. Excessive use of alcohol and drugs may be a complicating factor The disorder may be diagnosed if it occurs within six months of the trauma. In addition there must be repetitive intrusive recollection or re-enactment of the event in memories, daytime imagery or dreams. Conspicuous emotional detachment, numbing of feeling, and avoidance of stimuli that might arouse recollection of the trauma are often present but are not essential for the diagnosis. The autonomic disturbances, mood disorder, and behavioural abnormalities all contribute to the diagnosis but are not of prime importance

C. Persistent avoidance of
stimuli associated with the trauma
and numbing of general
responsiveness as indicated by
three of the following:
1. Avoidance of thought feelings or
conversations associated with the
trauma
2. Avoidance of activities, places or
people that arouse recollection of
the trauma
3. Inability to recall an important
aspect of the trauma
4. Markedly diminished interest
or participation in significant
activities
5. Restricted range of affect
6. Sense of foreshortened future

D. Persistent symptoms of
increased arousal as indicated by
two of the following:
1. Sleep difficulties
2. Irritability or outbursts of anger
3. Difficulty concentrating
4. Hypervigilance
5. Exaggerated startle response

E. Duration of disturbance longer
than 1 month

F. The disturbance causes clinically
significant distress and impairment of
social or academic functioning

Note: Adapted from DSM IV TR (APA, 2000a) and ICD 10 (WHO, 1992, 1996).

Interpersonal relationships are affected by different anxiety disorders in different ways. With simple phobias there may be minimal disruption although conflict with parents, teachers or peers may occur where the youngster refuses to conform or co-operate with routine activities so as to avoid the feared stimuli. For example, parent–child conflict may occur if a child refuses to get in an elevator at a shopping mall because of claustrophobia. With separation anxiety, selective mutism, panic disorder, generalized anxiety and PTSD, complete social isolation may occur and the youngster's peer relationships and school attendance may cease. A more detailed account of the assessment and treatment of these six types of anxiety disorder will be given below, after a consideration of aetiological theories and the assessment, formulation and management of anxiety disorders generally.

Table 12.8 Clinical features of anxiety in children

	Separation anxiety	Selective mutism	Phobias	Generalized anxiety disorder	Panic disorder	PTSD
Perception	• Separation is perceived as threatening	• Certain social situations such as school are perceived as threatening	• Specific objects, events or situations are perceived as threatening	• The whole environment is perceived as threatening • The child is hypervigilent scanning the environment for threats to well-being	• The recurrence of a panic attack is seen as threatening • Attention is directed inward and benign somatic sensations are perceived but misinterpreted as threatening	• Cues that remind the person of the trauma are perceived as threatening • Hallucinations or illusions may occur where aspects of the trauma are reperceived
Cognition	• The child believes that harm to the parent or the self will occur following separation	• The child believes that something threatening will happen if he or she speaks in unfamiliar situations	• The child believes that contact with the phobic object or entry into the phobic situation will lead to catastrophe	• The child catastrophizes about many minor daily events	• The youth believes that the panic attacks may lead to death or serious injury	• Recurrent memories of the trauma occur • The child tries to distract himself or herself from recalling these traumatic memories

Affect	• Intense fear or anger occurs when separation is anticipated, during separation or following separation	• Intense fear or anger is experienced if the child is urged to speak in unfamiliar situations	• Intense fear or anger is experienced if contact with the feared object or situation is anticipated or occurs	• A continual moderately high level of fear is experienced, often called free-floating anxiety	• During panic attacks, intense fear occurs, and between attacks a moderate level of fear of recurrence is experienced	• Against a background of hyperarousal, periodic intrusive episodes of intense fear, horror or anger like those that occurred during the trauma are experienced • The child feels emotionally blunted and cannot experience tender emotions • Depression may occur
Arousal	• Episodes of hyperarousal • Sleep problems	• Episodes of hyperarousal if forced to speak in unfamiliar situations	• Episodes of hyperarousal • Sleep problems	• Continual hyperarousal • Sleep problems	• Episodes of extreme hyperarousal against a background of moderate hyperarousal • Sleep problems	• Episodes of extreme hyperarousal against a background of moderate hyperarousal • Sleep problems

Continued

Table 12.8 continued

	Separation anxiety	Selective mutism	Phobias	Generalized anxiety disorder	Panic disorder	PTSD
Behaviour	• Separation is avoided or resisted. • The child refuses to go to school • The child refuses to sleep alone	• The child does not speak to others in school or other unfamiliar situations	• The phobic object or situation is avoided	• As worrying intensifies, social activities become restricted	• The youth may avoid public places in case the panic attacks occur away from the safety of home. This is secondary agoraphobia	• Young children may cling to parents and refuse to sleep alone • Teenagers may use drugs or alcohol to block the intrusive thoughts and emotions • Suicidal attempts may occur
Interpersonal adjustment	• Peer relationships may deteriorate • Academic performance may deteriorate	• The child's social development is constricted and the child may be bullied for being odd	• With simple phobias, interpersonal problems are confined to phobic situations • Agoraphobia may lead to social isolation	• Peer relationships may deteriorate • Academic performance may deteriorate	• If agoraphobia develops secondary to the panic attacks social isolation may result	• Complete social isolation may occur if the trauma was solitary • Where the trauma was shared, the child may confine interactions to the group who shared the trauma

AETIOLOGICAL THEORIES

Theories of anxiety may be divided into those which focus predominantly on biological variables and those that emphasize the role of psychological and psychosocial factors. A summary of the main theories of anxiety and the treatment approaches associated with them is presented in Table 12.9.

Biological theories

Biological theories have addressed the roles of genetic and temperamental factors and the dysregulation or a number of neurotransmitter systems in the aetiology of anxiety disorders.

The genetic hypothesis

This hypothesis entails the view that anxiety occurs where a person with an inherited vulnerability is exposed to threatening environmental stimuli at critical developmental stages when they are primed or prepared to develop fears (Boer & Lindhout, 2001). There is an ethological implication here that sensitivity to particular classes of stimuli at particular developmental stages has an adaptive function, and that this has evolved to protect the survival of the species (DeSilva Rachman & Seligman, 1977). The genetic hypothesis also entails the view that a dysfunctional biological factor which under-pins the process of detecting danger is genetically transmitted in families where anxiety disorders occur. For most measures of anxiety, about 30% of the variance is accounted for by genetic factors; about 20% by shared environmental factors, and about 50% by non-shared environmental factors (Eley & Gregory, 2004). There is considerable heterogeneity associated with age and gender, and whether anxiety is rated by parents or children (Boer & Lindhout, 2001; Eley & Gregory, 2004; Klein & Pine, 2002; Tharper & Scourfield, 2002). Heritability increases with age, is greater for girls than boys and anxiety rated by parents is more heritable than self-reported anxiety, suggesting that parents and children are rating different aspects of anxiety. There is also the evidence, mentioned earlier, that vulnerability to developing animal phobias and separation anxiety is highest during childhood, whereas social phobias, generalized anxiety disorder and panic disorder with agoraphobia more commonly emerge in adolescence (Öst & Treffers, 2001). The genetic hypothesis applies to all of the anxiety disorders, although probably has limited relevance for PTSD. Implicit in the genetic hypothesis is the view that pharmacological or psychological interventions should aim to help the person cope with a chronic lifelong disorder. Research efforts should focus on identifying the precise biological factors associated with deficits in threat perception that is genetically transmitted and the mechanisms of transmission.

Table 12.9 Theories and treatments for anxiety

	Theory	Theoretical principles	Principles of treatment
Biological theories	**Genetic theory**	Anxiety occurs when a person with an inherited vulnerability is exposed to threatening environmental stimuli at critical developmental stages	Pharmacological or psychological interventions to help the person cope with a chronic disorder
	Neurotransmitter hypotheses	Dysregulations of the noradrenergic system, the gamma-aminobutyric acid (GABA) system; and the serotonin system under-pin anxiety disorders	Psychopharmacological treatment with SSRIs, TCA or benzodiazepines rectify dysregulated neurotransmitter systems
	Behaviourally inhibited temperament hypothesis	A biologically based temperamental pre-disposition towards behavioural inhibition in unfamiliar situations renders children vulnerable to the development of anxiety disorders	Vulnerable children may be taught anxiety management strategies and exposed to novel situations until they cope with them
Psychological theories	**Psychoanalytic theories**	In anxiety disorders, defence mechanisms are used to keep unacceptable impulses and moral anxiety about their expression from entering consciousness. The unacceptable feelings and related moral anxiety are transformed into neurotic anxiety and displaced onto a phobic object which symbolizes the object about which the unacceptable impulses were felt	Individual psychodynamic psychotherapy in which the defence/ hidden feeling/ anxiety triangle of conflict is interpreted
		In generalized anxiety disorders, the defences break down and the person becomes overwhelmed with anxiety as the unacceptable impulses are displaced onto all available objects	

Cognitive theory	Anxiety occurs when life events involving threat reactivate threat-oriented cognitive schemas formed early in childhood during a threatening and stressful experience. These threat-oriented schemas contain assumptions about the dangerous nature of the environment or the person's health and cognitive distortions, such as minimizing safety-related events and maximizing threat-related negative events	Individual or group cognitive therapy in which clients are trained to monitor situations where anxiety related assumptions and distortions occur and to engage in activities that challenge their validity
Incubation theory	Anxiety develops through one-trial classical conditioning where a neutral object for which a person is prepared to develop an extinction-resistant fear (CS) is paired with a strongly feared object (UCS) and this object elicits anxiety (UCR). Repeated brief exposure to this previously neutral object (CS) leads to an increase in fear through a process of incubation. Incubation is a positive feedback process where fear itself reinforces fear of the phobic object. People who are constitutionally more neurotic and introverted are more likely to develop phobic anxiety through this incubation process	Behaviour therapy procedures in which the person is exposed gradually or completely to the phobic object in viva or imagination and helped through relaxation or some other method to remain until the anxiety subsides is the treatment of choice
Systems theory	Parents socialize children through modelling and reinforcement to interpret ambiguous situations in a threatening manner and to cope with fear through avoidance behaviour Family lifecycle transitions or stressful events precipitate the onset of anxiety disorders, which are inadvertently maintained by patterns of family interaction where anxiety is reinforced and parental child-focused behaviour allows parents to avoid facing marital and personal issues	Family work where parents learn to help the child manage anxiety

SSRI, selective serotonin re-uptake inhibitor; TCA, tricyclic anti-depressant.

Neurotransmitter hypotheses

Dysregulations of the noradrenergic system, the gamma-aminobutyric acid (GABA) system and the serotonin system within the lymbic system have all been proposed as under-pinning anxiety disorders, and there is some preliminary evidence for the effectiveness of psychopharmacological treatments (American Academy of Child and Adolescent Psychiatry, 1997c; Fonagy et al., 2002; Garland, 2002; Stein & Seedat, 2004). Psychopharmacological treatments aim to rectify dysregulated neurotransmitter systems. How they do so is the focus of much current research.

There is evidence for the efficacy of specific serotonin re-uptake inhibitors (SSRIs), such as fluoxetine and fluvoxamine, in the treatment of elective mutism, separation anxiety disorder, generalized anxiety disorder and social phobia. SSRIs increase low serotonin levels by preventing re-uptake, notably in neurons originating in the dorsal raphae nucleus of the brainstem.

There is some evidence for the efficacy of tricyclic anti-depressants (TCAs), such as imipramine, in the treatment of separation anxiety in children. TCAs are thought to ameliorate separation anxiety by affecting the noradrenergic neurons arising in the locus coeruleus.

Benzodiazepines, specifically clonazepam, have been found to improve panic disorder in adolescents. It is thought that benzodiazepines reduce anxiety by compensating for low GABA levels and by binding to GABA neuroreceptors. GABA is usually released automatically once arousal reaches a certain level and binds with GABA receptors on excited neurons; this underpins the experience of anxiety. This binding process causes inhibition, a reduction in arousal, and a decrease in experienced anxiety.

Behaviourally inhibited temperament hypothesis

This hypothesis attributes vulnerability to anxiety disorders to a biologically based temperamental pre-disposition towards behavioural inhibition (BI) in unfamiliar situations (Kagan et al., 1989). Children with BI show fearfulness, restraint, reticence and social withdrawal in novel situations, including those involving unfamiliar people, places and objects. There is growing evidence to support moderate heritability for BI, to indicate that children with BI have a lower threshold for limbic and sympathetic nervous system arousal and that BI is a risk factor for anxiety and the development of disorders (Hirshfeld-Becker, Biederman & Rosenbaum, 2004; Oosterlaan, 2001). Anxiety disorders in BI children may be prevented by identifying them early and giving them anxiety management training such as the FRIENDS programme (Barrett & Shortt, 2003) to allow them to cope better with unfamiliar situations.

Psychological theories

Psychoanalytic, cognitive, behavioural and family systems theories have been developed to explain how various anxiety problems develop, and how they can best be treated. What follows is an outline of an example of one theoretical formulation from each of these traditions.

Psychoanalytic theories

In anxiety disorders, according to classical psychoanalytic theory, defence mechanisms are used to keep unacceptable impulses (anger, sadness, sexual impulses) or feelings and moral anxiety about their expression from entering consciousness. The unacceptable feelings and related moral anxiety become transformed into neurotic anxiety and expressed as an anxiety disorder. In phobias, the unacceptable impulse is repressed and the neurotic anxiety into which it is transformed is displaced onto a substitute object, which symbolizes the original object about which the unacceptable impulses were felt. The key defence mechanism is *displacement*. Thus when children say that they are frightened of a particular object or situation, the psychoanalytic hypothesis is that they are frightened about something else, but have displaced their fear from the original taboo object or event onto a more socially acceptable target. In generalized anxiety disorders, the defences break down and the person becomes overwhelmed with anxiety as the unacceptable impulses continually intrude into consciousness and seek expression. In generalized anxiety disorder, anxiety about a taboo object is displaced onto every available target (McCullough-Vaillant, 1997).

In Freud's original statement of this hypothesis (the case of little Hans, who had a horse phobia), he argued that Hans' taboo fear was castration anxiety, and that fear of the father was displaced onto horses (Freud, 1909a).

Psychoanalytically based treatment is typically conducted within an individual, non-directive play therapy format with young children and individual psychodynamic psychotherapy with adolescents. In treatment, the aim is to interpret the defence, the hidden feelings which are being repressed and the associated neurotic anxiety. McCullough-Vaillant (1997) refers to these three elements (the defence, the hidden feeling and the associated anxiety) as the triangle of conflict. During treatment, the psychologist draws attention to the parallels between the way in which the youngster manages the current relationship with the therapist, the past relationship with the parents and current relationships with other significant people in their lives, such as their peers or teachers. McCullough-Vaillant (1997) refers to these three sets of relationships, which are at the heart of transference interpretations, as the triangle of person. Interpretations of the triangle of conflict and the triangle of person should be offered tentatively, at a stage in the therapy when a strong working alliance has been established, and within the context of a coherent psychodynamic case formulation.

The idea of displacement is clinically useful when working with anxious children. In my clinical experience, children worried about one thing may say that they are worried about another. However, there is no evidence to support the idea that all anxiety disorders represent displacement of anxiety associated with psychosexual developmental conflicts. There is some evidence that psychodynamic therapy is effective with children who have anxiety disorders (Fonagy et al., 2002).

Beck's cognitive theory

According to the theory that under-pins Beck's cognitive approach to therapy for anxiety disorders, anxiety occurs when life events involving threat re-activate threat-oriented cognitive schemas formed early in childhood during a threatening and stressful experience (Beck, Emery & Greenberg, 1985). These threat-oriented schemas contain assumptions about the dangerous nature of the environment or the person's health such as: 'The world is dangerous, so I must continually be on guard' or 'My health is ailing so any uncomfortable somatic sensation must reflect serious ill health'. They also entail cognitive distortions such as minimizing safety-related events and maximizing threat-related negative events. In a refinement of this original theory, Beck has more recently distinguished between three stages associated with the escalation of anxiety: (1) registration of a threat; (2) activation of primal threat mode; and (3) evocation of secondary elaborative checking (Beck & Clark, 1997). Individual or group cognitive therapy aims to help clients to challenge their assumptions about the dangerousness of the situations in which they feel anxiety. This involves them learning how to monitor their cognitions and anxiety levels and to test-out their cognitions by collecting information and engaging in experiences that allow the validity of their assumptions to be checked. Beck's theory is supported by evidence which shows that anxiety is associated with a threat-sensitive cognitive style and also by the results of treatment outcome studies with adults and children which support the efficacy of cognitive-behavioural approaches to treatment (Barrett & Shortt, 2003; Compton et al., 2004; Kendall, Aschenbrand & Hudson, 2003).

Incubation theory

The most elaborate conditioning model for phobias is Eysenck's (1979) incubation theory, which he developed to over-come the shortcomings of simpler behavioural formulations. Eysenck argued that anxiety initially develops through one-trial classical conditioning where a neutral object for which a person is biologically prepared to develop an extinction-resistant fear (CS) is paired with a strongly feared object (UCS) and this object elicits anxiety (UCR). Subsequent exposure to the previously neutral object (CS) elicits mild anxiety (CR). Repeated brief exposure to this previously neutral object (CS) leads to an increase in fear through a process of incubation. Brief exposure leads to anxiety (CR) which is effectively paired with the feared object and, on the next brief exposure, even more fear is elicited. Incubation is a positive feedback process where fear itself reinforces fear of the phobic object. This whole process occurs outside of cognitive control. Eysenck also argued that people who are constitutionally more neurotic and introverted are more likely to develop phobic anxiety through this incubation process. He also acknowledged, following Seligman, that phobias develop only to a limited group of stimuli and that humans have a preparedness, as a result of evolutionary processes, to develop phobias to these through a process of classical conditioning (DeSilva et al., 1977). Treatment for phobias according to this theory involves gradual or complete exposure to the phobic object or an image of it until the anxiety subsides. Thus both in vivo and imaginal desensitization or flooding procedures may be used to treat phobias, although the theory predicts that in vivo methods should be more effective. The use of relaxation skills or other coping strategies are only important insofar as they help the person tolerate remaining in the presence of the feared object. There is still controversy over details of the incubation theory as an explanation for the aetiology of phobias. However, a large body of research shows that exposure techniques such as desensitization and flooding, particularly in vivo, are very effective methods for treating specific phobias in children and adults (Barrett & Shortt, 2003; Compton et al., 2004; Kendall et al., 2003).

Family systems hypotheses

There is no well-articulated integrative theory about the role of the family and the socialization process in the aetiology of anxiety. However, a number of hypotheses from diverse sources may be drawn together to offer such explanation (Barrett & Shortt, 2003; Boer & Lindhout, 2001). Children probably develop anxiety problems when they are socialized in families where significant family members (particularly primary caretakers) elicit, model and reinforce anxiety-related beliefs and behaviours. Furthermore, family lifecycle transitions and stressful life events within the family may precipitate the onset of clinically significant anxiety problems. These problems are maintained by patterns of family interaction that reinforce the child's anxiety-related beliefs and avoidance behaviour.

Family belief systems that promote anxiety may involve the view that ambiguous situations should be routinely interpreted as threatening or dangerous; that the future will probably entail many hazards, catastrophes and dangers; that inconsequential events in the past will probably reap dangerous, threatening consequences at some unexpected point in the future; that fluctuations in autonomic arousal should be interpreted as the onset of full-blown anxiety attacks; that minor ailments are reflective of inevitable serious illness and that testing out the validity of any of these beliefs will inevitably lead to more negative consequences than continuing to assume that they are true. Through observing significant family members articulate these beliefs and engaging in family interactions premised on these beliefs, children may come to internalize them and develop a personal danger-saturated belief system.

When children observe significant family members cope with perceived threats by avoiding rather than confronting the perceived danger, they may adopt this coping strategy themselves.

Such anxiety-related beliefs and avoidant coping styles may be inadvertently reinforced when family members acknowledge their validity and do not challenge them.

Family lifecycle transitions, such as starting school, moving house, birth of a sibling and family stresses such as personal or parental illness, may precipitate the onset of a serious anxiety problem. In such situations, the child interprets the transition or stress as a major threat and copes by engaging in avoidant behaviour.

Parents, siblings and members of the extended family may all inadvertently maintain the child's anxiety-related beliefs and avoidance behaviour by sympathizing with the child's fears, accepting the child's danger-saturated view of the situation and condoning the avoidance behaviour as a legitimate coping strategy. The other family members' own danger-saturated belief systems and personal adjustment problems, if such are present, may prevent him or her from providing the child with opportunities to develop the skills required to confront and master feared situations. So, for example in families where there are marital problems, parental depression, parental alcohol abuse or some other difficulty, the parents may avoid facing these difficulties and focus their attention instead on reassuring the child or arranging extensive medical investigations for anxiety-related somatic complaints. The patterns of family interaction that evolve in such situations may inadvertently maintain the child's anxiety and reinforce the parents' avoidance of their own marital or personal difficulties. Commonly, the family members are not consciously aware of the secondary gains associated with these problem-maintaining patterns of interaction.

Family therapy for children with anxiety disorders aims to support the parents and child in creating opportunities within which the child can develop the skills required to confront and master feared situations. This may involve helping the parents and child interpret the feared situations in less threatening ways, helping the parents communicate with the child in a less intrusive and anxiety-laden way, showing the parents how to coach the child in relaxation skills and other anxiety management skills, showing the parents how to help the child expose him- or herself to the feared situation and arranging for the parent to reinforce the child for remaining in the feared situation until anxiety subsides.

There is evidence: (1) that the parents of a majority of children with anxiety disorders have anxiety disorders themselves and that other types of psychopathology, including depression, are over-represented in the families of youngsters with anxiety disorders; (2) that modelling and parenting style play an important role in the transmission of anxiety patterns from parent to children in at least some cases; and (3) that increased incidence of stressful life events and marital discord are associated with onset of anxiety disorders in some, but not all, anxious children (Boer & Lindhout, 2001; Klein & Pine, 2002). A small and growing body of research points to the effectiveness of family interventions in the treatment of anxiety disorders (Barrett & Shortt, 2003).

ASSESSMENT

In addition to the routine assessment protocol outlined in Chapter 4, the symptomatology associated with the diagnostic criteria set out in Tables 12.2, 12.3, 12.4, 12.5, 12.6 and 12.7 should be covered. The assessment instruments listed in Table 12.10 may be useful adjuncts in this process. In the differential diagnosis of anxiety disorders in children it is vital to exclude thyrotoxicosis (over-activity of the thyroid gland), the symptoms of which mimic anxiety. However, in thyrotoxicosis there is a raised early morning pulse, and T3 and T4 test results (which assess thyroxin levels) are typically abnormal. Referral to the family doctor or the paediatrician should be made to rule out thyrotoxicosis if it is suspected.

Aetiological factors to consider in the clinical assessment of cases where anxiety problems are a central concern are set out in Figure 12.3.

Pre-disposing factors

In cases of anxiety both personal and contextual pre-disposing factors may be present. Important personal pre-disposing factors to consider in the assessment of anxiety include possible genetic factors as indicated by a family history of anxiety. An inhibited temperament, low self-esteem and an external locus of control are other possible personal pre-disposing factors deserving consideration in assessment. Contextual factors that may pre-dispose youngsters to developing anxiety problems include anxious attachment to parents, exposure to parental anxiety and an anxiety-oriented family culture which privileges the interpretation of many environmental events as potentially hazardous.

Table 12.10 Psychometric instruments that may be used as an adjunct to clinical interviews in the assessment of anxiety

Construct	Instrument	Publication	Comments
DSM anxiety disorder diagnoses	Anxiety Disorder Interview Schedule for Children-IV-Children and Parent versions (ADIS-IV-C/P)	Silverman, W. & Albano. (1996). *The Anxiety Disorder Interview Schedule for Children-IV-Child and Parent Version.* Boulder, CO: Graywind	This structured interview yields reliable DSM IV diagnoses for anxiety disorders on the basis of either child or parent reports
	Screen for Child Anxiety Related Emotional Disorders (SCARED)	Birmaher, B., Brent, D., Chiappetta, L., Bridge, J., Monga, S. & Baugher, M. (1999). Psychometric properties of the Screen for Child Anxiety Related Emotional Disorders (SCARED): A replication study. *Journal of the American Academy of Child and Adolescent Psychiatry*, 38, 1230–1236	This 66-item inventory, for which parent and child report versions are available, yields scores for DSM IV anxiety categories: generalized anxiety disorder, social phobia, separation anxiety disorder, panic disorder, obsessive-compulsive disorder, post-traumatic stress disorder, and specific phobias
	Revised Anxiety and Depression Scales	Chorpita, B., Yim, L., Moffitt, C., Unemoto, L. & Francis, S. (2000). Assessment of symptoms of DSM IV anxiety and depression in children: A revised child anxiety and depression scale. *Behaviour Research and Therapy*, 38, 835–855	This self-report scale yields scores for DSM IV anxiety and depression categories: generalized anxiety disorder, social anxiety, separation anxiety, panic-agoraphobia, obsessive-compulsive disorder, injury phobia and depression
General anxiety	Multidimensional Anxiety Scale for Children (MASC)	March, J. (1998) *Multidimensional anxiety scale for children (MASC).* Toronto: Multihealth Systems	This 45-item self-report screening instrument yields a total anxiety disorder index and scores for social anxiety, physical symptoms, harm-avoidance and separation-panic
	Revised Children's Manifest Anxiety Scale	Reynolds, C. & Richmond, B. (1978). What I think and feel: a revised measure of children's manifest anxiety. *Journal of Abnormal Child Psychology*, 6, 271–280	This 37-item instrument, which is based on an adult scale, yields an anxiety score and a lie score which assesses social desirability response set

	Instrument	Reference	Description
	The State Trait Anxiety Inventory For Children	Spielberger, C. (1973). *Manual For The State Trait Anxiety Inventory For Children*. Palo Alto, CA. Consulting Psychologists Press	This 40-item instrument which is based on an adult scale yields a trait anxiety score and a situation-specific state anxiety score
	Hamilton Anxiety Rating Scale	Clark, D. & Donovan, J. (1994). Reliability and validity of the Hamilton Anxiety Rating Scale in an Adolescent Sample. *Journal of the American Academy of Child and Adolescent Psychiatry*, 33, 354–360	This 14-item rating scale is completed by clinicians following an interview. Items are scored on scales from 0 to 4. The instrument yields a global anxiety score, a psychic anxiety score and a somatic anxiety score
Separation anxiety	School Refusal Assessment Scale	Kearney, C. & Silverman, W. (1993). Measuring the function of school refusal behaviour: The school refusal assessment scale (SRAS). *Journal of Clinical Child Psychology*, 22, 85–96	A checklist to assess factors involved in school refusal
Specific fears	The Revised Fear Survey Schedule	Gullone, E. & King, N. (1992). Psychometric evaluation of a revised fear survey schedule for children and adolescents. *Journal of Child Psychology and Psychiatry*, 33, 987–998	This 75-item instrument, based on an adult instrument, yields information about specific fears, factor scores on 4 scales and an overall score
Social anxiety	Social Phobia and Anxiety Inventory for Children	Beidel, S., Turner, S. & Fink, C. (1996). Assessment of Childhood Social Phobia: Construct, convergent and discriminative validity of the Social Phobia Anxiety Inventory for Children (SPAI-C). *Psychological Assessment*, 8, 235–240	This 26-item inventory yields a total score and scores on five factors: assertiveness, conversation, physical and cognitive symptoms, avoidance and public performance. It accurately classifies cases with DSM diagnoses of social phobia
	Social Anxiety Scale for Children-Revised (SASC-R)	LaGreca, A. & Stone, W. (1998). *Social Anxiety Scales for Children and Adolescents: Manual and Instructions for the SASC, SASC-R, SAS-A*. Miami, FL: University of Miami, Psychology Department	This 22-item self-report inventory yields scores for (1) fear of negative evaluation, (2) generalized social avoidance and distress, and (3) social avoidance and distress with new peers
	Social Phobia and Anxiety Inventory for Adolescents	Clark, D., Turner, S., Beidel, D., Donovan, J., Kirisci, L. & Jacob, R. (1994). Reliability of the social phobia and anxiety inventory for adolescents. *Psychological Assessment*, 6, 135–140	For 45 social situations respondents rate cognitive, behavioural and physiological anxiety responses on 7-point scales and these yield scores for social phobia and agoraphobia

Continued

Table 12.10 continued

Construct	Instrument	Publication	Comments
Panic-related symptoms and beliefs	Childhood Anxiety Sensitivity Index	Silverman, W., Fleisig, W., Rabian, B. & Peterson, R. (1991). Childhood anxiety sensitivity index. *Journal of Clinical Child Psychology*, 20, 162–168	This 18-item questionnaire assesses the degree to which fear is caused by bodily signs of anxiety (e.g. tachycardia)
	Panic Attack Symptoms and Cognitions Questionnaire	Clum, G., Broyles, S., Borden, J., & Watkins, P. (1990). Validity and reliability of the Panic Attack Symptoms and Cognitions Questionnaire. *Journal of Psychopathology and Behavioural Assessment*, 12, 233–245	This self-report questionnaire yields an index of symptoms and maladaptive cognitions associated with panic attacks. Was developed for adults and may be used cautiously with adolescents
Agoraphobia	Agoraphobia Scale	Ost, L. (1990). The Agoraphobia Scale: An evaluation of its reliability and validity. *Behaviour Research and Therapy*, 28, 697–708	This self-report questionnaire assesses agoraphobic symptomatology. It was developed for adults and may be used cautiously with adolescents
	Agoraphobia Cognitions Questionnaire	Chambless, D., Caputo, C., Bright, P. & Gallagher, R. (1984). Assessment of fear in agoraphobics: the Body Sensations Questionnaire and the Agoraphobia Cognitions Questionnaire. *Journal of Consulting and Clinical Psychology*, 62, 1090–1097	This self-report questionnaire assesses agoraphobic cognitions and worries. It was developed for adults and may be used cautiously with adolescents
Post-traumatic stress related anxiety	Childhood PTSD Interview-Child Form	Fletcher K (1997), Childhood PTSD interview – child form. In E. Carlson (Ed.), *Trauma Assessments: A Clinician's Guide* (pp. 248–250). New York: Guilford	This semi-structured interview with good reliability yields DSM IV diagnoses of PTSD
	Clinician Administered PTSD Scale for Children (CAPS-C)	Nader, K., Blakem D., Kriegler, J., & Pynoos, R. (1994). *Clinician Administered PTSD Scale for Children (CAPS-C)*. Los Angeles: UCLA Neuropsychiatric Institute and National Centre for PTSD	This semi-structured interview with good reliability yields DSM IV diagnoses of PTSD

Instrument	Reference	Description
Child and Adolescent Trauma Survey (CATS)	March, J. (1999). Assessment of paediatric posttraumatic stress disorder. In P. Saigh & D. Bremner (Eds.), *Posttraumatic Stress Disorder* (pp. 199–218). Washington, DC: American Psychological Press	Normed self-report DSM IV PTSD scale for children
Change-sensitive PTSD Symptom Scale	March, J., Amaya-Jackson, L., Murray, M. & Schulte, A. (1998). Cognitive behavioural psychotherapy for children and adolescents with posttraumatic stress disorder following a single incident stressor. *Journal of the American Academy of Child and Adolescent Psychiatry*, 37, 585–593	Change-sensitive self-report DSM IV PTSD scale for children
Impact of Events Scale	Horowitz, M., Wilner, N. & Alverez, W. (1979). Impact of events scale. A measure of subjective stress. *Psychosomatic Medicine*, 41, 209–218	This 15-item measure of post-traumatic stress yields scores on intrusions and avoidance sub-scales as well as an overall score
Children's Post-traumatic Stress Disorder Inventory	Saigh, P. (1989). The development and validation of the Children's Post Traumatic Stress Disorder Inventory. *International Journal of Special Education*, 4, 75–84	This 17-item structured interview yields a PTSD diagnosis based on DSM criteria
Child PTSD Symptom Scale	Foa, E., Johnson, K., Feeney, N., Treadwell, K. (2001). The Child PTSD Symptom Scale: A preliminary examination of its psychometric properties. *Journal of Clinical Child Psychology*, 30, 376–384	This 24-item scale yields a PTSD diagnosis based on DSM IV criteria
Child Post-Traumatic Stress Disorder Reaction Index	Fredrick, C., Pynooss, R. & Nader, K. (1992). *The Child Post-Traumatic Stress Disorder Reaction Index*. Los Angeles, CA: UCLA Dept of Psychiatry and behavioural Sciences, 760 Westwood Plaza, LA, CA 90024	This self-report or interview instrument covers DSM symptomatology and yields an overall severity of symptomatology score
Child PTSD Interview	Pynoos, R. & Eth, S. (1986). Witness to violence: The child interview. *Journal of the American Academy of Child Psychiatry*, 25, 306–319	This is a set of guidelines for a semi-structured clinical interview and contains information on the use of drawings and other interview techniques

PRE-DISPOSING FACTORS

PERSONAL PRE-DISPOSING FACTORS

Biological factors
- Genetic vulnerabilities

Psychological factors
- Inhibited temperament
- Low self-esteem
- External locus of control

CONTEXTUAL PRE-DISPOSING FACTORS

Parent–child factors in early life
- Anxious attachment

Exposure to family problems in early life
- Parental anxiety
- Anxiety and threat-sensitive family culture

PERSONAL MAINTAINING FACTORS

Biological factors
- Dysregulation of GABA, serotonin, and noradrenergic systems
- Hyperarousal

Psychological factors
- Avoiding internal and external feared stimuli
- Approaching feared stimuli and withdrawing before anxiety subsides
- Threat and danger oriented cognitive set
- External hypervigilance and misinterpreting neutral events as threatening
- Internal hypervigilance and misinterpreting benign somatic sensations as signs of ill health

PERSONAL PROTECTIVE FACTORS

Biological factors
- Good physical health

Psychological factors
- High IQ
- Easy temperament
- High self-esteem
- Internal locus of control
- High self-efficacy
- Optimistic attributional style
- Mature defence mechanisms
- Functional coping strategies

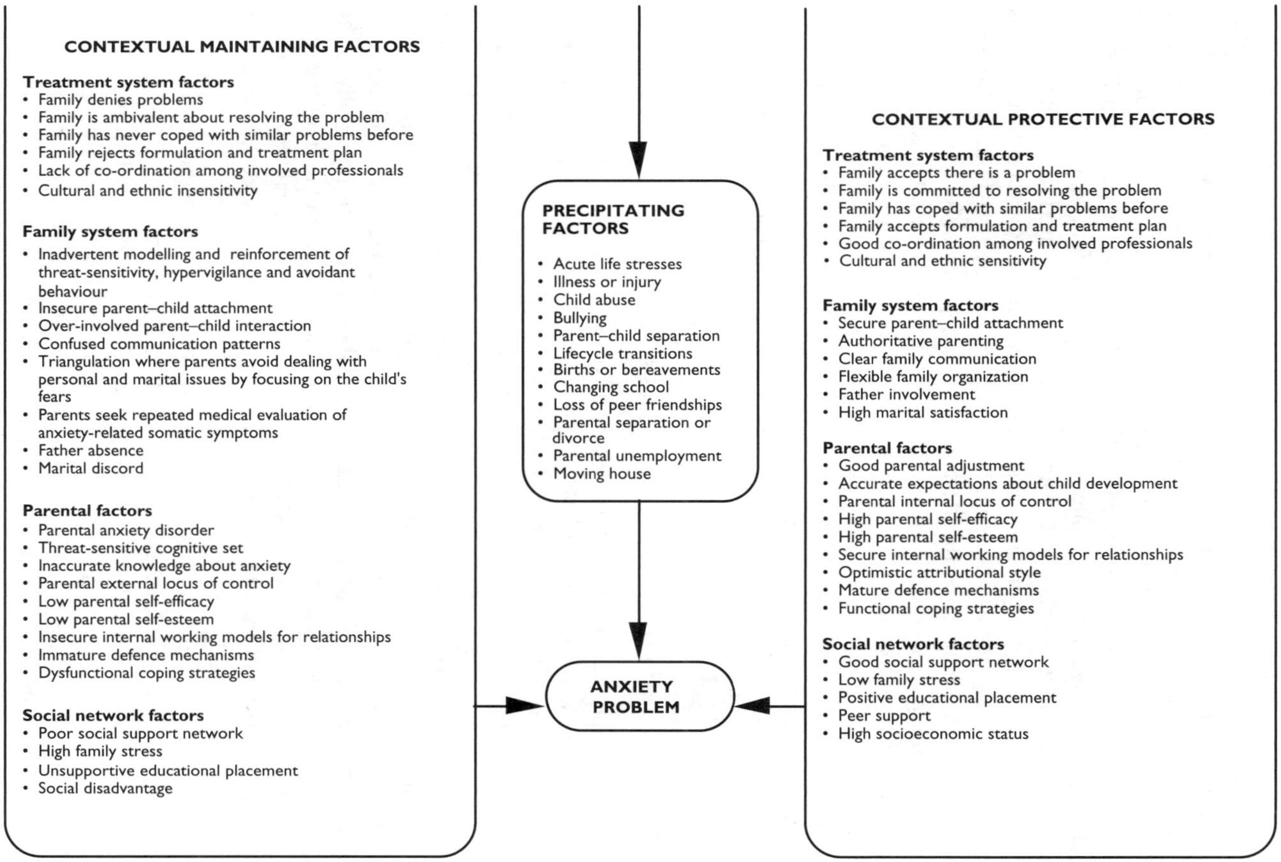

CONTEXTUAL MAINTAINING FACTORS

Treatment system factors
- Family denies problems
- Family is ambivalent about resolving the problem
- Family has never coped with similar problems before
- Family rejects formulation and treatment plan
- Lack of co-ordination among involved professionals
- Cultural and ethnic insensitivity

Family system factors
- Inadvertent modelling and reinforcement of threat-sensitivity, hypervigilance and avoidant behaviour
- Insecure parent–child attachment
- Over-involved parent–child interaction
- Confused communication patterns
- Triangulation where parents avoid dealing with personal and marital issues by focusing on the child's fears
- Parents seek repeated medical evaluation of anxiety-related somatic symptoms
- Father absence
- Marital discord

Parental factors
- Parental anxiety disorder
- Threat-sensitive cognitive set
- Inaccurate knowledge about anxiety
- Parental external locus of control
- Low parental self-efficacy
- Low parental self-esteem
- Insecure internal working models for relationships
- Immature defence mechanisms
- Dysfunctional coping strategies

Social network factors
- Poor social support network
- High family stress
- Unsupportive educational placement
- Social disadvantage

PRECIPITATING FACTORS
- Acute life stresses
- Illness or injury
- Child abuse
- Bullying
- Parent–child separation
- Lifecycle transitions
- Births or bereavements
- Changing school
- Loss of peer friendships
- Parental separation or divorce
- Parental unemployment
- Moving house

ANXIETY PROBLEM

CONTEXTUAL PROTECTIVE FACTORS

Treatment system factors
- Family accepts there is a problem
- Family is committed to resolving the problem
- Family has coped with similar problems before
- Family accepts formulation and treatment plan
- Good co-ordination among involved professionals
- Cultural and ethnic sensitivity

Family system factors
- Secure parent–child attachment
- Authoritative parenting
- Clear family communication
- Flexible family organization
- Father involvement
- High marital satisfaction

Parental factors
- Good parental adjustment
- Accurate expectations about child development
- Parental internal locus of control
- High parental self-efficacy
- High parental self-esteem
- Secure internal working models for relationships
- Optimistic attributional style
- Mature defence mechanisms
- Functional coping strategies

Social network factors
- Good social support network
- Low family stress
- Positive educational placement
- Peer support
- High socioeconomic status

Figure 12.3 Factors to consider in childhood anxiety problems

Precipitating factors

Personal or family illness or injury may precipitate the onset or exacerbation of anxiety problems, since they may be perceived as threats to the child's security or health. In conditions such as gastrointestinal illness, which involve significant abdominal discomfort, there is an added complication. The organically based abdominal pain may precipitate the onset of anxiety and, subsequently, when the organic factors that led to abdominal discomfort are no longer operative, anxiety-related abdominal discomfort may remain. Children with anxiety-related discomfort may become anxious because they interpret their anxiety-related discomfort as reflecting a dangerous illness. Lifecycle transitions such as going to school for the first time or having a sibling leave home; stressful life events such as parental separation, moving house, changing schools, losing friends or increased financial hardship within the family; and separation from the primary caregiver for a significant time period may all precipitate the onset or exacerbation of anxiety problems because these events all threaten the predictability of the child's world. For school-going children, both bullying by peers and victimization by teachers may precipitate anxiety problems, as may the occurrence of either intrafamilial or extrafamilial child abuse.

Maintaining factors

Personal and contextual factors may be involved in the maintenance of children's anxiety. At a personal level, ongoing avoidance of feared stimuli or a pattern of regularly approaching feared stimuli and then withdrawing before anxiety subsides may maintain or exacerbate the child's anxiety, since these behavioural patterns prevent habituation to anxiety-provoking stimuli. A threat- and danger-oriented cognitive set, where neutral or ambiguous stimuli are interpreted as threatening may also maintain anxiety problems. One important aspect of such a cognitive set is hypervigilance and frequent misinterpretation of non-threatening external events or internal bodily sensations as extremely hazardous. At a biological level, dysregulation of the serotonin, noradrenaline and GABA systems, and hyperarousal, may maintain anxiety, although in routine clinical practice thorough psychophysiological assessment is rarely necessary.

At a contextual level, children's anxiety may be maintained by parents interpreting ambiguous situations as threatening in their conversations with the child and inadvertently reinforcing the child for avoidant behaviour. Such interaction patterns may be characterized by over-involvement or confused communication, and either of these parent–child interaction styles tends to maintain rather than resolve problems. Parents' insistence on repeated medical evaluation of anxiety-related somatic complaints such as abdominal pains or headaches may also maintain the child's anxiety. Parents may be particularly prone to these types of anxiety-maintaining patterns of interaction when they cope with personal or marital difficulties by avoiding dealing with them and focusing instead on the child's problems. Parents who are worried about their own health may displace their anxiety about this onto the child and express intense concern about the child's well-being. Parents who experience marital discord and who have unresolved conflicts about intimacy or power within the marital relationship may avoid discussing these conflicts but routinely argue about how best to manage their anxious child. That is, they may become involved in a pattern of triangulation with the child. It is not unusual for such triangulation to involve intense interaction between the mother and child, with the father becoming increasingly peripheral as the problems progress.

Such patterns of parenting and family organization may be associated with parental anxiety and a threat-oriented cognitive set. Such parents may have insecure internal working models for relationships, low self-esteem, low self-efficacy, external locus of control, immature defences and poor coping strategies. Parents may also become involved in problem-maintaining interactions with their children if they have inaccurate knowledge about anxiety and related psychological processes.

Anxiety may be maintained by high levels of stress, limited support and social disadvantage within the family's wider social system, since these features may deplete parents' and children's personal resources for dealing constructively with anxiety. Poorly resourced educational placements, where teaching staff have little time to devote to contributing to school-based anxiety management interventions may maintain anxiety problems.

Within the treatment system, a lack of co-ordination and clear communication among involved professionals, including teachers, psychologists, paediatricians and so forth, may maintain children's anxiety-related problems. It is not unusual for various members of the professional network to offer conflicting opinions and advice on the nature and management of anxiety problems to children and their families. These may range from viewing the child as physically ill with secondary anxiety problems deserving careful management to seeing the child as healthy but malingering and deserving a disciplinarian management. Where co-operation problems between families and treatment teams develop, and families deny the existence of the problems, the validity of the diagnosis and formulation or the appropriateness of the treatment programme, then the child's difficulties may persist. Parents' lack of experience in dealing with similar problems in the past is a further factor that may compromise their capacity to work co-operatively with the treatment team and so may contribute to the maintenance of the child's anxiety. Treatment systems that are not sensitive to the cultural and ethnic beliefs and values of the youngster's family system may maintain anxiety by inhibiting engagement or promoting drop-out from treatment and preventing the development of a good working alliance between the treamtent team, the youngster and his or her family.

Protective factors

The probability that a treatment programme for anxiety will be effective is influenced by a variety of personal and contextual protective factors. It is important that these are assessed and included in the later formulation, since it is protective factors that usually serve as the foundation for therapeutic change. Good health, a high IQ, an easy temperament, high self-esteem, an internal locus of control, high self-efficacy and an optimistic attributional style are all important personal protective factors. Other important personal protective factors include mature defence mechanisms and functional coping strategies, particularly good problem-solving skills and a capacity to make and maintain friendships.

Within the family, secure parent–child attachment and authoritative parenting are central protective factors, particularly if they occur within the context of a flexible family structure in which there is clear communication, high marital satisfaction and both parents share the day-to-day tasks of child care.

Good parental adjustment is also a protective factor. Where parents have an internal locus of control, high self-efficacy, high self-esteem, internal working models for secure attachments, an optimistic attributional style, mature defences and functional coping strategies, then they are better resourced to manage their children's anxiety constructively. Of course, accurate knowledge about anxiety is also a protective factor.

Within the broader social network, high levels of support, low levels of stress and membership of a high socioeconomic group are all protective factors for children with anxiety problems. Where families are embedded in social networks that provide a high level of support and place few stressful demands on family members, then it is less likely that parents' and children's resources for dealing with anxiety-related problems will become depleted. A well-resourced educational placement may also be viewed as a protective factor. Educational placements where teachers have a clear understanding of anxiety-related problems and have sufficient time and flexibility to contribute to home–school anxiety management programmes contribute to positive outcomes for children with anxiety problems.

Within the treatment system, co-operative working relationships between the treatment team and the family and good co-ordination of multi-professional input are protective factors. Treatment systems that are sensitive to the cultural and ethnic beliefs and values of the youngster's family are more likely help families engage with, and remain in treatment, and foster the development of a good working alliance. Families are more likely to benefit from treatment when they accept the formulation of the problem given by the treatment team and are committed to working with the team to resolve it. Where families have successfully faced similar problems before, then they are more likely to benefit from treatment and, in this sense, previous experience with similar problems is a protective factor.

FORMULATION

Salient features from the assessment should be combined into a formulation which specifies the principal anxiety problems and the factors that maintain these. Background pre-disposing factors and specific events that precipitated the onset or exacerbation of the anxiety problems should be noted. Protective factors in the case should also be listed. Examples of formulations are given in the penultimate paragraphs of case studies set out in Boxes 12.1, 12.2, 12.4, 12.5 and 12.6.

GENERAL TREATMENT PRINCIPLES

Multi-systemic anxiety management programmes should aim to alter maintaining factors and capitalize upon protective factors. They should include some or all of the following elements:

- psychoeducation about the nature of anxiety and its treatment
- training in monitoring symptomatology
- relaxation skills training
- cognitive restructuring
- rehearsal following observation of a model for coping with exposure to feared stimuli
- exposure to feared stimuli until habituation occurs
- reward systems to increase motivation to follow through on exposure
- family involvement in treatment
- individual exploratory work
- school involvement in treatment where avoidance is school based
- liaison with other professionals, particularly medicine if there are anxiety-based somatic symptoms
- referral of parents for treatment of psychological and marital problems if appropriate.

A description of the principles of clinical practice for each of these elements follows. These descriptions are informed by the literature on effective treatments for anxiety disorders and on clinical experience (Allen & Rapee, 2005; American Academy of Child and Adolescent Psychiatry, 1997c, 1998b; Barrett & Shortt, 2003; Carr, 2004b; Compton et al., 2004; Kendall et al.,

2003; Morris & March, 2004; Ollendick & March, 2003; Silverman & Treffers, 2001).

Psychoeducation

When educating parents and children about anxiety it is useful to explain that anxiety has three different parts: thoughts about being afraid, physical feelings of being afraid and behaviour patterns that help the child avoid the situations of which they are frightened. This may then be elaborated as follows. It is the thoughts of being afraid and *the habit of seeing situations as dangerous* that are at the root of anxiety. A child who is afraid of dogs sees a dog as a danger because he or she automatically thinks of the possibility that the dog could bite him. There is, of course, an alternative. The dog could be seen as a child's best friend. If the child selected to see the dog this way then the child would have no thoughts of being afraid. The physical feelings that follow from the dangerous thoughts are the second part of anxiety. The thoughts of being afraid of a dangerous situation lead to the body getting ready to fight the danger or run from it. This physical part of anxiety (autonomic hyperarousal) involves adrenaline flowing into the blood-stream, the heart beating faster, a quickening of breathing and the muscles becoming tense. The faster breathing may lead to dizziness. The tense muscles may lead to headaches or stomach pains. Sometimes, these physical changes, like a racing heart beat, dizziness or pains are frightening themselves, and this leads to more physical changes. The thoughts of being afraid and the physical feelings that go with them lead the child to try to escape from the frightening situation or to avoid it. This is the third part of anxiety: the behaviour patterns that the child uses to avoid frightening situations. Children who are forced to face the situation without training may become so frightened that they kick and scream to try to escape. Parents and teachers might try this forceful approach to help the child face the situation until the fear dies, but then back off when they see how distressing it is for the child. After that, they allow the child to get into a habit of avoiding the frightening situation. Unfortunately, this makes the anxiety worse. What the child needs to learn to master the anxiety is to get into training so that he or she can handle rising anxiety and then go into the frightening situation and use all their training to cope with it. Treatment involves getting into training for handling anxiety and then facing the frightening situation until the anxiety dies. In the end, the only way to get rid of anxiety, dangerous thinking, anxiety feelings, pains, dizziness and avoidance behaviour patterns is to go into the frightening situation and stay there until the anxiety dies. Treatment cannot work the other way around. It is not possible to get rid of anxiety and then go into the frightening situation. A useful resource is *Helping your anxious child: a step-by-step guide for parents* (Rapee, Spense, Cobham & Wignal, 2000).

Monitoring

Monitoring cognitive, affective-somatic and behavioural aspects of anxiety, and monitoring the use of various coping skills in frightening situations, allows progress through treatment to be tracked by the child, the parents and the psychologist. At the simplest level, children may be trained to identify the affective and somatic experiences that contribute to their discomfort when they are in an anxiety-provoking situation. Each child has his or her own unique constellation of affective and somatic experiences that under-pin discomfort. Some feel anxiety in their stomachs and develop abdominal pains. Others find they hyperventilate and become light-headed. Still others become restless and move about in an agitated way. Careful interviewing and the use of drawings, puppets and metaphors may be used to help children articulate the core affective-somatic component of their anxiety experience. Once this has been identified, children may be invited to rate the intensity of this experience on a ten-point scale when they enter a frightening situation. This scale may also be used during relaxation training to indicate the impact of the relaxation exercises on the child's affective-somatic state.

Children may be trained to identify anxiety-provoking cognitions (*dangerous thoughts*) which occur in frightening situations. In family sessions, a series of situations that are ambiguous may be presented and family members may be invited to offer a range of possible threatening and non-threatening interpretations of these situations. This can open up a discussion about habits that family members have for interpreting situations in threatening or non-threatening ways and sensitize parents and children to the types of interpretations that they typically make. Both the Coping CAT (Kendall et al., 2003) and FRIENDs (Barrett & Shortt, 2003) programmes include workbooks for teaching cognitive self-monitoring skills (and other skills for anxiety management in children). These contain cartoons in which the protagonist appears in a range of ambiguous situations which are open to a wide variety of interpretations. The child is invited to write down (in the thought bubble over the cartoon character's head) what the character is thinking. The therapist uses these responses, and the fact that there are less danger-oriented alternatives, to help the child recognize the role of cognitive appraisal in generating anxiety. Once the child has grasped the idea that situations are open to a variety of interpretations, *dangerous thoughts* may be monitored along with fear ratings and description of the situations in which they occur. Later, children can be trained to challenge *dangerous thoughts*, to test out alternative interpretations and to reward themselves for doing so. The development of challenge–test–reward (CTR) skills is the central focus in the approach to cognitive restructuring for anxiety, which is described below in the 'Cognitive restructuring' section.

Approach and avoidance behaviour in frightening situations may be monitored by inviting the child or the parents to note which type of behaviour occurs in these situations. For example, with children who have a fear of the dark, whether children sleep in their own beds or their parents' beds may be recorded. For youngsters with agoraphobia, the distance they travel from the house each day may be recorded. For a child with a dental fear, the number of minutes they could tolerate sitting in the dentist's chair may be counted.

Coping responses, such as the use of relaxation skills, coping self-statements, self-reinforcement, support from parents, teachers or peers, or reinforcement from parents for approach behaviour may be monitored by asking the child or parent to name the coping strategy that was used in each situation where the child was exposed to the feared stimulus or anticipated such exposure.

A fear tracking form which allows situations, fear ratings, cognitions, approach or avoidance behaviours, and coping strategies to be monitored is presented in Figure 12.4. This form may be easily simplified by removing one or more columns and such simplified versions may be useful in the early stages of assessment and treatment, particularly with younger children.

Exposure

A central underlying feature of all effective psychological treatments for anxiety is exposure. That is, to overcome the anxiety, the child must be exposed to the feared stimulus until the anxiety subsides. This exposure may involve coping with a graded hierarchy of about ten increasingly threatening stimuli for relatively brief periods or facing a highly threatening situation for a protracted period. When the child is exposed to graded hierarchy of situations and is trained to cope with each situation by using relaxation skills to reduce anxiety, this is referred to as systematic desensitization. Flooding is the term used to describe treatment which involves prolonged exposure to highly feared stimuli. Desensitization sessions are far less stressful than flooding sessions, but usually a greater number of sessions are required for desensitization. The child may be exposed to the actual feared stimuli (in vivo) or to a cognitive representation of the feared stimulus (in imagination). In vivo exposure tends to be the most effective, although it requires more time and organization to set up.

Relaxation training

To manage exposure, the child may be trained in a variety of coping skills, particularly relaxation, cognitive restructuring and self-reinforcement. Relaxation skills allow the child to alter physiological arousal level. Relaxation skills may be taught by a psychologist or other professional, by a parent, by a peer or be learned from an audiotape. When relaxation is taught to children by their parents under a psychologist's supervision, it has the added benefit of disrupting anxiety-maintaining parent–child interactions. A set of

FEAR TRACKING FORM

When you have finished dealing with a frightening situation fill out one line of this form. This will help you to keep track of :
- the types of frightening situations you get into
- how frightened you become
- what you think about in those situations
- what you do in those situations and
- how you coped and how your parents teachers or friends helped you to cope

Day and time	Frightening situation	Fear rating	Thoughts	Actions	Coping responses
	Where was it? What was the most frightening thing about it?	1 = low 10 = high	Dangerous thoughts Coping thoughts	Avoid situation Face situation	Relaxation CTR (challenge–test–reward) Parental support Teacher support Friends support

Figure 12.4 Fear tracking form

relaxation exercises which parents may teach to children is presented in Figure 12.5. Customized relaxation tapes are a useful adjunct to direct instruction but relaxation tapes without instruction are of little clinical value.

When coaching parents in relaxation instruction, model the process first by going through the exercises with the child while the parents observe. Use a

RELAXATION EXERCISES

After a couple of weeks daily practice under your supervision, your child will have developed enough skill to use these exercises to get rid of unwanted body tension.

- Set aside 20 minutes a day to do these relaxation exercises with your child
- Try to arrange to be on good terms with your child when you do these exercises so your child looks forward to them
- Do them at the same time and in the same place every day
- Before you begin, remove all distractions (by turning off bright lights, the radio, etc.) and ask your child to loosen any tight clothes (like belts, ties or shoes)
- Ask your child to lie on a bed or recline in a comfortable chair with the eyes lightly closed
- Before and after each exercise ask your child to breath in deeply and exhale slowly three times while saying the word 'relax' to him or herself.
- At the end of each exercise praise your child by saying 'Well done' or 'You did that exercise well' or some other form of praise
- Repeat each exercise twice
- Throughout the exercises speak in a calm relaxed quiet voice

Area	Exercise
Hands	Close your hands into fists. Then allow them to open slowly Notice the change from tension to relaxation in your hands and allow this change to continue further and further still so the muscles of your hands become more and more relaxed
Arms	Bend your arms at the elbow and touch your shoulders with your hands Then allow them to return to the resting position. Notice the change from tension to relaxation in your arms and allow this change to continue further and further still so the muscles of your arms become more and more relaxed
Shoulders	Hunch your shoulders up to your ears. Then allow them to return to the resting position Notice the change from tension to relaxation in your shoulders and allow this change to continue further and further still so the muscles of your shoulders become more and more relaxed
Legs	Point your toes downwards. Then allow them to return to the resting position. Notice the change from tension to relaxation in the fronts of your legs and allow this change to continue further and further still so the muscles in the fronts of your legs become more and more relaxed. Point your toes upwards. Then allow them to return to the resting position Notice the change from tension to relaxation in the backs of your legs and allow this change to continue further and further still so the muscles in the backs of your legs become more and more relaxed
Stomach	Take a deep breath and hold it for three seconds, tensing the muscles in your stomach as you do so. Then breath out slowly Notice the change from tension to relaxation in your stomach muscles and allow this change to continue further and further still so your stomach muscles become more and more relaxed
Face	Clench your teeth tightly together. Then relax. Notice the change from tension to relaxation in your jaw and allow this change to continue further and further still so the muscles in your jaw become more and more relaxed Wrinkle your nose up. Then relax. Notice the change from tension to relaxation in the muscles around the front of your face and allow this change to continue further and further still so the muscles of your face become more and more relaxed Shut your eyes tightly. Then relax. Notice the change from tension to relaxation in the muscles around your eyes and allow this change to continue further and further still so the muscles around your eyes become more and more relaxed
All over	Now that you've done all your muscle exercises, check that all areas of your body are as relaxed as can be. Think of your hands and allow them to relax a little more Think of your arms and allow them to relax a little more Think of your shoulders and allow them to relax a little more Think of your legs and allow them to relax a little more Think of your stomach and allow it to relax a little more Think of your face and allow it to relax a little more
Breathing	Breath in . . . one . . . two . . . three . . . and out slowly . . . one . . . two . . . three . . . four . . . five . . . six . . . and again Breath in . . . one . . . two . . . three . . . and out slowly . . . one . . . two . . . three . . . four . . . five . . . six . . . and again Breath in . . . one . . . two . . . three . . . and out slowly . . . one . . . two . . . three . . . four . . . five . . . six
Visualizing	Imagine you are lying on a beautiful sandy beach and you feel the sun warm your body Make a picture in your mind of the golden sand and the warm sun As the sun warms your body you feel more and more relaxed As the sun warms your body you feel more and more relaxed As the sun warms your body you feel more and more relaxed The sky is a clear, clear blue. Above you, you can see a small white cloud drifting away into the distance As it drifts away you feel more and more relaxed It is drifting away and you feel more and more relaxed It is drifting away and you feel more and more relaxed As the sun warms your body you feel more and more relaxed AS the cloud drifts away you feel more and more relaxed (Wait for 30 seconds) When you are ready open your eyes ready to fact the rest of the day relaxed and calm

Figure 12.5 Relaxation exercises handout for parents and youngsters

slow calming tone of voice and repetition of instructions as required to help the child achieve a relaxed state. Before and after the exercises check out with the child how relaxed he or she feels on a ten-point scale where 1 reflects complete relaxation and 10 reflects extreme anxiety. Most children will report that even on their first trial, they achieve some tension reduction. This should be praised and interpreted to the child and the parents as an indication that the child has the aptitude for developing and refining his or her relaxation skills. The parents may then be invited to instruct the child in completing the exercises daily and to praise the child for completing the exercises.

For a minority of children, the relaxation exercises lead to increased tension. This may occur because the exercises make the child aware of body tension that is normally ignored. Alternatively, it may occur because focusing attention on somatic processes during the exercises induces anxiety. With youngsters who have had panic attacks, this is particularly common because they are sensitized to construing fluctuations in physiological functioning as signalling the onset of a panic attack. In such instances, work on only one or two muscle groups at a time and keep the training periods very short. Also request regular anxiety ratings from the child and when increases in anxiety occur, distract the child by asking him or her to engage in the visualization exercise described in Figure 12.5. With some such children it may be necessary to abandon the muscle-relaxation exercises completely and concentrate on training them in visualization or focusing on an external repetitive calming visual or auditory stimulus as a means of attaining a relaxed state. (For some of my clients I have used such stimuli as music, children's hanging mobiles, candlelight and a bowl of goldfish!) The important thing is to find a routine that the child can reliably use to reduce the subjective sense of anxiety as indicated by their status on a ten-point anxiety rating scale.

Some children find that the scene described for the visualization exercise given in Figure 12.5 is not relaxing. In such instances, ask the child to describe an alternative relaxing scene such as being in a wood or on top of a mountain and use this as an alternative.

Biofeedback-assisted relaxation is as effective as progressive muscle relaxation in reducing arousal in adults and this is also probably the case with children (Shapiro & Shapiro, 1982). Portable skin conductance biofeedback units are now widely available for this purpose. However, biofeedback equipment increases the cost of treatment. It also does not provide opportunities for enhancing parent–child relationships in the way that parent-assisted relaxation training does.

Cognitive restructuring

Cognitive restructuring or self-instructional coping skills are those required to reinterpret ambiguous situations in less threatening ways, to test out the validity of these alternative interpretations and to use self-reinforcement following such testing (Beck et al., 1985). The section on monitoring, above, described methods for coaching the child to identify *dangerous thoughts* (threat-oriented interpretations of situations). In CTR, self-instructional training children are invited to Challenge these dangerous thoughts by asking themselves what the other possible interpretations of the situation are, to Test out what evidence there is for the catastrophic outcome and the other less threatening outcomes and to Reward themselves for testing out the less catastrophic interpretation of the situation. So, a child who has a dog phobia who has been coached in CTR cognitive restructuring coping skills may carry out this internal dialogue:

'He's dangerous and will bite me' (dangerous thought)
'No, an alternative view is he wants to be my friend' (Challenge)
'I will not run away. There I didn't run and he didn't bite me. He did want to be friendly' (Test)
'Well done' (Reward).

CTR cognitive restructuring is derived from Beck's cognitive therapy for anxiety (Beck et al., 1985). Where CTR skills are taught within a family session, parents may be trained to prompt the child to use these coping skills in frightening situations and to offer support and reinforcement for using them effectively. Where family members, particularly parents, have anxiety problems, they can be coached in avoiding passing on their habits of *thinking dangerously* to their children by using CTR skills themselves.

Modelling and rehearsal

Rehearsal following observation of a model who used both relaxation and CTR cognitive restructuring skills to cope with exposure to feared stimuli enhances the learning process. The more like the child the model is, and the greater the esteem in which the model is held, the better. Because parents (or primary carers) are held in very high esteem and children identify with parents as part of the developmental process, parents may be coached in modelling good anxiety management skills for their children. Where parents have developed a threat- and danger-oriented family culture, helping them model good day-to-day anxiety management skills for their children may reduce the impact of the threat and danger oriented family culture on their children.

In addition to this family-based intervention, models who are similar to the child may be particularly effective in helping children develop anxiety management skills. Thus, a child who has had an anxiety problem but resolved it through using relaxation and cognitive restructuring skills during exposure is the ideal model. This type of modelling may be offered within a group therapy programme for children with anxiety problems which runs concurrently with family-based treatment sessions. Youngsters who have made progress in over-coming their fears may act as models for those who have not yet done so. Alternatively, a videotape of a child coping with exposure may be used as a model. This may be appropriate, for example, when dealing with anxiety associated with medical procedures. After observing the model the child may imitate the model's coping processes as a form of rehearsal.

Reward systems

To increase the child's motivation to follow through on the process of exposure to the feared stimuli, a reward system is a key part of most anxiety treatment plans. The child may receive praise and encouragement for each episode of exposure, along with some tangible reward. In addition, points may be given for each episode of exposure and accumulated to obtain items from a reinforcement menu. In developing such a system, a list of exposure situations should be drawn up and ranked in order of difficulty. Points may then be allocated to each situation, with the greatest number of points being earned by coping with the most difficult situation. Alongside this list of exposure situations, a list of desired rewards should be drawn up and rank-ordered in terms of their perceived value to the child. Then, the number of points required to earn each of these rewards on the reinforcement menu should be written down opposite the item. The numbers of points required to earn items from the reinforcement menu should be such that the child may accumulate enough points to earn something off the reinforcement menu by successfully coping with three or four anxiety-provoking situations. This type of long-range reward system, which yields weekly rewards, should be used in conjunction with an immediate reward system where praise and prizes are issued for managing each successful exposure to a feared situation. Once reward systems are in operation, parents may be coached in how to complement them with systematic ignoring of worry-talk, to help the child break the habit of ruminating about harmless events.

Family and school involvement

The chances of treatment gains being maintained are increased if the family is centrally involved in coaching the child in coping skills, managing the exposure process and implementing the reward system. This is because this process of family involvement challenges the family's threat-oriented culture if one is present, disrupts family-based interactional patterns which maintain the child's threat-oriented cognitive set and avoidance behaviour, makes full use of the parents' problem-solving potential and provides an outlet for parents' desire to help their child recover. School involvement is important where the child experiences anxiety in school or going to school. School staff may assist with supporting and rewarding the child for exposure to feared school-based situations. This issue will be discussed more fully below in the section on school refusal.

Individual exploratory work

Youngsters with generalized anxiety disorders or multiple co-morbid anxiety disorders sometimes have a small set of core underlying fears that their basic needs for safety, security and protection will not be met. These underlying fears may find expression in anxiety about multiple stimuli and situations. In cases where exposure and coping-skills training is ineffective, individual exploratory work may be conducted to identify these core danger-related beliefs or fear schemas. This type of work may progress from an initial exploratory review of children's multiple expressed fears. Common themes may be sought by the therapist and the child in a collaborative way so that eventually core underlying fears are identified. Drawing, art work, play and other media may be used to help youngsters conduct such explorations. This type of work may provide clearer targets for exposure work and for the use of challenge, test and self-reward skills.

Liaison with other professionals

Where anxiety-based somatic complaints (such as abdominal pains, headaches and dizziness) have led to involvement of medical professionals, liaison with these professionals is vital, so that the child and the family receive a unified message about the most useful way to conceptualize the somatic symptoms and the best way to manage them (Blagg, 1987). Difficulties usually occur when the paediatric physician's report indicates that there is no organic basis for the child's abdominal pains or headaches and the parents and child interpret this to mean that the child's experiences are imaginary or the child's reports are factitious. One way to handle this is to meet jointly with the paediatrician, the child and the parents. Then the psychologist and paediatrician may jointly explain that abdominal pains, headaches and dizziness are all distressing somatic manifestations of anxiety, and arise from autonomic nervous system hyperarousal. They are, in colloquial terms, *real*, not imaginary. Routine medical investigations such as physical examination, blood tests or X-rays are not designed to detect autonomic hyperarousal. They are designed to detect intestinal obstructions, lesions, tumours and disease processes which also cause abdominal pains and headaches. The negative results of the medical tests indicate that intestinal obstructions, lesions, tumours and disease processes were not detected.

Concurrent referral of parents

Referral for concurrent treatment of parental psychological problems or marital difficulties may be necessary in some cases, particularly where the parental behaviour that maintains the child's difficulties permits the parents to avoid dealing with their personal and marital problems.

TREATMENT OF SPECIFIC ANXIETY DISORDERS

The treatment programmes for specific types of anxiety disorder outlined below are premised on the general principles outlined in the previous section.

Management of separation anxiety and school refusal

Cases of separation anxiety are typically referred when the child refuses to attend school (Blagg, 1987; Heyne & King 2004; Heyne, King & Ollendick, 2005; Heyne & Rollings, 2002). The child's underlying belief when separation anxiety occurs is that a catastrophe will occur if the parent and child are separated, and this may lead to the parent or the child or both being harmed. This theme may pre-occupy the child when faced with the prospect of separation and also recur as a theme in night-mares. Some children experience intense episodes of separation anxiety when they awake from such nightmares and ask to sleep with their parents or siblings. When separation is anticipated or threatened, pronounced hyperarousal of the autonomic nervous system may occur resulting in tachycardia, stomachaches, headaches, nausea and vomiting. In some instances, children may faint. These physical symptoms commonly lead to many visits to the family doctor and occasionally to paediatric investigations. Children may feel misunderstood and disbelieved when such investigations fail to identify a discrete organic cause for these somatic complaints. Children and parents may interpret such findings to mean that the abdominal pains and headaches are being construed by the medical team to be either imaginary or factitious.

If physically forced to separate from the parent, the child usually becomes tearful and may cling to the parent or try to prevent separation by, for example, locking the car doors if the child has been driven to school. Attempts to force the child to separate may also lead to aggressive tantrums, kicking, screaming and other dramatic displays of anxiety. Commonly, such displays result in the child being allowed to remain with the attachment figure, and so the child's avoidance behaviour is negatively reinforced, thus making it more probable that it will recur. A number of such incidents will typically have occurred before the child is referred for psychological consultation. In other cases, the children will separate from the parents and go to school but be returned home when he or she appears to be ill with abdominal pains and headaches.

The management of separation anxiety and school refusal is complicated by the fact it may often begin when the child has a viral condition. Thus, parents and involved professionals may have difficulty interpreting the degree to which initial somatic complaints and those that occur during relapses have a viral basis or are due to anxiety or a combination of both. Also, simple formulations of the child's behaviour as a reflection of organic illness or misbehaviour may lead to polarization among parents and involved professional. Such polarization makes it difficult for parents and professionals to co-operate in helping the child return to school and manage the anxiety.

It is important to mention that not all cases of school refusal reflect separation anxiety. When school refusal occurs in five- or six-year-olds at the beginning of primary school it is most commonly associated with separation anxiety. When school refusal occurs at eleven or twelve years of age at the transition to secondary school both separation anxiety and other factors may be involved. For instance, the child may fear some aspect of the school experience, such as being bullied by peers, being victimized by teachers, entering into an unknown environment, fearing academic or athletic failure and so forth. Later in adolescence, if school refusal occurs it may reflect separation anxiety, avoidance of particularly threatening situations within the school, and also the onset of other psychological problems such as depression, obsessive-compulsive disorder, Tourette's syndrome or eating disorders. When a child refuses to go to school, all of these areas deserve careful assessment.

The most effective available treatment for school refusal is a behavioural problem-solving approach which involves all significant members of the child's social network, including parents, teachers and in some instances peers. This method, which is successful in over 90% of cases, involves first a thorough assessment of factors associated with the child, the family and the school, and the wider professional system that may be contributing to school non-attendance. A framework for assessing such factors is set out in Figure 12.6.

Child-related factors include separation anxiety, depression, other psychological adjustment problems and physical ill health, notably viral infections. Children may also refuse to go to school because of fear of specific events at school. Children with learning difficulties and attainment problems may develop a fear of academic failure and this may under-pin their school refusal. Children with physical disabilities or physical co-ordination problems that result in poor performance in athletics may refuse to go to school because of their fear of athletic failure. Children with physical characteristics about which they are embarrassed, such as delayed physical maturity or obesity, may refuse to go to school because of fears of being taunted by peers during athletics because of their physical characteristics.

Family factors that may contribute to school refusal include parental

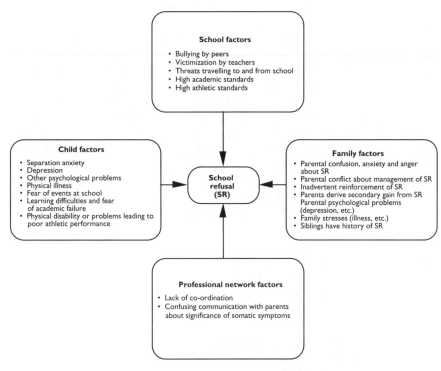

Figure 12.6 Factors to consider in the assessment of school refusal

confusion, anxiety or anger over the meaning of the child's school refusal and related somatic complaints and parental conflict about the management of the situation. Parents may inadvertently reinforce school refusal by insisting on school attendance but relenting when the child escalates his or her protests to a dramatic level. Parents may mismanage school refusal because they derive secondary gains from the child staying at home. For example, the child may provide the homemaker (usually the mother) with companionship. Parents may also mismanage school refusal because parental psychological adjustment problems may compromise their capacity to manage the child's difficulties. Such parental problems may include anxiety, depression, substance abuse or learning difficulties. Wider family stresses such as bereavement, unemployment, separation, birth of a child or moving house may place such demands on parents that they have few personal resources remaining to help their child develop a pattern of regular school attendance. Children from families in which siblings have a history of school refusal may develop school refusal themselves by imitating their older siblings behaviour.

School-based factors which may contribute to the development of school refusal include bullying by peers, victimization by teachers, threatening events occurring while travelling to or from school, poor academic performance and poor athletic performance.

Important factors in the wider professional system which may contribute to school refusal include poor co-ordination among members of the professional network in the management of the child's school refusal and poor communication between these professionals and the family.

The assessment of these factors should involve interviews with the child, the parents, the child's teachers and involved professionals. Such professionals may include the teacher, family doctor, paediatrician, school doctor, educational or school psychologist, and statutory school attendance officers. The School Refusal Assessment Scale, which is described in Table 12.10, maybe a useful adjunct to these interviews. Psychometric assessment of the child's abilities, attainments and symptomatology, where necessary using appropriate instruments (described in Chapter 8) may be conducted.

From this information, the factors that pre-disposed the child to develop school refusal may be identified. Those factors that precipitated the occurrence of the episode of school refusal may be pin-pointed. Finally, factors that are currently maintaining the condition may be clarified. An example of such a formulation is given in the penultimate paragraph of the case described in Box 12.1. When presenting such a formulation, it may be useful to also offer an explanation of the cognitive, affective-somatic, and behavioural components of anxiety, as outlined in the section on psychoeducation, above.

Where separation anxiety is present, the next step involves explaining to the child, the parents and the teacher that the somatic symptoms (headaches and stomachaches) and the associated worries that cause them can be resolved only by children proving to themselves that they are brave enough to attend school and tolerate the anxiety and discomfort that causes. It should be pointed out that a month or two of regular school attendance will resolve most of these symptoms. However, attempts to resolve the anxiety and somatic complaints first, and then return to school, will actually make the condition worse because the child will not overcome the fear that cause these symptoms without facing the feared situation, i.e. going to school.

Where factors at school, such as bullying, victimization or academic failure, are contributing to the school refusal these issues must be altered before return to school can be arranged. With bullying or teacher victimization, the bullies or teachers must be confronted and subsequently monitored so that a recurrence will not occur. With academic failure, additional remedial tuition may be provided. Where wider family factors such as parental psychological adjustment problems are a concern, referral to an appropriate agency for concurrent treatment may be arranged.

With this groundwork laid, the precise details of a return-to-school programme may be planned. This should specify the date and time at which the child will return; whether the child will have an immediate or gradual return, building-up from a few hours a day to a full day over a period of a week or two; who will escort the child to school; who will meet the child at school; which peers will be appointed as buddies to make the child feel welcome and which teacher will act as a secure base for the child if he or she experiences anxiety while in school. The child will require some opportunity to rehearse precisely how the return to school will be managed and to plan how he or she will cope with all major difficulties that may occur.

In addition to this return-to-school programme, a reward system should be set up to give the child an incentive to tolerate the anxiety that will inevitably be experienced during the first few days at school. This reward system should allow the child to earn a concrete daily reward that is received immediately following school each day. A point system which allows the child to accumulate points that may be used to obtain a more substantial reinforcer each week should also be implemented.

The mornings after holidays, illnesses and week-ends are times when relapses are most likely and specific plans for arranging an escort to school and a contingency management programme on these occasions needs to be made to prevent relapses. Ideally, the child should be accompanied to school and received by peers or a class teacher on arrival, and rewards should be given for managing any separation anxiety experienced on such occasions.

Elective mutism

Elective (or selective) mutism where the child is mute in social situations such as the school or peer group but speaks to a small circle of people usually involving family members may be a developmental precursor of social phobia (Carr, 1997; Freeman et al., 2004; Johnson & Wintgens, 2001; Sage & Sluckin, 2004). Elective mutism responds well to family-based behavioural treatment, where the child and a family member with whom the child will speak have planned conversations in those physical environments where the child is usually mute, such as the empty school classroom. Then, over a series of planned, graded steps, people in whose presence the child is normally mute, such as teachers and peers, join the child and family member who are conversing in the physical environment where the child is usually mute. Once the child can converse with the family member in the presence of peers and teachers, peers and teachers gradually join in with the child and family member's conversation. In the final steps of the programme, the distance between the child and the family member is increased so that eventually the child can converse with teachers and peers with the family member outside the classroom door. In the last step of the programme childen ask the family member, in the presence of the teacher and peers, to leave the school grounds and return to collect them at the end of the school day.

Phobias

The Fear Survey Schedule-Revised, described in Table 12.10, is useful for identifying specific fears. When it is clear that the child's anxiety is confined to a specific group of stimuli or situations, such as the dark, particular animals, dental treatment or a specific medical procedure, the child and the parents may be given an explanation of the cognitive, affective-somatic and behavioural components of anxiety. If no clear precipitating event caused the phobia, it is sufficient to say that being frightened of potentially dangerous situations is a good survival skill but that for some children it becomes over-developed and generalizes to situations which are not dangerous for reasons we do not understand. These fears become self-perpetuating when children enter feared situations briefly and then withdraw before their anxiety has reached a peak and begun to subside. The next time, the same situation will be even more frightening for them. Treatment following from this understanding of phobic anxiety involves exposure to feared situations until anxiety subsides (King, Muris & Ollendick, 2004; Ollendick et al., 2004).

Children may be offered the choice of flooding or systematic desensitization as potential treatment options. In both treatments children need to understand that they will be required to *confront their fear until it dies*. They also need to understand that this confrontation will not occur until they have learned the skills necessary to manage the anxiety they will feel in the frightening situation. The pros and cons of flooding versus systematic desensitization need to be explored with children and their parents. On the positive side, flooding is a relatively brief treatment and may involve a single three-hour session. However, it may be quite distressing. Systematic desensitization is typically far less distressing. However, it is a prolonged treatment and may require six or eight sessions.

Where children and parents opt for systematic desensitization, they first work with the psychologist to develop a hierarchy of frightening situations from the most frightening to the least frightening. The hierarchy should contain about ten steps. For darkness phobia, the hierarchy may include *in vivo situations* such as lying in bed in the dark with the door open and the landing light on. It may also include imaginal situations such as imagining lying in bed with the light out. Gradations may be included in the hierarchy. For example, lying in bed with the landing light on and the door fully open may be one feared situation. A more frightening gradation of the same situation may be lying in bed with the landing light on and the door half open.

Once the hierarchy has been established, relaxation and coping skills training (as described in the section on general treatment principles) may be conducted. Parental involvement, particularly in supervising home-based practice, is very useful. If it is feasible, children may be offered opportunities to observe a live or videotaped model using relaxation and coping skills to manage anxiety in situations similar to those in their hierarchy of frightening situations. Once this groundwork has been laid, a series of sessions are devoted to exposing the child to the feared situations in the hierarchy while in a relaxed state and monitoring their anxiety level on a ten-point scale. If children's anxiety increases noticeably while they are in a frightening situation, they should be prompted to use their relaxation skills and self-instructional skills to manage the anxiety and reduce it to a tolerable level. Social reinforcement should be offered for all efforts to master each of the steps in the hierarchy. In addition, a reward system may be used so that a certain number of points are earned for mastering each step in the hierarchy. These points may be accumulated and exchanged for an item from a reinforcement menu.

Home practice may supplement clinic-based treatment. For example, if a child with a fear of needles has managed handling a syringe and needle in the clinic, at home under parental supervision they may be given the task of spending twenty minutes per night handling the needle and syringe or engaging in some activity that involves handling this equipment, such as injecting a doll with water.

For young children, the process of desensitization may be transformed into a series of increasingly challenging games. For example, Mikulas and Coffman (1989) describe a desensitization programme for fear of darkness in which the child listens to a story about the adventures of Michael (a boy who is afraid of the dark) and Uncle Lightfoot who helps him to play games which progress from trying to find a toy dog while wearing a blindfold up to searching a dark house for a noisy toy animal. The child then plays this series of games with his or her parents under the supervision of the therapist as a playful type of desensitization.

Where children and their parents opt for flooding rather than systematic desensitization, extensive preparation should precede the flooding session. Training in relaxation and coping skills should be conducted and the child should be given an opportunity to observe a live or videotaped model managing the feared situation. Some time should be spent in cognitive rehearsal so that the child enters the flooding situation armed with both a well-rehearsed plan and a set of coping skills for managing the anxiety. In particular, the child and parents must be aware that anxiety will escalate during the flooding session, despite the use of coping strategies. It will then reach a peak and gradually decline and the session will end once a stable low level of anxiety has persisted for an agreed period of time, such as ten minutes. Adequate time should be scheduled for flooding sessions, since the process may extend over a number of hours and, if the child leaves the flooding sessions before the anxiety begins to subside, then the phobia may be exacerbated by the treatment.

Flooding may be completed within a single, long session; sometimes two or three such sessions are required. In each session the child is exposed to a highly feared stimulus and prompted to use relaxation skills and self-instructions to cope with the situation. Throughout each session anxiety is monitored regularly on a ten-point self-report rating scale. Within the flooding sessions, the child may receive social reinforcement or points at fixed intervals for enduring the anxiety and be prompted to use relaxation and self-instructional skills to cope with the anxiety. At the end of the session, if a points system has been used the child should be given an immediate opportunity to exchange the points earned for an item from a reinforcement menu established prior to the session.

Social phobias

The Social Phobia Anxiety Inventory for Children, the Revised Social Anxiety Scale for Children and the Social Phobia and Anxiety Inventory for Adolescents, all of which are described in Table 12.10, are useful in the clinical assessment of social anxiety. In assessing children with a social phobia it is worth taking into account the literature on shyness (Asendorpf, 1993). A distinction may be made between unsociability, temperamental shyness and social-evaluative shyness. These states are distinct from social non-acceptance due to excessive aggression. Unsociable children simply have a low need for interaction with others. They are not frightened of social situations but simply prefer a low level of interaction with others. Temperamentally shy children show behavioural inhibition in new social situations, but not with family members or peers whom they know well from an early age, a characteristic that is relatively stable over time. Adjustment of the temperamentally shy or unsociable children depends on the goodness-of-fit between their personality attributes and the culture. Children who show social-evaluative shyness are shy in familiar peer-group situations, have low self-esteem and fear non-acceptance by peers. Both temperamental shyness and social-evaluative shyness may pre-dispose youngsters to developing social phobia. Social phobia is an intense fear of particular social situations and an avoidance of these. The most common stimuli associated with social phobias are public speaking; interacting in social situations; eating, drinking and writing in public and using public toilets.

Cognitive and behavioural models of social phobia point to the complexity of the dynamics in this condition and its self-reinforcing nature (Beidel, Morris & Turner, 2004; Morris, 2004). At the heart of social phobia is the belief that one will behave in an embarrassing way in social situations and be negatively socially evaluated by others for doing so. This anxiety compromises youngsters' performance in social situations and confirms their expectations of behaving in an embarrassing way. That is, they blush, stammer, tremble, experience memory blanks and so forth and others respond to this in negative or ambiguous ways. The socially anxious youngster interprets these reactions of others as negative evaluation. In response to these types of experience they develop safety behaviours to either modify their embarrassing behaviour so as to create a good impression or create avenues for escaping from the scrutiny of others quickly, should they engage in embarrassing behaviours. Safety behaviours involve focusing largely on internal somatic and psychological events rather than outwards on the behaviour of others. So the youngsters' self-preoccupation precludes accurately interpreting positive responses of others to their behaviour. They selectively attend to the negative reactions of others and after each social interaction ruminate about these. This leads to a confirmation of their beliefs that they are socially inept and have once again been negatively evaluated by others. A vicious cycle develops where, in social situations, expectations to behave in embarrassing ways lead to anxiety. This is managed by engaging in safety behaviours and inaccurately monitoring the responses of others. In *post-mortems* of these events, social phobics interpret the reactions of others as confirming a view of the self as socially inept and likely to be negatively evaluated in the future. It is quite probable that with children and adolescents, this process is exacerbated by residing in a threat- and danger-oriented family culture and by advice from parents and others such as 'Concentrate on relaxing' or 'Think of what you are gong to say first and don't say the first thing that comes into your head'. These types of injunction encourage an inward focus and prompt the youngster to engage in safety behaviours.

Concurrent family and group sessions are probably the most useful format for treatment of youngsters with social phobias. In psychoeducational sessions the cognitive, affective-somatic and behavioural aspects of anxiety may be explained in general and then the specific model of social phobia outlined above may be described in family sessions. This provides a rationale for advising parents that they reward children for discarding safety behaviours and for all pro-active attempts to increase the number, duration and quality of their social interactions with peers and others. Where children have developed a constricted lifestyle, family-based sessions may be used as a forum within which to explore ways in which the child can have greater contact with peers by joining clubs, recreational classes and youth organizations.

Alongside a series of family sessions, a group-based treatment context is particularly useful for the treatment of youngsters' social phobias, since it provides the audience required for exposure to the feared stimulus (the expectation of negative evaluation by others). The core of the treatment is to provide the child with repeated exposure to situations in which they speak in front of the group without engaging in inwardly focused safety behaviours for managing anxiety associated with fear of negative evaluation. A hierarchy of ten increasingly threatening situations may be drawn up and youngsters may be offered opportunities to face these challenges in front of the group and to receive feedback on the adequacy of their performance. Where youngsters lack the social skills for initiating and maintaining social interactions they may be coached in these, so that they have the skills to perform in social situations. Often, one of the primary obstacles to performing well in social situations and receiving positive feedback is a predominantly internal focus and a pre-occupation with engaging in avoidant safety behaviours. One way to help children give up these inwardly-focused safety behaviours is to offer them videotaped feedback on the heightened social performance associated with not engaging in such inward-focused routines (Clark & Wells, 1995). Early in treatment, one of their episodes of talking to the group is video-taped. During this particular episode they are encouraged to engage in all of the inwardly focused safety behaviours they typically use to manage their fear of negative evaluation. Later in treatment, one of their talks to the group in which they do not use safety behaviours is videotaped. They then view and compare these two videotapes and see that the safety behaviours they use to manage anxiety detract from their social self-presentation and this challenges their beliefs about the value of engaging in such behaviours. As their beliefs in the importance of safety behaviours and their social ineptness weakens, they become freed to be outwardly focused, rather than inwardly focused when managing anxiety-provoking social situations and to be open to positive feedback from these more socially appropriate interactions.

Generalized anxiety disorder

With generalized anxiety disorder, the Multidimensional Anxiety Scale for Children, the Revised Fear Survey Schedule, the State Trait Anxiety Inventory, the Revised Children's Manifest Anxiety Scale and the Hamilton Anxiety Rating Scale, all of which are described in Table 12.10, contribute useful information to an initial assessment.

The meta-cognitive model offers a useful conceptual framework for understanding youngsters' experience of generalized anxiety disorder (Wells, 2005). In this model generalized anxiety disorder is characterized by both general worries about specific threats (type 1 worries) and negative thoughts about worry itself (type 2 worries) or worry about worrying. Children with generalized anxiety disorder believe that type 1 worries are useful coping strategies for managing threatening situations and so are motivated to engage in this type of worrying. However, they are also motivated to avoid type 1 worries because it leads them to engage in type 2 worries about: (1) the uncontrollability of the worrying process (e.g. 'I can't stop worrying'), and (2) the adverse consequences of worrying for personal well-being (e.g. 'This worrying is wrecking my life'). Thus they vacillate between trying to suppress type 1 worries and then, when such worries intrude unbidden into consciousness, actively worrying as a way of coping. This unbidden intrusion of type 1 worries into consciousness confirms type 2 worries that the process is out of control. Children may then seek reassurance from parents and family members that 'There is nothing to worry about' or avoid situations that might provide evidence that that their type 1 and type 2 worries are unfounded. These strategies for managing anxiety confirm and reinforce type 2 worries.

Treatment for generalized anxiety disorder, particularly where there is a threat- and danger-oriented family culture, may be predominantly family based and include many of the components of the anxiety management programme described in the section on general treatment principles (Flannery-Schroeder, 2004; Hudson, Hughes & Kendall, 2004). Within the context of family sessions, psychoeducation about anxiety may be offered. Parents may be coached in helping the child to challenge, test and reinforce non-threatening interpretations of situations using the CTR cognitive restructuring technique described earlier. Family sessions may also be used as a format for helping parents learn how to instruct their child in relaxation skills. Reward programmes may be set up within family sessions which provide a way for the parents to motivate their child to be more courageous. Parents may also be trained to use systematic ignoring of *worry-talk* to help children break the habit of consistently engaging in this type of threat-oriented discourse.

In addition to the core family-based treatment sessions, an individual or group treatment format may be used to help children explore the basis for their many fears and develop self-monitoring skills, self-instructional coping skills and relaxation coping skills following a structured format such as the Coping Cat (Kendall et al., 2003) or FRIENDs programmes (Barrett & Shortt, 2003). A useful focus for exploratory individual work is to help youngsters through explorations of their many expressed fears, identify and articulate their core underlying fears, which are often that their needs for safety, security and protection will not be met.

Panic disorder

The Childhood Anxiety Sensitivity Index and the Panic Attack Symptoms and Cognitions Questionnaire provide useful information in the assessment of panic attacks. The Panic Attack Symptoms and Cognitions Questionnaire was developed for use with adults but can be used cautiously with adolescents; it is probably unsuitable for use with children. For secondary agoraphobia, the Agoraphobia Scale and the Agoraphobia Cognitions Questionnaire may also be used cautiously in the assessment of adolescents. All of these instruments are described in Table 12.10.

Cognitive theories of panic disorder argue that panic attacks arise from catastrophic misinterpretation of bodily sensations associated with arousal (Barlow, 2002; Clark, 1986). Rapid heart rate may be misinterpreted as evidence of an impending heart attack. Breathlessness and choking sensations may be misinterpreted as evidence of immanent suffocation. Dizziness, derealization and depersonalization may be misinterpreted as evidence of loss of control or the onset of insanity. The disposition to make such catastrophic misinterpretations is referred to as anxiety sensitivity, which is measured with the Anxiety Sensitivity Index (Silverman, Fleisig, Rabian & Peterson,

1991) and has three factors: fear of somatic symptoms, fear of psychological symptoms and fear of publicly observable anxiety reactions.

There is probably a progression from separation anxiety through to panic disorder for some, but not all, children and the quality of panic attacks changes as the child matures from childhood to adolescence (Klein & Pine, 2002). Pre-adolescent children probably attribute panic to external rather than internal factors and so do not catastrophize like the adolescent who has the cognitive maturity to interpret physiological sensations in catastrophic terms. The child says 'When I do an exam my heart beats faster'. The adolescent says 'Even though I know I can do the exam, I notice my heart beating faster. I must be going mad or about to die!' In panic disorder youngsters are aroused by situations they interpret as threatening or by physical exertion and respond with hyperventilation. They perceive the somatic changes that go with hyperventilation as a sign of distress and focus inwardly on these. Their catastrophic cognitions about the somatic changes exacerbate arousal and hypersensitivity. The panic escalates. They develop expectations of recurrence and typically avoid unsafe situations. This normally evolves into secondary agoraphobia. If they do enter an unsafe situation they withdraw before their anxiety reaches a peak and so their avoidance behaviour is negatively reinforced. The youngster's family, friends and physician encourage an inward focus on somatic sensations and avoidance of feared situations. In doing so they maintain the panic attacks and secondary agoraphobia. This type of understanding of the condition is useful to include as part of psychoeducational input to parents and youngsters suffering from panic with secondary agoraphobia.

Treatment involves enlisting parental support to help youngsters develop relaxation and self-instructional coping skills so that they will be able to undergo exposure programmes for both feared internal somatic signs of hyperarousal and feared external stimuli such as being some distance away from the safety of the home (Mattis & Pincus, 2004).

Relaxation skills training with youngsters who have panic disorder is sometimes complicated by the fact that focusing-inward on changes in muscle tension may lead to increased tension rather than relaxation because of the tendency of youngsters with panic disorder to misperceive internal cues and catastrophize about them. Where this type of problem occurs, visualization may be used as an alternative to progressive muscle relaxation and youngsters invited to focus not on their somatic state but on relaxing imagery, such as that suggested in Figure 12.5.

With self-instructional training, much of the work involves helping youngsters see that misunderstanding the significance of fluctuations in arousal and construing them as dangerous, leads to the release of adrenaline and to an escalation of anxiety. In addition, hyperventilation leads to increased arousal. To overcome the fear of hyperarousal, the youngster should be given the opportunity to voluntarily enter into such a state by hyperventilating at a rate of thirty breaths per minute and then to wait and see if some catastrophic event occurs (Barlow & Cerny, 1988). When this is done on a number of occasions, the youngster learns that internal signs of arousal are not harbingers of doom. Youngsters may then be trained to change their breathing pattern to regular slow deep breaths (inhale for a count of three and breath out for a count of six). This pattern of slow breathing contributes to relieving the symptoms of hyperarousal. It is very useful if the parents are present and participate in supporting the youngster through these very taxing exposure sessions.

When exposure to internal arousal cues has been completed and these cues no longer arouse excessive anxiety, exposure to travelling away from the safety of the home may be conducted. It is most effective to conduct this type of treatment in vivo. A gradual desensitization or complete flooding approach may be used. The pros and cons of both may be discussed with the youngster and the parents. With desensitization the youngster and parents construct a hierarchy of about ten steps from *standing outside the front door of the home* to *being a few miles away from home*. Then arrangements are made for the youngster to enter these situations and remain in them until arousal reaches a peak and then drops to an acceptable level. Self-instructional coping skills and relaxation skills may be used to help the youngster reduce arousal in each of the situations. With flooding, the youngster agrees to travel a long way from the house and remain at this location until arousal reaches peak and subsides. For both gradual desensitization and flooding, the parents or psychologist or both may accompany the youngster on exposure treatment outings. In both flooding and desensitization sessions, anxiety is regularly monitored on a ten-point self-report rating scale.

Where panic disorder and secondary agoraphobia have led to a disruption of the youngster's schooling, liaison with school staff during assessment and when planning the return to school is vital. Those procedures that were described in the section on school refusal should be used for school liaison.

PTSD

The PTSD assessment instruments listed in Table 12.10 may be used to screen for and diagnose PTSD. In addition to the assessment protocol outlined earlier in this chapter, for victims of physical or sexual abuse, additional assessment procedures (given in Chapters 19 and 21) may be used. PTSD differs from other anxiety disorders in that the trauma violates more of children's safety assumptions than precipitating events in other anxiety disorders and it leads to more complex and wide-ranging effects (American Academy of Child and Adolescent Psychiatry, 1998b; Carr, 2004b; Enright & Carr, 2002; McKnight, Compton & March, 2004; Perrin, Smith & Yule, 2004). Following the traumatic event, the feared stimuli avoided by the youngster are both external and internal. The external stimuli may include people, places, objects and events that remind the child of the trauma. Repetitive intrusive memories, thoughts, images and emotions during wakefulness and trauma-related night-mares during sleep are the main internal anxiety-provoking stimuli. Reactions to these stimuli include hyperarousal and attempts at avoidance. At an intrapsychic level, an attempt to exclude trauma-related intrusions from consciousness through suppression or distraction is the principal avoidance reaction. At a behavioural level, youngsters avoid external stimuli associated with the traumatic event. They also attempt to avoid situations that will lead to intrapsychic trauma-related intrusions. For example, some children will not go to bed for fear of having night-mares; others will not separate from their parents or caregivers or sleep alone. A central concern for many traumatized youngsters who subsequently experience intrusions is the degree to which PTSD symptoms reflect the onset of psychosis. Such youngsters may ask 'Am I losing my mind?' 'Am I going mad?' Psycho-education about PTSD to address these concerns forms a central part of debriefing and treatment.

Children with PTSD engage in an ongoing approach-avoidance struggle with respect to stimuli that remind them of the trauma. Older children experience a pressure to talk about the trauma but have difficulty doing so. Younger children, while they may avoid talking about the trauma or external stimuli related to it, often engage in play activities, such as drawing or make-believe games, in which they repeatedly re-enact the trauma situation. This approach-avoidance conflict probably reflects competing drives to avoid further danger but also the need to process intense emotional information through exposure and rehearsal and to integrate this into one's overall world view.

More than any other anxiety disorder, PTSD has a profound effect on academic performance and so psychometric assessment of intelligence and attainments, along with an evaluation of the child's capacity to complete academic tasks, should form part of the overall assessment. (Guidelines for the psychometric assessment of abilities are set out in Chapter 8.)

The suddenness and degree of life-threateningness of the trauma are the two main trauma variables associated with the severity of symptomatology. The more sudden and life-threatening the trauma, the more severe the PTSD symptoms. Previous psychological difficulties and multiple family problems are important pre-disposing vulnerability factors. High ability and good problem-solving skills are significant protective factors.

Behavioural formulations of PTSD argue that, through classical conditioning, cues that were present at the time of the trauma and were paired with trauma experiences which elicited extreme trauma-related anxiety, later elicit similar post-traumatic anxiety and intrusive memories. Repeated exposure to these cues would lead to extinction but traumatized children avoid these cues, and this avoidance is negatively reinforced through instrumental conditioning. Negative reinforcement involves the strengthening of a response, which leads to a reduction in aversive stimulation. Behavioural treatment based on this formulation involves exposure to trauma-related cues and prevention of avoidance responses.

Ehlers and Clark (2000) argue that chronic PTSD is maintained by three sets of cognitive factors: (1) excessively negative appraisals of the trauma and its aftermath; (2) a disturbance of autobiographical memory characterized by poor elaboration and conceptualization of the trauma, strong associative memory and strong perceptual priming, which leads to rapid recollection of vivid emotional memories in response to trauma cues; and (3) the use of problematic avoidant coping strategies, which prevents adaptive modification of negative appraisals and vivid emotional traumatic memories. Brewin (2001) has argued that sensory, motor and physiological (but not verbal) aspects of traumatic memories are encoded (probably in the amygdala) with no input from the hippocampus and are triggered by cues associated with the trauma. Effective therapy involves accessing these situationally accessible memories (SAMs), and elaborating on them verbally, so they become encoded (probably in the hippocampus) as verbally accessible memories (VAMs). VAMs can be voluntarily retrieved, threatening aspects of these edited, and assimilated into the person's autobiographical memory and world view.

An extreme initial reaction to the trauma, significant additional stressful life events in the aftermath of the trauma, and the absence of adequate levels of parental or school support in the post-trauma period have all been found to determine the severity of PTSD symptoms. Where parents have been exposed to the same trauma as their children, the children's symptoms persist longer in cases where parents show protracted PTSD symptomatology. But where parents are skilled at processing their own emotions and managing their PTSD symptoms, they are better at helping their children do so, and this provides a rationale for a family-based approach to treatment.

Treatment for children with PTSD should aim to maximize family, school and peer support for the child and provide the child with opportunities to emotionally process the trauma through exposure to internal and external trauma-related stimuli. In the longer term, treatment may also aim to provide the youngster with opportunities to re-evaluate and reconstruct his or her view of their world. Family support may be maximized by making family sessions the core of a multi-systemic treatment programme. Within the sessions, the aim is to facilitate parental and sibling support of the traumatized child. Where all family members have been involved in the trauma (for example a house fire or an armed robbery) family members may each be given an opportunity to recount their recollections of the situation, and the parents may be coached during such sessions to support the children. Sometimes it is helpful to provide separate sessions for parents, within which they process their traumatic memories so that they will be better able to devote their energy to supporting their traumatized children within whole-family sessions.

Treatment may begin with psychoeducation, the aim of which is to provide a rationale for therapy and allay youngsters' and parents' fears that the child is 'going mad'. The three DSM IV TR clusters of symptoms should be described. The way avoidant strategies prevent traumatic memories from being processed may be explained. The need to bring these traumatic memories into consciousness, habituate to them and process them may then be presented as the rationale for exposure-based treatment. Other issues that may be covered in psychoeducation are the need to re-establish routines for daily living and sleeping; the need for the child to obtain support from family, friends and school staff; the need for parents to develop strategies for managing behavioural problems which have developed as result of traumatization and the need to address substance use in the way described in Chapter 15 if youngsters are using drugs or alcohol to manage PTSD symptoms.

Youngsters and/or parents may be invited to keep structured diaries in which they record the frequency and intensity of certain key symptoms. With re-experiencing symptoms, the number of flashbacks per day or the number of night-mares per night may be recorded. For hyperarousal symptoms, ratings may be made on a 100-point subjective units of discomfort (SUDs) fear thermometer which ranges from 0 = perfectly relaxed and calm, to 100 = the worst imaginable anxiety and distress. Ratings may be made either at fixed times during the day (9.00 in the morning, at 12.00 noon and at 9.00 at night) or at critical points such as during flashbacks or after awakening from night-mares. Also, youngsters may record intrusion recovery times, that is, how many minutes it took them to return to a rating of less than 50 SUDs after a flashback or night-mare. With avoidance symptoms, some index of the frequency or duration of exposure to trauma-related cues or memories may be recorded. For example, whether or not they spent five minutes per day talking to a parent about a frightening aspect of the trauma, the number of times they had the courage to walk past the scene of the trauma rather than avoiding it or the number of days they were able to overcome separation anxiety and go to school. Symptom-monitoring systems should be tailored to the unique requirements of each case. Symptom-monitoring diaries should be reviewed as the start of every session.

Where PTSD has led to disruption of normal daily and night-time routines, early in treatment youngsters may be invited, in collaboration with their parents, to plan normal daily routines including going to school, socializing with peers, engaging in regular pleasant recreational activities, getting regular physical aerobic exercise and regularizing their sleep–waking cycle. Sleep management involves setting fixed times for going to bed and getting up, agreeing on a system for gradually phasing out parental night-time contact in youngsters who have been coping with anxiety by sleeping with their parents and using relaxation exercise and audiotapes or soothing music to help them sleep when they go to bed initially and following night-mares which have awakened them. Coping-skills training may be offered to equip youngsters with ways of managing anxiety associated with flashbacks and night-mares and anxiety evoked during therapeutic exposure to trauma-related cues and memories. This type of training involves learning relaxation skills and cognitive coping skills described earlier in the chapter.

Graded exposure is the central therapeutic mechanism through which PTSD symptoms are resolved. Exposure procedures all involve recalling traumatic memories as vividly as possible, holding these in consciousness and tolerating the intense anxiety associated with them until habituation occurs. Exposure to trauma-related cues may be used to bring traumatic memories into consciousness. Video or audio recordings, or photographs of trauma-related stimuli, may be used and the site of the trauma may be visited. Visualization, writing, painting, drawing, drama and doll-play may all be used to help youngsters keep the traumatic memories in consciousness. Commonly, exposure is facilitated in a gradual way, with children being exposed to a graded hierarchy of increasingly anxiety-provoking situations. Situations may be graded, in terms of the amount of anxiety they evoke, with reference to the 100 SUDs fear thermometer. Where routine visualization evokes very high levels of anxiety, the amount of anxiety associated with visualizing traumatic scenes may be reduced by inviting youngsters to visualize these scenes as if viewing them from a distance or as if they were on TV.

Exposure sessions are carefully planned in a collaborative way with the youngster and parents. Youngsters are briefed that the aim of each exposure session is hold their traumatic memories vividly in consciousness until their SUD rating drops to an agreed level. They are informed that, initially, their SUDs will rise, then reach a peak and then gradually decrease. It should be made very clear to youngsters that to terminate exposure before habituation may sensitize them rather than help them to habituate to trauma-related memories. Because habituation can be a slow process, ninety-minute treatment sessions may be most appropriate. To facilitate habituation, youngsters may be invited to use their relaxation skills and cognitive coping skills or ask their parents to hold their hands, thereby providing social support. Each time youngsters complete an exposure exercise and habituate to the anxiety-provoking situation, they should be reinforced. They may be reinforced with praise and, if appropriate, with tokens or stars on a star chart, which can be accumulated and exchanged for valued prizes or treats on a reinforcement menu. Between exposure sessions, youngsters may be invited to listen to audiotapes of exposure sessions each day and/or to write a detailed account of the traumatic memories addressed in exposure sessions and read these accounts each day. These homework assignments consolidate habituation gains made during exposure sessions.

For imaginal exposure to traumatic memories or trauma-related night-mares, youngsters are invited to sit in a comfortable position with their eyes closed, to relax using relaxation and breathing exercises and to visualize the traumatic scene as vividly as possible. They are then asked to verbally recount their visualization of the traumatic scene or dream, in the first person, present tense. To enhance the vividness of the visualization, the therapist may request detailed accounts of what the youngster sees, hears, smells, tastes and feels. Throughout this process, at intervals of about five minutes, the therapist requests SUDs ratings. When the SUDs rating shows a marked increase, the therapist may ask the child to re-run that part of the scene (the 'hot spot') a number of times. This repeated exposure facilitates habituation. It is appropriate to progress from visualizing a less anxiety-provoking scene to visualizing a more anxiety-provoking scene after habituation to the former has occurred. When habituation to the most anxiety-provoking scene has occurred, it may be appropriate to progress to media-assisted exposure and in vivo exposure, particularly where residual PTSD symptoms remain.

For media-assisted exposure, traumatic memories are evoked using audiotapes, video recordings or photographs of trauma-related cues. Clips from TV or recorded films of trauma-related situations such as car crashes, bank raids, earthquakes, hurricanes that are particularly reminiscent of the actual trauma may be used. Audiotaped recordings of the sort of sounds that accompanied the trauma may be used, for example, a tape-recording of a howling wind for a hurricane survivor. Photographs of the trauma scene may also be used. During exposure to recordings or photographs of trauma-related cues, youngsters are invited to describe what the cues remind them of. Detailed sensory questioning is used to help them elaborate their memories. As with imaginal exposure, youngsters may be invited to verbally re-run 'hot spots' in these exposure sessions to facilitate habituation.

If parents have attended a number of imaginal or media-assisted exposure sessions and have observed the way the therapist has conducted these, then they may be invited to adopt the role of the therapist for in vivo exposure. The parents are invited to accompany the child to the trauma site, to encourage the youngster to verbalize memories it evokes and to use coping strategies to help them to habituate to being at the site of the trauma.

Where youngsters have been abused, confronting their victimizer either in imagination or in vivo is a critical part of the exposure process. This confrontation process involves staying in the presence of the imagined or actual abuser. Then, youngsters must clearly and forcefully state how the abuse has hurt them, how angry and betrayed they feel as a result of this and how they will never let the abuse recur because they now have the skills to protect themselves in future and the support of the non-abusing parent. Abuse survivors may be invited to imagine and rehearse this sort of conversation in therapy. As homework, they may also be invited to write detailed, emotionally charged letters to the abuser covering these points. However, only under carefully considered circumstances should such letters ever be sent. In the case of intrafamilial abuse, it may be appropriate in some instances for the therapist to facilitate a session in which the youngster, supported by the non-abusing parent, reads aloud a prepared confrontational letter to the abusing parent. A fuller discussion of family intervention where children have been traumatized by intrafamilial child sexual abuse is given in Chapter 21.

Grief work is necessary where youngsters with PTSD have experienced traumatic events which led to bereavement. Natural disasters, transportation accidents and shootings are examples of such events. Grief work involves movement through a series of processes including shock, denial, emotional turmoil, acceptance and resolution, as described in Chapter 24. These are not discrete stages, nor is progress through these process particularly orderly, and not all bereaved people experience all processes. However, to move towards resolution, imaginal exposure to memories of both positive and negative episodes of interaction with the deceased, and to memories of their death is necessary. This may be facilitated by media-assisted exposure, involving viewing photographs, videotapes, and other memorabilia that remind the bereaved of the deceased. In facilitating grief work in children with PTSD, it is appropriate to follow the procedures outlined above for imaginal and media-assisted exposure. In vivo exposure involving visiting the disaster site or the deceased's grave may also be incorporated into grief work. The goal of such grief work is to help the child develop a world view in which their valued relationship with the deceased as a living person is part of their past, but their valued memory of them lives on in the present. It should be acknowledged that the emotional pain associated with bereavement, takes time to resolve. This type of child-focused grief work is best offered within a family context, particularly where it is a family member who has died. Loss of a family member necessitates family reorganization. As the child makes progress in processing traumatic memories associated with bereavement, other family members may be invited to sessions to discuss the impact of the bereavement on family's rules, roles and routines. A full discussion of facilitating such family sessions is given in Chapter 24.

Safety skills may be required for survivors who have been victimized by others so that they will be equipped to prevent re-victimization. Safety-skills training is an essential part of treatment for survivors of abuse and violence. Youngsters need to be coached in anticipating and recognizing situations in which they may be victimized again. They also need to be coached in planning how to avoid or escape from potentially risky situations, by, for example, withdrawing from such situations as soon as they recognize them, saying 'No' assertively, calling for help and retaining a belief that they are in charge of their own lives.

Where survivors of sexual or aggressive victimization have difficulty controlling aggressive or sexual urges, they may need to be coached in socially appropriate ways to regulate and express these intense feelings. Relaxation skills, aerobic physical exercise and distraction through absorption in music or other activities may be used to regulate intense sexual and aggressive impulses. However, intense urges may also require expression. For managing strong sexual urges, youngsters may be helped to plan routines for private masturbation rather than public masturbation or inappropriate sexual interaction with others. For managing intense anger that is unresponsive to strategies already mentioned, youngsters may be helped to plan routines for expressing this privately in socially appropriate ways, by for example routinely scheduling time for hitting a punch bag.

Parents of traumatized children may be offered behavioural parent training to help them provide their children with appropriate support as they progress through an exposure programme, and also to manage trauma-related behavioural problems. These include separation anxiety, avoidance of routine social activities, sleep difficulties, aggression, defiance and over-sexualized behaviour. Parents and children may be coached in how to use reward programmes, as described in Chapter 4. This begins with pin-pointing behavioural goals. Common goals include completing daily therapeutic exposure homework assignments, school attendance (if separation anxiety has prevented school attendance), engaging in daily social interactions with peers (if they have become reclusive), sleeping in their own beds for some or all of each night (if, through separation anxiety they have been sleeping with parents), regulating intense anger using relaxation and breathing exercises (if they have problems with controlling aggression), and managing sexual urges in a socially appropriate way (if they display over-sexualized behaviour following child sexual abuse). At any one time, no more than three behavioural goals should be addressed. Large goals may be broken down into smaller and more easily achievable targets. Plans for reinforcing target behaviours need to be established. For rigid, entrenched problematic behaviour patterns, praise and approval may be insufficient reinforcement and a more formal system may be required. Token or star-chart systems are appropriate for young children; a points system may be used for adolescents. In collaboration with their children, parents may be helped to develop a reinforcement menu and arrive at an agreement about how an accumulation of tokens, stars or points may be periodically exchanged for a reward or privilege on the reinforcement menu.

Where youngsters occasionally have difficulty using the self-regulation skills mentioned in the previous section to control their sexual and aggressive impulses, parents may use time-out from reinforcement, as described in Chapter 4, to help them develop better self-control. Thus youngsters who display inappropriate aggression or sexual behaviour spend a brief period alone, under parental supervision, until they regulate their intense emotions and calm down. They then return to interacting with their parents and are reinforced for using time-out to successfully regulate their intense emotions. It is important that time-out is framed as a benign parental strategy for fostering self-regulation skills and not as a punishment, since this would amount to re-victimization.

Trying to help parents suffering from PTSD implement a behavioural programme for their child is likely to lead to a failure experience. This may impact negatively on both the parents' and the child's recovery. Therefore, where parents suffer from PTSD, they should be offered an opportunity to undergo their own exposure programme, to begin to resolve their own PTSD symptoms, before attempting to implement a child-focused behavioural programme.

School staff require psychoeducational input, of the type outlined earlier, when a pupil has been traumatized. A meeting between the school staff, child, parents and therapist may be convened. In this meeting, the profound effects of PTSD symptoms on academic performance should be highlighted. Teachers should be informed of the temporary need for the youngsters' workload to be tailored to take account of this. Arrangements should also be made for youngsters to have a designated member of the school staff to whom they can go if they become particularly distressed during school hours. This staff member should be briefed in how to facilitate the child in expressing concerns and informed that ventilating feelings and recounting trauma-related memories is a productive rather than a destructive process.

Traumatization may lead people to adopt catastrophic and pessimistic beliefs about the world, the future, the self and others. Common post-traumatic beliefs are that nowhere in the world is safe; a short life is inevitable; the traumatized person is going insane or losing their mind; the traumatized person is helpless, shameful, guilty, and stigmatized; and others are untrustworthy. In cognitive restructuring, youngsters with PTSD are invited to identify and articulate these post-traumatic beliefs. They are asked to accept that their new beliefs about the world are hypotheses deserving rigorous testing, rather than newly revealed truths. They may be invited to write down the beliefs they had about the world, the future, the self and others before the trauma and after the trauma. Then they may be invited, through Socratic questioning within therapy sessions and behavioural experiments outside therapy sessions, to collect evidence about each post-traumatic belief and evaluate the degree to which the belief is supported by evidence. As each new piece of evidence accumulates, for each belief they may be asked to rate their conviction that the belief is true on a 100-point scale ranging from 1 = 'I'm completely uncertain about how true this belief is', to 100 = 'I'm absolutely sure this belief is true'.

Relapse prevention involves helping youngsters and parents anticipate situations in which relapses may occur, planning strategies for detecting potential relapses early and writing out a relapse management plan. Relapses are more probable in situations where there are many trauma-related cues, where the person has little social support and a high level of other life stresses and when entry into the situation occurs unexpectedly or at a trauma anniversary. Relaxation skills, cognitive coping skills (especially retaining an optimistic perspective) and arranging social support from family, close friends or a therapist are useful elements to include in a relapse management plan.

SUMMARY

Fear is the natural response to a stimulus which is perceived as posing a threat to well-being, safety or security. This response includes cognitive, affective, physiological, behavioural and relational aspects. A distinction may be made between normal adaptive fears, which are premised on an accurate appraisal of the potential threat posed by a stimulus or situation, and maladaptive fears, which are based on an inaccurate appraisal of the threat to well-being. Children are referred for treatment of an anxiety problem when it prevents them from completing developmentally appropriate tasks, such as going to school or socializing with friends. As children's cognitive abilities develop, the stimuli that elicit normal fear and abnormal anxiety change from the predominantly concrete (e.g. animals) to the more abstract (e.g. negative evaluation). The overall prevalence for anxiety disorders in children and adolescents is approximately 6–10% and in clinical samples there is considerable co-morbidity among different anxiety disorders and between anxiety disorders and other problems such as those involving conduct or over-activity and attentional deficits. Distinctions are made in DSM IV TR and ICD 10 between separation anxiety, selective mutism, phobias, generalized anxiety, panic disorder and PTSD. These different anxiety problems vary in terms of the stimuli that elicit anxiety, the patterning of hyperarousal, the significance of differing aetiological factors in their development and their impact on interpersonal adjustment.

Biological, psychoanalytic, cognitive, behavioural and family systems formulations of anxiety disorders have been developed. Research and clinical accounts arising from these theories point to the complex, multi-determined nature of anxiety disorders in children. Biological and psychosocial factors may pre-dispose youngsters to developing anxiety disorders, precipitate their onset and maintain or exacerbate these conditions. Effective treatment programmes for youngsters with anxiety problems are based on a thorough assessment of symptomatology and aetiological factors, incorporate a high level of family involvement and begin with psychoeducational input about the complex nature of anxiety. Such orientation sessions are typically followed by training in monitoring of symptomatology and training in relaxation and cognitive restructuring skills. Treatment may also entail rehearsal following observation of a model coping with exposure to a feared stimulus; and exposure to feared stimuli until habituation occurs. Family- and school-based reward systems to increase motivation to follow through on exposure exercises are also included in most effective treatment programmes. School involvement in treatment where avoidance is school based and liaison with other professionals, particularly medicine, if there are anxiety-based somatic symptoms are important features of case management. Referral of parents for treatment of psychological and marital problems should also be made if appropriate.

EXERCISE 12.1

Conor is a fourteen-year-old boy who was referred in September because of strange behaviour at school. While his behaviour and attainments were broadly speaking normal last term, this term he is behaving oddly. He has been reluctant to go to school on a couple of occasions. In school, he tends to spend a lot of time pre-occupied and mixes little with his peers. His schoolwork is deteriorating. When asked to read in class he stammers and on one occasion ran out of the class-room crying. He is an only child and both of his parents are profes-sionals who work long hours. His parents say that he has been having night-mares but will not talk about them. His developmental history is unremarkable, although he was always a shy child, like his father and grandfather. He spent the summer at an adventure sports centre where he learned sailing, canoeing, horse-riding and rock climbing. Like the other children he learned to capsize and right a sailing dinghy and canoe. He fell off a pony while learning to jump and found the rock climbing very difficult. He didn't get hurt at that but slipped occasion-ally. His father, Kurt, was adamant that he attend the camp every sum-mer for the next three years to help him mature. His mother, Cynthia, is concerned that Conor may spend too long away from home and miss the stability of family life. Both parents are confused by their son's silence and odd behaviour.

- Draw a genogram and sketch in your hypotheses about family relationships.
- What are the main symptoms in this case and which of these suggest that they may reflect an anxiety problem?
- What do you suspect are the pre-disposing, precipitating, maintaining and protective factors?
- How would you proceed with the assessment and management of this case?

EXERCISE 12.2

Work in pairs and take turns practising the relaxation skills training protocol set out in Figure 12.5.

EXERCISE 12.3

Work in pairs taking the roles of therapist and client.

If you are taking the role of the client, imagine that you have generalized anxiety disorder. You are frightened of multiple situations and the fact that you can't stop worrying. Alternatively, you may imagine that you have panic disorder and are frightened to be in unsafe places where you might get a panic attack. Think your way into your role by imagining how your life in the role has been over the past ten days. Think about what has made you most frightened. Think about how has this affected your activity and relationships and how badly you want to be rid of this anxiety. In the role-play exercise assume you have a good relationship with the therapist and want to learn how to cope better with 'dangerous thinking'.

If you are taking the therapist role assume that there is a contract for therapy and the client wants help coping with anxiety:

- First, explain that the way we think affects how we feel with reference to a concrete example like the following. If you meet a dog on the street and think it is *dangerous*, you will feel *fear*. If you meet a dog on the street, and think it is *friendly*, you will feel *happy*. (So *dangerous thinking* – looking at ambiguous situations as if they were *dangerous* – causes *anxiety*.)
- Second, explain the CTR (challenge, test, reward) method with reference to an example like the following. One way to cope with anxiety is to begin to challenge dangerous thinking, test out this challenge, and then reward ourselves for doing this. Here is an example: Imagine you meet a dog on the street and think the following dangerous thought: *'He's dangerous and will bite me'*. You can **challenge** this by saying *'No, an alternative view is he wants to be my friend'*. You can **test** this alternative view out by looking for evidence to support it: *'I will not run away. There I didn't run and he didn't bite me. He did want to be friendly'*. If you find evidence to support your alternative to dangerous thinking praise yourself as a **reward**: *'Well done'*.
- Third, invite the client to use the CTR method in the following way: 'Think about a situation that occurred in the past ten days where you became anxious. What did you think? What was an alternative thought? How could you have tested that? How would you have rewarded yourself?'
- Finally, invite the client to use the CTR method for the next week.

FURTHER READING

Barrett, P., Lowry-Webster, H., & Turner, C. (2000a). *FRIENDS programme for children: Group Leader's Manual*. Brisbane: Australian Academic Press. http:// www.friends info.net

Barrett, P. Lowry-Webster, H., & Turner, C. (2000b). *FRIENDS programme for Youth: Group Leader's Manual*. Brisbane: Australian Academic Press. http://www.friends info.net

Heyne, D. & Rollings, S. (2002). *School Refusal*. Oxford: Blackwell.

Kendall, P.C. (2000). *Cognitive-Behavioural Therapy for Anxious Children: Therapist Manual* (Second Edition). Ardmore, PA: Workbook Publishing.

Kendall, P., Choudhurry, M., Hudson, J., & Webb, A. (2002). *The CAT Project Therapist Manual*. Ardmore, PA: Workbook Publishing. http://www.workbookpublishing.com

Morris, T. & March, J. (2004). *Anxiety Disorders in Children and Adolescents* (Second Edition). New York: Guilford.

Ollendick, T. & March, J. (2003). *Phobic and Anxiety Disorders in Children and Adolescents: A Clinical Guide to Effective Psychosocial and Pharmacological Interventions*. Oxford: Oxford University Press.

Sage, R. & Sluckin, A. (2004). *Silent Children: Approaches to Selective Mutism*. Leicester: University of Leicester. (*Video and book available from Mrs Lindsay Whittington, Secretary of SMIRA, +44-116-212-7411, e-mail smiraleicester@ hotmail.com*).

FURTHER READING FOR CLIENTS

Rapee, R., Spense, S., Cobham, V., & Wignal, A. (2000). *Helping Your Anxious Child: A Step-By-Step Guide for Parents*. San Francisco: New Harbinger.

Johnson, M. & Wintgens, A. (2001). *The Selective Mutism Resource Manual*. UK: Speechmark.

EQUIPMENT

GSR-2 basic relaxation system. Available: http://www.parinc.com

WEBSITES

Anxiety Disorders Association of America: http://www.adaa.org/Anxiety-DisorderInfor/ChildrenAdo.cfm

National Centre for PTSD: http://www.ncptsd.org/facts/treatment/fs_treatment.html

Paula Barrett's FRIENDS programme: http://www.friendsinfo.net

Philip Kendall's Coping Cat Workbooks: http://www.workbookpublishing.com

UCLA Child Anxiety Disorder Programme: http://www.npi.ucla.edu/caap/

Factsheets on worries and anxieties, school refusal and traumatic stress in children can be downloaded from the website for Rose, G. & York, A. (2004). *Mental Health and Growing Up. Fact sheets for Parents, Teachers and Young People* (Third edition). London: Gaskell: http://www.rcpsych.ac.uk

Chapter 13

Repetition problems

Obsessive-compulsive disorder (OCD), Tourette's syndrome, complex repetitive rituals, hair pulling (trichotillomania), nail biting, simple motor and vocal tics and isolated compulsions and obsessions collectively form part of a spectrum of psychological problems where the central psychological concern is the fact that adjustment is compromised by the execution of repetitive actions. The way in which these difficulties are classified in DSM IV TR (APA, 2000a) and ICD 10 (WHO, 1992, 1996) is presented in Figures 13.1 and 13.2. From these figures it is clear that, despite their similarity from a behavioural perspective, they have been classified within these systems as if they form discrete clusters of problems associated with anxiety, impulse control and childhood movement difficulties. Genetic evidence supports the view that these disorders probably fall along a continuum (Leckman & Cohen, 2002; Rapoport & Swedo, 2002; Shafran, 2001). For example, there is preponderance of OCD

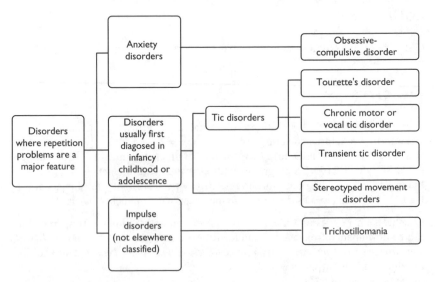

Figure 13.1 Classification of disorders where repetition is a central feature in DSM IV TR

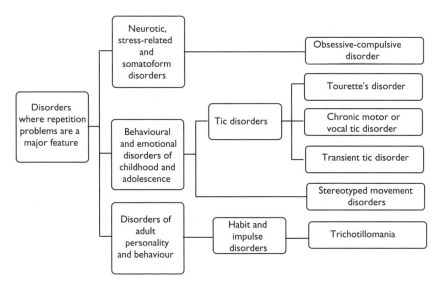

Figure 13.2 Classification of disorders where repetition is a central feature in ICD 10

and Tourette's syndrome within families where one or the other disorder is diagnosed. Hair pulling, an excessive grooming behaviour, has ethological similarities to compulsive cleansing behaviours associated with cases of OCD where obsessions about contamination are a central feature. The tics that characterize Tourette's syndrome are similar to those which occur in isolation, and the movements which typify chronic movement disorder are probably subserved by the same structures within the basal ganglia as those that under-pin compulsive behaviours and complex tics.

This chapter first gives special consideration to obsessive-compulsive disorder and then to Tourette's syndrome. These are particularly serious disorders. Tourette's syndrome is a troublesome, lifelong condition for which there is no permanent cure (Chowdhury, 2004; Leckman & Cohen, 2002). Between a third and a half of all paediatric cases of OCD continue to display significant symptomatology in adulthood that compromises social and vocational adjustment (Rapoport & Swedo, 2002; Shafran, 2001).

OBSESSIVE-COMPULSIVE DISORDER

Obsessive-compulsive disorder (OCD) is a condition typically characterized by distressing obsessional thoughts or impulses on the one hand and compulsive rituals which reduce the anxiety associated with the obsessions on the other. A case example of OCD is given in Box 13.1 and diagnostic criteria for OCD from DSM IV TR and ICD 10 are presented in Table 13.1.

Box 13.1 Case example of OCD

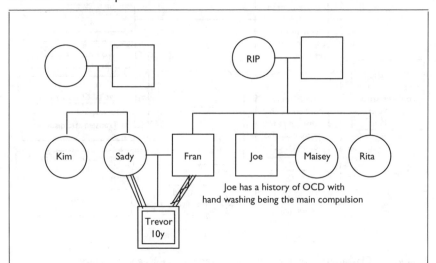

Joe has a history of OCD with
hand washing being the main compulsion

Referral. Trevor, an only child aged ten, was referred for consultation by the family doctor. Trevor was extremely unhappy because at school he was being ridiculed and rejected by his peers. They taunted him for being over-weight, poor at sports and overly clever. These, incidentally, were the principal ways in which he resembled his father, Fran. Trevor was also taunted at school for the foul odour that came from his clothing, which was usually saturated with saliva. His clothing was typically in this state because he felt compelled periodically to spit onto his hand and wipe the saliva onto his clothes.

History of the presenting problem. Usually, the impulse to spit arose when he thought about excrement, mucus, blood, semen or any substances that resembled these bodily products or swear words such as *shit* or *snot* or *fuck* associated with these body products. A range of stimuli made him think about these body products and swear words. For example, dog's excrement on the pavement, blood on his hand or congealed jelly in the pork pies that his father loved to eat, all reminded him of body products and swear words, although dog's excrement elicited far more vivid thoughts and images than other stimuli. Images or thoughts involving these bodily substances or associated swear words led Trevor to experience anxiety. The anxiety occurred because of the following conflict. Trevor prided himself on being a good boy and these thoughts or images were full of badness and so, according to his magical logic, made him bad. The anxiety was partially alleviated by the spitting because, for Trevor, the *badness* of the thoughts or images became contained in the saliva and spitting purified the body by providing an avenue through which the badness could be extruded.

Trevor's obsessions about body products and swear words and his compulsion to spit and wipe saliva on his clothes had progressively worsened over the two years prior to his referral. The problems had started following an incident where he fell off his bike at the end of the summer holidays just before returning to school to join a new class at the age of eight years. Trevor's mother, Sady, was very sympathetic to his condition and offered him a great deal of reassurance and support. Trevor's father, Fran, alternated between offering reassurance and attempting to curb Trevor's compulsive behaviour by criticizing him for engaging in it or withdrawing from contact with him. Trevor found that when his father was present he anticipated criticism and so was more likely to have intrusive thoughts.

Developmental and family history. Trevor's developmental history was well within normal limits. Both parents had been moderately strict with Trevor during his upbringing and he was a very obedient child. In the family history it was noteworthy that his uncle had OCD with hand washing as the principal ritual. There was also some marital discord and tension related to management of Trevor and also to the ways in which Trevor's parents perceived each other to have failed to live up to each other's expectations.

Formulation. Trevor was a ten-year-old boy with OCD. The principal obsessions were with bodily excretions and the principal compulsions with ridding himself of these by spitting. A positive family history of OCD suggested the possible presence of a genetic pre-disposition and the condition may have been maintained by the parents' inconsistent, over-intrusive and critical approach to the management of the condition.

Treatment. The condition was treated with family-based graded exposure and response prevention.

Table 13.1 Diagnostic criteria for OCD from DSM IV TR and ICD 10

DSM IV TR	ICD 10
A. Either obsessions or compulsions. Obsessions are defined by 1, 2, 3, and 4: 1. Recurrent or persistent thoughts impulses or images that are experienced as intrusive or inappropriate and cause marked anxiety or distress 2. The thoughts, images or impulse are not excessive worries about real-life problems 3. The person attempts to ignore or suppress these thoughts, impulses or images or to neutralize them with some other thought or action 4. The person recognizes that the thoughts images or impulses are the product of his or her own mind (and not imposed from without as in thought insertion) Compulsions are defined by 1 and 2: 1. Repetitive behaviours (e.g. hand washing, ordering, checking) or mental acts (e.g. praying, counting, repeating words silently) that the person feels driven to performing in response to an obsession or according to rules that must be applied rigidly 2. The behaviours or mental acts are aimed at preventing or reducing distress or preventing some dreaded event or situation. However, these behaviours or mental acts either are not connected in a realistic way with what they are designed to neutralize or prevent or are clearly excessive	The essential feature of this disorder is recurrent obsessional thoughts or compulsive acts Obsessional thoughts are ideas, images or impulses that enter the individual's mind again and again in a stereotyped form. They are invariably distressing either because they are violent or obscene or because they are senseless and the sufferer often tries unsuccessfully to resist them. They are recognized as the individual's own thoughts even though they are repugnant and/or involuntary Compulsive acts or rituals are stereotyped behaviours that are repeated again and again. They are not inherently enjoyable nor do they result in the completion of inherently useful tasks. The individual views them as preventing some objectively unlikely event often involving harm to, or caused by himself or herself. Usually this behaviour is recognized as pointless and repeated attempts are made to resist it

Continued

Table 13.1 continued

DSM IV TR	ICD 10
B. The person has at one time recognized that the obsessions or compulsions are unreasonable, but this condition does not apply to children	Autonomic anxiety symptoms are often present but distressing feelings of internal or psychic tension without obvious autonomic arousal are also common
C. The obsessions or compulsions cause considerable distress, are time consuming (more than 1 hour a day), and impair social and academic functioning	Depressive symptoms commonly accompany the condition
D. The content of the obsessions and compulsions is unrelated to another disorder if one is present	For a definite diagnosis obsessional symptoms or compulsive acts or both must be present on most days for at least two successive weeks and be a source of distress or interference with activities. The obsessional symptoms should have the following characteristics:
E. The disorder is not due to a medical condition or the effects of a drug	a. They must be recognized as the individual's own thoughts or impulses.
	b. There must be at least one thought or act that is still resisted unsuccessfully
	c. The thought of carrying out of the act must not be inherently pleasurable
	d. The thoughts, images or impulses must be unpleasantly repetitive

Note: Adapted from DSM IV TR (APA, 2000a) and ICD 10 (WHO, 1992, 1996).

Clinical features and epidemiology

The clinical features of OCD have been well described in the literature (e.g. American Academy of Child and Adolescent Psychiatry, 1997d; Barrett, Healey-Farrell, Piacentini & March, 2004; Beer, Karitani, Leonard, March & Swedo, 2002; Chowdhury, Frampton & Heyman, 2004; March, Frances & Carpenter, 1997; March, Franklin, Leonard & Foa, 2004; March & Mulle, 1998; Rapoport & Inoff-Germain, 2000; Rapoport & Swedo, 2002; Shafran, 2001; Thompsen, 1998). The two central features are obsessional anxiety-provoking thoughts and compulsive anxiety-reducing rituals. The most common obsessions are with dirt and contamination; harmful catastrophes such as fires, illness or death; symmetry, order and exactness; religious scrupulosity; disgust with bodily wastes or secretions such as urine, stools or saliva; unlucky or lucky numbers; unacceptable aggressive urges or ideas; forbidden sexual thoughts; and the need to tell, ask or confess. Obsessions are accompanied by anxiety and other affects including doubt, disgust and depression. Common anxiety-reducing compulsive rituals include washing, repeating an action, checking, removing contaminants, touching, ordering, collecting, counting and praying. Most youngsters have 'insight' and are aware that their obsessional ideas and related rituals are not sensible or socially acceptable. They therefore expend great effort to control their compulsions in public and keep them secret, but relinquish such control at home. This may lead parents to view the compulsions as under complete voluntary control and an expression of disobedience.

Obsessions and compulsions occur together in about 60% of cases, with the compulsion alleviating anxiety associated with the obsession. In 40% of cases compulsions occur in the absence of obsessions. The majority of cases have another co-morbid disorder, with the most common being tic disorders, including de la Tourette's syndrome, anxiety and depression. Other co-morbid disorders include, anorexia, bulimia, attention deficit hyperactivity disorder, developmental delays, elimination problems and schizophrenia. Most epidemiological studies including a recent national UK investigation confirm that about 1% of children and adolescents have OCD (Heyman et al., 2001). While it may appear as early as two years, the most common period of onset is late childhood or early adolescence. The condition may be chronic and continuous or episodic, with about one in three showing full recovery and one in ten cases having a continuous deteriorating course.

OCD is distinct from the normal rituals of childhood that are prominent in the pre-school years and wane by the age of eight or nine years, when hobbies involving collecting and ordering selected objects, toys and trinkets probably take their place.

OCD may be distinguished from tic disorders, where obsessions do not occur although there may be premonitory urges. OCD may also be distinguished from eating disorders where food-related rituals may occur, since these food-related rituals are not experienced as ego dystonic. The same may be said of gambling, repetitive sexual behaviour problems (such as exhibitionism) and drug abuse.

Theories

Biological and psychological hypotheses have been suggested to explain OCD and a summary of the main features of these positions is set out in Table 13.2.

Biological theories

There are four main theories about the biological basis for OCD and these point to genetic factors, a structural or functional abnormality of the basal ganglia, a low level of the neurotransmitter serotonin or inefficient functioning of the serotonergic system and a dysregulation of the immune system as

Table 13.2 Theories and treatments for OCD

Type	Theory	Theoretical principles	Principles of treatment
Biological theories	**Genetic hypothesis**	A pre-disposition to OCD is inherited and the condition develops in children exposed to particular environmental conditions, probably involving particular parenting styles, stressful life events or infections	Genetic counselling and family stress management
	Basal ganglia hypothesis	A structural problem in the basal ganglia under-pins OCD	Surgery to disconnect the basal ganglia from the frontal cortex will prevent the occurrence of obsessions and compulsions
	Serotonin hypothesis	OCD symptoms occur due to too rapid a re-uptake of serotonin or abnormally low level of serotonin	Administer clomipramine, a serotonin re-uptake inhibitor
	Autoimmune disorder hypothesis	PANDAS (Paediatric Autoimmune Neuropsychiatric Disorders Associated with Streptococcal Infections) occurs when a streptococcal infection triggers the production of antibodies, which cross-react with neuronal tissue to produce an autoimmune reaction within the basal ganglia resulting in obsessions, compulsions and tics	Treatment with immunomodulatory agents such as intravenous immunoglobulin and plasma exchange

	Neuroethological theory	Basal ganglia and serotonin abnormalities lead to the inappropriate release of fixed patterns of grooming or self-protective behaviour	
Psychological theories	**Psychoanalytic theory**	Repressed sexual-aggressive impulses associated with early parent–child conflict over toilet training are *displaced and substituted* by less unacceptable thoughts or impulses. When these intrude into consciousness, they are experienced as ego-alien because they have been disowned or *isolated* and cause anxiety. The anxiety is managed by carrying out a compulsive ritual to *undo* or cancel out the undesirable impulse	Individual psychodynamic psychotherapy to interpret the defences and work through the anxiety about the repressed impulses
	Behavioural theory	Through a process of classical conditioning, specific cues come to elicit anxiety, and compulsive rituals which develop to alleviate this anxiety are maintained by a process of negative reinforcement	Exposure to cues that elicit obsessions and response prevention where the person is prevented from carrying out the anxiety-reducing compulsive rituals
	Cognitive-behavioural theory	Normal intrusive thoughts, cued by exposure to specific stimuli, are mis-appraised such that youngsters believe that they will be fully responsible for serious harm to the self or others unless they engage in a	Exposure and response prevention coupled with cognitive therapy in which maladaptive beliefs about over-estimation of danger and over-responsibility for negative outcomes are challenged

Continued

Table 13.2 continued

Type	Theory	Theoretical principles	Principles of treatment
		specific compulsive activity or ritual. Engaging in these compulsive actions or rituals alleviates anxiety or distress, and so they are more likely to do so in future. Vulnerability to OCD arises from genetically determined hyperarousablity; depressed mood; socialization experiences that have led to the development of high moral standards; and a belief system involving thought–action fusion; over-responsibility; and self-doubt	
	Family systems hypothesis	Family lifecycle transitions precipitate the onset of OCD in individuals whose socialization has rendered them vulnerable to developing obsession and compulsions. The family become involved in patterns of interaction that maintain the child's compulsive ritualistic behaviour because of their beliefs about OCD, their beliefs about childcare, and because symptom maintaining patterns of interaction may meet their needs	Family work in which OCD is re-framed as a condition to be managed rather than an intrinsic characteristic of the child deserving parental punishment or over-intrusive concern Create opportunities for the family to break symptom-maintaining behavioural patterns and coach parents to use behavioural or other methods to help their child manage OCD

important in the aetiology of OCD (American Academy of Child and Adolescent Psychiatry, 1997d; Beer et al., 2002; Chowdhury, 2004; Rapoport & Inoff-Germain, 2000; Rapoport & Swedo, 2002; Shafran, 2001).

Genetic hypothesis

The genetic hypothesis argues that a pre-disposition to OCD is inherited and the condition develops in children exposed to particular environmental conditions, probably involving particular parenting styles, stressful life events or infections. Available evidence indicates that genetic factors may be important in the aetiology of a sub-group of cases of OCD (Eley, Collier & McGuffin, 2002). There is evidence for the aggregation of OCD and Tourette's disorder within families, and it is probable that what is transmitted is a pre-disposition to develop either disorder, which may most usefully be conceptualized as an OCD–tic disorder spectrum (Rapoport & Swedo, 2002).

Basal ganglia hypothesis

The basal ganglia hypothesis proposes that structural or functional abnormalities in the basal ganglia sub-serve the symptoms of OCD. In support of the basal ganglia hypothesis, there is considerable evidence that a strong association exists between basal ganglia disease and OCD (Beer et al., 2002; Rapoport & Swedo, 2002). For example, there is a very high incidence of OCD in cases of Sydenham's chorea, Huntington's chorea, Wilson's disease, Parkinson's disease and Tourette's syndrome. Furthermore, damage to the basal ganglia resulting from head injury may precipitate an episode of OCD. Also, surgery that disconnects the basal ganglia from the frontal cortex alleviates severe OCD. Finally, neuroimaging studies have shown that successful treatment of OCD with specific serotonin re-uptake inhibitors (SSRIs) or cognitive-behaviour therapy leads to functional changes in circuits linking the basal ganglia to the cortex (Rauch & Baxter, 1998; Schwartz, 1996).

Serotonin hypothesis

The serotonin hypothesis argues that the symptoms of OCD are sub-served by low serotonin levels or an inefficient seotonergic system. In support of the serotonergic hypothesis, both child and adult cases of OCD have been shown to respond to SSRIs such as clomiparamine, fluoxetine, fluvoxamine, paroxetine and sertraline (Beer et al., 2002). Also, OCD symptoms are exacerbated by serotonin agonists (Rapoport & Swedo, 2002).

Autoimmune disorder hypothesis

This hypothesis proposes that streptococcal infections trigger the production of antibodies, which cross-react with neuronal tissue to produce an autoimmune reaction within the basal ganglia, resulting in obsessions, compulsions and tics. The syndrome, PANDAS (Paediatric Autoimmune Neuropsychiatric Disorders Associated with Streptococcal Infections; Swedo et al., 1998) is characterized by abrupt pre-pubescent onset of OCD and or tic disorder following streptococcal infections, an episodic course of symptom severity and the presence of neurological abnormalities such as choreioform movements and motoric hyperactivity. Preliminary evidence suggests that children with this type of OCD may respond rapidly to immunomodulatory agents such as intravenous immunoglobulin and plasma exchange (Snider & Swedo, 2003).

Neuroethological theory

Neuroethological theories, inspired by evidence on basal ganglia and serotonin abnormalities, argue that in cases of OCD, relatively fixed adaptive behaviour patterns of grooming or self-protection are inappropriately released and these patterns are probably encoded in the basal ganglia (Rapoport & Swedo, 2002).

Psychological theories

Many psychological theories have been developed within psychoanalytic, cognitive-behavioural and family systems traditions. The main tenets of one theory from each of these traditions are set out in Table 13.2.

Psychoanalytic theory

From a psychoanalytic perspective, OCD is explained as the sequelae of toilet training battles (Freud, 1909b). According to psychoanalytic theory, during the anal phase of development children become angry with their parents' insistence that they use the toilet in an appropriate way. Attempts to express these aggressive impulses are met with sanctions from the parents and so the aggression is repressed. In later life these repressed sexual–aggressive impulses attempt to find expression but this causes anxiety. The aggressive impulses and thoughts are *displaced and substituted* by less unacceptable thoughts or impulses. When these intrude into consciousness, they are experienced as ego-alien because they have been disowned or *isolated*. The anxiety is managed by carrying out a compulsive ritual to *undo* or cancel out the undesirable impulse.

Surveys of people with OCD have invariably failed to identify a higher rate of such parent–child conflicts concerning toilet training in comparison with controls (Milby & Weber, 1991) and there is little evidence that children with OCD can benefit from interpretative psychoanalytic psychotherapy. However, the notion that compulsions reflect the use of the defence mechanism of undoing fits with both clinical observations and with the cognitive-behavioural explanation of OCD.

Behavioural theory

In behavioural theory it is proposed that, through a process of classical conditioning, specific cues (such as dirt) come to elicit anxiety, and compulsive rituals (such as washing), which develop to alleviate, escape from or avoid this anxiety, are maintained by a process of negative reinforcement (Mowrer, 1960). Treatment of OCD with exposure and response prevention (E/RP) is based on this theory. E/RP involves prolonged exposure to cues that elicit obsessions and related anxiety (such as dirt) coupled with prevention of compulsive rituals (such as hand washing). While E/RP continues to be the mainstay of effective psychological treatment of OCD, Mowrer's simple behavioural two-stage theory has been abandoned because of its failure to explain a number of phenomena. These include the absence of traumatic classical conditioning experiences in the history of many OCD patients, the small number of categories of stimuli that elicit obsessions and the fact that the expectation or over-prediction of fear, the expected absence of safety signals or the urge to feel 'just so' rather than cue-elicited fear are usually the main factors motivating compulsive behaviour (Rachman, 2002). The behavioural conditioning theory of OCD has been replaced by cognitive-behavioural explanations that give primacy to the role of appraisals and expectations in the OCD process.

Cognitive-behavioural theory

Cognitive-behavioural explanations of OCD argue that normal intrusive thoughts, cued by exposure to specific stimuli, are mis-appraised such that youngsters believe that they will be fully responsible for serious harm to the self or others unless they engage in a specific compulsive activity or ritual. Engaging in these compulsive actions or rituals alleviates anxiety or distress, and so they are more likely to do so in future (Salkovski, Forrester & Richards, 1998). A variety of factors contribute to this vulnerability, including genetically determined hyperarousability, depressed mood, socialization experiences that have led to the development of high moral standards, a belief system involving specific convictions about the relationships between thought and action, control and responsibility, and self-doubt or low self-efficacy (Barrett et al., 2004; Rachman, 2002). Youngsters who are vulnerable to OCD believe that intrusive and morally unacceptable obsessional thoughts will automatically translate into immoral action. They also believe that they are equally responsible for the occurrence of these thoughts and engagement in these actions. This is referred to as 'thought–action fusion'. They also believe that they should be able to control intrusive immoral obsessive thoughts and impulses. There is a conviction that they are reprehensible for having thoughts that may lead to actions that would harm others. Youngsters with OCD, because they have low self-efficacy, doubt the effectiveness of their actions in general, and also doubt the effectivness of their compulsive anxiety-reducing rituals in particular, and are therefore more likely to repeat them to reduce distress. According to cognitive-behavioural theories, episodes of OCD are usually precipitated by stressful life events, illness or family disruption. The cognitive-behavioural treatment of OCD is usually based on assessment of the stimuli which elicit obsessions, the anxiety associated with these and the compulsive rituals which reduce the anxiety. Treatment based on the cognitive-behavioural model, like that based in the behavioural model, typically involves exposure to those cues that elicit obsessional thoughts and response prevention where the person is prevented from carrying out the anxiety-reducing compulsive rituals. It may also involve cognitive therapy in which the youngster gathers evidence that challenges the 'OCD beliefs' about over-predicting danger and then notes the impact of this evidence on the degree to which he or she is certain that the belief are true. Substantial evidence exists for the vulnerability factors, precipitating factors and self-reinforcing nature of the vicious cycles of obsessions and compulsions that typify OCD in adults and a small body of evidence on children with OCD is now emerging (Barrett et al., 2004). In addition, there is some evidence that exposure and response prevention is a particularly effective treatment for the majority of children with OCD and a specific treatment module that incorporates this approach will be presented below (March & Mulle, 1998; Barrett et al., 2004).

Family systems theory

The family systems theory of OCD has been less well articulated than the positions taken within the psychoanalytic and cognitive-behavioural traditions (Dalton, 1983; O'Connor, 1983). Family systems approaches to OCD point to socialization experiences as the primary pre-disposing factors and family lifecycle transitions as the principle precipitating factors for OCD. Central to family systems explanations is the idea that the symptomatic child and other family members become involved in patterns of interaction that maintain the child's compulsive ritualistic behaviour. Beliefs about the best way to manage the child's condition specifically, or childrearing generally, may under-pin these patterns of interaction that inadvertently maintain the child's compulsive behaviour. Engaging in symptom-maintaining patterns of interaction may meet the needs of other family members. For example, it may meet a mother's need to be nurturent, a father's need to be a disciplinarian, a couples' need to avoid marital intimacy or a sibling's need to leave home.

Treatment premised on a family systems model aims to help the parents and child break the pattern of interaction in which the compulsive rituals are embedded and to alter the belief systems that under-pin these patterns. The belief systems may be altered by educating the family about OCD so that it is re-framed as a condition to be managed rather than an intrinsic characteristic of the child deserving either parental punishment or over-intrusive concern. Problem-maintaining patterns of family interaction may be disrupted by creating opportunities for the whole family to replace compulsive rituals and related family behaviours with alternative adaptive behaviours. Parents may be coached in how to break problem-maintaining behaviour patterns by using behavioural or other methods to empower their children. Response replacement, exposure and response prevention, anxiety management training and reward programmes may all be usefully employed by parents to empower their children to manage OCD.

A limited but growing body of evidence points to the importance of relatives' involvement in rituals and high levels of expressed emotion involving criticism and over-involvement as maintaining factors, and to the value of including family sessions as a routine part of cognitive-behavioural treatment programmes (Barrett et al., 2004; Hibbs et al., 1991).

Assessment

When assessing symptomatology in cases of OCD, particular attention should be paid to details of the specific stimuli that elicit the intrusive thoughts. For treatment planning these stimuli are ordered into a hierarchy. In addition, particular attention should be paid to the nature of the intrusive thoughts and the meaning of these for the child along with the precise way in which the compulsive rituals bring about relief. Patterns of family interaction in which these symptoms are embedded should also be clarified. Children may be asked to keep a daily diary, noting down the time and situations in which obsessions and compulsion occur, the amount of time they spend engaged in these, family involvement in rituals and the associated levels of distress on a ten-point scale. A reliable and valid standardized rating scale and a self-report assessment inventory for OCD are described included in Table 13.3 and may be used routinely to assess both the patterning of symptoms and the overall severity of the condition. Forms for assessing the impact of OCD on the child and family are also listed in Table 13.3. Aetiological factors deserving consideration in the clinical assessment of OCD are presented in Figure 13.3.

Pre-disposing factors

Figure 13.3 shows that both personal and contextual pre-disposing factors deserve consideration in the assessment of OCD. Genetic vulnerability is the main personal biological pre-disposing factor in cases of OCD and this may give rise to structural abnormalities in the basal ganglia and dysregulation of

Table 13.3 Psychometric instruments that may be used as an adjunct to clinical interviews in the assessment of OCD

Instrument	Publication	Comments
Children's Yale–Brown Obsessive Compulsive scale	Scahill, L., Riddle, M. A., McSwiggin-Hardin, M., Ort, S. I., King, R. A., Goodman, W. K., Cicchetti, D., & Leckman, J. F. (1997). Children's Yale-Brown Obsessive Compulsive Scale: Reliability and validity. *Journal of the American Academy of Child & Adolescent Psychiatry*, 36, 844–852. Reprinted in March, J. & Mulle, K. (1998). *OCD in Children and Adolescents: A Cognitive Behavioural Treatment Manual.* New York: Guilford	Four-point scales are used to rate 35 obsessions and 36 rituals on time spent, interference, distress, resistance and perceived control. This is the most widely used rating scale and may be used with children
Leyton Obsessional Inventory-Child Version:	Berg, C., Whitaker, A., Davies, M., Flament, M., Rapoport, J. (1988). The survey form of the Leyton Obsessional Inventory-Child Version: Norms from an epidemiological study. *Journal of the American Academy of Child and Adolescent Psychiatry*, 27, 759–763. Reprinted in March, J. & Mulle, K. (1998). *OCD in Children and Adolescents: A Cognitive Behavioural Treatment Manual.* New York: Guilford	Contains 20 statements concerning obsessions and compulsions which are rated on 5-point scales to indicate degree of interference in the child's life
Child OCD Impact Scale (COIS)	Piacentini, J., Jaffer, M., Bergman, R., McCracken, J., & Keller, M. (2001). Measuring impairment in childhood OCD. Psychometric properties of the COIS. *Proceedings of the American Academy of Child and Adolescent Psychiatry Meeting*, 48, 146	20 items are rated on 4-point Likert scales to indicate impact and impairment due to OCD in family, school, and peer-group situations. Child and parent forms are available
Family and Sibling Accommodation Scale	Barrett, P., Rasmussen, P. & Healy, L. (2001). The effect of obsessive compulsive disorder on sibling relationships in late childhood and early adolescence. Preliminary findings. *The Australian Educational and Developmental Psychologists*, 17, 82–102	13 items are rated by siblings or parents on 5-point Likert scales to indicate degree of family participation in rituals; consequences of this; and degree of related distress

the serotonergic system. A family history of OCD, tic disorders or Tourette's syndrome may all be taken as indicative of a genetic pre-disposition. Beliefs in over-responsibility, beliefs that negative thoughts automatically become negative actions, low self-esteem and depression are the principal psychological personal pre-disposing factors for OCD. Contextual pre-disposing factors include conditioning experiences where cues, such as dirt, that elicit anxiety-laden obsessional thoughts were paired with anxiety-provoking stimuli such as injury, threats or punishment. Socialization experiences with parents who espoused high, rigid moral standards may under-pin the beliefs in over-responsibility and the inevitability of negative thoughts leading to negative actions mentioned previously.

Precipitating factors

Psychosocial precipitating factors for OCD include stressful life events and family lifecycle transitions. At a biological level, OCD may be precipitated by head injury with frontal or temporal lobe lesions.

Maintaining factors

Personal and contextual factors may be involved in the maintenance of OCD. The anxiety-reducing effects of compulsive rituals when the youngster is exposed to cues that elicit anxiety-laden obsessions mean that OCD as a syndrome is intrinsically self-maintaining. Parental reassurance following the execution of a compulsive ritual may maintain the ritual through the process of inadvertent positive reinforcement. Parental criticism, on the other hand, may maintain OCD by eliciting obsessions. Both intrusive reassuring responses and punitive critical responses to the child are typically associated with parental beliefs that the OCD symptomatology are an essential rather than an accidental feature of the child. That is, parents come to see the child in a problem-saturated way, where the symptoms are not simply a minor aspect of the child but a central feature of his or her identity. The child comes to be treated as if he or she is essentially ill (in instances where parents adopt an over-involved reassuring position) or essentially disobedient or annoying (when parents adopt a punitive critical position). Parents who experience marital discord and who have unresolved conflicts about intimacy or power within the marital relationship may avoid discussing these conflicts but routinely argue about how best to manage their child's OCD problems. That is, they may become involved in a pattern of triangulation with the child. It is not unusual for such triangulation to involve intense interaction between the mother and child, with the father becoming increasingly peripheral as the problems progress.

Where parents themselves have OCD which goes untreated, their obsessional conversation and ritualistic actions may validate the child's symptoms

PRE-DISPOSING FACTORS

PERSONAL PRE-DISPOSING FACTORS

Biological factors
- Genetic vulnerability
- Structural abnormality in basal ganglia
- Dysregulation of serotonin system

Psychological factors
- Over-responsibility
- Belief that negative thoughts automatically become negative actions
- Low self-esteem
- Depressed mood

CONTEXTUAL PRE-DISPOSING FACTORS

Parent–child factors in early life
- Parents have high and rigid moral standards

Stresses in early life
- Conditioning experiences

PERSONAL MAINTAINING FACTORS

Psychological factors
- Compulsive behaviour is maintained by anxiety-reducing effects
- Anxiety is maintained by obsessional beliefs about danger associated with a class of stimuli

PERSONAL PROTECTIVE FACTORS

Biological factors
- Good physical health

Psychological factors
- High IQ
- Easy temperament
- High self-esteem
- Internal locus of control
- High self-efficacy
- Optimistic attributional style
- Mature defence mechanisms
- Functional coping strategies

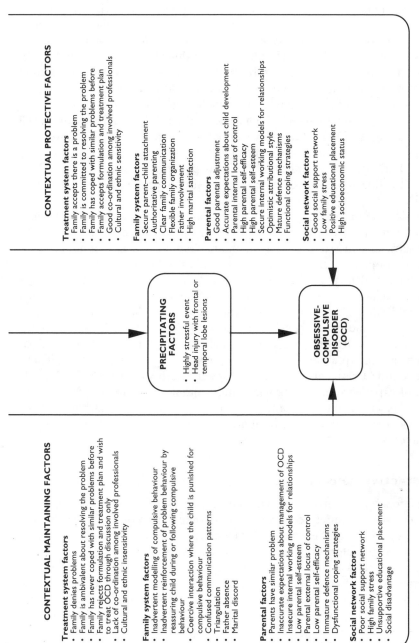

CONTEXTUAL MAINTAINING FACTORS

Treatment system factors
- Family denies problems
- Family is ambivalent about resolving the problem
- Family has never coped with similar problems before
- Family rejects formulation and treatment plan and wish to treat OCD through discussion only
- Lack of co-ordination among involved professionals
- Cultural and ethnic insensitivity

Family system factors
- Inadvertent modelling of compulsive behaviour
- Inadvertent reinforcement of problem behaviour by reassuring child during or following compulsive behaviour
- Coercive interaction where the child is punished for compulsive behaviour
- Confused communication patterns
- Triangulation
- Father absence
- Marital discord

Parental factors
- Parents have similar problem
- Inaccurate expectations about management of OCD
- Insecure internal working models for relationships
- Low parental self-esteem
- Parental external locus of control
- Low parental self-efficacy
- Immature defence mechanisms
- Dysfunctional coping strategies

Social network factors
- Poor social support network
- High family stress
- Unsupportive educational placement
- Social disadvantage

PRECIPITATING FACTORS
- Highly stressful event
- Head injury with frontal or temporal lobe lesions

OBSESSIVE-COMPULSIVE DISORDER (OCD)

CONTEXTUAL PROTECTIVE FACTORS

Treatment system factors
- Family accepts there is a problem
- Family is committed to resolving the problem
- Family has coped with similar problems before
- Family accepts formulation and treatment plan
- Good co-ordination among involved professionals
- Cultural and ethnic sensitivity

Family system factors
- Secure parent–child attachment
- Authoritative parenting
- Clear family communication
- Flexible family organization
- Father involvement
- High marital satisfaction

Parental factors
- Good parental adjustment
- Accurate expectations about child development
- Parental internal locus of control
- High parental self-efficacy
- High parental self-esteem
- Secure internal working models for relationships
- Optimistic attributional style
- Mature defence mechanisms
- Functional coping strategies

Social network factors
- Good social support network
- Low family stress
- Positive educational placement
- High socioeconomic status

Figure 13.3 Factors to consider in OCD

and the child's behaviour may be maintained by a process of modelling. Where parents have insecure internal working models for relationships, low self-esteem, low self-efficacy, an external locus of control, immature defences and poor coping strategies, they may lack the personal resources to deal constructively with their child's OCD and, in this sense, these parental attributes may maintain the child's problems. Parents may also become involved in problem-maintaining interactions with their children if they have inaccurate knowledge about OCD and related psychological processes.

OCD may be maintained by high levels of stress, limited support and social disadvantage within the family's wider social system, since these features may deplete parents' and children's personal resources for dealing constructively with OCD. Poorly resourced educational placements where teaching staff have little time to devote to home–school liaison meetings may also maintain OCD.

Within the treatment system, a lack of co-ordination and clear communication among involved professionals, including teachers, psychologists, paediatricians and so forth, may maintain children's OCD symptomatology. Where co-operation problems between families and treatment teams develop, and families deny the existence of the problems, the validity of the diagnosis and formulation or the appropriateness of the treatment programme, then the child's difficulties may persist. Treatment systems that are not sensitive to the cultural and ethnic beliefs and values of the youngster's family system may maintain OCD by inhibiting engagement or promoting drop-out from treatment and preventing the development of a good working alliance between the treatment team, the youngster and his or her family. Parents' lack of experience in dealing with similar problems in the past is a further factor that may compromise their capacity to work co-operatively with the treatment team and so may contribute to the maintenance of the child's OCD symptoms.

Protective factors

The probability that a treatment programme for OCD will be effective is influenced by a variety of personal and contextual protective factors. It is important that these be assessed and included in the later formulation, since it is protective factors that usually serve as the foundation for therapeutic change. Good health, a high IQ, an easy temperament, high self-esteem, an internal locus of control, high self-efficacy and an optimistic attributional style are all important personal protective factors. Other important personal protective factors include mature defence mechanisms and functional coping strategies, particularly good problem-solving skills and a capacity to make and maintain friendships.

Within the family, secure parent–child attachment and authoritative parenting are central protective factors, particularly if they occur within the context of a flexible family structure in which there is clear communication, high marital satisfaction and both parents share the day-to-day tasks of childcare.

Good parental adjustment is also a protective factor. Where parents have an internal locus of control, high self-efficacy, high self-esteem, internal working models for secure attachments, an optimistic attributional style, mature defences and functional coping strategies, then they are better resourced to manage their children's OCD constructively. Of course, accurate knowledge about OCD is also a protective factor.

Within the broader social network, high levels of support, low levels of stress and membership of a high socioeconomic group are all protective factors for children with OCD. Where families are embedded in social networks that provide a high level of support and place few stressful demands on family members, then it is less likely that parents' and children's resources for dealing with OCD will become depleted. A well-resourced educational placement may also be viewed as a protective factor. Educational placements where teachers have a clear understanding of OCD and have sufficient time and flexibility to attend home–school liaison meetings contribute to positive outcomes for children with OCD.

Within the treatment system, co-operative working relationships between the treatment team and the family and good co-ordination of multi-professional input are protective factors. Treatment systems that are sensitive to the cultural and ethnic beliefs and values of the youngster's family are more likely help families engage with, and remain in, treatment and foster the development of a good working alliance. Families are more likely to benefit from treatment when they accept the formulation of the problem given by the treatment team and are committed to working with the team to resolve it. Where families have successfully faced similar problems before, then they are more likely to benefit from treatment and, in this sense, previous experience with similar problems is a protective factor.

Formulation

Information from the intake interview, the standardized rating scale and inventory and self-monitoring form may be integrated into a formulation to guide treatment planning. A formulation in a case of OCD should link the pre-disposing factors to the occurrence of this episode of the condition via an identifiable precipitating event. In formulating the way symptoms are maintained, eliciting stimuli should be linked to intrusive thoughts and images and these in turn to anxiety and anxiety-reducing compulsions. Patterns of interaction that maintain these compulsions and involve parents, siblings, peers and school personnel should also be specified. An example of a formulation is given in the penultimate paragraph of the case example in Box 13.1.

Treatment

Effective treatment for OCD in children is multi-modal and includes psycho-logical intervention with a family-oriented exposure and response-prevention programme coupled with psychopharmacological interventions with SSRIs (such as clomipramine, fluoxetine, fluvoxamine, paroxetine and sertraline) if the psychological intervention programme alone is ineffective or if the symp-toms are particularly severe (American Academy of Child and Adolescent Psychiatry, 1997d). March and Mulle's (1998) and Barrett et al.'s (2004) psychological treatment protocols have both been empirically validated and draw together effective practices from the cognitive-behavioural and family systems traditions. They are conducted over about twelve- to eighteen-weekly, one-hour sessions in an individual or group format, with one to four later, follow-up sessions at intervals of approximately one, three, six and twelve months. The principal difference between the two approaches is the greater level of family involvement in Barrett's programme, where parallel parent and sibling sessions occur throughout the programme in addition to a couple of whole-family sessions. March and Mulle include parents in only four sessions. Barrett's programme is based on March and Mulle's and aims to retain the psychoeducational and exposure and response prevention components, while strengthening the family involvement component. The following are the key components of these programmes:

- psychoeducation
- externalizing the problem
- mapping OCD
- exposure and response prevention
- cognitive therapy
- family involvement
- relapse prevention and graduation.

Psychoeducation

Psychoeducation should be offered in the first treatment session, but it is also an underlying theme throughout treatment. The goal of psychoeducation is to help the child, parents and siblings understand OCD as a neurobehav-ioural disorder and to outline the rationale for the treatment programme. OCD as a neurobehavioural disorder entails two main problems. First, the nervous system mistakenly makes the child experience a great deal of fear, distress, doubt or discomfort in response to situations that should only elicit a low level of fear (such as touching something dirty). This may be explained metaphorically by saying that the *fear volume control* of the nervous system is damaged, and so where low levels of fear should be experienced, high levels of fear occur because the volume control knob is not working properly. The second problem with OCD as a neurobehavioural disorder is that it makes children carry out actions (compulsions) to reduce the fear, for example repeated hand washing. The more the child carries out these actions, the stronger OCD becomes.

An analogy may be made with a medical illness such as diabetes. In diabetes the pancreas fails to produce enough insulin, and so part of the treatment involves taking extra insulin. In OCD, the brain fails to produce enough serotonin, and so a drug that increases the level of serotonin in the brain (an SSRI) must be taken. Brain imaging studies by Jeff Schwartz and Lew Baxter in America have shown that after effective drug treatment and cognitive-behaviour therapy, the brain functions differently (Rauch & Baxter, 1998; Schwartz, 1996). In diabetes people have to make changes to their lifestyle by carefully controlling their diet and exercise. With OCD, people have to carefully carry out exercises in which they put themselves in situations that make them have uncomfortable OCD thoughts (obsessions), and then tolerate this discomfort without carrying out compulsive rituals until the discomfort subsides. With diabetes and OCD, not everyone gets completely better. So some people with diabetes and OCD attend long-term support groups or family therapy, to help them cope with the residual symptoms.

The psychological part of treatment aims to help the child *boss OCD back*. Treatment is a series of coaching sessions in which the child is taught the skills to fight OCD and run him off the child's land. Parent sessions aim to help parents understand this coaching process and support the child in overcoming OCD. Also, the amount of discomfort, fear or distress that particular situations evoke may be reduced by taking a serotonin re-uptake inhibitor (such as clomipramine or fluoxetine). This helps to increase the level of serotonin in the brain, which is a bit low in youngsters with OCD. It may be metaphorically explained to children that medication can have some impact on the *fear volume control* but it is their job to learn how to *boss OCD back*.

The effectiveness and costs and benefits of treatment may also be outlined in the first session. The family-based behavioural programme has been shown to be effective in approximately two out of three cases. Apart from the side effects of medication (dry mouth and constipation), there are no known negative effects of the programme. It is useful in the early sessions of treatment to give families information on support groups, websites and self-help literature. A good parent education package is contained in March and Mulle (1998).

Externalizing the problem

Externalizing the problem follows directly from psychoeducation and may be introduced in the first or second session. However, it is also a constant theme throughout treatment. With externalizing the problem, children and families are invited to construe OCD as a discrete oppressive neurobehavioural illness, which is distinct from the child and the source of the unusual behaviour that led to the referral for treatment (White & Epston, 1990). Children may be invited to give OCD a nasty nick-name like *Germy*; adolescents usually prefer to refer to the condition by its initials OCD. Once the problem has been externalized, OCD is referred to by its nick-name (in the case of children) or as OCD (in the case of teenagers) and so becomes externalized as a personified enemy to be defeated rather than a bad habit or naughty behaviour for which the youngster is fully responsible. When OCD is externalized and re-framed in this way, children and parents are less likely to view the compulsions as bad behaviours for which the child is accountable and for which the child can be blamed. Rather, children and parents are invited to join forces and *boss Germy off the child's land* or to manage OCD in an effective way. Thus, externalizing the problem and joining forces against it creates a context for forming an expert team. This team includes the child and family (who are experts on the specific ways in which OCD affects their unique family situation) and the mental health professionals who are experts on general principles for reducing the impact of OCD on children and families. The goal of this team is to reduce the influence of OCD on the child and family or, phrased in children's terms, *to boss OCD off the child's land*. The implication of this framing of the problem is that OCD is currently *bossing the child around*. The cues that make Germy or OCD try to boss the child around, or that elicit obsessions, are identified and rated on a scale from 1–10, where 1 = minimally distressing and 10 = maximally distressing. Self-monitoring homework is given to be reviewed in the next session. This involves keeping a daily diary in which the following are noted: the time and situations in which obsessions and compulsions occur, the amount of time devoted to these, family involvement in rituals, and the associated levels of distress on a 10-point scale.

Mapping

In the second or third session the self-monitoring data and material from the initial interview are used to help the child construct a hierarchy of cues that elicit OCD symptoms (an OCD ladder) using the form in Figure 13.4. The children are invited first to identify those situations where they can *beat Germy hands down*, or control OCD, and in which they may feel a mild level of anxiety (0–2 on a 10-point scale) but do not perform a ritual. These are 'win-all' situations. Next, the child is asked to name those situations where *Germy*, or OCD, always wins and in which they experience a lot of fear (6–10) and always conduct a ritual. These are 'lose-all' situations. Finally, they are asked to describe the transition zone, in which a third of the time the child wins and two-thirds of the time *Germy*, or OCD, wins. To identify the transition zone, it is useful to ask children about 'those exceptional circumstances in which you expected *Germy*, or OCD, to win but you managed to defeat him' (White & Epson, 1990). The transition zone contains 'win-some, lose-some'

Make an OCD ladder by listing the situations in which OCD affects you from those in which you find it easiest to boss back OCD to those in which you find it hardest.

For each situation do these four things.

In the first column give a rating from 1 to 10 which says how hard it would be to resist OCD

> If it's easy to resist OCD in the situation and you find these situations relaxing rate it as 1
> If it's very hard resist OCD in the situation and you get very tense in these situations rate it as 10

Very easy   1_____2_____3_____4_____5_____6_____7_____8_____9_____10   Very hard
Relaxed   Very tense

In the second column write down the SITUATION where OCD affects you
In the third column write down the OBSESSIONS (uncomfortable thoughts) you get in the situation
In the fourth column write down the COMPULSIONS (actions or thoughts) you find yourself doing to control your fear or bad feeling in the situation

Rating from 1 to 10	Situation	Obsession	Compulsion

Figure 13.4 OCD ladder

situations. This zone is the area from which targets should be selected for exposure and response prevention exercises. For this reason, it may also be referred to as the 'work zone', since much of the work of therapy involves exposure and response prevention (E/RP). And, like all forms of work such as homework or housework, E/RP work, or *bossing OCD back* work is hard and takes sustained commitment and effort.

Exposure and response prevention

For about ten sessions after the mapping session, children undergo an E/RP programme and learn anxiety management skills. Children are told that to increase the number of situations in which they and not *Germy*, or OCD, wins they must be exposed to those situations and prevent themselves from letting *Germy* or OCD make them do their rituals. They are exposed to increasingly more anxiety-provoking cues while concurrently being supported *to boss-back Germy or OCD* and refuse to engage in rituals. The anxiety-eliciting cues may be both real and imaginal situations. If obsessions occur without identifiable cues (e.g. the idea that a tidal wave may swamp the city) then the obsession may be written down and repeatedly read or recorded onto a closed-loop audiotape. Children must remain in each exposure situation and prevent themselves from carrying out their rituals until their anxiety subsides. This is critical, since engaging in anxiety-reducing behavioural or cognitive compulsions before the anxiety has peaked and begun to subside reinforces the compulsive behaviour. If total response prevention is too anxiety provoking, compulsions may be delayed, shortened, altered or done more slowly to reduce the power of OCD over the youngster. Anxiety levels can be monitored throughout each E/RP session on a 10-point self-report scale using the form in Figure 13.5. On this form, anxiety ratings are made at one-minute intervals for five minutes and thereafter at five-minute intervals until thirty minutes have elapsed. By reviewing the pattern of ratings on the form, children learn that E/RP leads to habituation and that, over time, anxiety initially increases and then decreases. Habituation may be explained with reference to a swimming analogy. If we go swimming in cold water, initially it feels very uncomfortable but the longer we stay in swimming the less uncomfortable it feels. Similarly with E/RP: initially, exposure to situations where it is hard to resist OCD make us feel very uncomfortable, but the longer we stay in these situations without performing compulsions, the less uncomfortable we feel. Children are invited to take charge of the speed at which they work through the hierarchy and to select new cues once they have *bossed-back Germy or OCD* in the presence of old cues that they have mastered. To manage the anxiety that this entails, the child is also taught relaxation skills, breathing skills and constructive self-talk in a manner similar to that outlined in Chapter 12. Each E/RP session begins with agenda or goal setting, a review of the previous week, giving information, practising exposure and response prevention or anxiety management skills and setting E/RP homework, which typically recapitulates the work conducted in the session. The form in Figure 13.5 may be used as a basis for giving E/RP homework and reviewed at each E/RP session.

For your homework, do this exposure and response prevention (E/RP) task

EXPOSURE means going into a situation where OCD makes you think OBSESSIONAL thoughts and want to do COMPULSIVE things

RESPONSE PREVENTION means using all your power to resist OCD by not doing your COMPULSIONS in these situations

E/RP TASK

_____

_____

_____

_____

PLAN FOR BOSSING OCD BACK

_____

_____

_____

Write the day in the first column. In the rest of the columns write down your rating from 1 to 10 which says how hard you are finding it to resist OCD.

If it's easy to resist OCD, give a rating of 1
If it's very hard to resist OCD, give a rating of 10

Very easy   1____2____3____4____5____6____7____8____9____10   Very hard
Relaxed   Very tense

Give one rating a minute for the first five minutes and then one rating every 5 minutes until 25 minutes have passed

Notice how your rating increases and then decreases as time passes

Day	Start	1 min	2 min	3 min	4 min	5 min	10 min	15 min	20 min	25 min	30 min

Figure 13.5 Exposure and response prevention homework sheet

Cognitive therapy

To be able to persevere with E/RP tasks, children require coping skills. Relaxation and breathing exercises (described in Chapter 12) are useful for reducing anxiety. However, cognitive strategies are required to counter pessimistic, catastrophic and overly responsible thinking. Children may be coached in actively _bossing OCD back_ by speaking aloud as if OCD were an external discrete enemy. Here are some useful constructive statements:

- 'This is difficult but I'll be able to handle this if I breath slowly and use relaxation skills'
- 'I've beaten you (OCD) before and I'll do it again'
- 'Go jump in the lake OCD, I'm the boss'
- 'Can't catch me this time, OCD'

Children may be coached in detaching from obsessional thinking by following these four steps, which may be written on an index card and used during E/RP exercise and at other times:

- Step 1: 'That's OCD talking again, not me'
- Step 2: 'I don't have to pay attention to OCD, because he makes no sense'
- Step 3: 'The discomfort in this situation will go away soon without me doing a ritual, if I just stick with it'
- Step 4: 'I'll think about something pleasant while I'm waiting to habituate'

During therapy sessions, children may be coached in challenging irrational beliefs about over-estimations of danger or over-responsibility. For example, where children have obsessional ideas involving over-estimation of danger associated with failure to wash their hands very frequently, they may be asked what the probability of death is due to not washing their hands according to OCD and then, according to themselves, based on their own observations of family members and friends who wash their hands a couple of times a day. They may then be invited to compare these two estimates, which might be 100% and 10%. They can use the information about this discrepancy between their own estimate and that of OCD to boss OCD back if they become anxious during an E/RP task involving exposure to dirt.

Where children have obsessional ideas about over-responsibility, for example they are 100% responsible for a family member dying in a plane crash, they may be invited to use a pie chart to identify the degree of responsibility held by all of the many people involved including the pilot, air traffic controller, mechanics and so forth, in the safety of the plane. They can then compare their percentage of the responsibility shown on the pie chart (which may be about 5%) to the 100% responsibility proposed by OCD, and use this discrepancy to boss OCD back.

Family involvement

Parents are briefed on the child's progress at every session. Family members are centrally involved in assessment and psychoeducational sessions and in sessions that focus on disengaging family members from children's compulsive rituals. Parents also participate in sessions on supporting the use of anxiety management skills and relapse prevention. At each briefing, parents are kept abreast of the child's progress and the fact that the child is in charge of the pacing of the treatment is emphasized. Parents are helped to avoid coercing their children into accelerating the rate at which they tackle increasingly anxiety-provoking cues. In mid-treatment sessions, parents and siblings work with the symptomatic child to identify situations which elicit OCD symptomatology and which also involve other family members. The family practises exposure and response prevention to these situations in therapy sessions and then repeat these family-involved E/RP exercises as homework. The challenge in these sessions is to help parents, symptomatic children and siblings negotiate E/RP tasks that the child can manage without being overwhelmed by anxiety, and to support parents to have the courage to refrain from involving themselves in their children's compulsive rituals.

In addition, parents are coached in how to help children to use anxiety management routines when exposed to anxiety-provoking cues. This is particularly important for those situations where parents typically reinforce their children's compulsive rituals. Parents are coached in how to use praise and reward systems, like those described in Chapter 4, to motivate their children to *boss Germy off their land*, or *to boss OCD out of their lives*. They are also coached in how to avoid criticism and punishment as a response to OCD rituals. Parents are advised to focus their attention on other aspects of their child's behaviour and positively reinforce developmentally appropriate activities. Where members of the child's wider social network, such as grandparents or school teachers, are involved in the maintenance of the OCD symptomatology, they are contacted and given similar coaching.

As gains are made, children may be given certificates for bravery and defeating OCD. They may also be invited to notify members of the extended family of their achievements.

Relapse prevention and graduation

Relapse prevention sessions focus on pin-pointing situations where relapses are likely to occur and planning how to manage these. Relapses are likely where usual routines are disrupted by going on holidays, changing class, moving house, starting a new job, going to college. Losses like failing an exam or falling out with friends may lead to relapses. So too may non-compliance with medication or development of infectious illness, especially in youngsters with the PANDAS sub-type of OCD. Plans for managing relapses should involve externalizing the problem, making a hierarchy of OCD-eliciting situations, re-running an E/RP programme with family support and therapist support as required, and recommencing SSRI treatment if it has been discontinued. Treatment ends with a graduation ceremony, receiving a certificate, an invitation to notify others in the social network of their achievements, and follow-up sessions at one, three, six and twelve months.

TIC DISORDERS

When children are referred with repetitive behaviours, it is important to distinguish between OCD on the one hand and tics and related conditions on the other, since the treatment implications are quite distinct (Chowdhury, 2004; Glaros & Epkins, 2003; Leckman & Cohen, 2002; Walkup, 2002). Sudden repetitive movements, gestures or utterances which mimic some fragment of normal behaviour are referred to as tics. Tics tend to last no more than a second or two and typically occur in bouts separated by tic-free intervals. They are experienced by young children as involuntary actions and by older children and adolescents as relief-bringing action preceded by irresistible premonitory urges. Thus they bear some phenomenological resemblance to obsessive-compulsive conditions. Tics are exacerbated by stressful situations and attenuated by absorbing activities such as reading. Tics may be suppressed for brief periods and are rarely present during sleep.

Simple motor tics include eye blinking, grimacing and shoulder shrugging. Touching, stamping, knee bending, smelling, echokinesis or echopraxia (imitation of another's movements), and copropraxia (making obscene gestures) are examples of complex motor tics. Snorting, barking, grunting and throat clearing are common simple vocal tics. Complex vocal tics include coprolalia (shouting obscene words), echolalia (repeating another's last phrase) and palilalia (repeating one's own last phrase).

Tics may occur alone or in clusters and be classified as transient or chronic, motor or vocal and as simple or complex. Figures 13.1. and 13.2 show that these distinctions are recognized within both ICD 10 and DSM IV TR. Both systems distinguish Tourette's disorder, which is characterized by chronic, multiple, complex motor and vocal tics, from other tic disorders. These other tic disorders are then sub-classified as chronic or transient and as motor or vocal and distinguished from other repetitive movement disorders such as trichotillomania and stereotyped movement disorders. A similar system has been developed by the Tourette Syndrome Classification Study Group (1993), which also includes diagnostic modifiers (probable, definite and history) to reflect diagnostic confidence.

Epidemiology

Epidemiological studies show that tics are common and that Tourette's syndrome is rare (Leckman & Cohen, 2002). Community surveys have shown that up to 13% of children have tics. Children are between five and twelve times more likely to have tics than adults. Boys are more likely to have tics than girls, although the ratio is less than 2:1. Tic disorders are rare, but there is extraordinary variability in prevalence estimates. The prevalence of Tourette's syndrome varies from 2.9 to 299 per 10,000 across studies, depending on the population studied and the methods used. The most common co-occurring disorders are ADHD (50–60%) and OCD (30–70%) (Walkup, 2002). Tic disorders are also relatively common among children on the autistic spectrum, with co-morbidity rates as high as 8% (Baron-Cohen, Mortimore & Moriarty, 1999).

Clinical features

Trichotillomania, stereotyped movement disorders and Tourette's disorder each have distinctive clinical features.

Trichotillomania

Grooming behaviours, such as adjusting one's hair, may sometimes constitute complex motor tics. However, habitual involuntary or compulsive grooming behaviour, which includes hair pulling, is distinguished from such tics and referred to in ICD 10 and DSM IV TR as trichotillomania. This condition holds some features in common with tic disorders and some features in common with OCD. Trichotillomania is a tic-like disorder in that obsessions are absent but a premonitory urge is present, which is relieved by hair pulling. However, trichotillomania is more like OCD in that there is considerable variability in the activity of hair-pulling. Hair may be pulled from any site, including the scalp, eyebrows and pubic area (Vitulano, King, Scahill & Cohen, 1992).

Stereotyped movement disorders

Some complex motor tics that occur alone or as part of Tourette's disorder may be self-injurious (such as biting oneself or punching oneself). However, a repetitive pattern of self-injurious behaviour such as head-banging, biting, skin-picking, eye-poking, hitting oneself or repetitive patterns of non-injurious non-functional rhythmic behaviour such as rocking, finger-flicking or hand-flapping are distinguished from tics and classified in DSM IV TR and ICD 10 as stereotyped movement disorders. Occasionally, children develop methods of self-restraint such as placing their hands inside their belts or clothing to prevent the repetitive movements from occurring. Stereotyped movement problems like these are most common among people with intellectual disabilities, particularly those with syndromes such as fragile X syndrome, de Lange syndrome and Lech–Nyhan syndrome, which is characterized by severe self-biting (Scott, 1994).

Tourette's disorder

Tourette's disorder is the most debilitating of all the tic disorders (Chowdhury, 2004; Gilles de la Tourette, 1885; Leckman & Cohen, 2002). It typically begins in early childhood with occasional simple motor tics and gradually evolves into a condition where multiple motor and vocal tics are present. These may include both simple and complex tics such as coprolalia, copropraxia, echolalia and echopraxia. Contrary to popular opinion, coprolalia is relatively rare in Tourette's syndrome and occurs in less than 6% of cases (Walkup, 2002). Speech fluency may be disrupted by vocal tics. By ten years, most children can recognize the premonitory urges that precede tics and this both increases the discomfort and distress caused by the condition, as well as permitting the youngster to suppress tics for brief periods of time. Typically, the child develops secondary adjustment difficulties which present as internalizing or externalizing behaviour problems; co-morbid obsessive-compulsive disorder or attention deficit hyperactivity disorder are common. Peer problems are quite common, perhaps because youngsters with Tourette's disorder are shunned by their peers because of their bizarre behaviour. During late adolescence and early adulthood, the severity of the condition may lessen. However, in middle and late adulthood, the condition worsens and becomes seriously debilitating. A typical case of Tourette's disorder is presented in Box 13.2 and diagnostic criteria for DSM IV TR and ICD 10 are set out in Table 13.4.

Box 13.2 A case example of Tourette's disorder

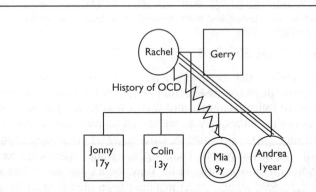

Referral. Mia was referred for treatment because of her frequent and uncontrolled swearing and behaviour problems at school. Specifically, Mia frequently stood-up during class and engaged in physical exercises, which involved pacing, squatting and jumping.

History of the presenting problem. The problems had developed over a twelve-month period following the birth of her sister Andrea. Initially her parents and teachers thought that the swearing and conduct problems were attention-seeking behaviours stemming from jealously towards her younger sister and grief at the loss of a privileged place within the family. Before the birth of her sister she was the youngest of three siblings and the only girl. Both of these factors allowed her to command the lion's share of her parents' attention. However, attempts by the parents and Mia's teachers to both offer her more attention, while at the same time set limits on her conduct problems, had little impact. Over the year prior to referral, her problems had steadily become more and more severe. This led to considerable conflict between Mia and her mother, particularly as her mother strongly disapproved of swearing. Her mother insisted that she pray for forgiveness and on more than one occasion washed out her mouth with soap. At the time of referral Mia had developed some depressive symptoms and also had periodic temper tantrums which her parents believed were completely out of character. Clinical interviews and evaluation confirmed that Mia's swearing and out-of-seat behaviour at school were coprolalia and complex motor tics rather than attention-seeking conduct problems. In addition, Mia displayed a number of simple motor and vocal tics including eyebrow twitching and throat clearing. Her depressive symptoms and tantrums appeared to be an emotional reaction to the conflict at home and at school that had arisen since the onset of Tourette's disorder.

Developmental and family history. Prior to the onset of symptoms a year before referral was made, Mia's development was essentially normal. There was a family history of OCD, with the mother, Rachel having been treated for this condition on two occasions.

Formulation. The positive family history for OCD suggested that Mia probably had a vulnerability to repetition disorders. The birth of her sibling and perceived stresses arising from this may have precipitated the onset of the symptoms. The mother, Rachel's, particularly strong dislike of swearing may have been a sub-clinical aspect of her obsessive-compulsive condition. Her obsessions included fear that she would utter obscenities herself and her cleansing and praying rituals helped her to reduce anxiety associated with these fears. She had therefore used similar rituals to attempt to deal with Mia's symptoms. Unfortunately, these measures appeared to have led Mia to develop secondary emotional and conduct problems.

Treatment. A family-based approach was taken to treatment comprising psychoeducation, tic monitoring and habit reversal. In addition, the paediatrician prescribed haloperidol for Mia.

There is now a consensus that biological factors are the main contributors to the aetiology of Tourette's disorder and that psychological factors such as life stress and coping resources play a role in determining the course of the disorder (Chowdhury, 2004; Leckman & Cohen, 2002). Twin and proband studies support the view that genetic factors play a major role in the genesis of Tourette's disorder. Abnormalities in the functioning of the basal ganglia and related cortical and thalamic structures have been identified as the possible neurobiological substrate for this disorder. There is some evidence that dysregulation of dopaminergic, noradrenergic and serotonergic systems and abnormalities in the functioning of endogenous opioid peptide systems may occur in Tourette's disorder. The higher incidence of the condition among boys has led to the hypothesis that androgenic steroids at key developmental periods may influence the emergence of Tourette's disorder. Adverse pre-natal and peri-natal factors including maternal stress or illness during pregnancy, pregnancy complications, and low birth weight have all been found to be associated with the condition.

The onset of Tourette's disorder or exacerbations of symptomatology

Table 13.4 Diagnostic criteria for Tourette's disorder from DSM IV TR and ICD 10

DSM IV TR	ICD 10
A. Both multiple motor and one or more vocal tics have been present at some time during the illness, although not necessarily concurrently. (A tic is a sudden, rapid, recurrent, non-rhythmic, stereotyped motor movement or vocalization.)	A form of tic disorder in which there are or have been multiple motor tics and one or more vocal tics, although these need not have occurred concurrently
B. The tics occur many times a day (usually in bouts) nearly every day or intermittently throughout a period of more than a year and during this period there was never a tic-free period of more than 3 consecutive months	Onset is almost always in childhood or adolescence. A history of motor tics before the development of vocal tics is common. The symptoms frequently worsen during adolescence and it is common for the disorder to persist into adult life
C. The disturbance causes considerable distress or significant impairment in social and academic functioning	The vocal tics are almost always multiple with explosive repetitive vocalizations, throat clearing, and grunting and there may be use of obscene words or phrases (coprolalia). Sometimes there is associated gestural echopraxia, which also may be of an obscene nature (copropraxia)
D. The onset is before 18	
E. The disorder is not due to a medical condition (e.g. Huntington's disease) or the effects of a drug (amphetamines)	
	Motor and vocal tics may be suppressed voluntarily for short periods, exacerbated by stress and disappear during sleep

Note: Adapted from DSM IV TR (APA, 2000a) and ICD 10 (WHO, 1992, 1996).

typically follow stressful life events. The likelihood that the disorder will find expression in a person with a genetic vulnerability is probably mediated by the supportiveness of the family environment, the wider school and peer network and the availability of coping strategies associated with such protective factors as high ability, self-esteem and self-efficacy. In children with ADHD, treatment with stimulant medication such as methylphenidate may precipitate the onset of a tic disorder.

Post-infectious autoimmune mechanisms contribute to the development of Tourette's syndrome in up to a fifth of cases (Leckman & Cohen, 2002). As was mentioned in the sub-section on PANDAS when discussing OCD above, autoimmune mechanisms deserve serious consideration as important aetiological factors in children who have had a streptococcal infection, who report an abrupt onset of Tourette's disorder following the infection, and who present with co-morbid OCD or ADHD. Referral to paediatrics for immunomodulatory treatments such as plasma exchange deserve consideration in such cases.

Assessment

Referral for a thorough paediatric medical assessment should always be made in cases where children present with repetitive behavioural problems, to rule out possible organic conditions such as Huntington's chorea, Wilson's disease and Sydenham's chorea. Once such conditions have been eliminated, in addition to the assessment protocol presented in Chapter 4, the standardized rating scales and self-report instruments presented in Table 13.5 may be useful in evaluating children who present with tics. Of these, the Yale Global Tic Severity Scale is the most widely used instrument in the field.

Table 13.5 Psychometric instruments that may be used as an adjunct to clinical interviews in the assessment of Tourette's syndrome

Instrument	Author & Date of Publication	Comments
Yale Global Tic Severity Scale	Leckman, J., Riddle, M., Hardin, M. et al. (1989). The Yale Global Tic Severity Scale: Initial Testing of a clinician-rated Scale of Tic Severity. *Journal of the American Academy of Child and Adolescent Psychiatry*, 28, 566–573	40 motor and phonic tics are rated on 5-point scales for number, frequency, intensity, complexity and interference. Overall impairment is rated on a 50-point scale. A global severity score is obtained by combining all ratings
Shapiro Tourette Syndrome Severity Scale (TSSS)	Shapiro, A. & Shapiro, E. (1984). Controlled study of pimozide vs. placebo in Tourette Syndrome. *Journal of the American Academy of Child Psychiatry*, 23, 161–173 Shapiro, A. Shapiro, E., Young, J. & Feinberg, T. (1988). *Gilles de la Tourette's Syndrome*. New York: Raven Press	Social disabilities associated with Tourette's syndrome are rated on 5 ordinal scales
Tourette Syndrome Global Scale	Harcherik, D., Leckman, J., Detlor, J. & Cohen, D. (1984). A new instrument for clinical studies of Tourette's Syndrome. *Journal of the American Academy of Child Psychiatry*, 23, 153–160	The frequency and disruption of simple and complex motor tics are assessed on 5-point scales along with ratings of behaviour, motor restlessness, school problems, and work problems on 25-point scales. Results are combined to give an overall score
Tourette Syndrome Questionnaire	Jagger, J., Prusoff, B., Cohen, D., Kidd, K., Carbonari, C. & John, K. (1982). The epidemiology of Tourette's syndrome. *Schizophrenia Bulletin*, 8, 267–278	A self-report or parent-report questionnaire which provides information on developmental history, the course of tic behaviours and the impact of Tourette's syndrome on the child's life

Continued

Table 13.5 continued

Instrument	Author & Date of Publication	Comments
Tourette's Syndrome Symptom List	Cohen, D., Leckman, J. & Shaywitz, B. (1985). The Tourette syndrome and other tics. In D. Shaffer, A. Ehrhard, L. Greenhill (eds.), *The Clinical Guide to Child Psychiatry* (pp. 77–88). New York: Free Press	A self-report or parent-report questionnaire focusing on symptomatology
Motor Tic, Obsessions and Compulsions, Vocal Tic Evaluation Survey (MOVES)	Gaffney, G., Sieg, K. & Hellings, J. (1994). The MOVES: A self-rating scale for Tourette's syndrome. *Journal of Child and Adolescent Psychopharmacology,* 44, 269–280	A self-report or parent-report questionnaire focusing on symptomatology
National Hospital Interview Schedule (NHIS)	Robertson, M. & Eapen, V. (1996). The National Hospital Interview Schedule for the assessment of Gilles de la Tourette Syndrome. *International Journal of Methods in Psychiatric Research,* 6, 203–226	A structured interview schedule for diagnosing Tourette's syndrome
Hopkins Motor and Vocal Tic Scale	Walkup, J. Rosenberg, L., Brown, J. & Singer, H. (1992). The validity of instruments measuring tic severity in Tourette's syndrome. *Journal of the American Academy of Child and Adolescent Psychiatry,* 30, 472–477	An instrument that combines self-report and clinician rating data for measuring tic severity

A functional analysis of the antecedents and consequences of tics over the course of a number of days should be conducted in the child's natural environment. For infrequently occurring tics, every single tic that occurs during each of a number of days should be recorded along with the antecedents and consequences. For frequently occurring tics, the number of tics occurring in the first ten minutes of each hour may be counted and the antecedents and consequences of these periods noted using the tic recording form presented in Figure 13.6. This monitoring may be conducted by parents, teachers or the children themselves. Where parents and children are unable to do this, a professional observer may be trained to conduct this part of the assessment. This aspect of the assessment throws light on the naturally occurring antecedents and consequences of the child's tics that increase or decrease their frequency. It also highlights times during the day when high and low rates of tics are emitted.

Two daily recording intervals of about 10-minutes duration which are representative of periods when particularly high and particularly low numbers of tics typically occur should be selected on the basis of the data supplied by this part of the assessment. Parents or children may be trained to count the number of tics or tic clusters occurring during these periods. These frequency counts may be graphed by the child to monitor progress. A tic recording form for this purpose is presented in Figure 13.7. This approach to assessment, which is far less time consuming than the all-day approach, may be used to establish a baseline during an extended assessment period and to monitor progress during treatment.

Treatment

Information from the paediatric evaluation, psychological assessment and assessments conducted by professionals from other disciplines may be pooled to arrive at a diagnosis of the tic disorder and any co-morbid or secondary conditions. Multi-systemic management of tic disorders may include some or all of the following components:

- psychoeducation
- environmental manipulation
- management of secondary conditions
- habit reversal
- contingent negative practice
- medication.

Psychoeducation

If offering psychoeducation, a primary goal is first to convey the ideas that tics are involuntary and expressions of a clear neurodevelopmental disorder which has a major genetic component in most cases and which is probably based in the basal ganglia. It should be stressed that tics are not expressions of unconscious conflicts or family dysfunction, although they can cause the child and family considerable distress. It should also be emphasized that tics are never intentional, although they can be suppressed for brief periods with great effort, and that stress – particularly criticism or punishment – makes them worse. This type of information may help parents and teachers minimize the exposure of the child to punitive criticism. This may be a very significant intervention in cases where the child has developed complex motor tics or coprolalia which are disruptive in school and distressing for family members at home and have led to the child being regularly punished, criticized or ostracized.

A second goal of psychoeducation is to offer a diagnosis with some indication of the degree of confidence with which the diagnosis may be made. This is important since it has major implications for prognosis. As far as we know, only Tourette's disorder has a chronic lifelong course in the vast majority of cases. Where children present with tics for less than a year,

Time slot	What happened just before the time slot ?	How many tics occurred in the time slot ?	What happened immediately after the time slot?
6.00–6.10			
7.00–7.10			
8.00–8.10			
9.00–9.10			
10.00–10.10			
11.00–11.10			
12.00–12.10			
13.00–13.10			
14.00–14.10			
15.00–15.10			
16.00–16.10			
17.00–17.10			
18.00–18.10			
19.00–19.10			
20.00–20.10			
21.00–21.10			
22.00–22.10			
23.00–23.10			

Figure 13.6 Tic recording form for assessing antecedents and consequences throughout the day

no matter how pervasive or complex they are, a diagnosis of Tourette's disorder should not be given, although it should be mentioned that it may be a possibility. However, once there is certainty that Tourette's disorder is present, the diagnosis should be made to permit the child and parents to

This chart is for recording the number of tics that occur during a specific time period each day.

The type of tic you are to count is:_____

Begin counting at this time each day:_____

Each time a tic occurs mark a stroke in the tally box.

Stop counting at this time each day:_____

Add up the strokes in the tally box and put the number in the right box on the graph.

For example, if on Monday you counted 48 tics, you would put 48 in the box with the x in it.

		Monday	Tuesday	Wednesday	Thursday	Friday	Saturday	Sunday
	50							
	48	X						
	46							
	44							
	42							
	40							
	38							
	36							
	34							
	32							
	30							
	28							
	26							
	24							
	22							
	20							
Number	18							
of tics	16							
	14							
	12							
	10							
	8							
	6							
	4							
	2							
	Tally box							

Figure 13.7 Tic recording form for assessing the number of tics in a single time slot over a week

develop reasonable plans about adjusting to it. The final diagnosis should be offered by a full multi-disciplinary team that can offer an authoritative psychosocial and paediatric summary of the outcome of a thorough evaluation.

Environmental manipulation

Environmental changes which may make the child's tic disorder more manageable may be suggested by the information recorded on the form in Figure 13.6. Antecedents or consequences associated with frequent tics may be removed or modified. Arrangements may be made for children to have relatively isolated quiet *time* following daily transitions from home to school or school to home, or between classes at school during which they can relax and cease attempting to control their tics.

Arrangements may be made with school staff for the child to sit exams separately from the class, particularly in cases where there are vocal tics. Ideally, the degree to which the tics interfere with exam performance should be taken into account when grading the child's oral, written and practical work. Time pressure should be minimized in exam situations and youngsters should be permitted to take occasional rests during exams to reduce the frequency of tics (Harrington, 1998).

Management of secondary problems

Evaluation and treatment should be offered for secondary adjustment problems and co-morbid difficulties. The sensitive management of children's and parents' grief reactions to the diagnosis and prognosis in cases of Tourette's disorder may be based on an understanding of grief processes as described in Chapter 24. Co-morbid depression, anxiety, conduct problems, attention deficit hyperactivity disorder, obsessive-compulsive disorder and school-based learning problems may be managed following the guidelines set out for these problems elsewhere in this text.

Habit reversal

Habit reversal has been shown to significantly reduce tic frequency in Tourette's disorder and in transient and chronic tic disorders, and also to be effective in reducing the frequency of hair-pulling in trichotillomania (Azrin & Nunn, 1973; Azrin & Peterson, 1990; Vitulano et al., 1992). Habit reversal includes awareness training, competing response training, relaxation training and contingency management.

The aim of awareness training is to increase the child's awareness of the nature of the tics, their frequency, and the antecedents and consequences which effect the frequency of the tics. First, the child is taught how to describe the tic in detail. A mirror or videotape may be used over a number of sessions to give immediate accurate feedback on the nature and occurrence of the tics. The psychologist may also alert the child to each occurrence of the tic during training periods. This procedure helps the child to describe the tics, increases motivation to control them and also helps the child to develop awareness of early warning signs that the tic is about to occur. This awareness of early warning signs is used as a cue for carrying out a competing response, which will be described below. Another aspect of awareness training is coaching the child in using the tic recording forms in Figures 13.6 and 13.7. The form in Figure 13.6 may be used by the child for three or four days to learn about the antecedents and consequences in the child's natural environment which effect tic frequency. When using this form, the child notes the number of tics that occur in the first ten minutes of each hour throughout the day and the associated antecedents and consequences. The form in Figure 13.7 may be used over an extended period of weeks or months to help the child retain awareness of fluctuations in tic frequency. With this form, the child is trained to count the number of tics occurring during a set ten-minute period each day.

The child is also trained to carry out a competing response for two minutes contingent on the occurrence of the tic or contingent on recognizing an early warning sign that the tic is about to occur. Competing responses should be incompatible with the tic, be capable of being maintained for two minutes, be inconspicuous, strengthen the muscles antagonistic to the tic or habit and produce a heightened awareness through tensing the muscle. For tics, it is recommended that the competing response should involve the isometric tensing of the muscles opposite to those involved in the tic movement. For eye blinking, the competing response is opening the eyes wide, for shoulder jerking the competing response is the isometric tensing of the shoulder depressors, for trichotillomania the competing response is fist clenching.

Relaxation training is included in the habit reversal programme so that children can lower their arousal level in stressful situations and so reduce the frequency with which tics occur. A relaxation training routine is described in Chapter 12.

Whereas self-monitoring, the use of competing responses and relaxation training directly affect the frequency with which tics occur, contingency management aims to increase the child's motivation to use these three sets of skills. Contingency management begins with a habit inconvenience review. Here children are helped to list all of the embarrassing and inconvenient consequences of the tics or habits on one side of an index card and all of the advantages of reducing the frequency of the tics on the other. They should carry this card at all times and review it frequently to remind them of the benefits of complying with the treatment programme. Parents may be trained to praise the child and to use a reward system, like that described in Chapter 4, to reinforce the child for using the competing response and relaxation skills in appropriate ways. In cases where there is a very high rate of tics, the reward system may be confined to a specific period each day and the duration of this period may be gradually lengthened as the child gains more control over the tics or habits.

Contingent negative practice

Levine and Ramirez (1989) have shown that as an alternative to carrying out a competing response contingent on the occurrence of a tic, the child may be instructed to carry out the tic itself consistently for thirty seconds every time the tic occurs in the child's natural home and school environments. The child is also instructed not to try to prevent the tics from happening. This procedure is known as contingent negative practice and is distinct from massed practice, where the tic is practised consistently for periods of up to thirty minutes in the consulting room. There is good evidence for the effectiveness of contingent negative practice, with tics but not for massed practice, where relapses are common (Levine and Ramirez, 1989).

Medication

Referral to a physician may be made to assess the appropriateness of including medication in the overall treatment programme (Leckman & Cohen, 2002; Walkup, 2001). Up to 70% of children with Tourette's disorder achieve significant symptom reduction when treated with dopamine-blocking agents, of which haloperidol was the first to be widely used. However, haloperidol has troublesome short-term side effects (e.g. akathesia, and akinesia) and irreversible long-term side effects, particularly tardive dyskinesia. Other neuroleptic medications which, like haloperidol, affect the dopamine system but have fewer short-term side effects include fluphenazine, pimozide, respiridone, sulpiride and tiapride. Because of their uncomfortable short-term side effects and irreversible long-term side effects, these medications are used in low doses, and only in moderate to severe cases of Tourette's disorder. Alpha-adrenergic agonists, notably clonidine and guanfacine, are sometimes effective in suppressing tics and have minimal side effects. Clonidine also has a positive impact on ADHD symptoms, so is a first choice of medication in young children with co-morbid ADHD and tic disorders.

SUMMARY

In obsessive-compulsive disorder (OCD), Tourette's disorder, trichotillomania and other tic disorders, the central psychological concern is the fact that adjustment is compromised by the execution of repetitive actions. Collectively, these conditions form part of a spectrum of psychological problems with a common genetic diathesis, and basal ganglia dysfunction has been implicated in their aetiology. Psychoanalytic theories of OCD, which implicate parent–child conflict over toilet-training in the aetiology of the condition have not been empirically supported. Family systems frameworks for understanding OCD have not been fully developed, although there is evidence that families may play a role in the maintenance of OCD. Cognitive-behavioural explanations of OCD argue that specific environmental stimuli are appraised in a way that triggers anxiety-provoking obsessional thoughts. Compulsive rituals are used to neutralize these intrusive, obsessional thoughts. Some people have a particular vulnerability to developing intrusive, unacceptable obsessive thoughts. The treatment of choice for OCD in children is built around exposure and response prevention procedures and offered in a way that maximizes parental involvement in helping the child reduce symptomatology. Tourette's disorder, a lifelong debilitating condition involving multiple motor and vocal tics, may be distinguished from more circumscribed and transient tic disorders and from trichotillomania and stereotyped movement disorders. Tourette's disorder cannot be cured and management programmes include psychoeducation, environmental manipulation at home and at school to minimize stressful events that exacerbate the tics, evaluation and treatment of secondary or co-morbid conditions, habit reversal and contingent negative practice to reduce the frequency of tics and medication, the most effective of which is dopamine-blocking agents. Habit reversal and contingent negative practice may also be used with more circumscribed tic disorders and trichotillomania.

EXERCISE 13.1

Work in pairs, with one person taking the role of the interviewer and the other taking the role of Trevor described Box 13.1. The interviewer is invited to explain OCD to Trevor and invite him to give it a nick-name. Then the interviewer may help Trevor construct a hierarchy of situations that elicit obsessional anxiety.

EXERCISE 13.2

Work in pairs. Develop an assessment management plan for the case of Mia, presented in Box 13.2.

FURTHER READING

Barrett, P., Healy, L., & March, J. (In Press). *FOCUS: Freedom from Obsessions and Compulsions Using Skills. Therapist Manual and Workbooks*. Mount Gravatt, Brisbane: Griffith University.

Chowdhury, U. (2004). *Tics and Tourette Syndrome*. London: Jessica Kingsley.

Leckman, J. & Cohen, D. (1998). *Tourette Syndrome, Tics Obsessions, Compulsions: Developmental Psychopathology and Clinical Care*. New York: Wiley.

March, J. & Mulle, K. (1998). *OCD in Children and Adolescents: A Cognitive-Behavioural Treatment Manual*. New York: Guilford.

FURTHER READING FOR PARENTS AND CHILDREN

Foa, E. & Wilson, R. (1991). *Stop Obsessing*. New York: Bantam.

Rapoport, J. (1991). *The Boy Who Couldn't Stop Washing*. New York: Penguin.

Carroll, A. & Robertson, M. (2000). *Tourette Syndrome. A Practical Guide for Teachers, Parents and Carers*. London: David Fulton.

Wever, C. (1994). *The Secret Problem*. Sydney, Australia: Shrinkwarp Press. (*A children's book on OCD*.)

WEBSITES

OCD Action UK: http://www.ocdaction.org.uk/

OCD and TS websites: http://www.homestead.com/westsuffolkpsych/resources.html

OCD Foundation: http://www.ocfoundation.org/

OCD Resources Centre: http://www.ocdresource.com/

OCD websites: http://www.geonius.com/ocd/

Tourette Syndrome Association UK: http://www.tsa.org.uk/

Tourette Syndrome Association USA: http://www.tsa-usa.org/

Tourette Syndrome page: http://www.mentalhealth.com/dis/p20-ch04.html

Tourette Syndrome webpage for educators: http://www.tourettesyndrome.net/

Factsheets on OCD can be downloaded from the website for Rose, G. & York, A. (2004). *Mental Health and Growing Up. Fact sheets for Parents, Teachers and Young People* (Third edition). London: Gaskell: http://www.rcpsych.ac.uk

Chapter 14

Somatic problems

Children and adolescents may be referred for psychological consultation with the central focus being a somatic complaint. Somatization or conversion symptoms, chronic fatigue syndrome, pain, adjustment to chronic illness and preparation for anxiety-provoking medical and dental procedures are among the more common reasons for referral. This chapter addresses common childhood problems in each of these areas. Other conditions where somatic factors are involved, such as enuresis and encopresis, sensory impairment, head injury, eating disorders, drug abuse and injuries arising from physical abuse are discussed in other chapters. The anticipatory grieving process associated with life-threatening illness such as cancer is discussed in Chapter 24. However, before addressing specific somatic presentations, a consideration of the development of children's concepts of illness and pain will be given, and some frameworks within which to conceptualize somatic problems will be presented. From a clinical perspective, the assessment and management of somatization problems and the management of chronic childhood illness must take account of children, conceptions of illness and pain which evolve as children mature. The wider psychosocial context within which illness occurs must also be taken into account.

DEVELOPMENT OF THE CONCEPTS OF ILLNESS

The development of the child's concept of illness is determined by both cognitive maturation and experience of, or exposure to, illness (Bibace, 1981; Bibace & Walsh, 1979). Children's understanding of the causes of illness progresses through a series of stages that is, broadly speaking, consistent with Piaget's theory of cognitive development. Below three years, illness is defined by children in terms of a single symptom, and the cause of illness is understood to be remote. For example, a child may say that tummyaches are caused by the man on the television. Between three and five years children still conceive of illness in single-symptom terms but use the concept of contagion to explain the aetiology of the diseases. So a five-year-old may explain that you catch measles if you go too near another child who has them. Magical thinking may also occur during this stage and children may wonder if something that they did caused their illness or if the illness is a punishment for wrong-doing. Such magical ideas may persist as a feature of children's thinking into teenage years and, since it can cause unnecessary distress, deserves clinical exploration. With the transition that occurs between five and seven years to concrete operational thinking, most children develop a more sophisticated idea about the symptomatology and aetiology of illness. Most illnesses are construed at this stage as entailing multiple symptoms and being caused by internal processes such as ingesting germs. So children at this stage begin to develop health-related behaviours, such as washing their hands before eating to remove germs or exercising to keep their body healthy. As children approach adolescence and the onset of formal operational thought, they can give detailed physiological explanations of illnesses. So an eleven-year-old may say that lung cancer is caused by cells growing too quickly and this in turn is due to being covered in tar from cigarette smoke. Teenagers can offer sophisticated psychophysiological explanations for the aetiology of illnesses. For example, diabetic teenagers may explain that their blood sugar level is affected by their diet, insulin intake, level of physical activity and stress level.

DEVELOPMENT OF THE CONCEPT OF PAIN

The development of the child's concept of pain is affected by both cognitive maturation and the child's experience of pain (McGrath, 1995). Prior to eighteen months, children can indicate that they are in pain by crying or simple verbalizations but are unable to conceptualize or verbalize different levels of pain intensity. Rating scales rather than self-report scales are probably the best way to assess changes in pain levels in children at this stage of development (McGrath et al., 1985). Children of eighteen months can verbalize the fact that pain hurts. They can localize pain in their own bodies and they can identify pain in others. They can understand that their experience of pain may be alleviated by asking for medicine or receiving hugs and kisses from carers. They may also try to alleviate pain in others by offering to hug them. At about two years, more elaborate descriptions of pain occur and children can more clearly attribute pain to external causes. By three or four years of age children can differentiate between differing intensities and qualities of pain and verbalize these. So in assessing children as young as three, it is possible to ask them about how much pain they feel and how stingy or hot or throbby it feels. Poker chips or counters may be used as concrete symbols of pain and children as young as three years may be asked to indicate the intensity of their pain using such concrete symbols (Hester, Foster & Kristensen, 1990). By three years children are also aware that specific strategies such as distraction may be used to cope with pain. So children at this age may be aware that playing when they have hurt themselves may make them feel better by distracting them from the pain. Between five and seven years, children become more proficient at distinguishing between differing levels of pain intensity and may be able to use face scales to indicate fluctuations in pain experiences (Bieri, Reeve, Champion & Addicoat, 1990). On face scales, children indicate the intensity of their pain by selecting a face from an array of faces expressing a variety of levels of pain, which most closely reflects their own experience of pain. Between the ages of seven and ten years, children can explain why pain hurts and once they reach adolescence they can explain the adaptive value of pain for protecting people from harm.

CLASSIFICATION OF SOMATIZATION PROBLEMS

Somatization refers to the expression of psychological distress through somatic symptoms (Garralda, 1999). When children somaticize psychological distress, their somatic symptoms are not fully explicable in terms of organic factors such as infection or tissue damage and it is assumed that psychological factors play a significant role in the aetiology or maintenance of their complaints. Single-symptom or multi-symptom somatization may occur, although multi-symptom presentations are the most common. Where multi-symptom presentations occur they typically cluster around a central complaint, the most common of which are head, stomach and limb pains. With recurrent abdominal pain (RAP), stomach pains are the central complaint but these may be accompanied by nausea, a lump in the throat, a bad taste in the mouth and gastrointestinal difficulties of various sorts. Where headaches are the chief complaint, they may occur in conjunction with chest pain, breathlessness, a pounding heart and dizziness. Where limb pains are the main concern, they may be accompanied by an abnormal gait, paralysis and occasionally areas of limb anaesthesia which do not conform to the anatomical distribution of sensory nerves. However, the clinical picture for each of the central complaints may include multiple symptoms in unrelated bodily systems.

Multi-variate studies of the Child Behaviour Checklist and other ASEBA instruments have identified a somatic complaints syndrome as a narrow-band factor falling within the broader dimension of internalizing behaviour problems (Achenbach & Rescorla, 2000, 2001). Items in the syndrome for toddlers and older children are presented in Table 14.1. The identification of a somatic complaint factor in many factor-analytic studies supports the idea of a single somatic complaint syndrome which may find expression in a variety of ways, with one symptom, such as headaches, pre-dominating in one case and another symptom, such as abdominal pain, being prominent in another case.

A number of disorders with somatic complaints as the central concern are classified within DSM IV TR (APA, 2000a) and ICD 10 (WHO, 1992, 1996),

Table 14.1 ASEBA Somatic Complaints syndrome for 1.5- to 5 and 6-18-year-olds.

ASEBA *1.5- to 5-year-olds*	ASEBA *6- to 18-year-olds*
Pain	**Pain**
Stomachaches (P&T)	Stomachaches (P&T&C)
Headaches (P&T)	Headaches (P&T&C)
Aches (P&T)	Aches (P&T&C)
Nausea and vomiting	**Nausea and vomiting**
Nausea (P&T)	Nausea (P&T&C)
Vomits (P&T)	Vomits (P&T&C)
Doesn't eat well (P)	
Bowel problems	**Bowel problems**
Constipated (P)	Constipated (P)
Diarrhoea (P)	
Painful bowel movements (P)	
Other anxiety symptoms	**Other anxiety symptoms**
Can't stand things out of place (P&T)	Night-mares (P&C)
Too concerned with neatness or cleanliness (P&T)	Over-tired (P&T&C)
	Feels dizzy (P&T&C)
	Eye problems (P&T&C)
	Skin problems (P&T&C)

Note: Adapted from Achenbach & Rescorla (2000, 2001). Items marked (P) are on the parent report CBCL. Items marked (T) are on the Teacher Report or Caregiver and Teacher Report form. Items marked (C) are on the Youth Self-Report form.

chief among these being somatization disorder (Figures 14.1 and 14.2). However, the diagnostic criteria for somatization disorder in DSM IV TR (four pain symptoms, two gastrointestinal symptoms, one sexual symptom and one pseudoneurological symptom) are probably of little relevance to children, who tend to have simpler presentations than adults. Polysymptomatic somatization disorder is distinguished from monosymptomatic pain disorder in both ICD 10 and DSM IV TR, and probably most children who present with recurrent abdominal pain and persistent headaches would be categorized as having a monosymptomatic pain disorder. Where motor or sensory symptoms such as paralysis, convulsions or anaesthesia for which no neurological basis can be found occur within DSM IV TR and ICD 10, a diagnosis of conversion disorder is given. Within ICD 10 where exhaustion following little effort is the central symptom, a diagnosis of neurasthenia is given (which excludes chronic fatigue syndrome). However, in clinical practice most children that present with fatigue as the core symptom in the absence of a current identifiable physical illness receive diagnosis of chronic fatigue syndrome (Garralda & Rangel, 2002).

In the absence of symptoms, where a fear of ill health persists despite negative findings from a medical examination, a diagnosis of hypochondriasis

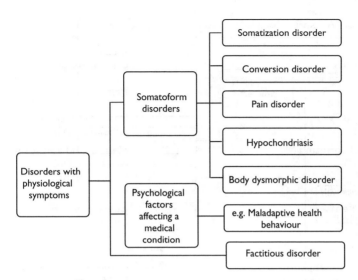

Figure 14.1 The classification of psychological conditions with pre-dominantly physiological symptoms in DSM IV TR

is given. 'Factitious disorder' is the term used to describe those circumstances where people intentionally produce symptoms so that they can assume a sick role. In DSM IV TR, factitious disorder by proxy is included as a category warranting further study. Here, the parent (usually the mother) deliberately induces symptoms in the child. Preliminary data suggest that this typically occurs in pre-school children. This condition, also known as Munchausen syndrome by proxy, is addressed in Chapter 19 on physical abuse.

In clinical practice it may be useful to conceptualize paediatric difficulties referred for psychological consultation as falling along two dimensions, as set out in Figure 14.3. Thus in any case, the child's symptomatology may be viewed as falling along a continuum from the physiological to the psychological. The aetiology of the condition may also be viewed as falling along such a continuum. This dimensional approach allows the clinician to avoid falling into the trap of over-simplification and of classifying somatic complaints as organic or psychological.

EPIDEMIOLOGY

Epidemiological data for somatization problems is sketchy (Campo & Fritsch, 1994; Eminson, Benjamin, Shortall & Woods, 1996; Garralda, 1999). Prevalence rates for somatization in children and adolescents vary between 2 and 10%, depending on the methods used to identify cases and the populations studied.

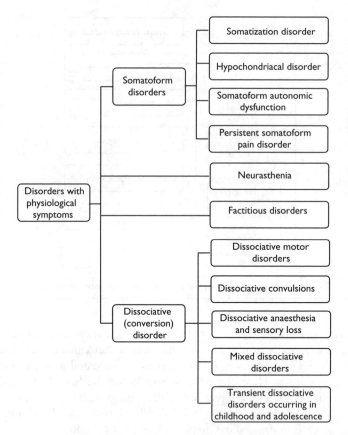

Figure 14.2 The classification of psychological conditions with pre-dominantly physio-logical symptoms in ICD 10

Table 3.4 (p. 86) shows that there is considerable co-morbidity between the somatic complaints syndrome of the Child Behaviour Checklist on the one hand and other types of behaviour problems such as aggression, attentional difficulties, anxiety and depression on the other. In community samples, co-morbidity rates vary from 12 to 20%, depending on the problem types and whether the child or the parent is the informant. In clinical samples, co-morbidity rates vary from 23 to 32%, with the highest rate of co-morbidity being with child-reported anxiety and depression.

Prevalence rates for chronic physical disorders in which psychological adjustment may be a central concern are presented in Table 14.2. In order of decreasing prevalence these are: asthma, seizure disorder, diabetes mellitus and leukaemia. Reliable prevalence rates for adjustment problems among children with these difficulties are unavailable.

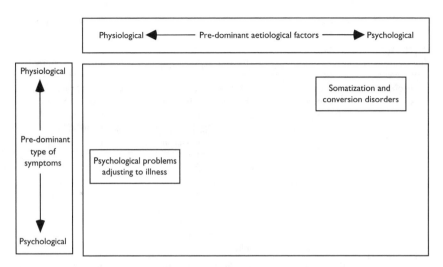

Figure 14.3 Psychological and physiological dimensions along which the aetiology and symptomatology of typical paediatric presentations fall

Table 14.2 Prevalence of most common illnesses in children aged 0–10 in the USA in 1980

Disorder	Prevalence estimates per 1000
Asthma	30–120
Seizure disorder	5.0
Diabetes mellitus	2.0
Leukaemia (acute lymphocytic)	0.5

Note: Adapted from Goodman (2002) and Mrazek (2002).

THEORETICAL FRAMEWORKS

This section considers theoretical accounts of the role of biological and psychosocial factors in pain, conversion symptoms and adjustment to chronic illness. A summary of central tenets of the main theories that offer explanations of these conditions and related treatment principles are presented in Table 14.3.

Biological perspectives

Two types of biological theory about the role of somatic factors in illness and pain are of particular relevance to paediatric clinical psychology. The first type of theory focuses on children's personal vulnerabilities to somatic

Table 14.3 Psychological theories and treatments for somatization problems, conversion problems and problems of adjustment to illness

Theory		Theoretical principles	Principles of treatment
Biological theories	**Biological vulnerability theory**	Children, because of their genetic heritage or developmental history, may have specific organs or biological systems that are vulnerable to dysfunction. When exposed to stress and/or infection, they develop symptoms associated with their biological vulnerability	Children are trained to avoid stressors or stimuli to which they are vulnerable
	General adaptation syndrome theory	A build-up of stress, regardless of the type, leads to a generalized stress response (General Adaptation Syndrome, GAS) The syndrome begins with an alarm stage characterized by autonomic arousal, followed by the resistance stage, during which physiological hyperarousal is maintained and concludes with the exhaustion stage, during which the body's immune system functions poorly and vulnerability to stress and infections is greatly increased	Reduce the build-up of stress
Intrapsychic theories	**Psychoanalytic theories**	Anxiety aroused by an unconscious conflict is converted into physical symptoms which are more tolerable than the anxiety	Individual psychotherapy, in which transference develops so that feelings associated with unresolved conflict are projected onto the therapist

		The primary gain derived from conversion symptoms is anxiety reduction and the secondary gain is that they allow the child to avoid unpleasant activities and solicit kindness from others	Conflictual feelings, primary gains and secondary gains are interpreted and worked through
	Psychosomatic theory	Conversion symptoms and chronic pain allow children to communicate distressing emotions to others	Psychotherapy, in which the communicative function of the symptom is explored and then interpreted
		Children who have difficulty acknowledging and expressing their emotions and who have experienced illness themselves or observed it in their immediate social network learn to somaticize to express distress	Hypnotherapy, in which suggestion is used to modify the symptom
Interpersonal theories	**Behavioural theory**	Conversion symptoms, chronic pain and adjustment problems associated with chronic illness are reinforced by rewards associated with these illness behaviours	Behaviour modification programmes, in which well behaviours are rewarded and sick-role behaviours are extinguished
	Cognitive-behavioural theory	Pain has biological, sensory, cognitive, emotional and behavioural or interpersonal dimensions which are inter-related in complex ways	Relaxation training to reduce arousal Cognitive skills training to aid distraction and interpretation of the pain as controllable Life stress reduction and enhancement of social support
	Stress and coping	Adjustment to the chronic strains entailed by an illness depends on the balance of risk and resistance factors	Counselling and psychoeducation to help the child and family maximize adherence to the medical treatment regime to minimize illness-related parameters

Continued

Table 14.3 continued

Theory	Theoretical principles	Principles of treatment
	Risk factors include illness-related parameters; functional independence; and psychosocial stressors Resistance factors fall into three categories: interpersonal factors such as competence, easy temperament and problem-solving abilities; socio-ecological factors including family environment, social support, material and economic resources; and stress-processing factors, such as cognitive appraisal and coping strategies	Self-management skills training to maximize the child's functional independence Stress management training to reduce life stress and improve stress-processing resources Arranging membership of self-help groups to increase social support
Family systems theory	Specific maladaptive family processes determine the extent to which children develop somatization or conversion symptoms or develop adjustment problems to chronic illness. These processes include enmeshment, disengagement, overly rigid or flexible boundaries, triangulation, marital discord and responsivity to illness The severity of symptoms will also depend on the child's personal psychophysiological reactivity. The specific symptoms displayed will be determined by the child's physiological vulnerabilities	Family therapy, which aims to modify maladaptive family processes

complaints, whereas the second is concerned with the characteristics of stressors that precipitate the onset of the illnesses or symptoms.

Biological vulnerability theory

Biological vulnerability theory argues that different people, because of their genetic heritage or developmental history, have specific organs or biological systems that are vulnerable to dysfunction. When exposed to stress and/or infection, they develop symptoms associated with their biological vulnerability (Lask & Fosson, 1989). For example, this theory predicts that children with a family history of asthma and allergies inherit an atopic constitution and bronchial hyperactivity, which makes them vulnerable to developing asthma. Other children, with a family history of migraine, have a genetically inherited reactive cerebral vascular system. When exposed to stress, the theory predicts that individuals with bronchial reactivity will develop asthma and those with reactive cerebral vascular systems will develop headaches. These symptoms will have been precipitated by stress but the nature of the symptoms will have been determined by the biological vulnerability. Available evidence partially supports this position (Llewelyn & Kennedy, 2003).

General adaptation syndrome theory

Theories that focus on the characteristics of the stressor in explaining the development of somatic complaints argue that a build-up of stress, regardless of the type, leads to a generalized stress response. Selye (1976) was the first to propose a General Adaptation Syndrome (GAS), which he suggested occurred in response to chronic stress of any type. The syndrome he proposed begins with an alarm stage characterized by autonomic arousal and preparation for fight or flight. This is followed by the resistance stage, during which physiological arousal drops somewhat but does not return to normal. During this resistance phase the body is attempting to adapt to chronic stress and so its resources for dealing with infections or new stressors are greatly depleted. During the resistance phase the body is vulnerable to many illnesses, including asthma, ulcers, hypertension and diseases that result from impaired immune functioning. Finally, there is the exhaustion stage, during which the body's immune system functions poorly and vulnerability to stress and infections is greatly increased.

While Selye's notion of the General Adaptation Syndrome is supported by a large body of research (Selye, 1976), his formulation fails to explain why some stressors produce different responses than others and why different people show different responses to the same stressor. That is, there is evidence that sudden intense acute stressors and gradually increasing chronic stressors each produce different patterns of arousal (Sarafino, 2001). There is also evidence (mentioned earlier) that there is considerable variability in different people's responses to the same stressors, which may be partly accounted for by variability in biological vulnerability (Lask & Fosson, 1989); it may also be partly accounted for by differences in psychological vulnerability and coping strategies (Turk, Meichenbaum & Genest, 1983).

Psychosocial theories

Psychological explanations of somatic complaints have been developed within the psychoanalytic and psychosomatic traditions. These emphasize the role of intrapsychic factors and the behavioural, cognitive-behavioural, stress and coping, and family systems traditions, which place greater emphasis on interpersonal factors.

Psychoanalytic theory

A significant portion of Freud's (1894) cases presented with somatic symptoms for which an organic basis could not be found and this led to the development of his theory of conversion hysteria. According to this theory, anxiety aroused by an unconscious conflict is converted into physical symptoms, which are more tolerable than the anxiety. The unconscious conflict in classical psychoanalytic theory usually stems from an unresolved Oedipus or Electra complex. In modern psychodynamic theory, it is argued that anxiety may stem from any conflict (McCullough-Vaillant, 1997). The *primary gain* derived from conversion symptoms is that they keep repressed, unresolved conflicts out of awareness and reduce anxiety associated with these conflicts. The *secondary gain* derived from conversion symptoms is that they allow the person to avoid unpleasant activities and they elicit kindness from others.

The treatment of choice, according to the psychoanalytic model, is individual psychodynamic psychotherapy in which transference from patient to therapist develops. Feelings associated with the unresolved conflict are projected onto the therapist and these are interpreted, as are the primary and secondary gains associated with the symptoms, and worked through within the context of a long-term, intensive, therapeutic relationship.

While evidence for pure conversion symptoms in children, in the absence of a pre-existing organically based complaint, is lacking, there is a small but growing body of evidence that intensive individual psychodynamic psychotherapy can have a dramatic effect on the adjustment of children with brittle diabetes and that this effect is related to the emergence and interpretation of unconscious material (Fonagy & Moran, 1990).

Psychosomatic theory

In early versions of psychosomatic theory it was suggested that specific physical symptoms or conditions reflected particular personality types. These different personality types were thought to have difficulties expressing specific emotions (Alexander, 1950). For example, wheezing associated with asthma, was thought to be a stifled cry and an expression of guilt about unresolved dependency needs. Hypertension, on the other hand, was thought to reflect repressed hostility. This type of theory has received little empirical support. If anything, there are more similarities than differences between people who develop different psychosomatic complaints. A meta-analysis of studies of adults with asthma, headaches, heart disease, ulcers and other psychosomatic conditions found that in each instance there were significant relationships between the presence of the condition and three major affective states, i.e. anxiety, depression and anger (Friedman & Boothby-Kewley, 1987).

Modern revisions of psychosomatic theory argue that in all illnesses the role of physiological and psychosocial factors are inextricably linked (Garralda, 1999; Gledhill & Garralda, 2000; Lask & Fosson, 1989; Lipowski, 1987). Conversion symptoms and chronic pain are a way that people communicate or express distressing emotions, such as anger, jealousy, envy, guilt, anxiety and depression. Individuals who have difficulty acknowledging and expressing their emotions and who have experienced illness themselves, or observed it in their immediate social network, learn the language of bodily symptoms. This learning process usually happens outside of awareness. The types of symptom that develop depend on the person's unique physiological vulnerabilities. So, for example, a child with hyper-reactive respiratory system will develop asthma, whereas, a person with gastrointestinal difficulties may develop recurrent abdominal pain.

Psychosomatic theory argues that individual or family psychotherapy in which the communicative function of the symptom is explored and interpreted may help to reduce the role the psychological process plays in maintaining or exacerbating physiological processes that more directly under-pin the physical symptoms. Offering children skills to control their symptoms and express their feelings and helping families to develop healthier communication patterns are other approaches to treatment that derive from the psychosomatic model.

Behavioural theory

The kernel of behavioural theory is that conversion symptoms, chronic pain and adjustment problems associated with chronic illness elicit behaviour from members of the child's family and network that reinforce the symptoms, illness behaviour or sick-role behaviour (Fordyce, 1976). These reinforcers may include keeping the child out of difficult relationships, helping the child avoid difficult work or school situations and eliciting attention that might otherwise be withheld. With physical illnesses that develop into conversion disorders, children may be shaped into sick-role behaviour during episodes of illness when members of the child's network inadvertently reinforce illness behaviours. In other cases, children consciously or unconsciously imitate the behaviour of ill family members and then this sick-role behaviour is reinforced inadvertently by members of the child's network. In all instances, specific environmental or interpersonal cues may develop into discriminative stimuli, which initiate the onset of episodes of illness behaviour.

Clinical management of conversion symptoms, chronic pain and adjustment problems associated with chronic illness based on a behavioural theory begins with a functional analysis of the antecedents and consequences of the symptoms or sick-role behaviours of the child within hospital, home and school environments. On the basis of the results of the functional analysis a behaviour modification programme is developed in which specific well behaviours are reinforced and sick-role behaviours are extinguished. Typically, such programmes are implemented by nursing staff in hospitals, by parents within the child's home and by teachers within the child's school. Behavioural methods, particularly family-based contingency management programmes, have been found to be particularly effective with conditions such as recurrent abdominal pain and with adherence problems in the management of chronic illnesses such as asthma and diabetes (Brinkley, Cullen & Carr, 2002; Farrell, Cullen & Carr, 2002; Murphy & Carr, 2000b).

Cognitive-behavioural theory

Pain has been conceptualized within a cognitive-behavioural framework as a multi-dimensional response to actual or threatened tissue damage or irritation (McGrath & Goodman, 2005; McGrath & Hiller, 1999). Pain, according to the cognitive-behavioural perspective, has biological, sensory, cognitive, emotional and behavioural or interpersonal dimensions. At a physiological level, actual or anticipated noxious stimulation leads to the release of algogenic substances at the injury site, which causes a message to be sent to the brain via afferent nerves. However, Melzak and Wall (1989) have shown that this input may be modulated by descending nerve pathways from the cortex and there is not a clear correspondence between the amount of tissue damage and the perceived intensity of pain. At a sensory level, pain varies in quality (e.g. pounding, stabbing, crushing, searing, smarting, or dull), intensity (e.g. mild or excruciating) and duration (e.g. acute or chronic). At a cognitive level, pain intensity and duration is related to the degree to which attention is focused on the injury site and the appraisal of pain as threatening and beyond personal control. At an emotional level, anxiety is associated with acute pain and subsides when the pain is alleviated. Depression, helplessness and hopelessness are associated with chronic pain. At a behavioural and interpersonal level, pain is associated with avoidance of situations that place additional demands on coping resources, irritability in interpersonal situations and loss of peer relationships. Pain behaviour leads to the transformation of remaining relationships into ones where pain behaviour is reinforced. Pain behaviour may be maintained by contingencies such as the possibility of a successful insurance claim or the possibility of compensation.

According to cognitive-behavioural theory, psychological interventions may be directed at a number of levels to alleviate pain. At a physiological level, tension and arousal that compound irritation of injury sites may be reduced through tension reduction and anxiety management procedures. These include relaxation, autohypnosis or biofeedback. At a cognitive level, children may be helped to reduce the intensity of pain through interventions that help them to distract themselves from pain sensations and also by interventions that help them to construe pain as controllable rather than overwhelming. Distraction, cognitive restructuring and self-instructional training are examples of such procedures. At a behavioural and interpersonal level, interventions that reduce life stress and increase social support for the child within the family and peer group, and that reinforce well behaviour while extinguishing pain behaviour, may all modify pain experiences. Broadly speaking, these treatment predictions derived from cognitive-behavioural theory have been borne out by treatment studies (Murphy & Carr, 2000b).

Stress and coping theory

Children's adjustment to chronic illness has been conceptualized by Wallander's group within a stress and coping framework (Varni, Katz, Colegrove & Dolgin, 1996; Wallander, Thompson & Alriksson-Schmidt, 2003; Wallander & Varni, 1992, 1998). Chronic childhood illnesses such as cystic fibrosis, cancer or asthma are conceptualized as sources of chronic strains, for both children and their parents, which repeatedly interfere with the performance of role-related activities. For example, children with cancer experience such chronic strains as treatment-related pain, nausea, hair-loss, school absence and reduced peer contact. Their parents experience the chronic threat of bereavement, demands for numerous hospital visits and so forth. According to Varni's model, adjustment to the chronic strains entailed by an illness depends on the balance of risk and resistance factors. Risk factors include illness-related parameters such as the severity of the illness or the salience of the handicaps it entails, functional independence and psychosocial stressors including major stressful life events and daily hassles. Resistance factors fall into three categories. First, there are personal factors such as competence, easy temperament and problem-solving abilities. Second, there are socio-ecological factors including family environment, social support and economic resources. Third, there are stress-processing factors, such as cognitive appraisal and coping strategies. For modifiable strains, problem-focused strategies which aim to alter the strains may be most appropriate. For uncontrollable sources of stress, emotion-focused coping strategies such as seeking support, relaxation, re-framing the situation or distraction may be more appropriate. The model is well supported by available evidence (Wallander et al., 2003).

Intervention based on this model aims to reduce modifiable risk factors and increase modifiable resistance factors. Here are some examples of how risk factors may be reduced: illness-related parameters such as the degree of the child's handicap may be modified by helping the child and family maximize adherence to the medical treatment regime. Functional independence may be maximized by training the child in self-management skills or providing the child with prostheses that increase independence. Stressors, such as daily hassles associated with frequent hospital attendance, may be reduced through providing community-based treatment.

Some examples of how resistance factors may be increased follow: children's problem-solving skills for dealing with their illness may be enhanced through psychoeducation. The quality of the child's family environment may be improved through family work which focuses on enhancing the support and autonomy the parents and siblings offer the ill child. Extrafamilial social support may be enhanced through facilitating increased peer contact and through membership of self-help support groups for children with the same illness. Stress-processing resources may be enhanced through stress management training. All of these types of intervention have been shown to enhance adjustment in youngsters with chronic illness (Carr, 2000a; 2002a).

Family systems theory

A variety of family systems models have been developed concerning illness in families (e.g. Altschuler, 1997; Kazak, Rourke & Crump, 2003; Minuchin, Rosman & Baker, 1978; Rolland, 2003; Wood & Miller, 2003). Of these, Wood's (1994, 1996; Wood & Miller, 2003) is one of the best validated and so will be summarized here. Specific maladaptive family processes determine the extent to which children develop somatization or conversion symptoms or develop adjustment problems to chronic illness. The more of these processes that are present, the greater the probability that the child will be symptomatic. These maladaptive processes are:

- extreme emotional enmeshment and over-involvement, or disengagement and estrangement
- extremely rigid authoritarian or flexible *laissez-faire* generational hierarchy
- negative parental relationship or marital discord
- triangulation, where there is a cross-generational coalition or detouring of marital conflict through the child by engaging in conflict about the management of the child's symptoms
- an extremely high or low level of family responsivity to the child's symptoms.

The severity of symptoms will also depend on the child's personal psychophysiological reactivity, with highly reactive children showing greater symptoms. The specific symptoms displayed will be determined by the child's physiological vulnerabilities.

Assessment based on this model aims to evaluate the status of the child's illness and psychophysiological reactivity and the family's status on each of the process dimensions, listed above. Intervention involves family therapy, which aims to reduce family reactivity and triangulation and to optimize proximity and hierarchy. Adjunctive marital work may also be necessary to reduce marital discord.

A growing body of evidence supports the links between family processes and disease processes (Wood & Miller, 2003). There is also growing evidence that family and marital intervention may improve somatization symptoms and children's adjustment to chronic illness (Carr, 2000a; 2002a).

Wood's model has been extended to cover the wider social context in which the child lives. Within this extended multi-systemic framework, which incorporates the school, healthcare providers and peer contexts, Wood (1996) argues that process problems similar to those that occur in families may arise and maintain somatic difficulties. Thus children's problems may be maintained or exacerbated if they become involved in enmeshed or disengaged relationships with peers, school staff or healthcare professionals; if they find themselves in rigid authoritarian or flexible *laissez-faire* hierarchical relationships with teachers or healthcare professionals; and if their parents, teachers and health professionals develop negative relationships. Children's somatic complaints may also be maintained if they become triangulated between parents and teachers or parents and healthcare professionals, or if members of these wider systems are highly responsive to their somatic complaints.

Multi-systemic consultation based on this broader model involves identifying and resolving problems associated with proximity, hierarchy, negativity in relationships, triangulation and reactivity in the wider system, including the child, the family, the school, the peer group and the healthcare system. Guidelines for convening such wider systems meetings are given in Chapter 4. The goal of such meetings is for parents, teachers, peers and healthcare professionals to share the same understanding of the child's illness. A second goal is for parents, teachers and healthcare professionals to form positive alliances and offer the child a unified and supportive message about management of the somatic problem. This position should offer the child age-appropriate responsibility in management of the complaint.

ASSESSMENT

Specific categories of pre-disposing, precipitating, maintaining and protective factors deserving assessment when somatic complaints and adjustment to chronic illness are the central concern are set out in Figure 14.4 (Roberts,

PRE-DISPOSING FACTORS

PERSONAL PRE-DISPOSING FACTORS

Biological factors
- Physiological vulnerability
- Psychophysiological reactivity
- History of physical illness

Psychological factors
- Suggestibility
- Perfectionistic
- High achievement orientation
- Anxious to please adults and peers
- Low intelligence
- Difficult temperament
- Low self-esteem
- External locus of control

CONTEXTUAL PRE-DISPOSING FACTORS

Exposure to family problems in early life
- Parental history of physical illness
- Parental history of psychological problems
- Family culture in which distress is expressed somatically
- Family culture in which sick-role behaviour elicits care
- Chaotic family culture where adherence to directions is not fostered

PERSONAL MAINTAINING FACTORS

Biological factors
- Autonomic hyperarousal
- Poorly functioning immune system

Psychological factors
- Focused on physical sensations
- Somatic attributions
- Sick-role behaviour
- Non-adherence
- External health locus of control
- Cognitive distortions (catastrophizing)
- Immature defence mechanisms (denial)
- Dysfunctional coping strategies

PERSONAL PROTECTIVE FACTORS

Biological factors
- Low psychophysiological reactivity
- With somatization problems, an acute condition

Psychological factors
- High IQ
- Easy temperament
- High self-esteem
- Internal locus of control
- High self-efficacy
- Optimistic attributional style
- Mature defence mechanisms
- Functional coping strategies

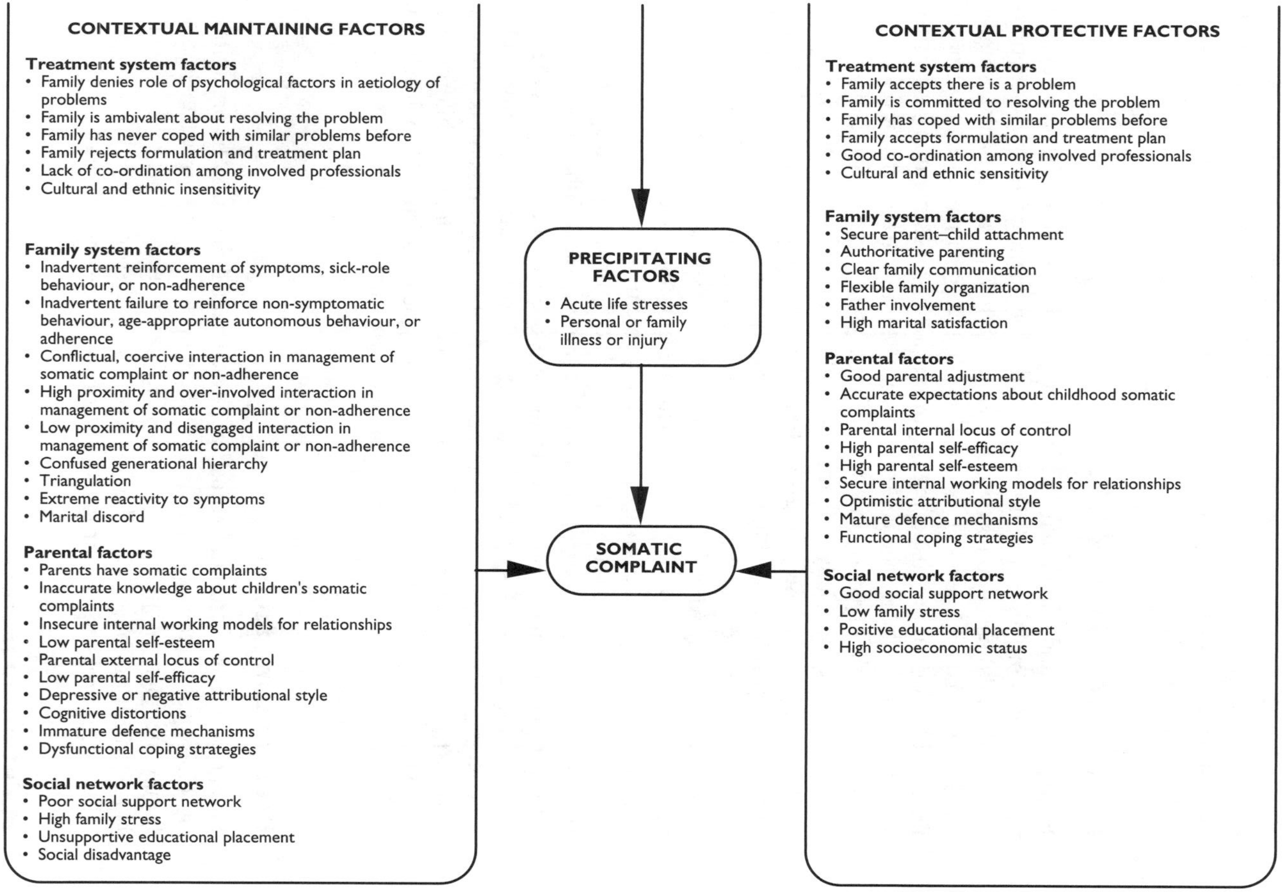

CONTEXTUAL MAINTAINING FACTORS

Treatment system factors
- Family denies role of psychological factors in aetiology of problems
- Family is ambivalent about resolving the problem
- Family has never coped with similar problems before
- Family rejects formulation and treatment plan
- Lack of co-ordination among involved professionals
- Cultural and ethnic insensitivity

Family system factors
- Inadvertent reinforcement of symptoms, sick-role behaviour, or non-adherence
- Inadvertent failure to reinforce non-symptomatic behaviour, age-appropriate autonomous behaviour, or adherence
- Conflictual, coercive interaction in management of somatic complaint or non-adherence
- High proximity and over-involved interaction in management of somatic complaint or non-adherence
- Low proximity and disengaged interaction in management of somatic complaint or non-adherence
- Confused generational hierarchy
- Triangulation
- Extreme reactivity to symptoms
- Marital discord

Parental factors
- Parents have somatic complaints
- Inaccurate knowledge about children's somatic complaints
- Insecure internal working models for relationships
- Low parental self-esteem
- Parental external locus of control
- Low parental self-efficacy
- Depressive or negative attributional style
- Cognitive distortions
- Immature defence mechanisms
- Dysfunctional coping strategies

Social network factors
- Poor social support network
- High family stress
- Unsupportive educational placement
- Social disadvantage

CONTEXTUAL PROTECTIVE FACTORS

Treatment system factors
- Family accepts there is a problem
- Family is committed to resolving the problem
- Family has coped with similar problems before
- Family accepts formulation and treatment plan
- Good co-ordination among involved professionals
- Cultural and ethnic sensitivity

Family system factors
- Secure parent–child attachment
- Authoritative parenting
- Clear family communication
- Flexible family organization
- Father involvement
- High marital satisfaction

Parental factors
- Good parental adjustment
- Accurate expectations about childhood somatic complaints
- Parental internal locus of control
- High parental self-efficacy
- High parental self-esteem
- Secure internal working models for relationships
- Optimistic attributional style
- Mature defence mechanisms
- Functional coping strategies

Social network factors
- Good social support network
- Low family stress
- Positive educational placement
- High socioeconomic status

PRECIPITATING FACTORS
- Acute life stresses
- Personal or family illness or injury

SOMATIC COMPLAINT

Figure 14.4 Factors to consider in the assessment of somatic complaints

2003). These areas should be covered within the context of the assessment protocol set out in Chapter 4. For specific conditions, such as recurrent abdominal pain, headaches, asthma and so forth, more detailed guidance on assessment is contained later in the chapter.

Pre-disposing factors

Both personal and contextual factors may pre-dispose youngsters to developing somatic complaints and illness-related adjustment problems. Genetic or constitutionally based physiological vulnerability to a particular somatic condition and a high level of psychophysiological reactivity are the principal personal biological pre-disposing factors requiring assessment in cases where somatic complaints are the central concern. At an intrapsychic level, a high level of suggestibility may pre-dispose some youngsters to developing somatic complaints, especially if their family culture is illness-oriented. Low intelligence may pre-dispose youngsters to mismanage complex medical regimes. Difficult temperament and low self-esteem may render youngsters vulnerable to developing conduct and emotional problems in response to somatic complaints and illness. An external locus of control, especially for health-related matters, may pre-dispose youngsters to developing adherence problems if they develop illnesses requiring strict management.

At a contextual level, two aspects of family culture may pre-dispose youngsters to developing somatization problems or adjustment difficulties in coping with chronic somatic conditions through a process of modelling. In the first, children observe that sick-role behaviours of other family members elicit excessive care and concern. In the second, emotional expression is inhibited and distress is communicated through somatic complaints. Children who come from a chaotically organized family may be pre-disposed to developing adherence problems, since following-through on plans is not part of the family culture.

Precipitating factors

Somatization problems and adjustment to chronic illness may be precipitated by biological factors such as personal illness or injury, or when another family member is injured or becomes ill. Major stressful life events such as bereavement or abuse, and a build-up of small stressors, may also precipitate adjustment problems to chronic illness or somatization difficulties.

Maintaining factors

Somatic complaints and adjustment problems may be maintained by a range of personal and contextual factors. Somatic complaints may be maintained by an external health locus of control, i.e. beliefs that somatization symptoms or complaints associated with chronic illness or treatment side effects are uncontrollable. These types of belief may prevent youngsters from developing coping strategies for managing symptoms and from adhering to medical treatment regimes. Thus youngsters may lapse into sick-role behaviour patterns or behaviour patterns where non-adherence is a central feature. With chronic illness, the use of immature defences such as denial of the nature and severity of the condition may lead to non-adherence to treatment regimes and this may maintain adjustment problems. With somatization problems, denial of the role of suggestion in producing the symptoms may maintain the somatic complaints. Such denial may also entail a primary gain, since it permits the youngster to avoid anxiety-provoking issues which would have to be faced if the somatization symptoms were resolved. Dysfunctional coping strategies, such as seeking questionable advice from unqualified people about illness management, wishful thinking and drug abuse, may all maintain somatic complaints and illness-related adjustment problems. In all somatic conditions, cognitive distortions involving catastrophizing about aspects of the condition may contribute to the maintenance of the symptoms by increasing autonomic arousal and eventually reducing the efficiency of the immune system. This is more likely to occur where children are characterized by a high level of physiological reactivity. In this way, biological and psychological maintaining factors are closely linked.

With respect to contextual maintaining factors, members of the child's family, school, peer group and healthcare system may inadvertently reinforce or give the child secondary gains for somatization symptoms, non-adherence to medical treatment regimes and behaviour associated with the sick role. They may also inadvertently fail to selectively reinforce behaviours associated with a non-symptomatic role, adherence to medical treatment regimes and age-appropriate autonomy. These contingencies are more likely to occur in family, school, peer group and healthcare contexts characterized by extreme emotional enmeshment or disengagement, an extremely rigid authoritarian hierarchy or an extremely *laissez-faire* lack of hierarchy, conflictual relationships, triangulation where conflicts are detoured through the child, or in which the child has a covert alliance with one authority figure against another, and systems which are highly reactive to the child's condition.

Such patterns of parenting and family organization may be partially maintained by parents' personal experience of somatic complaints or psychological difficulties. Where parents have insecure internal working models for relationships, low self-esteem, low self-efficacy, an external locus of control, immature defences and poor coping strategies, their resourcefulness in managing their children's difficulties may be compromised. Parents may also become involved in problem-maintaining interactions with their children if they have inaccurate knowledge about the role of psychological factors in the genesis and maintenance of somatic complaints and illness-related adjustment difficulties.

Somatic complaints and illness-related adjustment problems may also be maintained by high levels of stress, limited support and social disadvantage within the family's wider social system, since these features may deplete parents' and children's personal resources for dealing constructively with illness. Educational placements which are poorly resourced and where teaching staff have little time to devote to home–school liaison meetings may also maintain illness-related adjustment problems and somatic complaints.

Within the treatment system, a lack of co-ordination and clear communication among involved professionals, including family physicians, paediatricians, nurses, teachers, psychologists and so forth, may maintain children's somatic problems. It is not unusual for various members of the professional network to offer conflicting opinions and advice on the nature and management of somatic complaints to children and their families. These may range from viewing the child as physically ill with secondary psychological problems deserving careful management to seeing the child as healthy but malingering and deserving a disciplinarian management. Where co-operation problems between families and treatment teams develop, and families deny the existence of the problems, the validity of the diagnosis and formulation or the appropriateness of the treatment programme, then the child's difficulties may persist. Treatment systems that are not sensitive to the cultural and ethnic beliefs and values of the youngster's family system may maintain somatic problems by inhibiting engagement or promoting drop-out from treatment and preventing the development of a good working alliance between the treatment team, the youngster and his or her family. Parents' lack of experience in dealing with similar problems in the past is a further factor that may compromise their capacity to work co-operatively with the treatment team and so may contribute to the maintenance of the child's difficulties.

Protective factors

The probability that a treatment programme will be effective is influenced by a variety of personal and contextual protective factors. It is important that these are assessed and included in the later formulation, since it is protective factors that usually serve as the foundation for therapeutic change. At a biological level, physical fitness and low psychophysiological reactivity are protective factors. It may also be useful to consider acute somatization presentations as having a better prognosis than chronic presentations. A high IQ, an easy temperament, high self-esteem, an internal locus of control, high self-efficacy and an optimistic attributional style are all important personal protective factors. Other important personal protective factors include mature defence mechanisms and functional coping strategies, particularly good problem-solving skills and a capacity to make and maintain friendships.

Within the family, secure parent–child attachment and authoritative parenting are central protective factors, particularly if they occur within the context of a flexible family structure in which there is clear communication, high marital satisfaction and both parents share the day-to-day tasks of childcare.

Good parental adjustment is also a protective factor. Where parents have an internal locus of control, high self-efficacy, high self-esteem, internal working models for secure attachments, an optimistic attributional style, mature defences and functional coping strategies, then they are better resourced to manage their children's difficulties constructively. Accurate knowledge about the role of psychological factors in illness is also a protective factor.

Within the broader social network, high levels of support, low levels of stress and membership of a high socioeconomic group are all protective factors for children with somatic complaints and illness-related adjustment difficulties. Where families are embedded in social networks that provide a high level of support and place few stressful demands on family members, then it is less likely that parents' and children's resources for dealing with health-related problems will become depleted. A well-resourced educational placement can also be viewed as a protective factor. Educational placements where teachers have sufficient time and flexibility to attend home–school liaison meetings if invited to do so contribute to positive outcomes for children with somatic complaints and illness-related adjustment problems.

Within the treatment system, co-operative working relationships between the treatment team and the family and good co-ordination of multi-professional input are protective factors. Treatment systems that are sensitive to the cultural and ethnic beliefs and values of the youngster's family are more likely to help families engage with, and remain in, treatment and foster the development of a good working alliance. Families are more likely to benefit from treatment when they accept the formulation of the problem given by the treatment team and are committed to working with the team to resolve it. With somatization problems, this requires parents and children to be able to accept a complex multi-factorial account of symptoms rather than a simple dichotomous division of symptoms into those due to organic factors and those due to psychological factors. With adherence problems, the child's ability to follow and internalize rules and the parents' willingness to use contingency management programmes are protective factors. With adjustment to chronic illness, the families' openness to the grieving process and to using support is a protective factor. Where families have successfully faced similar problems before, then they are more likely to benefit from treatment and, in this sense, previous experience with similar problems is a protective factor.

FORMULATION

At the conclusion of the assessment phase it is useful to draw together salient points from the history and presentation into a formulation which explains the somatization difficulty or adjustment problem with reference to specific pre-disposing, precipitating and maintaining factors. Protective factors may also be highlighted and management plans should take account of these strengths. Examples of formulations are given in the relevant sections later in the chapter.

MANAGEMENT

Certain general principles for the management of somatic problems may be educed from the treatment outcome literature and clinical experience. (e.g. Carr, 2000a, 2002a; Roberts, 2003); these will be elaborated in this section. In subsequent sections, guidance will be given on how these general principles may be adapted for specific types of somatic problem, such as headaches or diabetes. A psychological approach to somatic complaints may include one or more of the following elements:

- close liaison with referring physician
- careful contracting for assessment
- thorough child and family assessment
- careful contracting for treatment
- family-based approach
- psychoeducation
- monitoring of symptoms
- relaxation skills training
- cognitive restructuring and self-instructional skills training
- coaching parents in contingency management
- relapse management training
- arranging family membership of a support group.

Liaison with referring physician

Work closely with the referring physician and other members of the medical team, including the family physician, the paediatrician, nurses, physiotherapist and so forth. If possible, clarify the precise question to which the referrer requires an answer. In some instances these questions will be highly specific, for example, a request to help a youngster with diabetes improve adherence to a self-care regime. In others, requests may be more global, for example, a request to offer an opinion on the management of a child with recurrent abdominal pains and headaches. If possible, clarify the referrer's views of the somatic problem. For children to resolve somatization and conversion symptoms, to manage pain, or adhere to complex regimes in managing chronic illness, they need a clear consistent message from all members of the family and healthcare network. Often they receive conflicting and confused messages, with one parent or healthcare professional emphasizing the primary role of physiological factors while the other parent and other health-care professionals may define the problem in intrapsychic terms. Given the child's need for clarity and the potential for confusion, it is essential that the referring physician and the psychologist understand each other's positions clearly and work towards a shared view of the problem and a shared management plan.

Contracting for assessment

Parents and children may have difficulty understanding the relevance of a psychological consultation when the chief complaint is somatic. This difficulty may be based on a belief that symptoms are either due to organic factors or psychological factors. Thus, part of process of offering a contract for assessment involves inviting families to accept the view that, in all ill-nesses, both psychological and physiological factors contribute to the development of symptoms, the perception of symptoms, adherence to management plans, and adjustment to illness-related stresses. It is useful to use concrete examples to illustrate these points. For example:

- Stresses like changing jobs or going into a new class reduces the efficiency of the immune system in fighting infections.
- If people are engrossed in an activity like playing rugby, they may not perceive pain associated with injuries.
- If youngsters are sad, angry or confused about their illness and its treatment, they may not follow their treatment programme properly and so become worse.
- Illnesses may place a strain on all family members, and it may be useful to explore the best way to manage this stress.

If the parents remain confused about the relevance of a psychological assessment, include the referring physician in a further contracting meeting and invite her or him to explain why a purely medical approach to the problem is not in the child's best interests.

Assessment

Unless a highly specific, and focused, referral question has been asked, conduct a thorough assessment of the child and family following the protocol set out in Chapter 4. Supplement this protocol with assessment procedures that have been developed for the specific somatic complaint with which the child presents. Details of areas of inquiry for clinical interviews for a variety of somatic complaints such as recurrent abdominal pain, headaches, asthma, and diabetes are given later in the chapter. Specific assessment instruments for various condition are listed in Table 14.4.

If these assessment procedures suggest the presence of other difficulties, such as learning problems, mood problems, risk of self-harm, possibility of child abuse or anticipatory grief associated with a life-threatening illness, extend the assessment to cover these issues (which are described in other chapters).

Following assessment, construct a formulation outlining the pre-disposing, precipitating, maintaining and protective factors for the core problem. Then construct a psychological case management plan based on the formulation. This plan will usually include feedback to the referring physician and appropriate members of the treatment team, feedback to the family and contracting for further treatment.

Contracting for treatment

If the assessment sessions have been used as an opportunity to build a good working alliance with the child and the parents, and if a shared position has been developed by the psychologist and the other members of the multi-disciplinary team, particularly the referring physician, then contracting for further treatment is less likely to be problematic. The most common problem which occurs at this point in the psychological consultation process is that the parents or the child are unable to accept a multi-factorial explanation of the presenting problems, which includes both biological and psychosocial factors. The main pitfall to avoid when this happens is becoming involved in a heated argument. Rather, it is most helpful to adopt a position of respectful curiosity, and inquire about the conditions under which they would be able to accept a multi-factorial explanation for the problem. In some instances, such acceptance will not be possible, particularly with conversion symptoms, because the loss of secondary gains to the entire family may not be worth giving up the symptom for. If the family accepts the formulation and a contract for further treatment, this may include psychoeducation, individual work for the child focusing on self-monitoring skills and symptom management strategies and family sessions focusing on coaching the parents in contingency management and optimizing family support for the child.

Family-based treatment approach

A family-based approach to illness management aims to help family members communicate clearly and openly about the illness, symptoms and related issues; to make clearer family boundaries and increase the autonomy of the

Table 14.4 Psychometric instruments that may be used as an adjunct to clinical interviews in the assessment of somatic complaints

Construct	Instrument	Author & date of publication	Comments
Pain	The Varni-Thompson Paediatric Pain Questionnaire	Varni, J. Thompson, K. & Hanson, V. (1987). The Varni-Thompson Paediatric Pain Questionnaire: 1. Chronic-musculo-skel-etal pain in juvenile rheumatoid arthritis. *Pain*, 28, 27–38. Available from NFER Nelson, UK	Parent and child versions of this questionnaire are available and they include visual analogue scales to assess pain intensity; a body outline to assess pain location; and adjectives to assess sensory, affective and evaluative aspects of pain. In addition, there is a disease-activity rating scale
	Children's Comprehensive Pain Questionnaire	McGrath, P. (1987). The multidimensional assessment and management of recurrent pain syndromes in children. *Behaviour Research and Therapy*, 25, 251–262	A comprehensive pain assessment questionnaire
	Procedure Behaviour Checklist	Le Baron, S. & Zeltzer, L. (1984). Assessment of acute pain and anxiety in children and adolescents by self-reports, observer reports and a behaviour checklist. *Journal of Consulting and Clinical Psychology*, 52, 729–738	Simple numerical and face scales for assessing pain from the child's viewpoint and a method for assessing pain from an observer are reported in this paper
	The Faces Pain Scale	Bieri, D. Reeve, R. Champion, G. & Addicoat, L. (1990). The faces pain scale for the self-assessment of the severity of pain experienced by children: Development,	Children are asked which of a series of drawn faces reflects how they feel

Continued

Table 14.4 continued

Construct	Instrument	Author & date of publication	Comments
		initial validation and preliminary investigation for ratio scale properties. *Pain*, 41, 139–150	Children are asked which of a series of drawn faces reflects how they feel
	Pain Ladder and the Poker Chip Tool	Hester, N., Foster, R. & Kristensen, K. (1990). Measurement of pain in children: Generalizability and validity of the pain ladder and the poker chip tool. In D. Tyler & E. Krane (eds.), *Paediatric Pain. Advances in Pain Research and Therapy* (Volume 15, pp. 79–84). New York: Raven	Concrete symbols (poker chips and ladder rungs) are used to asses how many pieces of hurt are present for children under 5
	Children's Hospital Eastern Ontario Pain Scale (CHEOPS)	McGrath, P., Johnson, G., Goodman, J., Schillinger, J., Dunn, J., & Chapman, J. (1985). CHEOPS: A behavioural scale for rating post-operative pain in children. In H. Fields, R. Dubner & F. Cerveero (eds.), *Advances in Pain Research and Therapy* (Volume 9, pp 395–401). New York: Raven	This 6-item, time sampling scale includes items measuring cry, facial behaviour, verbal behaviour, torso movement, leg movement, and touching the affected area
Headaches	Childhood Headaches Questionnaire	Labbé, E., Williamson, D. & Southard, D. (1985). Reliability and validity of children's reports of migraine headache symptoms. *Journal of Psychopathology and Behavioural Assessment*, 7, 375–383	This 35-item self-report questionnaire assesses migraine symptomatology

	Headache Symptom Questionnaire	Mindell, J. & Andrasik, F. (1987). Headache classification and factor analysis with a paediatric population. *Headache*, 27, 96–101	This is a 20-item self-report questionnaire
Somatiz-ation	Somatic Symptom Checklist	Eminson, M., Benjamin, S., Shortall, A. & Woods, T. (1996). Physical symptoms and illness attitudes in adolescents: An epidemiological Study. *Journal of Child Psychology and Psychiatry*, 37, 519–528	This 37-item self-report checklist covers symptoms typically characterizing somatization disorder
	Illness Attitudes Scale	Kellner, P. (1987). *Abridged Manual of the Illness Attitudes Scale.* Albuquerque, New Mexico: Department of Psychiatry. Contained in Eminson, M., Benjamin, S., Shortall, A. & Woods, T. (1996). Physical symptoms and illness attitudes in adolescents: An epidemiological Study. *Journal of Child Psychology and Psychiatry*, 37, 519–528	This 31-item scale yields scores for the following sub-scales: worry about illness; concern about pain; health habits; hypochondriacal beliefs; thanatophobia; disease phobia; bodily preoccupations; treatment experience; effects of symptoms
Hypnotiz-ability	Stanford Hypnotic Scale for Children	Morgan, A. & Hilgard, J. (1979). Stanford Hypnotic Scale for Children. *American Journal of Clinical Hypnosis*, 21, 155–169	This 7-item hypnotic induction scale may be administered to children 6–16. The items are administered following trance induction and include hand lowering; arm rigidity; visual and auditory hallucination; dream; age regression; and response to a post-hypnotic suggestion

Continued

Table 14.4 continued

Construct	Instrument	Author & date of publication	Comments
Asthma	Childhood Asthma Questionnaires	Christie, M., French, D., Sowden, A. & West, A. (1993). Development of child centred disease specific questionnaires for living with asthma. *Psychosomatic Medicine,* 55, 541–548 French, D., Christie, M. & Sowden, A. (1994). The reproducibility of the childhood asthma questionnaires. *Quality of Life Research. An International Quarterly Journal of Quality of Life Aspects of Treatment, Care and Rehabilitation,* 3, 215–224	These self-report measures assess quality of life and symptom distress in paediatric asthma
	Life Activities Questionnaire for Childhood asthma	Creer, T., Wigal, J., Kotses, H. Hatala, J. et al. (1993). A. life activities questionnaire for childhood asthma. *Journal of Asthma,* 30, 467–473	This self-report questionnaire assesses activity restriction in chronic asthma
	Self-efficacy in Asthma	Schlosser, M. & Havermans, G. (1992). A self-efficacy scale for children and adolescents with asthma: Construction and validation. *Journal of Asthma,* 29, 99–108	This 22-item self-report scale measures efficacy expectations concerning medical treatment, the environment and problem-solving skills
	Asthma Self-Management Interview	Taylor, G., Rea, H., McNaughton, S., Smith, L. et al (1991). A tool for measuring the asthma self-management competence of families. *Journal of Psychosomatic Research,* 35, 483–491	In this structured family interview respondents indicate how they would respond to three asthma management scenarios and transcripts of their responses may be rated using a coding system

Diabetes	Diabetes Knowledge Scale	Beeney, L., Dunn, S. & Welch, G. (1994). Measurement of diabetes knowledge. The development of the DKN scales. In C. Bradley (ed.), *Handbook of Psychology and Diabetes* (pp. 159–190). Chur, Switzerland: Harwood	There are three equivalent versions of this 15-item knowledge test
	Summary of Diabetes Self-care Activities Questionnaire	Tootbert, D. & Glasgow, R. (1994). Assessing diabetes self-management: The summary of diabetes self-care activities questionnaire. In C. Bradley (ed.), *Handbook of Psychology and Diabetes* (pp. 351–378). Chur, Switzerland: Harwood	This 12-item inventory covers diet, exercise, glucose testing and medication usage
	Barriers to Diabetes Self-care Scale	Glasgow, R. (1994). Social environmental factors in diabetes: Barriers to diabetes self-care. In C. Bradley (ed.), *Handbook of Psychology and Diabetes* (pp. 335–350). Chur, Switzerland: Harwood	This 31-item self-report instrument yields an overall barriers score and sub-scale scores for barriers in the areas of diet, exercise, glucose testing and medication usage
	Adjustment to Diabetes Scale (ATT39)	Welch, G. (1994). The ATT39: A measure of psychological adjustment to diabetes. In C. Bradley (ed.), *Handbook of Psychology and Diabetes* (pp. 291–334). Chur, Switzerland: Harwood	This 39-item self-report instrument yields an overall score which indicates adjustment to diabetes and sub-scale scores in the areas of stress, coping, guilt, alienation, illness conviction and tolerance for ambiguity

Continued

Table 14.4 continued

Construct	Instrument	Author & date of publication	Comments
	Perceived Control of Diabetes Scale	Bradley, C. (1994). Measures of perceived control of diabetes. In C. Bradley (ed.), *Handbook of Psychology and Diabetes* (pp. 291–334). Chur, Switzerland: Harwood	This instrument contains a series of eight scenarios about diabetes control problems. Respondents indicate the cause of the control problem and the degree to which the problem was controllable on seven dimensions
	Diabetes Quality of Life Measure	Jacobson, A. (1994). The diabetes quality of life measure. In C. Bradley (ed.), *Handbook of Psychology and Diabetes* (pp. 65–88). Chur, Switzerland: Harwood	This 60-item questionnaire yields an overall quality of life score and sub-scale scores for satisfaction, impact, diabetes-related worry and social/vocational worry
	Diabetes Family Behaviour Checklist	Schafer, L., McCaul, K., & Glasgow, R. (1986). Supportive and non-supportive family behaviours: Relationships to adherence and metabolic control in persons with Type 1 diabetes. *Diabetes*, 9, 179–185	This 16-item self-report scale assesses the degree to which families are perceived to support adherence to the diabetic's regime
Adjustment to chronic illness	Impact on Family Scale	Stein, R. & Riessman, C. (1980). The development of an impact-on-family scale: Preliminary Findings. *Medical Care*, 18, 465–472. Contained in Bennett Johnson, S. (1989). Chronic illness and Pain. In E. Mash & L. Terdal. (eds.) *Behavioural Assessment of Childhood Disorders* (pp. 491–527). New York: Guilford	This 24-item scale may be used to determine the effects of a child's chronic illness on a family. It yields scores on four factors: financial burden; familial and social impact; personal strain; and mastery

Child Attitude Toward Illness Scale	Austin, J. & Huberty, T. (1993). Development of the Child Attitude Toward Illness Scale. *Journal of Paediatric Psychology*, 18, 467–480	This self-report instrument assesses the degree to which children have a favourable or unfavourable attitude to their chronic illness

child in symptom management; to decrease the emotional intensity of parent–child interactions related to the symptom; to encourage joint parental problem-solving with respect to the symptom; to optimize the parent's support of the ill child and siblings and to optimize parents' use of healthcare resources and support groups.

To achieve these aims, some treatment sessions may be conducted with children to help them develop symptom management skills such as relaxation exercises, breathing exercises, visualization, distraction and self-instruction. However, other treatment sessions should involve the parents and siblings, who may become marginalized as family life becomes organized around the ill child.

Where fathers are unavailable during office hours, it is worthwhile making special arrangements to schedule at least a couple of family sessions which are convenient for the father, since the participation of fathers in family therapy is associated with a positive outcome (Carr, 2000b). Where parents are separated or divorced, it is particularly important to arrange some sessions with the non-custodial parent, since it is vital that both parents adopt the same approach in understanding and managing the child's somatic difficulties.

Psychoeducation

In psychoeducational sessions parents, ill children and their siblings are given both general information about the illness and specific information about the symptomatic child's particular illness. Information on clinical features, pre-disposing, precipitating, maintaining and protective factors should be given along with its impact on cognition, behaviour, family adjustment, school adjustment and health over the lifespan. Details of the medical treatment programme covering medication, exercise, physiotherapy, diet, tests and medical crisis management and so forth should be given both orally and in written form in a way that is comprehensible to the parents and the child. Psychoeducation may be offered in individual sessions, family sessions or group sessions. For many illnesses such as diabetes, interactive instructional software programs are available that permit children to learn about their illness at their own pace. These have the advantage of being highly motivating for children and exciting to use. However, such programs should always be supplemented with individual consultations to answer the child's specific questions. Family psychoeducation sessions allow the family to develop a shared understanding of the illness. Group psychoeducation offers a forum where children and parents can meet others in the same position and this has the benefit of providing additional support for family members.

Monitoring of symptoms

For all somatic complaints, it is useful to train children and/or parents to regularly record information about the symptom, the circumstances surrounding its occurrence and treatment adherence. Intensity ratings, frequency counts, durations and other features of symptoms may be recorded regularly. Intrapsychic and interpersonal events that happened before, during and after the symptoms may also be noted. The amount of medication used, particular foods that were eaten, particular exercises that were completed and results of tests (such as blood sugar or peak-flow meter readings) may all be monitored in standard ways on a regular basis. When inviting parents and children to use a monitoring system, the chances of them co-operating is better if a simple system is used to start out with. Later, more complex versions of it may be developed. For example, children with headaches may record the intensity of their pain three times a day for a week to start out with. Later, when they have become used to the practice of self-monitoring, they may be invited to also record information about medication usage. A page from a pain diary, which can be used with headaches, abdominal pains and other types of pain, is presented in Figure 14.5. Simplified versions of this may be used earlier in the monitoring process. A self-monitoring chart for physical illness is presented in Figure 14.6. It may be used to monitor fluctuations in symptomatology and adherence to healthcare regimes involving medication, diet and exercise programmes.

Relaxation skills training

Stressful events which increase physiological arousal may precipitate, maintain or exacerbate many symptoms, including pain, asthma attacks, epileptic seizures and changes in diabetic blood sugar levels. For this reason, training in tension reduction skills is a core element of most treatment programmes described in this chapter. The progressive muscle relaxation exercise, breathing exercises and visualization skills described in Chapter 12 may be taught to children who present with somatic complaints.

PAIN DIARY		
	Fill in this column in the middle of the day	Fill in this column in the evening
What day is it?	Sun Mon Tues Wed Thurs Fri Sat Sun	Sun Mon Tues Wed Thurs Fri Sat Sun
Have you had a pain since you last filled in your pain diary?	Yes No	Yes No
What time did you have the pain?		
How long did the pain last?		
Where were you?		
Where was the pain?	Head Stomach _____	Head Stomach _____
How sore was it ?	1 2 3 4 5	1 2 3 4 5
What happened before the pain started and what were you thinking and feeling?		
What happened while you had the pain and what were you thinking and feeling?		
Did you miss school?	Yes No	Yes No
How much medicine did you take?		
What happened after the pain ended and what were you thinking and feeling?		

Figure 14.5 Pain diary

Cognitive coping strategies

The degree to which children focus their attention on their symptoms, the way in which they evaluate them and the behavioural and interpersonal patterns that they develop related to their symptoms all influence children's

			Monitoring Chart				
	Name_____Age_____Condition_____						

Day	Time	Symptom	Medication	Diet	Exercises	Situation	Thoughts
	(Indicate the period to which the monitoring applies)	(Indicate intensity, frequency, duration or other aspects)	(Indicate name and quantity)	(Indicate what was eaten)	(Indicate if prescribed exercises were completed)	(Indicate who was present and your role in what was happening)	(Indicate what you thought about)

Figure 14.6 Self-monitoring system for physical illnesses

overall psychological adjustment to somatic complaints. In certain situations, it may be appropriate for children to learn to distract themselves from their symptoms by thinking about something else or becoming engrossed in an activity that prevents them from thinking about their condition. Distraction may be useful in coping with various types of pain, particularly recurrent abdominal pain, which may arise from focusing on minor fluctuations in internal physiological states and catastrophizing about these. Children may be helped to develop their own distraction routines, such as listening to their favourite music or story on a personal stereo, playing with a favourite toy or reciting favourite poems.

Where children have developed a habit of catastrophizing about symptoms or misinterpreting benign bodily sensations, they may be trained to challenge these negative thoughts in the way described in Chapter 12. In CTR self-instructional training, children are invited to Challenge these catastrophic thoughts by asking themselves what the other possible interpretations of the situation are, to Test out what evidence there is for the catastrophic outcome and the other less threatening outcomes, and to Reward themselves for testing out the less catastrophic interpretation of the situation.

Where children have developed debilitating behaviour patterns and inter-personal routines in response to their symptoms, they may be helped to break out of the sick role by planning alternative ways of acting and managing their interpersonal relationships. That is, they may be invited to plan ways to replace illness behaviour or pain behaviour with well behaviour.

Contingency management

Contingency management programmes may be conducted on a hospital ward or in the child's home. For home-based programmes, parents require guid-ance on using reward systems, such as that described in Chapter 4, to reinforce the child's well behaviour. Ideally, this reward system should be set up with the full participation of the child. A reward chart for use with chil-dren who present with somatic complaints is presented in Figure 14.7. With frequently occurring symptoms or illness behaviours, well behaviour should be rewarded more frequently, so briefer time slots need to be written into the left-hand column of the chart. In addition to the reward system, parents may be advised to ignore non-verbal illness behaviours and use children's com-plaints about symptoms as opportunities to prompt them to use symptom management skills.

Relapse management training

Recurrence of illness-related adjustment problems is inevitable with chronic conditions such as asthma, diabetes, epilepsy and migraine. Planning how such recurrences will be managed should be covered in the final sessions of a time-limited episode of psychological intervention. The child and parents may be helped to envisage how they will use the symptom management skills, contingency management procedures and clear communication to manage such relapses.

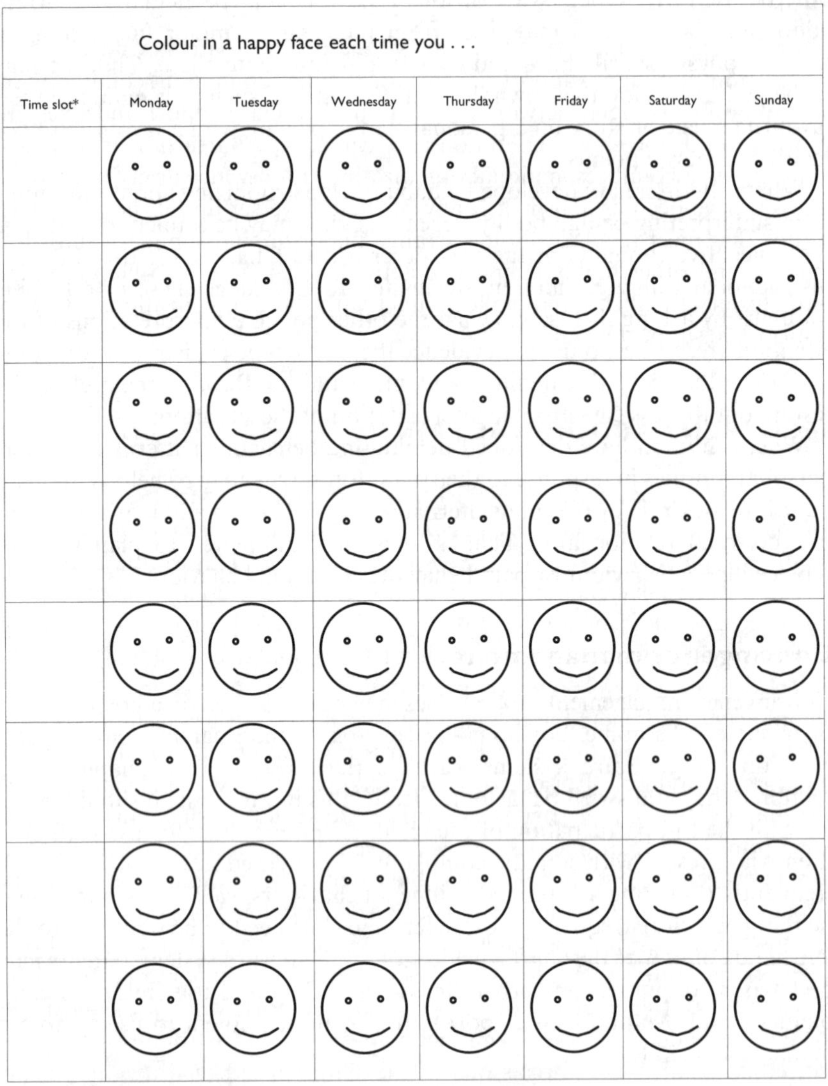

Time slot*	Monday	Tuesday	Wednesday	Thursday	Friday	Saturday	Sunday

Colour in a happy face each time you . . .

Figure 14.7 Child's star chart for use with somatic complaints

* Write in the time period in this column. For symptoms of sick-role behaviour that occur 3–4 times a week or less, a day is a useful time period to use for winning a smiling face for well behaviour. For symptoms of sick-role behaviour that occur 9–10 times a week, a half day is a good time period to use. For very frequent symptoms of sick-role behaviour, an hour may be the appropriate time period.

Support groups

For most chronic illnesses like epilepsy or asthma, parents and children benefit from joining a support network of families containing children with similar problems. Such networks provide both social support and relevant information of the child's condition and available resources for its management. In most countries, national organizations for a wide variety of chronic illnesses have been established. Many of these have set up self-help support groups that meet regularly. Some arrange major annual summer camps for children and other highly supportive activities. It is useful to help families with chronically ill children make contact with these organizations and join appropriate support groups.

RECURRENT ABDOMINAL PAIN

In recurrent abdominal pain (RAP), repeated stomachaches are the central complaint (Banez & Cunningham, 2003; Garralda, 1999; Murphy & Carr, 2000). A typical case of RAP is presented in Box 14.1. RAP may occur as part of a wider constellation of somatic complaints including nausea, vomiting, headache, limb or joint pains. In Table 14.1, Achenbach's empirically derived somatic syndromes for pre-school and school-aged children and adolescents illustrates this type of presentation. RAP occurs in 10–20% of school-aged children and accounts for 2–4% of paediatric consultations. It is most common in the five- to twelve-year age group and is equally common among boys and girls. Episodes of abdominal pain may vary in length from a few minutes to a couple of hours and the frequency of such episodes may vary from more than one daily to a couple of times a month. Episodes of pain may occur at any time of the day but rarely at night. Sometimes episodes of pain occur in anticipation of separation from parents or going to school. In these instances, it is probable that separation anxiety is the central difficulty (separation anxiety is discussed in Chapter 12). Laboratory investigations and a full paediatric examination must be normal for a diagnosis of RAP to be made. RAP often begins with an episode of gastrointestinal illness with abdominal discomfort as one of the symptoms. There are three main courses for the condition. About a third of children with RAP have a good prognosis. About a third develop chronic tension or migraine headaches and about a third continue to have recurrent abdominal pain.

The causes of RAP are still unclear and available evidence has not identified a single constellation of aetiological factors. However, clinical observations and the results of small, uncontrolled studies have led to many interesting hypotheses (Banez & Cunningham, 2003; Garralda, 1999). Abnormal physiological processes which have been suggested to make children vulnerable to the condition include decreased gastrointestinal motility,

Box 14.1 A case of recurrent abdominal pain

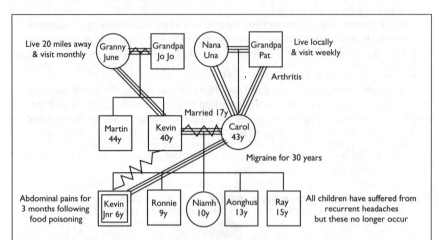

Referral. Kevin was referred by his family doctor because of recurrent abdominal pain. The pains had occurred regularly for three months following an episode of food poisoning. A paediatric evaluation had been conducted and all medical investigations were negative. The family doctor requested a psychological assessment of the condition with a view to psychological treatment. There was a good relationship between the psychologist and the family doctor, who was quite psychologically minded and adopted a similar approach to recurrent abdominal pain as that set out in this chapter.

Presenting problems. In an intake assessment interview with Kevin and his parents, it became clear that the pains were worst in the evening and prevented Kevin from sleeping. His mother would sit with him and rub his stomach to ease the pain. Usually the rest of the family would be watching TV or doing their homework. Eventually Kevin would nod off to sleep. Occasionally he would awake in the night and sometimes the pains would recur. In these instances he would get into his mother's bed and the father, Kevin Senior, would sleep in the son's bed. Carol was supported in her management of the problem in this way by her parents but not by the paternal grandparents.

Often Kevin Senior and Carol would have heated discussions about the problem, its cause and the best way to manage it. Carol believed that the pain was due to residual food poisoning or a viral condition. The original poisoning occurred while on holiday in Spain. The holiday was a disaster. The hotel had not been fully built. The rooms were cramped and Kevin Senior had numerous rows with the management, the other guests and Carol. The holiday had been Carol's idea. The father believed that Kevin's pains were a sham much of the time, but occasionally took the view that they may have been 'abdominal migraine', since all of the other children had suffered from headaches at one point or another in the past and Carol suffered from migraine.

Developmental history and child assessment. Kevin Junior had an unremarkable developmental history. He showed no food intolerances and abdominal X-rays were normal. He was a high achiever at school, meticulous in his work and had a small number of close friends. He was in his second year of primary school when referred. He regularly ate a balanced diet and got regular exercise. He believed that his pains were due to some undiagnosed organic illness and worried about this at night.

Psychometric assessment showed that he was of exceptionally high intelligence and that his problems were quite circumscribed. On a short form of the WISC-III he obtained a FSIQ of 124 and on the WRAT-R his reading quotient was 130. On the CBCL, his scores on all scales fell within the normal range, with the exception of the somatic complaints sub-scale which was within the abnormal range.

Family history. Kevin's mother, Carol, had migraine and Kevin's four siblings had a history of headaches. On the mother's side there was an illness-oriented family culture and the grandfather suffered from arthritis. Carol's family lived nearby and were very close. They also visited regularly and conversed a good deal about Kevin's condition. The father's family lived further away, were less close than the mother's family, visited less frequently and viewed Kevin's difficulties as a minor event that would resolve with the passage of time.

Formulation. Kevin is a very bright six-year-old boy with a three-month history of recurrent abdominal pain, the onset of which was precipitated by an episode of food poisoning. The mother's history of migraine and the siblings' history of headaches suggest that he may be biologically and/or psychosocially pre-disposed to developing pain problems. The pain is currently being maintained by Kevin's anxiety that some organic disease process has not been detected and by his parents' inadvertent reinforcement of his sick-role behaviour. This in turn may be maintained by the parents' difficulty in reaching agreement on how best to manage Kevin's reports of recurrent pain, so that Kevin becomes triangulated between his parents. Differing family cultures and experiences of illness may under-pin this process. Protective factors include the child and parent's wish to work with the team to resolve the problem; the family's success in managing headaches in the past; the high level of support that Kevin obtains from his family and peers; and his high intelligence.

Treatment. Treatment in this case involved a series of family sessions in which the formulation was explained and family members' doubts about it were aired. Kevin's parents were coached in training him in relaxation skills to help him manage episodes of pain. In addition, a reward system was set up, where Kevin earned smiling faces on a face chart for sleeping in his own bed for more than six hours per night. Six faces could be exchanged for a trip to the zoo. The six-session programme led to a resolution of his problems over a period of two months. The tension between Kevin Senior and Carol decreased as treatment progressed.

---

chronic stool retention, lactose intolerance and irritable colon. Stressful life events have been posited as a possible aetiological factor for RAP. Anxiety, depression, difficult temperament, fastidiousness, high-achievement orientation, dependency and inadequate coping strategies are the principal personal characteristics that have been observed in some instances to characterize children with RAP. Hypotheses implicating parental anxiety, depression, pre-occupation with health concerns, a family history of illness and patterns of family interaction that reinforce illness behaviour have also been mentioned in the literature.

Assessment

A full medical paediatric examination should be conducted in all cases of recurrent abdominal pain. Medical conditions which may cause the abdominal pain need to be excluded. These include appendicitis, mesenteric adenitis, urinary tract infection and Crohn's disease.

The protocol set out in Chapter 4 and the framework given in Figure 14.4 may be used to assess youngsters where RAP is the central complaint. Structured self-report questionnaires such as the Varni–Thompson Paediatric Pain Questionnaire (Varni et al., 1987) listed in Table 14.4 may be useful adjuncts to assessment. Pain diaries (such as that presented in Figure 14.5) may be used to monitor fluctuations in pain over the course of assessment and treatment. The child or parent is invited to complete the diary between one and four times per day. On each occasion the severity, duration and location of the pain is recorded along with events that preceded and followed the episode of pain, including medication usage. In such diaries pain intensity may be evaluated using visual analogue scales (such as the five-point scale given in Figure 14.5) for children aged seven and older; the faces pain scale is appropriate for children in the five to seven age range (Bieri et al., 1990). Concrete pain rating methods such as poker chips may be used for younger children (Hester et al., 1990).

Specific issues deserving assessment in the case of RAP are the location, frequency, duration and intensity of the pain and associated features such as nausea, vomiting and other symptoms. A family history of illness, medical and surgical history, previous treatment for abdominal pain and its effectiveness all require evaluation. Children should be asked about the coping strategies they spontaneously use and the effectiveness of these. These may include various forms of distraction or the spontaneous use of tension reduction routines such as deep breathing or relaxation. The consequences of the abdominal pains and the pattern of social interaction that typically occurs with parents, teachers, friends and significant others requires careful scrutiny to assess the degree to which members of the child's family and network are inadvertently reinforcing the pain behaviour and related pain experiences.

Treatment

Results of the assessment should be integrated into a concise formulation where pre-disposing, precipitating, maintaining and protective factors are specified. A case management plan based on the formulation may then be developed. Such an intervention plan should be family based and may include psychoeducation, pain management skills training and contingency management. Well-designed controlled treatment outcome studies using such a package have shown that this type of behavioural family therapy is more effective in the management of RAP than routine paediatric care (Murphy & Carr, 2000). Such family-based behavioural programmes may usefully be supplemented with increased dietary fibre. A controlled trial of increased fibre showed that it can lead to a significant reduction in RAP (Feldman, McGrath, Hodgson, Ritter & Shipman, 1985). Such dietary interventions should be arranged in consultation with a dietician.

Psychoeducation

Psychoeducation should begin by affirming the reality or validity of the child's experience of pain and dispelling the idea that because no current identifiable physiological basis for the child's pain can be found, the pain is therefore not real, feigned, imaginary or a sign of serious psychological disturbance. All pain has both a physical basis and a psychological basis. Physical factors that cause pain include muscle tension, tissue damage and infection. Psychological factors include the attention we give to the pain and our reactions to the sensations we perceive. The following example can be used to explain the role of physical and psychological factors in pain perception: A sailor who is injured while sail-boarding in high winds may feel no pain because he pays little attention to the sensation caused by the tissue damage. The same person may experience excruciating pain for weeks following a stomach upset, because he expects to feel such pain and directs attention to the stomach. Thus, children with RAP have usually begun with a pain determined largely by gastrointestinal infection, tension or tissue damage. This pain then persists because they expect it to, and the expectation may cause tension, which leads to further pain and patterns of behaviour that are used to deal with the pain, like focusing on the pain, talking about it and not engaging in distracting activities like playing or going to school. RAP and the patterns of behaviour associated with it, both the child's and the parents', are like bad habits. RAP can therefore be managed like a habit. The child may be trained in skills to reduce tension and be distracted from the pain. The parents may be coached in how to reward the child for using these pain management skills.

Pain management skills

Pain management skills include self-monitoring, progressive muscle relaxation, breathing exercises, visualization, positive self-instructions and distraction by engaging in competing activities. With self-monitoring, the child is taught how to use a pain diary of the type set out in Figure 14.5. This allows the youngster to see the links between the occurrence of the stomach pains, precipitating specific situations and possible reinforcing events that follow from the occurrence of the pains. They also learn what internal dialogues are associated with the occurrence of the pains.

The muscle relaxation, breathing and visualization exercises described in Chapter 12 for anxiety control may be used with children who have RAP. Youngsters may be trained to use the CTR approach to cognitive restructuring (also described in Chapter 12) to help them cope with pain-inducing cognitions. They may also learn to praise themselves when they cope with pain successfully, by relaxing, challenging pain-inducing thoughts or distracting themselves. Finally, youngsters may be helped to plan lists of competing activities in which they may engage when they experience pain.

Contingency management

Parents may be trained to reinforce all well behaviour with praise and a structured reward chart points system such as that presented in Figure 14.7. They can also be trained to ignore non-verbal pain behaviour and respond to verbal complaints of RAP pain by prompting the child to use pain management skills. With non-RAP pain, parents should be encouraged to respond with appropriate care and attention.

Relapse management

In the final sessions, relapse management may be discussed and families may be encouraged to plan strategies for managing recurrences of abdominal pains.

Sanders, Shepard, Cleghorn & Woolford (1994) found that two key sets of skills that parents and children learned from behavioural family therapy using a programme like this predicted a positive response to treatment. These were the children's use of pain control skills and parents' use of contingency management skills.

When RAP occurs as part of a school-refusal syndrome, and extreme anxiety accompanies early morning episodes of abdominal pain, the approach to assessment and treatment set out in Chapter 12 for school refusal is more appropriate than the protocol offered here.

HEADACHES

Reviews of epidemiological data concur that headaches are common among children and adolescents (Connelly, 2003; Eminson et al., 1996; Garralda, 1999). A conservative estimate based on community surveys is that occasional headaches occur in up to 70% of children and adolescents, and the frequency with which they occur increases with age. Headaches tend to be more common and more severe among girls than boys. Severe recurrent headaches may interfere with psychosocial and academic adjustment and so it is not surprising that headaches account for 1–2% of paediatric consultations. A distinction may be made between tension or migraine headaches. Approximately 11% of five- to fifteen-year-olds in a UK community study met the International Headache Society's diagnostic criteria for migraine (Abu-Arefeh & Russell, 1994). Approximately 30–40% of children show spontaneous remission from headaches within one year. A case example of a child with severe headaches is presented in Box 14.2.

Box 14.2 A case of severe migraine

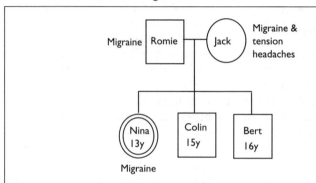

History and presentation. Nina, aged thirteen, who suffered from migraine, was referred by her family doctor for stress management training. The referral occurred at the request of both parents, who also suffered from migraine themselves and the mother in addition suffered from tension headaches which often developed into migraine. Both parents had attended a day-long stress management training programme for adults as part of a staff development programme in a major financial institution where they both held senior positions. Nina's migraine had developed gradually. She had very occasional headaches up until the age of eight and thereafter the frequency and severity of the headaches had increased. She now had one or two a month and found that they interfered with schoolwork, hockey and her social life. The headaches usually occurred on the right side of the head and were preceded by an aura. On some occasions they were precipitated by excitement or stress associated with important hockey matches. On others, they were precipitated by eating chocolate during a period of excitement, for example at Christmas or Easter. Nina's parents were very understanding of her difficulties and encouraged her to withdraw from social interaction when she was having a migraine attack. She would lie in her room and listen to quiet music and take ergotamine. The episodes would typically subside after a night's sleep but sometimes persisted for 48 hours.

Formulation. Nina was a thirteen-year-old who had bimonthly migraine attacks over a four-year period. There was a positive family history for migraine on both the mother and the father's side of the family, so she probably had a biological pre-disposition to developing the condition. Attacks were precipitated by sustained periods of stress and excitement and also by some foods, notably chocolate. She coped well with the attacks using medication and rest and was well supported in this approach by her parents who took an unintrusive approach to her condition.

Treatment. An explanation of migraine following a simplified version of the model set out in Figure 14.8 was given to Nina and her parents. Nina was trained in relaxation and visualization skills in a series of four sessions. She audiotaped these sessions and used the tapes to help her practise the exercises at home. She was also trained to keep a pain diary similar to that presented in Figure 14.5. She was subsequently seen, by arrangement, for two further sessions, each following a migraine attack to review the precipitating events and the effectiveness of the relaxation and visualization skills for pain management. Nina was able to use the relaxation skills to make the pain more bearable. She also found that she tended to catastrophize while in pain and was taught to challenge these stress-inducing thoughts using the CTR method described in Chapter 12 and focus her attention on visualization and relaxation. At follow-up the headaches occurred less frequently and interfered less in her schoolwork and leisure activities.

Tension headaches are very frequent, bilateral, accompanied by dizziness and are experienced as a tight band, a heavy weight or a fullness in the head. Tension headaches are usually associated with stressful, anxiety-provoking situations at home or school. This leads to muscular tension in the muscles of the neck, shoulders and head, which in turn leads to pain.

Migraine is periodic, severe and unilateral accompanied by a visual aura, nausea, vomiting and photophobia. The exact incidence in unknown. A family history of migraine among children with migraine is very common. Migraine attacks usually follow a clear precipitant such as excitement, stress, eating certain foods such as chocolate or cheese, or exposure to stroboscopic effects, e.g. TV, cinema or strobe lights.

Three phases may be distinguished in an episode of migraine (Williamson, 1993). In the first phase, vasoconstriction of the innervated cerebral vascular system and extracranial arteries occurs and leads to decreased oxygenation within these systems and increased serotonin levels in certain areas of the brain. This increase in serotonin is probably what under-pins the prodromal symptoms of migraine. The vasoconstriction which occurs in the first phase of a migraine attack may be caused by any stimuli that lead to intense emotional experiences, by certain foods such as chocolate or cheese, or by stroboscopic effects. In the second phase, rebound extracranial vasodilatation occurs in the non-innervated cerebral vascular system and the extracranial arteries. This is associated with the release of histamine and polypeptides that produce oedema and a reduction in pain threshold. These changes lead to distended arteries and inflammation of the nerves of the blood vessel so that with each pulse of blood through the artery there is a sharp throbbing pain. In the third phase, vascular and biochemical changes return to normal but there may be temporary swelling and tenderness for some hours or days after the headache has ceased.

The perceived intensity of headaches is moderated by three important psychological factors. First, exposure to people who model pain behaviour influences the level of perceived pain. Where children have grown up in families in which one or more members suffered from headaches, or other painful conditions, and displayed pronounced pain-related behaviours, youngsters will experience more intense migraine headaches. Second, the level of perceived pain is influenced by the coping strategies the youngster uses. Youngsters who use active coping strategies to reduce pain experience less intense migraines than youngsters who passively endure the pain. Third, the intensity of experienced pain is influenced by the amount of social reinforcement provided within the family, school and peer group for pain-related behaviour and complaints. Youngsters whose parents, friends and teachers express intense concern about migraine headaches experience more intense pain than those who receive less attention.

Distinguishing between migraine and tension headaches is usually difficult and in some instances both types of headache co-occur or children with tension headaches later develop migraine as well. The onset of migraine rarely occurs before nine years, while tension headaches can occur in very young children. Some theorists reject the categorical classification of head-aches and argue that tension and migraine headaches reflect two ends of a continuum (Williamson, 1993). The model of headaches set out in Figure 14.8 accommodates important aetiological factors that have been identified for both migraine and tension headaches and combined migraine and tension headaches and integrates aspects of previous models of the aetiology of headaches (Andrasik, 1986; Connelly, 2003; Williamson, 1993). It is a useful guide for assessment, formulation and psychoeducation.

Assessment

A full medical paediatric evaluation is essential for children who present with headaches to exclude medical conditions which may under-pin the head-aches. These include infections, head trauma, intracranial pressure, toxic conditions, meningitis, encephalitis and a variety of neurological conditions.

An assessment following the protocol contained in Chapter 4 and the framework given in Figure 14.4 should be conducted and supplemented with information from structured self-report questionnaires such as the Childhood Headaches Questionnaire (Labbé, Williamson & Southard, 1985) or the Revised Headache Symptom Questionnaire (Mindell & Andrasik, 1987), which are described in Table 14.4. Headache diaries, such as that presented in Figure 14.5, may be used to monitor fluctuations in pain over the course of assessment and treatment. With such diaries, the child or parent is invited to make an entry between one and four times per day. On each occa-sion the severity, duration and location of the pain is recorded, along with events that preceded and followed the episode of pain including medication usage.

Specific issues deserving assessment in the case of headaches are the

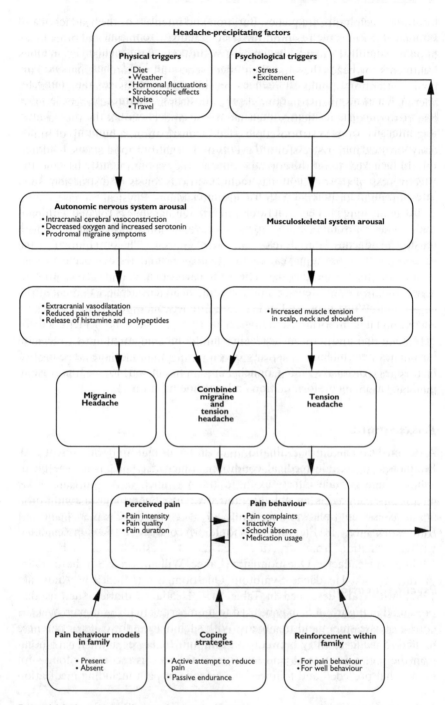

Figure 14.8 Aetiological factors for headaches

location, precipitants, frequency, duration and intensity of the headaches and associated features such as prodromal signs, nausea, vomiting and other areas of pain. A family history of headaches, medical and surgical history, previous treatments for headaches and their effectiveness all require evaluation. Particular attention should be paid to precipitants such as weather changes, allergic reactions, menstruation, changes in sleeping habits, changes in exercise pattern, dietary factors such as cheese and chocolate in the case of migraine, exposure to stroboscopic effects, constipation, a build-up of minor daily stresses, major stressful life events and negative mood states. Children should be asked about the coping strategies they spontaneously use and the effectiveness of these. These may include various forms of distraction, such as solitary play or playing with friends and siblings. Physical exercise, eating and sleeping may also be used by children to regulate pain. To cope with pain some children spontaneously use tension reduction routines such as deep breathing, relaxation to music and autohypnosis. These require routine evaluation. The consequences of the headaches and the pattern of social interaction that typically occurs with parents, teachers, friends and significant others requires careful scrutiny to assess the degree to which members of the child's family and network are inadvertently reinforcing the pain behaviour and related pain experiences.

Information from the assessment should be integrated into a concise formulation in which pre-disposing, precipitating, maintaining and protective factors are specified. A case management plan based on this formulation may then be developed.

Treatment

Results of treatment outcome studies of headaches and other types of childhood pain suggests that effective treatment for tension headaches in children should be based on a multi-modal family-based approach which includes psychoeducation; a reduction of environmental stresses within the family, school and peer group; family-based contingency management and pain management skills training (McGrath & Hiller, 1999; Williamson, 1993).

Psychoeducation

For psychoeducation, a simplified version of the explanation of tension headaches or migraine headaches (presented above) and in Figure 14.8 may be offered to the child and parents. This input may be made when explaining the formulation of the child's problem.

Stress reduction

Stress reduction within the family, school and peer group involves targeting those stresses identified during the assessment and exploring ways that these stresses may be reduced in meetings with relevant members of the child's social network.

Contingency management

In setting up a home-based contingency management programme, parents require guidance on using praise and a reward system such as that described in Chapter 4 to reinforce the child's well behaviour. Ideally, this reward system should be set up with the full participation of the child. The older the child, the more important this participation becomes. In addition to the reward system, an agreement should be reached with the parents and child that non-verbal pain behaviours will be ignored and children's complaints about experiencing pain should be used as opportunities to prompt them to use pain management skills.

Pain management skills

For tension headaches, children may be taught the progressive muscle relaxation, deep breathing skills and visualization techniques described in Chapter 12. EMG biofeedback may also be used to reduce tension but it is no more effective than technologically unaided tension reduction methods. In addition to these tension reduction techniques, youngsters may be coached in the use of cognitive strategies such as distraction, engaging in competing activities and positive self-instructions.

For migraine, a similar programme may be used but with some modifications. Particular attention should be paid to eliminating dietary and other triggers, such as exposure to stroboscopic effects. Migraine-specific medication, such as ergotamine, and thermal biofeedback may also be incorporated into the overall management plan.

CONVERSION SYMPTOMS

Conversion symptoms are motor or sensory symptoms which occur in the absence of a clearly identifiable underlying organic pathology or injury (Garralda, 1992; Pehlivantuerk & Unal, 2002). Conversion symptoms usually follow an injury, illness or accident in which a sensory or motor function was impaired. The loss of function continues despite the absence of an organic basis for the continued dysfunction. The presentation mimics the child's conception of a disorder. Children who develop conversion symptoms have often been sensitized to health problems through family- or school-based experiences. The dysfunction may not correspond to the known anatomical pattern of innervation of the affected organs. For example, children may present with *glove* or *stocking* anaesthesia. Common examples of conversion disorder in children include limb pain with gait abnormalities, numbness or paralysis (following limb injury or accident), chronic cough (following influenza) and pseudoseizures (with epilepsy). Both parents and children are usually strongly opposed to a psychological explanation for the physical symptoms and point to the genesis of the disorder in a well-founded organic illness or physical injury. Thus conversion symptoms are often maintained by the way in which the child is treated by family members and other members of the child's social network, and by the pay-offs associated with the conversion symptoms for the child. Thus, the parents and other members of the child's social network may inadvertently reinforce the child's illness behaviour by offering the child subtle privileges for behaving in a way consistent with a physical illness. The child may unconsciously adopt the symptoms to avoid feared, conflictual or challenging situations and so reduce negative affect. For example, symptoms may permit the expression of socially unacceptable aggression or dependency, without having to reap the consequences of expressing such emotions. Conversion disorder has a favourable outcome but residual mood and anxiety disorders may persist after recovery from conversion symptoms. A history of severe physical or sexual abuse and hypnotic suggestibility are both pre-disposing risk factors for developing conversion symptoms (Roelofs et al., 2002a,b). Children with a high level of hypnotic susceptibility have a greater ability to dissociate. They or their parents can suggest that they have physical complaints and the children genuinely experience these physical symptoms. However, they lack insight that the symptoms arise from suggestion rather than a pre-dominantly physical aetiology. Children exposed to abuse who later develop conversion symptoms probably used dissociation as an effective short-term method for coping with trauma-related negative affect, and in later life continue to unconsciously use dissociation and conversion to cope with challenging situations to reduce negative affect. However, many children with conversion symptoms have not experienced abuse. An example of a case of conversion hysteria is presented in Box 14.3.

Assessment

Close liaison between the clinical psychologist, the family doctor and all members of the paediatric medical team is essential in the management of cases of conversion disorder. A thorough paediatric medical evaluation should be conducted and a full child and family assessment following the guidelines set out in Chapter 4 and the framework given in Figure 14.4. Specific attention should be paid to the avoidance function of the symptom,

Box 14.3 A case of conversion symptoms

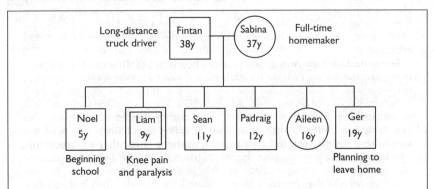

Referral. Liam was referred by a paediatrician because of persistent knee pain and paralysis of the right leg. The pain followed an incident where his brother Ger, aged 18 at the time, jumped on him accidentally while at the swimming pool. This incident occurred about 6 months before he was referred to the psychology service. There was initially some bruising and the possibility of some torn ligaments. However, the family doctor saw it as a minor injury and was surprised when Liam returned to him repeatedly with the condition becoming gradually worse, until finally, Liam could no longer walk without a crutch and found the leg was hypersensitive to touch.

History of medical treatment. Both parents, Fintan and Sabina, were convinced that Liam had a serious injury requiring orthopaedic attention. A referral was made in the first instance to a paediatrician, and subsequently to an orthopaedic surgeon and physiotherapist, who all took the view that physiological factors could not account for the extent of disability. Throughout this process, the parents became more and more convinced that some important investigation had been over-looked, or that the results of X-rays and the physiotherapist's assessment had been inaccurate or misinterpreted. The case was subsequently referred back to the paediatrician and then on to psychology. Both parents strongly opposed the referral.

Developmental history. Liam's developmental history was essentially normal and his current academic and peer-group adjustment were within normal limits. At school, he missed playing football and hoped that he would recover and be able to play again soon. He attended a local primary school with his brother Noel, aged 5 years.

Family situation. At home, Liam and Noel were the central focus for their mother's attention. The father, Fintan, was a long-distance lorry driver and spent little time at home. Also the siblings spent much of the time away from home. Sean, aged 11 years; Padraig, aged 12 years; and Aileen aged 16 years were all at secondary school and commuted a long distance each day so they left home early and did not arrive home until seven in the evening. Ger commuted to university and was due to leave home within a few months to live on campus because the travelling was very tiring. Sabina, the mother, would collect Liam and Noel from school each day and drive them home. A regular topic of conversation was the inadequate medical care that Liam had received. However, there was no talk of suing the swimming-pool management for compensation. All family members were fit and healthy. Within the wider extended family, there were no major physical or psychological problems.

Responsivity of the symptom to suggestion. During a family assessment interview, Liam was invited to relax and visualize the hot-air balloon scene described elsewhere in the chapter. Once in a light trance he was invited to anaesthetize the pain in his leg and walk unaided, which he did without any problem, to the surprise of his parents and siblings. Once out of the trance the pain and paralysis returned as expected.

Formulation. Liam was a nine-year-old boy who presented with conversion symptoms: specifically a pain in his left knee and related paralysis, which prevented him from walking unaided. Liam may have been pre-disposed to developing these symptoms because of his high level of suggestibility. The onset of the symptoms was precipitated by a knee injury which subsequently healed satisfactorily. The symptoms have probably been maintained by Liam's interactions with significant members of his network including parents, siblings and healthcare professionals, who have conflicting views about the role of tissue damage or disease processes in the aetiology of the symptoms. Because of the health professional's lack of certainty about the cause of the symptoms, his parents have stated their beliefs that a physical illness or injury has gone unnoticed in very strong terms repeatedly in Liam's presence. With his high level of suggestibility, this has led to the persistence of his pain experience. Protective factors in this case include the family support available to Liam, and the willingness of his parents to participate in a psychological assessment process about which they have serious reservations.

Treatment. There were three subsequent family meetings in which Liam and his parents were presented with the formulation and offered an opportunity to discuss their doubts about it. Both parents were trained to help Liam enter a light trance, anaesthetize his leg and walk unaided and they conducted this procedure at home with Liam on a regular basis, gradually extending the distance walked. Liam discarded his crutch and began to walk with a stiff leg within a month of the first consultation. At follow-up a year later he was playing football again.

the communicative function of the symptom and patterns of social interaction that maintain the symptoms.

As part of the assessment process, the degree to which the child's symptoms may be altered through suggestion may be evaluated. The child is helped to enter a trance and then to perform actions that involve either losing the symptom (for example, moving a paralysed limb) or making the symptom occur (for example, having a pseudoseizure) while in the trance. This may be accomplished by helping the child achieve a relaxed state, using the relaxation and visualization routine described in Chapter 12 and then helping them enter a light trance using the *hot-air balloon method*. Here, the child is invited to imagine that he or she is in a hot-air balloon and, as this rises up off the ground and flies higher and higher into the sky, the child's trance deepens. Once children can clearly visualize that they are in the balloon and stationary over their own house or school, they should indicate this by moving the index finger. The child may then be invited to do an action within the hot-air balloon that involves them losing their conversion symptom. For example, a child with an arm paralysis may be asked to wave to the people below the balloon on the ground. A child with leg paralysis may be invited to stand up and look over the edge of the balloon's basket so that he or she can see the house below. A child who has pseudoseizures may be invited to lie down on the floor of the hot-air balloon basket and have a seizure and then to terminate the seizure at will (Levine, 1994). Particular care needs to be taken in this type of assessment to ensure the child's safety. At the end of the assessment, the child may be asked to land the balloon gently and open his or her eyes.

My own practice is to conduct this part of the assessment in a family interview, so the parents and siblings can see the degree to which the symptoms are influenced by suggestion. However, it should be stressed to parents that this is only an assessment, not treatment. Any alteration in conversion symptoms that occurs during such assessment exercises is temporary.

A comprehensive formulation in which pre-disposing, precipitating, maintaining and protective factors are specified should be drawn up on the basis of salient features drawn from the assessment. A treatment plan based on the formulation may then be developed.

Treatment

Once the team has reached agreement on the diagnosis of conversion disorder and developed a formulation, arrangements should be made to communicate this diagnosis and formulation and the team's agreement about it to the child and family.

Presenting the formulation

This feedback process should be arranged so that a number of goals are met. First, the child's experience of the symptoms as real (rather than imaginary or feigned) should be affirmed. There should be no argument about the fact that children experience the paralysis or seizures or whatever the symptoms may be, as outside their control. Second, the parents' management of the symptoms should be affirmed. Thus, they need to be told that they have done a good job of coping with a confusing set of symptoms that have baffled other healthcare professionals. Third, the organic basis for the physical illness that preceded the development of the conversion symptoms should be highlighted. Fourth, the fact that the infection, tissue damage, muscle tension or other organic factors that under-pinned these symptoms are now absent should be made clear and the fact that this is very good news and bodes well for the child's recovery. Fifth, the current symptoms may be described as an after-effect of the organic illness that has persisted as a set of habits and that the child's body needs to learn how to break these habits by gradually resuming a normal lifestyle. Sixth, the parents' role in helping the child assume this lifestyle may be defined in light of the formulation, although explicit reference to it may not be necessary or appropriate in all cases.

Contingency management

The parents' role, it may be explained, is to supervise and reward the child for developing a symptom-free lifestyle. This involves them encouraging the child to achieve age-appropriate autonomy and to express concern about issues that trouble them, since bottling these up may cause stress and make the symptoms return. These issues, it may be explained, probably include the child's perception of parental conflict or the child's perceptions of parental expectations for achievement. The importance of discussing the discrepancy between children's perceptions of such issues and parental perceptions of such issues should be noted. A series of sessions of psychological consultation may be offered to the parents and the child in which discussions of these discrepancies are facilitated and which have the explicit aim of supporting the parents in achieving these goals of helping the child give up the sick role, communicating more clearly and drawing age-appropriate boundaries between parents and children.

Parent–child tasks

Within subsequent sessions, for motor conversion symptoms and paralysis, parents may be invited to supervise the child carrying out daily exercises prescribed by the physiotherapist. Parents may be advised to use a reward system to motivate their child to complete their daily exercises. Successive approximations to asymptomatic behaviour may be rewarded. For pseudo-seizures, parents may be trained to help their children to gain control over these. Daily practice sessions may be arranged within which the parent helps the child to plan to have seizures by closing their eyes and willing the seizure to occur after a count of three and then wakening from the seizure after a further count of three. Once children learn to induce the seizures, they have a sense of control over them and so can learn to prevent them.

Pitfalls

The main pitfall with this type of approach is to offer the family the opinion of the team before there is complete agreement among members of all disciplines that the diagnosis is a conversion disorder. Lack of consensus on the part of team members may fuel the family's confusion about the condition and entrench the patterns of interaction that maintain the child's problems. A second pitfall is to offer to conduct further medical investigations when all team members are confident that the results will be negative. If the team has reached an opinion based on a thorough multi-disciplinary assessment then the family should not be confused by being told that on the one hand the team is certain and on the other team members want to do more tests. A third pitfall is to enter into a symmetrical battle with the parents or the child about the reality of the symptoms or the validity of the diagnosis. The team should adopt a clear position that the symptoms are real (not imaginary or feigned) and the diagnosis is valid, but respect the family's right to reject this viewpoint and to seek a second opinion. Attempts to convince the family of the validity of the diagnosis, or to coerce them into accepting it, tend to confuse and upset parents and children. For a proportion of cases it will not be possible for parents and children to accept a diagnosis of conversion disorder and the child will become socialized into the role of a chronic invalid.

In a minority of cases where conversion symptoms occur as a reaction to child sexual abuse, local child protection procedures should be followed. The management of child sexual abuse is described in Chapter 21.

CHRONIC FATIGUE SYNDROME

Chronic fatigue syndrome is characterized by persistent physical and mental fatigue, which is made worse by exercise, accompanied by a range of other symptoms including low activity levels, social withdrawal from peer-group activities, school non-attendance, low mood, headaches and muscle pains, sore throat and flu symptoms, insomnia or hypersomnia, and loss of appetite (Chalder, 2005; Garralda & Rangel, 2002; Lines, 2004; Richards, 2000). The condition occurs in 0.19% of eleven- to fifteen-year-olds and about 50% of cases meet the diagnostic criteria for anxiety or depression. In the past, the condition has been known as chronic fatigue immune dysfunction syndrome, fatigue dysphoria syndrome, post-viral-fatigue syndrome, myalgic encephalomyelitis, epidemic neuromyasthenia and neurasthenia, although in ICD 10 neurasthenia is distinguished from chronic fatigue syndrome. The degree of disability shown by children suffering from fatigue syndrome is extraordinary and may exceed that shown by children with juvenile arthritis or cystic fibrosis. Chronic fatigue syndrome usually develops during a viral illness but remains after the illness has cleared. So viral illness is the most common precipitating factor. Typically, medical and laboratory investigations are negative. A personal coping style characterized by emotional sensitivity, anxiety, rigidity, over-dependency and over-conformity with parental authority; a build-up of life stresses at home, school and in the peer group, and with which the child has difficulty coping using these strategies; and consequent immunosupression are possible pre-disposing factors. The build-up of stresses may involve fear of academic, athletic or social failure. These fears may be associated with inappropriately high personal or family expectations. The absence of good personal and family coping skills, exclusively biological attributions for the child's experience of chronic fatigue and related symptoms, fear that the condition may deteriorate further and consequent avoidance of activity which exacerbates fatigue, inadvertent parental reinforcement of children's inactivity and poor co-ordination and lack of consistency in the formulation and management offered by the professional network are possible maintaining factors. Better outcome occurs in cases of high socioeconomic status, where there is a clear precipitating factor, when the onset occurs in the autumn, when the duration of fatigue is less than a year and where active coping that counters the cycle of avoidance, such as carefully planned home tuition, are present and where the professional network offers a clear coherent formulation and management plan. Best clinical practice involves thorough multi-disciplinary assessment and the implementation of family-based treatment programmes, which include psychoeducation, self-monitoring of activity and of rest and sleep patterns; graded increase in activity levels and regularization of the sleep–waking cycle; contingency management; home–school liaison and coping skills training. Recovery occurs in over two-thirds of cases.

Assessment

Close liaison between the clinical psychologist, the family doctor and all members of the paediatric medical team is essential in the management of cases of chronic fatigue syndrome to avoid giving children and families mixed messages about the diagnosis and management plan. A thorough paediatric medical evaluation should be conducted and a full child and family assessment following the guidelines set out in Chapter 4 and the framework given in Figure 14.4. Specific attention should be paid to the role of the pre-disposing precipitating, maintaining and protective factors mentioned in the previous section. A comprehensive formulation in which pre-disposing, precipitating, maintaining and protective factors are specified should be drawn up on the basis of salient features drawn from the assessment. A treatment plan based on the formulation may then be developed.

Treatment

Once the multi-disciplinary team has reached agreement on the diagnosis of chronic fatigue syndrome and developed a formulation, arrangements should be made to communicate this diagnosis and formulation and to highlight the team's agreement about it to the child and family. In light of this, a management plan may be offered (Chalder, 2005).

Psychoeducation and presentation of the formulation

This feedback process should be arranged so that a number of goals are met. First, the child's experience of fatigue should be affirmed as distressing, and the lack of engagement in activities as understandable. Second, the parents' management of the symptoms should be affirmed. Their tendency to support the child's inactivity because of the apparent negative consequences of exercise and academic and social activities should be described as understandable and a legitimate response to the condition. Parents need to be told that they have done a good job of coping with their child's fatigue and related symptoms. Third, the build-up of stresses in the school, the peer group and at home, and the ways in which these were coped with by the child and the probable under-functioning of the child's immune system should be proposed. Fourth, the key role of viral infection in triggering the flu-like symptoms and fatigue should be identified as the starting point of the chronic fatigue syndrome. Fifth, the current symptoms may be described as an after-effect of the viral infection and under-functioning of the immune system, which is partly maintained by lack of exercise, lack of engagement in school and peer-group activities, and a disrupted sleep–waking cycle. Sixth, the slow and gradual return to a normal lifestyle involving a regular sleep pattern and a gradual increase in activity should be presented as the central focus of the management plan. An analogy may be drawn with an athlete who has become unfit after an injury and who requires a careful programme of graded exercise to regain peak fitness. Seventh, the parents' role in supporting the child's gradual and graded return to normal activity level may be highlighted. An analogy may be drawn with the role of a coach in helping an unfit athlete return to peak fitness through facilitating a gradual daily increase in exercise and a gradual regularization of sleep and dietary patterns. The programme may be offered as a series of fifteen to twenty family sessions spaced at weekly, fortnightly and later monthly intervals over a period of nine to twelve months. Self-help reading material may be given to the family (Chalder, 1995; Chalder & Hussain, 2002).

Self-monitoring and goal setting

Children and parents may be invited to keep a daily diary in which a detailed record is kept of the child's daily activity, rest and sleeping patterns. This diary should be kept throughout treatment to monitor progress. Following a one- or two-week baseline period, an estimate may be made of the amount of time spent each day engaging in activities, resting and sleeping. In light of this information, overall long-term treatment goals may be set, as well as short-term weekly targets. Weekly targets should aim to gradually increase the amount of time engaged in specific physical, academic and peer-group activities and decrease the amount of time resting each day by a specified set amount. The longer-term goal should be to restore a reasonable level of daily activity with short rest periods. Weekly targets for regularizing the sleep–waking cycle should also be set, with the long-term aim of helping the child establish a pattern of sleeping eight to ten hours per night with regular retiring and waking times.

Graded increased activity scheduling

Over the course of treatment, daily targets should be set to gradually increase activity levels, decrease rest periods, eliminate cat-naps and routinize the timing and duration of night-time sleep. Specific daily targets should cover physical exercise (e.g. walking for 10 minutes twice a day and keeping going even when this is very challenging), academic activity (e.g. attending school for an hour a day or doing thirty minutes supervised study per day), peer-group activities (e.g. having friends round for an hour a day), resting (e.g. resting without cat-napping during the day) and sleeping (e.g. retiring at 11 p.m. and rising at 8 a.m. each day).

Contingency management

The parents' role, it may be explained, is to supervise and reward the child for developing a lifestyle that includes gradually increasing levels of activity, shorter rest periods, a regular sleep–waking cycle and a reduced conversational focus on health issues. Smiling face charts like that in Figure 14.7, a points system or a token system may all be used to reward children regularly for achieving daily activity targets, rest and sleep targets. These daily points, tokens or smiling faces may be accumulated and exchanged for valued rewards on a weekly basis.

Home–school liaison

Meetings involving the child, parents and relevant school staff and home tutors (if such tutors are involved) should be set up to plan a gradual increase in the child's school attendance and activity level while in school.

Coping skills training

Children with chronic fatigue syndrome may have developed avoidant coping strategies (such as avoiding exercise) and hold unhelpful beliefs such as 'My fatigue is due to biological factors and so requires a medical cure', 'I can't increase my activity levels or I will become exhausted', 'I must be very good at sports or schoolwork otherwise I will be failure', 'I'm so far behind in my schoolwork, there is no point in returning now'. In place of avoidant coping strategies, children may be encouraged to carefully plan a graded increase in activity. Maladaptive beliefs may be countered using the Challenge Test Reward (CTR) method described in Chapter 12 (p. 514). Where children have co-morbid anxiety or depression, treatment protocols described in Chapters 12 and 16 may be used.

PREPARATION FOR PAINFUL MEDICAL AND DENTAL PROCEDURES

In a paediatric setting, clinical psychologists may be asked to consult to cases where children are undergoing painful medical procedures. These include routine injections but also more complex painful procedures, such as the management of burns, bone marrow aspirations and lumbar punctures. In dental settings, fear of pain associated with drilling and extractions may lead to a referral to psychology (Blount, Piira & Cohen, 2003; Murphy & Carr, 2000; Sarafino, 2001).

A number of psychological interventions have been shown to be useful to help children to manage painful medical and dental procedures. All of these have maximum benefit when learned and used within the context of a supportive network, which ideally includes the child's parents as well as the psychologist and other members of the treatment team. The specific pain-control techniques include preparatory psychoeducation, modelling, giving the child some degree of control over the procedure, giving the child permission to cry and express distress, distraction, relaxation, visualization, auto-hypnosis, re-framing and self-instruction, desensitization, reward systems and parental involvement.

Psychoeducation

With preparatory psychoeducation, the central feature of treatment is giving children both objective procedural information about the specific medical or dental procedure they will undergo and subjective sensory information about the sensations they will experience when undergoing the procedure. With an injection, procedural information includes the fact that the skin will first be disinfected, the needle will be inserted, the plunger of the syringe will be pushed slowly, the needle will be withdrawn, and a small piece of cotton wool will be placed over the little needle-hole and will be secured with an elasto-plaster. Sensory information about the same event would be that the disinfectant will be cold, the insertion of the needle will be like a small pinch, they will not feel much when the plunger is being depressed but when the needle is withdrawn and a bandage put on the injection site it will feel a bit tight for a few minutes. It is crucial that the psychologist be fully familiar with the procedure in order to give children accurate sensory and procedural information. Pictures, diagrams and videotapes may be used to give this procedural and sensory information to the child.

An important issue is the most effective way to give sensory and procedural information to children. While there is little literature on this issue for paediatric populations, the literature on pain management in adults indicates that people tend to have a preference for one of two broad coping strategies when faced with painful medical and dental procedures. With the first of these, the patients actively seek information about the anticipated procedure and use this information to rehearse the way in which they will cope with the painful event. The second strategy is to passively avoid information and engage in distracting activities. A series of studies reviewed by Sarafino (2001) suggests that prospective patients who habitually use a passive, avoidant coping style, require more frequent and intensive exposure to procedural and sensory information to desensitize them to it and equip them to use more active coping strategies when they face a painful medical procedure. Brief psych-oeducational interventions with people who habitually use a passive avoidant coping style may sensitize them to the painful medical procedure and they may actually experience more pain than if they were given no information! The implications of this interpretation of available data on coping styles for the management of children is as follows. A careful assessment of whether children typically use an active or a passive coping style should be incorpor-ated into the psychoeducational intervention. Where children indicate that they would rather not think about the procedure, additional time may be scheduled to allow them to overcome this avoidance and to familiarize themselves extensively with the relevant procedural and sensory information.

Modelling and rehearsal

With modelling, child are offered an opportunity to see another child or surrogate going through the medical procedure for which they are being pre-pared. Videotapes of other children going through similar procedures, puppets or dolls may be used as models. It is important for the models used in demonstrations of the procedures to make statements about their sensory experiences and to give an account of their coping strategies. Modelling is usefully coupled with rehearsal where the child role-plays going through the procedure using coping strategies to manage the pain. An alternative to role-play is for the child to enact the procedure with dolls or puppets and verbalize the experiences and coping strategies used by the doll or the puppet. For example, injection procedures may be modelled using a doll and a toy syringe set. Following this, the child may re-enact the injection procedure and take the role of the nurse giving the doll the injection and instructing the doll in how to cope with the procedure (Ioannou, 1991).

Giving control

Giving children a sense of control over some aspect of the procedure reduces pain. The psychologist may find out from the members of the medical or dental team what aspects of the procedure may be placed under the child's control and incorporate this into control training. For example, children facing a painful dental procedure may be informed that there is a red button on the arm of the dentist's chair and that if they push this the drill will stop.

Thus, they can be reassured that they will never have to face more discomfort than they can withstand.

Another way in which children may be offered control is to give them permission to cry as loud as they wish and to express as much distress as they wish without fear of embarrassment or disapproval.

Distraction

Helping the child to focus on something other than the medical or dental procedure and the related pain sensations is the key feature of distraction. It is important that the distracting stimuli be complex and interesting enough to hold the child's attention and that the stimuli are age appropriate. Pre-schoolers may be distracted by nursery rhymes, particularly those involving distracting sensory routines such as round-and-round-the-garden-goes-the-teddy-bear. Also for pre-schoolers, toys that engage the child's attention for a few minutes at a time and require little activity, such as a jack in the box, are useful distracters. Story books with pictures are also useful distracters for the younger child. With school-going children hand-held videogames are sufficiently engrossing to distract many youngsters from painful medical procedures. Number games, such as counting by 5s or doing mental arithmetic are also possible distracters.

Relaxation

An approach to teaching children progressive muscle relaxation, breathing and visualization skills is presented in Chapter 12, which deals with anxiety. Youngsters who are facing painful medical procedures may be coached using similar techniques.

Autohypnosis

There is substantial evidence to show that hypnosis may be used to manage acute and chronic pain and related anxiety (Hart & Hart, 1996; Olness & Gardner, 1988). The more hypnotizable the child, the better the outcome for acute pain. Hypnotizability may be assessed using the Stanford Hypnotic Scale for Children (Morgan & Hilgard, 1979). There are many induction techniques. With pre-adolescent children, I use a technique where children close their eyes and imagine themselves going on a journey in a hot-air balloon and leaving the pain and anxiety behind. The suggestion of rising in the balloon and flying further away is used to help youngsters deepen their trance. They are then invited to imagine that the particular area where the pain will be localized has become as cold as ice and then that it has become completely numb. This suggestion is repeated a number of times. This procedure can induce a marked degree of anaesthesia. Significant skill in inducing such anaesthesia may be learned in a couple of pre-procedural sessions and taperecording therapy sessions may be used to help children develop self-hypnosis skills which they can then use during painful medical and dental procedures.

Re-framing and self-instruction

With re-framing, the child is coached in how to imagine that the painful procedure is occurring within a context that is less pain inducing than the medical or dental setting (such as receiving an injury while scoring a goal in a football match) or that the experience is not pain but some other sensation (such as tightness). Children may be shown how to use self-instructions to redirect their attention (e.g. 'I'm thinking about my holidays'), to define themselves as coping adequately (e.g. 'I'm doing well. I'm brave') and to reward themselves for coping (e.g. 'Great! I did it').

Desensitization

For children who show high levels of fear and avoidance of dental or medical procedures, a hierarchy of approximations to the procedure may be developed and the child may be offered an opportunity to cope with each of these using relaxation and other coping skills. For example, with a needle phobia, the steps of the hierarchy may include:

- looking at an encased needle
- touching an encased needle
- touching a needle which has been removed from its case
- placing the needle on the skin
- piercing the top layer of tough skin of the index finger with the needle
- placing the tip of the needle at the injection site
- receiving an injection.

Throughout each desensitization session, the child should be instructed to regularly report his or her anxiety level on a ten-point scale. Children may progress from one step in the hierarchy to the next when their anxiety level has reached a peak and then declined significantly. If children attempt to cope with a step in the hierarchy but then withdraw before their anxiety has reached a peak and begun to decline, they become sensitized to the feared stimulus and the treatment programme actually makes their anxiety increase rather than decrease. In light of this, it is critical to explain all this to parents and children before contracting to complete a desensitization programme. Children should feel confident that they have mastered relaxation, distraction and self-instructional coping skills before beginning a desensitization session.

Reward systems

Throughout the process of psychoeducation, coaching children in pain management prior to a painful procedure and managing pain during the procedure, children may be rewarded for all approximations to adequate coping with praise and approval. Where children have particularly strong fears of the procedure and desensitization is necessary, a reward system may be used to reward the child with points or tokens for each step in the desensitization programme, and these points may be used for obtaining valued reinforcers. Finally, a highly valued prize may be awarded for having the courage to complete the medical or dental procedure. This type of reward will have maximum benefit as a pain management strategy if the child selects the prize before the event and is encouraged to anticipate receiving it during the procedure.

Family involvement

Except in instances where parents are very anxious about medical or dental procedures, complete parental involvement in pain management programmes is advised, since available research shows that for children the presence of parents is rated as the single most effective pain control strategy (Lansdown & Sokel, 1993). Parents may attend all sessions and be shown how to engage the child in practising the skills learned in the sessions at home.

ASTHMA

Asthma is a reversible reactive airway disease (Sarafino, 2001). About 3% of children have asthma and 80% of all asthmatics have their first episode in childhood; 50% of asthmatic children grow out of their condition by adulthood. However, there is no way to tell who will grow out of asthma and who will not. A small but significant proportion of children die from asthma and this number is increasing every year. A case example of asthma is presented in Box 14.4.

The central feature of an asthma attack is bronchial constriction. Asthma attacks begin when the immune system produces antibodies that cause the bronchial tubes to release histamine. Histamine causes the smooth muscles in the walls of the smaller air passages of the lungs (the bronchi and bronchioles, which are controlled by the autonomic nervous system) to become inflamed, contract and produce mucus. These secretions accumulate and the walls of the air passages swell. Tissue damage may occur as a result of this swelling and make future attacks more likely. The child has difficulty breathing and cannot cough-up the secretions. The lungs tend to become over-filled with air and the chest cavity becomes over-expanded. As the attack continues, the child has more and more difficulty breathing. Wheezing occurs. Less and

Box 14.4 A case of asthma

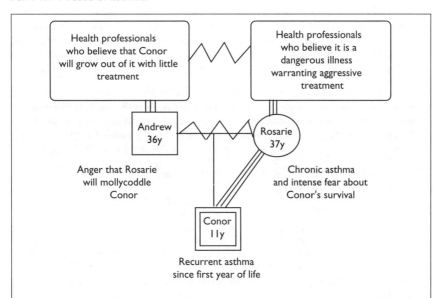

Referral. Conor, an eleven-year-old boy, with a lifelong history of asthma, was referred because the frequency of his attacks had increased to two a month over the preceding year. Conor was an only child of high average ability, who had an outstanding academic record. He was also an accomplished chess player. Despite his interest in soccer, his asthma prevented him from playing. However, when he did play he was very talented.

History of the problem. His attacks occurred when he developed chest infections (which he often did) and when he engaged in physical exercise. He avoided situations where he would be exposed to dust and cats or dogs, since he was allergic to them. His mother, Rosarie, usually treated his attacks with oral corticosteroids and salbutimol delivered by inhaler or a nebulizer. She would sleep in his bed, or keep an all-night vigil to ensure that he continued to breath. She feared that he would have a hypoxic seizure. The father, Andrew, tolerated this approach but occasionally argued with Rosarie about it, since he thought that she was mollycoddling Conor and preventing him from becoming an athlete. On some of these occasions the couple would refer to conflicting advice given by the various child health professionals that they had consulted regarding Conor's condition. A stalemate would develop. Usually, Rosarie brought Conor to the family doctor or the hospital alone, and Andrew would withdraw into his work responsibilities.

Family history. During a family assessment interview, it became clear that Rosarie's fears about Conor were based on the experience of the exacerbation of her own asthma, which occurred during her pregnancy with Conor. She had a bad attack and on one occasion almost passed out from lack of oxygen. Andrew's views were based on the belief that illness is made worse by too much attention and that illness is a sign of weakness. These were views held strongly by both of Andrew's parents.

Formulation. The formulation in this case was that Conor was pre-disposed to asthma because of a genetically inherited physiological vulnerability and also because of the anxiety-laden and illness-sensitive family environment into which he was born. Episodes of asthma were precipitated by exercise-related arousal and infection. They were maintained by the emotionally intense interaction pattern of triangulation involving Conor and his parents. This in turn was maintained by conflicting views about the management of asthma given by other involved health professionals.

Treatment. The formulation was presented to Conor and his parents in a family session and subsequently the boy and the parents were seen separately for four sessions each. Conor was trained to independently manage his asthma on a day-to-day basis: to use his inhalers, to avoid precipitants; to check his peak-flow meter and to keep a diary of these activities. Concurrently his parents were invited to explore ways that they could allow Conor to have increased independence in managing his asthma and ways in which they could minimize the degree to which they exposed Conor to their intense feelings of concern about his condition. They agreed to ban all talk of asthma in his presence unless he reported that his peak-flow meter fell below a level set by the family doctor. Once this limit was breached, Andrew was to bring him to the family doctor for an immediate assessment. This plan was discussed and agreed with the family doctor and paediatrician. In addition, Rosarie was encouraged to join a support group for parents of children with asthma, and use that forum to discuss her intense feelings about Conor's condition. The family doctor, some months later, reported that a reduction in the frequency of asthma attacks occurred.

less oxygen is taken in. The child becomes pale and the lips take on a blue tinge. If the attack persists without treatment, the child becomes unconscious, develops seizures due to lack of oxygen and may suffer brain damage due to hypoxia; severe attacks of asthma may be fatal. In recent years, fatalities due to asthma have increased; deaths are associated with hypoxic seizures, previous respiratory arrest, non-adherence to medication regime, poor self-care and family dysfunction (Mrazek, 2002).

Both physiological and psychosocial pre-disposing factors have been identified for asthma. At a physiological level, children may be genetically pre-disposed to developing asthma. Such children typically have relatives who have suffered from asthma, allergies, hay-fever or eczema. All of these conditions reflect the presence of an atopic constitution. Evidence is growing that immunoglobulin E (IgE) plays a central role in the mechanism under-pinning symptom expression in asthma and that the regulation of IgE antibody level is under genetic control. A history of viral respiratory infections in infancy may also pre-dispose youngsters to developing asthma. Such infections may damage the respiratory system, rendering it sensitive to certain triggering conditions. At a psychological level, parental beliefs about asthma may lead them to interact with their children and other family members in anxiety-provoking ways (Miller & Wood, 1991). High levels of family anxiety may pre-dispose youngsters, particularly those with a genetic vulnerability to developing asthma. Parents who have suffered from asthma themselves, or who have watched their siblings or parents cope with asthma, may have developed inaccurate and unhelpful beliefs about the condition. For example, many mothers with severe asthma experience a worsening of their condition during pregnancy. This first-hand experience of severe asthma may lead such mothers to believe that their child is in constant danger of respiratory arrest and therefore warrants continual monitoring and very close supervision. On the other hand, parents who have not experienced asthma themselves, but who have grown up in families where siblings have suffered from asthma, may harbour considerable hostility towards the siblings for claiming the lion's share of parental attention. When they find that their own children suffer from asthma they may adopt a critical stance and view the symptoms as a sign of weakness or attention-seeking behaviour. Suggestibility may also be a pre-disposing factor, since there is clear evidence that bronchodilation and constriction can be influenced by suggestion, particularly in suggestible youngsters (Isenberg, Lehrer & Hochron, 1992).

Asthma attacks may be precipitated by allergy, infection, physical exercise, cold air or psychological factors that lead to autonomic arousal. Common allergens that cause asthma attacks are dust, pollen, cat and dog hair, air pollution and house-dust mites. Psychological factors which may lead to hyperarousal and precipitate an asthma attack include stresses within the family, school or peer group that pose an immediate threat to the person's perceived safety or security and so cause anger or anxiety. These stresses include rigid repetitive patterns characterized by enmeshment or over-involvement with a highly anxious parent; triangulation, where the child is required, usually covertly, to take sides with one or other parent in a conflict; or a chaotic family environment where parents institute no clear rules and routines for children's daily activities or medication regime when asthma attacks are likely to occur.

The child's breathing difficulties during an attack can be extremely distressing, both for the child and the parents. The distressing nature of the respiratory symptoms and the fact that asthma may be fatal, may lead some children and their parents to respond to asthma with considerable anxiety, which in turn may exacerbate or maintain the symptoms. Alternatively, where parents view asthma as a sign of weakness or attention seeking, the child's anticipation of the parents' punitive or neglectful response to the attacks may exacerbate or maintain the attacks. There is also considerable variability in the ways in which family physicians and paediatricians respond to asthma. Some intervene early with aggressive treatment whereas others intervene later with a less intensive approach. Such variability may be confusing for parents, who themselves are uncertain how to proceed when an attack begins. This confusion fuels parental anxiety, which in turn increases the child's arousal level and exacerbates or maintains the condition.

Asthma, particularly if it is poorly controlled, may lead to learning difficulties (Annett & Bender, 1994; Celano & Geller, 1993). Factors that contribute to such difficulties in children with asthma include the iatrogenic effects of oral steroids, poor management of the disease and stress associated with having a chronic illness.

Routine paediatric treatment of asthma includes the administration of steroids (such as Becotide®) and bronchodilators (such as Ventolin®) in relatively high doses during an attack. Bronchodilators open the constricted airways; steroids reduce inflammation. Asthma is an episodic condition and, between attacks, in addition to avoiding situations that may trigger attacks and a regime of gentle exercise, maintenance doses of steroids and broncho-dilators are typically prescribed. These are usually self-administered or administered by the parents using an inhaler. However, both have side effects. Excessive use of steroids renders the body vulnerable to infections and excessive use of bronchodilators leads to disinhibition.

Assessment

Where children with asthma have severe and frequent attacks, they may be referred for a psychological consultation. In assessing such cases, pre-disposing, precipitating and maintaining factors outlined above should be added to the routine assessment protocol set out in Chapter 4 and Figure 14.4. A number of structured instruments that may be useful in assessing asthma symptomatology, its impact on quality of life, self-efficacy beliefs relevant to the management of asthma and family competence in managing asthma are set out in Table 14.4. Following formulation, where pre-disposing, precipitating, maintaining and protective factors relevant to the specific case are specified, a case management plan may be developed.

Treatment

Case management for asthma should be family based and may include psy-choeducation, relaxation training, self-management skills training, a reward programme to improve adherence and family work to disrupt patterns of interaction that maintain the condition (Brinkley et al., 2002; Guevara, Wolf, Grum & Clark, 2003; McQuaid & Walders, 2003).

Psychoeducation

Within the psychoeducational aspect of treatment, the symptoms of asthma and the pre-disposing, precipitating and maintaining factors that may under-pin the condition should be explained. In light of this, the specific factors relevant to the case should be described within the context of a formulation. The importance of self-monitoring of respiratory functioning, avoiding trig-gers, using medication appropriately and practising relaxation should be highlighted.

Self-management skills

Self-management skills of particular importance for youngsters with asthma are self-monitoring, environmental control, relaxation and cognitive restructuring. For self-monitoring, the chart presented in Figure 14.6 may be adapted, so that youngsters can record the medication that they have taken, the status of their symptoms, the situations in which the symptoms occur with particular reference to allergens and emotionally arousing family interactions, and the thoughts (both anxiety-generating and anxiety-reducing) that they have in these situations. Daily peak-flow meter readings are a reliable index of symptomatology. A peak-flow meter is a device that assesses the efficiency of the child's lungs. Increases in peak-flow meter readings are an objective index of improvement in respiratory functioning.

With respect to environmental control, youngsters should be encouraged to learn, from their self-monitoring charts, those situations that lead them to have respiratory difficulties and those that do not. They should then be helped to plan to avoid physical environments that precipitate asthma attacks, such as dusty rooms or gardens where there are high levels of pollen. There may also be psychosocial situations that precipitate attacks, such as becoming involved in intense three-way interactions with both parents. These may be dealt with in family sessions specifically aimed at disrupting such transactions.

The relaxation and cognitive restructuring skills, described in Chapter 12 for anxiety management, may be incorporated into treatment programmes for asthmatic youngsters. Youngsters may be trained how to use progressive muscle relaxation, breathing exercises and visualization to reduce physiological arousal and manage asthma symptoms. Cognitive restructuring may be used to modify the anxiety-provoking thoughts that increase arousal and exacerbate asthma symptoms.

Family work

Family intervention should aim to disrupt interaction patterns that maintain symptoms (Lask & Fosson, 1989). Broadly speaking, these fall into two categories. First, there are those interaction patterns that increase autonomic arousal, which in turn leads to bronchial constriction and eventually to asthma attacks. Second, there are interaction patterns that do not facilitate adherence to the medication regime and the avoidance of environments that constrain allergens that precipitate asthma attacks.

Intense, intrusive emotional interactions between an over-involved parent and an asthmatic child may increase arousal. Such interactions often occur as part of a pattern of triangulation, where the child is involved in an intense relationship with one parent and a distant relationship with another, and the parents have a weak interparental alliance. In such instances, the less-involved parent may be invited to take on the role of managing the child's asthma, with the rationale that this may give the other parent a well-deserved break (Minuchin et al., 1978). Alternatively, both parents may be invited to spend thirty minutes each night, without the child present, reviewing the child's progress and planning how to manage the next day. Both of these types of intervention reduce the emotional intensity of the asthma-related inter-actions in which the child is engaged. They also create opportunities to dis-cuss the beliefs that under-pin the over-involved parent's intense emotional reactions within family sessions. Providing opportunities for parents to express their worst fears about their child's fate as a victim of asthma, and the ways in which these fears have evolved, within family sessions sets the stage for altering these anxiety-provoking belief systems. Within family sessions, parents may be invited to re-evaluate these catastrophic beliefs, and to develop low-anxiety strategies for managing asthma attacks. With families that display such emotionally intense interaction patterns, adherence and avoidance of allergenic environments are rarely major problems. So planning low-anxiety strategies for asthma management should focus on giving the child more autonomy for the self-management of asthma. That is, using self-monitoring, relaxation, and cognitive restructuring to reduce arousal and decrease the probability of asthma attack. It is therefore useful to engage the child in concurrent individual sessions to teach these skills and foster increased autonomy.

Interaction patterns that do not facilitate adherence to the medication regime and the avoidance of environments that contain allergens which pre-cipitate asthma attacks tend to occur in chaotic or neglectful families. In these families, raising awareness that asthma can be fatal is a useful way to help parents and children focus their efforts on avoiding precipitants and increas-ing compliance. Here, it is useful to explain the formulation in detail and to logically outline how starving the body of oxygen can eventually lead to hypoxic seizures, respiratory arrest, unconsciousness and death. Where par-ents have difficulty understanding just how debilitating asthma can be, simu-lation exercises may be set up to help them empathize with their children. For example, parents may be given a straw to breathe through and then be invited to do some gentle exercise like jogging on the spot for a couple of minutes, while only breathing through a straw. The breathlessness that this exercise induces, and the sense of oxygen starvation, allows parents to understand the sort of discomfort their children are suffering during an asthma attack.

Next, the parents and children may be helped to construct a poster for the kitchen with a list of Dos and Don'ts on it. In the Dos column, this poster may include: Do take 3 puffs of Ventolin 3 times a day. Do remember to take puffer to school. Do get a smiling face on the reward chart each night you do this. Do call your parents if you get a tight chest at night. In the Don'ts column, the following list may appear: Don't stroke cats or dogs. Don't go into dusty places. Don't play in the hayfield. Don't say 'It will go away if I ignore it'. Along side the Do's and Don'ts poster, a reward chart should be set up like that presented in Figure 14.7. Each time children take their medication as prescribed, they colour in a smiling face, and a number of these can be cashed in for a prize at the end of the week.

Finally, an emergency routine needs to be established, stating each person's responsibility when an acute attack occurs. The family should be helped to write this routine on a poster to be hung in the kitchen. The routine should be rehearsed a couple of times in family sessions.

SEIZURE DISORDER

Epilepsy is a condition marked by recurrent seizures that result from electrophysiological disturbances in the cerebral cortex (Cull & Goldstein, 1997; Goodman, 2002). The period of abnormal electrical activity is referred to as the *ictus*. Typically, a diagnosis is reached on the basis of full clinical examination in conjunction with EEG results. Epileptic seizures are distinguished from febrile convulsions, which occur during a febrile illness; hypoglycaemic seizures associated with diabetes; and hypoxic seizures that occur during a breath-holding or asthma attack. Epileptic seizures are also distinguished from fainting and pseudoseizures, which mimic epileptic seizures but are not accompanied by EEG abnormalities. However, it should be kept in mind that co-morbid epileptic seizures and pseudoseizures are not uncommon. Epilepsy occurs in about 1 in 200 children and is more common among those with intellectual disability.

Epileptic seizure disorders have been sub-classified in various ways. Traditionally, a distinction has been made between grand mal and petite mal seizures. 'Grand mal' (or tonic-clonic) seizures is the term given to a condition where the seizures of a couple of minutes duration are preceded by an aura in which unexplained sounds, smells or other sensations occur. During the subsequent very brief tonic phase of the seizure, breathing ceases and consciousness is lost. In the clonic phase which follows, twitching and muscle spasms occur. In the last stage the person drifts into a relaxed comatose state until awakening.

During a petite mal attack, there is a momentary *absence* which involves diminished consciousness. During this no movement occurs or it may be accompanied by slight facial twitching. After the attack, children carry on with whatever they were doing before-hand, often not noticing that they have been absent.

While the distinction between petite mal and grand mal seizures is still widely used clinically, the Commission on Classification and Terminology of the International League Against Epilepsy (1989) has argued that a more sophisticated classification system is required, which takes account of the aetiology and underlying electrophysiological basis for seizures rather than classifying on the basis of observable symptomatology alone. With respect to aetiology, the Commission also makes distinction between symptomatic epilepsies in children with structural brain disease, cryptogenic epilepsy in which the pathology is presumed but unproven, and idiopathic epilepsies, which occur in the absence of structural brain damage. With respect to underlying brain activity as assessed by EEG, the Commission makes a basic distinction between generalized seizures and partial seizures. Generalized seizures do not have a focal onset but rather have a broad bilateral origin, whereas partial seizures have a clearly identifiable focal point of origin in the brain. In partial seizures children may retain consciousness but some functions such as speech may be temporarily impaired. Thus both petite mal and grand mal seizures are classified as generalized by the Commission. Partial seizures are further sub-divided into those with simple or complex symptomatology. Simple seizures are associated with simple sensory or motor abnormalities. Complex partial seizures usually begin in the temporal or frontal lobes and are associated with complex motor and sensory abnormalities. Higher cognitive functions may also be affected giving rise to experiences such as *déjà vu*. Included under complex partial seizures are more traditional categories such as temporal lobe epilepsy, psychomotor seizures and frontal lobe epilepsy.

Temporal lobe epilepsy (complex partial seizures originating in the temporal lobe) are of concern to clinical psychologists because this disorder may be associated with more pronounced psychological adjustment problems, particularly anger control, inattention and over-activity. Temporal lobe epilepsy begins with an epigastric aura, dizziness and flushing. In children these are rarely accompanied by *déjà vu* distorted perceptions and hallucinations. The aura is typically experienced as extremely frightening. The seizures are of the grand-mal, tonic-clonic variety. While many children with temporal lobe epilepsy develop into well-adjusted adults, temporal lobe epilepsy is a risk factor for a schizophrenia-like condition (inter-ictal psychosis) in adult life, with up to 10% developing this psychotic condition. Also, boys with temporal lobe epilepsy are likely to be sexually inactive and remain unmarried (Goodman, 2002).

Frontal lobe epilepsy (complex partial seizures originating in the frontal lobe) are of interest to psychologists because they may be misdiagnosed as pseudoseizures or parasomnias. These seizures, which occur primarily during sleep, are characterized by complex movements including punching with the arms, cycling with the legs, torso twisting and vocalizations including shouting or swearing. The seizures begin and end abruptly, tonic-clonic movements are absent and there is a rapid return to responsiveness. Frontal lobe seizures are often mistaken for pseudoseizures because of the complexity of the movements, the vocalizations and the abrupt return to responsiveness.

The evaluation of children with epilepsy invariably involves an EEG in addition to a routine paediatric neurological evaluation. Treatment involves a long-term regime of anti-convulsant medication. Common anti-convulsants include phenobarbitone, phenytoin, primidone, carbamexapine, ethsuximide, sulthiame and sodium valporate (Goodman, 2002).

Epilepsy may cause high levels of psychosocial difficulties for all family members, including stigmatization, stress, psychological problems, family conflict and restriction of social activities (Ellis, Upton & Thompson, 2000). The quality of family support may be an important intervening factor between epilepsy and the child's overall adjustment.

Assessment

Children with seizure disorders may be referred for psychological consultation to help with the differential diagnosis of seizures and pseudoseizures, to assess cognitive impairment associated with epilepsy or anti-convulsant medication and to help youngsters and their families adjust to the seizure disorder, avoid situations that may precipitate seizures and adhere to treatment regimes.

Differential diagnosis of pseudoseizures

Making the differential diagnosis of pseudoseizures poses a diagnostic challenge because most youngsters with pseudoseizures also present with epileptic seizures, both types of seizure are typically precipitated by a build-up of stress and both may be associated with personal and family-based adjustment problems. However, with video-EEG telemetry and careful history taking, a differential diagnosis of seizures and pseudoseizure may be made. Goodman (2002) has listed a number of criteria which may distinguish between seizures and pseudoseizures: they occur on video in the absence of EEG abnormalities, they occur when the child is being observed but not when the child is alone, the onset is gradual rather than abrupt, quivering and flailing occur but not a true clonus, dramatic screaming accompanied by semi-purpositive movements occur, painful stimuli are avoided, serious injury does not occur and they end abruptly with a complete return to an alert state of consciousness. It is also possible to induce pseudoseizures through suggestion while the child is in a light trance (Levine, 1994). Where children have pseudoseizures, they may be managed following the guidelines set out for conversion symptoms in an earlier section of this chapter.

Assessment of cognitive impairment

Children with seizure disorders often show cognitive impairment on intelligence, attainment and memory tests (Cull & Goldstein 1997; Goodman, 2002; Svoboda, 2004). Specific learning difficulties are also more common among children with epilepsy. However, anti-convulsant medication may impair cognitive functioning. Where children with epilepsy are referred for psychological assessment of cognitive abilities, a full assessment of attainment, intelligence and memory may be conducted while on anti-convulsant medication. Appropriate standardized tests for assessing these functions are described in Chapter 8. However, if the concern is the impact of the medication on academic performance, an assessment during a low-stress medication holiday should be arranged. Sufficient time should be allowed to pass for the anti-convulsants to wash out of the child's system. Where possible, parallel forms of cognitive and attainment test should be used to minimize learning effects from the first to the second assessment.

Treatment

Psychoeducation, illness management and the provision of support or arrangement for support group membership are the principle components of psychological treatment packages for children with epilepsy and their families.

Psychoeducation

Children with epilepsy and their parents require an opportunity to be given up-to-date and accurate information about medical, psychosocial, legal and historical aspects of epilepsy. At a medical level, information should be given on the specific form of epilepsy that the child has, the EEG results and aspects of the history that have been taken into account in making the diagnosis, the factors that may precipitate seizures, the appropriate use of medication and possible cognitive and other side effects of medication. A clear distinction between epilepsy and psychosis needs to be made since many myths about epilepsy and madness are propagated through folklore and the media. Information on the law relating to epilepsy, driving and operating heavy machinery should be given. In most countries, people with a diagnosis of epilepsy are not permitted to drive a car unless they have been seizure free for a period of months. Also, some career options, such as being an aircraft pilot, are closed to people with epilepsy. It may also be useful to reduce negative impact of the diagnosis by pointing to the many talented people who have had epilepsy, including Dostoevsky, the Russian novelist.

Illness-management skills

Children with epilepsy and their parents require training in monitoring the occurrence of the seizures, the precipitants of the seizures, adherence to the medication regime and the side effects of medication including drowsiness and impaired cognitive or academic performance. The monitoring chart presented in Figure 14.6 may be useful for this. Where increased arousal precipitates seizures, training in relaxation skills, such as those outlined in Chapter 12, may be conducted to equip children to reduce arousal in situations where seizures occur. Reward systems (described in Chapter 4) may be used by parents to help children adhere to their medication regimes and avoid situations that precipitate seizures.

Support groups

Youngsters and their parents may be given information on local and national epilepsy support groups and organizations. Contact with such organizations reduces the sense of stigmatization and isolation that children and families may feel as a result of the seizure disorder.

DIABETES MELLITUS

Juvenile-onset insulin-dependent diabetes mellitus is a complex condition which affects under 0.2% of school-age children and adolescents (Bradley, 1994a; Farrell et al., 2002; Mrazek, 2002; Wysocki, Greco & Buchloh, 2003). A case example of diabetes is presented in Box 14.5. Diabetes has changed, as a result of advances in medical management, from being a brief fatal condition to being a chronic illness requiring careful management if long-term

Box 14.5 A case of poorly controlled diabetes

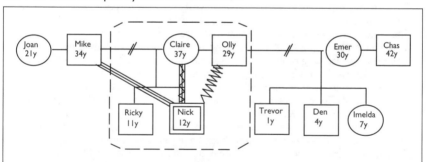

Referral. Nick, a twelve-year-old boy, was referred because of poor diabetic control. He refused to regularly test his blood sugar level, preferring to assess this by intuition alone. He also violated his diet frequently. These difficulties had emerged in the six-month period before his parents' separation. The referral was made about a year following the separation, and was precipitated by a hospital admission following a hyperglycaemic crisis. Nick was shocked by the crisis but his anxiety about the episode was coupled with anger at his mother and step-father. He blamed them for the crisis. He was angry at his mother for not reminding him about his diet and angry at Olly, his mother's live-in boyfriend, for living in his house and occupying the centre of his mother's attentions.

Child's development and current status. Nick's developmental history had been normal and he and his parents had managed the control of his diabetes quite well until he was about ten years old. His school performance and peer relationships had also been well within normal limits until that time. A psychometric evaluation using the WISC-III, the WRAT-III and the Child Behaviour Checklist and the Teacher Report Form showed that Nick was of high average intelligence and his basic academic skills were within the normal range, but he displayed clinically significant internalizing and externalizing behaviours at home and at school. On a series of diabetes-related assessment instruments he showed adequate knowledge of the condition but little belief that he could control the condition and a strong sense that this mother and step-father were unsupportive of his attempts to manage his condition.

Family development. When Nick was ten, his mother Claire, found out that Nick's father, Mike, was having a clandestine affair with Joan, a 19-year-old woman. An episode of intense marital conflict ensued which culminated in a separation after about 6 months. Nick and his younger brother Ricky remained living with their mother, and visited their father on a regular basis. Nick idolized his father and blamed the parental separation on his mother. When Olly, his mother's boyfriend, appeared on the scene and moved into Nick's house within a few months, Nick became extremely angry at him and his mother. This coincided with a radical deterioration in his diabetic control and academic performance.

Nick's parents each took a different approach to the issue of adhering to the diabetic self-care regime. His father, Mike, saw the regime as Nick's responsibility and so rarely even mentioned it. From time to time, without thinking, Mike would allow Nick to violate his diet. The mother, Claire, in contrast worried about Nick's lax approach to adherence and regularly reminded him to do his tests and take his insulin. This often led to conflict between Nick and Claire. The ongoing acrimony between Claire and Mike prevented them from taking a concerted approach to helping Nick develop better control over his condition.

Formulation. Nick was a bright twelve-year-old boy with poor diabetic control. This poor control was due to Nick's personal beliefs about the uncontrollability of the condition and difficulties his separated parents and their new partners had in taking a consistent, non-conflictual and supportive approach to helping him develop good diabetic self-care routines.

Treatment. Treatment in this case involved both individual and family sessions. A series of sessions with Nick and his father, Nick and his mother and one session with Nick and both of his parents were held. Within these sessions, the focus was on helping both parents develop non-conflictual ways to check Nick's adherence to his regime regularly. The joint session focused on establishing a way for both parents to communicate with each other about Nick's adherence when he made transitions from one household to another. Within the individual sessions Nick was given space to ventilate his intense feelings about his parents' separation and to explore how these feelings interfered with adequate self-management of his diabetes. He also learned stress management skills to reduce arousal which adversely affected his diabetic control.

negative sequelae are to be avoided. The disease affects islet cells of the pancreas and is characterized by a deficiency in insulin production, a deficiency that may now be corrected through careful monitoring of blood sugar levels and a regular intake of insulin. In the short term, failure to adequately monitor blood sugar levels and take appropriate amounts of insulin may lead to a coma induced by hyperglycaemia or hypoglycaemia. In the long term, poorly controlled diabetes may lead to neuropathy and retinopathy, with increased risk of heart disease, kidney disease, blindness and lower limb infections leading to gangrene. In such instances amputation may be necessary. Men with a history of poorly controlled diabetes are at risk for impotence associated with neuropathy. A significant proportion of people with diabetes develop obesity in adulthood.

Routine medical treatment for diabetes involves: (1) regular blood-sugar tests; (2) regular intake of insulin by tablet or injection; (3) a low-sugar, low-fat, high-fibre diet; and (4) a moderate amount of daily exercise at times that will not have a negative effect on blood sugar levels (Wysocki et al., 2003).

Psychological factors influence the course of diabetes (Bradley, 1994a; Farrell et al., 2002; Mrazek, 2002; Wysocki et al., 2003). Certain psychological characteristics of children and their families are associated with adherence to the diabetic regime and to good glycaemic control. Extensive empirical research has shown that these personal and family characteristics tend to be highly specific to diabetes and that more general indices of personal and family functioning are only associated with glycaemic control in extreme cases. Personal characteristics associated with glycaemic control and adherence include knowledge about diabetes, diabetes self-care skills, beliefs about the controllability of diabetes through the careful use of self-care skills and anxiety usually associated with fear of short- and long-term consequences of poor glycaemic control. The developmental stage of the child also has a bearing on glycaemic control, with adolescents showing more adherence problems and poorer control. Parent–adolescent conflict about autonomy-related issues may become focused on adherence to the diabetic regime and poor glycaemic control may result from this unfortunate state of affairs.

Family characteristics associated with good adherence and glycaemic control include parental support of the child, the absence of extreme anxiety about diabetes and good joint parental problem-solving skills with specific reference to diabetes management. These skills include monitoring adherence-related behaviours; promoting the use of appropriate diabetic self-care skills in the areas of diet, exercise, testing and insulin administration; offering positive reinforcement and praise for using self-care skills and avoiding nagging, threatening, catastrophizing and criticizing for poor adherence.

High levels of adherence and glycaemic control are associated with characteristics of the wider healthcare network. Specifically, good adherence is associated with congruence between physicians', parents' and children's treatment regime adherence goals. This type of congruence is associated with psychoeducational strategies that take account of parents' beliefs about diabetes and children's level of cognitive development. A build-up of life stress, either through exposure to many daily hassles or a smaller number of major life changes, may precipitate episodes of poor glycaemic control.

Diabetes affects many areas of life (Bradley, 1994a; Farrell et al., 2002; Mrazek, 2002; Wysocki et al., 2003). It may affect children's view of themselves, their cognitive abilities and academic achievements, their family relationships, their peer relationships and their leisure activities. As with all chronic illnesses, the child is at risk for developing a negative self-image and low self-esteem because of their illness and the constraints it places on them. This may be reinforced by critical or over-protective parental attitudes. Poor glycaemic control is associated with cognitive impairment and the development of learning difficulties. Thus, some youngsters with diabetes have attainment problems in school. Because exercise and diet must be carefully controlled in diabetes, youngsters with the condition may encounter problems in peer-group situations and leisure activities where there are pressures to, for example, eat sugar-based sweets or candy and engage in excessive physical exercise. In late adolescence and adulthood, diabetes may also have an impact on vocational adjustment and, for men, diabetes-related impotence may have a negative effect on sexual functioning in intimate relationships.

Assessment

Psychological consultation to youngsters with diabetes and their families should begin with thorough assessment of psychosocial, cognitive and academic functioning following the guidelines set out in Chapters 4 and 8 and the framework given in Figure 14.4. Additionally, instruments listed in Table 14.4 for assessing the following areas may be used: quality of life related to diabetes, knowledge about diabetes, beliefs about the controllability of diabetes, family diabetic-related behaviours and adherence to the diabetes self-care regime. Salient features from the assessment may be integrated into a concise formulation in which pre-disposing, precipitating and maintaining factors are specified along with protective factors and family strengths that may be relevant to disease management.

Treatment

Effective psychological interventions for diabetes involve psychoeducation for the child and family, self-monitoring training, stress-management training and family work aimed at helping the parents support the child in developing autonomous control over the self-care regime (Farrell et al., 2002).

Psychoeducation

Parents and children need a simple explanation of the complex relationship between blood sugar levels and insulin intake, diet and exercise. The short- and long-term effects of poor glycaemic control need to be highlighted. The importance of regular blood-sugar testing as a way of optimizing control should be clarified; educational interactive software programs are available to help youngsters master this information.

Self-monitoring

Youngsters with diabetes are typically required by the paediatric clinic to regularly complete a self-monitoring chart on which they record the results of their blood-sugar tests and the times at which they took insulin injections or tablets. Where youngsters have problems with glycaemic control, it is critical that they are trained in accurate self-monitoring and in some instances a reward system may be used by parents to motivate them to take on the responsibility of self-monitoring.

Stress management

A high level of physiological arousal can reduce glycaemic control, which in turn may lead to further anxiety and arousal. So for some youngsters with diabetes a vicious cycle develops. One way to empower youngsters to break this cycle is to teach them the relaxation, breathing and visualization skills described in Chapter 12. However, relaxation can markedly reduce blood sugar, so exercises should not be practised when blood sugar is below 4 mmol/l (Bradley, 1994a). Where youngsters catastrophize about their diabetes, they may be taught to challenge these arousal producing cognitions using the CTR method described in Chapter 12.

Family work

The principal aims of family work in cases where children have poorly controlled diabetes are to increase the child's degree of autonomy in managing the illness, reducing the emotional intensity of parent–child interactions related to illness, coaching parents and children in using clear supportive communication and helping all family members develop effective problem-solving routines for managing illness-related stress. Guidelines for training in communications and problem-solving skills are given in Chapter 4.

CANCER

Leukaemia and brain tumours are the most common types of paediatric cancer. In recent years, with advances in treatment methods, survival rates from childhood cancer have increased to 60–70% (Mrazek, 2002; Vannatta & Gerhardt, 2003; Varni et al.,1996). For children with a poor prognosis, the central psychological issue is the process of anticipatory grieving through which the child and family pass prior to the child's death. Grief and loss are discussed in Chapter 24; this chapter is concerned with psychological strategies for improving the quality of life of paediatric cancer survivors.

Leukaemia is a malignancy of the bone marrow characterized by unregulated rapid proliferation of malignant white blood cells (lymphoblasts). Lymphoblasts gradually replace healthy white blood cells and this results in anaemia, infection and haemorrhage. The most common overt signs are fatigue, fever, bruising and bone pain. Painful bone marrow aspirations are conducted to assess if lymphoblasts are present in the bone marrow. A lumbar puncture (spinal tap) is conducted to assess if there are lymphoblasts in the cerebrospinal fluid.

Treatment is conducted over three phases. In the first phase (remission induction) over a six-week period, the child receives intensive chemotherapy which aims to destroy all lymphoblasts. The second phase (maintenance chemotherapy) involves a thirty-month period of chemotherapy. In the third phase (prophylactic central nervous system treatment), chemotherapy is injected into the spinal canal (intrathecal therapy). This may be combined with cranial irradiation to destroy leukaemia cells in the brain. Progress is monitored over a five-year period and cases in remission at five years are considered cured.

The prognosis for brain tumours is not as good as that for leukaemia. Initial symptoms include headaches, nausea and vomiting. Later symptoms vary, depending on the site of the tumour. With cerebellar tumours, which are the most common in childhood, loss of balance may occur. Diagnosis is made on the basis of CT or MRI scans and a biopsy to determine the characteristic of the tumour. Treatment typically involves resection of the tumour followed by chemotherapy and/or cranial radiation therapy.

Chemotherapeutic agents interrupt the reproduction of cancer cells but also have major side effects, including abdominal pain, nausea, vomiting and hair loss. Many children undergoing chemotherapy develop anticipatory nausea and vomiting. Radiation therapy may also cause nausea, vomiting, inflammation, oedema and hair loss. In the longer term, it may lead to neuropsychological deficits and infertility.

Paediatric cancer may be conceptualized within the stress and coping conceptual framework outlined earlier as a condition entailing many chronic strains for both the child and parents (Varni et al., 1996). These include treatment-related pain, nausea and vomiting; visible treatment side effects, such as hair loss, weight alteration and physical disfigurement; and repeated absence from school and peer-group situations. Adjustment to these strains may be influenced by risk factors such as degree of disability, degree of functional independence and degree of stress. Adjustment may also be influenced by personal and contextual protective factors. Personal protective factors include coping strategies, easy temperament and problem-solving abilities. Contextual protective factors include intrafamilial and extrafamilial support.

Children who survive cancer show a higher incidence of depression, anxiety, drug abuse, school attendance problems and learning difficulties, and their families have more adjustment problems (Mrazek, 2002; Vannatta &

Gerhardt, 2003). The stress of chronic, life-threatening illness and the pain and discomfort associated with its treatment lead to mood and drug-abuse problems and family adjustment difficulties. Learning difficulties may arise from both extended school absence and the impact of treatment, specifically, cranial radiation therapy and intrathecal chemotherapy.

Assessment

In cases of paediatric cancer, where improving the child's quality of life is the central concern, a routine child and family assessment following the protocol described in Chapter 4 and the framework given in Figure 14.4 may be conducted and supplemented with inquiries about the impact of the diagnosis and illness-related stresses on family life and the child's adjustment. Deterioration in cognitive abilities due to treatment should be monitored through routine attainment and ability testing, as described in Chapter 8. Educational intervention for learning problems should be arranged where appropriate. Formulation should take the child's central psychological difficulties such as pain control, mood regulation or educational problems and identify the pre-disposing, precipitating, maintaining and protective factors for these problems. Psychological management plans should focus on altering problem-maintaining factors.

Treatment

Best-practice guidelines indicate that treatment programmes may include psychoeducation and support for the child and family, pain management skills training for the child, support group membership for parents and children and remedial educational input to compensate for time lost at school and learning difficulties that have developed due to treatment (Noll & Kazak, 1997).

Psychoeducation

Psychoeducational sessions may focus on the nature of the child's illness, the medical treatment plan and the prognosis. Psychologists need to liaise closely with medical colleagues about such issues to minimize ambiguity and confusion about such information. Some families find it helpful to audiotape consultations with the oncologist so that they may replay them repeatedly and clarify important information about the child's condition.

Family work

In family sessions, one part of the psychologist's role is helping family members communicate clearly with each other about practical issues and plans related to the child's care. Guidelines for communication training are given in Chapter 4. The other part is to help family members process the complex grief-related emotions that occur in response to living in a state of chronic uncertainty about the child's survival. Grief work is discussed in Chapter 24.

Pain management

Pain management skills training for medical and dental procedures has been discussed in an earlier section and is appropriate for helping youngsters with cancer cope with pain (McGrath & Hiller, 1999; Murphy & Carr, 2000).

Support group membership

National cancer organizations and many paediatric hospitals have set up self-help support groups for children with cancer and their parents. These groups are invaluable in the support they provide for children and parents, who may become isolated as a result of changes in routines brought about by the illness and by the difficulty many parents have in accepting support from those who have not had first-hand experience of cancer.

Remedial education

Youngsters with cancer may need remedial education to catch up on school-work following extensive absences during their treatment. They may also require remedial tuition to compensate for learning difficulties that have developed as a result of treatment.

SUMMARY

Abdominal pain, headaches, polysymptomatic somatization or conversion symptoms; chronic fatigue syndrome; preparation for anxiety-provoking medical and dental procedures and adjustment to chronic illness are among the more common somatic complaints referred to clinical psychologists. Management of these problems should take account of the development of children's concepts of pain and illness, which is influenced by both cognitive maturity and exposure to illness and pain either personally or within the child's immediate social network. A number of disorders with somatic complaints as the central concern are classified within DSM IV TR and ICD 10, chief among these being somatization disorder, but the diagnostic criteria for somatization disorder in DSM IV TR (four pain symptoms, two gastro-intestinal symptoms, one sexual symptom, one pseudoneurological symptom) are probably of little relevance to children, who tend to have simpler presentations than adults. In clinical practice it may be useful to conceptualize the factors involved in the aetiology of any somatic complaint as falling on a continuum from largely psychological to largely physiological, and for symptomatology as falling along a similar continuum. Prevalence rates for somatization in children and adolescents vary between 2 and 10%, depending on the methods used to identify cases and the populations studied. Co-morbidity rates for somatization problems with other emotional and behavioural problems vary from 12 to 20% in community samples and from 23 to 32% in clinical samples, with the highest rate of co-morbidity being with anxiety and depression. Reliable prevalence rates for adjustment problems among children with chronic illnesses such as asthma, diabetes, epilepsy and cancer are unavailable.

Biological theories which explain the development of somatic complaints in terms of physiological vulnerability to particular illnesses or general adaptation to a build-up of life stress are of special relevance to paediatric clinical psychology. Psychological explanations of somatic complaints have been developed within the psychoanalytic and psychosomatic traditions, which emphasize the role of intrapsychic factors, and also within the behavioural, cognitive-behavioural, stress and coping, and family systems traditions, which place greater emphasis on the role of interpersonal factors.

When assessing somatic complaints, particular attention should be paid to certain pre-disposing, precipitating, maintaining and protective factors. Physiological vulnerability, a high level of psychophysiological reactivity, exposure to the sick-role behaviours of other family members, inhibited emotional expression and a high level of suggestibility may pre-dispose youngsters to develop somatization problems or adjustment difficulties when faced with chronic illness. Precipitating factors for these conditions include personal or familial illness or injury, major stressful life events or a build-up of small stressors. Maintaining factors include beliefs about the controllability of symptoms, the use of problematic coping strategies such as denial or catastrophizing; inadvertent reinforcement of sick-role behaviours and a family environment characterized by extremities of proximity, hierarchy, conflict, triangulation and reactivity. Important protective factors include acceptance of the formulation, commitment to resolving the problems, self-efficacy, low stress and high support.

A psychological approach to somatic complaints should ideally be family based and include close liaison with the referring physician so that medical aspects of the case are adequately managed. Psychological consultation should involve careful contracting for assessment, thorough child and family assessment, clear formulation and careful contracting for treatment. Where appropriate, treatment may include psychoeducation, monitoring of symptoms, relaxation skills training, cognitive restructuring, coaching parents in contingency management, relapse management training and arranging membership of a support group. In planning a treatment programme the unique features of the child's somatic complaints should be taken into account.

EXERCISE 14.1

Fay, an eleven-year-old girl whose parents separated a year ago, has found that her asthma has become worse over the summer months. She has also found that she develops persistent headaches, a problem she never had in the past. She visits her mother every week and lives with her father and her older brother. She dislikes her mother's new partner, Kevin. Fay's developmental history is normal. Her asthma was well controlled until she moved house a year ago. There is, however, a family history of both asthma and headaches. Fay has not changed school as a result of the separation but is due to go to secondary school in a few weeks. She will attend a different secondary school than her best friend. Her mood and behaviour are within normal limits and her schoolwork is satisfactory.

- Work in teams. Write a preliminary formulation for this case outlining probable pre-disposing, precipitating, maintaining and protective factors.
- Write an assessment plan to check out the validity of the preliminary formulation. State who you would interview and the lines of interviewing you would follow and any additional assessment procedures you would use.

EXERCISE 14.2

Role-play the first assessment interview.

FURTHER READING

Roberts, M. (2003). *Handbook of Paediatric Psychology* (Third edition). New York: Guilford Press.

FURTHER READING FOR CLIENTS

Davis, M., Robbins-Eshelman, E., & McKay, M. (2000). *The Relaxation and Stress Reduction Workbook (Fifth Edition)* Oakland, CA: New Harbinger Publications.

WEBSITES

American Psychological Association's Division 54 – Paediatric Psychology website offers links to sites for all of the conditions covered in this chapter: http://www.apa.org/divisions/div54/

Factsheets on unexplained physical symptoms, chronic physical illness, chronic fatigue syndrome and coping with stress can be downloaded from the website for Rose, G. & York, A. (2004). *Mental Health and Growing Up. Fact sheets for Parents, Teachers and Young People* (Third edition). London: Gaskell: http://www.rcpsych.ac.uk

Section IV

Problems in adolescence

Chapter 15

Drug abuse

Habitual drug abuse in adolescence is of particular concern to clinical psychologists because it may have a negative long-term effect on the adolescent and an intergenerational effect on their children (American Academy of Child and Adolescent Psychiatry, 1997e; Chassin, Ritter, Trim & King, 2003; Crome, Ghodse, Gilvarry & McArdle, 2004; Rutter, 2002b). For the adolescent, habitual drug abuse may negatively affect: mental and physical health, criminal status, educational status, the establishment of autonomy from the family of origin and the development of long-term intimate relationships. The children of habitual teenage drug abusers may suffer from drug-related problems such as fetal alcohol syndrome, intrauterine addiction or HIV infection.

Cases of drug abuse vary widely in their presentation. Examples of two very different types of cases are presented in Boxes 15.1 and 15.2. The first is a chronic and complex case of polydrug abuse while the second involves only recreational or experimental use of two drugs. These cases differ along a number of dimensions, including: the pattern of drug-using behaviour, the types of drug used, the impact of the drugs used, the overall personal adjustment of the teenager and the presence of other personal or family-based problems. Clearly, drug abuse itself is not always a unidimensional problem and it may occur as part of a wider pattern of life difficulties. The definition and classification of drug abuse is therefore a complex challenge. In this chapter, after considering the classification, epidemiology and clinical features of drug abuse, a variety of theoretical explanations concerning their aetiology will be considered along with relevant empirical evidence. The assessment of drug abuse and a family-based approach to treatment will then be given. The chapter will conclude with some ideas on how to prevent drug abuse in populations at risk.

CLASSIFICATION

To deal with the extraordinary complexities of defining and classifying drug-related problems, in DSM IV TR (APA, 2000a) and ICD 10 (WHO, 1992,

Box 15.1. A case of polysubstance abuse

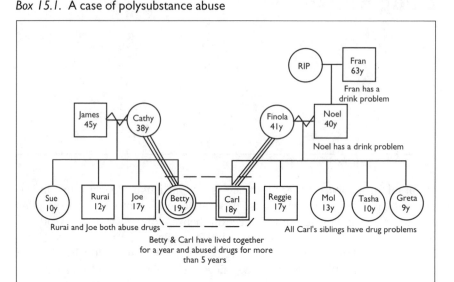

Fran 63y

Fran has a drink problem

RIP

James 45y

Cathy 38y

Finola 41y

Noel 40y

Noel has a drink problem

Sue 10y

Rurai 12y

Joe 17y

Betty 19y

Carl 18y

Reggie 17y

Mol 13y

Tasha 10y

Greta 9y

Rurai and Joe both abuse drugs

All Carl's siblings have drug problems

Betty & Carl have lived together for a year and abused drugs for more than 5 years

Referral. Carl, eighteen, and Betty, nineteen, referred themselves for treatment to an inner-city drug clinic. Both were polydrug abusers and had developed physiological dependence to opiates at the time of referral.

History of the presenting problem. They both had been using drugs since primary school, beginning with cigarettes at the ages of about 10 years as part of peer-group-based experimental drug abuse. They stole the cigarettes from their parents who smoked. At 12 they both began drinking and stole beer from Carl's father and later wine from a supermarket. They began using benzodiazepines, which they stole from Betty's mother who had been prescribed these for anxiety and sleep problems by the family doctor. They then used cannabis, various solvents; a variety of stimulants but mainly dextroamphetamines. They progressed to opiates about a year before they first attended the clinic. They had got to the stage where they could no longer finance their drug-taking habits and had a series of bad debts. They requested evaluation for placement on a methadone maintenance programme.

The couple lived together on welfare in a two-room apartment. They financed their drug habits through theft and, occasionally, prostitution. They were part of a group of drug users who lived in Dublin's inner city. Their whole lifestyle centred around getting and using any drugs they could find, but mainly opiates.

Developmental and family history. Betty and Carl had known each other from childhood. Both had a history of academic and conduct problems at school. Their families were very close but disapproved of the teenage couple when they began living together about six months previously. However, in both of the families their mothers were very loyal to them and occasionally gave them financial assistance when it was clear that they were showing withdrawal symptoms and needed a fix. Carl's grandad lived with his parents and both he and Carl's dad had serious drink problems for which they had been unsuccessfully treated over many years.

Carl had four siblings, all of whom had drug problems. Betty had three siblings, all but one of whom were using drugs. However, Carl and Betty had the most serious drug problems of the two families. They were both oldest children.

Formulation. Betty and Carl's habitual drug abuse had evolved gradually out of an earlier pattern of pre-adolescent experimental drug abuse. Both were predisposed to develop substance abuse problems because of the family role models, their academic difficulties, lack of career opportunities and other conduct problems. These problems were maintained at a physiological level by addiction and at a psychosocial level through involvement in a lifestyle which revolved around obtaining and using drugs to the exclusion of almost all other activities.

Treatment. The treatment plan for Betty and Carl involved detoxification followed by residential treatment in a therapeutic community.

Box 15.2. A case of early drug experimentation

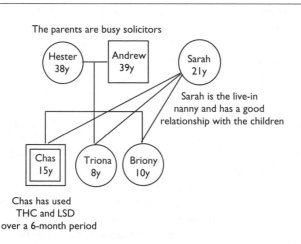

The parents are busy solicitors

Hester 38y — Andrew 39y   Sarah 21y

Sarah is the live-in nanny and has a good relationship with the children

Chas 15y   Triona 8y   Briony 10y

Chas has used THC and LSD over a 6-month period

Referral. Chas, aged fifteen, was referred for treatment to a private family therapy institute when his parents found that he had been smoking cannabis (THC) with his school friends at a party. He had smoked cannabis a couple of dozen times over a six-month period and had also taken LSD once. His drug use occurred within the context of a peer group who were experimenting with a range of drugs and associated drug use with listening to and playing music.

Developmental history. His developmental history was unremarkable. He was a fine student in the top stream in his school and had come second in his class in the junior certificate. He was an able sportsman, an avid chess player and musician. He loved to push himself to the limit in all of his leisure activities and was clearly a risk-taker. He had excellent social skills, a wide circle of friends including a girlfriend with whom he had being having a relationship for about four months. He had particularly good relationships with his parents.

Family history. Neither of his parents smoked or drank alcohol and both were solicitors. They worked long hours, but on a matter of principle would not send Chas to boarding school, believing strongly in the importance of family life. There was a live-in nanny in their house who cared for Chas and his two younger sisters Triona (aged 8 years) and Briony (aged 10 years). The parents were guilt ridden when they brought the family for the intake interview. Both were of the view that Chas's drug abuse resulted from a failure to be sufficently available for him during his adolescence due to their heavy work schedule.

Formulation. Chas presented with experimental rather than habitual drug abuse. The onset of the drug abuse was precipitated by availability of the drug and Chas was pre-disposed to become involved in experimental drug abuse because of his tendency for sensation seeking and risk taking. The drug use was maintained through involvement in a drug-using peer group.

Treatment. In a series of sessions involving Chas and his parents, the risks of abusing various types of drugs were discussed. Other recreational channels into which Chas could direct his energy were explored. As part of this process, Chas and his father arranged a weekend at an adventure sports centre in Donegal together. The parents were supported in setting strict limits on drug use while Chas lived in their house. In later sessions the focus moved to Chas's career plans.

1996) drug problems are classified on axis 1 on the basis of the following three parameters:

- the behavioural pattern of use
- the effects of the drug when it is taken or unavailable
- the type of drug used.

Related life stresses and overall level of adjustment are rated on other axes. Details of these multi-axial systems are given in Chapter 3. Within both ICD 10 and DSM IV, a distinction is made between drug dependence and drug abuse. While drug abuse refers to drug taking that leads to personal harm, drug dependence refers to those situations where there is a compulsive pattern of use involving physiological changes associated with tolerance and withdrawal. Definitions of abuse and dependence are given in Table 15.1. Both DSM IV TR and ICD 10 make distinctions between the effects of drugs that occur immediately after they are taken (intoxication), when they are unavailable after habitual use (withdrawal) and when they lead to certain types of symptom (for example, delirium, anxiety or psychosis). These clinical conditions are listed in Table 15.2. Each drug leads to characteristic intoxication and withdrawal syndromes. These are not documented in the ICD 10. The list of such syndromes presented in Table 15.3 is based on the DSM IV TR.

EPIDEMIOLOGY

Illegal drug use across the lifespan is common. In an Irish national survey of over 8000 fifteen- to sixty-four-year olds in 2002, the lifetime prevalence of illegal drug use was 19% (National Advisory Committee on Drugs and the Drug and Alcohol Information and Research Unit, 2004). In a UK national survey of over 9000 eleven- to fifteen-year-olds in 2001, the lifetime prevalence for illegal drug use was 29% (National Centre for Social Research and the National Foundation for Educational Research, 2002). In both surveys

Table 15.1 DSM IV TR and ICD 10 diagnostic criteria for drug abuse and dependence

DSM IV TR	ICD 10
Substance abuse A. A maladaptive pattern of substance use leading to clinically significant impairment or distress as manifested by one or more of the following occurring within a 12-month period: 1. Recurrent substance abuse resulting in a failure to fulfil major obligations at work, school or home. 2. Recurrent substance abuse in situations in which it is physically hazardous 3. Recurrent substance-related legal problems 4. Continued substance use despite having persistent or recurrent social or interpersonal problems caused by or exacerbated by the effects of the substance B. The symptoms have never met the criteria for substance dependence for this type of substance	**Harmful use** A pattern of psychoactive substance abuse that is causing harm to health. The damage may be physical (as in cases of hepatitis from the self-administration of injected drugs) or mental (e.g. episodes of depressive disorder secondary to heavy consumption of alcohol) The fact that pattern of use of a particular substance is disapproved of by a culture or may have led to socially negative consequence such as arrest or marital arguments is not in itself evidence of harmful use
Substance dependence A maladaptive pattern of substance abuse, leading to clinically significant impairment or distress, as manifested by three or more of the following occurring at any time in the same 12-month period: 1. Tolerance defined by either: (a) a need for markedly increased amounts of the substance to achieve intoxication (b) markedly diminished effect with continued use of the same amount of the substance 2. Withdrawal as manifested by either of the following: (a) the characteristic withdrawal syndrome for the substance (b) the same substance is taken to relieve or avoid withdrawal symptoms 3. The substance is taken in larger amounts over a longer period than was intended 4. There is a persistent desire or unsuccessful efforts to cut down or control substance use 5. A great deal of time is spent in activities necessary to obtain the substance, use the substance or recover from its effects 6. Important social, occupational or recreational activities are given up or reduced because of substance use	**Dependence syndrome** A cluster of physiological, behavioural and cognitive phenomena in which the use of a substance or a class of substances takes on a much higher priority than other behaviours that once had greater value. Three or more of the following in a 12-month period: (a) A strong desire or sense of compulsion to take the substance (b) Difficulty in controlling substance-taking behaviour in terms of onset, termination or levels of use (c) A physiological withdrawal state when substance use has ceased or been reduced as evidenced by: the characteristic withdrawal syndrome for the substance; use of the substance to avoid withdrawal symptoms (c) Evidence of tolerance such that increased doses of the substance are required in order to achieve the effects originally produced by lower doses (e) Progressive neglect of alternative pleasures or interests because of psychoactive substance use, increased amount of time necessary to obtain or take the substance or to recover from its effects

Continued

Table 15.1 continued

DSM IV TR	ICD 10
7. The substance use is continued despite knowledge of having a persistent or recurrent physical or psychological problem that is likely to have been caused or exacerbated by the substance Specify with or without physiological dependence	(f) Persisting with substance use despite clear evidence of overtly harmful consequences such as harm to the liver through excessive drinking, depressive mood states consequent to periods of heavy substance abuse, or drug-related impairment of cognitive functioning

Note: Adapted from DSM IV TR (APA, 2000a) and ICD 10 (WHO, 1992, 1996).

cannabis was the most commonly used drug and prevalence was highest amongst older male teenagers.

Experimentation with drugs in adolescence is common (Chassin et al., 2003; Weinberg, Harper & Brumback, 2002). Major US and UK surveys concur that, by nineteen years of age, approximately 80% of teenagers have drunk alcohol, 60% have tried cigarettes, 50% have used cannabis, 20% have tried other street drugs such as solvents, stimulants, hallucinogens or opiates and 20–40% have used multiple drugs. Between 5 and 10% of teenagers under nineteen have drug problems serious enough to require clinical intervention.

CLINICAL FEATURES

Because of the heterogeneity of states, stages and types of drug abuse, outlining a concise set of salient clinical features is problematic. However, some guidelines may be offered on the behavioural, physiological, affective, perceptual, cognitive and interpersonal features deserving attention in the assessment of cases of substance abuse (American Academy of Child and Adolescent Psychiatry, 1997e; Chassin et al., 2003; Crome et al., 2004; Myers, Brown & Vik, 1998; Pagliaro & Pagliaro, 1996; Rutter, 2002b; Vik, Brown & Myers, 1997; Weinberg et al., 2002). These are summarized in Table 15.4.

Drug abuse is associated with a wide variety of behaviour patterns. These patterns may be described in term of the age of onset, the duration of drug abuse, the frequency of use, the range of substances used and the amount used. Thus useful distinctions may be made between adolescents who began abusing drugs early or later in their development; between those who have recently begun experimenting with drugs and those who have a chronic history of drug abuse; between daily users, week-end users and occasional users; between those who confine their drug abuse to a limited range of substances, such as alcohol and Cannabis (THC), and those who use a wide range of substances; and between those who use a little and those who use a great deal

Table 15.2 Classification of clinical conditions arising from the effects of drug abuse listed in DSM IV TR and ICD 10

Clinical condition	Clinical features of the condition
Intoxication	The development of a substance-specific syndrome due to recent ingestion of the substance and clinically significant maladaptive psychological changes due to the substance
Withdrawal	The development of a substance-specific syndrome due to cessation of prolonged substance use which causes clinically significant distress or impairment of social or occupational functioning
Flashbacks	Re-experiencing, following cessation of use of a hallucinogen, perceptual abnormalities such as hallucinations, flashes of colour, intensified colour, trails of images of moving objects, halos around objects and objects appearing larger or smaller than they are
Intoxication delirium	During intoxication, reduced ability to focus, sustain or shift attention; disorientation; memory deficit or language disturbance
Withdrawal delirium	During withdrawal following sustained drug use reduced ability to focus, sustain or shift attention; disorientation; memory deficit or language disturbance
Dementia	Impaired ability to learn new information or recall previously learned information; aphasia (language disturbance); apraxia (impaired ability to carry out motor function); agnosia (failure to recognize familiar objects); disturbance in executive functioning (planning, organizing, sequencing and abstracting)
Amnestic disorder	Impaired ability to learn new information or recall previously learned information leading to a decline in social or occupational functioning
Psychotic disorder	Hallucinations or delusions
Mood disorders	Depressed mood or markedly diminished interest or pleasure in almost all activities, or elevated expansive or irritable mood
Anxiety disorders	Prominent anxiety, panic attacks or obsessions and compulsions pre-dominate the clinical picture
Sexual dysfunctions	Clinically significant sexual dysfunction that results in marked distress or interpersonal difficulty and may included impaired desire, impaired arousal, impaired orgasm or sexual pain
Sleep disorders	A prominent disturbance of sleep sufficiently severe to warrant clinical attention and may include insomnia, hypersomnia, parasomnia or a mixed type

Note: Substance-abuse-related dementia, mood disorders, anxiety disorders, sexual dysfunctions and sleep disorders are listed in DSM IV TR (APA, 2000a) but not ICD 10 (WHO, 1992, 1996).

Table 15.3 Intoxication and withdrawal syndromes for substances listed in DSM IV TR

Substance	Intoxication	Withdrawal syndrome: Other associated clinical conditions
Alcohol	Elation; impaired judgement; impaired social or occupational functioning; slurred speech; inco-ordination; unsteady gait; nystagmus; impairment of attention and memory; stupor or coma	Withdrawal involves autonomic hyperactivity; hand tremor; insomnia; nausea and vomiting; visual; tactile or auditory hallucinations; psychomotor agitation; anxiety; grand mal seizures
		Associated clinical conditions include delirium; dementia; amnestic syndrome; psychosis; depression; anxiety; sexual dysfunction; and sleep disorder
Amphetamines	Euphoria, sociability, impaired judgement, impaired social or occupational functioning tachycardia or bradycardia; papillary dilation; elevated or lowered blood pressure; perspiration or chills; nausea or vomiting; evidence of weight loss; psychomotor retardation or agitation; muscular weakness, respiratory depression, chest pain, or cardiac arrhythmias, confusion, seizures, dyskinesis or coma	Withdrawal involves dysphoric mood; fatigue; vivid unpleasant dreams; insomnia or hypersomnia; increased appetite; psychomotor retardation or agitation
		Associated clinical conditions include delirium; psychosis; depression; anxiety; sexual dysfunction; and sleep disorder
Caffeine	Excitement; period of inexhaustibility; restlessness; nervousness; insomnia; flushed face; diuresis; gastrointestinal disturbance; muscle twitching; rambling flow of thought and speech; tachycardia; and psychomotor agitation	No withdrawal syndrome
		Associated clinical conditions include anxiety and sleep disorder
Cannabis	Euphoria; sense of slowed time; impaired judgement; impaired motor co-ordination; social withdrawal; increased appetite; dry mouth; tachycardia	No withdrawal syndrome
		Associated clinical conditions include delirium; psychosis; and anxiety
Cocaine	Euphoria, sociability, impaired judgement, impaired social or occupational functioning tachycardia or bradycardia; papillary dilation; elevated or lowered blood pressure;	Withdrawal involves dysphoric mood; fatigue; vivid unpleasant dreams; insomnia or hypersomnia; increased appetite; psychomotor retardation or agitation

	perspiration or chills; nausea or vomiting; evidence of weight loss; psychomotor retardation or agitation; muscular weakness, respiratory depression, chest pain, or cardiac arrhythmias, confusion, seizures, dyskinesis or coma	Associated clinical conditions include delirium; psychosis; depression; anxiety; sexual dysfunction; and sleep disorder
Hallucinogens	Hallucinations; illusions; intensification of perception; depersonalization; derealization; ideas of reference; paranoid ideation; anxiety or depression; impaired judgement; impaired social or occupational functioning; papillary dilation; tachycardia; sweating; palpitations; blurring of vision; tremors; inco-ordination	No withdrawal syndrome Associated clinical conditions include flashbacks; delirium; psychosis; depression; and anxiety
Inhalants	Euphoria, belligerence; impaired judgement; impaired social or occupational functioning; dizziness; nystagmus; inco-ordination; slurred speech; unsteady gait; lethargy; depressed reflexes; psychomotor retardation; tremor; muscle weakness; blurred vision; stupor; coma	No withdrawal syndrome Associated clinical conditions include dementia; delirium; psychosis; depression; and anxiety
Nicotine	None	Withdrawal involves depressed mood; insomnia; irritability; anxiety; concentration problems; restlessness; decreased heart rate; increased appetite or weight gain
Opioids	Initial euphoria followed by apathy; dysphoria; psychomotor agitation or retardation; impaired judgement; impaired social and occupational functioning	Withdrawal involves dysphoric mood; nausea and vomiting; muscle aches; lacrimation; papillary dilation; sweating; diarrhoea; yawning; fever; insomnia Associated clinical conditions include delirium; psychosis; depression; sexual dysfunction; and sleep disorder

Continued

Table 15.3 continued

Substance	Intoxication	Withdrawal syndrome: Other associated clinical conditions
Phencyclidine (PCP or angel dust)	Euphoria; hallucinations; belligerence; impulsivity; psychomotor agitation; impaired judgement; impaired social and occupational functioning; nystagmus; tachycardia; numbness; ataxia; dysarthria; muscle rigidity; seizures; coma	No withdrawal syndrome Associated clinical conditions include delirium; psychosis; depression; and anxiety
Sedatives, hypnotics and anxiolytics	Apathy; impaired judgement; impaired social or occupational functioning; slurred speech; inco-ordination; unsteady gait; nystagmus; impairment of attention and memory; stupor or coma	Withdrawal involves autonomic hyperactivity; hand tremor; insomnia; nausea and vomiting; visual, tactile or auditory hallucinations; psychomotor agitation; anxiety; grand mal seizures Associated clinical conditions include delirium; dementia; amnestic syndrome; psychosis; depression; anxiety; sexual dysfunction; and sleep disorder

Note: Substance-abuse-related intoxication and withdrawal syndromes are listed in DSM IV TR (APA, 2000a) but not ICD 10 (WHO, 1992, 1996).

of drugs. Chronic and extensive daily polydrug abuse with an early onset is associated with more difficulties than experimental, occasional use of a limited number of drugs with a recent onset. The former usually entails a constricted drug-focused lifestyle and multiple associated physical and psychosocial problems, whereas the latter does not. A consistent finding is that only a minority of youngsters progress from experimental to habitual drug abuse and from the use of a single legal drug to multiple legal and illegal drugs.

Behavioural patterns of drug abuse evolve within specific contexts and drug-using behaviour often comes to be associated with particular locations, times, modes of administering the drug, physiological states, affective states, control beliefs and social situations. With recreational experimental drug use, weekly oral drug taking at peer-group gatherings while in a positive mood state may occur and youngsters may have strong beliefs that they are in control of their drug-taking behaviour. With habitual drug abuse, solitary daily injections to prevent withdrawal and alleviate negative mood may occur. This type of drug abuse may be accompanied by strong feelings of being unable to control the frequency of drug abuse or to cut down on the amount taken.

Physiological features of drug abuse may be grouped into those associated with intoxication, those that follow intoxication, those associated with

Table 15.4 Clinical features of drug abuse

Domain	Features
Behaviour	**Drug-using behaviour** • Age of onset • Duration of drug abuse • Frequency of use • Range of substances used • Amount used • Change in pattern over time **Context of drug-using behaviour** • People present • Locations • Times • Modes of administering the drug (oral, nasal or injection) • Physiological state (during withdrawal) • Affective state (positive or negative) • Beliefs about ability to control drug use
Physiological effects	**Intoxication** • Physical problems due to hyperarousal (e.g. arrhythmias or dehydration) • Physical problems due to hypoarousal (e.g. stupor) **Following intoxication** • Exhaustion • Dehydration • Sleep and appetite disturbance • Sexual dysfunction **Withdrawal** • Nausea, vomiting, muscle aches and discomfort following opioid use • Sleep and appetite disturbance following stimulant use • Seizures following sedative use **Long-term medical complications** • Poisoning and over-dose Infections including hepatitis and HIV • Liver and kidney damage
Affect	**During intoxication** • Fear and anxiety due to unexpected effects of drugs (particularly hallucinogens) **Following intoxication and during withdrawal** • Depressed mood • Irritability and anger • Anxiety
Perception	**During intoxication** • Hallucinations (with hallucinogens and some stimulants)

Continued

Table 15.4 continued

Domain	Features
	Following intoxication • Brief flashbacks and protracted psychotic states (with hallucinogens and some stimulants)
Cognition	• Impaired cognitive functioning • Declining academic performance
Interpersonal adjustment	• Adolescent–parent conflict • Adolescent–teacher conflict • Induction into drug using peer sub-culture • Social isolation • Conflict with juvenile justice system • Conflict with healthcare system

withdrawal following the development of dependence and medical complications which arise from drug abuse. A full list of intoxication and withdrawal syndromes for commonly abused drugs is set out in Table 15.3. From this it may be seen that, broadly speaking, stimulants and hallucinogens lead to physiological changes associated with increased arousal, such as tachycardia and blood-pressure changes. In cases of extreme intoxication, cardiac arrhythmias and seizures may occur. On the other hand, extreme intoxication following the use of alcohol, sedatives, solvents and opioids leads to physiological changes associated with reduced arousal such as drowsiness, stupor and coma. Withdrawal from dependence-producing stimulants entails significant disruption of sleep and increased appetite. Withdrawal from sedatives and alcohol is particularly dangerous because, as part of a syndrome of autonomic hyperactivity, grand mal seizures may occur. Withdrawal from opioids leads to a syndrome characterized by nausea, vomiting, diarrhoea and muscle aches. A wide variety of medical complications is associated with drug abuse and these range from injuries sustained while intoxicated, to liver or kidney damage due to the toxicity of substances abused, to infections including hepatitis and HIV arising from non-sterile injections. With all street drugs there is a risk of death by intentional or accidental over-dose or poisoning due to impurities in the drug.

A central reason for many forms of drug abuse is to pharmacologically induce a pleasant affective state. It is therefore not surprising that for many drugs, including alcohol, stimulants, hallucinogens and opioids, elation is a central feature of initial intoxication. With sedatives, in contrast, intoxication leads to apathy. Many polydrug abusers refer to drugs by their primary mood-altering characteristics. Thus, a distinction is made between *uppers* and *downers*, and particular cocktails of drugs or sequences of drugs are used to regulate mood in particular ways. Negative mood states typically follow intoxication, for most classes of drugs. This is particularly true for drugs such as opioids or cocaine, which lead to tolerance and dependence. The intense negative mood states which characterize withdrawal syndromes associated with such addictive drugs motivate habitual drug abuse. The health problems, financial difficulties and psychosocial adjustment problems that evolve as part of habitual drug abuse may also contribute to frequent and intense negative mood states and paradoxically motivate drug abusers to use more drugs to improve their mood state. Negative mood states typically include some combination of depression, anxiety and anger.

At a perceptual level, some types of drug, but particularly hallucinogens, lead to pronounced abnormalities during intoxication and withdrawal. In the current decade, widely used hallucinogens include MDMA (known as *Ecstasy* or *E*) or LSD (known as *acid*). The hallucinations and perceptual distortions that occur during intoxication are not always experienced as pleasant; in some situations they lead to great distress. Brief flashbacks or enduring psychotic states which involve hallucinations and perceptual distortions may occur following intoxication and these invariably are experienced as distressing.

With respect to cognition, all of the drugs listed in Table 15.3 and most other street drugs lead to impaired concentration, reasoning and judgement during intoxication and withdrawal. Long-term regular drug abuse in many instances leads to impaired cognitive functioning. The nature, extent and reversibility of this impairment varies, depending on the pattern of drug abuse. In teenagers, the impaired cognitive functioning associated with regular drug abuse may lead to a decline in academic performance.

Drug abuse may have an impact on interpersonal adjustment. Within the family, drug abuse often leads to conflict or estrangement between adolescents and their parents. At school, drug abuse may lead to conflict between the adolescent and teachers, both because of declining academic performance and because of anti-social behaviour such as theft or aggression associated with drug abuse. Youngsters who abuse drugs within a peer-group situation may become deeply involved in a drug-oriented sub-culture and break ties with peers who do not abuse drugs. Some youngsters develop a solitary drug-using pattern and become more and more socially isolated as their drug-using progresses. Within the wider community, drug-related anti-social behaviour such as aggression, theft and selling drugs may bring youngsters into contact with the juvenile justice system. Drug-related health problems and drug dependency may bring them into contact with the health service. Conflict between drug abusers and healthcare professionals may arise in situations where youngsters expect to be offered prescribed drugs (such as methadone) as a substitute for street drugs (such as heroin) and this does not occur.

Drug abuse often occurs with other co-morbid psychological problems, including conduct disorder, ADHD, specific learning difficulties, mood disorders, anxiety disorders, schizophrenia and bulimia. The relationship between these co-morbid psychological problems and drug abuse is complex.

Any or all of them may precede drug abuse and contribute in some way to the development of drug-using behaviour. In addition, drug abuse may precipitate or maintain these other psychological problems. For example, the use of hallucinogens may precipitate the onset of schizophrenia. Chronic polydrug abuse may lead to learning difficulties and chronic alcohol use can lead to amnesic syndrome. Amphetamine usage may lead to anxiety problems. Drug dependence may lead to chronic conduct problems such as assault and theft. Negative drug-related experiences such as losses and drug-related accidents may lead to mood disorder, which in turn may lead to further drug use. Drug abuse is also an important risk factor for suicide in teenagers.

THEORIES

The many explanations for drug abuse that have been developed fall broadly into seven categories:

- First, biological theories of drug abuse focus on specific genetic predisposing factors, temperamental attributes that are known to be strongly genetically determined and the role of physiological mechanisms in development of tolerance, dependence and withdrawal.
- Second, intrapsychic deficit theories point to the importance of personal psychological vulnerabilities in the development of drug-using behaviour patterns.
- Third, cognitive-behavioural theories underline the significance of certain learning processes in the genesis of drug problems.
- Fourth, family systems theories emphasize the importance of parental drug-using behaviour, parenting style and family organization patterns in the aetiology and maintenance of drug abuse.
- Fifth, the role of societal factors such as social disadvantage, neighbourhood norms concerning drug use and abuse and drug availability are the central concerns of sociological theories of drug abuse.
- Sixth, multiple risk factor theories highlight the roles of factors at biological, psychological and social levels in the aetiology of drug abuse.
- Finally, change process theories offer explanations for how recovery and relapse occur.

Some of the more important theoretical formulations falling into each of these seven categories are listed in Table 15.5.

Biological theories

Biological formulations point to the role of genetic pre-disposing factors in drug abuse, the association between temperamental attributes that are known

Table 15.5 Theories of drug abuse

Type of theory	Explanatory variables	Hypotheses	Interventions
Biological theories	Genetic factors	Genetic factors pre-dispose some males to develop specific types of drug problems such as alcohol abuse	Emphasize the disease model of alcoholism and the importance of abstinence as a treatment goal for children of parents with alcohol problems
	Temperament and risk taking	Difficult temperament, high risk-taking and low harm-avoidance pre-dispose youngsters to drug abuse	Help youngsters with difficult temperaments and risk-taking tendencies to refocus their energy into demanding and risky pro-social leisure or work activities
	Tolerance and dependence	For certain classes of drugs such as opioids, cocaine and alcohol physiological changes occur with habitual drug use that lead to tolerance, dependence and withdrawal and this maintains further drug abuse	Include detoxification in treatment programmes for youngsters who have developed dependence and offer methadone maintenance as a substitute for opioids
Intrapsychic deficit theories	Stress and coping	Early and current life normative stresses and traumatic events including neglect; physical emotional and sexual child abuse; exposure to life-threatening violence; involvement in natural disasters; bereavement; relationship difficulties; and work difficulties lead to distressing intrapsychic states. Drugs are used as an avoidant coping strategy to pharamcologically suppress or regulate these distressing intrapsychic states	Provide psychotherapy to help resolve early life issues and work through current life issues that under-pin negative affective states

Continued

Table 15.5 continued

Type of theory	Explanatory variables	Hypotheses	Interventions
	Academic failure	Children who are unable to achieve in school do not develop a strong commitment to achieving academic goals and turn to drug abuse as an alternative lifestyle	Provide school curriculum appropriate to the youngsters' ability level and a participative ethos that includes youngsters and their parents in school activities
	Drive for autonomy	Participation in a drug-using sub-culture is one of a wide range of lifestyles explored in search of an adult identity and autonomy from parental control	Work with parents and youngsters to facilitate individuation and explore alternatives to drug taking as a route to autonomy
Behavioural theories	Operant conditioning	Drug-taking behaviour is maintained initially by positive reinforcement associated with mood elevating effects of drugs and later (in the case of dependence-producing drugs) by negative reinforcement, where drugs prevent withdrawal symptoms	Arrange for detoxification so drugs are not required for their negative reinforcement value. Then highlight costs and dangers of continued drug use and provide reinforcement for alternatives to drug-using behaviours
	Classical conditioning	Certain cues (CS) in the environments of opioid addicts elicit withdrawal, because in the past they have been associated with withdrawal symptoms (UCS)	In cue exposure treatment, expose the youngster to withdrawal-eliciting cues and reinforce them for not engaging in drug-taking behaviour
Family systems theories	Parental drug abuse	Drug-using behaviour is learned and maintained through observation and imitation of parents' drug-using behaviour and co-dependent behaviour	Provide inpatient or community-based treatment for parents or place the child in foster or residential care away from deviant parental role models
	Parenting style	Lack of clear rules prohibiting drug abuse, consistent parental supervision, and consistent consequences for rule-breaking leads to drug abuse	Train parents in behavioural parenting skills

	Family disorganization	Parental psychological problems, interparental conflict; interparental conflict avoidance; parent–child conflict; lack of clear communication, hierarchies, boundaries, rules, roles and routines; lack of emotional cohesion; and the occurrence or immanence of lifecycle transitions such as leaving home maintain drug abuse	Help family clarify communication, rules, roles, routines hierarchies and boundaries; resolve conflicts; increase emotional cohesion; and manage lifecycle transition
Sociological theories	Social disadvantage	Neighbourhoods characterized by poverty, low socioeconomic status, high population density and high crime rates create a context within which drug abuse can flourish	Provide financial support to specific families; initiate community development projects; increase law enforcement
	Alienation	Alienation from mainstream societal values; tolerance for deviance; rejection of authority; low religiosity; high independence; and membership of a peer group in which drug abuse is an accepted behaviour leads to the development of positive attitudes to drug abuse and to drug-using behaviour	Provide community interventions that offer alternatives to drug abuse for youngsters and their peers. Provide residential peer-group-based treatment where the rejection of drug abuse is part of the sub-culture
	Drug availability	Lenient laws or inadequately enforced laws about teenage use of nicotine, alcohol and street drugs increase the probability of drug abuse	Make drug-related legislation stricter and enforce laws more vigorously
	Social norms	Social norms contribute to the development of drug abuse	Arrange media-based campaigns which aim to modify norms concerning drug taking

Continued

Table 15.5 continued

Type of theory	Explanatory variables	Hypotheses	Interventions
Multiple risk factor theories	Accumulation of risk factors	The greater the number of biological risk factors; personal deficit risk factors; family systems risk factors and sociological risk factors, the greater the risk of drug abuse	Develop multi-systemic intervention programmes which target biological, psychological, family and social factors that maintain drug abuse
Theories of recovery and relapse	Process of change	Recovery involves progression through stages of pre-contemplation, contemplation, preparation, action and maintenance. Addictive behaviour is maintained by factors at 5 levels: situational, conscious cognitive, interpersonal, family systems, and intrapsychic conflict	In the early stage of change provide support; in the middle stages facilitate belief system exploration; and in the later stages provide consultancy on behavioural change. Target the systemic levels that will maximize recovery
	Relapse processes	Relapses occur in stressful high-risk situations when individuals have low self-efficacy and poor relapse-management skills	Offer relapse-prevention training where individuals learn to identify and manage high relapse risk situations

to be strongly genetically determined and drug-taking behaviour and the role of physiological mechanisms in development of tolerance, dependence and withdrawal.

Genetic hypothesis

Genetic theories of drug abuse are partly supported by the findings of twin and adoption studies (Rutter, 2002b). These show that a pre-disposition to drug and alcohol abuse and dependence is moderately heritable, particularly in males, but that genetic influences on experimentation and recreational drug use are less pronounced. Over half of the variance in the genetic pre-disposition to drug, alcohol and nicotine abuse is shared, and not drug-specific. However, genetic factors do influence individual differences in sensitivity to, and tolerance for, specific drugs. For example, some males are genetically pre-disposed to developing alcohol problems; the characteristic that is transmitted may be a low physiological and subjective response to alcohol (Schuckit, 1994). The self-help organization Alcoholics Anonymous has drawn on the genetic hypothesis and supporting evidence to underline the view that alcoholism is a disease that can be managed but not cured. Complete abstinence and regular attendance at self-help meetings, where a 12-step programme is pursued, are the corner-stones of managing the disease according to this viewpoint. The twelve AA steps are set out in Table 15.6. While there is little doubt that the AA approach to managing alcohol abuse may be effective for some people (probably adults with more severe problems) controlled studies of the effectiveness of AA with teenagers have not been conducted (Chiauzzi & Liljegren, 1993).

Temperament hypothesis

The temperament hypothesis holds that youngsters who develop drug and alcohol problems do so because they have particular temperamental

Table 15.6 The twelve steps of AA

Step	Principle
Step 1	We admitted we were powerless over alcohol and that our lives had become unmanageable
Step 2	Came to believe that a power greater than ourselves could restore us to sanity
Step 3	Made a decision to turn our will and our lives over to God *as we understood him*
Step 4	Made a searching and moral inventory of ourselves
Step 5	Admitted to God, to ourselves and to other human beings the exact nature of our wrongs
Step 6	Were entirely ready to have God remove all these defects of character
Step 7	Humbly asked him to remove our shortcomings
Step 8	Made a list of all persons we had harmed, and became willing to make amends to them all
Step 9	Made direct amends to such people whenever possible, except when to do so would injure them or others
Step 10	Continued to take personal inventory and when we were wrong, admitted it
Step 11	Sought through prayer and meditation to improve our conscious contact with God *as we understood him* praying only for knowledge of his will for the power to carry that out
Step 12	Having had a spiritual awakening as a result of these steps, we tried to carry this message to alcoholics, and to practise these principles in all our affairs

Note: Adapted from AA (1986) *The Little Red Book.* City Centre, MN: Hazelden.

characteristics, which are partially biologically determined, that pre-dispose them to developing drug problems. In support of this hypothesis, difficult temperament in early childhood, sensation-seeking and a low level of harm avoidance in adolescence have been found consistently to be related to drug abuse (Hawkins, Catalano & Miller, 1992; Rutter, 2002b). Youngsters with these temperamental characteristics engage in dangerous novel experiences and risky rule-breaking behaviour, of which drug abuse is just one example. Other related risky behaviours include driving fast cars or motor bikes, play-ing high-contact sports, fighting and theft. Available evidence shows that there is a relationship between engaging in all of these types of activities and heavy drug abuse (Wills & Filer, 1996). Treatment programmes influenced by this position may aim to train youngsters in self-control skills so that they can regulate their tendencies to pursue novel and dangerous experiences, includ-ing intoxication. Alternatively, they may help such youngsters refocus their energy into demanding and risky pro-social leisure or work activities. For a minority of youngsters with drug-abuse problems, self-control training or participation in group residential programmes, where the youngsters are challenged to take risks and master skills such as horse riding, sailing or mountain climbing, may be effective.

The temperamental hypothesis is a refined version of the addictive person-ality hypothesis, which argues that a particular type of personality is prone to addiction. The search for such a personality type has not been fruitful (Chiauzzi & Liljegren, 1993).

Tolerance and dependence

Pharmacological theories argue that, with habitual drug use tolerance, dependence and withdrawal develop. With tolerance, a gradual increase in drug dosage is required for intoxication to occur. This increase in dosage in turn leads to physiological dependence and the related phenomenon of unpleasant or hazardous withdrawal symptoms when drug taking ceases abruptly. An attempt to avoid this withdrawal syndrome maintains further drug abuse. Extensive pharmacological evidence supports the hypothesis that for certain classes of drugs, tolerance, dependence and withdrawal occur. In particular these phenomena are associated with habitual use of alcohol, opioids, stimulants and sedatives, but not for hallucinogens (Mirza, 2002; Weinberg et al., 2002). Summaries of withdrawal syndromes associated with a number of widely abused drugs are presented in Table 15.3. Pharmaco-logical theories have led to the inclusion of detoxification in treatment pro-grammes for youngsters who have developed dependence. Pharmacological theories have also informed the development of methadone maintenance programmes. In such programmes, youngsters who have developed opioid dependency are prescribed a daily dose of methadone as a substitute for street opioids (Mirza, 2002).

Intrapsychic deficit theories

Many hypotheses account for drug abuse in terms of specific intrapsychic vulnerabilities and deficits. Among the more important are those that highlight the stress and coping processes, those that underline the role of academic failure and those concerned with lack of autonomy and the process of identity formation.

Stress and coping through self-medication

Stress and coping formulations of drug-taking behaviour argue that drugs are used to alleviate negative affective states. This is often referred to as the self-medication hypothesis (Khantzian, 1985; Weinberg et al., 2002). Thus drugs are conceptualized as a strategy for coping with responses to current life stresses, such as bereavement, or the sequelae of early life stresses, such as problematic parent–child relationships or abuse. For example, psychoanalytic theorists have argued that low levels of care and high levels of criticism from primary caregivers in early childhood may lead to insecure attachment, unmet dependency needs, harsh super-ego development and low self-esteem. Drugs are used, according to this hypothesis, to alleviate the negative mood states that arise from these detrimental formative experiences (Wieder & Kaplan, 1969). This, like temperament theory, is a refined version of the addictive personality hypothesis.

Another variant of the intrapsychic deficit hypothesis argues that where youngsters have suffered sexual abuse or exposure to other traumatic events, drugs may be used to pharmacologically suppress intrusive trauma-related memories and affect (Chiaveroli, 1992). According to these formulations, intervention may focus on resolving the issues or processing the negative emotions that under-pin the drug abuse. Alternatively, treatment may focus on helping youngsters develop other less harmful coping strategies for regulating negative affect.

Response to academic failure

Another intrapsychic deficit which has been suggested to pre-dispose youngsters to developing drug abuse is learning difficulties. According to this position, children who have attainment difficulties at school do not develop a strong commitment to achieving academic goals and turn to drug abuse as an alternative lifestyle (Hawkins et al., 1992). Interventions which derive from this perspective aim to provide youngsters with a school curriculum appropriate to their ability levels and a participative ethos that includes youngsters and their parents in school activities so as to enhance commitment to academic goals.

Drive for autonomy

The lack of an established identity during adolescence is a normative intra-psychic deficit according to some lifespan development theories, such as that proposed by Erikson (1968). Erikson argues that participation in a drug-using sub-culture is one of a wide range of lifestyles explored during the search for adult identity and autonomy from parental control. Treatment programmes deriving from this position focus on working with parents and youngsters to facilitate individuation and exploring alternatives to drug taking as a route to autonomy.

Evidence reviewed by Wills and Filer (1996) and Hawkins et al. (1992) offers partial support for these hypotheses. A high level of early and current life stress is associated with persistent rather than experimental drug abuse. Persistent drug use in a significant proportion of cases represents a way to cope with current and past life stresses, particularly those that elicit the experiences of helplessness and anger, when other non-pharmacological coping strategies are unavailable. Non-pharmacological active coping strategies are more commonly used by children who have a high level of social support from parents and high levels of academic and social competence. However, there is little evidence that specific early life experiences, specific personality structures arising from these or specific current life stresses in all instances lead to drug abuse. There is also little evidence that specific learning difficulties or the search for an adult identity will inevitably lead to drug abuse. However, drug abuse is more likely to happen where some or all of these factors are present in conjunction with other risk factors, such as parental drug abuse or deviant peer-group membership.

Individual outpatient psychotherapeutic or educational approaches to the management of drug abuse premised on the intrapsychic deficit hypothesis have only limited effect on adolescent drug abusers' problems (Pagliaro & Pagliaro, 1996).

Behavioural theories

Behavioural theories focus on the role of classical and operant conditioning processes in the maintenance of drug abuse.

Operant conditioning theories

Solomon (1980) has argued that drug abuse is maintained initially by positive reinforcement associated with the mood elevating effects of drugs and later, in the case of dependence-producing drugs, by negative reinforcement, where drugs prevent withdrawal symptoms. Treatment programmes based on this formulation include initial detoxification so drugs lose their negative reinforcement value; exploration of the costs and dangers of continued drug use to reduce their positive reinforcement value; and the provision of positive reinforcement for alternatives to drug-using behaviours.

Classical conditioning theories

Wikler (1973) has offered an explanation of relapse following detoxification in people who have developed tolerance and dependence using a classical conditioning framework. According to this position, certain conditioning stimuli (CS) or cues in the environments of drug abusers elicit withdrawal symptoms and craving (a conditioned response, or CR) because, in the past, these cues have been associated with withdrawal symptoms which are conceptualized as unconditioned stimuli (UCS). In cue exposure treatment, which is based on this formulation, exposure to withdrawal- and craving-eliciting cues (CS) without engaging in drug taking leads to extinction of the CR, particularly the craving. In cue exposure treatment, the youngster may enter the situations that elicit craving, observe video or audiotapes of such situations, or undergo imaginal exposure to such situations and concurrently use a variety of coping strategies to avoid drug taking. There is some evidence that cue exposure treatment is effective for a sub-group of drug abusers (Chiauzzi, & Liljegren, 1993).

Family systems theories

Family systems theories of drug abuse implicate parental use of drugs, poor parenting skills or wider family disorganization in the aetiology and maintenance of drug abuse.

Parental drug abuse

In families where parents abuse drugs, empirical studies show that a greater proportion of children abuse drugs compared to families where parental drug abuse does not occur (Hawkins et al., 1992). A variety of mechanisms have been suggested to explain why youngsters develop drug-using behaviour (Brook, Brook, Gordon, Whiteman & Cohen, 1990). It may be that youngsters learn drug-abusing behaviour patterns directly through a process of modelling. Alternatively, they may acquire positive attitudes towards drugs through exposure to their parents' permissive attitudes to drugs and this in turn may lead them to avail of drugs when they become available. Finally, it may be that parents' drug-using behaviour and the responses of their spouses to this chronic and difficult problem compromises their capacity to provide a well-organized family environment and this in turn leads to the development of drug abuse. A variation of this latter mechanism is central to co-dependency theory, which argues that living in a family where a drug-abusing parent and a parent who inadvertently reinforces the drug-abusing parent to persist with drug abuse by engaging in *enabling behaviours*, leads to the intergenerational transmission of drug abuse (Cullen & Carr, 1999; Hands & Dear, 1994). In late adolescence, children from such households, it is argued, either develop drug-using behaviour patterns like their parents or enabling interactional styles which foster drug dependence in their partners. Thus within intimate relationships they replicate the interactional patterns which characterized their parents' marriage.

Treatment derived from theories of drug abuse that give primacy to parental drug-using behaviour may focus on altering the parents' drug abuse, the child's internalization of the parental drug-related attitudes and behaviour or the family interaction patterns that involve the misuse of drugs. Family-based intervention programmes which aim to change current patterns of family interaction that maintain adolescent substance abuse are particularly effective (Cormack & Carr, 2000).

Parenting style

Theories that explain drug abuse in terms of parenting style argue that the lack of clear rules prohibiting drug abuse, the lack of consistent parental supervision and the lack of consistent consequences for rule-breaking leads initially to experimental drug use and later to habitual drug taking (Drummond & Fitzpatrick, 2000; Kandel & Andrews, 1987). According to this position, intervention should focus on helping parents develop the parenting skills they lack and supporting them in using these to help their youngsters avoid drug abuse. Parent training is an important part of a number of programmes that have been shown to be effective in helping adolescent drug abusers (Cormack & Carr, 2000; Rowe & Liddle, 2003).

Family disorganization

Some theorists have argued that adolescent drug abuse evolves as part of a broader pattern of family disorganization, which includes parental psychological problems; interparental conflict; parent–child conflict; lack of clear communication, hierarchies, boundaries, rules, roles and routines; lack of emotional cohesion and the occurrence or immanence of lifecycle transitions such as leaving home (Cormack & Carr, 2000; Drummond & Fitzpatrick, 2000; Rowe & Liddle, 2003). Within such disorganized families, drug abuse may serve an organizing function, since it introduces certain predictable routines into family life and provides a focus for parental concern, which may increase family cohesion and prevent parental separation. Intervention with these families should help family members clarify communication, rules, roles, routines, hierarchies and boundaries; resolve conflicts; increase emotional cohesion and manage lifecycle transitions. The results of controlled trials of family intervention with adolescents shows highly structured approaches to family engagement and family therapy are effective in treating youngsters with drug problems (Cormack & Carr, 2000; Rowe & Liddle, 2003).

Sociological theories

Social disadvantage, alienation and drug availability are the principal variables included in the more important sociological theories of drug abuse.

Social disadvantage

Social disadvantage theories argue that neighbourhoods characterized by poverty, low socioeconomic status, high population density and high crime rates create a context within which drug abuse can flourish. This is because drugs offer an escape from the multiple stresses associated with this type of social environment, they are available in these environments and they are socially sanctioned within a crime-oriented sub-culture (Fagan, 1988; Rumball & Crome, 2004). Intervention programmes based on social disadvantage theories provide financial support to vulnerable families, initiate community development projects which provide an alternative to a drug-oriented deviant drug sub-culture and increase law enforcement so as to reduce drug availability. There is a great need for careful research to evaluate the effects of such programmes.

Alienation

Alienation theories posit a link between the rejection of mainstream societal values and membership of a peer group to drug abuse. Problem-behaviour theory is a particularly prominent alienation theory. Jessor and Jessor (1977) argue that substance abuse, precocious sexual behaviour and delinquency are inter-related and reflect adherence to deviant or unconventional attitudes. Usually, youngsters engage in these behaviours to achieve personal goals, such as acceptance from a deviant peer group and excitement. Youngsters are pre-disposed to developing problem behaviours if they are alienated from mainstream society and this may be reflected in their weak attachments to parents, their rejection of authority, their valuing independence more than academic achievement and their lack of religiosity. A wealth of survey data supports this theory (Rumball & Crome, 2004; Wills & Filer, 1996).

Winick's (1962) Role Strain theory is another explanation of drug abuse which focuses on the centrality of alienation in the genesis of drug abuse. Winick argues that drug abuse is most likely to occur when role strain or role deprivation occurs. Role strain is the difficulty experienced when taking on a new role, and role deprivation occurs when a familiar and valued role is terminated. Role Strain theory argues that drug abuse declines when availability is lessened, when negative attitudes to drug abuse become salient and when there is a reduction in role strain or deprivation. Data from studies of alienated youth, soldiers, physicians and nurses support this formulation (Pagliaro & Pagliaro, 1996).

Treatment programmes based on alienation theory provide residential peer-group-based treatment, within the context of a therapeutic community, where the rejection of drug abuse is part of the therapeutic community's subculture. Therapeutic communities are highly effective for youngsters who complete treatment and positive outcome rates of 75% for programme completers have been reported. However, more than 75% of cases who enter treatment drop out before completion (Pagliaro & Pagliaro, 1996).

Availability

Hypotheses about availability suggest that lenient laws or inadequately enforced laws about teenage use of nicotine, alcohol and street drugs increase the probability of drug abuse. This type of theory has few treatment implications but suggests important avenues for prevention. Prevention programmes, according to this view, should promote stricter drug-related legislation and the enforcement of laws affecting availability of drugs to teenagers. The availability hypothesis has largely been supported by empirical tests, and prevention programmes based on it have been moderately effective (Hawkins et al., 1992).

Social norms

That social norms may contribute to the development of drug abuse is a widely held view. One implication of this is that media-based campaigns which aim to modify norms concerning drug taking will be effective in reducing drug abuse. Unfortunately, media-based campaigns to modify teenage drug abuse have had equivocal results (Schinke, Botvin & Orlandi, 1991).

Multiple risk factor theories

Multiple risk factor theories argue that biological and psychological personal characteristics, family environment factors, factors within the peer group and features of the broader social context within which the youngster lives may contribute to the development and maintenance of drug abuse. One such theory, grounded in a thorough review of empirical research on risk factors and drug abuse, has been developed by Hawkins et al. (1992). They list seventeen categories of risk factor for which there is substantial evidence and argue that the greater the number of these that are present in any given case, the greater the risk of drug abuse. These factors are: temperament and genetic pre-disposition, early and persistent problem behaviours, academic failure, low commitment to school, family drug-taking behaviour, parenting skills, family conflict, low family bonding, peer rejection in early childhood, deviant peer-group membership in adolescence, alienation and rebelliousness, favourable attitudes to drug use, early onset of drug use, laws and norms favourable to drug use, drug availability, poverty and neighbourhood disorganization.

It follows from multiple risk factor theory that treatment and prevention programmes should target the biological, psychological, family and social factors that maintain drug abuse. For both treatment and prevention, available evidence suggests that multi-systemic programmes that target more than one risk factor are probably most effective (Cormack & Carr, 2000; Rowe & Liddle, 2003).

Theories of recovery and relapse

Two important theories of drug abuse, focus not on aetiology but on the process of recovery and relapse. These are Prochaska, DiClement & Norcross's (1992) theory of the change process and Marlatt and Gordon's (1985) relapse prevention theory.

Change processes

Prochaska et al.'s (1992) data from an analysis of twenty-four schools of psychotherapy, identified five stages of therapeutic change: pre-contemplation, contemplation, preparation, action and maintenance. They also found, by surveying clients and therapists engaged in therapy, that specific techniques were maximally effective in helping clients make the transition from one stage of change to the next. The list of a dozen techniques identified by Prochaska and colleagues fall into the categories of support, belief exploration and consulting to behavioural change.

In the pre-contemplation stage, the provision of support creates a climate within which clients may ventilate their feelings and express their views about their drug problem and life situation. Such support may help clients move from the pre-contemplation phase to the contemplation phase. By facilitating an exploration of belief systems about the evolution of the drug problem and its impact on the youngster's life, in addition to providing support, the psychologist may help the youngster move from the contemplation to the planning stage.

Motivational interviewing is an evidence-based technique for facilitating movement from pre-contemplation through contemplation to planning (Miller & Rollnick, 2002; Schmidt, 2005). Here, the therapist empathizes with the client to convey understanding of the problem, elaborates the discrepancy between the client's deeply held values and the problematic drug-using behaviour, meets resistance to change with reflection and understanding rather than confrontation and supports self-efficacy by highlighting evidence that shows change is possible.

In the transition from planning to action, the most helpful role for the psychologist to adopt is that of consultant to the clients' attempts at problem solving. In addition to providing support and an opportunity to explore belief systems, the psychologist helps youngsters examine various action plans that may help disrupt destructive behavioural patterns. The psychologist also facilitates the development of an emotional commitment to change. This role of consultant to the client's attempts at behavioural change is also appropriate for the transition from the action phase to the maintenance phase, where the central concern of the youngster is relapse prevention.

Prochaska et al. (1992) noted that different schools of therapy place particular emphasis on one or more of these common change processes, but most schools of therapy have something to say about each and in practice therapists tend to move through a progression from support to belief-system exploration to behavioural change consultation. Furthermore, naturalistic studies of a wide variety of substance abusers show that maturation out of substance abuse, when it occurs without treatment, involves life events that help people move from pre-contemplation through the various stages to maintenance. Thus, those who recover change daily routines, enlist social support, achieve a non-drug-related purpose in life and avoid cues that trigger relapse (Chiauzzi & Liljegren, 1993).

Prochaska et al. (1992) argue that five principal categories of factor are involved in symptom maintenance:

- situational symptom-maintaining factors
- maladaptive cognitions
- interpersonal conflicts
- family conflicts
- intrapsychic conflicts.

These five factors are hierarchically organized, with earlier factors being more responsive to change than later factors. Effective therapy in the addictions may follow one of three strategies once the person has passed through to the action stage. The first strategy is to target the situation which maintains the symptom only and, if symptom relief does not occur, a shift to the cognitive level should be made. Shifts to other levels within the hierarchy should only be made when symptom relief does not occur. The second strategy is to focus on the key level within the hierarchy that assessment shows is involved in problem maintenance. With teenager drug users this is most likely to be at the family systems level. A third strategy is to target all levels by, for example, offering individual work to alter maladaptive cognitions and intrapsychic conflicts, peer-group work and social skills training to target interpersonal conflicts and family work to address family conflicts and drug-abuse-maintaining family interaction patterns.

Relapse prevention theory

Marlatt and Gordon (1985) argue that, in high-risk situations, drug users who have well-rehearsed coping strategies and use them effectively develop increased self-efficacy beliefs and a decreased probability of relapse. Those who have no coping strategies are driven to relapse by their low self-efficacy beliefs in their capacity to avoid substance use and their expectations of a high from drug use. This leads to the abstinence violation effect (AVE), where guilt and a sense of loss of control pre-dominate. This failure experience in turn leads to an increased probability of relapse. The central component of treatment based on this model is the development and rehearsal of coping strategies for managing situations where there is a high risk of relapse and also managing the AVE, so that a minor slip, like taking one drink, does not snowball into a major relapse.

ASSESSMENT

In addition to the routine assessment procedures outlined in Chapter 4, assessment of adolescents or children with drug-related problems should cover the clinical features and diagnostic criteria outlined in Tables 15.1, 15.2, 15.3 and 15.4 and the aetiological and protective factors outlined in Figure 15.1. A number of psychometric instruments that may be a useful adjunct to a clinical interview are listed in Table 15.7. In addition, referral for a full physical examination and regular urinalysis for the duration of assessment and treatment are essential. Physical examination allows for the identification and treatment of drug-related physical complications and to determine if conditions such as hepatitis or HIV infection are present. Awareness of the extent of physical problems may have an important motivating effect for the youngster and family to become fully engaged in treatment. Regular urinalysis provides reliable information on relapse, which is critical for effective treatment of habitual but not experimental drug abusers.

In assessing the families of youngsters with drug problems, child protection issues should be kept in mind. Parents who abuse drugs act as deviant role models for their children and expose their children to a variety of other life stresses (Coleman & Cassell, 1995; Drummond & Fitzpatrick, 2000). These include psychological unavailability due to intoxication or drug-related illnesses, especially AIDS; neglect and unresponsive parenting; poverty, due to the costs of maintaining their drug abuse; exposure to aggression associated with bad debts or anger-regulation problems while intoxicated or in withdrawal; exposure to criminal activities such as prostitution and physical child abuse due to poor frustration tolerance. Teenagers who abuse drugs and have children may require assessment from a child protection viewpoint, and reference should be made to Chapters 19, 20 and 21 in conducting such

PRE-DISPOSING FACTORS

CONTEXTUAL PRE-DISPOSING FACTORS

Parent–child factors in early life
- Attachment problems
- Inconsistent parental discipline
- Lack of intellectual stimulation
- Authoritarian parenting
- Permissive parenting
- Neglectful parenting

Exposure to family problems in early life
- Parental alcohol and substance abuse
- Parental psychological problems
- Parental criminality
- Marital discord or violence
- Family disorganization
- Deviant siblings

Stresses in early life
- Bereavements
- Separations
- Child abuse
- Social disadvantage
- Institutional upbringing

PERSONAL PRE-DISPOSING FACTORS

Psychological factors
- Conduct problems
- Emotional problems
- Specific learning disabilities
- Positive beliefs about drug abuse
- Risk taking and sensation seeking
- Difficult temperament
- Low self-esteem
- External locus of control

PERSONAL PROTECTIVE FACTORS

Biological factors
- Good physical health

Psychological factors
- High IQ
- Easy temperament
- High self-esteem
- Internal locus of control
- High self-efficacy
- Optimistic attributional style
- Mature defence mechanisms
- Functional coping strategies

PERSONAL MAINTAINING FACTORS

Biological factors
- Physiological dependence
- HIV, hepatitis and other drug-related illnesses may cause negative mood states which maintain drug abuse

Behaviour
- Academic and vocational problems arising from drug abuse may cause negative mood states which maintain drug abuse
- Involvement in justice system due to theft or drug abuse may cause negative mood states which maintain drug abuse
- Positive beliefs about drug abuse
- Sensation seeking and risk taking
- Low self-efficacy
- Immature defence mechanisms
- Dysfunctional coping strategies

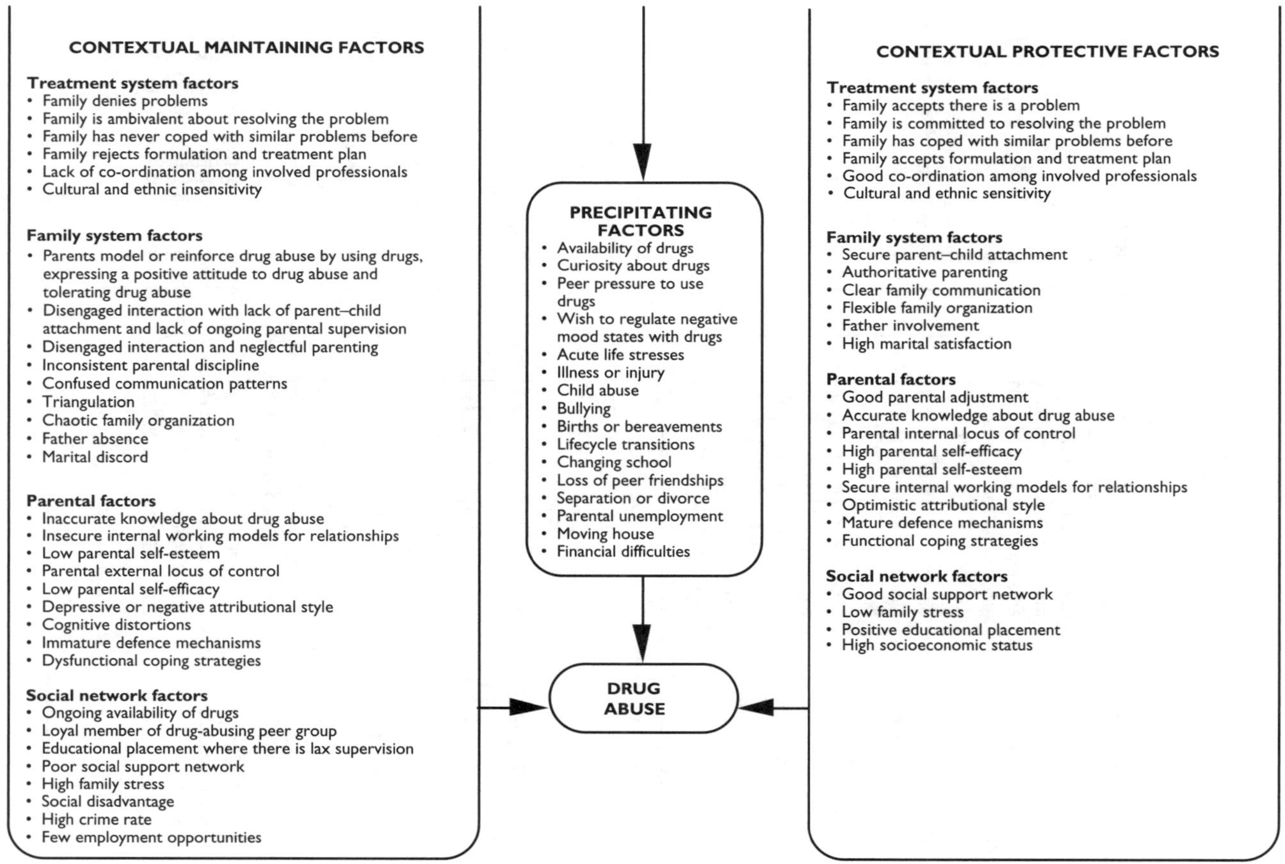

CONTEXTUAL MAINTAINING FACTORS

Treatment system factors
- Family denies problems
- Family is ambivalent about resolving the problem
- Family has never coped with similar problems before
- Family rejects formulation and treatment plan
- Lack of co-ordination among involved professionals
- Cultural and ethnic insensitivity

Family system factors
- Parents model or reinforce drug abuse by using drugs, expressing a positive attitude to drug abuse and tolerating drug abuse
- Disengaged interaction with lack of parent–child attachment and lack of ongoing parental supervision
- Disengaged interaction and neglectful parenting
- Inconsistent parental discipline
- Confused communication patterns
- Triangulation
- Chaotic family organization
- Father absence
- Marital discord

Parental factors
- Inaccurate knowledge about drug abuse
- Insecure internal working models for relationships
- Low parental self-esteem
- Parental external locus of control
- Low parental self-efficacy
- Depressive or negative attributional style
- Cognitive distortions
- Immature defence mechanisms
- Dysfunctional coping strategies

Social network factors
- Ongoing availability of drugs
- Loyal member of drug-abusing peer group
- Educational placement where there is lax supervision
- Poor social support network
- High family stress
- Social disadvantage
- High crime rate
- Few employment opportunities

PRECIPITATING FACTORS
- Availability of drugs
- Curiosity about drugs
- Peer pressure to use drugs
- Wish to regulate negative mood states with drugs
- Acute life stresses
- Illness or injury
- Child abuse
- Births or bereavements
- Lifecycle transitions
- Changing school
- Loss of peer friendships
- Separation or divorce
- Parental unemployment
- Moving house
- Financial difficulties

DRUG ABUSE

CONTEXTUAL PROTECTIVE FACTORS

Treatment system factors
- Family accepts there is a problem
- Family is committed to resolving the problem
- Family has coped with similar problems before
- Family accepts formulation and treatment plan
- Good co-ordination among involved professionals
- Cultural and ethnic sensitivity

Family system factors
- Secure parent–child attachment
- Authoritative parenting
- Clear family communication
- Flexible family organization
- Father involvement
- High marital satisfaction

Parental factors
- Good parental adjustment
- Accurate knowledge about drug abuse
- Parental internal locus of control
- High parental self-efficacy
- High parental self-esteem
- Secure internal working models for relationships
- Optimistic attributional style
- Mature defence mechanisms
- Functional coping strategies

Social network factors
- Good social support network
- Low family stress
- Positive educational placement
- High socioeconomic status

Figure 15.1 Factors to consider in adolescent drug abuse

Table 15.7 Psychometric instruments that may be used as an adjunct to clinical interviews in the assessment of drug abuse

Instrument	Publication	Comments
Adolescent Alcohol Involvement Scale	Mayer, J. & Filstead, W. (1979). The adolescent alcohol involvement scale: An instrument for measuring adolescent use and misuse of alcohol. *Journal of Studies in Alcohol*, 40, 291–300	A brief self-report screening inventory
Drug Abuse Screening Test	Skinner, H. (1982). The drug abuse screening test. *Addictive Behaviour*, 7, 363–371	A 20-item self-report screening test
Personal Experience Screening Questionnaire	Winters, K. (1991). *Personal Experience Screening Questionnaire*. Los Angeles, CA: Western Psychological Services. http://www.wpspublish.com/	A 40-item screening instrument which is a scaled-down version of the Personal Experience Inventory
Adolescent Diagnostic Interview	Winters, K. & Henly, G. (1989). *Adolescent Diagnostic Interview*. Los Angeles, CA: Western Psychological Services. http://www.wpspublish.com/	A structured interview which yields DSM diagnoses and indices of social and cognitive functioning and life stress
Personal Experience Inventory	Winters, K. & Henly, G. (1989). *Personal Experience Inventory*. Los Angeles, CA: Western Psychological Services. http://www.wpspublish.com/	A 276-item self-report inventory that assesses drug use, personal, family and school-related adjustment for use in treatment planning
Drug use Severity Inventory	Tarter, R. (1990). Evaluation and treatment of adolescent substance abuse: A decision tree method. *American Journal of Drug and Alcohol Abuse*, 16, 1–46	A 149-self-report instrument that yields a profile which highlights treatment needs
Teen Addiction Severity Index	Kaiminer, Y., Wagner, E., Plummer, E., Seifer, R. (1993). Validation of the Teen Addiction Severity Index (T-ASI): Preliminary Findings. *The American Journal of Addictions*, 3, 250–254	An extensive interview that yields information on drug abuse, family, peer group, school/employment, psychiatric and legal status

assessments. These chapters may also be consulted in cases where the parents of referred children are engaged in habitual drug abuse that compromises the child's parenting environment. A summary of pre-disposing, precipitating, maintaining and protective factors to consider in the assessment of cases of drug abuse is presented in Figure 15.1 (American Academy of Child and Adolescent Psychiatry, 1997e; Chassin et al., 2003; Crome et al., 2004; Myers et al., 1998; Pagliaro & Pagliaro, 1996; Rutter, 2002b; Vik et al., 1997; Weinberg et al., 2002).

Pre-disposing risk factors

Both personal and contextual factors may pre-dispose youngsters to developing drug abuse. Personal pre-disposing factors include pre-existing conduct problems or emotional problems; specific learning difficulties, attention problems and academic difficulties; a propensity for risk taking and positive attitudes and values concerning drug use. Difficult temperament, low self-esteem and an external locus of control may also pre-dispose youngsters to engage in drug abuse. Early onset of drug abuse is a personal risk factor for later persistent drug abuse. Contextual pre-disposing factors deserving particular attention include a poor relationship with parents, often associated with attachment problems or a problematic parenting style; little supervision from parents and inconsistent discipline; parental drug abuse; and family disorganization with unclear rules, roles and routines. Parental criminality or psychological problems, marital discord or the presence of deviant siblings within the family home are other possible contextual pre-disposing factors. Early life stresses may render youngsters vulnerable to developing drug problems. Included here are abusive experiences, bereavements, separation, social disadvantage and an institutional upbringing.

Precipitating factors

Adolescent drug abuse in Western society tends to follow a progression from early use of cigarettes and alcohol, to problem drinking, to the use of hallucinogenic drugs (such as THC) to polydrug abuse (Wills & Filer, 1996). Not all adolescents progress from one stage to the next. Progression is dependent on the presence of precipitating factors and pre-disposing risk factors. However, at all stages, availability of drugs is a precipitating factor when coupled with some personal wish such as the desire to experiment to satisfy curiosity, the wish to conform to peer pressure or the wish to control negative mood states. These negative mood states may arise as a response to recent life stresses such as child abuse, bullying, changing schools, loss of peer friendships, parental separation, bereavement, illness, injury, parental unemployment, moving house or financial difficulties. Involvement in a deviant peer group, parental cigarette and alcohol use and minor delinquent activities are the main risk factors which precede initial cigarette and alcohol use. Progression to problem drinking is more likely to occur if the adolescent develops beliefs and values favouring excessive alcohol use. A further progression to the use of hallucinogenic drugs (such as THC) requires the availability of such drugs and exposure to peer use. A host of pre-disposing risk factors, listed in the previous section, predict the progression towards the final step of polydrug abuse; the more of these factors that are present, the more likely the adolescent is to progress to polydrug abuse.

Maintaining factors

Once a pattern of drug abuse has become established it may be maintained by both personal and contextual factors. At a personal level, drug abuse may be maintained by physical and psychological dependence and by a wish to regulate negative mood states that arise from physical, economic and psychosocial complications of drug abuse. Thus drug abuse may be maintained by depressed mood or anxiety arising from hepatitis, HIV infection, lack of money, relationship problems, academic and vocational difficulties, involvement in the justice system for drug-related crimes and so forth. Positive beliefs about drugs and the need to engage in risk-taking behaviour may also maintain drug abuse. Drug abuse may be maintained, on the one hand, by low self-efficacy, that is, the belief that the youngster cannot be effective in controlling drug use. On the other hand, drug abuse may be maintained by the use of immature defences, such as denial of the severity of the problems or the degree of dependence. Dysfunctional coping strategies such as wishful thinking may all maintain drug abuse by preventing youngsters from taking responsibility for planning a strategy for managing the problem.

At a contextual level, drug abuse may be maintained by parental modelling of drug abuse, expressing positive attitudes about drug abuse and reinforcement of drug abuse through failing to consistently prohibit drug use and failing to adequately supervise youngsters. These difficulties are more likely to occur in families where there is a lack of attachment between parents and children, and where there is inconsistent discipline, confused communication, and chaotic family organization. Marital discord and limited involvement of the father in routine care and supervision of the adolescents may also maintain adolescent drug abuse. Often this involves a process of triangulation. Here, parental conflicts are de-toured through the child, so the parents chronically and inconclusively argue about how to manage the drug abuse rather than resolving their dissatisfactions with each other and then working as a co-operative co-parental team. In these instances the adolescent may engage in a covert alliance with one parent against the other. Such patterns of parenting and family organization may be partially maintained by parent personal psychological difficulties. Where parents have insecure internal working models for relationships, low self-esteem, low self-efficacy, an external locus of control, immature defences and poor coping strategies their resourcefulness in managing their children's difficulties may be compromised. Parents may also become involved in drug-abuse-maintaining interactions with their children if they have inaccurate knowledge about adolescent drug abuse and its management.

Drug abuse may be maintained by high levels of stress, limited support and social disadvantage within the family's wider social system, since these features may deplete parents' and children's personal resources for dealing constructively with the drug problem. Educational placements where teaching staff have little time to devote to home–school liaison meetings and closely supervising youngsters so that they do not abuse drugs at school may also maintain drug problems. Drug problems may be maintained through the adolescent's attachment to a deviant peer group in which drug abuse and positive attitudes towards drugs are present. Adolescents are more likely to continue to use drugs if they live in an area where there is high availability, a high crime rate, few alternatives to drug abuse and few employment opportunities.

Within the treatment system, a lack of co-ordination and clear communication among involved professionals, including family physicians, paediatricians, psychiatrists, drug treatment counsellors, nurses, teachers, psychologists and so forth may maintain adolescents' drug problems. It is not unusual for various members of the professional network to offer conflicting opinions and advice on the nature and management of drug problems to adolescents and their families. These may range from viewing the adolescent as mentally or physically ill and therefore not responsible for drug-using behaviour on the one hand, to seeing the youngster as healthy but deviant and deserving punitive management, on the other. Where co-operation problems between families and treatment teams develop, and families deny the existence of the problems, the validity of the diagnosis and formulation, or the appropriateness of the treatment programme, then the adolescent's difficulties may persist. Treatment systems that are not sensitive to the cultural and ethnic beliefs and values of the youngster's family system may maintain drug abuse by inhibiting engagement or promoting drop-out from treatment and preventing the development of a good working alliance between the treatment team, the youngster and his or her family. Parents' lack of experience in dealing with similar problems in the past is a further factor that may compromise their capacity to work co-operatively with the treatment team and so may contribute to the maintenance of the adolescent's difficulties.

Protective factors

The probability that a treatment programme will be effective is influenced by a variety of personal and contextual protective factors. It is important that these be assessed and included in the later formulation, since it is protective factors that usually serve as the foundation for therapeutic change. At a biological level, physical health and the absence of drug-related conditions such as HIV infection or hepatitis may be viewed as protective factors which may contribute to recovery. Where health problems are present, these may lead to demoralization and treatment drop-out. A high IQ, an easy temperament, high self-esteem, an internal locus of control, high self-efficacy and an optimistic attributional style are all important personal protective factors. Other important personal protective factors include mature defence mechanisms and functional coping strategies, particularly good problem-solving skills and a capacity to make and maintain non-deviant peer friendships.

Within the family, secure parent–adolescent attachment and authoritative parenting are central protective factors, particularly if they occur within the context of a flexible family structure in which there is clear communication, high marital satisfaction and both parents share the day-to-day tasks of caring for, and supervising the adolescent.

Good parental adjustment is also a protective factor. Where parents have an internal locus of control, high self-efficacy, high self-esteem, internal working models for secure attachments, an optimistic attributional style, mature defences and functional coping strategies, then they are better resourced to manage their adolescent's difficulties constructively. Accurate knowledge about drug abuse is also a protective factor.

Within the broader social network, the lack of availability of drugs, high levels of support, low levels of stress and membership of a high socio-economic group are all protective factors. Where families are embedded in social networks that provide a high level of support and place few stressful demands on family members, then it is less likely that parents' and children's resources for dealing with drug-related problems will become depleted. A well-resourced educational placement may also be viewed as a protective factor. Educational placements where teachers have sufficient time and flexibility to attend home–school liaison meetings and offer close supervision to prevent drug taking at school contribute to positive outcomes for adolescents with drug-related problems.

Within the treatment system, co-operative working relationships between the treatment team and the family and good co-ordination of multi-professional input are protective factors. Treatment systems that are sensitive to the cultural and ethnic beliefs and values of the youngster's family are more likely help families engage with, and remain in treatment, and foster the development of a good working alliance. Families are more likely to benefit from treatment when they accept the formulation of the problem given by the treatment team and are committed to working with the team to resolve it. Where families have successfully faced similar problems before, then they are more likely to benefit from treatment and in this sense previous experience with similar problems is a protective factor.

FORMULATION

Following assessment, a formulation should be constructed that integrates and systematizes salient features from assessment interviews, psychometrics and physical examinations into a coherent explanation for the aetiology and maintenance of the youngster's drug problem. A clear position should be reached on whether the drug problem reflects transient experimentation or a more entrenched pattern of habitual drug abuse. Pre-disposing, precipitating and maintaining factors should be specified and important strengths or protective factors noted. Co-morbid problems should be mentioned and their association with the drug problem explained. In light of the formulation, a series of treatment options and the preferred treatment plan should be specified. This plan should aim to modify the youngster's pattern of drug abuse primarily by addressing significant maintaining factors and building on personal and family strengths.

TREATMENT

A multi-systemic approach to drug abuse involving family-based intervention and individual therapy is the most effective available treatment for adolescent drug abusers (Cormack & Carr, 2000; Rowe & Liddle, 2003). Multi-systemic family-based approaches have been shown to be effective for engaging abusers and their networks in therapy, for reducing drug abuse, for improving associated behaviour problems, for improving the overall family functioning and for preventing relapse.

A central assumption of family-based intervention is that drug abuse is maintained by inappropriate patterns of family functioning. For example, in some of the best-controlled studies of family therapy for adolescent drug abusers, Szapocznik and Kurtines (1989) found that drug abuse was associated with a lack of clear parental alliance and intergenerational boundaries between the drug abuser and the parents, a lack of flexibility in problem-solving strategies or chaotic problem-solving strategies, a lack of conflict-resolution skills, extreme enmeshment or disengagement, difficulty negotiating a lifecycle transition such as a family member leaving home and a family perception of the drug abuser as a problem independent of the pattern of interaction around him. These patterns may include criticism, over-protection, excessive nurturance, excessive attention or denial of all other problems. Family-based intervention aims to reduce drug abuse by engaging families in treatment and helping family members change these patterns of family functioning in which the drug abuse is embedded.

Effective family-based treatment programmes for adolescent drug abuse involve the following processes which, while overlapping, may be conceptualized as stages of therapy (Cormack & Carr, 2000; Liddle & Hogue, 2001; Rowe & Liddle, 2003; Stanton & Heath, 1995):

- engagement, problem definition and contracting
- becoming drug free
- facing denial and creating a context for a drug-free lifestyle
- family reorganization
- disengagement.

What follows is an outline of how to work with adolescents and their families using this framework.

The engagement stage

During the engagement phase, the goal is to develop a strong working alliance with a sufficient number of family members to help their adolescent change his or her drug-using behaviour. The engagement process begins with whoever comes for treatment concerned that the adolescent stop using drugs. From their account of the drug abuser's problem and the pattern of interaction in which it is embedded, other family members who are central to the maintenance of the problems or who could help with changing these problem-maintaining patterns may be identified. The psychologist may then ask about what would happen if these other people attended treatment. This line of questioning throws light on aspects of resistance to engagement in treatment.

Often those family members who attend initially (for example, the mother or the drug abuser or the sibling) are ambivalent about involving other family members in treatment. They fear that something unpleasant will happen if other family members join the treatment process. Adolescents may fear that their parents will punish them. Mothers may fear that their husbands will not support them or that they will punish the adolescent. Fathers may fear that their wives will mollycoddle the adolescent and disregard their attempts at being firm. The task of the psychologist is to frame the attendance of other family members in a way that offers reassurance that the feared outcome will not occur. The seriousness of the problem may always be offered as a reason why other family members will not do that which is feared. So the psychologist may say:

> Joey isn't here. But from what you say, at some level, he is very concerned about this drug problem too. Because we all know that there is a risk of death here. Death from over-dose, AIDS, or assault is very, very common. Most families I work with are like you and Joey. They put their differences to one side to prevent the death of one of their own. So let's talk about the best way to invite Joey to come in.

The discussion then turns to the most practical way to organize a meeting. This may involve an immediate phone call, a home visit, an individual appointment for the resistant family member outside office hours or a letter explaining that the psychologist needs the family member's assistance to prevent further risk to the drug-abusing adolescent.

In each meeting with each new member of the network, the psychologist adopts a non-blaming stance and focuses on building an alliance with that family member and recruiting them into treatment to help deal with the drug abuse. Many parents are paralysed by self-blame and view family-based treatment as a parent-punishing process. Often, this self-blame is heightened as it becomes apparent that patterns of family interaction are maintaining the drug-using behaviour. The psychologist must find a way to reduce blame while at the same time highlighting the importance of the family being engaged in treatment. Here is one way to do this:

> You asked me are you to blame for Sam's addiction. No you are not. Are there things you could have done to prevent it? Probably. But you didn't know what these were. Say you don't know this part of Dublin and you park below the bridge and when you go back to your car, there is a dent in it. Are you to blame for the dent? No. Because you didn't know it's a rough area down there. But the next time, you are responsible, because you know parking there is bad news. Well, it's the same with drug abuse. You're not to blame for what happened. But you are partly responsible for his recovery. That's a fact. Drug abuse is a family problem because your child needs you to help recover. You can help him recover. You can reduce the risk of his death. I know you sense this and that's why you're here.

The engagement phase concludes when important family members have agreed to participate in a time-limited treatment contract with the goal of the adolescent becoming drug free.

To engage youngsters and parents in treatment, begin by identifying the youngster's and parents' agendas, which may be quite different. Youngsters may wish to be understood and taken seriously, to learn better street-survival skills or to resolve parent–adolescent conflicts. Parents may wish their youngsters to stop taking drugs, pursue their education and conform to parental house rules. Concreteness and specificity in identifying such agendas or goals is critical. Assume that youngsters and parents will have difficulty forming a good working alliance and engaging in treatment with very good reason. Youngsters with extensive treatment histories and parents with a history of failing to help their youngster may be wary of being pathologized, judged and misunderstood. Thus, an approach that privileges their viewpoint and the identification of their strengths and potential and de-emphasizes their deficits will facilitate engagement. Engagement of parents is enhanced by allowing ample time to ventilate emotions. This allows parents to feel understood. However, during ventilation, be vigilant for instances where parents express an emotionally charged wish to help their child escape from a drug-abusing lifestyle just one more time. Such expressions may be amplified and expanded as a motivational platform from which parents may become committed to following through on treatment. Engagement of parents is also enhanced through psychoeducation. This involves giving them accurate information on adolescent development, drug abuse and ways in which individual, family, school and peer-group interventions can alter drug-taking behaviour.

Becoming street-drug free

Once the family agrees to participate in treatment, the psychologist tells the family that for treatment to be effective, drug use must stop first and, once that has happened, alternatives to a drug-based lifestyle can be discussed, not vice versa. If alternatives to a drug-based lifestyle and changes in family relationships are discussed first, with the expectation that this will lead to drug use stopping, then treatment will probably fail.

If the adolescent is not physically dependent on drugs, then a date for stopping should be set in the near future and a drug-free period of 10 days after that date set, during which the parents take responsibility for round-the-clock surveillance of the adolescent, to both comfort him and prevent drug use. If the adolescent is physically dependent on drugs, plans for detoxification should be made. Home-based detoxification with medical back-up may be possible in some cases. Home-based detoxification requires the family to agree a 24-hour rota to monitor the adolescent and administer medication periodically under medical direction. Alternatively, hospital-based detoxification may be arranged. However, home-based detoxification has the advantage of giving the family a central role in the recovery process. Following home-based detoxification, family members will be less likely to become involved in patterns of behaviour that maintain drug abuse in the future. They will also be less likely to blame the treatment team when relapses occur during the recovery process and more likely to take some responsibility for dealing with these relapses.

In some instances, where opiate-dependent drug-abusers are unwilling to become drug-free, participation in a methadone maintenance programme is an alternative to detoxification. Methadone is typically prescribed for people addicted to heroin as an alternative to either detoxification or continued use of street drugs. Family-based treatment in conjunction with methadone maintenance has been shown to lead to a significant reduction in the use of street drugs in comparison with methadone maintenance alone (Stanton and Todd, 1982). However, a problem with methadone maintenance is that drug dependence (albeit prescribed-drug dependence) continues to be central to the adolescent's lifestyle and to the organization of the family.

Confronting denial and creating a context for a drug-free lifestyle

Where adolescents have developed a drug-oriented identity and lifestyle, participation in self-help programmes such as Nar-Anon is essential. These programmes provide the unique combination of peer support and confrontation required to erode the denial that characterizes many adolescents who have become habitual drug users. Such drug users deny their physical and psychological dependence on drugs, the impact of their drug-related behaviour on their emotional and social development, the impact of their drug-related behaviour on their family relationships and their drug-related crimes.

If access to a self-help group is unavailable, such groups may be set up and facilitated by a psychologist. In this type of group, each member must begin by stating congruently and honestly their experience of being dependent on drugs and not in control of their lives. Members must describe repeatedly and congruently the ways in which their use of drugs has effected their relationships with all significant people in their lives and their evaluation of themselves. They must make an inventory of everyone they have wronged as a result of their drug abuse and make reparation. They must make commitment to an alternative drug-free lifestyle. The role of the facilitator is to encourage group members to confront each other's denial when they engage in various distortions, minimizations and rationalizations for their drug-related behaviour. The facilitator must also encourage members to support each other when they have shown courage and honesty in owning up to the destructive drug-related behaviour for which they have been responsible.

As group members give up denial and accept the support of the group, unresolved personal issues related to emotional development and identity formation may emerge. These include unresolved grief associated with losses and bereavements, or reactions to trauma such as physical or sexual abuse. Guidelines for working with grief and loss are given in Chapter 24. Reactions to trauma are discussed under PTSD in Chapter 12 and child abuse and neglect are covered in Chapters 19, 20 and 21.

Adolescents who have experimented with drugs or been involved in mild recreational drug use do not usually require group work, where the focus is on denial. Rather, they require individual or group work to help them develop assertiveness skills for avoiding peer pressure to engage in further drug use or social anxiety management training to help them deal with social pressure if this under-pins their recreational drug taking.

Family reorganization

The central task in family reorganization is to help the family disrupt the patterns of interaction which have evolved around the adolescent's drug-related behaviours. These drug-related behaviours include obtaining money and resources to get drugs, anti-social actions carried out when under the influence of drugs and conduct problems such as breaking rules about curfew times, school non-attendance, homework non-completion, theft, destruction of property and so forth. To alter interactional patterns around drug abuse and drug-related deviant behaviour, family members must be helped to set very clear, observable and realistic goals both with respect to the adolescent's behaviour and with respect to the parents' behaviour. Broadly speaking, the goals for the adolescent will amount to conforming to a set of house rules which specify minimum behavioural standards at home. The main goal for the parents will be to retain a parental alliance with respect to enforcing the house rules. Resolving conflict about the precise behaviour expected of the adolescent, the consequences for compliance and non-compliance and the way in which both parents will work jointly to support each other is a central part of this work. Communication training, problem-solving training and the use of points-based reward systems in the manner described for adolescent conduct disorders in Chapter 10 may be incorporated into this stage of treatment as appropriate.

Parents should be asked to err on the side of treating adolescents as somewhat younger than their years during the early part of this phase of treatment. They should agree to relax the house rules by negotiation, as their adolescents show that they have the maturity to remain drug-free and follow the house rules.

Concurrently, the psychologist should hold a number of sessions with the parents in the absence of the teenager and siblings to help them draw a boundary around their marital system by planning time together without the children. The goal here is to foster mutual support between the parents and to detriangulate the adolescent, who may have been stuck in the position of a go-between with one parent looking to the child rather than their spouse for support.

Disengagement

Once a stable drug-free period has elapsed and new routines have been established within the family which disrupt drug-abuse-maintaining family patterns, disengagement may occur. Relapse prevention is central to the disengagement process. It involves identifying situations which may precipitate relapse and helping the youngster and family members identify and develop confidence in their coping strategies for managing these. Dangerous situations tend to be those where there is high stress, low mood, lessened vigilance and greater opportunity for drug availability and use. Coping strategies include positive thinking, distraction, avoidance and seeking social support.

One-person family treatment

Not all youngsters are lucky enough to have families who are willing or able to engage in conjoint family treatment. Unfortunately, individual supportive or exploratory psychotherapy is of little benefit for adolescent substance abusers and in some instances these types of intervention may exacerbate drug abuse by helping the adolescent find historical reasons to account for his or her current problems. An alternative to traditional individual approaches is one-person family treatment (Szapocznik & Kurtines, 1989). In one-person family treatment, during the engagement phase, the psychologist identifies the part of the client that wants to recover and develops an alliance with that part. Treatment goals and a time-frame for the treatment contract is agreed. Then, to clarify the patterns of interaction in which the drug-related behaviours are embedded, the psychologist invites the adolescent to describe the roles other family members take with respect to him or her when he or she engages in drug-related behaviour. When the psychologist has a good idea of what these behaviours are, he or she can role-play one or more family members and check out how the adolescent responds to the mother, father, siblings and so forth, and which aspects of their behaviour is maintaining the drug-using behaviour. This will yield a fairly accurate description of the pattern of interaction around the presenting problem.

To change the drug-abuse-maintaining patterns of family interaction, the psychologist maps out these patterns on paper with the adolescent and coaches him or her to act differently at home to change the family's behaviour. For example, if a regular interaction involves the adolescent being called 'a good-for-nothing junkie' by the father, and this is followed by the mother attacking the father and calling him a 'waster and a lush', the adolescent might be coached to say:

> We're all in this together. We always fight with each other. It solves nothing and I'm stopping right now.

Of if the mother has confided to the adolescent that she knows her husband is having an affair and this hurts her deeply, the adolescent might be coached to say:

> Mum, talk to him about it. Don't bring that stuff to me.

These changes in the adolescent's behaviour will disrupt patterns of behaviour associated with drug-using behaviour. Each treatment session begins with a review of the way in which changes in the adolescent's behaviour affected drug-using related interaction patterns within the family. For one-person family treatment to be effective it is useful if it is coupled with attendance at a drug abuser's self-help programme such as Nar-Anon (NA) and regular urinalysis to objectively monitor drug abstinence.

PREVENTION

Many approaches to preventing drug abuse have been shown to be ineffective (Essau, 2004; Schinke et al., 1991). These include giving factual information only, giving factual information coupled with anxiety-provoking information or moral appeals and offering alternative interpersonal or risky activities so that adolescents can get a natural high rather than a drug-induced high. The most promising preventive interventions are school-based skills training programmes coupled with community-based parent training programmes embedded in a multi-agency and multi-professional community-wide co-operative network (Coughlan, Doyle & Carr, 2002; Crome & McArdle, 2004). In the most effective school-based skills training programmes, youngsters are targeted during their pre-teens and are trained in an array of social and interpersonal skills necessary to resist inducements to smoke, drink alcohol or use street drugs. These skills include identifying and avoiding situations where there is a risk of being pressurized into drug abuse, assertiveness skills to resist peer pressure, cognitive skills to resist media persuasion to smoke and drink, interpersonal problem-solving skills to look for alternatives in complex social situations where drugs are being used, communication skills, self-control skills, self-monitoring and self-instructional skills for building confidence, and self-regulation and relaxation skills for reducing tension. These skills are taught through live or videotape demonstration, instruction, rehearsal, feedback, reinforcement and home practice. Parent groups may be run concurrently with school-based skills training. The parents' groups aim to network parents into a cohesive organization, keep them informed of the skills training curriculum in which the children are engaged, and coach them in how to support the children in using the skills taught in the school-based classes. To be maximally effective, child-focused skills training and parent training should be conducted within the context of a co-operative multi-agency and multi-professional community-wide network. Within this network, policy and guidelines for practice should be developed to reduce drug availability and treat youngsters who become involved in drug abuse at an early stage. This network should include professionals and representatives from law enforcement, justice, education, health services, social services, probation, child protection, self-help organizations such as AA and NA and other relevant agencies within the public and private domains.

SUMMARY

Habitual drug abuse in adolescence is of particular concern to clinical psychologists because it may have a negative long-term effect on adolescents and an intergenerational effect on their children. A conservative estimate is that between 5 and 10% of teenagers under 19 have drug problems serious enough to require clinical intervention. A distinction is made between drug dependence and drug abuse. While drug abuse refers to using drugs in such a way that the person is harmed, drug dependence refers to those situations where there is a compulsive pattern of use that may involve physiological changes that accompany the phenomena of tolerance and withdrawal. Drug abuse is associated with a wide variety of behaviour patterns which may be described in terms of the age of onset, the duration of drug abuse, the frequency of use, the range of substances used, and the amount used. Physiological features of drug abuse may be grouped into those associated with intoxication, those that follow intoxication, those associated with withdrawal following the development of dependence and medical complications which arise from drug abuse. At an affective level, negative mood states typically follow the euphoria of intoxication for most classes of drugs. At a perceptual level, some types of drugs, but particularly hallucinogens, lead to pronounced abnormalities during intoxication and withdrawal. With respect to cognition most street drugs lead to impaired concentration, reasoning and judgement during intoxication and withdrawal. Long-term regular drug abuse in many instances leads to impaired cognitive functioning. Drug abuse may have an impact on interpersonal adjustment leading to family-, school- and peer-group-based difficulties. Drug abuse often occurs with other co-morbid psychological problems, including conduct disorder, ADHD, specific learning difficulties, mood disorders, anxiety disorders, schizophrenia and bulimia. The relationship between these co-morbid psychological problems and drug abuse is complex. Explanations for drug abuse have focused on biological pre-disposing factors, intrapsychic deficits, cognitive-behavioural learning processes, family systems factors, societal factors, multiple risk factors and the change process involved in recovery and relapse. Research conducted to test these various theories have led to the identification of biological, psychological and social factors which increase vulnerability to drug abuse, which may precipitate its onset or maintain habitual drug abuse. Because of the complex aetiology of drug abuse, a multi-systemic approach to assessment and treatment is essential. Effective treatment programmes for adolescent drug abuse are typically family based and progress through a series of stages. These include engagement, becoming drug free, facing denial and creating a context for a drug-free lifestyle, family reorganization and disengagement. Effective prevention programmes involve child-focused skills training and the parent training conducted within the context of a co-operative multi-agency and multi-professional community wide network.

EXERCISE 15.1

Luke is a fifteen-year-old who was caught stealing money from his mother's purse at home. Both of his parents suspect that he wanted the money for drugs. They suspect that he uses cannabis and possibly LSD or E occasionally. Their suspicions are based on his unusual behaviour over the past year, particularly at week-ends. Luke is the eldest of three boys. His parents are separated and he lives with his mother three days a week and with his father four days a week. His parents separated about three years ago and have a reasonably good co-parenting relationship. Luke's development has been normal, although he has a specific learning difficulty and so has never done as well as he thinks he should at school. He is a good tennis player but has given that up in the past year. He goes out with his friends every night and comes home late. His parents find him impossible to control. Luke's brothers Ted and Ben both have some conduct problems. Luke's mother, Maria, works in a supermarket and his dad, Shay, mends cars in a back-street garage.

* Work in pairs and develop a preliminary formulation and interview plan for intake interview. Specify who you would invite and what lines of inquiry you would follow.

EXERCISE 15.2

Assign roles (two interviewers, five family members and the remainder observers) and role-play the intake interview. Refine the preliminary formulation in the light of the information gained in this interview.

FURTHER READING

Liddle, H. A. (2005). *Multidimensional Family Therapy for Adolescent Substance abuse*. New York: Norton. A version of this book is available at: http://www.chestnut.org/LI/cyt/products/MDFT_CYT_v5.pdf

Szapocznik, J. & Kurtines, W. (1989). *Breakthroughs In Family Therapy With Drug Abusing Problem Youth*. New York: Springer.

Szapocznik, J., Hervis, O. & Schwartz, S. (2002). *Brief Strategic Family Therapy for Adolescent Drug Abuse*. Rockville, MD: National Institute for Drug Abuse. Available at: http://www.drugabuse.gov/TXManuals/bsft/BSFTIndex.html

WEBSITES

Gilbert Botvin's Life Skills Drug Abuse Prevention Programme: http://www.lifeskillstraining.com/
Howard Liddle's Multidimensional Family Therapy: http://www.miami.edu/ctrada/
José Szapocznik's Brief Strategic Family Therapy: http://www.cfs.med.miami.edu/
National Substance Abuse Web Index: http://www.health.org/dbases/nsawi.aspx
The Central East Addiction Technology Transfer Centre: http://www.ceattc.org/nidacsat_bpr.asp?id=MDFT
Websites for Addictions: http://www.well.com/user/woa

Factsheets on drugs and alcohol can be downloaded from the website for Rose, G. & York, A. (2004). *Mental Health and Growing Up. Fact sheets for Parents, Teachers and Young People* (Third edition). London: Gaskell: http://www.rcpsych.ac.uk

Chapter 16

Mood problems

Depression in childhood or adolescence is a particularly distressing experience for both the young person and other family members, particularly parents. This is illustrated by the case presented in Box 16.1. Unfortunately, the outcome for depression in childhood and adolescence is not favourable. Available evidence suggests that while the majority of youngsters recover from a depressive episode within a year, they do not *grow out of* their mood disorder (American Academy of Child and Adolescent Psychiatry, 1998c; Goodyer, 2001a; Hammen & Rudolph, 2003; Harrington, 2002; Park & Goodyer, 2000). Major depression is a recurrent condition and depressed youngsters are more likely than their non-depressed counterparts to develop episodes of depression as adults, although they are no more likely to develop other types of psychological problems. Double depression, that is an ongoing persistent mood disorder (dysthymia) and an episodic major depressive condition, severe depressive symptoms, maternal depression, co-morbid conduct or drug abuse, family problems and social adversity have all been shown in longitudinal studies to be predictive of worse outcome.

After discussing the classification, epidemiology and clinical features of mood disorders, this chapter considers a variety of theoretical explanations concerning the aetiology of these types of problems, along with relevant empirical evidence. An approach to the assessment of childhood depression and its treatment will then be given. Bipolar disorder, which is characterized by episodes of both depression and mania or hypomania, is then considered. This is followed by a discussion of the management of suicide risk. The chapter concludes with a consideration of prevention of depression in at-risk populations.

DIAGNOSIS AND CLASSIFICATION

Diagnostic criteria for episodes of major depression from the DSM IV TR (APA, 2000a) and ICD 10 (WHO, 1992,1996) classification systems are presented in Table 16.1. Table 16.2 contains items from the ASEBA (Achenback

Box 16.1 A case of adolescent depression

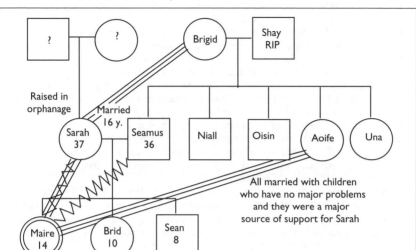

Referral. The O'Connors phoned and requested an urgent appointment at the Clanwilliam Institute after Maire admitted to shoplifting, lying and truanting from school. Seamus described his daughter on the phone as 'right out of control'.

History of the presenting problems. In the intake interview the following history of the presenting problem emerged. Sarah, while cleaning Maire's room, had found some bottles of perfume in her drawer and confronted her about this. Eventually Maire admitted to stealing them. A couple of days later, the principal from Maire's school, phoned to ask her whereabouts, and from this her parents concluded she was truanting. When confronted by her father she admitted to truanting with a girl, Julie, who was known as a troublemaker in the school. She agreed to follow house and school rules and was apparently well behaved for the next week but was found by her mother on the way home from school smoking with Julie and a gang of four youths who were in their late teens or early twenties. When grounded following this incident, she locked herself in her room for 24 hours and wailed or cried periodically and made threats of self-harm.

Developmental history. Maire was born and bred in Sligo, but moved to Dublin with the family 12 months before the referral. Maire's birth was without complications but her mother suffered post-partum depression for about 6 months following her birth. During this period Maire was cared for by her Aunt Aoife in Sligo. Aoife was one of Seamus' four married siblings. Maire's pre-school development was unremarkable but she did have trouble settling into junior school and used to be very clingy when her mother left her at school in the morning. Sometimes she refused to go into her classroom unless her mother slapped her. She occasionally had night-mares during this period. In junior school Maire was in the top half of the class and on the school junior hockey team. She had two close friends and many acquaintances. The transition to secondary school was relatively uneventful. Maire expressed some anxieties to her mother about managing in the new school. The fact that her two close friends went to secondary school with her made the process fairly easy for her. However, she found that she was physically maturing more rapidly than her two friends and felt awkward about this.

During her first two years at secondary school she formed a close friendship with an older girl was particularly wild. This girl, Tricia, lived in a single-parent family and spent a lot of time unsupervised since her mother worked shiftwork and was often at work or sleeping while Tricia and Maire were in the house. Marie occasionally became involved in conflicts with her mother because of her relationship with Tricia and the fact that she often stayed out later than permitted at Tricia's and had begun smoking.

When the O'Connors moved to Dublin, Sarah was hopeful that the rift that had opened between herself and her daughter would close and in fact this began to happen during the early months in Dublin. Maire would confide that she had few close friends at school and felt excluded by her class-mates. She would cry and confess to strong feelings of loneliness and stay in bed for whole days at the week-end but have difficulty sleeping at night. However, then she met Julie and the gap between herself and her mother widened. She became irritable around the house. She had tantrums and would not keep house rules. This was the lead-in to the presenting problems described above.

Family history. Sarah and Seamus had been married for 16 years. They met on holiday in England. Seamus was working there as a driver at the time and Sarah was in secretarial work. After about a year they were married and moved to Sligo, Seamus' home town, where he got work as a distribution manager in a computing manufacturing firm and Sarah also found a secretarial position in the same firm.

Sarah was happy to do this because she had no family ties in the UK. She had been brought up in an orphanage and a series of foster homes. She was pleased to move into a district where Seamus' family of origin lived. Seamus's mother and his four married siblings accepted her and formed good friendships with her.

Seamus and Sarah had three children, Maire, in their third year of marriage, Brid four years later and Sean two years after that. After each child, Sarah experienced post-partum depression. The first episode following Maire's birth was the worst and lasted six months. All Seamus's family were very supportive during these episodes and Aoife (Seamus's eldest sibling) in each instance took care of the new-born child while Sarah recovered.

Sarah took a break from work during the children's early years but went back to work full time two years before the family moved to Dublin. The move to Dublin was prompted by a lucrative job offer for Seamus. The job, with a foreign computing manufacturing company, was highly stressful and involved long hours, unpredictable interruptions of home life during the evenings and weekends and an aggressive work ethic. It left Seamus relatively unavailable for family life and, when available, he was irritable and exhausted.

In Dublin Sarah found herself isolated through the absence of Seamus's family of origin and Seamus's own absence from family life because of his long working hours. This isolation led to a recurrence of her depression and she was on medication for this at the time of referral.

Sarah found herself having to manage the crisis with Maire without input from Seamus because of his work commitment. She oscillated between a harsh critical stance towards Maire's theft, smoking, truanting and defiance and a highly empathic, concerned and tolerant stance towards Maire's loneliness and sense of despair. Seamus criticized her for adopting such an ambiguous position.

Maire's presentation. Maire's scores on both the internalizing and externalizing scale of the Child Behaviour Checklist, Teacher Report Form and Youth Self-Report Form were in the clinical range. On the Childhood Depression Inventory, Maire also scored above the clinical cut-off. In individual interviews, Maire reported suicidal ideation without intent. She described herself as lonely much of the time and hated living in Dublin. She missed her friends from the west and dreaded going to school, where she was ostracized and humiliated. She had become engaged in shoplifting to obtain gifts for Tricia who had befriended her. Later she stole goods and sold them to get money for cigarettes for herself and Tricia. She did not believe that she would ever fit into her new school or do well in exams despite her excellent previous school record. She thought that there was something wrong with her and that was the reason why the other girls excluded her. She described herself as ugly, boring and horrible. She found that she could not concentrate on her work and often drifted into depressing day-dreams. She looked back on her life in the west as if it belonged to someone else and said that she knew things would only get worse and nothing she would do could change this. She had thought of killing herself from time to time but had no firm plan. She had difficulty sleeping through the night and often awoke at 5 a.m. and couldn't go back to sleep. She felt tired most of the time and rarely felt like eating more than tea and toast.

Formulation. Maire shows affective, cognitive, behavioural and somatic features consistent with a diagnosis of depression. The current episode has lasted about a year. In addition she shows a variety of conduct problems which began in early adolescence and have fluctuated since then.

Pre-disposing factors for her mood disorder include a probable genetic pre-disposition and an early separation experience during her mother's post-partum depression.

The current episode was precipitated by the move to Dublin, which involved the loss of important friendships and a school context in which she was accepted and was performing above average.

Her depressed state is maintained by her self-defeating style of thought, the fact that she has now resigned herself to an isolated position in school, and the fact that she and her parents have developed a style of interacting that is either critical or over-involved.

These immediate maintaining factors occur within a wider social context where both of her parents find themselves virtually unsupported and under high levels of stress. For Seamus the main stresses are work related and for Sarah isolation is the main source of stress. The high stress and low support has begun to erode the good working relationship that Seamus and Sarah enjoyed as parents and marital partners before the move to Dublin.

The conduct problems appear to be secondary to the depression. They reflect an attempt to cope with isolation by mixing with deviant peers.

There are a number of important protective factors in this case which suggest that there may be a positive outcome. These included Maire's high overall level of academic ability and problem-solving skills; Maire's ability in the past to make and maintain friendships; Seamus and Sarah's demonstrated capacity to maintain a good marital relationship over many years and in the face of three major episodes of depression; and the parent's and Maire's commitment to resolving the problem.

Treatment. Treatment in this case involved family work to improve the level of support offered to Maire by her parents; liaison with the school, which aimed to increase Maire's involvement in structured activities such as sports and drama; and individual cognitive therapy work which aimed to help Maire challenge her negative beliefs and improve her problem-solving skills.

Table 16.1 Criteria for a major depressive episode

DSM IV TR	ICD 10
A. Five or more of the following symptoms have been present during the same two-week period nearly every day and represent a change from previous functioning; at least one of the symptoms is either (1) depressed mood or (2) loss of interest or pleasure. Symptoms may be reported or observed:	In a typical depressive episode the individual usually suffers from depressed mood, loss of interest and enjoyment and reduced energy leading to increased fatigueability and diminished activity. Marked tiredness after only slight effort is common. Other common symptoms are:
1. Depressed mood. In children and adolescents can be irritable mood 2. Markedly diminished interest or pleasure in almost all daily activities 3. Significant weight loss or gain (of 5% per month) or decrease or increase in appetite. In children consider failure to make expected weight gains 4. Insomnia or hypersomnia 5. Psychomotor agitation or retardation 6. Fatigue or loss of energy 7. Feelings of worthlessness, excessive guilt 8. Poor concentration and indecisiveness 9. Recurrent thoughts of death, suicidal ideation or suicide attempt	a. reduced concentration and attention b. reduced self-esteem and confidence c. ideas of guilt and unworthiness d. bleak and pessimistic views of the future e. ideas or acts of self-harm or suicide f. disturbed sleep g. diminished appetite The lowered mood varies little from day to day and is often unresponsive to circumstances and may show a characteristic diurnal variation as the day goes on
B. Symptoms do not meet criteria for mixed episode of mania and depression	Some of the above symptoms may be marked and develop characteristic features that are widely regarded as having special significance for example the *somatic symptoms* which are: loss of interest or pleasure in activities that are normally enjoyable; lack of emotional reactivity to normally pleasurable surroundings; waking in the morning 2 hours or more before the usual time; depression worse in the mornings; psychomotor retardation or agitation; marked loss of appetite or weight; marked loss of libido. Usually the somatic syndrome is not regarded as present unless at least four of these symptoms are present
C. Symptoms cause clinically significant distress or impairment in social occupational, educational or other important areas of functioning	
D. Symptoms not due to the direct effects of a drug or a general medical condition such as hypothyroidism	
E. The symptoms are not better accounted for by uncomplicated bereavement	*Atypical presentations* are particularly common in adolescence. In some cases anxiety, distress, and motor agitation may be more prominent at times than depression and mood changes may be masked by such features as irritability, excessive consumption of alcohol, histrionic behaviour and exacerbation of pre-existing phobic or obsessional symptoms or by hypochondriacal pre-occupations
	A duration of two weeks is required for a diagnosis

Note: Adapted from DSM IV TR (APA, 2000a), ICD 10 (WHO, 1992, 1996).

Table 16.2 ASEBA Anxious-Depressed and Withdrawn-Depressed syndromes for 1.5 to 5 and 6 to 18-year-olds

	ASEBA 1.5- to 5-year-olds	*ASEBA 6- to 18-year-olds*
Anxious–depressed syndrome	**Depression** Sad (P&T) Looks unhappy (P&T) Feels hurt (P&T)	**Depression** Talks or thinks of suicide (P&T&C) Feels worthless (P&T&C) Feels unloved (P&T&C) Feels too guilty (P&T&C) Must be perfect (P&T&C) Anxious to please (C) Afraid to make mistakes (C) Feels hurt when criticized (T)
	Anxiety Fearful (P&T) Nervous (P&T) Self-conscious (P&T) Upset by separation (P&T) Clings (P&T)	**Anxiety** Fearful and anxious (P&T&C) Nervous (P&T&C) Self-conscious (P&T&C) Has many fears (P&T&C) Fears school (P&T&C) Fears doing bad things (P&T&C) Worries (P&T&C) Cries a lot (P&T&C)
Withdrawn–depressed syndrome	**Depression** Shows little interest (P&T) Shows little affection (P&T) Unresponsive to affection (P&T)	**Depression** Sad (P&T&C) Enjoys little (P&T&C) Lacks energy (P&T&C)
	Social withdrawal Withdrawn (P&T) Avoids eye contact (P&T) Doesn't answer when spoken to (P&T) Refuses to play active games (P&T) Day-dreams (T) Acts too young (P&T) Apathetic (T)	**Social withdrawal** Withdrawn (P&T&C) Shy (P&T&C) Secretive (P&T&C) Would rather be alone (P&T&C) Refuses to talk (P&T&C)

Note: Adapted from Achenbach and Rescorla (2000, 2001). Items marked (P) are on the parent report CBCL. Items marked (T) are on the Teacher Report or Caregiver and Teacher Report form. Items marked (C) are on the Youth Self-Report form.

& Rescorla, 2000, 2001) Anxious/depressed and Withdrawn/depressed syndrome scales for toddlers and school-aged youngsters. There are marked similarities between these three diagnostic systems. All three include depressed mood, depressive cognition and suicidal ideation as central to a depressive episode. However, the DSM and ICD systems include vegetative or somatic features, which are absent from Achenbach's system. It is noteworthy that the ASEBA empirically derived syndromes, in addition to excluding vegetative features, include anxiety. The co-occurrence of anxiety and depression is dealt with in the DSM and ICD systems by making co-morbid diagnoses.

The ways various conditions which involve depressed mood have been classified in DSM IV TR and ICD 10 are set out in Figures 16.1 and 16.2. Both systems make a distinction between primary mood disorders and other conditions where affective symptoms are a secondary feature. Within the primary mood disorders, both systems make distinctions between unipolar and bipolar mood disorders and between severe episodic disorders and the milder but more persistent conditions of dysthymia and cyclothymia, which in earlier classification systems may have been termed depressive neuroses. Both systems provide a category for schizoaffective disorder for cases that

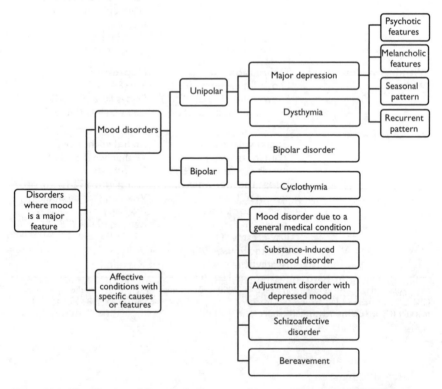

Figure 16.1 Classification of disorders where mood is major feature in DSM IV TR

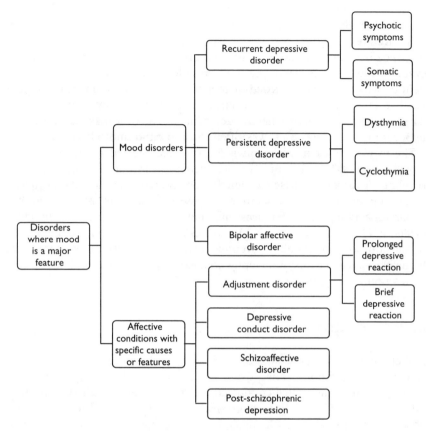

Figure 16.2 Classification of disorders where mood is major feature in ICD 10

show features of schizophrenia and depression, although only ICD 10 provides a specific category for post-psychotic depression. Both systems also provide a category for adjustment disorder with depressed mood. ICD 10 is unique in recognizing depressive conduct disorder as a distinct syndrome. Children who show features of major depression and conduct disorders would receive a dual diagnosis within the DSM IV TR system.

The distinctions between primary and secondary mood problems, between unipolar and bipolar conditions, and between recurrent and persistent disorders have replaced distinctions used in earlier classifications systems. These include:

• endogenous and reactive
• overt and masked
• neurotic and psychotic.

Reviews of the classification of mood disorders identify the following reasons for abandoning these earlier distinctions (Farmer & McGuffin, 1989; Kendell, 1976; Kolvin & Hartwin-Sadowski, 2001). The endogenous–reactive distinction has been abandoned because evidence from stressful life event research shows that almost all episodes of depression, regardless of quality or severity, are preceded by stressful life events and in that sense are reactive. The recognition that youngsters with depression may show co-morbid conduct disorders has rendered the concept of masked depression unnecessary, since the term was often used in child and adolescent psychology to classify depressed youngsters who masked their low mood with angry outbursts of aggressive or destructive behaviour. The neurotic and psychotic distinction, based originally on inferred psychodynamic aetiological factors has been discarded because evidence for inferred psychodynamic aetiological differences has not been supported by empirical evidence. However, both the ICD and DSM systems permit a diagnosis of depression with observable psychotic features, such as mood congruent hallucinations and delusions. Depression with psychotic features is associated with a poorer prognosis.

EPIDEMIOLOGY

For children and adolescents, the reliability of diagnoses of depression in epidemiological studies range from. 36 to .9 (see Table 3.2, p. 84). Thus, it appears from the better conducted studies that even with standardized interview schedules and clear diagnostic criteria, it is often difficult to diagnose depression reliably. Depression is not a rare condition (Angold & Costello, 2001; Harrington, 2002). In community samples prevalence rates of depression in youngsters under 18 range from 2 to 9%. About 2% of youngsters under 19 have severe depression and about 4% have mild to moderate depression. Depression is more common among adolescents than pre-adolescents. Depression is more common in pre-adolescent boys than girls, but more common in adolescent girls than boys. This greater preponderance of depression among teenage girls compared to boys is similar to the sex distribution of depression among adults. Depression is very common among clinic referrals. In clinic studies about 25% of referrals have a major depression.

Depression quite commonly occurs in conjunction with other disorders, particularly in children referred for treatment. In community studies of childhood depression, co-morbidity rates of 10–17% have been found for conduct disorder, anxiety disorders and attention deficit disorder (see Table 3.4, p. 86). In a community population study of the CBCL anxious-depressed syndrome, co-morbidity rates of 15–28% were found for the CBCL aggressive behaviour, attention problems and somatic symptoms syndromes (see Table 3.5, p. 87). In contrast, the co-morbidity rates for the same syndromes were much higher: 30–43% in a clinic population study of the CBCL anxious-depressed syndrome (see Table 3.4, p. 86).

It has been mentioned that in ICD 10 children who show both serious conduct problems and depression are given a diagnosis of depressive conduct disorder. This is because these children have a distinct profile. Children with depressive conduct disorder or who meet DSM diagnostic criteria for both conduct disorder and depression have greater mood variability, a worse response to imipramine, and have higher rates of substance abuse in adulthood (Harrington, 1993).

CLINICAL FEATURES

The main features of depression are presented in Table 16.3 (American Academy of Child and Adolescent Psychiatry, 1998c; Goodyer, 2001a; Hammen & Rudolph, 2003; Harrington, 2002; Park & Goodyer, 2000). These features may be linked by assuming that the depressed child has usually suffered a loss

Table 16.3 Clinical features of depression in children and adolescents

Perception	• Perceptual bias towards negative events • Mood-congruent hallucinations*
Cognition	• Negative view of self, world and future • Excessive guilt • Suicidal ideation* • Mood-congruent delusions* • Cognitive distortions • Inability to concentrate
Affect	• Depressed mood • Inability to experience pleasure • Irritable mood • Anxiety and apprehension
Behaviour	• Psychomotor retardation or agitation • Depressive stupor*
Somatic state	• Fatigue • Disturbance of sleep • Aches and pains • Loss of appetite or overeating • Change in weight* • Diurnal variation of mood (worse in morning) • Loss of interest in sex
Interpersonal adjustment	• Deterioration in family relationships • Withdrawal from peer relationships • Poor school performance

* These features occur in severe episodes of depression.

of some sort. Either a loss of an important relationship, a loss of some valued attribute such as athletic ability or health, or a loss of status.

With respect to perception, having suffered a loss, depressed children tend to perceive the world as if further losses were probable. Depressed children selectively attend to negative features of the environment and this in turn leads them to engage in depressive cognitions and unrewarding behaviour patterns, which further entrench their depressed mood. In severe cases of adolescent depression, youngsters may report mood-congruent auditory hallucinations. We may assume that this severe perceptual abnormality is present when youngsters report hearing voices criticizing them or telling them depressive things. Auditory hallucinations also occur in schizophrenia, which is discussed in Chapter 18. However, the hallucinations that occur in schizophrenia are not necessarily mood congruent.

With respect to cognition, depressed children describe themselves, the world and the future in negative terms. They evaluate themselves as worthless and are critical of their academic, athletic, musical and social accomplishments. Often, this negative self-evaluation is expressed as guilt for not living up to certain standards or letting others down. They see their world, including family, friends and school as unrewarding, critical and hostile or apathetic. They describe the future in bleak terms and report little, if any, hope that things will improve. When they report extreme hopelessness, and this is coupled with excessive guilt for which they believe they should be punished, suicidal ideas or intentions may be reported. Suicide will be discussed in detail in a later section of this chapter (p. 776). Extremely negative thoughts about the self, the world and the future may be woven together in severe cases into depressive delusional systems. In addition to the content of the depressed youngsters' thought being bleak, they also display logical errors in their thinking and concentration problems. Errors in reasoning are marked by a tendency to maximize the significance and implications of negative events and minimize the significance of positive events. Concentration and attention difficulties lead to difficulties managing schoolwork or leisure activities demanding sustained attention.

With respect to affect, low mood is a core feature of depression. Depressed mood is usually reported as a feeling of sadness, loneliness or despair and an inability to experience pleasure. Alternatively, irritability, anxiety and aggression may be the main features, with sadness and inability to experience pleasure being less prominent. This is not surprising since normal grief is characterized by sadness at the absence of the lost object, anger at the lost object for abandoning the grieving person and anxiety that further losses may occur. These grief processes are discussed in detail in Chapter 24. Depressed children and adolescents may show some cocktail of all three emotional processes, i.e. depressed mood, irritability and anxiety.

At a behavioural level, depressed youngsters may show either reduced and slowed activity levels (psychomotor retardation) or increased but ineffective activity (psychomotor agitation). They may show a failure to engage in activities that would bring them a sense of achievement or connectedness to family or friends. Where youngsters become immobile, this is referred to as depressive stupor; fortunately, this is rare.

Somatic or vegetative features such as loss of energy, disturbances of sleep and appetite, weight loss or failure to make age-appropriate weight gain, abdominal pains or headaches and diurnal variation in mood are all associated with more severe conditions. Teenagers may also report losing interest in sex. These features of depression are consistent with findings that dysregulation of neurophysiological, endocrine and immune functions are associated with depression and that sleep architecture is also affected. This material will be mentioned in more detail in the section on biological theories of depression.

At an interpersonal level, depressed children report a deterioration in their relationships with family, friends, teachers and other significant figures in their lives. They describe themselves as lonely and yet unable or unworthy of taking steps to make contact with others.

THEORIES

Theoretical explanations for depression fall into three main categories: those which focus on the role of biological factors, those which address psychological processes and those which focus on social factors in the genesis and maintenance of mood disorders. A number of influential theories from each of these areas will be briefly reviewed below.

Biological theories

Hypotheses about six classes of biological factors involved in the aetiology and maintenance of depression are set out in Table 16.4. Much of the work on the biology of depression is extremely complex and still in its early stages. The positions set out represent simplifications of this vast literature. It is also important to mention that most research on the psychobiology of mood disorders has been conducted with depressed adults rather than with children or adolescents, and in many instances biological abnormalities detected in adults with mood disorders have not been found in children and adolescents (Goodyer, 2001a).

Genetic theories

Results of twin, adoption and family studies suggest that a pre-disposition to mood disorders is genetically transmitted (Jones et al., 2002; Rice, Harold & Thapar, 2002; Strober, 2001). Precisely what biological characteristics are

Table 16.4 Theories of depression

Type	Theory	Theoretical principles	Principles of assessment and treatment
Biological theories	**Genetic theories**	Some vulnerability to abnormalities in the neurophysiological or endocrine systems which are dysfunctional in mood disorder is inherited and a polygenetic mechanism of transmission is involved	Genetic counselling
	Amine dysregulation theories	Depression occurs when there is a dysregulation of the amine systems in those centres of the brain which subserve reward- and punishment-related experiences. Noradrenalin and serotonin are the main neurotransmitters involved	Anti-depressant medication
	Endocrine dysregulation theories	Depression is due to: (1) a drop in thyroxin levels associated with a dysregulation of the hypothalamic-pituitary-thyroid axis and (2) raised cortisol levels associated with dysregulation of the hypothalamic-pituitary-adrenal axis following chronic stress	Use the dexamethasone suppression test to aid diagnosis of mood disorders
	Immune system dysfunction theories	Exposure to chronic stress or acute loss such as bereavement leads to both impaired immune system functioning and depressive symptoms. Impaired immune system functioning increases susceptibility to infections and consequent illnesses may maintain or exacerbate depression	Reduce life stress so that immune system functioning improves
	Circadian rhythm de-synchrony theories	Depression occurs when there is a de-synchrony in the circadian rhythms which governs the sleep–waking cycle	Assess REM onset latency to diagnose depression Temporarily relieve depression through partial or complete sleep deprivation

	Seasonal rhythm dysregulation theories	Depression occurs in winter when reduced daylight leads to increased secretion of melatonin by the pineal gland and this results in hibernation-like features of fatigue, over-sleeping an increase in appetite and weight gain	Treat seasonal affective disorder by: (1) administering light therapy to artificially lengthen the day and reduce melatonin secretion and (2) by altering the time at which melatonin is secreted through administering melatonin orally at key times during the day
Psychoanalytic	**Freud's introjected anger theory**	Depression occurs when a person turns anger towards the self. This usually follows the loss of a loved caregiver and the anger is directed at a part of the self that represents the lost object	Individual psychodynamic psychotherapy in which transference develops so that self-directed hostility, self-criticism, and ideas of abandonment or loss of autonomy are projected onto therapist
	Bibring's low self-esteem theory	Depression occurs when low self-esteem develops as a result of perceiving a gap between the actual and ideal self. The wide gap results from an unrealistic ideal self based on internalizations of early parental injunctions, which were probably highly critical or perfectionistic	This transference is interpreted and worked through so that more realistic standards for self-evaluation and more trusting internal working models for relationships are developed
	Blatt's attachment and autonomy theory	There are two types of depression associated with two distinct types of early parent–child relationships which engender vulnerability to depression when faced with two distinct types of stresses in later life: • *Loss of attachment* relationships may precipitate depression in those who experienced neglecting or over-indulgent parenting • *Loss of autonomy* may lead to depression in those who experienced critical punitive parenting	

Table 16.4 continued

Type	Theory	Theoretical principles	Principles of assessment and treatment
Behavioural	**Lewinsohn's behavioural theory**	People with depression avoid situations where they can receive response-contingent positive reinforcement (RCPR) because they lack the social skills required for eliciting rewarding interactions from others	Social-skills training which aims to train clients in skills necessary for receiving response-contingent positive reinforcement and to arrange the environment so that there are many opportunities for using these social skills
	Rehm's self-control theory	Depression occurs when a person selectively monitors the occurrence of negative events to the exclusion of positive events; selectively monitors immediate rather than long-term consequences of actions; sets overly stringent criteria for evaluating actions; makes negative attributions for personal actions; engages in little self-reinforcement for adaptive behaviours; and engages in excessive self-punishment	Training which aims to improve the skills required for more effective self-monitoring, self-evaluation and self-reinforcement
Cognitive	**Beck's cognitive theory**	Depression occurs when life events involving loss occur and reactivate negative cognitive schemas formed early in childhood as a result of early loss experiences. Negative schemas give rise to negative automatic thoughts and cognitive distortions which maintain a depressed mood	Cognitive therapy which aims to train clients to monitor situations where depressive automatic thoughts and distortions occur; to evaluate the validity of depressive assumptions and distortions; and to engage in activities that provide evidence to refute the negative assumptions
	Reformulated learned helplessness theory	Depressions occurs when a person repeatedly fails to control the occurrence of aversive stimuli and makes internal global stable attributions for these failures (and external, specific, unstable attributions for success)	Attributional retraining where clients learn to attribute failure to external, specific, unstable factors and success to internal, global, stable factors Change the environment so that the likelihood of successful experiences greatly outweighs the likelihood of failure experiences

Social theories		Train youngsters to reduce preferences for highly preferred successes that are beyond their ability
	Family systems theory	Depression occurs when the structure and functioning of the family prevents the child from completing age-appropriate developmental tasks	Family therapy in which family members develop supportive relationships with the depressed child and facilitate them in completing age-appropriate developmental tasks, such as individuation, in adolescence
		Bereavement, parental discord, divorce, abuse and placement in care all disrupt family structure and may lead to depression	
		In childhood, excessive parental criticism, offering attention only when failure occurs and ignoring success may lead to depression	
		In adolescence, family enmeshment and related parent–child conflict over individuation may be associated with depression	
	Interpersonal theory	Depression is multi-factorially determined but interpersonal difficulties maintain depressive symptoms	Interpersonal therapy for adolescents which addresses the specific focal interpersonal factors that maintain the youngster's depressive symptoms
		The five categories of interpersonal factors that maintain adolescent depression and are addressed in interpersonal therapy are: (1) grief, (2) role disputes, (3) role transitions, (4) interpersonal deficits, and (5) problems living in a single-parent family	

genetically transmitted and the mechanisms of transmissions are unknown. However, the results of studies conducted on amine dysregulation, endocrine abnormalities, immune system dysfunction, circadian rhythm abnormalities and the seasonal occurrence of depression in some cases suggests that a biological vulnerability to dysregulation of one or more of these systems is probably inherited (Goodyer, 2001a; Harrington, 2002). It is also probable that the vulnerability is polygenetically transmitted, since the results of family studies cannot easily be accounted for by simpler models of genetic transmission.

Amine dysregulation theories

Amine dysregulation theories argue that hypoactivity of the amine systems in neuroanatomical centres associated with reward and punishment is central to depression (Liddle, 2001; Schulz & Remschmidt, 2001). Available evidence shows that depression occurs when there is a dysregulation of the amine systems in the medial forebrain bundle (reward system) and the periventricular system (punishment system), which affect drives for seeking pleasure and appetite. Noradrenaline and serotonin are the main neurotransmitters involved. Originally, depletion of these neurotransmitters was thought to cause depression but now a more complex dysregulation of the system involving a reduction in the sensitivity of post-synaptic receptor sites is hypothesized to be the critical difficulty.

Amine dysregulation theories predict that psychopharmacological treatment which increases the sensitivity of the dysfunctional post-synaptic membranes or increases the amount of serotonin or noradrenaline in the reward and punishment centres of the brain will lead to recovery. Three main classes of anti-depressant medication have been used to test these predictions. Tricyclic antidepressants (TCAs), like imipramine/Tofranil®, increase the sensitivity of dysfunctional receptor sites to neurotransmitters, particularly noradrenaline. Monoamine oxidase inhibitors (MAOIs), like phenelzine/Nardil®, prevent the enzyme monoamine oxidase from breaking down neurotransmitters in the synaptic cleft, and lead to an increase in amine levels. Selective serotonin re-uptake inhibitors (SSRIs), like fluoxetine/Prozac®, prevent serotonin from being re-absorbed into the pre-synaptic membrane and so increase levels of this neurotransmitter. Results of treatment trials show that all three classes of anti-depressant are effective in alleviating depression in up to two-thirds of adult cases, but that only SSRIs are effective in alleviating depression in children or adolescents (Ryan, 2002; Schulz & Remschmidt, 2001), so only these are routinely used in the treatment of depression in youngsters under 18 years of age.

Endocrine dysregulation theories

In endocrine dysreglation theories, abnormalities in cortisol, thyroxin, growth hormone, melatonin and prolactin systems are implicated in the development or maintenance of depression (Solokov & Kutcher, 2001). Research guided by endocrine dysregulation theories is still at an early stage of development, but there have been some important breakthroughs. For example, the occurrence of depression following exposure to chronic stress is associated with elevated cortisol levels and abnormal cortisol circadian rhythms. Thus the cortisol system may mediate the impact of adversity on mood. In comparison with non-depressed individuals, people with depression show a more rapid recovery over a 24-hour period to dexamethasone (a synthetic cortisol-like compound). Research continues on using the dexamethasone suppression test (DST) as a biological aid to diagnosing major depression (Harrington, 2002).

Immune system dysfunction theories

Various theorists have argued that there is a link between the functioning of the immune system and the occurrence of depression (Kiecolt-Glaser & Glaser, 2002; Kronfol, 2002). A growing body of evidence, largely based on studies of adults, shows that exposure to chronic stress or acute loss, such as bereavement, leads to both impaired immune system functioning and depressive symptoms. Impaired immune system functioning increases susceptibility to infections and consequent illnesses, which may be perceived as additional life stresses. These in turn may maintain or exacerbate depression.

Circadian rhythm de-synchrony theories

These theories argue that depression occurs when there is a dysregulation or de-synchrony in the circadian rhythms which govern the sleep–waking cycle. In support of these theories, sleep studies of depressed people show that they have abnormal circadian rhythms characterized by shortened rapid eye movement (REM) onset latency, broken sleep, early morning waking and difficulties with sleep onset (Brooks-Gunn, Auth, Petersen & Compas, 2001; Kupfer and Reynolds, 1992). The neuroanatomical basis for this de-synchrony may lie in the reticular activating system, which has been shown to govern arousal and the sleep–waking cycle. This line of research has shown that in some instances depression in adults may be diagnosed by assessing REM onset latency, which is reduced in those with depression. Furthermore, some depressed people temporarily recover following sleep deprivation, and this has led to the exploration of REM deprivation as a potential treatment for depression. While these findings have not been replicated in adolescents, Armitage et al. (2002) found that youngsters who showed low temporal coherence of their sleep electroencephalogram (EEG), were slower to recover from depression and relapsed more quickly.

Seasonal rhythm dysregulation theories

It has also been found that some people show depressive symptoms in winter time (Wehr & Rosenthal, 1989). This condition is known as seasonal affective disorder, and has rarely been studied in children and adolescents. One hypothesis about seasonal affective disorder is that this is a phylogenetic derivative of hibernation. Symptoms of fatigue, over-sleeping and increased appetite are under the control of melatonin, which is secreted by the pineal gland during periods of diminished daylight. Artificially lengthening the day using light therapy is the most important treatment to derive from this line of research and it has been shown to improve the mood of adolescents with seasonal affective disorder (Swedo et al., 1997). There is also a line of research at present investigating the effects of administering melatonin at key times to alter the time of its release from the pineal gland and thereby ameliorate depressive symptoms.

Psychological theories

The main propositions central to some of the more important examples of psychoanalytic, behavioural, and cognitive theories of depression are set out in Table 16.4. What follows is a brief summary of the central tenets of each of these theories along with a consideration of their treatment implications.

Psychoanalytic theories

Of the many psychoanalytic theories of depression that have been developed, reference will be made here to Freud's (1917) original position, Bibring's (1965) ego-psychological model and Blatt's object-relations formulation (Blatt, 2004). These theories have been selected because they are illustrative of psychodynamic explanations, and Blatt's model has been singled out for attention because, unlike many psychodynamic theories, considerable effort has gone into testing it empirically.

Freud's classical psychoanalytic theory

Freud's (1917) psychoanalytic theory argued that, following object loss, regression to the oral stage occurs, during which a distinction between self and the lost object is not made and the lost person is introjected. Subsequent aggression at the introject of the lost object for bringing about a state of abandonment is experienced as self-directed anger, or the self-hatred which characterizes depressed people. People whose primary caregivers either failed to meet their dependency needs during the oral phase, or who were over-indulgent, are pre-disposed to developing depression as described within this model. This is because they devote much of their energy to desperately seeking love by working hard or devoting themselves to helping others at great personal cost. When they lose a loved one, they feel the loss more acutely and are more likely to regress, introject the lost object and experience retroflexive anger. Freud also made provision for losses such as unemployment, which could symbolize object losses within his theory. Because, the super-ego, which is not fully developed in children, is the psychological structure necessary for directing anger at the ego, the traditional psychoanalytic position entails the view that children are unable to experience depression. This view is unsupported by available epidemiological data presented in Chapter 3. However, Freud's position was important in drawing attention to the significance of self-directed anger in the maintenance of depression in some cases. Freud also pointed out the importance of early life experiences in creating a vulnerability to depression, an idea which is central to modern psychodynamic and cognitive theories of depression.

Bibring's ego-psychology theory

Bibring (1965), a later psychodynamic ego psychologist, explained depression as the outcome of low self-esteem, which resulted from perceiving a large discrepancy between the self as it is and the ideal self. Internalization of harsh critical parental injunctions or perfectionistic parental injunctions during early childhood accounted for the development of a particularly unrealistic ego-ideal. A substantial body of evidence supports the view that low self-esteem is an important correlate and in some instances precursor of depression and in some but not all cases this is associated with a history of critical or punitive parenting (Blatt, 2004).

Blatt's object-relations theory

Blatt (2004) argues that there are two types of depression associated with two distinct types of early parent–child relationship which engender vulnerability to depression when faced with two distinct types of stresses in later life. A vulnerability to stresses involving *loss of attachment* relationships is central to one type of depression and this has its roots in early experiences of neglectful or over-indulgent parenting. A vulnerability to stresses involving *loss of autonomy* and control is central to the other type of depression and this has its roots in early experiences of critical, punitive parenting. This distinction between depression associated with disruption of interpersonal relationships and that associated with threats to mastering important achievement-oriented tasks has been made by many psychodynamic object-relations theorists, and indeed by cognitive theorists including Beck, whose theory will be discussed below, but has found its clearest articulation in Blatt's (2004) work. A growing body of evidence shows that, in adults, these sub-types of depression are associated with the recall of different childhood experiences, which presumably have led to the development of different types of depressive object-relations, which are activated in later life by different types of stressful life events. According to Blatt (2004), children who receive either neglectful or over-indulgent parenting develop internal working models for later life relationships in which expectations of abandonment are a central feature. For such individuals, denial and repression are the most common defence mechanisms employed to deal with perceived threats. These individuals are particularly vulnerable in later life to stressful life events that involve the disruption of relationships, such as rejection or bereavement. When they develop a mood disorder it is characterized by a pre-occupation with the themes of abandonment, helplessness and a desire to find someone who will provide love. On the other hand, children exposed to critical and punitive parenting develop internal working models for relationships in which the constructs of success and failure or blame and responsibility are central organizing features. Projection or reaction formation are the most common defences used by such individuals. In teenage years and adulthood such individuals are particularly vulnerable to experiences of criticism, failure or loss of control. Their mood disorders are characterized by a sense of self-criticism, inferiority, worthlessness and guilt.

Within the psychodynamic tradition, individual psychodynamic psychotherapy or classical psychoanalysis are the treatments of choice (McCullough-Vaillant, 1997). In such therapies, transference develops so that self-directed hostility, self-criticism and ideas of abandonment or loss of autonomy are projected onto the therapist. This transference is interpreted. The therapist points out parallels between the patient–parent relationship and the patient–analyst relationship. Also, parallels between these relationships and those that patients have with other significant people in their lives are noted. This process of interpretation helps patients learn to identify when they are falling into problematic relationship habits in future. The analytic relationship also provides patients with a forum where they can ventilate and work through the intense depressive and angry feelings that under-pin their problematic ways of managing relationships. This frees them to explore more realistic standards for self-evaluation and to develop more trusting internal working models for relationships. Evidence from an uncontrolled trial suggests that psychodynamic therapy can alleviate childhood depression (Target & Fonagy, 1994).

Behavioural theories

Of the many behavioural theories of depression, those of Lewinsohn (Lewinsohn, Clarke, Hops & Andrew, 1990; Lewinsohn, Hitch & Walker,

1994) and Rehm (Kaslow, Morris & Rehm, 1998) are particularly important because they have led to a considerable amount of research on the effectiveness of behavioural treatments for mood disorders.

Lewinsohn's behavioural theory

Lewinsohn's behavioural theory argues that depression is maintained by a lack of response-contingent positive reinforcement (RCPR). This may occur because people with depression lack the social skills required for eliciting rewarding interactions from others (Lewinsohn et al., 1990, 1994). Treatment programmes based on this model include individual or group social-skills training, which aims to train clients in skills necessary for receiving response-contingent positive reinforcement and to arrange the environment so that there are many opportunities for using these social skills. Controlled evaluations of such programmes with adults and analogue adolescent clients support their effectiveness (Clarke, DeBar & Lewinsohn, 2003).

Rehm's self-control theory

While Lewinsohn's theory focuses on the roles of environmental contingencies in depression, Rehm, bases her model of depression on a consideration of internal contingencies. According to Rehm's self-control theory, depression arises from deficits in self-monitoring, self-evaluation and self-reinforcement (Kaslow et al., 1998). Specifically, depression arises when a person selectively monitors the occurrence of negative events to the exclusion of positive events, selectively monitors immediate rather than long-term consequences of actions, sets overly stringent criteria for evaluating actions, makes negative attributions for personal actions, engages in little self-reinforcement for adaptive behaviours and engages in excessive self-punishment. Treatment programmes derived from this model aim to improve the skills required for more effective self-monitoring, self-evaluation and self-reinforcement. Controlled evaluations of such programmes with adults and analogue adolescent clients support their effectiveness (Kaslow et al., 1998).

Cognitive theories

Beck (1976) and Seligman's (Abramson et al., 1978) cognitive theories of depression are among the most important and influential in the field.

Beck's cognitive theory

According to Beck's (1976) theory, and Brent's adaptation of this theory for youngsters under 18 years (Weersing & Brent, 2003), depression occurs when life events involving loss occur and re-activate negative cognitive schemas formed early in childhood as a result of early loss experiences. These negative schemas entail negative assumptions such as 'I am only worthwhile if everybody likes me'. When activated, such schemas under-pin the occurrence of negative automatic thoughts, such as 'No one here likes me', and cognitive distortions, such as *all or nothing thinking*.

Negative schemas have their roots in loss experiences in early childhood including:

- loss of parents or family members through death, illness or separation
- loss of positive parental care through parental rejection, criticism, severe punishment, over-protection, neglect or abuse
- loss of personal health
- loss or lack of positive peer relationships through bullying or exclusion from peer group
- expectation of loss, e.g. where a parent was expected to die of chronic illness.

According to Beck, two negative schemas, which contain latent attitudes about the self, the world and the future, are of particular importance in depression. The first relates to interpersonal relationships and the second to personal achievement; he referred to these as sociotropy and autonomy. Individuals who have negative self-schemas where sociotropy is the central organizing theme define themselves negatively if they perceive themselves to be failing in maintaining positive relationships. Thus their core assumption about the self may be 'If I am not liked by everybody, then I am worthless'. Individuals who have negative self-schemas where autonomy is the central organizing theme define themselves negatively if they perceive themselves to be failing in achieving work-related goals. Thus their core assumption about the self may be 'If I am not a success and in control, then I am worthless'.

When faced with life stresses, individuals vulnerable to depression because of early loss experience and the related development of negative self-schemas become prone to interpreting ambiguous situations in negative, mood-depressing ways. The various logical errors that they make are referred to by Beck as cognitive distortions and these include the following:

- *All or nothing thinking*: thinking in extreme categorical terms, for example, 'Either I'm a success or a failure'.
- *Selective abstraction*: selectively focusing on a small aspect of a situation and drawing conclusions from this, for example, 'I made a mistake so every thing I did was wrong'.
- *Over-generalization*: generalizing from one instance to all possible instances, for example, 'He didn't say hello so he must hate me'.
- *Magnification*: exaggerating the significance of an event, for example, 'He said she didn't like me so that must mean she hates me'.

- *Personalization*: attributing negative feeling of others to the self, for example, 'He looked really angry when he walked into the room, so I must have done something wrong'.
- *Emotional reasoning*: taking feelings as facts, for example, 'I feel like the future is black so the future is hopeless'.

Depressed individuals interpret situations in terms of their negative cognitive schemas and so their automatic thoughts are characterized by these depressive cognitive distortions. Automatic thoughts are self-statements which occur without apparent volition when an individual attempts to interpret a situation so as to respond to it in a coherent way.

Cognitive-behavioural therapy (CBT) aims to train clients to monitor situations where depressive assumptions and distortions occur, to evaluate the validity of these depressive assumptions and distortions and to engage in activities that provide evidence to refute the negative assumptions. With adults, cognitive therapy is as effective as anti-depressant medication in alleviating depressive symptoms and more effective in relapse prevention than medication. With clinically depressed adolescents referred for treatment, David Brent and his team found that after treatment 60% of cases treated with CBT had improved, compared with about 38% of cases treated with family therapy or non-directive therapy, but these group differences disappeared at two-year follow-up (Weersing & Brent, 2003).

Seligman's reformulated learned helplessness theory

According to Seligman, depression arises when a person repeatedly fails to control the occurrence of aversive stimuli or failure experiences and makes internal, global, stable attributions for these failures and external, specific, unstable attributions for success (Abramson et al., 1978). Attributional retraining (Fösterling, 1985) in which clients learn to attribute failure to external, specific unstable factors and success to internal global stable factors is the principal treatment to emerge from this model. In addition, the youngster's environment may be modified so that the likelihood of non-aversive successful experiences greatly outweighs the likelihood of aversive failure experiences. Adolescents may also be trained to reduce their preferences for success experiences that are beyond their abilities.

Social theories

The main propositions central to two of the main social theories of depression are set out in Table 16.4. What follows is a brief summary of the central tenets of each of these theories along with a consideration of their treatment implications.

Family systems theory

According to family systems theory, depression occurs when the structure and functioning of the family, often in response to stressors, prevents the child from completing age-appropriate developmental tasks (Cottrell, 2003), a position supported by considerable evidence (Goodyer, 2001b; McCauley, Pavlidis & Kendall, 2001). Bereavement, parental discord, divorce, abuse and placement in care all disrupt family structure and may lead to depression. Excessive parental criticism, offering attention only when failure occurs and ignoring success may lead to depression. In adolescence, parental over-involvement, family enmeshment and related parent–child conflict over indi-viduation may be associated with depression. Family therapy aims to help family members develop supportive relationships with the depressed child, co-operative family problem-solving skills, short- and long-term goals with a focus on solutions, and to help families create a context within which young-sters can complete age-appropriate developmental tasks such as individu-ation in adolescence (Cottrell, 2003). This is achieved through a series of whole-family meetings. There is some evidence that family therapy and inter-personal therapy may be effective in alleviating depression in adolescents (Cottrell, 2003; Mufson & Pollack, 2003).

Interpersonal theory

Interpersonal therapy (IPT), which has developed within the tradition founded by Harry Stack Sullivan (1953), is based on an interpersonal theory of depression. Within this empirically supported theory it is assumed that depression is multi-factorially determined, but that interpersonal difficulties play a central role in the maintenance of depressive symptoms (Mufson, Dorta, Moreau & Weissman, 2004; Mufson & Pollack, 2003). Within IPT for depressed adolescents, it is assumed that five categories of interpersonal difficulties are of particular importance in maintaining depression: (1) grief associated with the loss of a loved one; (2) role disputes involving family members and friends; (3) role transitions such as starting or ending relation-ships within family, school or peer-group contexts, moving houses, gradu-ation, or diagnosis of an illness; (4) interpersonal deficits, particularly poor social skills for making and maintaining relationships; and (5) relationship difficulties associated with living in a single-parent family. In IPT for adoles-cents, the specific focal interpersonal factors that maintain the youngster's depressive symptoms are addressed within a series of individual child-focused and conjoint family sessions. Where grief is the central concern, the aim is to facilitate mourning and then help the youngster find relationships and activities to compensate for the loss. Where role disputes are a central factor maintaining depression, the aim is to develop and implement a plan for resolving these conflicts. Where role transitions are a central factor maintaining depression, the aim is to help the youngster mourn the loss of the old role, appreciate the benefits of the new one and develop a sense of mastery concerning the demands of the new role. Where depression is maintained by difficulties making and maintaining significant relationships the aim is to help youngsters reduce social isolation and form new relationships. Where depression is maintained by single-parent family situations, the aim is to help the youngster understand their new family situation, let go of inappropriate guilt feelings concerning parental separation and develop new role-relationships appropriate to the new family situation.

ASSESSMENT

In the management of mood problems, the first priority is to assess risk of self-harm. A structured approach to the assessment and formulation of suicide risk is presented later in this chapter (p. 776). Once suicide risk has been managed, it is appropriate to begin a more thorough assessment.

A second priority is to determine if the depression is a response to a child abuse situation, which requires a child protection intervention such as those described in Chapters 19, 20 and 21. Where children are exposed regularly to physical, sexual or emotional abuse, or to neglect, offering a contract for treatment outside of a statutory child-protection framework may reinforce the pattern of abuse. This issue is discussed more fully in Chapter 21.

The third priority in cases where children or adolescents present with mood disorders is to clarify the nature and extent of symptomatology. The diagnostic criteria in Table 16.1 and the clinical features in Table 16.3 offer a useful basis for interviewing in this area. Standardized self-report instruments and rating scales that may supplement clinical interviewing are listed in Table 16.5. For research purposes, the standardized diagnostic interview schedules listed in Chapter 3 are particularly useful.

The fourth priority is to establish the context within which the depression has arisen. The framework set out in Figure 16.3 may be used as a template for identifying important pre-disposing, precipitating, maintaining and protective factors that emerge in interviews with the child, the parents, other family members, school staff and significant members of the child's network. What follows is a discussion of the elements contained in that framework; these are drawn from the empirical and clinical literature on depression in adolescents and children (American Academy of Child and Adolescent Psychiatry, 1998c; Clarke et al., 2003; Compton et al., 2004; Cottrell, 2003; Goodyer, 2001a; Hammen & Rudolph, 2003; Harrington, 2002; Kaslow et al., 1998; Mufson & Pollack, 2003; Park & Goodyer, 2000; Weersing & Brent, 2003; Weisz, Southam-Gerow, Gordis & Connor-Smith, 2003). These areas should be covered within the context of the assessment protocol set out in Chapter 4.

Table 16.5 Psychometric instruments that may be used as an adjunct to clinical interviews in the assessment of depression

Construct	Instrument	Publication	Comments
DSM diagnostic interviews	Washington University in St. Louis Kiddie Schedule for Affective Disorders and Schizophrenia (WASH-U-KSADS)	Geller, B., Williams, M., Zimerman, B., Frazier, J. (1996). *Washington University in St. Louis Kiddie Schedule for Affective Disorders and Schizophrenia (WASH-U-KSADS)*. St Louis: Washington University	This structured interview has good psychometric properties for rating diagnoses of unipolar and bipolar mood disorder
Depression as reported by the child	Childhood Depression Inventory	Kovacs, M & Beck, A. (1977). An empirical clinical approach towards definition of childhood depression. In J. Schulterbrandt et al (Eds.) *Depression in Children.* (pp. 1–25). New York: Raven	This 27-item self-report child and adolescent version of the Beck Depression Inventory is useful for screening and assessing change in symptom intensity
	Depression Self-Rating Scale	Birleson, P. (1981). The validity of depressive disorder in childhood and the development of a self-rating scale: A research report. *Journal of Child Psychology and Psychiatry, 22,* 73–88

Birleson, P. Hudson, I., Buchanan, D. & Wolff, S. (1987). Clinical evaluation of a self-rating scale for depressive disorder in childhood (Depression Self-Rating Scale). *Journal of Child Psychology and Psychiatry, 28,* 43–60 | This 18-item self-report inventory yields a single depression score |
| **Depression as reported by the parent** | Children's Depression Rating Scale | Polanski et al. (1984). Preliminary studies of the reliability and validity of the Children's depression rating scale. *Journal of the American Academy of Child Psychiatry, 23,* 191–197 | Child and adolescent version of the Hamilton Rating Scale. Useful in assessing change in symptom intensity |

Cognitive distortions	Children's Negative Cognitive Error Questionnaire	Leitenberg, H., Yost, L., Carroll-Wilson, M. (1986). Negative cognitive errors in children: Questionnaire development, normative data, and comparisons between children with and without self-reported symptoms of depression, low self-esteem and evaluation anxiety. *Journal of Consulting and Clinical Psychology*, 54, 528–536	A self-report instrument which assesses cognitive distortions in children based on Beck's model
Depressive attributional style	Children's Attributional Styles Questionnaire	Seligman, M., Peterson, C., Kaslow, N., Tanenbaum, R. Alloy, L. & Abramson, L. (1984). Attributional style and depressive symptoms among children. *Journal of Abnormal Psychology*, 93, 235–238	A self-report measure of depressive attributional style based on the reformulated helplessness model
Self-esteem	Battle Culture-free Self-esteem Inventory	Battle, J. (1992). *Culture-Free Self-Esteem Inventories*. Examiner's Manual. Austin, TX: Pro-ed	A multi-dimensional measure of self-esteem. Yields scores on academic, social, parental and general self-esteem and includes a lie scale
Hopelessness	Hopelessness Scale for Children	Kazdin, A., French, N. et al. (1983). Hopelessness, depression and suicidal intent among psychiatrically disturbed inpatient children. *Journal of Consulting and Clinical Psychology*, 51, 504–510 Kazdin, A. Colbus, D. & Rogers, A. (1986). Assessment of depression and diagnosis of depressive disorder among psychiatrically disturbed children. *Journal of Abnormal Child Psychology*, 14, 499–515	17-item self-report hopelessness scale

Continued

Table 16.5 continued

Construct	Instrument	Publication	Comments
Social skills	Matson Evaluation of Social Skills for Youths	Matson, J., Rotatori, A. & Helsel, W. (1983). Development of a rating scale to measure social skills in children: The Matson evaluation of social skills for youths (MESSY). *Behavioural Research and Therapy*, 41, 335–340	A 64-item teacher report scale which measures social competence and behaviour problems. There is also a parallel self-report scale
Suicidal ideation	Beck's Suicidal Ideation Scale	Beck, A. and Steer, R. (1991). *Beck Scale for Suicide Ideation*. New York: The Psychological Corporation	A psychometric measure of suicidal ideation for use with adults but can be used with adolescents cautiously
Suicidal intent	Suicide Interview Schedule	Reynolds, W. (1991). Development of a semistructured clinical interview for suicidal behaviour in adolescents. *Psychological Assessment: A Journal of Consulting and Clinical Psychology*, 2, 382–390	A semi-structured interview for assessing suicidal risk
Mania	Young Mania Rating Scale	Gracious, B., Youngstrom, E., Findling, R. & Calabrese, J. (2002). Discriminative validity of a parent version of the Young Mania Rating Scale. *Journal of the American Academy of Child and Adolescent Psychiatry*, 41, 1350–1359 http://www.bpkids.org/learning/reference/articles/08–20–03.htm	This 11-item scale for rating mania can be completed by parents and clinicians

Pre-disposing factors

Both personal and contextual factors may pre-dispose youngsters to developing depression. A genetic vulnerability as indexed by a family history of mood disorders, early loss experiences, exposure to non-optimal parenting experiences and parental depression are among the more important predisposing risk factors for mood disorders. Loss experiences may include health-related losses, such as difficulties associated with pre- or peri-natal complications and early illness or injury. Psychosocial losses may include bereavements, separations, institutional care, social disadvantage and loss of trusting relationships through abuse. A punitive, critical and authoritarian non-optimal parenting style, where the parent focuses on the child's failures rather than his or her successes, may render the child vulnerable to depression. The child, as a result of such parenting, may be sensitized to failure experiences and threats to his or her autonomy. Neglectful parenting, on the other hand, may sensitize the child to loss of relationships and threats of abandonment. Neither of these types of parenting fosters secure attachment and the development of secure internal working models for trusting intimate relationships. Parental depression or drug or alcohol abuse may sub-serve these problematic parenting styles. Marital discord and family disorganization may also create a context where these types of non-optimal parenting occur. Personal characteristics of the adolescent, such as low intelligence, difficult or inhibited temperament, low self-esteem and an external locus of control, may pre-dispose adolescents to developing depression. Low intelligence may be associated with failure to achieve valued academic goals. Difficult or inhibited temperament may compromise the youngster's capacity to regulate mood and this in turn may interfere with the development of supportive relationships. Negative self-evaluative beliefs and the belief that important sources of reinforcement are beyond personal control may render youngsters vulnerable to self-criticism and helplessness which are part of the depressive experience.

Precipitating factors

Loss experiences associated with the disruption of significant relationships and loss experiences associated with failure to achieve valued goals all may precipitate an episode of depression in children and adolescents. Relationships may be disrupted through illness, parent–child separations, parental divorce, moving house, moving school, bullying or abuse. Failure to achieve valued goals and threats to autonomy may occur with exam failure and illnesses or injuries that prevent success in sports or leisure activities.

PRE-DISPOSING FACTORS

PERSONAL PRE-DISPOSING FACTORS

Biological factors
- Genetic vulnerabilities
- Pre- and peri-natal complications
- Early insults, injuries and illnesses

Psychological factors
- Low intelligence
- Difficult temperament
- Low self-esteem
- External locus of control

CONTEXTUAL PRE-DISPOSING FACTORS

Parent–child factors in early life
- Attachment problems
- Lack of intellectual stimulation
- Authoritarian punitive parenting
- Permissive parenting
- Neglectful parenting
- Parental focus on failure

Exposure to family problems in early life
- Parental psychological problems, especially depression
- Parental alcohol and substance abuse
- Marital discord or violence
- Family disorganization

Stresses in early life
- Bereavements
- Separations
- Child abuse
- Social disadvantage
- Institutional upbringing

PERSONAL PROTECTIVE FACTORS

Biological factors
- Good physical health
- Regular exercise

Psychological factors
- High IQ
- Easy temperament
- High self-esteem
- Internal locus of control
- High self-efficacy
- Optimistic attributional style
- Mature defence mechanisms
- Functional coping strategies
- Absence of double depression
- Presence of co-morbid problems

PERSONAL MAINTAINING FACTORS

Biological factors
- Dysregulation of amine system governing reward and punishment processes
- Dysregulation of endocrine and immune systems governing defence against illness
- De-synchrony of sleep–waking cycle

Psychological factors
- Depressive attributional style
- Negative cognitive distortions
- Negative automatic thoughts
- Negative self-monitoring
- Self-criticism
- Low self-efficacy
- Self-defeating behaviour and poor social skills leading to little response-contingent positive reinforcement
- Low level of self-reinforcement
- High level of self-punishment
- Self-harming behaviour
- Drug abuse
- Immature defence mechanisms

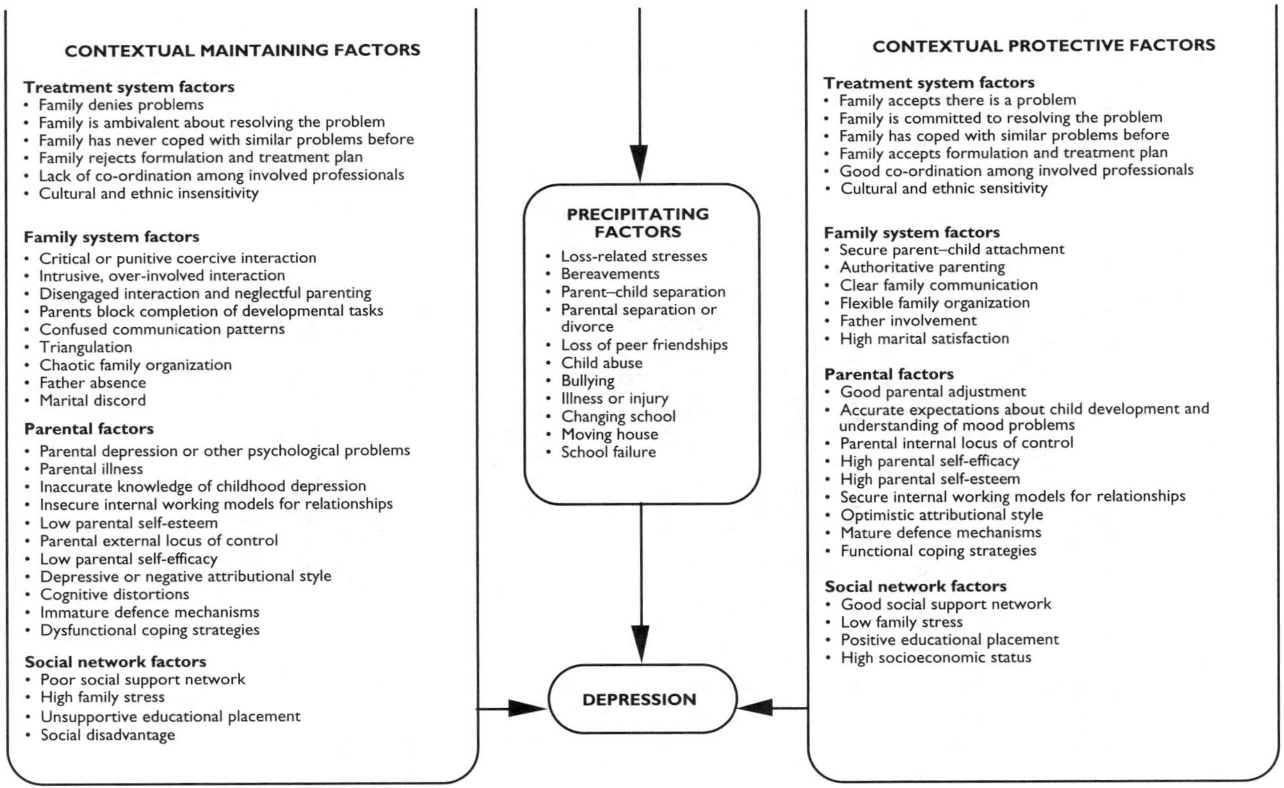

CONTEXTUAL MAINTAINING FACTORS

Treatment system factors
- Family denies problems
- Family is ambivalent about resolving the problem
- Family has never coped with similar problems before
- Family rejects formulation and treatment plan
- Lack of co-ordination among involved professionals
- Cultural and ethnic insensitivity

Family system factors
- Critical or punitive coercive interaction
- Intrusive, over-involved interaction
- Disengaged interaction and neglectful parenting
- Parents block completion of developmental tasks
- Confused communication patterns
- Triangulation
- Chaotic family organization
- Father absence
- Marital discord

Parental factors
- Parental depression or other psychological problems
- Parental illness
- Inaccurate knowledge of childhood depression
- Insecure internal working models for relationships
- Low parental self-esteem
- Parental external locus of control
- Low parental self-efficacy
- Depressive or negative attributional style
- Cognitive distortions
- Immature defence mechanisms
- Dysfunctional coping strategies

Social network factors
- Poor social support network
- High family stress
- Unsupportive educational placement
- Social disadvantage

PRECIPITATING FACTORS
- Loss-related stresses
- Bereavements
- Parent–child separation
- Parental separation or divorce
- Loss of peer friendships
- Child abuse
- Bullying
- Illness or injury
- Changing school
- Moving house
- School failure

DEPRESSION

CONTEXTUAL PROTECTIVE FACTORS

Treatment system factors
- Family accepts there is a problem
- Family is committed to resolving the problem
- Family has coped with similar problems before
- Family accepts formulation and treatment plan
- Good co-ordination among involved professionals
- Cultural and ethnic sensitivity

Family system factors
- Secure parent–child attachment
- Authoritative parenting
- Clear family communication
- Flexible family organization
- Father involvement
- High marital satisfaction

Parental factors
- Good parental adjustment
- Accurate expectations about child development and understanding of mood problems
- Parental internal locus of control
- High parental self-efficacy
- High parental self-esteem
- Secure internal working models for relationships
- Optimistic attributional style
- Mature defence mechanisms
- Functional coping strategies

Social network factors
- Good social support network
- Low family stress
- Positive educational placement
- High socioeconomic status

Figure 16.3 Factors to consider in the assessment of depression

Maintaining factors

Both personal and contextual factors may maintain depression. Personal cognitive factors that maintain low mood include negative automatic thoughts and cognitive distortions that arise from negative cognitive schemas, particularly those associated with threats to attachment and autonomy. A depressive attributional style where internal, global stable attributions are made for failure experiences and external, specific and unstable attributions are made for success can also maintain depression. Low mood may be maintained by high levels of self-criticism and low self-efficacy beliefs. Other important cognitive factors that maintain depression include selectively monitoring negative aspects of one's actions, engaging in high levels of punitive self-talk or punishment; and engaging in little positive self-talk or self-reinforcement. Self-defeating behavioural patterns that arise from social skills deficits, particularly engaging others in depressive conversations which lead them to avoid future interactions, may maintain depressed mood. Depression may be maintained or exacerbated by using dysfunctional coping strategies, particularly substance abuse and self-harming gestures. Immature defences for dealing with perceived threats such as denial or reaction formation may also maintain depressed mood. At a biological level, depression may be maintained by dysregulation of the amine system governing reward and punishment processes; dysregulation of the endocrine system and the immune system governing defence against illness and de-synchrony of the sleep–waking cycle.

Within the youngster's family or school context, a variety of factors maintain mood problems. These include ongoing inescapable abuse, bullying or punishment in the absence of adequate support or being in an unsupportive educational placement. Ongoing interactions with parents or primary carers characterized by excessive criticism, neglect or excessive over-involvement may maintain depression, as may family circumstances where the youngster is blocked from achieving developmental tasks, such as autonomy. These parenting patterns may be sub-served by confused family communication, family disorganization and triangulation, where the depressed youngster is caught between the conflicting parental demands. These types of difficulties may arise in family contexts where parents have high levels of stress including social disadvantage, low levels of social support, marital discord, low father involvement and physical illness or psychological problems including depression. Where parents have insecure internal working models for relationships, low self-esteem, low self-efficacy, an external locus of control, immature defences and poor coping strategies, their resourcefulness in managing their children's depression may be compromised. Parents may also become involved in problem-maintaining interactions with their children if they have inaccurate knowledge about the role of psychological factors in the genesis and maintenance of depression.

Within the treatment system, a lack of co-ordination and clear communication among involved professionals, including family physicians, paediatricians, nurses, teachers, psychologists and so forth, may maintain adolescents' depression. It is not unusual for various members of the professional network to offer conflicting opinions and advice on the nature and management of adolescent depression. These may range from viewing the child as psychiatrically ill and deserving inpatient care, anti-depressant medication and permissive management to seeing the child as delinquent and requiring strict behavioural control. Where co-operation problems between families and treatment teams develop, and families deny the existence of the problems, the validity of the diagnosis and formulation or the appropriateness of the treatment programme, then the adolescent's difficulties may persist. Treatment systems that are not sensitive to the cultural and ethnic beliefs and values of the youngster's family system may maintain mood problems by inhibiting engagement or promoting drop-out from treatment and preventing the development of a good working alliance between the treatment team, the youngster and his or her family. Parents' lack of experience in dealing with similar problems in the past is a further factor that may compromise their capacity to work co-operatively with the treatment team and so may contribute to the maintenance of the adolescent's difficulties.

Protective factors

The probability that a treatment programme will be effective is influenced by a variety of personal and contextual protective factors. It is important that these be assessed and included in the later formulation, since it is protective factors that usually serve as the foundation for therapeutic change. Youngsters with less severe mood disorders which are clearly episodic and who also show co-morbid conduct problems are less at risk than those with double depression (severe episodic mood disorder superimposed on a persistent milder mood problem) and no conduct problems. At a biological level, physical fitness and a willingness to engage in regular physical exercise are protective factors. A high IQ, an easy temperament, high self-esteem, an internal locus of control, high self-efficacy and an optimistic attributional style are all important personal protective factors. Other important personal protective factors include mature defence mechanisms and functional coping strategies, particularly good problem-solving skills and a capacity to make and maintain friendships.

Within the family, secure parent–child attachment and authoritative parenting are central protective factors, particularly if they occur within the context of a flexible family structure in which there is clear communication, high marital satisfaction and both parents share the day-to-day tasks of managing home life.

Good parental adjustment is also a protective factor. Where parents have an internal locus of control, high self-efficacy, high self-esteem, an internal working model for secure attachments, an optimistic attributional style, mature defences and functional coping strategies, then they are better resourced to manage their children's difficulties constructively. Accurate knowledge about the role of psychological factors in recovery from depression is also a protective factor.

Within the broader social network, high levels of support, low levels of stress and membership of a high socioeconomic group are all protective factors for depressed adolescents. Where families are embedded in social networks that provide a high level of support and place few stressful demands on family members, then it is less likely that parents' and children's resources for dealing with health-related problems will become depleted. A well-resourced educational placement may also be viewed as a protective factor. Educational placements where teachers have sufficient time and flexibility to attend home–school liaison meetings if invited to do so contribute to positive outcomes for depressed adolescents.

Within the treatment system, co-operative working relationships between the treatment team and the family and good co-ordination of multi-professional input are protective factors. Treatment systems that are sensitive to the cultural and ethnic beliefs and values of the youngster's family are more likely help families engage with, and remain in treatment, and foster the development of a good working alliance. Families are more likely to benefit from treatment when they accept the formulation of the problem given by the treatment team and are committed to working with the team to resolve it. Where families have successfully faced similar problems before, then they are more likely to benefit from treatment and, in this sense, previous experience with similar problems is a protective factor.

FORMULATION

Following thorough assessment interviews, a case formulation may be drawn up to link pre-disposing, precipitating, maintaining and protective factors to depressive symptomatology; potential treatment goals and possible plans for reaching these.

TREATMENT

Thorough assessment typically reveals that a youngster's mood problems are maintained by personal factors, family-based factors, school-based factors and possibly factors within the child's wider network. While it is useful for the core intervention to target the child in his or her family, interventions with the school or ward staff in hospitalized cases, or focusing on the parents in multi-problem families may be necessary. In the treatment protocol given here, I have attempted to integrate those techniques which have been shown to be effective in the cognitive-behavioural literature, with well established systemic, interpersonal and social-learning based approaches to working with families along with the literature on pharmacological treatment of depression in children and adolescents (American Academy of Child and Adolescent Psychiatry, 1998c; Brent, Gaynor & Weersing, 2002; Clarke et al., 2003; Compton et al., 2004; Cottrell, 2003; Friedberg & McClure, 2002; Kaslow et al., 1998; Kovacs & Sherrill, 2001; Moore & Carr, 2000; Mufson & Pollack, 2003; NICE, 2005; Park & Goodyer, 2000; Ryan, 2002; Schulz & Remschmidt, 2001; Stallard, 2002; Weersing & Brent, 2003; Weisz et al., 2003). The following elements are contained in this approach to treatment:

- psychoeducation
- self-monitoring
- interventions focusing on activity
- interventions focusing on changing family relationships
- interventions focusing on cognition
- social skills and social problem-solving skills training
- school interventions
- medication
- management of parental mood problems
- relapse management.

Psychoeducation

Psychoeducational input is appropriately offered early in the consultation process so that the adolescent and his or her family share a common understanding of depression with the treatment team. However, throughout therapy it is necessary to remind clients from time to time about various aspects of this way of conceptualizing depression. Depression is explained as a complex condition involving changes in mood, biological functioning, thinking, behaviour and relationships. Vulnerability to depression may be due to genetic factors or early loss experiences. Current episodes of depression arise from a build-up of recent life stress. These activate the vulnerability, which then comes to be maintained by depressed thinking, action and relationships. Genetic vulnerability may be explained as a nervous system that goes slow under pressure and disrupts sleep, appetite and energy. This going-slow process leads to depressed mood. Early loss-related vulnerability may be explained as a set of memories about loss that have been filed away, but are taken out when a recent loss occurs. The files inform the youngster that more and more losses will occur and this leads to depressed mood. Treatment centres on helping youngsters and their families learn how to control and change patterns of thinking, action and relationships that maintain depression. It is important to highlight that the youngster's thinking processes or beliefs, behavioural routines and ways of managing relationships which maintain depressed mood are under conscious control, so treatment will focus on coaching the youngster to change these three things. The role of the family is to help the youngster develop new beliefs, routines and ways of managing relationships which protect him or her from becoming stuck in low moods. Within this context, protective factors, particularly social support from the family, may be mentioned. This allows the youngster and the family to view themselves as a problem-solving team. A model of this explanation of depression is presented in Figure 16.4 and may be photocopied and given to clients as part of the psychoeducational input.

Somatic state has also been included in the model. Although TCAs are

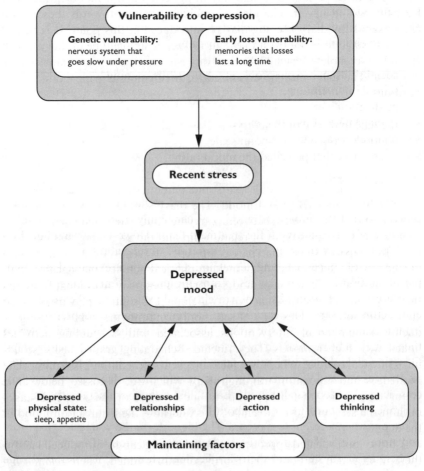

Figure 16.4 Model of depression for psychoeducation

ineffective in the treatment of depression in youngsters, there is evidence that SSRI anti-depressant medication may be used to regulate sleep and appetite and increase energy levels in adolescents.

As part of psychoeducation, parents may be invited to read *Coping with Depression in Young People. A Guide for Parents* (Fitzpatrick, 2004).

Self-monitoring

Self-monitoring and goal setting may be introduced together in the earliest stages of therapy. The youngster and the family are invited to set very small achievable goals, which, if reached, would clearly demonstrate that improvement was occurring, for example, having at least one period in the day when the youngster's mood rises at least one point on a ten-point scale, or having three periods of a half day in a week when a mood rating of at least five was achieved. The idea of tracking progress towards these mood change goals by diary keeping may be introduced at this point. It is best at this early stage to invite the adolescent to keep a simple type of diary, which should be completed each time the youngster notices a significant change in mood. The diary may be organized as three columns with the following headings

- the date and time of the entry
- a mood rating on a ten-point scale
- the activity that preceded the mood rating.

This type of diary helps adolescents and parents develop an awareness of the link between activity and mood. The diary should be reviewed in each session and links made between carrying out particular activities or engaging in particular types of relationship and mood. Youngsters may find from this type of diary that particular type of events are associated with higher moods. Such events may include physical activity, manageable challenges, co-operative activities and so forth. They may also identify events that lower mood, such as inactivity, watching TV, solitary playing of video games and so forth. This type of self-monitoring provides a basis for introducing a number of interventions associated with scheduling activities linked with higher moods. These include scheduling graded tasks, scheduling physical exercise, scheduling pleasant events, scheduling age-appropriate challenges and relaxation training, all of which are discussed below. The youngster may be invited to complete one or more of these types of tasks both in the session and between sessions and note their impact on mood in the diary.

A more sophisticated approach to diary keeping can be introduced later in therapy, in which an additional fourth column is added, where *relationship events* which preceded a mood rating are made. In particular, the person to whom the youngster was most recently talking and the degree to which that relationship or conversation was experienced as supportive or stressful may be noted. This diary should include the following columns.

- the date and time of the entry
- a mood rating on a ten-point scale
- the activity that preceded the mood rating
- the relationship that preceded the mood rating.

Reviews of this type of diary allow teenagers and their parents to track the relationship between mood and certain types of social interaction that commonly occur within the family or peer group. It is not unusual for parents to learn that conversations intended to cheer their child up actually depressed him or her further, whereas fairly neutral exchanges led to improvements in mood. Family members may also become aware of the negative impact of conflict and triangulation on the teenager by reviewing this type of diary. This type of information provides a basis for relationship-focused interventions including family communication training, family problem-solving training, providing support and renegotiating role relationships. The impact of using these skills in family conversations on the youngster's mood may be tested in treatment sessions and also between sessions and the results noted in the diary.

Later, a new column may be added to the diary in which youngsters record the thoughts or ideas that went through their minds and which contributed to their mood rating. Training in capturing negative automatic thoughts and understanding cognitive distortions should precede this self-monitoring assignment and this will be discussed below. In this type of self-monitoring task the following five columns should be included in the diary:

- the date and time of the entry
- a mood rating on a ten-point scale
- the activity that preceded the mood rating
- the relationship that preceded the mood rating
- the thoughts that the person had about the activity or relationship that contributed to the mood rating.

Reviewing this type of diary allows the adolescent and family members to see that the youngster's interpretation of events contributes to negative mood. This provides a rationale for teaching the challenge test reward (CTR) routine for challenging negative automatic thoughts (described in Chapter 12 and below). Conducting this type of training in family sessions is particularly important in families where a parent suffers from depression, since it provides such parents with a strategy for being less critical of their depressed child. Many depressed parents attribute negative intentions and qualities to their children, who subsequently develop depression and, unless this process can be modified, youngsters may find that it contributes to relapses.

Once youngsters have become proficient in using diaries that allow the impact of activities, relationships and thoughts on mood to be tracked, two additional columns may be added in which coping strategies used to alter mood and the impact of these on mood are noted. A full seven-column diary form is presented in Figure 16.5.

Interventions focusing on activity

Through psychoeducation and diary keeping, adolescents and their families discover that activity directly affects mood. Small tasks, pleasant tasks and age-appropriate challenges all improve mood, whereas large tasks, unpleasant events and being blocked from facing age-appropriate challenges lead to a depressed mood. Physical exercise and relaxation also promote a positive mood. In light of this there are certain interventions which help youngsters develop activity patterns that improve mood. These include:

- scheduling graded tasks
- scheduling pleasant events
- remembering pleasant events
- scheduling age-appropriate challenges
- scheduling physical exercise
- using relaxation skills.

Scheduling graded tasks

Depressed youngsters may report that there are things that they feel they should do or want to do but believe that they cannot because the tasks appear to be overwhelmingly demanding. In scheduling graded tasks, the youngster is invited to break large insuperable tasks into small manageable tasks, complete these and receive reinforcement for doing so. Parents and youngsters may be invited to work together in a treatment session and break a big task into smaller tasks and agree on a reward system using points or tokens, whereby the adolescent will be reinforced for completing each small component of the large task. Reward systems are discussed in Chapter 4.

Scheduling pleasant events

Parents and youngsters may be invited to draw up lists of pleasant events, such as going for a walk together or watching a film, which the adolescent believes are associated with improved mood, and plan to carry these out.

Column 1	Column 2	Column 3	Column 4	Column 5	Column 6	Column 7
Day and time	Mood rating 1 = low mood 10 = high mood	Activity before mood rating	Relationship before mood rating	Thought about activity or relationship before mood rating	Coping response **Changed activity** • Pleasant event • Challenging event • Relaxation • Physical exercise **Changed relationship** • Stopped depressed talk • Asked about person and listened • Spoke about positive events • Asked for listening time **Changed thought** • Challenge Test Reward • Reattribution • Focused on positive	Mood after coping 1 = low mood 10 = high mood

Figure 16.5 Self-monitoring form for depression

Remembering pleasant events

Parents may be shown how to schedule a period each evening to help young-sters review their day and remember all the positive things that have happened, list these and post them on the fridge door or the child's bedroom wall.

Scheduling age-appropriate challenges

Where adolescents and their parents have become entrenched in patterns of interaction appropriate to the pre-adolescent stage of development, fam-ilies may be invited to arrange for adolescents to gradually work towards dealing with age-appropriate challenges. These may include travelling independently to meet with friends, shopping for their own clothes, planning to stay overnight at a friend's house and so forth.

Scheduling physical exercise

Youngsters and their parents may be invited to gradually increase the amount of daily physical exercise the teenager takes, since inactivity maintains low mood and regular exercise, particularly aerobic exercise, improves mood.

Using relaxation skills

Youngsters may be trained either directly or through their parents in using the relaxation, breathing and visualization skills described in Chapter 12. These skills are particularly useful where the youngster experiences irritability and anxiety as part of their mood disorder. They may also be used with sleep problems. Parents may be shown how to help their children practise relaxation exercises at bedtime to facilitate sleep onset.

Interventions focusing on family relationships

Both preliminary assessment interviews and the results of self-monitoring tasks typically provide evidence that the adolescent's mood is influenced by family relationships, notably those characterized by confusing communica-tion, conflict, criticism, over-involvement and triangulation. Furthermore role-relationship difficulties associated with family transitions including the onset of adolescence, parental separation, bereavements and so forth may contribute to depression. On the other hand, parental support, clear com-munication, non-conflictual approaches to solving relationship problems and clear roles tend to be associated with positive moods. The interventions which may be used to promote the types of family relationships which improve mood are:

- family communication training and problem-solving training
- facilitating support
- re-negotiating role relationships.

Family communication training and problem-solving training

Guidelines for training family members in communications skills and problem-solving skills are given in Chapter 4. With communication training, where the core skills are turn-taking, making points unambiguously, listening, summarizing and checking the accuracy of what was heard, a central difficulty that many families containing depressed teenagers have is avoiding mind-reading. That is, it is not unusual during communications training for depressed parents to attribute negative intentions and ideas to their depressed adolescents, and vice versa. The challenge in communication training is to coach family members in avoiding this pitfall, by listening carefully and accepting what is said on face value. With problem-solving training, where the main steps are defining problems in small solvable terms, brain-storming options uncritically and then selecting the best option, a difficulty in families with depressed members is the premature criticism of possible solutions, which creates a culture within which no one ventures new ideas lest they be criticized. Family members require careful coaching in the skill of delaying evaluation of options until a large number have been generated. Without this creative approach, solutions to family problems which maintain the adolescent's depression may be more difficult to find.

Facilitating support

Supportive conversations may be scheduled for time-limited periods, such as 30 minutes at a set time each day. The role of the supporting family member is to use listening skills learned in the communications training exercise and do no more than summarize what the depressed adolescent has said and check that they have understood the adolescent correctly. No attempt should be made by the supporting family member to cheer depressed adolescents up or to make suggestions about how they might solve their problems. Family members require coaching in this very difficult skill, since even the most patient parent or sibling will have urges to talk the adolescent out of his or her depression.

Re-negotiating role relationships

Role relationship difficulties which maintain depression may be characterized by over-involvement, criticism and problems associated with divided loyalties. What follows are some strategies for re-negotiating these problematic role relationships. Where parents have become over-involved with their child and regularly engage in intrusive interactions, this non-supportive pattern may be disrupted by offering them the opportunity of having a break from caring for the depressed child by passing the responsibility of caring for the depressed adolescent over to the less involved parent. This type of intervention may be particularly useful in families where the over-involved parent is inadvertently blocking the adolescent's completion of age-appropriate developmental tasks such as developing autonomy and maintaining privacy. In such instances, often the more the peripheral parent argues for the over-involved parent to allow the adolescent some space, the more over-intrusive the over-involved parent becomes. This intervention of placing the peripheral parent in charge of the adolescent's welfare disrupts this pattern of triangulation.

Where one parent has become highly critical of the youngster and his or her depressive behaviour, the parent and child may be encouraged to join forces to defeat or overcome the depression which may be externalized and personified as a black knight, a dragon, a monster or some other mythological entity. The central feature of the intervention is that the parent and child join in a strong alliance against the depression, so the child feels supported by the parent. I have found this intervention particularly useful in families where one parent (typically the father) has become very critical of the child, while the other parent (typically the mother) sympathizes with the child's position.

In families where parents are separated or divorced, depressed adolescents often find the experience of divided loyalties very distressing. They feel that they must choose between being loyal to one parent or to the other, but both of these positions entails the loss of a relationship with a parent. This experience of divided loyalties is exacerbated when a parent expresses anger and disappointment concerning the ex-partner to the adolescent. In such instances, with coaching from the psychologist, the adolescent may be helped to explain to the parents the extraordinary anguish that this type of triangulation causes and to ask the parents to make a commitment never to ask the teenager to take sides again because he or she is loyal to both parents and will remain so. Where adolescents have difficulty facing their parents and saying this, they may write them a letter containing these sentiments and read it out to the parents in the session. The parents, in reply may be coached to agree to the adolescent's request. Where parents cannot consent to this, it is vital that they understand the consequences of this for the adolescent, i.e. chronic psychological problems including depression. A fuller discussion of the impact of chronic parental divorce-related conflict on children's development is contained in Chapter 23, which deals with divorce.

Interventions focusing on cognition

The techniques described in this section are family-based variations of interventions developed for use with individual adults in cognitive therapy.

Because children's belief systems are inextricably bound up with their parent's belief systems, I have found that this family-based approach to cognitive therapy is particularly useful with adolescents. Interventions which focus on cognitions begin by teaching both parents and youngsters to identify automatic thoughts and their impact on mood. The adolescent and parents may be asked to give a current mood rating on a ten-point scale and then identify the thought they are telling themselves that accounts for that rating. A challenge may then be posed to the youngster to complete a difficult arithmetic problem or puzzle. After trying to solve the problem for a minute or so, the psychologist may then ask the adolescent to give a mood rating and the automatic thought that under-pins it. Usually, there will be a drop in mood associated with a negative thought arising from failure to solve the puzzle. In this way the link between automatic thoughts and mood is established. It may be pointed out that the automatic thought (for example 'Because I can't do it quickly I'm stupid') could conceivably be replaced with another thought ('If I had a calculator I'd be finished now') that might lead to a less depressed mood rating. The adolescent may be invited to keep track of automatic thoughts and related mood states using the self-monitoring system described earlier. Reviewing self-monitoring forms throws light on situations that led to mood changes and the automatic thoughts that occurred in these situations. Parents and adolescents may be helped to develop specific routines for challenging or neutralizing negative automatic thoughts. Three methods deserve particular mention:

- the challenge test reward (CTR) method
- re-attribution training
- focusing on positives.

Challenge-test-reward (CTR) method

Challenging negative automatic thoughts involves generating alternative self-statements that could have been made in a specific situation in which a negative automatic thought occurred and then looking for evidence to *test* the validity of this alternative. Finally, when this task has been completed and the youngster shows that the depressive automatic thought was invalid, he or she engages in self-*reward* or self-reinforcement. So, for example, one alternative to the automatic thought 'He didn't talk to me so he doesn't like me' is 'He didn't talk to me because he is shy'. 'If there is evidence that the person in question never injured me before and on a couple of occasions smiled at me, then the more valid statement is that the person is shy. I may reward myself for challenging and testing this automatic thought by telling myself that I have done a good job of testing my automatic thought.'

The CTR method may be taught within family sessions and the family may be asked to think about how much evidence there is for each of a series of negative automatic thoughts and possible alternatives. They may then be coached in praising themselves for testing out the alternatives efficiently. Parents may be invited to prompt adolescents to use their CTR skills, in situations where low mood occurs.

Re-attribution training

Challenging depressive attributions is a second strategy for reducing the impact of negative automatic thoughts. In particular failure situations, which have led to automatic thoughts, the parents and the youngster are asked to rate the degree to which the negative automatic thought reflects an internal, global, stable attribution. For example, the automatic thought 'I couldn't do the problem because I've always been completely stupid' might receive the following ratings:

Internal		**External**
Due to me	(1) 2 3 4 5 6 7 8 9 10	Due to circumstances
Global		**Specific**
To do with many situations	1 (2) 3 4 5 6 7 8 9 10	To do with this situation
Stable		**Unstable**
Is permanent	(1) 2 3 4 5 6 7 8 9 10	Is temporary

An alternative self-statement 'I couldn't do the problem because it's very hard and I'm having a bad day' might receive the following ratings, which characterize an optimistic rather than a depressive cognitive style:

Internal		**External**
Due to me	1 2 3 4 5 6 7 8 9 (10)	Due to circumstances
Global		**Specific**
To do with many situations	1 2 3 4 5 6 7 8 (9) 10	To do with this situation
Stable		**Unstable**
Is permanent	1 2 3 4 5 6 7 8 9 (10)	Is temporary

Youngsters and their parents may be trained to ask of each internal, global, stable explanation for failure, if alternative external, specific or unstable alternative explanations may be offered which fit the available evidence.

Focusing on positives

Where adolescents selectively attend to negative aspects of their situation and then criticize themselves, they and their parents may be shown how to complete mildly challenging activities, like making a meal or watering the plants, while modelling positive self-monitoring, self-evaluation and self-reinforcement by verbalizing their thoughts and giving a running commentary on how they are monitoring themselves, evaluating their performance and reinforcing themselves through using self-praise. They and their parents may then be invited to jointly complete this type of routine at home.

Social skills and social problem-solving skills training

Group activity programmes and a group therapy format may be used to help teenagers develop social skills so that they can initiate and maintain positive interactions with peers. Common problems with depressed teenagers include avoidance of initiating conversations, engaging in depressive, self-critical or pessimistic talk which other teenagers find aversive and withdrawing from complex social situations. These difficulties in turn lead to exclusion from peer-group activities. Social skills training should aim to help youngsters learn strategies for tracking peer-group conversations, identifying opportunities for contributing, and making contributions to conversations and activities that benefit themselves and others and generating solutions to complex social situations. Youngsters may be coached in social skills by first being given a rationale for the skill and second by observing a model of the appropriate skill and then practising it and receiving verbal or videotaped corrective feedback and reinforcement.

A useful rationale is to explain that most peer groups want new members that are going to give something good (like companionship or good humour) rather than take something away (like replacing a good mood with a bad mood). When you are depressed, this takes some planning because the depression forces you to give nothing and take away any good mood there is. Coaching in social skills is a way of beating depression by planning to give companionship and good humour rather than taking it away. In the long run, using social skills may lead to getting some friendship back.

Following this type of rationale, the psychologist may show a videotape of an appropriate and inappropriate way of initiating a conversation or a conversation in which a youngster gives good humour or engages in depressive talk. In some of our groups I have taped clips from TV programmes to use as models. In others, myself and my colleagues modelled the interactions ourselves.

With rehearsal, youngsters are invited to imitate the behaviour demonstrated by the model. It is important that all approximations to positive social skills be praised and suggestions for improvement be made tactfully. Videotaped feedback, in my clinical experience, is only useful when significant improvement has been made which can clearly be pointed out to the youngster viewing the tape. If their performance is poor, the process of watching themselves engage in poor social skills on videotape may exacerbate their depression.

Once basic social skills such as joining, initiating and maintaining conversations have been mastered, training in social problem-solving may begin. Here, youngsters generate a list of difficult social situations that they fear handling, such as being criticized, snubbed, laughed at or embarrassed and are asked to generate as many possible alternative ways of dealing with these problems as possible. Positive and negative possible outcomes of all these options may be explored and the group may then be coached in how to implement the most favourable solution. Again, video clips from soap operas and group members' favourite TV programmes may be used to illustrate difficult peer-group interactions and solutions to these interpersonal problems.

School interventions

Work with the school should help the child's teacher understand the formulation and develop supportive patterns of interaction with the child. Where children have become withdrawn, teachers may be helped to create opportunities where the depressed child can interact with peers.

Medication

In cases where psychosocial interventions alone have been ineffective, SSRIs should be included as a key element in a multi-modal treatment programme. Prescription of anti-depressants and the monitoring of side effects is usually the responsibility of a physician (GP, psychiatrist or paediatrician) who shares the care of a client with a clinical psychologist.

Management of parental mood problems

Interventions which focus on parental mood problems, a reduction of parental stress and the amplification of parental support should be prioritized if it is clear from the formulation that these factors will compromise the parent's capacity to help the adolescent recover. Many youngsters referred for treatment come from families where one or both parents are depressed. In such instances, it is important to insure that depressed parents are referred immediately for treatment, if they are to be able to engage effectively in family work to help their youngsters recover.

Where particular life stresses and support deficits such as marital conflict, conflict within the extended family, social isolation, inadequate accommodation, financial difficulties, work-related difficulties and so forth are severe enough to prevent any therapeutic progress, in a minority of instances it may be necessary to address these first. However, where possible, the focus of the work should be on helping the family to help the child to recover. Success with this goal, may increase parental self-efficacy so that they are empowered to tackle their other life difficulties with greater confidence. A protocol for the treatment of adult depression is given in Carr and McNulty (in press c).

Relapse management

Depression is a recurrent disorder and while 90% of episodes may resolve with intensive short-term intervention within twelve months, most children relapse. Therefore brief therapy must be offered within the context of a longer-term care programme. Children and parents may be trained to identify and cope with relapses and invited to re-contact the clinical psychology service in the event of a further episode of depression.

Managing resistance

A central guideline for working with depressed adolescents is to set tasks where there is a very high chance of success. So psychoeducational input should be pitched at the youngster's ability level. Easy self-monitoring tasks should be given before progressing to more complex ones. Simple and small homework assignments focusing on activities, relationships and cognitions should be given first before moving on to more challenging invitations. Where youngsters have difficulty completing tasks, responsibility for this should be taken by the psychologist, who probably asked more of the youngster and the family than they were ready for. It is very easy when working with depressed youngsters from families in which one of the parents is depressed to fall into a pattern of criticism and blaming the family for lack of progress. The challenge is to establish and maintain a good working alliance and find a pace of work which suits the family.

BIPOLAR DISORDER

Bipolar disorder is characterized by episodes of mania or hypomania and by episodes of depression (American Academy of Child and Adolescent Psychiatry, 1997f; Clark, 2001; Findling, Kowatch & Post 2003; Geller & DelBello, 2003; James & Javaloyes, 2001; Kusumakar, Lazier, MacMaster & Santor, 2002; Lofthouse & Fristad, 2004). The ICD 10 and DSM IV TR diagnostic criteria for bipolar disorder are given in Table 16.6. For a DSM IV TR diagnosis, an episode of elevated manic or hypomanic mood is required and for an ICD 10 diagnosis, two episodes of mood disorder are required involving either elevated or depressed mood. A distinction is made between cases characterized by at least one manic or mixed episode (bipolar I) and cases characterized by both depressive and hypomanic episodes, but without manic or mixed episodes (bipolar II). Bipolar I disorder is the classic prototype of what was historically known as manic depression.

Table 16.6 Definitions of bipolar disorder

DSM IV TR	ICD 10
Bipolar I Disorder. At least one manic, hypomanic or mixed episode	Bipolar disorder is characterized by repeated (i.e. at least two) episodes in which the patient's mood and activity levels are significantly disturbed, this disturbance consisting on some occasions of an elevation of mood and increased energy and activity (mania or hypomania), and on others of a lowering of mood and decreased energy and activity (depression). Characteristically, recovery is usually complete between episodes, and the incidence in the two sexes is more nearly equal than in other mood disorders. As patients who suffer only from repeated episodes of mania are comparatively rare, and resemble (in their family history, pre-morbid personality, age of onset, and long-term prognosis) those who also have at least occasional episodes of depression, such patients are classified as bipolar. Manic episodes usually begin abruptly and last for between 2 weeks and 4–5 months (median duration about 4 months). Depressions tend to last longer (median length about 6 months), though rarely for more than a year, except in the elderly. Episodes of both kinds often follow stressful life events or other mental trauma, but the presence of such stress is not essential for the diagnosis. The first episode may occur at any age. The frequency of episodes and the pattern of remissions and relapses are both very variable, though remissions tend to get shorter as time goes on and depressions to become commoner and longer lasting after middle age
Bipolar II Disorder. One or more episodes of both major depression and hypomania, but no manic or mixed episodes	
A seasonal pattern or rapid cycling should be specified for both bipolar I and II	
A seasonal pattern represents a course of illness where the major depressive episodes occur consistently at a particular time of year	
Rapid cycling involves at least four episodes of a mood disturbance (major depression, mania, mixed, or hypomania) over a 12-month period	
Criteria for a manic episode	**Manic episode**
A. A distinct period of abnormally and persistently elevated, expansive, or irritable mood (or any duration if hospitalization is necessary)	Distinctions are made between hypomania, mania, mania with psychotic symptoms, mixed episodes, and depressive episodes (described in Table 16.1)
B. During the period of mood disturbance, three (or more) of the following symptoms have persisted:	**Mania.** Mood is elevated out of keeping with the individual's circumstances and may vary from carefree joviality to almost uncontrollable excitement. Elation is accompanied by increased energy, resulting in over-activity, pressure of speech, and a decreased need for sleep. Normal social inhibitions are lost, attention cannot be sustained, and there is often marked distractibility. Self-esteem is inflated, and grandiose or over-optimistic ideas are freely expressed. Perceptual disorders may occur, such as the appreciation of colours as especially vivid (and usually beautiful), a pre-occupation with fine details of surfaces or textures, and subjective hyperacusis. The individual may embark on extravagant and impractical schemes, spend money recklessly, or become aggressive, amorous, or facetious in inappropriate circumstances. In some manic episodes the mood is irritable and suspicious rather than elated.
1. inflated self-esteem or grandiosity	
2. decreased need for sleep	
3. more talkative than usual or pressured speech	
4. flight of ideas or racing thoughts	
5. distractibility	
6. increased goal-directed activity or psychomotor agitation	
7. excessive involvement in pleasurable reckless activities (e.g. buying sprees or sexual indiscretion)	

Continued

Table 16.6 continued

DSM IV TR	CD 10
C. The mood disturbance is not part of a mixed manic-depressive episode D. The mood disturbance causes marked impairment in educational, occupational or social functioning. This may include the need for hospitalization, or the presence of psychotic symptoms E. The symptoms are not due to the direct effects of a substance (e.g. drug abuse, anti-depressant medications), or to a general medical condition **Hypomanic episode.** A hypomanic episode has similar symptoms as a manic episode, but differs in the severity and duration criteria. The symptoms must be present for at least 4 days, and must produce an unequivocal change in the patient's functioning that is observable by others. However, by definition, there is no marked deterioration in functioning, need for hospitalization, or psychotic symptoms; otherwise, a manic episode is diagnosed **Mixed episode.** A mixed episode is diagnosed when the criteria are met for both a manic episode and a major depressive episode (Table 16.1.) over at least a 1-week period. The requirement for significant impairment, and the exclusion of organic causes are the same as for a manic episode	The first attack occurs most commonly between the ages of 15 and 30 years, but may occur at any age. The episode should last for at least 1 week and should be severe enough to disrupt ordinary work and social activities more or less completely. The mood change should be accompanied by increased energy and several of the symptoms referred to above (particularly pressure of speech, decreased need for sleep, grandiosity, and excessive optimism) **Hypomania.** Hypomania is a lesser degree of mania, in which abnormalities of mood and behaviour are too persistent and marked to be included under cyclothymia but are not accompanied by hallucinations or delusions. There is a persistent mild elevation of mood (for at least several days on end), increased energy and activity, and usually marked feelings of well-being and both physical and mental efficiency. Increased sociability, talkativeness, over-familiarity, increased sexual energy, and a decreased need for sleep are often present but not to the extent that they lead to severe disruption of work or result in social rejection. Irritability, conceit, and boorish behaviour may take the place of the more usual euphoric sociability. Concentration and attention may be impaired, thus diminishing the ability to settle down to work or to relaxation and leisure, but this may not prevent the appearance of interests in quite new ventures and activities, or mild over-spending. Hypomania covers the range of disorders of mood and level of activities between cyclothymia and mania. The increased activity and restlessness (and often weight loss) must be distinguished from the same symptoms occurring in hyperthyroidism, anorexia nervosa, and early states of 'agitated depression', which may bear a superficial resemblance to hypomania of the irritable variety **Mania with psychotic symptoms.** The clinical picture is that of a more severe form of mania as described above. Inflated self-esteem and grandiose ideas may develop into delusions, and irritability and suspiciousness into delusions of persecution. In severe cases, grandiose or religious delusions of identity or role may be prominent, and flight of ideas and pressure of speech may result in the individual becoming incomprehensible. Severe and sustained physical activity and excitement may result in aggression or violence, and neglect of eating, drinking, and personal hygiene may

Continued

result in dangerous states of dehydration and self-neglect. One of the most common problems is differentiation of this disorder from schizophrenia, particularly if the stages of development through hypomania have been missed and the patient is seen only at the height of the illness when widespread delusions, incomprehensible speech, and violent excitement may obscure the basic disturbance of affect. Patients with mania that is responding to neuroleptic medication may present a similar diagnostic problem at the stage when they have returned to normal levels of physical and mental activity but still have delusions or hallucinations

Mixed episode. Although the most typical form of bipolar disorder consists of alternating manic and depressive episodes separated by periods of normal mood, it is not uncommon for depressive mood to be accompanied for days or weeks on end by over-activity and pressure of speech, or for a manic mood and grandiosity to be accompanied by agitation and loss of energy and libido. Depressive symptoms and symptoms of hypomania or mania may also alternate rapidly, from day to day or even from hour to hour

Note: Adapted from DSM IV TR (APA, 2000a), ICD 10 (WHO, 1992, 1996).

Epidemiology

The lifetime prevalence of bipolar disorder is 1% and it affects both genders equally (James & Javaloyes, 2001). Around 20% of all bipolar patients have their first episode during adolescence, with a peak age of onset between 15 and 19 years of age. Co-morbid disruptive behaviour disorders, including conduct disorder and ADHD, are common and occur in over half of all cases. Typically, onset of episodes of mania or hypomania is rapid, e.g. from two weeks to three months. About 50% of cases have a favourable outcome. Better outcome is associated with high IQ, good pre-morbid adjustment, and a condition characterized largely by manic episodes. Poorer outcome occurs where the principal characteristic of the condition is mixed manic depressive episodes and where the condition follows a rapid cycling course. Suicide and attempted suicide occur in up to 40% of cases and is more common in those with mixed and depressive episodes, a family history of depression, and co-morbid substance abuse.

Clinical features

Unlike adults, children and adolescents with bipolar disorder may present with symptoms that do not closely conform to the ICD and DSM criteria set out in Table 16.6 (Kusumaker et al., 2002). In pre-adolescence, bipolar disorder rarely presents with the classic adult pattern of discrete episodes of mania and depression. Rather, children present with mixed episodes involving depression and agitation or irritability, rather than elation; with rapid cycling and with sub-threshold biphasic mood dysregulation, in which they do not meet the full diagnostic criteria for either hypomanic or depressive episodes. Because the clinical picture differs from the classic adult presentation, it may be mistaken for ADHD or conduct disorder. Adolescents with bipolar disorder typically present with depressive episodes before manic episodes occur. If treated with anti-depressants during a depressive episode, bipolar adolescents may rapidly develop manic symptoms and may then require short-term anti-psychotic medication to treat these manic states.

Aetiology

Results of twin, adoption and family studies confirm the important role of genetic factors in the aetiology of bipolar disorder in adults (Jones et al., 2002). Averaging across well-conducted studies, the concordance rate for monozygotic twins is about 50%, suggesting that environmental factors are as significant as genetic factors in the aetiology of bipolar disorder. There is some evidence that stressful life events and unsupportive family relationships affect the course of bipolar disorder in adults, with build-up of stresses and negative family interactions precipitating relapses (James & Javaloyes, 2001).

Differential diagnosis

The main alternatives to include the differential diagnosis of bipolar disorder are ADHD, conduct disorder, schizophrenia, drug abuse, endocrinopathies such as hyperthyroidism, and neurological conditions such as temporal lobe epilepsy (American Academy of Child and Adolescent Psychiatry, 1997f; Clark, 2001; James & Javaloyes, 2001). Youngsters with bipolar disorder, like those with ADHD, may show distractibility, impulsivity and over-activity. However, ADHD has an earlier onset than bipolar disorder; the symptoms of distractibility, impulsivity and over-activity are persistent, not episodic; and elated mood rarely occurs in ADHD. Children with bipolar disorder, like those with conduct disorder, may show oppositional behaviour, tantrums, defiance, sexual promiscuity and a pattern of rule-breaking and socially deviant behaviour. However, in bipolar disorder, this overall pattern of behaviour is episodic rather than persistent and there is usually a family history of mood disorder. With bipolar disorder, guilt or remorse may be expressed for rule-breaking, which is rare in conduct disorder. Neither flight of ideas nor pressured speech are present in conduct disorder or ADHD, but both occur in bipolar disorder. Delusions and hallucinations may occur during manic episodes, making children with this type of presentation difficult to distinguish from youngsters with schizophrenia. In such cases, extended periods of observation may be required. A family history of schizophrenia rather than mood disorder and an insidious onset of current difficulties suggest a diagnosis of schizophrenia rather than bipolar disorder. Youngsters who abuse amphetamines or hallucinogenic drugs may present with hypomanic-like behaviour. However, this typically abates over time. A thorough medical and neurological assessment (including an EEG if seizure disorder is suspected) is essential to rule out endocrinopathies, such as hyperthyroidism, and neurological conditions, such as temporal lobe epilepsy, which can contribute to a hypomanic-like presentation.

Assessment

Multi-disciplinary assessment involving a range of disciplines including psychiatry and psychology is essential for cases where bipolar disorder is suspected. Structured clinical interviews such as the Diagnostic Interview for Children and Adolescents (DICA; Reich, 2000), the Schedule for Affective Disorders and Schizophrenia for School-Age Children (KSADS; Ambrosini, 2000), and the Diagnostic Interview Schedule for Children (DISC; Shaffer, Fisher, Lucas, Dulcan & Schwabe-Stone, 2000) all of which are listed in Table 3.11 (p. 103) may be used for diagnosis. The Mania Rating Scale (Fristad, Weller & Weller, 1992) may also be incorporated into the overall assessment protocol given in Chapter 4. Because of the association between suicide and bipolar disorder, a suicide risk assessment, following the guidelines given later in this chapter, should be routinely conducted.

Treatment

A multi-modal intervention programme including psychopharmacological and psychological treatment is the treatment of choice (American Academy of Child and Adolescent Psychiatry, 1997f; Clark, 2001; Findling et al., 2003; Geller & DelBello, 2003; James & Javaloyes, 2001; Kusumakar et al., 2002; Lam & Jones, in press; Lofthouse & Fristad, 2004). Psychopharmacological intervention involves acute treatment of manic or depressive symptoms and long-term prophylaxis. Psychological treatment includes family psychoeducation, family-based problem-solving and communication skills training to strengthen family support for bipolar children, adherence training to prevent non-adherence to the prophylactic medication regime, cognitive-behaviour therapy to facilitate mood control and relapse prevention, family support group membership and school liaison to optimize the youngster's educational environment. In many cases, hospitalization during acute manic episodes may be essential.

Medication

With pharmacological therapy of severe acute manic or mixed episodes, an anti-psychotic (such as chlorpromazine) or an atypical anti-psychotic (such as olanzapine or risperidone) may be prescribed for a brief period until the youngster's over-active and expansive behaviour comes under control. It is worth noting that atypical anti-psychotics may lead to severe weight gain, a side effect that may interfere with later compliance of adolescents with prophylaxis. Benzodiazepines such as clonazepine or lorazepam may also be used where severe agitation is present. For acute depression, anti-depressants in conjunction with lithium are usually prescribed. An anti-depressant taken alone is associated with the risk of rapidly switching from a depressive to a manic episode. TCAs carry a greater risk of precipitating this switch to mania than other anti-depressants such as SSRIs, so SSRIs are preferred. For long-term prophylaxis, lithium, sodium valporate or carbamezapine are usually prescribed and some combination of these medications prevents rapid relapse in about 70% of cases. Non-adherence to prophylactic medication regimes leads to rapid relapse in over 90% of cases. Youngsters may show non-adherence problems because prophylaxis, especially with lithium, may have unpleasant side effects including weight gain, skin rashes and cognitive dulling. Lithium levels require careful three-monthly monitoring because excessive levels can have adverse effects on renal functioning. Lithium should be discontinued during pregnancy because of potentially negative effects on fetal development. Rapid withdrawal of lithium can precipitate an episode of mania. Sodium valporate may be preferred for prophylaxis in adolescents because it has fewer toxic side effects and because it may be more effective alone and in combination with carbamezapine for mixed manic-depressive episodes and rapid cycling bipolar disorder.

Psychological therapy

Psychoeducation, is the cornerstone of psychological intervention. Families need to know about the diagnostic criteria for bipolar disorder, as set out in Table 16.6, and the information on the epidemiology, aetiology and treatment of bipolar disorder outlined above. The analogy of diabetes may be used in explaining the importance of adherence to long-term prophylactic medication regimes. Just as the diabetic requires insulin to remain healthy, so the youngster with bipolar disorder requires lithium, sodium valporate or carbamezapine to remain healthy. As part of psychoeducation parents may be invited to read *The Bipolar Child* (Papolos & Papolos, 2002). Psychoeducation helps youngsters and parents to externalize the problem. That is, it helps them to attribute troublesome manic and depressive behaviour to bipolar disorder rather than to negative intentions of the child. This process of externalizing the problems helps parents to treat children with bipolar disorder less critically and more sympathetically.

Families may also be helped to counteract tendencies to be overly critical or hostile towards the youngster with bipolar disorder through using the problem-solving and communication skills described in Chapter 4 and earlier in this chapter to address day-to-day difficulties.

Families can be helped to facilitate the youngsters' engagement in regular daily routines, which includes taking medication regularly at pre-set times; adhering to regular times for eating meals, retiring at night and rising in the morning; and avoiding alcohol and recreational drug use. If necessary, reward programmes may be used to reinforce regular adherence to medication, eating and sleeping routines, and avoidance of drugs and alcohol.

Youngsters may be helped to recognize their manic and depressive pro-dromes and to develop good coping strategies to prevent the development of full-blown episodes of mania or depression. Prodromes for mania include sleeping less, feeling driven to engage in risky goal-directed behaviour, irrit-ability, increased sociability, racing thoughts and increased optimism. Good coping strategies include restraining oneself, delaying acting on potentially risky plans until they have been discussed with parents or the therapist, doing relaxation exercises, setting aside time to sleep, and talking to parents about calming down. Prodromes for depression include feeling sad, loss of interest in normal activities, being unable to stop worrying and sleep problems. Good coping strategies include getting support from parents, engaging in pleasant activities, challenging negative thoughts following the procedures outlined earlier in this chapter and keeping regular times for retiring and rising in the morning.

Because bipolar disorder places a chronic strain on families, it is important for families to develop a supportive network to help them cope with this long-term stress. Within this context, families may be introduced to long-term support groups for families containing a youngster with bipolar disorder and given information about bipolar disorder websites, such as that for the Child and Adolescent Bipolar Foundation: http://www.bpkids.org/

Bipolar disorder compromises youngsters' capacity to address edu-cational challenges. Within this context, liaison with youngsters' schools is critical. School staff need psychoeducation about bipolar disorder. Schools should adapt youngsters' educational programmes to take account of their absence from school during periods of hospitalization or home-based recovery. Also, in some instances it is appropriate to lessen educational demands and stresses on youngsters to prevent relapse associated with such pressures.

SUICIDE

Suicide rates increase from childhood to adolescence; in late adolescence two to five times more males than females commit suicide (World Health Organization, 1997–1979). In Ireland, the UK, Australia, New Zealand, Canada and the USA, childhood suicide (for children under 14 years) is rare with rates in the late 1990s being under 2 per 100,000. In these same countries, for fifteen- to twenty-five-year-olds, rates for males ranged from 11 to 37 per 100,000 and for females from 2 to 13 per 100,000.

Parasuicide, or attempted suicide, is a common event. A mean parasuicide event rate of 195/100,000 per year was found in a WHO twelve-centre study covering much of Europe, and parasuicide repetition was found to be common (Platt, 1992). While completed suicide is more common among adolescent males, suicidal ideation and attempted suicide is more common among adolescent females. This pattern probably occurs because adolescent males who complete suicide typically are impulsive, aggressive risk takers with a history of conduct disorder and substance abuse who respond to precipitating stresses with intense self-harming reactions such as hanging or shooting themselves. In contrast, females with high rates of suicidal ideation and suicide attempts typically have a history of mood or anxiety disorders and respond to precipitating stresses by contemplating suicide or engaging in far less intense self-harming reactions, such as taking an over-dose (Shaffer & Gutstein, 2002).

Risk and protective factors for suicide

Assessment of suicide risk is necessary when youngsters have attempted suicide recently, when youngsters threaten self-harm or where they show signs of severe depression. Suicide risk assessment involves assessing the degree to which a range of risk and protective factors are present in a particular case and making a judgement about the probability that a suicide attempt will be made. This is not an exact science. It involves careful interviewing and clinical judgment informed by what is known about risk and protective factors in suicide. Risk and protective factors for adolescent suicide are set out below and summarized in Table 16.7. Assessment of suicide risk should cover the following domains:

* suicidal ideation and intention
* method lethality
* precipitating factors
* motivation
* personality-based factors
* disorder-related factors
* historical factors

- family factors
- demographic factors.

The factors listed in Table 16.7, and discussed below, are drawn from thorough literature review (American Academy of Child And Adolescent Psychiatry, 2001a; Berman & Jobes, 1996; Brent, 1997; Carr, 2002b; de Wilde, Kienhorst & Diekstra, 2001; Shaffer & Gutstein, 2002).

Suicidal intention and ideation

Suicidal intention may be distinguished from suicidal ideation. Suicidal intention is characterized by:

- advanced planning
- precautions against discovery
- lethal method
- absence of help seeking
- a final act.

Thus, when youngsters' attempted suicides are characterized by suicidal intention, there is evidence that they have engaged in advanced planning about taking their own lives and have taken precautions against discovery. There is also evidence that they have used a potentially lethal method, such as hanging, self-poisoning, using a gun or jumping from a very dangerous height, and have not sought help after making the suicide attempt. Youngsters with suicidal intentions typically have also completed a final act such as writing a suicide note. Where youngsters show all of these features of suicidal intention, there is a high risk of suicide.

With suicidal ideation, in contrast, adolescents report thinking about self-harm and possibly engaging in non-lethal self-harm such as superficial wrist-cutting but have no clear plans about killing themselves. Suicidal intention and ideation probably reflect two ends of a continuum, with states that approximate suicidal intention reflecting a higher level of risk and those approximating suicidal ideation reflecting a lower level of risk.

The absence of suicidal intentions may be considered a protective factor. The acceptance by the adolescent of a verbal or written contract during a suicide risk assessment, not to attempt suicide, is also a protective factor. The commitment on the part of the parents of carers to monitor the adolescent constantly until all suicidal intention and ideation have abated is a further important protective factor to consider in this domain. This commitment may take the form of an oral or written contract between the clinician and the parents or carers.

Table 16.7 Risk and protective factors for suicide

Risk factors	Domain	Protective factors
• Suicidal intention • Advanced planning • Precautions against discovery • Lethal method • Absence of help seeking and • A final act	**Suicidal intention and ideation**	• Suicidal ideation (not intention) • Acceptance by adolescent of no-suicide contract • Acceptance by parents and carers of suicide monitoring contract
• Availability of lethal methods	**Method lethality**	• Absence of lethal methods
• Loss of parents or partner by death, separation or illness • Conflict with parents or partner • Involvement in judicial system • Severe personal illness • Major exam failure • Unwanted pregnancy • Imitation of other suicides	**Precipitating factors**	• Resolution of interpersonal conflict with parents or partner that precipitated attempted suicide • Acceptance and mourning of losses that precipitated attempted suicide • Physical and psychological distancing from peers or others who precipitated attempted imitative suicide
Suicide attempted to serve the function of: • Escaping an unbearable psychological state or situation • Gaining revenge by inducing guilt • Inflicting self-punishment • Gaining care and attention • Sacrificing the self for a greater good	**Motivation**	Capacity to develop non-destructive coping styles or engage in treatment to be better able to: • Regulate difficult psychological states • Modify painful situations • Express anger assertively • Resolve conflicts productively • Mourn losses • Manage perfectionistic expectations • Solicit care and attention from others • Cope with family disorganization
• High level of hopelessness • High level of perfectionism • High level of impulsivity • High levels of hostility and aggression • Inflexible coping style	**Personality-based factors**	• Low level of hopelessness • Low level of perfectionism • Low level of impulsivity • Low levels of hostility and aggression • Flexible coping style
• Depression • Alcohol and drug abuse • Conduct disorder	**Disorder-related factors**	• Absence of psychological disorders • Absence of physical disorders

• Anti-social personality disorder • Borderline personality disorder • Epilepsy • Chronic painful illness • Multiple co-morbid chronic disorders		• Absence of multiple co-morbid chronic disorders • Capacity to form therapeutic alliance and engage in treatment for psychological and physical disorders
• Previous suicide attempts • Loss of a parent in early life • Previous psychiatric treatment • Involvement in the juvenile justice system	**Historical factors**	• No history of previous suicide attempts • No history of loss of a parent in early life • No history of previous psychiatric treatment • No history of involvement in the juvenile justice system
• Family history of suicide attempts • Family history of depression • Family history of drug and alcohol abuse • Family history of assaultive behaviour • Disorganized, unsupportive family • Family denies seriousness of suicide attempts • Family has high stress and crowding • Family has low social support and is socially isolated	**Family factors**	• No family history of suicide attempts • No family history of depression • No family history of drug and alcohol abuse • No family history of assaultive behaviour • Well-organized supportive family • Family has low stress • Family has high social support
• Male • Social class 5 • White (not black) in USA • Weak religious commitment • Early summer	**Demographic factors**	• Female • Social classes 2, 3 or 4 • Black (not white) in USA • Strong religious commitment

Method lethality

The lethality of the method used or threatened is an important factor to consider in assessing risk with more lethal methods being associated with greater risk in some instances. Using a firearm, hanging, jumping from a great height and self-poisoning with highly toxic drugs are considered to be more lethal than cutting or over-dosing on non-prescription drugs. Within this domain, the availability of a lethal method, such as access to a firearm or highly toxic drugs, constitutes an important risk factor for suicide. Self-harm, particularly superficially cutting of the wrists and arms, should be distinguished from potentially lethal incomplete suicide attempts. Non-lethal self-harm of this sort is sometimes associated with an attempt to relieve tension or gain attention following an interpersonal crisis. This type of self-harming is sometimes preceded by a sense of emptiness or depersonalization (a sense of not being oneself). It is common among adolescents with a history of abuse or neglect and among adolescents with a history of repeated parasuicidal episodes.

However, the degree of suicidal intention cannot always be judged from the lethality of the method used. Where adolescents misunderstand the degree of lethality associated with a particular method, apparently minor parasuicidal gestures may be a significant risk factor for actual suicide.

The unavailability of lethal methods such as firearms and toxic drugs is an important protective factor. This protective factor can be put in place by inviting parents to remove guns, drugs and other lethal methods from the household or placing the adolescent in a place where there is no access to lethal methods.

Precipitating events

Suicide attempts are commonly precipitated by interpersonal conflict or loss involving a parent or romantic attachment. Ongoing conflict with parents, particularly if this entails child abuse, is strongly associated with completed suicide. More severe abuse, combined physical and sexual abuse and chronic abuse are all associated with higher risk. Conflict over disciplinary matters, rule-breaking, particularly if this involves court appearance and imprisonment, are all associated with suicide attempts. For imprisoned adolescents, the risk of suicide attempts is greater during the early part of detention. Loss of parents or a romantic partner through death, long-term separation, or severe chronic illness may precipitate attempted suicide. Other loss experiences, such as diagnosis of severe personal illness (e.g. being HIV positive) or exam failure, may precipitate self-harm. Adolescent pregnancy may also precipitate attempted suicide and may reflect a loss of innocence and a potential focus for intense parent–adolescent conflict.

Suicide arising from imitation of others may be precipitated by suicides within the peer group, school or locality or media coverage of suicides.

Repeated attempted suicide (as distinct from completed suicide) is associated with impulsive separation following romantic relationship difficulties or recent court appearance associated with impulsive or aggressive anti-social behaviour.

Protective factors in this domain include the resolution of interpersonal conflict with parents or romantic partner that precipitated attempted suicide, acceptance and mourning of losses that precipitated attempted suicide and physical and psychological distancing from peers or others who precipitated attempted imitative suicide.

Motivation

Youngsters may be motivated to attempt suicide for a wide variety of reasons. Suicide is usually perceived by youngsters as the only feasible solution to a difficult problem involving interpersonal loss or conflict. In this respect, the act of suicide may be construed as fulfilling one or more functions including:

- escaping an unbearable psychological state or situation
- gaining revenge by inducing guilt
- inflicting self-punishment
- gaining care and attention
- sacrificing the self for a greater good.

Suicide may be construed by youngsters as a means of escaping from the psychological pain entailed by loss or conflict. From this perspective, death may be seen as a state that will bring relief from pain. Suicide may alternatively reflect an attempt to obtain revenge, to express aggression, to retaliate or punish a parent or romantic partner for their hostility or for leaving them through death, separation or illness. Here the sentiment is 'You have hurt me, but I will get my revenge by hurting you through killing myself and causing you to feel guilt'. Revenge motives may be over-emphasized by some clinicians because these cases are so difficult to help. In other instances, suicide represents self-punishment arising from guilt for not living up to perfectionistic self-expectations or expectations that youngsters perceive parents or others to have of them. For example, youngsters who fail exams or become unintentionally pregnant may see suicide as a way of atoning for their failure to meet academic or moral standards. Attempted suicide may represent a way of obtaining care and attention, particularly for adolescents who repeatedly make self-harming gestures. Finally, youngsters from disorganized conflictual families may view their suicide as a necessary sacrifice that must be made to preserve the integrity of their family. That is, they may fantasize that their suicide will serve as a rallying point, which will unite a fragmented family.

The potential for finding alternative ways of fulfilling the functions of attempted suicide is a protective factor. Thus flexibility about developing new coping styles for solving the problem for which the suicide attempt was a destructive solution places adolescents at lower risk for suicide. Understanding suicidal motives and the functions that suicidal gestures are intended to fulfil are important in treatment planning. When the functions of an attempted suicide are understood, the treatment plan should help the youngster find other ways to fulfil these functions. That is, treatment plans should help youngsters find less destructive ways for regulating difficult psychological states, modifying painful situations, expressing anger assertively, resolving conflicts productively, mourning losses, managing perfectionistic expectations, soliciting care and attention from others and coping with family disorganization.

Personality-based risk factors

Personality traits which place adolescents at risk for suicide include hopelessness, perfectionism, impulsivity, hostility, aggression and an inflexible coping style. Youngsters who attempt suicide view themselves as incapable of changing their situation and so the future, to them, looks hopeless. Perfectionism is a risk factor for suicide probably because it leads to heightened self-expectations which may be difficult to achieve. Suicidal adolescents tend to be inflexible in their coping styles and have difficulties drawing on memories of successfully solving problems in the past and so have a limited repertoire of coping strategies to draw on. Thus they resort to strategies which may be ineffective. Their aggression and impulsivity may lead them to engage in self-directed aggression with little reflection on other possible alternatives for solving their difficulties.

Low levels of personality traits which place adolescents at risk for suicide are protective factors in this domain, i.e. low levels of hopelessness, perfectionism, impulsivity, hostility and aggression. It has already been noted (in the previous section) that the potential for flexibility in finding alternatives to suicide as a way of coping is also a protective factor.

Disorder-related risk factors

Among adolescents, and particularly among males, who constitute a large proportion of completed suicides, disorders which are risk factors for suicide include alcohol and drug abuse, conduct disorder, anti-social or borderline personality disorders. All of these are more common among impulsive individuals and impulsivity has been already been mentioned as a personality-based risk factor for suicide. The presence of depression is a highly significant health-related risk factor for future suicide. Depression is strongly associated with hopelessness, which paves the way for suicide. Major depression (a recurrent episodic mood disorder) is strongly associated with completed suicide whereas dysthymia (a chronic milder non-episodic mood disorder) is associated with repeated suicide attempts. Epilepsy and chronic painful illness are the two physical illnesses which place adolescents at increased risk of suicide. Increased suicide risk is strongly associated with multiple co-morbid chronic psychological and physical disorders.

The absence of psychological or physical disorders and the absence of multiple co-morbid chronic psychological and physical disorders are important protective factors in this domain. So, too, is the capacity to form a good therapeutic alliance and engage in a contract for treatment of disorders, including depression, alcohol and drug abuse, conduct disorder, anti-social or borderline personality disorders, epilepsy and chronic painful illness.

Historical risk factors

A history of previous suicide attempts is the single strongest historical risk factor for future suicide. Other historical risk factors include loss of a parent in early life, previous psychiatric treatment and a history of involvement in the juvenile justice system. These three factors are particularly strongly associated with repeated suicidal attempts or parasuicide.

The absence of these historical events is a protective factor as is a history of good pre-morbid adjustment.

Family risk factors

A family history of a range of problems, notably suicide attempts, depression, drug and alcohol abuse and assaultive behaviour, place youngsters at risk for suicide. In addition, youngsters are placed at increased risk of suicide if their families are socially isolated, live in stressful, over-crowded conditions and if they deny the seriousness of the youngster's suicidal intentions or are unsupportive of the youngster.

A family history that does not entail suicide attempts, depression, drug and alcohol abuse, and assaultive behaviour is a protective factor. Where the family is well organized and supportive of the youngster, and where there are low levels of stress and high levels of social support for the family as a whole, these may be considered as protective factors.

Demographic risk factors

Male adolescents are at greater risk for completed suicide, whereas female adolescents are at greatest risk of parasucide. Males tend to use more lethal methods (guns and hanging) whereas females use less lethal methods (cutting or self-poisoning). Membership of social class 5 (unskilled workers with low incomes and educational levels) is a risk factor for completed suicide and repeated parasuicide, while membership of social class 1 (professional and higher managerial employees) is a risk factor for completed suicide only. With respect to ethnicity, in the USA suicide rates are higher for white than black adolescents. With respect to religion, adolescents from communities with lower levels of religious practice are at greater risk for suicide. With respect to seasonality, completed suicide is most common in early summer.

Protective demographic factors include being female; membership of social classes 2, 3 and 4; being black (not white) in the USA; and having a strong commitment to religious values and practices.

Assessment of suicide risk

Family-focused, social-learning-theory-based interventions for the management of suicide risk emphasize the importance of adopting a structured problem-solving approach that takes account of the child's or adolescent's personal features and the social context within which the suicide attempt was made (American Academy of Child And Adolescent Psychiatry, 2001a; Berman & Jobes, 1996; Brent, 1997; Carr, 2002b; Lerner & Clum, 1990; Shaffer & Gutstein, 2002; Richman, 1984; Rotherham-Borus et al., 1994, 1996). The over-riding objective of a family consultation where suicide has been threatened or attempted is to prevent harm, injury or death from occurring. Certain broad principles for assessment may be followed. First, offer immediate consultation. Second, use the consultation process to develop a comprehensive understanding of the situation surrounding the suicide threat or attempt. Third, during the consultation process, establish or deepen your working alliance with all significant members of the network. Fourth, assess all of the factors mentioned below and listed in Table 16.7. Check if the factors were present in the past, the extent to which they were present during the recent episode, and whether they are immediately present. Where possible, obtain information relating to risk factors from as many members of the network as possible. This includes the youngster who has threatened self-harm or attempted suicide, key members of the family, and previously involved professionals. Fifth, identify people within the youngster's social network and the professional network that may be available to help implement a management plan. Sixth, draw the information you obtain into a clear formulation on which a management plan can be based. The formulation must logically link the risk factors identified in the case together to explain the occurrence of the episode of self-injurious behaviour and the current level of risk. It is important to specify pre-disposing factors and triggering factors that led to an escalation from suicidal ideation to intention or from suicidal intention to self-injury. The management plan must specify the short-term action to be taken in the light of the formulation. The plan must logically indicate that the changes it entails will probably lower the risk of self-harm. It is also vital that until the risk of suicide has reduced, the youngster and the parents make a contract at the conclusion of each session to return to meet the clinician at a specified time. For the youngster, this contract involves making a commitment to not make further suicide attempts. For the parents or carers, the contract involves making a commitment to monitor the youngster so as to prevent further suicide attempts.

Multi-systemic interviews

With children and adolescents it is useful to conduct at least three different interviews: one with the parents, guardians or foster parents alone; one with the child alone and one whole-family interview. The separate parent and child interviews provide opportunities to obtain different perspectives on the presence or absence of risk factors. The family interview may be used to explore differences between parent and child views of the situation and to observe patterns of whole-family interaction.

For example, in one case the parents reported that their child continually displayed attention-seeking behaviour and that the self-injurious behaviour was just one more example of that attention-seeking process. The child asserted that he felt neglected and occasionally abused by the parents and that his self-injurious behaviour was an attempt to escape from that abuse. Later, in a whole-family interview, the pattern of interaction in which the parents and child engaged was explored and the differences between their views of the situation were examined. This case also shows that with children and adolescents it is crucial to interview the child alone at some point during the evaluation. If the child's concerns are being discounted by the parents, they will be less inhibited to talk about them in a one-to-one situation. Also if neglect or abuse is occurring, this can best be explored in an individual interview. Child protection issues are covered in Chapters 19, 20 and 21. Family interviews offer a forum within which parents can be invited to view suicidal behaviour and ideation as reflecting a broad contextual problem rather than a difficulty which is intrinsic to the child.

In custody and access cases, foster-care cases and cases where a child is in a residential school or institution, key people involved in the child's network must all be interviewed individually if necessary. These key people will include the person legally responsible for the child, the child's primary caretaker, the person most concerned that the referral be made, the teachers or careworkers who see the child on a day-to-day basis and other professionals who have been involved in case management, including social workers paediatricians and the GP. Other complications and issues associated with cases where parents have separated or where the child is in foster or residential care are discussed in Chapters 22 and 23.

Child-centred interviewing

When conducting the child-centred interview it is important first to let the child know the duration of the interview and what will follow on from it. If hospitalization or some other protective intervention is an option, it is better to mention that this is a possible outcome than to conceal it. It is also crucial to be accurate about the limits of confidentiality. You must let children and adolescents know that you will not break a confidence that they ask you to keep unless it is necessary for ensuring their safety. Initially, to establish rapport, it may be useful to start by inquiring about some relatively unthreatening area like schoolwork or friendships. Once you have established a working relationship with the youngster, move into the central part of the interview.

In cases where a suicide attempt has been made, obtain a detailed description of the self-destructive behaviour that led to the referral and all related suicidal ideation and intentions. Specifically, note if the behaviour was dangerous and the strength of the child's will to die. Note the presence of a detailed plan, the taking of precautions to avoid discovery and the carrying-out of a final act like making a will or writing a note. If you are re-assessing a youngster who has been hospitalized with a view to discharging the case, or if you are assessing a case where suicide is suspected but no self-injurious behaviour has occurred, ask these questions.

- Have you thought of harming yourself?
- How strong is the urge to harm yourself?
- Have you a plan to harm yourself?
- What preparations have you made to harm yourself?
- Suppose, you harmed yourself and died, what do you hope your family/your mum/your dad/your brother/your sister would think/do/feel?
- Suppose, you harmed yourself but didn't die, what do you hope your family/your mum/your dad/your brother/your sister would think/do/feel?
- Do you want to escape from something or some situation?
- Do you want to punish somebody by harming yourself?

Note if the plan includes specific details of a dangerous method, precautions against discovery and a final act such as writing a suicide note or a will. The Beck Scale for Suicide Ideation, Childhood Depression Inventory, the Hopelessness Scale for Children and Reynold's Semistructured Interview are useful adjuncts to a clinical interview and are listed in Table 16.5. Invitations to engage in writing, drawing or painting offer other avenues for understanding youngsters' world views, especially where they are particularly reluctant to engage in conversation.

In cases where an attempt has been made, build up a picture of the immediate circumstances surrounding the episode and the events that happened before, during and after the episode. Clarify if this is an escalation of an entrenched pattern of interaction around previous suicidal ideas or intentions. In cases where no self-injury has occurred but where suicidal ideation is present, ask the youngster to describe the sequence of events that led up to and followed on from episodes of suicidal ideation.

Identify the youngsters' perception of their network and of the roles of significant people in the recent episode and previous episodes of suicidal ideation or self-injurious behaviour. The aim here is to obtain a coherent account of how the youngster came to view his or her life situation as hopeless and selected self-harm as a solution to this experience of hopelessness. Include a full discussion of the youngster's family, friends and involved professionals in this assessment. The procedures for constructing and elaborating a genogram and lifeline, described in Chapter 4, may be useful here. It is also useful to take account of empirically identified risk and triggering actors that may have been included in the sequence of events that led to the child experiencing hopelessness and attempting or considering suicide.

The following questions may be useful in eliciting information about risk and protective factors listed in Table 16.7. All of these questions should be followed-up with probes and linked together with alliance-building reassurance:

- Can you tell me about the things that were happening before you tried to (threatened to) harm yourself?
- What was going wrong in your life?
- How did you reach the decision to end your life?
- How exactly did you harm yourself?
- What happened afterwards and how did you survive?
- In what way did you believe that ending your life would solve the difficulties you faced?
- When you look back on that episode, do you think now that there were other things you could have done, besides harming yourself to deal with the difficulties you faced?
- When you look into the future now, are you hopeful about changing your situation so that it will become more bearable?
- To what extent do you think that the high expectations that you have of yourself may push you towards self-harm again?
- To what extent do you think that you acted on impulse, without thinking, when you harmed yourself?
- Do you expect that you may act on impulse, without thinking, and harm yourself again?
- Have you had problems with low mood in the past?
- Have you tried to harm yourself before?
- Can you tell me about that episode, how it started, what happened, how it ended?
- Have you been in trouble at school or with the courts because of rule-breaking in the past?
- Have you been using drugs or alcohol much in the past?
- Have you attended a clinic for help with any problems like low mood, being in trouble, or using drugs or alcohol in the past?
- Have you been treated for any painful health problems or illnesses?
- Are you on medication for any conditions such as epilepsy?
- Has anyone in your family had problems with low mood, getting in trouble with the law or using too many drugs or too much alcohol?
- In your family, who do you feel you can turn to now for help with the difficulties you face?

Integrate the youngster's story, check its accuracy and agree a plan for discussing this account with parents or legal guardian and significant members of the adolescent's network.

Management of suicide risk

In assessing risk factors it is important to determine if factors identified in the assessment interviews were present or absent before and during the episode of self-injurious behaviour, if they are present or absent now, and if there is any available resource that can modify risk factors that are still present. For example, if social isolation was a risk factor and it is still present, it might be modified by arranging for the patient to stay with relatives.

In assessing overall risk it is important to distinguish between high, immediate suicide risk and long-term risk associated with parasuicide. Immediate focused intervention based on clear formulation and a coherent management plan can reduce immediate suicide risk. Individuals who engage in repeated self-injurious behaviour are at high long-term risk for suicide and have difficulty deriving sustained significant benefit from immediate focused intervention or indeed long-term counselling or therapy.

The principal focused interventions in cases of suicide risk are home-based care or referral for hospital-based or residential care.

Home-based care

With home-based care, the clinician and other relevant team members make a no-suicide contract with the adolescent and a monitoring contract with the parents or carers.

No-suicide contract

The no-suicide contract is an agreement, either oral or written between the adolescent and clinician not to attempt suicide before the next appointment. The contract should also include the steps that the adolescent will take if the circumstances that triggered the previous suicidal threat or attempt recur or if suicidal intentions develop. Such steps may include disengaging from conflict with parents, partners, peers or others; avoiding catastrophizing about loss experiences; engaging in supportive conversation with a parent or carer; engaging in a distracting or soothing activity such as reading or listening to restful music and phoning the clinic's 24-hour on-call service as a last resort if strong suicidal ideation and intentions persist.

Monitoring contract

The parents or carers are invited to agree to a monitoring contract. This entails developing a family rota for keeping the youngster under 24-hour supervision to prevent the youngster from attempting suicide; agreeing that the person on the rota will only engage in supportive and non-conflictual conversation with the youngster and phoning the clinic's 24-hour on-call service as a last resort if strong suicidal ideation and intentions persist.

24-hour on-call service

Ideally, the no-suicide and monitoring contract are offered as part of a thera-peutic plan in which the adolescent and parents are given a 24-hour on-call phone number that they can call to contact a member of the treatment team if strong suicidal ideation and intentions persist. This has been shown to significantly reduce the number of suicide attempts and threats (Brent, 1997).

Treatment plan

The no-suicide and monitoring contract are offered as part of a therapeutic plan, which involves the adolescent and parents being invited to attend a series of sessions aimed at planning ways to modify risk or triggering factors which contributed to the suicide attempt or threat. The treatment plan should address the functions of an attempted suicide and help the youngster, in collaboration with the parents, find other ways for regulating difficult psycho-logical states, modifying painful situations, expressing anger assertively, resolving conflicts productively, mourning losses, managing perfectionistic expectations, soliciting care and attention from others and coping with family disorganization. The treatment plan should also aim to treat the underlying depression and related difficulties, such as conduct problems and drug abuse. The treatment programme described for depression in the first part of this chapter is appropriate here.

Active follow-up

Adolescents who attempt or threaten suicide are at risk for not attending fol-low-up appointment and so an active approach to follow-up is a vital part of the no-suicide contract and the parents' monitoring contract. The adolescent and parents should be given a definite appointment after the initial consult-ation and this should be within a couple of days of the first meeting. The family should be contacted by phone to remind them about the appointment and to inquire about non-attendance if this occurs. The number, duration and agenda for therapeutic sessions should be made clear to both the parents and the adolescent from the outset and the importance of follow-up for preventing further suicide threats and attempt should be highlighted.

Hospital-based care

With hospital-based and residential care, while actively suicidal, 24-hour constant observation should be arranged in consultation with nursing or residential care staff. As part of the admission contract, the parents or legal guardians should be invited to attend a series of sessions aimed at planning ways to modify risk or triggering factors which contributed to the crisis and which when modified would create a safe context for discharge from hospital or residential care unit. Thereafter, the protocol outlined above for home-based care should be followed.

PREVENTION

School-based programmes to prevent depression in children should help youngsters develop the cognitive and social skills necessary to reduce their vulnerability to depression. In particular such programmes may include the following components:

- A model for understanding depression which outlines the roles of psychological, social and biological factors.
- Attribution training to help youngsters develop learned optimism (rather than learned helplessness).
- Self-instructional training to help youngsters develop positive self-monitoring, self-evaluative and self-reinforcement skills.
- Social problem-solving skills.
- Planning pleasant events.
- Relaxation training.

Analogue treatment studies including these components show that youngsters can benefit from such training (Harrington et al., 1998). Such programmes may be offered to unscreened populations or to children screened for depressive symptoms or cognitive styles using instruments such as those listed in Table 16.5. Parent training programmes, particularly for parents identified by their family doctors as suffering from mood problems, which emphasize the development of supportive parent–child relationships are a second avenue for the prevention of childhood depression. Child abuse prevention programmes discussed in Chapters 19, 20 and 21 are a further possible way of preventing childhood depression.

   While such programmes may go some way towards preventing some children who are at suicide risk, broader preventative strategies are required here. These fall into three categories (Hickey & Carr, 2002; Shaffer & Gutstein, 2002):

- education
- case finding
- hotlines.

With education, school-based programmes targeting children and community-based programmes targeting parents may offer information on the signs of suicide and parasuicide, suicide risk factors and the type of help that is available from teachers, GPs, counsellors and others within the community. With case finding, educational programmes may also outline how a concerned peer, teacher or parent should refer a child suspected of being at risk for suicide to suicide prevention health services. Telephone hotlines offer a third avenue for suicide prevention.

SUMMARY

Mood disorders in children and adolescents constitute a serious problem because of the high rate of relapse. While equal numbers of children develop mood problems, in adolescence there is a sharp rise in the prevalence of depression among girls. The prevalence of depression for two- to eighteen-year-olds is 2–9%. Within DSM IV TR and ICD 10, the main distinctions are between primary and secondary mood disorders, recurrent major and persistent minor mood problems, and unipolar and bipolar mood disorders. Major and minor unipolar disorders are probably the most commonly seen in clinical practice. A low mood, negative cognitive set, self-defeating behavioural patterns, disruption of sleep and appetite, and conflict or social withdrawal from important relationships at home and at school are the main clinical features. Psychoanalytic theories of depression point to the importance of early separation or bereavement and critical parenting styles in developing a vulnerability to depression. Behavioural theories point to lack of reinforcement or poor self-reinforcement skills in the maintenance of depression. Cognitive theories highlight the role of negative interpretation of ambiguous events in the maintenance of depression. Systems theory underlines the role of problematic family relationships in maintaining low mood. Biological theories point to the importance of genetic factors, dysregulation of the neurotransmitter systems in the reward and punishment centres of the brain, endocrine dysfunction, immune system dysregulation, disruption of the sleep–waking cycle and, in some instances, seasonal biological changes in the aetiology of depression. Because of the complexity of mood problems and the uniqueness of each case, intervention programmes should be based on a comprehensive case formulation arising from a thorough multi-systemic assessment. Available evidence suggests that, with children and adolescents, multi-systemic intervention based on the principles of cognitive-behaviour therapy, family systems therapy and social leaning theory is the treatment of choice. SSRI anti-depressant medication should be considered if psychological therapy has been ineffective.

Bipolar disorder is characterized by episodes of mania or hypomania and by episodes of depression, but children often present with mixed episodes and rapid cycling. Co-morbid disruptive behaviour disorders are common; 20% of all bipolar patients have their first episode during adolescence. ADHD, conduct disorder, schizophrenia, drug abuse, hyperthyroidism and temporal lobe epilepsy should be included in the differential diagnosis. Best practice involves multi-disciplinary assessment and multi-modal intervention, including psychopharmacological and psychological treatment.

Where adolescents present with threats of self-harm or self-injurious behaviour the youngster and significant network members should be interviewed. This should be followed with an exploration of the details of the adolescent's suicidal ideation, suicidal intention and self-injurious behaviour. Then the circumstances surrounding the episode require clarification and risk factors in the social network may be explored. Demographic, historical and health-related risk factors and protective factors should also be identified. These should be integrated into a formulation and a plan for risk reduction developed and implemented.

EXERCISE 16.1

Paula Black is a sixteen-year-old only child who was referred for assessment after her mother found a bottle of assorted pills hidden in her chest of drawers. Recently, her school performance has deteriorated; she has also stopped playing hockey. She is tearful from time to time and very moody. Her mother has tried to talk her round but she becomes mute or throws a tantrum. Her mother has never had patience for that type of moodiness. Up until the beginning of last summer (four months ago) her behaviour was within normal limits. Her developmental history is unremarkable, with sensorimotor, cognitive and social development all within the normal range. She had all the normal childhood illnesses and recovered from all of these admirably. A full family history is unavailable. This is what may be gleaned from the GP's letter: her maternal grandparents live locally and have a supportive relationship with her. Paula's only aunt lives abroad but comes back to Dublin regularly, although she missed her trip last summer because she was in hospital. Paula never knew her father, who was killed in a road traffic accident when she was two weeks old. Her paternal grandparents, who live in Athlone and are farmers, have little contact with her although they did offer to take her on holiday this year and she refused. Paula plans to sit her leaving cert. in 18 months. In the long term Paula wants to study veterinary medicine and has the ability to do so according to her teachers. She obtained nine honours in her junior cert., including seven A's. Paula has never had any romantic attachments, to her mother's or her GP's knowledge, but goes to dances and outings with her two close girl-friends who have recently begun dating boyfriends occasionally.

- Develop a preliminary formulation for this case in which you clearly identify possible pre-disposing, precipitating, maintaining and protective factors.
- What would your top three priorities be in a preliminary interview with Paula and her mother?
- Role-play this interview.

EXERCISE 16.2

Use the model for formulating suicide risk contained in Table 16.7 to decide if the risk of suicide is higher in the case of Maire O'Connor, which was presented in Box 16.1, or Paula Black, which was presented in exercise 16.1. List the reasons for your judgement.

FURTHER READING

Friedberg, R. & McClure, J. (2002). *Clinical Practice of Cognitive Therapy with Children and Adolescents*. New York: Guilford.

Geller, B. & DelBello, M. (2003). *Bipolar Disorder in Childhood and Early Adolescence*. New York: Guilford Press.

Mufson, L., Dorta, K., Moreau, D., Weissman, M. (2004). *Interpersonal Psychotherapy for Depressed Adolescents* (Second Edition). New York: Guilford.

Stallard, P. (2002). *Think Good – Feel Good: A Cognitive Behaviour Therapy Workbook for Children and Young People*. Chichester, UK: Wiley.

Wodarski, J., Wodarski, L & Dulmus, C. (2002). *Adolescent Depression and Suicide: A Comprehensive Empirical Intervention for Prevention and Treatment*. Springfield, IL: Charles C Thomas.

FURTHER READING FOR CLIENTS

Fitzpatrick, C. (2004). *Coping with Depression in Young People. A Guide for Parents.* Chichester, UK: Wiley.

Papolos, D. & Papolos, J. (2002). *The Bipolar Child: The Definitive and Reassuring Guide to Childhood's Most Misunderstood Disorder* (Second Edition). New York: Broadway.

WEBSITES

American Foundation for Suicide Prevention (AFSP): http://www.afsp.org

Child & Adolescent Bipolar Foundation: http://www.bpkids.org/

David Brent's therapy manuals: http://www.wpic.pitt.edu/research/star/ or BrentDA@upmc.edu

John Weisz's therapy manuals: e-mail:weisz@psych.ucla.edu

Manual for Coping with Depression Course: http://www.kpchr.org/public/acwd/acwd.html

National Self-Harm Network: info@nshn.co.uk: http://www.nshn.co.uk

Suicide awareness. Voice of education: http://www.save.org

Suicide Prevention Advocacy Network (SPAN): http://www.spanusa.org

Young People and Self Harm information resource website: http://www.selfharm.org.uk

Factsheets on depression, bipolar disorder, suicide and self-harm can be downloaded from the website for Rose, G. & York, A. (2004). *Mental Health and Growing Up. Fact sheets for Parents, Teachers and Young People* (Third edition). London: Gaskell: http://www.rcpsych.ac.uk

Chapter 17

Anorexia and bulimia nervosa

In our Western industrial culture, where food is plentiful, it is ironic that self-starvation and a pattern of bingeing and purging are major problems affecting teenage girls. An example of a typical eating disorder case is presented in Box 17.1. The outcome for eating disorders is poor, but early intervention and evidence-based treatment can improve outcome (American Psychiatric Association (APA), 2000b; Gowers & Bryant Waugh, 2004; Neiderman, 2000; NICE, 2004; Steinhausen, 2002a,b; Stice, 2002). For anorexia nervosa, about half of all cases have a good outcome, a third have moderate outcome and a fifth have a poor outcome. At 20 years follow-up, the mortality rate is about 6% (with a range from 0 to 21% across studies). Poor prognosis is associated with lower weight, a more chronic condition, the absence of a clear precipitating stressful life event, bulimic symptoms, co-morbid obsessive-compulsive disorder, problematic family relationships, dropping out of treatment and lower social class. For bulimia nervosa, about half of all cases have a good outcome, a quarter have a moderate outcome and the remaining quarter have a poor outcome. Poor prognosis in bulimia is associated with later onset, a more chronic condition, more frequent bingeing and vomiting, greater body dissatisfaction, higher perfectionism, co-morbid substance abuse, impulsive personality disorders and lower social class. After discussing the classification, epidemiology and clinical features of eating disorders, this chapter considers a variety of theoretical explanations concerning their aetiology, along with relevant empirical evidence. The assessment of eating disorders is followed by an outline of a family therapy approach to the treatment of anorexia and a cognitive-behavioural approach to the treatment of bulimia. The chapter concludes with some ideas on how to prevent eating disorders in populations at risk.

CLASSIFICATION

An excessive concern with the control of body weight and shape, along with an inadequate and unhealthy pattern of eating are the central manifestations

Box 17.1 A case of anorexia nervosa

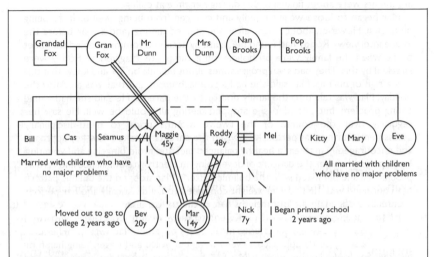

Married with children who have no major problems

All married with children who have no major problems

Moved out to go to college 2 years ago

Began primary school 2 years ago

Referral. Mar, a fourteen-year-old girl was referred for treatment because her weight had continued to fall since she was about twelve years. When assessed she was 37 kg (80% of her expected weight), had amenorrhoea, a highly restrictive eating pattern of two-years duration and a daily routine involving episodes of intensive exercise. Mar had gone through an episode of self-induced vomiting after meal-times for about three months but this had ceased a year previously.

Presentation. In the intake interview she expressed a fear of becoming fat and experienced her hips, buttocks, stomach and thighs to be considerably larger than their actual size. She continually thought of food and the number of calories associated with all aspects of her diet. Her mood was generally low and she had on occasion experienced suicidal thoughts, but had never had frank suicidal intentions. On the Eating Disorder Inventory, Mar obtained extreme scores on the drive for thinness and body dissatisfaction sub-scales. She also obtained extreme scores on the ineffectiveness, perfectionism, maturity fear sub-scales. Mar held a range of rigid beliefs about the importance of controlling her body shape. She also had a distorted body image, believing herself to be markedly larger than her actual size.

Developmental history. Her personal developmental history was well within normal limits. Language and cognitive development, if anything, were rapid and Mar had always been in the top 10% of her class. She was a model child at home showing no behavioural or emotional problems. She had good peer relationships and a circle of four to six good friends in her neighbourhood. The transition to secondary school had been uneventful, as had her menarche. She continued to do well in school but towards the end of her first year in secondary school became despondent about her weight. She was, according to her mother, 'well built'. Mar began dieting shortly before her thirteenth birthday. Her own view was that she felt like she wasn't fitting in with her friends, who by now were going to discos and beginning to take an interest in boys. Her mother's view was that she had been hurt by some comments made by girls at her school about her weight.

History of the presenting problem. What began as innocent dieting, that was wholeheartedly supported by Maggie and Roddy, the parents, gradually became more and more intense around the time that Bev, Mar's older step-sister went to college and her younger brother Nick began school. Also at that time there was increased conflict between Seamus (Bev's father) and Maggie. Most of the arguments were about financing Bev during her time at college.

Mar began to loose weight rapidly and changed from being 'well built' to being quite slim. However, about a year after she started dieting (and a year before the intake interview), Roddy had found her, quite by accident, vomiting behind the toilet block, when the family were on holiday on a camp site. Maggie and Roddy were shocked by this. They had seen programmes about bulimia on TV and knew that this was a sign of bulimia. Mar said she had a stomach upset and that was all. After the holiday, Mar was taken to the family doctor by the parents. He said she had a mild eating problem, but provided she stopped dieting all would be well. He saw her regularly over the course of the twelve months prior to multi-disciplinary assessment. During that period, he advised the parents to take a low-key approach and encouraged Mar to eat a healthy balanced diet and avoid bingeing and vomiting. He impressed on her the dangers of developing an electrolyte imbalance and cardiac problems if she persisted with the bulimic pattern. Mar stopped the bulimic pattern but continued with dieting. Her weight continued to fall drastically and her periods eventually stopped about four months before the assessment.

Roddy and Maggie were at their wits' end to know what to do. Maggie, who loved to cook made increasingly sumptuous meals to try to tempt Mar away from her diet. She took a softly-softly approach, never raising her voice and never being harsh or punitive. She looked to her mother Mrs Fox, for support and gradually felt more and more guilt. She was convinced that the eating problem was a reflection of some mistake she had made as a parent. Roddy left the management of the problem to Maggie, although occasionally, he tried to convince Mar to eat. These conversations usually ended in a row so they now happened less frequently. Meal-times had become a night-mare, according to Roddy. He said he now frequently played a round of golf after work and ate a bar-meal with his brother Mel afterwards.

Family history. Roddy's brother and three sisters and Maggie's two brothers were all married with children and none had any significant psychological problems or eating disorders. Bill and Cas tended to deny the reality of Mar's problem or to say it was something she would grow out of. Mel, Roddy's brother saw Mar's behaviour as defiance that required strict discipline. Kitty, Mary and Eve thought that it was a personal problem and Eve thought it might have something to do with having an older step-sister.

Formulation. Mar was a fourteen-year-old girl who presented with anorexia nervosa and a history of bulimia, the onset of which was precipitated by Mar's entry into adolescence, Mar's dissatisfaction with her weight, critical comments made by peers about her weight and increased family stress associated with her step-sister's move to college and her younger brother's entry into primary school. The restrictive eating was maintained at an interpersonal level by the inconsistent way in which Mar's parents managed her refusal to maintain a normal body weight and at an intrapsychic level by Mar's distorted body image, maturity fears and need for control coupled with a sense of being powerless.

Treatment. Family-based treatment was offered which focused on helping the parents to disengage from intrusive and inconsistent interaction with Mar concerning food while encouraging Mar to take responsibility for attaining a healthy target body weight and developing a less food-focused lifestyle.

of eating problems in children and adolescents (Lask & Bryant-Waugh, 2000). The sub-classification of such eating problems has been managed in similar ways in both the DSM IV TR (APA, 2000a) and ICD 10 (WHO, 1992, 1996). In both systems, a distinction has been made between anorexia nervosa and bulimia nervosa, with the former being characterized primarily by weight loss and the latter by a cyclical pattern of bingeing and purging. Diagnostic criteria from both systems for these disorders are set out in Tables 17.1 and 17.2. The ICD and DSM criteria for anorexia, while suitable for older teenagers or young adults, are not suitable for children. The body mass index of 17.5 specified in the ICD 10, is within the normal range for children under 15 and the criterion of 85% of expected body weight for age and height, specified in DSM IV TR, may be an inappropriate criterion to use where growth retardation has occurred as a result of restricted food intake. Alternative diagnostic criteria proposed by Lask and Bryant-Waugh (1993) are included in Table 17.1.

The distinction made between anorexia nervosa and bulimia nervosa, while descriptively useful, does not take full account of variations in eating problems seen in clinical practice. Many anorexic patients present with bulimic symptoms and many bulimic patients, such as Mar described in Box 17.1, develop anorexia. For this reason, in DSM IV TR, a distinction is made between two sub-types of anorexia: the restricting type and the binge–purge type.

Eating problems seen in clinical practice but which do not meet the criteria for anorexia or bulimia include food avoidance emotional disorder, selective eating, restrictive eating, food refusal, functional dysphagia and pervasive food refusal syndrome (Bryant-Waugh, 2000). In food avoidance emotional disorder, the child avoids food and shows signs of anxiety, depression and obsessive-compulsive features. With selective eating, only a narrow range of foods are eaten. With restrictive eating, smaller amounts of food than is usual are eaten. With food refusal, situationally bound episodes of not eating occur. With functional dysphagia, a fear of swallowing, choking or vomiting leads to food avoidance. With pervasive refusal syndrome, not only do children refuse to eat but they also refuse to engage in any other social or self-care activity. No abnormal pre-occupation with weight or shape occurs with any of these disorders, and this distinguishes them from anorexia and bulimia nervosa.

EPIDEMIOLOGY

Anorexia nervosa and bulimia nervosa are most common among female adolescents (Doyle & Bryant-Waugh, 2000; Gowers & Bryant-Waugh, 2004; Steinhausen, 2000a; Wilson, Black-Becker & Heffernan, 2003). About 1–2% of the adolescent female population suffer from eating disorders. Anorexia is

Table 17.1 Diagnostic criteria for anorexia nervosa

DSM IV TR	ICD 10	Lask & Bryant-Waugh
A. Refusal to maintain body weight at or above a minimally normal weight for age and height (weight loss or failure to gain weight in a growth period leading to body weight less than 85% of that expected) B. Intense fear of gaining weight or becoming fat even though under-weight C. Disturbance in the way in which one's body weight or shape is experienced, undue influence of body weight or shape on self-evaluation, or denial of seriousness of the current low body weight D. In post-menarcheal females, amenorrhoea (the absence of at least three consecutive menstrual cycles) Specify restricting type or binge-eating–purging type	For a definitive diagnosis the following are required: A. Body weight is maintained at least 15% below that expected (either lost or never achieved) or a Quetelet's body mass index of 17.5 or less (BMI = weight (kg)/ (height (m²)). Pre-pubertal patients may show failure to make the expected weight gain during the period of growth B. The weigh loss is self-induced by the avoidance of fattening foods, self-induced vomiting, self-induced purging, excessive exercise, use of appetite suppressants or diuretics C. There is a body image distortion in the form of a specific psychopathology whereby a dread of fatness persists as an intrusive, over-valued idea and the patient imposes a low weight threshold on him- or herself D. A widespread endocrine disorder involving the hypothalamic–pituitary– gonadal axis is manifest in women as amenorrhoea and in men as a loss of sexual interest and potency. There may also be elevated levels of growth hormone, raised cortisol levels, changes in the peripheral metabolism of the thyroid hormone and abnormalities of insulin secretion	1. Determined food avoidance 2. Weight loss or failure to gain weight during the period of pre-adolescent growth (10–14 years) in the absence of other physical or mental illness 3. Any two of the following: a. Pre-occupation with body weight b. Pre-occupation with energy intake c. Distorted body image d. Fear of fatness e. Self-induced vomiting f. Extensive exercising g. Purging or laxative abuse

Continued

Table 17.1 continued

DSM IV TR	ICD 10	Lask & Bryant-Waugh
	E. If the onset is pre-pubertal, the sequence of pubertal events is delayed or arrested (growth ceases; in girls breasts do not develop and there is a primary amenorrhoea; in boys the genitals remain juvenile). With recovery, puberty is often completed normally but the menarche is late	

Note: Adapted from DSM IV TR (APA, 2000a), ICD 10 (WHO, 1992, 1996), Lask and Bryant-Waugh (1993).

Table 17.2 Diagnostic criteria for bulimia nervosa

DSM IV TR	ICD 10
A. Recurrent episodes of binge eating. An episode of binge eating is characterized by both of the following: 1. Eating, in a discrete period of time (e.g. within a 2-hour period), an amount of food that is definitely larger than most people would eat during a similar period of time and under similar circumstances 2. A sense of lack of control over eating during the episode (e.g. a feeling that one cannot stop eating or control what or how much one is eating) B. Recurrent inappropriate compensatory behaviour in order to prevent weight gain, such as self-induced vomiting; misuse of laxatives; diuretics; enemas; or other medications; fasting or excessive exercise C. The binge eating and inappropriate compensatory behaviours both occur, on average, at least twice a week for 3 months D. Self-evaluation is unduly influenced by body shape and weight E. The disturbance does not occur exclusively during episodes of anorexia nervosa Specify purging or non-purging type	For a definitive diagnosis all of the following are required: A. There is a persistent pre-occupation with eating and an irresistible craving for food; the patient succumbs to episodes of over-eating in which large amounts of food are consumed in short periods of time B. The patient attempts to counteract the fattening effects of food by one or more of the following: self-induced vomiting; purgative abuse; alternating periods of starvation; use of drugs such as appetite suppressants, thyroid preparations or diuretics. When bulimia occurs in diabetic patients they may choose to neglect their insulin treatment C. The psychopathology consists of a morbid dread of fatness and the patient sets herself or himself a sharply defined weight threshold, well below the pre-morbid weight that constitutes the optimum or healthy weight in the opinion of the physician. There is often but not always a history of an earlier episode of anorexia nervosa, the interval between the two disorders ranging from a few months to several years. This earlier episode may have been fully expressed or may have assumed minor cryptic form with a moderate loss of weight and/or a transient phase of amenorrhoea

Note: Adapted from DSM IV TR (APA, 2000a) and ICD 10 (WHO, 1992, 1996).

less common than bulimia. The prevalence of anorexia nervosa among teenage girls is about 0.5%; the prevalence of bulimia nervosa is about 1%. The female:male ratio for anorexia and bulimia is about 9:1 in adolescents and 4:1 in pre-adolescents. The peak age of onset for anorexia and bulimia is during mid to late adolescence. Community studies show that, contrary to earlier data from clinical studies, there is not a significant relationship between eating disorders and social class. Since 1960 there has been an increase in the incidence of anorexia but not bulimia. While eating disorders may be more common in Western industrialized countries, there is growing evidence of eating disorders in non-Westernized cultures. In clinical rather than community populations, co-morbid mood disorders and obsessive-compulsive disorders are common in cases of anorexia, and for bulimia co-morbid drug abuse and borderline personality disorder are relatively common.

CLINICAL FEATURES

Clinical features of eating disorders are presented in Table 17.3 (Gowers & Bryant-Waugh, 2004; Lask & Bryant-Waugh, 2000; Steinhausen, 2002a; Wilson et al., 2003). With respect to perception, in most clinical cases of eating disorder there is a distortion of body image. The patient perceives the body – or parts of the body, such as the stomach, buttocks, thighs and so forth – to be larger than they are.

With respect to cognition, there is a pre-occupation with food. In cases where bingeing is occurring, there is a belief that the bingeing behaviour is out of control. There may also be conflict concerning dependence and maturity. On the one hand, there may be a wish to remain a dependent child and a fear of maturity and independence; on the other, there may be a wish to escape from parental control and the lack of autonomy and privacy that this entails. Low self-esteem, low self-efficacy and perfectionism are also common. Thus, many youngsters with eating disorders view themselves as worthless because they construe themselves as failing to meet high perfectionistic standards and, in addition, they believe themselves to be powerless to ever achieve these standards.

With respect to emotional status, there is an intense fear of fatness and in some instances a depressive mood. The fear of fatness in conjunction with the distorted perception of the body as larger than it actually is and perfectionistic strivings to achieve thinness may under-pin a sense of failure and associated depressive affect.

At a behavioural level, restrictive eating is typical of anorexia; a cycle of restrictive eating, bingeing and compensatory behaviours is typical of bulimia. These compensatory behaviours may include vomiting, using diuretics and laxatives or excessive exercising. Usually, particular classes of

Table 17.3 Clinical features of eating disorders in children and adolescents

Perception	• Distorted body image
Thought	• Pre-occupation with food • In bulimia a belief in lack of control over bingeing • Conflict about individuation • Perfectionism • Low self-esteem and low self-efficacy
Emotion	• Intense fear of becoming fat • Depressive affect
Behaviour	• In anorexia, restricted food intake • In bulimia, bingeing • In bulimia, vomiting, using laxatives and excessive exercise to prevent weight gain • In bulimia, self-harm or substance abuse
Interpersonal adjustment	• Poor school performance • Withdrawal from peer relationships • Deterioration in family relationships
Physical complications	• Endocrine disorder affecting the hypothalamic–pituitary–gonadal axis manifested by amenorrhoea • Starvation symptomatology such as reduced metabolic rate, bradycardia; hypotension; hypothermia; and anaemia • Lanugo hair on the back • Delayed gastric emptying • Electrolyte abnormalities • Renal dysfunction • Zinc deficiency • In bulimia, erosion of dental enamel due to vomiting and lesions on the back of the dominant hand due to use for initiating vomiting

situations that are interpreted as threatening or stressful lead to a negative mood state and it is these that precipitate a bout of bingeing. Such situations include interpersonal conflicts, isolation and small violations of a strict diet, such as eating a square of chocolate. While bingeing brings immediate relief, it also leads to physical discomfort and to guilt for not adhering to a strict diet. Purging relieves both guilt and physical discomfort but may also induce shame and fear of negative consequences of the binge–purge cycle. In addition to abnormal eating patterns, youngsters with eating disorders may display a variety of self-destructive behaviours, including self-injurious behaviour, suicide attempts and drug abuse. These self-destructive behaviours are often construed as self-punishments for not living up to perfectionistic standards or as attempts to escape from conflicts associated with self-worth and individuation.

With respect to interpersonal adjustment, poor school performance, withdrawal from peer relationships and deterioration in family relationships may all occur during the development of eating problems. Many youngsters who develop eating disorders are described by their parents as model children, like Mar in Box 17.1, prior to the onset of the eating problems. This good pre-morbid adjustment is often, although not always, in stark contrast to the family- and school-based relationship difficulties that arise once eating disorders become entrenched.

A wide variety of physical complications may also occur when children or adolescents develop eating disorders. These include an endocrine disorder affecting the hypothalamic–pituitary–gonadal axis and manifested by amenorrhoea or delayed onset of puberty; starvation symptomatology such as reduced metabolic rate, bradycardia, hypotension, hypothermia, and anaemia; lanugo hair on the back; delayed gastric emptying; electrolyte abnormalities; renal dysfunction and zinc deficiency. In bulimia, erosion of dental enamel may occur due to vomiting, and lesions on the back of the dominant hand may develop if the hand is used to initiate vomiting. With both anorexia and bulimia, a particularly serious concern is that the youngster may develop electrolyte abnormalities, which may lead to a fatal arrhythmia. With anorexia, there is a long-term concern that 20% of cases die.

AETIOLOGICAL THEORIES

Theoretical accounts of eating disorders focus on different aspects of aetiology. Genetic and neurotransmitter theories focus primarily on biological pre-disposing factors. Cultural and social pre-disposing factors are the central concern of sociocultural theories. Theories concerned with lifecycle transitions and stresses attempt to explain the way various precipitating factors lead to the onset of eating disorders within the context of certain pre-disposing factors. Psychoanalytic, cognitive-behavioural and family systems theories all focus largely on intrapsychic or interpersonal factors that maintain eating disorders, although all three classes of theory also address pre-disposing factors. Starvation theories are concerned primarily with the way in which the biological sequelae of self-starvation contribute to the maintenance of abnormal eating patterns. This section outlines some examples of each of these types of theory, along with a brief consideration of relevant evidence. A summary of the central features of each of these types of theory is presented in Table 17.4, along with the key implications of each for treatment.

Genetic theories

Genetic theories hold that a biological pre-disposition to eating disorders is genetically transmitted and that individuals with this pre-disposition, when exposed to certain environmental conditions, will develop an eating disorder.

Table 17.4 Theories of eating disorders

Theory	Theoretical principles	Principles of treatment
Genetic theories	Genetic factors under-pin a specific pre-disposition to anorexia nervosa and a general pre-disposition to bulimia which has links with substance abuse, obesity and affective disorders	Education about pre-disposition
Neurotransmitter theories	A dysregulation of neurotransmitters (especially serotonin) associated with mood and appetite under-pin eating disorders	Anti-depressant medication
Starvation theories	Anorexia and bulimia are partly maintained by neuroendocrine and gastric changes that result from starvation	Re-feeding, rehydration and management of medical complications
Sociocultural theories	Cultural norms that value slimness and promote dieting in societies where food is plentiful pre-dispose people to eating disorders	Education about sociocultural pressures
Lifecycle transition and stress theory	A build-up of stressful life events during individual or family lifecycle transitions precipitate anorexia and bulimia	Support individuals and families in management of stresses related to lifecycle transitions
Psychoanalytic theories	Children with eating disorders have difficulty learning how to interpret need-related internal physiological states and developing a coherent sense of self because their mothers adopt a parenting style in which parental needs for control and compliance take primacy over the child's needs for self-expression and autonomy. In adolescence the fear of fatness, obsession with food, and guilt for eating are part of an attempt to manage a central conflict related to the attainment of autonomy and a coherent sense of self	Psychodynamic psychotherapy that facilitates insight into the way early relationships affect current relationships with the therapist and significant others, with particular reference to autonomy and individuation issues
Cognitive-behavioural theories	Psychologically vulnerable youngsters with negative core beliefs and assumptions exposed to stressful events engage in dieting behaviour in response to critical comments from others	Contingency management so that weight gain is reinforced Cognitive therapy in which alternatives to cognitive distortions are learned Exposure and response prevention for bulimia

	Weight loss becomes positively reinforcing and the avoidance of fatness and criticism for being over-weight is negatively reinforcing	
	Negative automatic thoughts and cognitive distortions also maintain these destructive eating patterns	
	The impact of both the reinforcement contingencies and these cognitive factors on the youngster's eating behaviour becomes more pronounced when the eating disorder becomes entrenched and the physiological sequelae of starvation develop	
	With bulimia, extreme hunger resulting from dieting in conjunction with triggering events that elicit negative affect lead to bingeing. Binges are followed by distorted cognitions and related negative affect which in turn leads to purging. Purging initially is reinforcing since it brings relief. Later, guilt and fear about the effects of purging leads to increased dietary restraint until the cycle repeats	
Family theories	Where children have a biological vulnerability and dieting occurs, organizational features of the family may maintain eating disorders. These include enmeshment, rigidity, conflict avoidance, and triangulation. Family values such as an ethic of self-sacrifice, the rejection of personal leadership by the parents, blame-shifting and the use of unclear communication may also maintain eating disorders	Family therapy where parents take an active role in re-feeding the youngster and then develop boundaries and roles appropriate to the adolescent's stage of development. The family are helped to let the adolescent develop age-appropriate autonomy

Evidence from twin and family studies show unequivocally that genetic pre-disposing factors contribute moderately to the aetiology of eating disorders (Eley et al., 2002; Lask, 2000). There is some evidence that an appetite and satiety dysregulation renders children vulnerable to the development of eating disorders and that this vulnerability may be polygenetically determined (Stice, Agras & Hammer, 1999). Collier and Treasure (2004) propose that genetic factors contribute to temperamental dispositions that under-pin the development of personality traits associated with eating disorders. These may be conceptualized as falling along a continuum from restrictive-anorexia-like disorders to disinhibited-bulimia-like disorders. The pre-disposing personality traits of perfectionism, harm avoidance and depression may be the personality traits which place people at risk for developing both restrictive-anorexia-like and disinhibited-bulimia-like eating disorders. Compulsivity and inflexibility may be the personality traits that place people at specific risk for developing restrictive-anorexia-like disorders. Impulsivity and novelty seeking may be the personality traits that place people at specific risk for developing disinhibited-bulimia-like eating disorders. The assumption in this proposal is that the biological basis for each of these personality traits is polygenetically determined, and that through interaction with the environment the traits develop and pre-dispose the person to developing an eating disorder. Thus, central to this hypothesis is the assumption that environmental factors play a key role in the aetiology of eating disorders.

Neurotransmitter theories

Neurotransmitter theories propose that eating disorders arise from a dys-regulation of neurotransmitters, notably serotonin, in those centres of the brain that govern mood and appetite. It has been proposed that eating disorders are an expression of a mood disorder, which is often present in the family histories of people with eating disorders, along with other mood regulation difficulties such as substance abuse. This theory has led to controlled trials of anti-depressants for eating disorders, mainly conducted with young adults. These show that anti-depressants (both SSRIs and TCAs) lead to short-term improvements in bulimia but have no impact on anorexia nervosa (Wilson & Fairburn, 2002). Systematic reviews of child, adolescent and adult literature conclude that when CBT for bulimia nervosa is ineffective, anti-depressants may be considered as an adjunct (Gowers & Bryant-Waugh, 2004; Wilson & Fairburn, 2002).

Starvation theories

Starvation theories argue that eating disorders are maintained by biological and psychological changes that arise from the neuroendocrine abnormalities which accompany starvation. Evidence from studies of people with anorexia and bulimia, and participants in starvation laboratory experiments show that the neuroendocrine abnormalities and changes in gastric functioning that arise from experimentally induced starvation are similar to those observed in patients with eating disorders (Frichter & Pirke, 1995). The evidence also shows that more pronounced changes occur in anorexia than in bulimia. Most of the starvation-related neuroendocrine changes occur in the hypothalamic–pituitary–gonadal axis, which governs reproductive functioning, and in the hypothalamic–pituitary–adrenal axis and the hypothalamic–pituitary–thyroid axis, which governs mood, appetite, arousal and other vegetative functions. There is also evidence that starvation leads to delayed gastric emptying and that this reduces hunger perception. One implication of starvation theories is that a distinction should be made between re-feeding programmes, which initially aim to reverse the starvation process by helping youngsters regain weight to help them become accessible to psychological therapy, and later therapy that aims to help youngsters maintain normal body weight and eating patterns. This distinction is central to effective forms of family therapy for early-onset anorexia nervosa (Lock, LeGrange, Agras & Dare, 2001).

Sociocultural theories

Sociocultural theories highlight the role of broad cultural factors such as the idealization of female thinness specific to particular societies, notably those prevalent in Western industrialized nations, in pre-disposing individuals to developing eating disorders (Nasser & Katzman, 2003). Evidence to support the sociocultural position allows the following conclusions to be drawn (Szmukler & Patton, 1995): epidemiological studies consistently show that eating disorders are more prevalent in Western societies where food is plentiful; thinness is valued and dieting is promoted. Also, there has been a concurrent increase in the idealization of thinness and the promotion of dieting on the one hand and the prevalence of eating disorders on the other since 1960. This has been most pronounced in the case of bulimia. Furthermore, eating disorders are more prevalent among groups exposed to greater pressure to achieve the slim aesthetic ideal, such as dancers. Finally, the prevalence of eating disorders is higher in ethnic groups that move from a culture that does not idealize the thin female form to cultures that do engage in such idealization.

While these findings point to the importance of sociocultural factors in pre-disposing individuals to developing eating problems, not all dieters develop anorexia or bulimia. Precipitating factors such as stressful life events and the presence of other individual psychological or family factors probably contribute to the development of eating disorders.

Lifecycle transition and stress theories

These theories argue that a build-up of stresses at particular points in the lifecycle may precipitate the onset of an eating disorder or prevent the rapid resolution of a potential eating disorder, particularly in cases where biological and psychosocial pre-disposing factors are already present (e.g. Crisp, 1983;

Dare, 1985; Serpell & Troup, 2003). At an individual level, Crisp (1983) argues that when youngsters have particular difficulties dealing with the physical and emotional changes that coincide with the transition to adolescence, an eating disorder may occur since it allows youngsters to avoid the challenges posed by adolescence. At a family level, Dare (1985) argues that the co-occurrence of a number of critical transitional stresses, such as an older sibling leaving home, the youngster with anorexia entering puberty or loss of a grandparent, may place excessive demands on family members to develop new roles, routines and support systems. The development of an eating disorder provides families with a period of respite, where routines, roles and supports appropriate to a previous stage of the family lifecycle may continue to be used so that families may maintain the status quo rather than negotiating changes appropriate to the next stage of the family lifecycle. Serpell and Troup (2003) propose that four background pre-disposing factors render people vulnerable to developing eating disorders: (1) childhood helplessness; (2) childhood adversity; (3) low self-esteem; and (4) rigid perfectionism. In response to sociocultural pressures for thinness, these four factors give rise to four intermediate pre-disposing factors: (1) dietary restraint; (2) low shape- and weight-based self-esteem; (3) disgust of food and food-related body stimuli; and (4) bodily shame. When stressful life events that involve managing complex interpersonal situations and relationships arise in people who have these vulnerability factors, an eating disorder may occur.

Empirical research confirms that the peak age of onset for anorexia and bulimia is in mid-adolescence, and a build-up of stressful life events often precipitates the onset of anorexia and bulimia. Typically, this is more common among youngsters with a number of vulnerability factors, as suggested by lifecycle transition and stress theories (Gowers & Bryant-Waugh, 2004; Serpell & Troup, 2003; Steinhausen, 2002a).

Psychoanalytic theories

Hilda Bruch (1973) argued that the psychodynamics which under-pin anorexia arise from early childhood experiences. According to Bruch, the mothers of anorexic girls adopt a parenting style in which parental needs for control and compliance take primacy over the child's needs for self-expression and autonomy. The child has difficulty learning how to interpret need-related internal physiological states and in developing a coherent sense of self separate from caregivers. In adolescence, the fear of fatness, obsession with food, and guilt for eating are part of an attempt to manage a central conflict related to the attainment of autonomy and a coherent sense of self. The youngster experiences a fear of separation from parents and a fear of being overly controlled by the parents; a fear of maturation, sexuality, intimacy and independence; and a fear of having little control over the self or body size (as a symbol of self). This conflict about autonomy is characterized by negative self-evaluative beliefs (low self-esteem) coupled with perfectionistic strivings to improve the self. There is ample evidence for distorted body image, maturity fears, perfectionistic strivings, low self-esteem and low self-efficacy among teenagers with eating disorders (Lask & Bryant-Waugh, 2000). Evidence pointing to the centrality of a dysfunctional parent–child relationship is lacking. However, early stressful life events, such as loss of a parent through bereavement, or child sexual abuse, are more common among children and teenagers with eating disorders, particularly bulimia (Eisler, 1995).

Psychoanalytic theories offer a way for making sense of the phenomenology of eating disorders (Dare & Crowther, 1995a,b). In a series of controlled trials of psychodynamic psychotherapy with young adults, the Maudsley group, working within the context of Malan's (1995) psychodynamic therapy model, has found that a unique psychodynamic focal hypothesis may be formed for each patient and that Bruch's (1973) themes typically characterize these focal hypotheses.

Psychoanalytic psychotherapy, as practised by the Maudsley group, aims to help the patient gain insight into the way in which the psychodynamics of past relationships with parents under-pin the transference–countertransference patient–therapist relationship and the relationships that the patient has with other significant people in her life. In addition, the therapist facilitates the patient's search for less destructive ways to assert autonomy from the parents and develop a strong sense of personal identity. This type of therapy is effective with older adolescents and adults with anorexia but not children (Szmukler & Dare, 1991).

Cognitive-behavioural theories

Stewart's (2005) CBT model of child and adolescent eating disorders represents a synthesis of models from the adult literature (Wilson & Fairburn, 2002) and important concepts from developmental psychology (Lask & Bryant-Waugh, 2000). The model assumes that youngsters are rendered vulnerable to eating disorders by pre-disposing individual and environmental factors. Individual factors include low self-esteem, perfectionism and past obesity. Environmental factors include physical and sexual abuse; neglect; parental under-involvment or over-protection; parental criticism and high expectations; parental conflict; a family history of depression, substance abuse or eating disorders; and societal and family pressures to be thin. These pre-disposing factors contribute to the development of negative beliefs such as 'I am worthless', 'I am unlovable' or 'I am unattractive'. These core beliefs lead to the development of assumptions such as 'I must be thin to be attractive, successful or happy', 'I must do everything perfectly for people to love me' or 'I must punish myself to be good'. Although these beliefs and assumptions develop during childhood, they do not have a significant effect on the youngster's life until they are activated by a series of critical stressful demands associated with the transition to adolescence and other life stresses.

Demands associated with adolescence include adjusting to the biological changes associated with puberty, developing independence, coping with the increased complexity of peer-group and romantic relationships, managing the challenges of school and work pressures and developing an identity. Additional demands that occur within the context of these normative pressures which trigger negative beliefs and assumptions include negative comments about weight and shape, exposure to peer rejection, academic failure, family conflict and abuse. Once core beliefs and assumptions have been activated, in specific types of day-to-day situation, they give rise to negative automatic thoughts conducive to dieting. For example, when dressing or looking in the mirror, the youngster may think 'I'm too heavy, too fat and too ugly'; or when hungry or eating the youngster may think 'I'm not in control'.

Negative automatic thoughts typically involve cognitive distortions. The following examples of cognitive distortions are typical of youngsters with eating problems:

- *All or nothing thinking*: thinking in extreme categorical terms, for example 'If I'm not in complete control, then I have no control whatsoever'.
- *Selective abstraction*: selectively focusing on a small aspect of a situation and drawing conclusions from this, for example 'I will only be good if I am thin and nothing else matters'.
- *Over-generalization*: generalizing from one instance to all possible instances, for example 'I ate too much last night, so I will always eat too much'.
- *Magnification*: exaggerating the significance of an event, for example 'I gained a pound, so I know that I will never be able to wear a mini-skirt again'.
- *Personalization*: attributing negative feeling of others to the self, for example 'If people see me, I will ruin their day because I'm fat'.
- *Emotional reasoning*: taking feelings as facts, for example 'I feel fat so I am fat'.

Cognitively distorted negative automatic thoughts lead to the development of an entrenched behavioural pattern of dietary restraint.

Once negative automatic thoughts about shape, weight and the need for control, and the related behaviour pattern of dietary restriction have become a routine part of a youngster's life, they come to be maintained by emotional factors, behavioural factors, family factors, social factors, avoidance, the starvation state, and binge eating and purging. The emotional factors that maintain restricted eating include the associated sense of mastery and control for eating little, the sense of being special for becoming thin, the associated increase in self-esteem for achieving perfectionistic weight and shape goals, and the alleviation of low mood and high anxiety that such increases in self-esteem may bring. Behavioural factors such as weighing and checking the size of body parts increases the salience of perceived deficits in body weight and shape, which in turn increases motivation for restrained eating. Family factors that maintain restricted eating include family approval and attention for weight loss, the sense of having control within the family that dietary restriction brings and the continued dependence on the family that comes with excessive weight loss, which may be particularly reinforcing for youngsters who fear independence. Peer approval for weight loss is a social factor that maintains dietary restriction. By providing a predictable and regimented lifestyle, dietary restriction allows youngsters to avoid anxiety about the complexity and uncertainty of normal adolescent life. The starvation state may maintain restricted eating patterns because it entails a loss of appetite, lack of energy, constricted lifestyle and cognitive rigidity, all of which make changing restrictive eating patterns difficult. In youngsters with bulimia, the binge–purge cycle may be self-maintaining. Bingeing may offer short-term relief from negative affect associated with specific situations, but later it induces guilt and negative self-evaluation, which in turn may be alleviated by purging. Hunger arising from dietary restriction in conjunction with triggering events that elicit depression, anger or anxiety give way to bingeing. Binges are followed by distorted cognitions about the significance of the bingeing and the negative implications of bingeing both for body shape and self-evaluative beliefs. These cognitions and related negative affect in turn lead to purging, laxative use, diuretic use or excessive exercise. Purging initially is reinforcing since it brings relief. However, later guilt and fear about the long-term physical and psychological consequences occurs. This is followed by increased dietary restraint until the cycle repeats (Wilson & Pike, 2001).

For older adolescents and young adults with bulimia, cognitive-behavioural therapy is the treatment of choice (Wilson & Fairburn, 2002). This therapy helps patients to map out the binge–purge cycle, to monitor eating patterns and related cognitions and contingencies and use cognitive and behavioural strategies to disrupt the cycle and manage relapses. These include avoiding trigger situations or habituating to them through exposure and response prevention routines similar to those used for obsessive-compulsive disorder. A second set of strategies involves using cognitive therapy to help patients interpret potential trigger situations in ways that do not lead to negative affect and bingeing. A third strategy involves helping patients avoid persisting with bingeing once it starts by coaching them in countering self-deprecatory cognitions and related negative mood states that occur one bingeing starts.

Family theories

Family systems theories of anorexia point to a number of organizational features that may be pre-disposing or maintaining factors for eating disorders. For example, Minuchin et al. (1978) characterized the families of teenagers with anorexia as enmeshed and rigid with a strongly over-protective attitude towards the child. He also argued that there was a lack of conflict resolution and an involvement of children in parental conflicts. Selvini Palazzoli (1988) pin-pointed the following features as typical of the anorexic family: an ethic of self-sacrifice, the rejection of personal leadership by the parents, blame-shifting since everything is done for the good of others, unclear communication and secret alliances between parents and the child, which go hand-in-hand with covert marital dissatisfaction. Weber and Stierlin (1981) suggest that a process occurs where individuation in adolescence is complicated by the child's fantasy that the parents will have nothing left in common when the child matures and gains autonomy. The youngster copes by playing the role of a model child but eventually the parents become interested in another child or pursuit. The child retaliates by doggedly pursuing autonomy through self-starvation, which achieves the twin gains of providing a type of pseudo-autonomy centring on control of the shape of the body and eliciting parental attention which has been lost.

Available empirical evidence clearly shows that there is not a single dysfunctional family constellation (a psychosomatic family) that causes anorexia and bulimia (Eisler, LeGrange & Aisen, 2003; Lock et al., 2001). Rather, various different patterns of family organization can be associated with eating disorders. For example, using cluster analysis Vandereycken, Kog & Vanderlinden (1989) found that a range of family types could be identified with differing levels of enmeshment, rigidity and conflict-avoidance. Families of youngsters with anorexia tend to be more controlled and organized, while families of bulimic adolescents tend to be more chaotic, conflicted and critical (Steiger, Leung & Houle, 1992). These patterns of organization probably reflect families' attempts to cope with eating disorders (Eisler et al., 2003; Nielsen & Bará-Carril, 2003). Unfortunately, it is quite likely that, in many instances, these patterns of family organization inadvertently maintain the dysfunctional eating habits. The various patterns of family organization that have been found in studies of youngsters with eating disorders probably reflect extreme forms of relational styles that preceded the onset of eating disorders. Families that value closeness may find that the experience of coping with a chronic eating disorder is an isolating process, and this may lead them to strive for greater closeness. Families in which predictable routines are valued may become extremely rigid in response to a youngster's self-starvation. Consistent with these hypotheses is the finding that members of families with an anorexic child in a questionnaire study that examined the difference between the actual and desired family structure, described themselves as isolated and constrained by overly rigid expectations within their families (Eisler, 1995). That families which deal with conflict by occasional conflict avoidance may cope with eating disorders by showing extreme conflict avoidance is supported by the results of expressed emotions studies. These consistently show that families with eating disorders are characterized by very low levels of expressed emotion, including both criticism and emotional over-involvement, compared with families containing teenagers or adults with other psychological problems such as schizophrenia (Eisler, 1995). Furthermore, the families of youngsters with eating disorders that show the highest levels of criticism, tend to contain youngsters with more chronic eating disorders and are more likely to drop out of treatment.

Controlled treatment outcome studies of family therapy for anorexia nervosa show that one to six years following treatment, 60–90% are fully recovered and at present it is the treatment of choice for young adolescents with anorexia (Eisler et al., 2003; Mitchell & Carr, 2000). With older adolescents and young adults with anorexia and bulimia there is some evidence that individual therapy may be more effective than family therapy. In the Maudsley group's evidence-based family therapy for adolescent eating disorders, treatment progresses from re-feeding the patient, to negotiating a new pattern of family relationships, and finally to addressing adolescent individuation issues and therapy termination (Lock et al., 2001).

ASSESSMENT

Assessment in cases of anorexia nervosa should include a full physical examination and appropriate medical investigations. Where any of the following features are present, inpatient treatment is indicated (APA, 2000b; Lask & Bryant-Waugh, 2000; NICE, 2004; Royal College of Psychiatrists, 2002):

- weight is less than 70% of that expected
- marked dehydration
- electrolyte imbalance
- circulatory failure
- uncontrolled vomiting
- gastrointestinal bleeding
- self-injurious behaviour
- severe depression
- lack of response to outpatient treatment
- intolerable family situation.

Details of a weight restoration programme for use with hospitalized anorectic youngsters are described below. Height and weight measurements may be used to chart changes in children's body mass index (Cole, Freeman

& Preece, 1995). Precautions must be taken to ensure that adolescents do not increase their weight artificially by putting weights in their pockets or drinking excess fluid prior to weighing. Some psychometric instruments that may be useful in the assessment of youngsters with eating disorder are listed in Table 17.5. Assessment should include family and individual interviews addressing all areas routinely covered in a thorough intake interview as set out in Chapter 4. Particular attention should be paid to those factors outlined in Figure 17.1.

Table 17.5 Psychometric instruments that may be used as an adjunct to clinical interviews in the assessment of eating disorders

Construct	Instrument	Publication	Comments
Body weight	Body mass index (BMI) tables	Cole, T., Freeman, J., & Preece, M. (1995). Body mass index reference curves for the UK, 1990. *Archives of Disease in Childhood*, 73, 25–29. Charts are available from Harlow Printing http://www.harlowprinting.co.uk/	Gives BMI centiles for children and centile rankings
Screening instruments for eating disorders	Setting Conditions for Anorexia Nervosa Scale (SCANS)	Slade, P. & Dewey, M. (1986). Development and preliminary validation of SCANS: A screening instrument for identifying individuals at risk of developing anorexia and bulimia nervosa. *International Journal of Eating Disorders*, 5, 517–538 Slade, P., Dewey, M., Kiemle, G. & Newton, T. (1990). Update on SCANS: A screening instrument for identifying individuals at risk of developing an eating disorder. *International Journal of Eating Disorders*, 9, 583–584	This 40-item instrument may be used to screen children and adolescents at risk for eating disorders. It assesses dissatisfaction and loss of control, social and personal anxiety, perfectionism, adolescent problems, and need for weight control. It was standardized in the UK on large samples of children and adolescents
	Kids Eating Disorder Survey (KEDS)	Childress, A., Brewerton, T., Hodges, E. & Jarrell, M. (1993). Kids Eating Disorder Survey (KEDS). A study of middle school children. *Journal of the American Academy of Child and Adolescent Psychiatry*, 32, 843–850	With this 14-item scale children rate drawings of male and female bodies ranging from underweight to over-weight and indicate their satisfaction with their perceived body size

Children's Version of the Eating Attitudes Test (ChEAT)	Maloney, M., McGuire, J. & Daniels, S. (1988). Reliability testing of the Children's Version of the Eating Attitudes Test. *Journal of the American Academy of Child and Adolescent Psychiatry*, 27, 541–543	Scores above 20 on this 26-item screening self-report instrument suggest that a child between 8 and 13 may have anorexia or bulimia
Eating Attitudes Test (EAT)	Garner, D., Olmsted, M., Bohr, Y. & Garfinkle, P. (1982). The Eating Attitudes Test, psychometric features and clinical correlates. *Psychological Medicine*, 12, 871–878	Scores above 40 on this 26-item screening self-report instrument suggest that a teenager over 13 may have anorexia or bulimia
Questionnaire for Eating Disorder Diagnoses (Q-EDD)	Mintz, L., O'Halloran, M., Mulholland, A. & Schneider, P. (1997). Questionnaire for eating disorder diagnoses. Reliability and validity of operationalizing DSM-IV criteria into a self-report format. *Journal of Counselling Psychology*, 44, 63–71	This 50-item self-report inventory yields DSM IV eating disorder diagnoses in adolescents and adults
Body Shape Question-naire (BSQ)	Cooper, P., Taylor, M., Cooper, Z., & Fairburn, C. (1987). The development and validation of the Body Shape Questionnaire. *International Journal of Eating Disorders*, 6, 485–494	This 34-item self-report inventory assesses body weight and shape dissatisfaction
Body Satisfaction Scale (BSS)	Slade, P., Dewey, M., Newton, T., Brodie, D., Kiemle, G. (1990). Development and preliminary validation of the body satisfaction scale (BSS). *Psychology and Health*, 4, 213–220	On this 16-item scale, respondents rate satisfaction with 16 body parts and the scale yields an overall body satisfaction score
Revised Bulimia Test (BULIT-R)	Thelen, M., Farmer, J., Wonderlich, S. & Smith, M. (1991). A revision of the bulimia test: The BULIT-R. *Psychological Assessment*, 3, 119–124	A self-report inventory based on DSM II R criteria for bulimia
Bulimia Investigatory Test Edinburgh (BITE)	Henderson, M. & Freeman, C. (1987). A self-rating scale for bulimia: the 'BITE'. *British Journal of Psychiatry*, 150, 18–24	A self-report scale for screening for bulimia

Continued

Table 17.5 continued

Construct	Instrument	Publication	Comments
Eating attitudes, behaviour and related personality and family dimensions	Third Edition of the Eating Disorder Inventory (EDI-3)	Garner, D. (2005). *Eating Disorder Inventory-2 (EDI-3)*. Psychological Assessment Resources, PO Box 998, Odessa: FL 33556	This 91-item inventory yields scores on 12 primary scales, consisting of 3 eating-disorder-specific scales and 9 general psychological. It also yields six composites: Eating Disorder Risk, Ineffectiveness, Interpersonal Problems, Affective Problems, Over-control, General Psychological Maladjustment. Norms for groups of US high-school and college students and anorexia and bulimia patients are available. Computer administration and scoring are available
	Stirling Eating Disorder Scales (SEDS)	Williams, G., Power, K., Miller, H., Freeman, C., Yellowlees, A., Dowds, T., Walker, M. & Parry-Jones, W. (1994). Development and validation of the Stirling Eating Disorder Scales. *International Journal of Eating Disorders*, 16, 35–43	This 80-item inventory yields scores on 8 scales: anorexic dietary behaviour, anorexic dietary cognitions, bulimic dietary behaviour, bulimic dietary cognitions, external locus of control, low assertiveness, low self-esteem, and self-directed hostility
	Parent–Adolescent Relationship Questionnaire (PARQ)	Robin, A., Koepke, T. & Moye, A. (1990). Multidimensional assessment of parent adolescent relations: Psychological assessment. *Journal of Consulting and Clinical Psychology*, 2, 451–459	Versions of the PARQ are completed by adolescents and parents. They yield (among other indices), a score for parent–adolescent conflict over eating and a general parent–adolescent conflict score; these are particularly relevant to the assessment of families containing teenagers with eating disorders

Clinical interviews for diagnosing eating disorders	Eating Disorder Examination (EDE)	Cooper, Z. & Fairburn, C. (1987). The Eating Disorder Examination. A semistructured interview for the assessment of the specific psychopathology of eating disorders. *International Journal of Eating Disorders*, 6, 1–8 Bryant-Waugh, R., Cooper, P., Taylor, C. & Lask, B. (1996). The use of the Eating Disorder Examination with Children. A Pilot Study. *International Journal of Eating Disorders*, 19, 391–398	An interview schedule for use with adolescents and adults developed in the UK and widely considered to be the gold standard in the area. It has been adapted for use with children by Rachel Bryant-Waugh
	Clinical Eating Disorder Rating Instrument (CEDRI)	Palmer, R., Christie, M., Cordle, C., & Kendrick, J. (1987). The clinical eating disorder rating instrument (CEDRI): A preliminary description. *International Journal of Eating Disorders*, 6, 9–16	An interview schedule for use with adolescents and adults
	Structured Interview for Anorexia and Bulimia Nervosa (SIAB)	Fichter, M., Elton, M., Engel, K., et al. (1990). The structured interview for anorexia and bulimia nervosa (SIAB): development and characteristics of a (semi-) standardized instrument. In M. Fichter (ed.), *Bulimia nervosa: Basic Research Diagnosis and Therapy* (pp. 57–70). Chichester: Wiley	An interview schedule for use with adolescents and adults
	Interview for the Diagnosis of Eating Disorders (IDED)	Williamson, D. (1990). *Assessment of Eating Disorders. Obesity, Anorexia and Bulimia Nervosa*. Elmsforth, NY: Pergamon	An interview schedule for use with adolescents and adults
Outcome of eating disorders	Morgan–Russell Outcome Assessment Schedule	Morgan, A. & Hayward, A. (1988). Clinical assessment of anorexia nervosa: the Morgan–Russell outcome assessment schedule. *British Journal of Psychiatry*, 152, 367–371	A schedule for assessing outcome as good, intermediate or poor depending upon their status on five scales; nutritional status; menstrual function; mental state; psychosexual; and socioeconomic adjustment

PRE-DISPOSING FACTORS

PERSONAL PRE-DISPOSING FACTORS

Biological factors
- Genetic vulnerability

Psychological factors
- Conflict about autonomy and dependence
- External locus of control and helplessness
- Perfectionism
- Low shape and weight-based self-esteem
- Bodily shame
- Disgust about food-related bodily stimuli
- History of obesity
- History of dietary restraint

CONTEXTUAL PRE-DISPOSING FACTORS

Cultural factors
- Wide availability of food in a culture that values thinness and promotes dieting

Stresses in early life
- Parental eating disorders, substance abuse or depression
- High parental expectations and criticism
- Marital discord
- Bereavements
- Child abuse or neglect

PERSONAL PROTECTIVE FACTORS

Eating problems
- Recent onset and short duration

Biological factors
- Good physical health

Psychological factors
- High IQ
- Easy temperament
- High self-esteem
- Internal locus of control
- High self-efficacy
- Optimistic attributional style
- Mature defence mechanisms
- Functional coping strategies

PERSONAL MAINTAINING FACTORS

Biological factors
- Dysregulation of neuroendocrine system due to starvation leading to low appetite and cognitive rigidity
- Delayed gastric emptying

Psychological factors
- Severe body image distortion
- Negative food-related cognitive distortions
- In anorexia, sense of mastery, esteem, and 'being special' arising from extreme dietary restraint
- In anorexia, reinforcement of dietary restraint arising from frequent weighing and checking body shape
- In bulimia, negative mood regulation by bingeing and guilt alleviation by purging

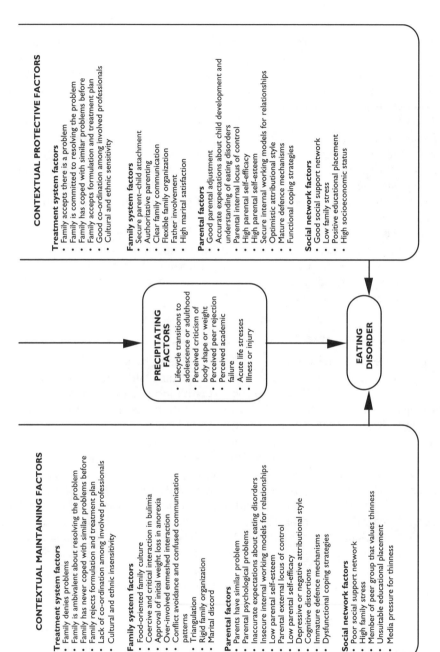

CONTEXTUAL MAINTAINING FACTORS

Treatment system factors
- Family denies problems
- Family is ambivalent about resolving the problem
- Family has never coped with similar problems before
- Family rejects formulation and treatment plan
- Lack of co-ordination among involved professionals
- Cultural and ethnic insensitivity

Family system factors
- Food-oriented family culture
- Coercive and critical interaction in bulimia
- Approval of initial weight loss in anorexia
- Over-involved enmeshed interaction
- Conflict avoidance and confused communication patterns
- Triangulation
- Rigid family organization
- Marital discord

Parental factors
- Parents have similar problem
- Parental psychological problems
- Inaccurate expectations about eating disorders
- Insecure internal working models for relationships
- Low parental self-esteem
- Parental external locus of control
- Low parental self-efficacy
- Depressive or negative attributional style
- Cognitive distortions
- Immature defence mechanisms
- Dysfunctional coping strategies

Social network factors
- Poor social support network
- High family stress
- Member of peer group that values thinness
- Unsuitable educational placement
- Media pressure for thinness

PRECIPITATING FACTORS
- Lifecycle transitions to adolescence or adulthood
- Perceived criticism of body shape or weight
- Perceived peer rejection
- Perceived academic failure
- Acute life stresses
- Illness or injury

EATING DISORDER

CONTEXTUAL PROTECTIVE FACTORS

Treatment system factors
- Family accepts there is a problem
- Family is committed to resolving the problem
- Family has coped with similar problems before
- Family accepts formulation and treatment plan
- Good co-ordination among involved professionals
- Cultural and ethnic sensitivity

Family system factors
- Secure parent–child attachment
- Authoritative parenting
- Clear family communication
- Flexible family organization
- Father involvement
- High marital satisfaction

Parental factors
- Good parental adjustment
- Accurate expectations about child development and understanding of eating disorders
- Parental internal locus of control
- High parental self-efficacy
- High parental self-esteem
- Secure internal working models for relationships
- Optimistic attributional style
- Mature defence mechanisms
- Functional coping strategies

Social network factors
- Good social support network
- Low family stress
- Positive educational placement
- High socioeconomic status

Figure 17.1 Aetiological and protective factors to consider in the assessment of eating disorders

Pre-disposing factors

The principal biological pre-disposing factor to consider is a genetic pre-disposition to eating disorders. A family history of anorexia may suggest that such a pre-disposition is present for restrictive eating; a family history of bulimia, obesity or mood disorders, drug abuse or alcohol problems may suggest that a broader genetic pre-disposition to bulimia and these related disorders is present. Relatively enduring broad personal psychological characteristics that may pre-dispose a youngster to developing an eating disorder include a conflict about individuation, external locus of control and helplessness, and perfectionistic strivings. Relatively personal food-related psychological characteristics that may pre-dispose a youngster to developing an eating disorder include low shape- and weight-related self-esteem, bodily shame, disgust about food-related bodily stimuli, and a personal history of obesity or dietary restraint. Cultural pressures for thinness and dieting along with the easy access to food are important pre-disposing psychosocial factors for eating disorders. Other historical psychosocial pre-disposing factors include high parental expectations and criticism, parental marital discord and a history of early trauma or stressful life events, but particularly bereavement or sexual abuse.

Precipitating factors

An episode of eating disorder can be precipitated by a build-up of stress. Typically, such stresses occur at the transition from childhood to adolescence or at the transition from adolescence to adulthood at the stage where the youngster is about to leave home. These stresses may include pressures that impinge directly on the youngster such as academic challenges or exam failure; difficulties with peers, such as teasing, bullying or rejection; perceived criticism of body shape or weight by peers; and personal illness, injury or bereavement. Stresses which affect the youngster indirectly by impinging of parents and siblings may precipitate eating disorders if they are construed by youngsters to place stressful demands on them. These stresses include family bereavements that are deeply felt by the parents or siblings, parental illness or injury, and changes in the household composition that are experienced as particularly demanding by parents or siblings, such as the transition of younger siblings from being at home to being in school or the transition of older siblings from living at home to living away from home.

Maintaining factors

Once an episode of anorexia has begun it may be maintained by both personal and contextual factors. At a biological level, delayed gastric emptying and starvation-related neuroendocrine changes may maintain abnormal eating problems by compromising the youngster's ability to accurately perceive hunger and satiety signals, by exacerbating the youngster's preoccupation with food and by exacerbating the youngster's cognitive distortions about food-related issues, or indeed any significant personal issues. At a psychological level, a distorted body image may also maintain abnormal patterns of eating, since the youngster will strive to reduce perceived body size rather than actual body size. In anorexia, the sense of mastery and 'feeling special' that arises from extreme dietary restraint may maintain restrictive eating. Restrained eating may be reinforced in anorexia by feedback which occurs during frequent weighing and checking body parts. In bulimia, bingeing may be reinforced by the way it alleviates negative mood states, and vomiting may be reinforced by inaccurate beliefs that it prevents weight gain and by the way it may alleviates guilt for bingeing.

Parents and children become involved in a range of interaction patterns centring on food preparation and eating that maintain abnormal eating habits. Often, these patterns reflect an accentuation of the family's normal style of interaction. Families that value closeness may find that the experience of coping with a chronic eating disorder leads to entrenched enmeshment, which may lead the youngster to attempt to define his or her autonomy and separateness through controlling food intake. Families in which routines are valued may become extremely rigid, so that parents have difficulty breaking out of repetitive patterns, such as ineffective gentle cajoling at mealtimes, that maintain eating problems. Families that tend to ignore conflict about minor issues may deal with eating disorders by engaging in extreme conflict avoidance through denial of the existence or severity of the problem. Periodically, this process of denial may give way to bouts of extreme criticism, especially in cases of bulimia, which undermine the child's self esteem and self-efficacy. Families in which generational boundaries are not clearly drawn may triangulate youngsters with eating disorders into parental conflicts which are overtly denied. So youngsters may find that their abnormal eating pattern is opposed by one parent and supported by the other parent, and this conflict about child management may be part of a wider pattern of interparental disagreement or marital discord. However, the entire process of triangulation is not openly acknowledged and discussed, so parents are unable to jointly develop a plan for helping children to develop normal eating patterns. Families where communication is commonly a little unclear may develop extremely confused communication patterns when an adolescent develops an eating disorder. All of these interactional patterns are more likely to maintain abnormal eating habits in food-oriented family cultures, where food preparation and eating meals are used to symbolize affection or power. In such family cultures, preparing a meal may symbolically mean 'I care about you and/or control you' and refusing to eat may symbolize a rejection of parental affection or control.

Such patterns of parenting and family organization may be partially maintained by parents' personal experience of similar eating disorders or psychological difficulties. Where parents have insecure internal working models for relationships, low self-esteem, low self-efficacy, an external locus of control, immature defences and poor coping strategies, their resourcefulness in managing their children's difficulties may be compromised. Parents may also become involved in problem-maintaining interactions with their children if they have inaccurate knowledge about the role of psychological factors in the genesis and maintenance of eating disorders.

Eating disorders may also be maintained by high levels of stress, limited support and social disadvantage within the family's wider social system, since these features may deplete parents' and children's personal resources for dealing constructively with eating problems. Within the adolescent's ecological context both peer-group pressure and media pressure for thinness may maintain abnormal patterns of eating. Educational placements which are poorly resourced and where teaching staff have little time to devote to home–school liaison meetings may also maintain eating problems.

Within the treatment team and multi-agency system, a lack of co-ordination and clear communication among involved professionals, particularly family physicians, paediatricians, nurses, psychologists and other staff, may maintain adolescents' eating problems. It is not unusual for various members of the professional network to offer conflicting opinions and advice on the nature and management of eating disorders to adolescents and their families. These may range from viewing the child as physically ill and deserving routine nursing for the treatment of starvation to seeing the child as healthy but disobedient and deserving punitive management. Where co-operation problems between families and treatment teams develop, and families deny the existence of the problems, the validity of the diagnosis and formulation, or the appropriateness of the treatment programme, then the child's difficulties may persist. Treatment systems that are not sensitive to the cultural and ethnic beliefs and values of the youngster's family system may maintain eating disorders by inhibiting engagement or promoting drop-out from treatment and preventing the development of a good working alliance between the treatment team, the youngster and his or her family. Parents' lack of experience in dealing with similar problems in the past is a further factor that may compromise their capacity to work co-operatively with the treatment team and so may contribute to the maintenance of the child's difficulties.

Protective factors

The probability that a treatment programme will be effective is influenced by a variety of personal and contextual protective factors. It is important that these be assessed and included in the later formulation, since it is protective factors that usually serve as the foundation for therapeutic change. Youngsters with an eating disorder of recent onset and short duration have a better prognosis than those with more entrenched abnormal eating patterns. A high

IQ, an easy temperament, high self-esteem, an internal locus of control, high self-efficacy and an optimistic attributional style are all important personal protective factors. Other important personal protective factors include mature defence mechanisms and functional coping strategies, particularly good problem-solving skills and a capacity to make and maintain friendships.

Within the family, secure parent–child attachment and authoritative parenting are central protective factors, particularly if they occur within the context of a flexible family structure in which there is clear communication, high marital satisfaction and both parents share the day-to-day tasks of child care.

Good parental adjustment is also a protective factor. Where parents have an internal locus of control, high self-efficacy, high self-esteem, internal working models for secure attachments, an optimistic attributional style, mature defences and functional coping strategies, then they are better resourced to manage their children's difficulties constructively. Accurate knowledge about eating disorders is also a protective factor.

Within the broader social network, high levels of support, low levels of stress and membership of a high socioeconomic group are all protective factors for children with eating disorders. Where families are embedded in social networks that provide a high level of support and place few stressful demands on family members, then it is less likely that parents' and children's resources for dealing with eating problems will become depleted. A well-resourced educational placement may also be viewed as a protective factor. Educational placements where teachers have sufficient time and flexibility to attend home–school liaison meetings if invited to do so contribute to positive outcomes for children with eating disorders.

Within the treatment system, co-operative working relationships between the treatment team and the family and good co-ordination of multi-professional input are protective factors. Treatment systems that are sensitive to the cultural and ethnic beliefs and values of the youngster's family are more likely help families engage with, and remain in, treatment, and foster the development of a good working alliance. Families that are more likely to benefit from treatment are those that accept the formulation of the problem given by the treatment team and are committed to working with the team to resolve it. Where families have successfully faced similar problems before, then they are more likely to benefit from treatment and, in this sense, previous experience with similar problems is a protective factor.

FORMULATION

On the basis of the assessment, a preliminary formulation may be drawn up. This should link pre-disposing, precipitating and maintaining factors to the abnormal eating pattern and specify protective factors that may be drawn on during treatment.

TREATMENT

Currently, the treatment of choice for anorexia in young adolescents is family therapy (Lock et al., 2001); for bulimia in older adolescents it is cognitive-behaviour therapy (CBT; Fairburn, 1997; Fairburn, Marcus & Wilson, 1993; Stewart, 2005). A description of each will be given below, following procedures outlined in relevant treatment manuals. Two main modifications to the manualized procedures have been made. First, ways in which family therapy for anorexia may be adapted to address bulimic symptoms have been included. Second, guidelines on how to include parents in CBT for bulimia are given.

Family therapy for anorexia

The treatment of young adolescents with anorexia should begin with inpatient care to address physical complications of starvation in severe cases with high medical risk. This should be followed-up with outpatient family therapy. In lower risk cases, treatment may begin with outpatient family therapy.

Inpatient management of anorexia

Most children and teenagers can be treated effectively in outpatient family-based treatment. Where an adolescent's medical condition is dangerous enough to warrant inpatient treatment, this should be offered in conjunction with family-based treatment, which is described in some detail below. The goals of inpatient treatment are managing the immediate threat to the child's physical or mental health, weight restoration and providing a context for the first stage of family-based treatment.

Once the paediatric medical team is satisfied that threats to the adolescent's physical health have been managed, inpatient weight restoration may begin. The psychologist should work closely with the paediatric nursing staff and arrange a behavioural weight-gain programme (Carr, 1997). The details of the patient's diet may be agreed in conjunction with the nursing staff and the dietician. The patient is confined to bed with no privileges except for a brief visit from the parents each day. An overall target weight is set at about the 40th percentile for the adolescent's height and age or a body mass index of about 20–22 kg/m^2. In addition, intermediate weekly weight gain targets of about 1–1.5 kg are set. As these intermediate targets are met, the adolescent may select privileges and freedoms from a list agreed during the first days of hospitalization. When the patient's weight reaches the 40th percentile and remains stable for three days, she may be discharged home.

Daily or thrice-weekly weighing routines may be established on the ward. Nursing staff without specialist training may require considerable support in dealing with youngsters with eating disorders. Helping them to avoid the pitfalls of being either too punitive or too protective is essential since such attitudes may simply replicate family responses to the condition and further maintaining the child's eating problems. Nursing staff need to be briefed on weight targets, meal-time routines, specific privileges that have been earned and specific limits that must be kept. For meal-time routines, at the outset, the youngster may be given a set time period, such as an hour, within which to consume a meal, otherwise finishing the meal may be supervised by a nurse. In supervising eating, nurses sit with the youngster and sympathetically but firmly insist that they eat, in some instances cutting their food for them and feeding them (as if they were truculent pre-school children). Nurses need to be briefed on setting limits and constantly supervising patients who hide food, vomit or exercise excessively. The over-riding position taken by the nursing staff is one of supporting the adolescent in her fight against the disorder.

Weekly family-based treatment sessions are held while the patient is hospitalized following the guidelines set out below. At discharge, the patient is instructed to be responsible for maintaining her own weight while living at home and, before each family-based treatment meeting, she is weighed. If her weight falls below the 40th percentile for height and age, the patient is told that she will be re-hospitalized without privileges within ten days unless her target weigh is restored. Concurrently with this achievement of the overall target weight, discussion of food and weight is prohibited both at home and in the family-based treatment sessions. The family-based treatment sessions then focus on issues described below in the second phase of outpatient family therapy before progressing to the disengagement phase.

Where inpatient weight restoration spans a number of weeks, arrangements may be made for schoolwork to be brought to the hospital, or for hospital-based tuition.

Outpatient family therapy for anorexia

The Maudsley group's evidence-based, manualized outpatient family therapy programme for anorexia nervosa for young adolescents makes a distinction between three distinct phases: (1) engagement and re-feeding; (2) negotiating a new pattern of family relationships; and (3) addressing adolescent issues and therapy termination (Lock et al., 2001).

Phase I. Engagement and re-feeding

The aim of the first phase is to establish a strong positive working alliance with all family members and to maximize their motivation to co-operate with re-feeding the youngster with an eating disorder. This is done by raising their anxiety about the seriousness of the child's condition and highlighting that co-operation with therapy, in which the parents will have a central and authoritative role, will lead to recovery.

Before the first session, usually in a phone conversation, the psychologist communicates that there is a crisis because there is a mortality rate of 6% and a morbidity rate of 30% for patients with anorexia, and many bulimic youngsters become anorexic. The authority of the parents is supported, by acknowledging that they want the best for their child and so must use their authority to insist on all household members attending family sessions. With bulimic patients, the dangers of the fasting–bingeing–purging cycle are highlighted. Of these the most important are the potentially fatal arrhythmias, which may occur as a result of an electrolyte imbalance. Other dangers include gastrointestinal bleeding and erosion of the teeth.

The patient should be weighed privately outside the family-based treatment room just before the first and subsequent sessions, and the body mass index (BMI) or height and weight charts brought into the session as evidence of the severity of the child's condition. In the first session the idea must be conveyed that anorexia or bulimia are extremely dangerous conditions and that the psychologist is concerned for the patient and the parents, and will go the extra mile to help them bring the youngster back to health. The loyalty and concern of the family, shown by their attendance at the interview and their willingness to be involved in treatment, may be acknowledged. Each family member may be asked their understanding of the problem and invited to give an account of all that has been tried by the family and other professionals to solve it and the way in which all previous attempted solutions have been unsuccessful. If patients have received inpatient care, they probably gained weight but relapsed as soon as they returned home. If therapy is beginning just after an inpatient weight-gain programme, this pattern of instant relapse should be predicted since it happens in almost all cases. This process should be used to establish a strong alliance with all family members by empathizing with their despondency about the problem and by modelling an uncritical and supportive attitude to the patient.

At the same time, the psychologist should attempt to raise the level of concern and anxiety experienced by the parents and by the patient about the problem by highlighting the failure of other professionals to help the youngster to maintain a safe weight. The climax of the first session occurs when the psychologist says that it will be down to the whole family, who know and understand the patient best, to use their loyalty and resourcefulness to help the patient take control of her symptomatic behaviour and begin to eat, gain weight, stop bingeing and vomiting and avoid excessive exercise. The family's protests should be met with a statement that all other alternatives have failed or are going to fail and that, in 90% of cases, families who work together with a psychologist over eighteen sessions spread across a year find a way to empower the child to restore her health, but the solution resides within the family. In cases of anorexia, the parents are asked to bring a picnic lunch to the next session with as much food for the patient as they think the patient should eat given that the patient is suffering from starvation.

The finding that parental criticism of the anorexic teenager is associated with drop-out deserves special attention in our discussion of engagement (Szmukler & Dare, 1991). When such criticism occurs (and it is more common in bulimic and chronic cases), it may reflect parental guilt. That is, parents may endure their child's self-starvation for extended periods and show great tolerance and sympathy, but when their experience of guilt reaches a critical level, they may flip over into criticism. Such criticisms typically convey the message that 'I as parent have tried everything to help you, so it's not my fault you are starving, it's your own'. For the anorexic youngster, this blaming process may lead to self-blame, hopelessness and further entrench the low sense of self-esteem and self-efficacy that characterizes youngsters with eating problems.

The engagement phase described here is specifically designed to neutralize parental guilt by highlighting that the parents are not to blame for their child's condition but that they have a central role to play in helping their child recover. By neutralizing guilt it is expected that they will not flip into criticism and exacerbate their youngster's low self-esteem and self-efficacy. Parents who ask whether they caused their child's eating disorder can be told that we can never be sure, but that parents can contribute to their child's recovery. Family-based treatment is not about blaming families for causing problems but is a way of helping families use their wisdom and loyalty to help youngsters recover. The only way in which families can contribute to their child's eating disorders is by inadvertently maintaining the youngster's eating habits through trying and failing to help them eat. The solution to this is to use family-based treatment as a way of breaking these patterns of interaction.

After the engagement process, the family is helped to create a culture within which the adolescent is expected to follow a normal eating pattern. In early-onset short-duration anorexia, most families have developed a series of symptom-maintaining patterns of interaction which involve the parents having difficulty working as a united goal-directed team in insisting that the child eat. They have also typically developed a belief that they are powerless to help their youngster re-learn how to eat normally and retain a normal weight. Often, this pattern is associated with strongly held family beliefs and myths about parental roles, feeding, managing conflict and power. It may also be associated with marital discord or parental mood problems. In this part of therapy, which begins with the picnic lunch, the parents' problem-maintaining interaction patterns and beliefs are challenged.

At the outset of the session, the psychologist acknowledges the whole family's commitment to resolving the serious problem. The failure of professionals to offer a long-term solution is re-iterated, as is the dire prognosis for the condition. It is pointed out that this is a highly stressful session and may take a few hours and that the session ends when the patient eats one more mouthful than she wants to under her parents' guidance. This is a symbolic statement that a family culture has been created within which the child is expected to eat.

The parents may ask that conflict be avoided and suggest that family relationships or self-esteem be improved and that this may lead to the child's recovery. The psychologist may say that this has been tried in other cases and that it actually makes things worse, since much effort is expended in pursuing an inappropriate treatment that leads to further failure.

The psychologist then asks the parents to sit one on each side of the daughter and make sure she eats a good meal. The psychologist may urge them to insist that the daughter eat in the same way that they would insist that a toddler would take her medicine if she were ill. The parents will engage in their routine patterns of breaking their coalition to avoid conflict with the girl and fall into helplessness. But the psychologist must continue to urge them to feed the girl lest she die.

It is important for the psychologist concurrently to support the girl and acknowledge that she has a right to independence and freedom and to her own space, so she must resist being fed by her parents and the humiliation of this until she can find some other way to express her desire for independence.

Eventually, with urging and coaching, the parents join forces and insist that the child eat one more mouthful and she does so. The psychologist acknowledges that the family is strong and may have turned the corner on the long, difficult road to helping the girl recover. The role of siblings throughout this ordeal is to support the patient (not the symptoms) and not to interfere with the parents' joint concerted control of the symptoms.

With separated parents, both parents and their partners in separate sessions may require training in managing symptoms. With single parents, the help of a grandparent or other family member may be co-opted to help control symptoms.

During the three or four sessions that follow the family lunch session, the focus is on supporting the parents in re-feeding the child so that her weight reaches a target weight at or above the 40th percentile for her height at a rate of between 1 and 1.5 kg per week. Decisions are made by the parents about a balanced diet and menus for four meals a day containing between 1500 and 3000 calories, depending on the child's stage of recovery.

The parents are given absolute control over this although, if they require help, an appointment can be made for them to consult with a dietician. The parents are encouraged to create a rotational system so that one of them is at home supervising the patient throughout the weight-gain programme and the patient is confined to the house or, if weight gain is slow, the patient may be confined to bed. Increasing levels of freedom may be given to adolescents as they show steady weight gain.

Symptoms of bingeing and purging in bulimic cases must also be controlled by the parents. How this is to be achieved is negotiated within the treatment sessions. Some examples of strategies used by parents in the Maudsley group's studies include supervising the adolescent eating all of her meals or snacks, making food unavailable between meals by locking the kitchen, limiting the adolescent's access to money to buy food or laxatives and arranging parental supervision of the child for two hours after each meal to prevent purging (Dodge et al., 1995). A critical part of the therapy is empowering the parents to negotiate a plan for controlling the symptoms without triangulating the child into their discussion and then following through on this plan in a co-operative way. The psychologist must balance support for the parents in this co-operative effort, while at the same time supporting the youngster, who may feel embarrassed by her bingeing and purging and powerless to change the tyranny of the binge–purge cycle.

As regular eating habits develop, the youngster is coached in recognizing the triggers that precipitate the binge–purge cycle and helped to develop autonomous strategies for disrupting this cycle, so that eventually self-control may replace parental control of the binge–purge cycle. Self-help manuals for youngsters (Cooper, 1995; Fairburn, 1995; Treasure & Schmidt, 1993) and their parents (Bryant-Waugh & Lask, 1999; Lock & LeGrange, 2004; Treasure, 1997) may be a useful adjunct to therapy at this point.

Phase II. Negotiating a new pattern of family relationships

During the transition into this phase of treatment, an agreement is reached between the psychologist and the family that as soon as the youngster reaches the target weight or demonstrates an ability to avoid bingeing and purging, parental control of feeding will stop. Adolescents then become fully responsible for their own weight. They are weighed privately before each family session and the issue of their weight is only brought into the session if they fall below their target weight. After this point is reached, food, feeding and weight are not discussed in the family sessions by agreement with the family. The family is also advised to avoid food- and weight-related conversations at home.

Family members are invited to explore ways in which the adolescent may express their wish for independence, autonomy and privacy within the family and to negotiate age-appropriate freedoms and responsibilities. Issues such as curfew times, homework, pocket-money, locks on bedroom doors and so forth dominate the *content* of the sessions. The *process* of these sessions is concerned with helping the parents and teenager communicate their wishes clearly, to listen to each other without mind-reading or interruption and learn how to use problem-solving skills to resolve conflicts of interest. Communication and problem-solving training, as described in Chapter 4, may occur during this phase of treatment. Sessions are scheduled less frequently, i.e. for every third or fourth week. Typically, families report that the teenager is showing greater autonomy and independence and spends more time with peers and less time engaged in family activities.

Phase III. Adolescent issues and termination of treatment

In the disengagement phase, the psychologist helps the family review the progress made. The way in which early-onset eating disorders may coincide with a family lifecycle transition from childhood to adolescence is discussed. The possibility of relapse is mentioned and the way in which the parents can use the re-feeding system, which began in the picnic lunch session, to manage relapses is discussed.

The therapy now focuses on the management of the next lifecycle transition. The adolescent's career plans and the issue of leaving home are discussed. The ways in which the parents spend time together as a couple separate from the children is explored. Often in these families there is a belief that the couple's raison d'être is to offer parental care to the children and that without children to care for, the parents' lives would be meaningless. In the disengagement phase, this issue must be raised. However, it is not necessary to resolve it; it is sufficient for the children to know that this is an issue that the parents recognize and are well capable of managing.

Cognitive-behavioural treatment of bulimia

Manualized CBT, typically conducted over ten to twenty sessions, aims to disrupt the binge–purge cycle and modify the belief systems which under-pin this cycle (Fairburn, 1997; Fairburn et al.,1993; Stewart, 2005). In the first stage, the youngster and parents are helped to understand the cognitive-behavioural view on the maintenance of bulimia and the implications of this for resolving the eating problems. Behavioural techniques are employed to help the youngster begin to replace the binge eating pattern with a more normal eating pattern. In the second stage, attempts are made to establish healthy eating habits with a particular focus on eliminating dieting. It is during this stage that youngsters learn to challenge the beliefs and values concerning shape, weight and self-worth that maintain their eating disorder. Maintenance of therapeutic gains and relapse prevention are the focus of the third stage of therapy.

Stage I. Rationale for CBT treatment of bulimia and addressing binge eating

The two main goals of the first stage are to establish the rationale for a CBT approach to treatment and to replace binge eating with a regular eating pattern. The psychologist initially develops therapeutic relationships with the youngster and parents through the process of history taking, presenting a CBT formulation of the youngster's binge–purge cycle, and offering a contract for treatment. This stage spans eight weekly sessions, some of which may be conducted conjointly with parents and some with the youngster alone. With history taking, in addition to the usual areas outlined in Chapter 4, detailed information is gathered on the youngster's attitudes to shape and weight (including the importance attached to shape and weight; desired weight; and cognitive, emotional and behavioural reactions to comments about shape and weight); eating habits (including daily eating pattern, dieting and bingeing); weight-control methods (including self-induced vomiting; use of laxatives, purgatives and diuretics; and exercise); and current medical status, particularly the status of the youngster's electrolytes.

Rationale and formulation

In presenting the formulation, Figure 17.2 is used. Usually, binge eating is presented as the central concern. The youngster wishes to stop bingeing but feels out of control. With this in mind, certain key points should be made in presenting the formulation. First, dieting maintains binge eating because it leads to feelings of intense hunger and negative affect. Second, this negative affect is intensified in specific trigger situations. Youngsters interpret these trigger situations (such as noticing that they are not slim) in a negative way (due to perfectionism, black and white thinking or other cognitive distortions) and these negative appraisals intensify negative mood states. For example, they may think 'I want to be slim, I never will be, I feel terrible, eating is the only thing that will comfort me'. Binge eating is a short-term way of improving the negative mood states associated with these negative automatic thoughts. Third, vomiting and purging also maintain binge eating because youngsters hold the mistaken belief that these are effective methods for calorie control, and the act of vomiting brings relief because of these erroneous beliefs. For example, a youngster may hold the following beliefs 'I've stuffed myself and I will get very fat unless I get this food out of my system now. I must be perfectly thin or I'm no good, I feel completely guilty for having eaten so much and having no will power, so I'll vomit. That's a relief, now that I've vomited. I will diet from now on.' Fourth, the belief that high self-worth will arise from a slim shape and low weight promotes extreme dieting, partly because youngsters adopt a perfectionistic thinking style and tend to think in black and white terms. For example, youngsters may hold beliefs such as 'I must be the perfect shape otherwise no one will like me' or 'Either I'm thin or I'm fat, good or bad, there is no middle ground'. Fifth, over-concern about shape and weight is linked to long-standing negative self-evaluation. This may include beliefs that the youngster has little intrinsic worth as a person and has very little power to change this, except through maintaining a slim shape and low weight. While these five general issues should be addressed in presenting the formulation, it should be customized in each case to the unique circumstances and beliefs of the youngster in question. It is useful to draw the formulation, as given in Figure 17.2, for the youngster and parents working from the bottom of the diagram (the bingeing

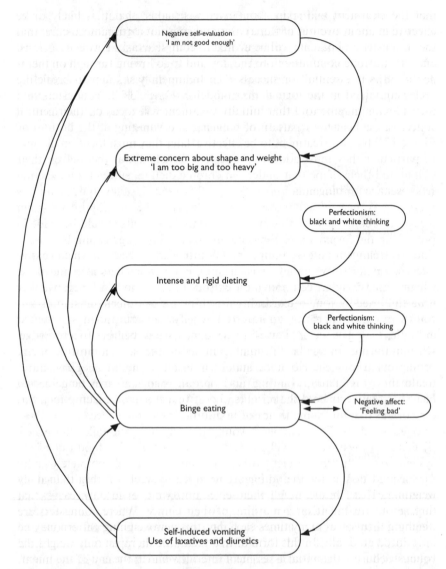

Negative self-evaluation
'I am not good enough'

Extreme concern about shape and weight
'I am too big and too heavy'

Perfectionism:
black and white thinking

Intense and rigid dieting

Perfectionism:
black and white thinking

Binge eating

Negative affect:
'Feeling bad'

Self-induced vomiting
Use of laxatives and diuretics

Figure 17.2 CBT model of the maintenance of bulimia nervosa

Note: Adapted from Fairburn, C. (1997). Eating disorders. In: D. Clark & C. Fairburn (Eds.), *The Science and Practice of Cognitive Behaviour Therapy* (p. 212). Oxford: Oxford University Press.

and vomiting cycle) upwards. The formulation may be revisited regularly throughout the process of treatment.

When youngsters and parents understand this CBT formulation they may be offered a contract for treatment. The youngster and parent are informed that the treatment will span about twenty sessions; that it is likely to be effective in about two out of three cases and so is not a guaranteed cure; that the youngster and parents will be invited to complete tasks between sessions; and that a strong commitment to therapy and to following through on thera-peutic tasks is essential for success. The treatment tasks aim to break the cycles contained in the formulation model in Figure 17.2. Youngsters and their parents may be told that initially treatment will focus on their central concerns, the behaviour pattern of bingeing and vomiting at the bottom of Figure 17.2 but, for treatment to be effective, later they must focus on dieting. In particular they must address youngsters' beliefs about themselves, their weight and their shape that under-pin chronic dieting, since chronic dieting sets the stage for bingeing.

Self-monitoring

The first treatment task is to complete self-monitoring sheets in which young-sters record exactly what they eat each day, the time when it is eaten, the place, whether the youngster considered the episode of eating to be a binge, whether it was followed by vomiting or laxative use, and the overall circumstances and context under which the eating occurred. A self-monitoring form is presented in Figure 17.3. The second and all subsequent sessions begin with a review of self-monitoring forms. In the final column of the self-monitoring form, youngsters record the situation and their thoughts about it. Throughout treatment, by regularly reviewing this material, youngsters may be helped to identify negative automatic thoughts, cognitive distortions, assumptions and core beliefs that under-pin their eating disorder.

Weekly weighing

The second task is for the youngster to agree to weekly rather than daily weighing. They should weigh themselves once, and once only, each week throughout treatment on a morning of their choice. Where youngsters are weighing themselves many times each day, this new weighing pattern may be introduced gradually. In this form of treatment, the therapist only weighs the youngster during the initial assessment interview and at the end of treatment, to avoid the therapy becoming over-focused on weight-related issues.

Reading self-help books

The third task is for the youngster and parents to read bulimia self-help books, a process that should continue throughout treatment (Cooper, 1995; Fairburn, 1995; Treasure & Schmidt, 1993). Detailed instructions on under-standing eating disorders, completing self-monitoring, and all other CBT tasks are given in these self-help books. With younger teenagers, parents may

To understand your eating habits, it is important for you to keep a detailed daily record of **everything** you eat and drink and the related circumstances.

In the first column write down the time of day, e.g., 9.15 a.m.

In the second column write down what you ate and drank, e.g., 3 slices of toast and marmalade and 3 cups of coffee with milk and two sugar.

In the third column write down where you ate them, e.g., in the kitchen.

In the fourth column put an X if you think this was binging (eating too much).

In the fifth column put an X if you vomited after you ate the food.

In the sixth column put a D if you took a diuretic, put an L if you took a laxative, put an E if you did some exercise to burn off the food you ate.

In the seventh column write down your comments on the situation and what you were thinking, e.g. I was upset because I thought I looked fat in the mirror in my school uniform. I said this to my mum and she started to argue with me. I thought 'I'm so fat. No one likes me.' Then I ate a lot to make me feel better. Then I made myself sick. I felt a bit of relief then.

In the seventh column write down your weight on the one morning a week you weigh yourself.

Complete this form every day and bring all forms you complete to every meeting to review with your therapist.

Date

Time	Food and drink consumed	Place	Binge	Vomit	Laxative Diuretic Exercise	The situation and what you thought

Figure 17.3 Self-monitoring form for bulimia

be invited to supervise CBT tasks. With older teenagers, the tasks may be conducted autonomously.

Psychoeducation

Psychoeducation about bulimia is also covered in the first stage of treatment. This should be given orally and appropriate chapters of self-help books should be given as homework assignments. Youngsters and their parents are informed about how to calculate the body mass index (BMI) and to set a weight goal using BMI tables that does not involve dieting. Psychoeducation also covers the physical consequences of bingeing and vomiting; the ineffectiveness of vomiting, laxative and diuretic use as means of weight control; and the fact that dieting inevitably leads to intense hunger, loss of control and bingeing. The negative consequences of bingeing, vomiting and using purgatives that should be stressed include electrolyte imbalance, salivary gland enlargement (leading to a chubby face), erosion of dental enamel, intermittent oedema and menstruation irregularities.

Prescribing a regular eating pattern

Youngsters should be given the following advice on eating habits. First, eat three meals per day, and two or three planned snacks, spaced no more than three hours apart. Meals should not be followed by vomiting, the use of diuretics, purgative or intense exercise and other unplanned eating should be avoided. Where eating habits are severely disturbed, this regular pattern should be introduced gradually. This task aims to both regularize eating habits and show youngsters that the eating pattern does not result in weight gain.

Stimulus control

Stimulus control techniques may be introduced to help youngsters adhere to a regular eating pattern. These include not engaging in other activities (such as watching TV) while eating, savouring their food, confining eating to one place and formalizing the eating process by setting the table, limiting the supply of food available while eating by putting out the required amount and putting the packet away before the meal starts, practising leaving food on the plate, throwing away left-overs, keeping as little 'danger food' such as chocolate in the house as possible, planning shopping lists when not hungry and sticking to them, and avoiding finishing food on plates of other family members. Particularly with younger adolescents, the implementation of these stimulus control techniques should be discussed in detail with parents.

Planning alternatives to bingeing and vomiting

Youngsters may be invited to predict trigger situations where they are at risk of bingeing and vomiting, and to develop lists of alternative behaviours in which they can engage to avoid bingeing and vomiting. Such behaviours may include talking to a parent, phoning a friend, playing a computer game, playing music, taking gentle exercise or having a bath.

Managing vomiting

To reduce the frequency of vomiting, youngsters may be invited to select meals or snacks which induce a lower urge to vomit, and to carefully plan to engage in distracting activities for an hour following eating to avoid vomiting.

Managing laxative and diuretic use

To reduce the frequency of laxative and diuretic use, the ineffectiveness of these drugs in preventing food absorption should be explained. Then youngsters may be invited to discard their supply of such drugs in one step or a series of gradual steps. Sometimes there is a brief temporary rebound effect after ceasing diuretic use, during which weight increases, and youngsters should be warned of this.

Stage II. Reducing dieting, improving problem solving and challenging cognitive distortions

Throughout stages II and III, processes begun in stage I are continued. The three main goals of the second stage, which spans about eight weeks, are to reduce dieting, improve problem-solving skills and challenge the beliefs about shape, weight and self-worth that maintain the eating disorder.

Reducing dieting

With bulimia, most youngsters practise three types of dieting: (1) abstaining from eating for long periods of time; (2) avoiding specific 'forbidden' foods; and (3) restricting the amount of food eaten. Youngsters attempt to follow strict rules about when to eat, which forbidden foods to avoid and how much to eat. Following these rules leads to intense hunger. In stressful trigger situations, this hunger leads to bingeing, which is interpreted as evidence for poor-self control and low self-worth rather than unrealistic dietary rules. A central strategy for resolving bulimia, therefore, is reducing or eliminating dieting. In stage I, the prescription of a regular eating pattern of three meals and two snacks a day, with intervals no longer than three hours addressed the first type of dieting, i.e. avoiding eating for long time periods.

To address the second type of dieting, youngsters may be invited to visit a supermarket, identify and list all the 'forbidden' foods they can see, and then classify these into four categories from the least to the most forbidden. Over the following weeks, the youngster, alone or with parents, is invited to plan and eat meals or snacks in which these forbidden foods are incorporated in small or normal amounts into the meals, starting with the least forbidden and working gradually towards the most forbidden foods. These meals or snacks containing forbidden foods should only be planned for low-stress periods when the youngster is likely to experience a high degree of self-control. This gradual and graded introduction of forbidden foods into the youngster's diet should be continued until the youngster no longer feels anxious about eating them. After that, youngsters may return to a narrower diet that may not often include them. In some situations, youngsters may be so anxious about eating certain foods because they fear over-eating or vomiting, that desensitization to them should be conducted in the clinic using an exposure and response prevention format. These sessions should be carefully planned. The meal or snack containing the forbidden food is eaten early in the session and the youngster is helped by the therapist for the remainder of the session to cope with the urges to over-eat the forbidden food or to vomit. For youngsters with strong food avoidance, a number of such sessions may be necessary.

To address the third type of dieting – restrictive dieting – the youngster should be helped to move from a restricted diet to a diet containing 1500 calories per day. Inspection of self-monitoring sheets will indicate current calorific intake and this information may be used to plan a gradual increase in food consumption. Youngsters may also be invited to eat a more varied diet.

Problem solving

To deal with problematic situations, especially trigger situations that precede bingeing, youngsters may be coached in using systematic problem-solving skills. Invite youngsters to first break big vague problems into many smaller specific problems to be tackled one at a time. Second, define each of these in solvable terms. Third, focus on solving the specific problem at hand, not attacking the person or people involved in the problem, or simply leaving the problem unresolved. Fourth, generate many possible solutions to the problem in hand. Fifth, when all solutions are generated, examine the pros and cons of each, and select the best. Sixth, implement this solution, review progress, and modify the solution if it's not working. Finally, repeat this sequence as often as is necessary to solve the problem and celebrate success. Inspection of self-monitoring forms will usually show that many binge-triggering situations involve difficult interpersonal problems. Through addressing these in therapy sessions, as they arise, youngsters gradually learn systematic problem-solving skills.

Cognitive restructuring

From the formulation in Figure 17.2 it is clear that dieting and the bingeing and vomiting cycle are driven by negative mood states that arise from negative beliefs about shape and weight (such as 'I'm too big and too heavy') and negative self-evaluative beliefs (such as 'I'm not good enough' or 'I've no self-control'). In specific triggering situations, these beliefs give rise to specific negative automatic thoughts, which are typically distorted by a range of cognitive processes of which perfectionism and black and white thinking are often the most salient. For example, when a youngster notices that her weight has increased by two pounds as she steps on the scales she may have the negative automatic thought 'I'm a tub of lard!'. This negative automatic thought is under-pinned by the core beliefs 'I'm no good' and 'I'm too fat'. This negative automatic thought is also under-pinned by perfectionism insofar as only perfection is acceptable, and by black and white thinking, insofar as the thought does not reflect the fact that a minor gain in weight has occurred, but rather that the youngster is either 'a tub of lard' or not.

With cognitive restructuring, the first step is for the youngster to write down the actual situation and the specific negative automatic thought that occurred in the situation (not a summary or rephrasing of it). These thoughts may be identified in the final columns of self-monitoring sheets within and outside treatment sessions. The following situations usually elicit relevant automatic thoughts: looking in a mirror, weighing themselves, reacting to a comment about their appearance or appetite, situations where urges to binge or vomit occur, or seeing themselves in a swimming costume or tight clothes. The following is an example of a situation and the negative automatic thought: 'I stepped on the scales on Tuesday morning and was 8 stone 2 when I should have been 8 stone. I thought "I'm a tub of lard! I'm really fat!" '.

The second step in cognitive restructuring is to accurately list the evidence that supports the thought. For example, 'My weight increased by two pounds over a period of ten days'.

The third step is to help youngsters list arguments or evidence which cast doubt on the validity of the negative automatic thought. Here, Socratic questioning may be used: 'How would you know if any person was fat?' 'What clothes size do you have to have to be fat?' 'Would you judge someone in your class at school who was 8 stone 2 pounds to be fat?' 'Are you applying one set of standards to yourself and another set to other people?' 'Have you gained two pounds because your body has accumulated more fat due to over-eating or because you are retaining fluid due to being in the premenstrual stage of your monthly cycle?'. Youngsters may be taught to recognize the cognitive distortions listed earlier in the section on CBT theories of eating disorders and invited to identify which of these are present in their negative automatic thoughts.

The fourth and final step of cognitive restructuring is to help youngsters reach a reasoned conclusion which they may then use to guide their behaviour as an alternative to the negative automatic thought. For example, 'I put on two pounds but my weight is within the normal range'.

It is not essential for youngsters to fully accept the validity of their reasoned conclusion. The point is that they become aware, through repeatedly challenging, of their negative automatic thoughts in therapy sessions and, as homework, that they have a limited number of such thoughts which drive their dieting, bingeing and vomiting behaviour, and that these thoughts are not absolutely true. Also, the negative automatic thoughts become less automatic and more conscious as youngsters become more practised at challenging them.

As more examples of negative automatic thoughts are addressed in therapy, certain extreme, rigid, underlying assumptions, of which youngsters are usually not conscious and which they hold with great tenacity, become clear. Examples include: 'If I am thin and light, then I will be loved by others, happy, successful and worthwhile', 'If I am fat and heavy, I will be abandoned by others, a failure, sad and worthless', 'If I have self-control I am strong, good and a success', 'If I show any sign of lack of control, I am completely powerless, bad and a failure'. These underlying assumptions may tentatively be suggested to youngsters and they may be challenged using the four steps for cognitive restructuring outlined above. In addition, youngsters may be invited to complete behavioural experiments, to disconfirm their beliefs that they will be ostracized if others see their bodies. For example, youngsters may be invited to wear more close-fitting clothes, to go to exercise classes where they wear leotards, or to go swimming.

Stage III. Relapse prevention

Throughout stage III, processes begun in stages I and II are continued. The main goal of the third stage, which involves three fortnightly sessions, is relapse prevention. A distinction should be made between a complete relapse (a rare event) and a minor lapse or slip (which is a common event). Bingeing as a response to stress may be described as the youngster's Achilles' heel. Youngsters' mastery of bulimia is strengthened by coping well with slips, where they occasionally binge in response to stress. To equip them to cope with slips, youngsters and their parents may be invited to predict the sorts of situations that might trigger such slips, and to develop plans for managing lapses when they occur. Such plans should include acknowledging that the temporary slip is not a permanent relapse; that a slip is an opportunity for gaining strength rather than a sign of weakness; that planning regular daily eating patterns with three meals, two snacks and no dieting is crucial for success; that problem-solving skills should be used to address complex social problems that trigger urges to binge; that negative automatic thoughts and assumptions must be continually challenged; and that parental support is essential for the youngster's success. The youngster should be given a home-work assignment of writing out a plan to manage lapses and this plan should be reviewed in the final session.

PREVENTION

Eating disorders have the highest mortality rate (6% at 20 years) of all psychological problems. For this reason alone, the development of prevention programmes is essential, although, to date, little work in this area has been conducted (Slade, 1995). The target group with highest priority for primary prevention is young teenage girls and their families. If resources demand a focused approach, a screening questionnaire such as the Children's Eating Attitudes Test (ChEAT; Maloney, McGuire & Daniels, 1988) or the Setting Conditions for Anorexia Nervosa Scale (SCANS; Slade & Dewey, 1986; Slade, Dewey, Kiemle & Newton, 1990) may be used to identify adolescents who are particularly at risk for eating disorders. School- or community-based educational programmes with parallel parent meetings focusing on the following points deserve exploration:

- identifying and questioning the value of the thin ideal female body shape
- the illusory correlation between slimness and happiness
- dieting, bingeing and purging
- the short- and long-term dangers of eating disorders
- common academic, psychological, social and biological demands and challenges that adolescents (and their parents) face
- fears that adolescents must deal with in developing an independent sense of identity
- eating disorders as a solution to demands of the transition to the adolescent phase of the lifecycle
- other solutions to the demands of the transition to adolescence and adulthood.

SUMMARY

About 1–2% of teenage girls have eating disorders. Anorexia is characterized by self-starvation and bulimia by a pattern of dieting, bingeing and purging. Clinical features include a fear of fatness, a distorted body image, a preoccupation with food, a belief that bingeing behaviour is out of control, concerns about individuation, low self-esteem, low self-efficacy, perfectionism, depressive affect, self-destructive behaviour, poor interpersonal adjustment and neuroendocrine abnormalities related to starvation. Important pre-disposing factors include a genetic pre-disposition, cultural pressures for thinness, early trauma, perfectionism, low self-esteem, low self-efficacy and unresolved conflicts about individuation. Stresses associated with lifecycle transitions to adolescence or young adulthood may precipitate the onset of eating disorders and they are maintained by the neurophysiological sequelae of starvation in conjunction with belief systems characterized by distorted cognitions and enmeshed, rigid and conflict-avoiding patterns of family interaction. There is a better prognosis for less chronic and severe conditions, and protective factors include the youngster's problem-solving and inter-personal skills and the family and peer group's capacity to support the youngster with the abnormal eating pattern. For anorexic children and teen-agers the treatment of choice is a highly structured family-based treatment programme in which the parents are empowered to re-feed the child and later the child is helped to individuate. In severe cases hospitalization for re-feeding may be necessary. Manualized CBT over ten to twenty sessions, which aims to disrupt the binge–purge cycle and modify the belief systems which under-pin this cycle is the treatment of choice for bulimia. Educational prevention pro-grammes should target teenage girls scoring above the cut-off point on a screening instrument such as the Children's Eating Attitude Test.

EXERCISE 17.1

Divide the class into a family team and a treatment team. Class members in the family team should take the roles of family members Maggie, Roddy, Bev, Mar and Nick listed in Box 17.1. Imagine that it is the hour before the second family session in which a picnic lunch will occur. Draw up a list of the top three hopes and top three fears that each family member would have going into a family lunch session. Class members in the treatment team should draw up their plan for the session, the things they hope to achieve and their best guess about how family members will respond to this plan. Both groups should present their findings to each other and explore the degree to which the family and treatment teams' expectations match up.

FURTHER READING

Fairburn, C. & Wilson, G. (1993). *Binge Eating: Nature, Assessment & Treatment.* New York: Guilford.

Garner, D. & Garfinkle, P. (1997). *Handbook of Treatment for Eating Disorders* (Second edition). New York: Guilford.

Lock, J., LeGrange, D., Agras, W., & Dare, C. (2001). *Treatment Manual for Anorexia Nervosa. A Family Based Approach.* New York: Guilford.

Treasure, J. & Schmidt, U. (1993). *Clinician's Guide to Getting Better Bit(e) by Bit(e).* Hove, UK: Lawrence Erlbaum Associates Ltd.

FURTHER READING FOR CLIENTS

Bryant-Waugh, R. & Lask, B. (1999). *Eating Disorders: A Parent's Guide*. London: Penguin.

Cooper, P. (1995). *Bulimia Nervosa: A Guide to Recovery*. London: Robinson Publishing.

Crisp, A., Joughin, N. Halek, C., & Bower, C. (1996). *Anorexia Nervosa: The Wish to Change. Self-help and Discovery, the Thirty Steps* (Second Edition). Hove, UK: Psychology Press.

Fairburn, C. (1995). *Overcoming Binge Eating*. New York: Guilford.

Fox, C. & Joughin, C. (2002). *Eating Problems in Children. Information for Parents*. London: Gaskell.

Lock, J. J. & Le Grange, D. (2004). *Help Your Teenager Beat an Eating Disorder*. London: Brunner Routledge.

Treasure, J. (1997). *Anorexia Nervosa. A Survival Guide for Families Friends and Sufferers*. Hove, UK: Psychology Press.

Treasure, J. & Schmidt, U. (1993). *Getting Better Bit(e) by Bit(e): A Survival Kit for Sufferers of Bulimia Nervosa and Binge Eating*. Hove, UK: Lawrence Erlbaum Associates Ltd.

WEBSITES

Eating Disorders Association: http://gurney.co.uk/eda
Eating Disorders Resources: http://edr.org.uk/
Eating Disorders Shared Awareness: http://eating-disorder.com

Factsheets on eating disorders and worries about weight can be downloaded from the website for Rose, G. & York, A. (2004). *Mental Health and Growing Up. Fact sheets for Parents, Teachers and Young People* (Third edition). London: Gaskell: http://www.rcpsych.ac.uk

Chapter 18

Schizophrenia

Schizophrenia is a diagnosis usually given to individuals who present with seriously debilitating problems, as may be seen from the case study of Julian, a nineteen-year-old adolescent, presented in Box 18.1. Research on schizophrenia follows from two principal traditions, the first represented by Kraepelin (1896) and the second by Bleuler (1911). Whereas Kraepelin defined the presentation now called schizophrenia as principally character-ized by a large constellation of observable symptoms (such as delusions, hallucinations and thought disorder), an underlying degenerative neuro-logical cause and a chronic course, Bleuler proposed that schizophrenia was a circumscribed set of inferred psychological processes, which often led to the sorts of presentations to which Kraeplein had referred as 'dementia praecox'. Bleuler speculated that the capacity to associate one thought with another, to associate thoughts with emotions and the self with reality, were impaired or *split*. Hence the term 'schizophrenia' (from the Greek words for *split* and *mind*). Bleuler argued that observable symptoms such as delusions and hal-lucinations were secondary to these central disrupted psychological processes and reflected the person's attempt to cope with the world despite the dis-rupted psychological processes. Up until the late 1970s, Bleuler's tradition, associated with a broad definition of schizophrenia, pre-dominated in the USA, whereas in the UK, Ireland and Europe, Kraepelin's narrower defin-ition held sway. Following the landmark US–UK diagnostic study (US–UK Team, 1974), which highlighted the extraordinary differences between the way schizophrenia was defined in the USA and Britain, there has been a gradual move towards developing an internationally acceptable set of diag-nostic criteria, as can be seen from Table 18.1.

Today, particularly within mainstream research and practice, a theme that has increasing acceptance is that schizophrenia is a complex and as yet poorly understood condition with a pre-dominantly neurobiological basis, with profound psychological and psychosocial features, and for which, in the long-term, a pre-dominantly pharmacological cure will be found which will be offered within the context of a multi-modal programme involving psychological intervention (American Academy of Child and Adolescent

Box 18.1. A case of schizophrenia: Julian the boy who walked east

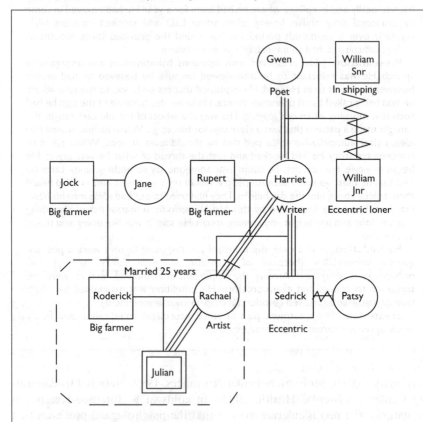

Referral. Julian was referred for assessment and advice by his GP in Norfolk in the summer of 1987. His parents were worried about him because he had been behaving strangely since returning to the family home after studying in London for a year. Julian had failed his exams and came home, he said 'to sort his head out'. He lacked concentration and his conversation was incoherent much of the time. Also, his behaviour was erratic. He had gone jogging one morning the previous week and not returned. His parents had found him in his training shoes and running shorts 35 miles away later that day. He was exhausted and dehydrated. He explained that he was on his way to the car ferry to Holland on a secret mission.

Developmental and family history. He was the nineteen-year-old son of a prominent local farmer. His father was devoted to his work and had a positive, if distant relationship with Julian. His mother was a painter and also a prominent local figure. She was a warm flamboyant woman who retained strong anti-establishment beliefs. She responded to Julian in the interview setting with intense concern and protectiveness. There was no family history of psychological disorder but some members of the mother's family were well-to-do but odd or eccentric, especially her brother Sedrick and her uncle William Junior. William's eccentricities led him into serious conflict with his father and Sedrick's odd behaviour under-pinned his highly conflictual childless marriage to Patsy.

Julian grew up on the farm and went to the local school. His development was essentially normal. He was excellent at cricket and did well at school. He had many friends locally and in college where he had been for a year. He had engaged in some experimental drug abuse, having taken some LSD and smoked cannabis fairly regularly over a six-month period. He had found the previous three months at college difficult and had an intense fear of exam failure.

Presentation. Julian presented with delusions, hallucinations and disorganized speech. He was reluctant to be interviewed because he believed he had urgent business to attend to in Holland. He explained that his path was to the east where he was being called by an unknown source. He knew this because of the sign he had seen that morning when out jogging. The way the wheel of the old cart caught the sunlight made a pattern that was a clear sign for him to go. When he questioned this idea, a clear authoritative voice said that he should leave at once. When asked to continue his story he had blocked and lost the thread of what he was saying. He began to giggle. He said that he could hear someone say something funny. Later he said that he must go soon because people would try to prevent him. He had heard them talking about him the day before. They had tried to put bad ideas into his head. He described being frightened by this and by periodic sensations that everything was too loud and too bright and coming at him. He said 'It was like doing acid (LSD) all the time . . .'

Formulation. In this case, the principal pre-disposing factors were a possible genetic vulnerability (because of eccentric maternal family history) and hallucinogenic drug use. Among the important precipitating factors were his transition to college and exam pressure. His condition was maintained by a high level of maternal expressed emotion (principally over-involvement).

Treatment. The treatment plan included neuroleptic medication and family work to reduce parental expressed emotion.

Psychiatry, 2001b; McEvoy, Scheifler & Frances, 1999; National Collaborating Centre for Mental Health, 2003). In contrast to this neo-Kraepelian perspective, the neo-Bleulerian view is that the psychological processes that under-pin hallucinations and delusions are on a continuum with normal experiences of loud thoughts and compelling beliefs, and that these processes are best understood and treated psychologically on a symptom-by-symptom basis (Bentall, 2004; British Psychological Society Division of Clinical Psychology, 2000). The neo-Krapelian position privileges the idea of under-standing and treating schizophrenia as a syndrome; the neo-Bleulerian position favours understanding and treating each of the symptoms of schizophrenia as extreme versions of normal processes. Both traditions continue to generate valuable knowledge and treatment possibilities and valuable debate about the validity and ethical implications of the construct of schizophrenia (e.g. Bentall, 2004; Boyle, 2002).

After discussing the classification, epidemiology and clinical features of the construct of schizophrenia, this chapter considers a variety of theoretical explanations concerning the aetiology of the conditions subsumed under this label, along with relevant empirical evidence. An approach to the assessment of schizophrenia and its treatment will then be given.

Table 18.1 Definitions of schizophrenia

DSM IV TR	ICD 10
A. Characteristic symptoms. Two or more of the following, each present for a significant portion of time during a 1-month period (or less if successfully treated): (1) delusions (2) hallucinations (3) disorganized speech (e.g. frequent derailment or incoherence) (4) Grossly disorganized or catatonic behaviour (5) Negative symptoms, affective flattening, alogia or avolition Only one criterion A symptom required if delusions are bizarre or hallucinations consist of a voice keeping up a running commentary on the person's behaviour or thoughts, or two or more voices conversing with each other	A minimum of one very clear symptom (or two or more of less clear cut) belonging to any one of the groups (a) to (d) and at least two of the symptoms (e) to (i) should have been present most of the time during a period of 1 month or more: (a) thought echo, thought insertion or withdrawal and thought broadcasting (b) delusions of control, influence, or passivity, clearly referred to body of limb movements or specific thoughts (c) hallucinatory voices giving a running commentary on the patient's behaviour, or discussing the patient among themselves, or other types of hallucinatory voice coming from some part of the body (d) persistent delusions of other kinds that are culturally inappropriate and completely impossible, such as religious or political identity, or superhuman powers and abilities
B. Social/occupational dysfunction. For a significant portion of the time since the onset of the disturbance, one or more major areas of functioning such as work, interpersonal relations, or self-care are markedly below the level achieved prior to onset or with children a failure to achieve the expected level of interpersonal, academic or occupational achievement	(e) persistent hallucinations in any modality, when accompanied either by fleeting or half-formed delusions without clear affective content, or by persistent over-valued ideas, or when occurring every day for weeks or months on end
C. Duration. Continuous signs of the disturbance persist for at least 6 months	(f) breaks or interpolations in the train of thought, resulting in incoherence or irrelevant speech or neologisms
D. Not due to schizoaffective or mood disorder	(g) catatonic behaviour, such as excitement, posturing, or waxy flexibility, negativism, mutism or stupor
E. Not due to substance use or general medical condition	(h) negative symptoms such as marked apathy, paucity of speech, and blunting or incongruity of emotional responses, usually result in social withdrawal and lowering of social performance
F. If there is autism or a pervasive developmental disorder, then prominent delusions and hallucinations of 1 month's duration must be present	(i) a significant and consistent change in the overall quality of some aspects of personal behaviour, manifest as loss of interest, aimlessness, idleness, a self-absorbed attitude and social withdrawal

Note: Adapted from DSM IV TR (APA, 2000a) and ICD 10 (WHO, 1992, 1996).

DIAGNOSIS AND CLASSIFICATION

The narrowing of the gap between the North American and European definitions of schizophrenia is reflected in the marked similarity between the diagnostic criteria for the disorder contained in ICD 10 (WHO, 1992, 1996) and DSM IV TR (APA, 2000a). These criteria are presented in Table 18.1. The two definitions include delusions and hallucinations, disorganized speech or thought disorder, and negative symptoms. The DSM IV TR system is more cautious in requiring evidence of deterioration in social or occupational functioning and proof that the symptoms have persisted for six months before a diagnosis can be made. With ICD 10, a diagnosis may be made after a month and there is no requirement for evidence of deterioration in social or occupational functioning. While the DSM IV TR and ICD 10 diagnostic criteria have been developed for use with adults, a growing body of studies has shown that these systems may be used reliably with children (Asarnow, Thompson & McGrath, 2004).

The marked variability among people with schizophrenia in symptomatology, course, treatment response and possible aetiological factors has led to the development of a variety of sub-classification systems. Also, many psychotic conditions which closely resemble schizophrenia have been identified. In ICD 10 and DSM IV TR, symptomatology, rather than inferred biological or psychological aetiological factors, is used as a basis for sub-typing the schizophrenia. Sub-types of schizophrenia and of other related psychotic disorders classified in ICD 10 and DSM IV TR are presented in Figures 18.1 and 18.2. In both sub-typing systems where paranoid delusions pre-dominate, a diagnosis of paranoid schizophrenia is given. Cases where psychomotor abnormalities, such as excitability or negativism, pre-dominate are classified as catatonic. Cases are classified as hebephrenic in the ICD 10 and disorganized in the DSM IV TR when inappropriate of flat affect are the principal features and where there is disorganization of behaviour and speech. Both ICD 10 and DSM IV TR classify cases that do not fall into the three categories just mentioned as undifferentiated. Beyond these four principal sub-types, various other categories have been proposed to take account of unclassifiable cases. For example, 'simple schizophrenia' refers to cases where negative symptoms are present in the absence of positive symptoms.

In an appendix to DSM IV TR, an alternative three-dimensional system for coding symptoms is proposed (reflecting the influence of Liddle's (2001) three-dimensional theory, described below in the section in theories of schizophrenia). The psychotic dimension covers positive symptoms such as hallucinations and delusions. The negative symptoms dimension covers restricted behaviour, blunted affect and impoverished speech. The third dimension covers disorganization in affect, speech and behaviour, and includes bizarre behaviour and thought disorder. This approach, where dimensionally assessed processes are profiled, may prove in future to be more

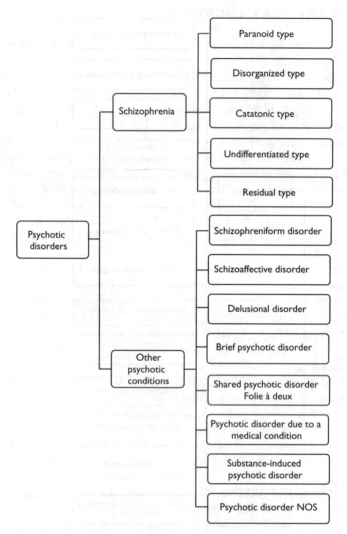

Figure 18.1 Classification of schizophrenia and other psychotic disorders in DSM IV
     TR

clinically useful than the current sub-typing system, which has little clinical validity.

The boundaries between schizophrenic disorders and other disorders, notably mood and personality disorders, are by no means clear cut, probably because aspects of the disorders are dimensionally rather than categoric-ally distributed within the population. Nevertheless, within the ICD and DSM systems, imperfect attempts have been made to manage this boundary problem by constructing new categories to accommodate cases that straddle

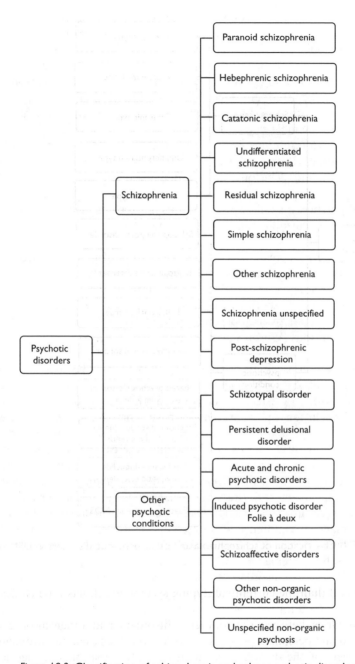

Figure 18.2 Classification of schizophrenia and other psychotic disorders in ICD 10

category borders. The boundaries between schizophrenic disorders and mood disorders have been dealt with in the ICD and DSM systems by proposing mixed disorders such as schizoaffective disorder or post-psychotic depression. Where aspects of symptomatology are insufficient for a diagnosis of schizophrenia, ICD 10 and DSM IV TR indicate that diagnoses of personality disorders may be given, although these can only be given to youngsters over eighteen years of age. A marked pattern of social withdrawal and aloofness, which may resemble negative symptoms of schizophrenia, but in the absence of positive symptoms, is the primary characteristic of the schizoid personality disorder. People showing eccentricities which fall just short of thought disorder and delusions may be diagnosed as having schizotypal personality disorder.

In clinical practice, the following conditions may be included in the differential diagnosis of schizophrenia in children and adolescents (Hollis, 2002):

- mood disorders (depression, schizoaffecive disorder, bipolar disorder)
- personality disorders (particularly schizoid and schizotypal)
- pervasive developmental disorders (such as autism)
- drug-induced psychoses (involving drugs such as ecstasy or LSD)
- temporal lobe epilepsy (complex partial seizures)
- organic conditions (Wilson's disease).

Mood disorders with psychotic features may in some cases be distinguished from schizophrenia by taking account of the content of delusions and hallucinations, which are usually mood congruent in affective disorders. So in depression, the delusions and hallucinations have depressive content, whereas in mania they have grandiose content. Also, the onset of schizophrenia tends to be insidious in many children and adolescents, whereas the onset of major depression with psychotic features tends to be acute. Despite all this, some cases meet the criteria for schizoaffective disorder and about a third of children who meet the diagnostic criteria for schizophrenia also meet the criteria for depression (Asarnow et al., 2004). Diagnoses of personality disorders are not usually made in children and adolescents. However, a proportion of youngsters show psychotic symptomatology insufficiently severe for a diagnosis of schizophrenia, but which meets the criteria for schizoid or schizotypal personality disorder. Youngsters with extreme levels of social withdrawal and aloofness in conjunction with some mild negative symptoms may meet the criteria for schizoid personality disorder. Youngsters showing eccentricities which fall just short of thought disorder and delusions may meet the criteria for schizotypal personality disorder. To rule out transient psychoses arising from the use of hallucinogenic drugs such as ecstasy of LSD, extended periods of observation and a referral for toxicological tests is appropriate. Autism may be distinguished from schizophrenia by the absence of sustained delusions and hallucinations and by the child's inability to engage in reciprocal communication. However, children with autism and schizophrenia both typically have a history of early language delay. Those with schizophrenia also typically show a delay in fine and gross motor development (Asarnow & Karatekin, 2001). Referral for an EEG can rule out temporal lobe epilepsy as a cause of psychotic sympomatology, although in a small proportion of cases co-morbid schizophrenia and seizure disorder occur. Referral for a thorough paediatric medical assessment is appropriate to exclude possible organic factors, for example Wilson's disease, as the source of psychotic symptoms.

EPIDEMIOLOGY

The prevalence of schizophrenia is 1% in populations over eighteen years of age (Kuipers et al., in press). This international cross-cultural finding was replicated in Ireland by NíNualláin et al. in the 1980s; prior to NíNualláin's (NíNualláin et al. 1990) work, methodologically flawed studies had suggested that the incidence of schizophrenia in Ireland was higher than in other countries. There are few reliable data on the epidemiology of schizophrenia in youngsters under eighteen years of age, but the consensus is that childhood onset schizophrenia is far rarer than schizophrenia with an adolescent onset (Asarnow & Asarnow, 2003; Gillberg, 2000). Among children and teenagers, there are more male cases than females but in adulthood equal numbers of both gender are affected. This suggests that the age of onset is earlier for males.

Among children and adolescents with schizophrenia, about a fifth have a single episode with a good outcome, about a third have a poor outcome involving persistent psychosis or multiple episodes with incomplete remission between episodes and the remainder (just under half) have a moderate outcome with two or more episodes with complete remission between episodes (Hollis, 2002). The following characteristics may be predictive of a good outcome (Asarnow et al., 2001, 2004; Asarnow & Asarnow, 2003; Hollis, 2002; Jablensky, 2000; Merry & Werry, 2001):

- low incidence of family psychopathology
- adolescent (rather than child)
- female (rather than male)
- good pre-morbid adjustment
- rapid onset in response to a precipitating stressful life event
- family history of affective disorder (rather than schizophrenia)
- additional affective features in the presentation of the case
- absence of negative symptoms
- absence of ongoing co-morbid drug abuse
- early treatment

- good initial response to neuroleptic medication
- supportive, non-critical, family and school placement.

Medication adherence is also an important prognostic factor. For adults, non-adherence ranges from about 40–50% and is associated with the following factors (Lacro, Dunn, Dolder, Leckband & Jeste, 2002):

- previous non-adherence
- poor insight
- negative attitude or subjective response towards medication
- substance abuse
- shorter illness duration
- inadequate discharge planning
- unsupportive after-care environment
- poorer therapeutic alliance.

CLINICAL FEATURES

The clinical features of schizophrenia are presented in Table 18.2 (American Academy of Child and Adolescent Psychiatry, 2001b; Hollis, 2002; McEvoy et al, 1999; National Collaborating Centre for Mental Health, 2003; Remschmidt, 2001). Psychotic episodes may last from one to six months, although some extend to a year. They are usually preceded by a prodromal period of a number of weeks, and in children there is usually a protracted insidious onset. Psychotic episodes may be shortened and the severity of symptomatology ameliorated through early detection and the use of pharmacological and psychological treatment as outlined below. Interepisode functioning may vary greatly and better interepisode functioning is associated with a better prognosis. The duration of remission between episodes may be lengthened through the use of maintenance medication, family intervention to reduce the amount of stress to which the adolescent is exposed and the use of stress-reducing coping strategies.

At a perceptual level, adolescents with schizophrenia describe a break-down in perceptual selectivity with difficulties focusing on essential information or stimuli to the exclusion of accidental details or background noise. In a florid psychotic state, internal stimuli (or thoughts) are interpreted as originating from another source and experienced as auditory hallucinations. Adolescents may perceive voices to vary along a number of dimensions. Voices may be construed as benign or malevolent, controlling or impotent, all-knowing or knowing little about the person, and the person may feel compelled to do what the voice says or not. Hallucinations that are perceived to be malevolent, controlling, all-knowing and which the adolescent feels compelled to obey are far more distressing than those which are not construed as having

Table 18.2 Clinical features of schizophrenia

Perception	• Breakdown in perceptual selectivity • Hallucinations
Thought	• Formal thought disorder • Delusions • Impaired judgement and reality testing • Confused sense of self
Emotion	• Prodromal anxiety and depression • Inappropriate affect • Flattened affect and impoverished affect • Post-psychotic depression
Behaviour	• Prodromal sleep disturbance • Prodromal impulsivity • Prodromal repetitive compulsive behaviour • Impaired goal-directed behaviour • Catatonia, negativism and mutism
Interpersonal adjustment	• Poor school performance • Withdrawal from peer relationships • Deterioration in family relationships

these attributes. Challenging those beliefs about voices which make them distressing to youngsters is central to the cognitive-behavioural treatment of hallucinations (Kuipers et al., in press).

At a cognitive level, formal thought disorder occurs in schizophrenia and is characterized by a difficulty following a logical train of thought from A to B. Judgement may be impaired and unusual significance accorded to unrelated events, so that delusions occur. Delusions, from a cognitive-behavioural perspective are beliefs or inferences that have been drawn to explain why a particular set of events has occurred. Delusions may vary in the degree of conviction with which they are held (from great certainty to little certainty), the degree to which the person is pre-occupied with them (the amount of time spent thinking about the belief) and the amount of distress they cause. From a cognitive-behavioural perspective these are the three main dimensions along which delusions and changes in delusional beliefs are assessed (Chadwick, Birchwood & Trower, 1996).

Particular sets of delusions may entail a confused sense of self, particularly paranoid delusions, where adolescents believe that they are being persecuted or punished for misdeeds, or delusions of control, where there is a belief that one's actions are controlled by others.

At an emotional level, during the prodromal phase anxiety or depression may occur in response to initial changes on perceptual selectivity and cognitive inefficiency, and a key part of relapse prevention is learning how to identify and manage prodromal changes in affect. During the florid phase, high arousal levels may occur in response to the experience of delusions and hallucinations. Inappropriate affect may be present particularly, in hebephrenic schizophrenia, where the youngster responds not to the external social context but to internal stimuli such as auditory hallucinations. Flattened affect may also occur, particularly in chronic cases where high levels of medication have been taken for extended time periods. In response to an episode of psychosis, the sense of loss may give rise to post-psychotic depression.

At a behavioural level, during the prodromal phase, sleep disturbance, impulsive behaviour and compulsive behaviour may be present. During psychotic episodes, goal-directed behaviour is impaired and in chronic cases, negativism, mutism and catatonia may occur.

At an interpersonal level, a deterioration in relationships with family members may occur. Social withdrawal from interaction with peers may occur and at school there is usually a marked decline in academic performance and participation in sports and non-academic activities such as music and drama.

THEORIES

Modern research on schizophrenia has been guided by two broad groups of theory. The first has been concerned largely with the role of biological factors in the aetiology and maintenance of the disorder. The second group of theories has addressed the role of psychological factors in schizophrenia. In addition, an increasing number of integrative diathesis–stress models of schizophrenia have been developed, which attempt to offer explanations for the interplay of a myriad of biological and psychological factors in the development and course of this very puzzling condition. Brief summaries of representative hypotheses from each of these groups of explanations will be presented below, along with comments on the degree to which the various positions are supported by available evidence. Salient points from this discussion are given in Table 18.3. Virtually all of the research that has been conducted to throw light on aetiological factors in schizophrenia has involved late adolescents or adults, not children (Asarnow & Asarnow, 2003; Hollis, 2002; Remschmidt, 2001). Caution is therefore required when making generalizations about schizophrenia in children and adolescents on the basis of this literature. However, the similarities between schizophrenia as it presents in children and adults suggest that there is considerable continuity from childhood to adulthood for this condition, and therefore it is quite likely that similar biological and psychological processes under-pin the disorder in both populations.

Table 18.3 Biological and psychosocial theories of schizophrenia

Type	Theory	Theoretical principles	Principals of treatment
Biological	**Genetic hypothesis**	A genetic pre-disposition renders some youngsters vulnerable to schizophrenia	Genetic counselling and medication
	Neurodevelopmental hypothesis	Pre- and peri-natal adversities which cause neuroanatomical abnormalities lead to schizophrenia in genetically vulnerable cases	Custodial care
	Dopamine hypothesis	Excessive activity in the mesolymbic dopaminergic system causes the symptoms of schizophrenia	Neuroleptic medication to rectify dopamine dysregulation
	Two-syndrome hypothesis	Type I schizophrenia is genetically determined and leads to positive symptoms associated with dysregulation of the dopamine system Type 2 schizophrenia is due to pre- or peri-natal brain damage and leads to negative symptoms	Use of neuroleptic medication to treat positive symptoms and supportive or operant rehabilitative interventions to treat negative symptoms
	Three-dimension hypothesis	Positive and negative symptoms and disorganization constitute the three dimensions of schizophrenia and each dimension is associated with a specific localized neurobiological deficit involving either the dopamine system or the connectivity of the CNS	Use of neuroleptic medication to treat positive symptoms and disorganization and supportive or operant rehabilitative interventions to treat negative symptoms

Continued

Table 18.3 continued

Type	Theory	Theoretical principles	Principals of treatment
Psychosocial theories	**Cognitive deficit hypothesis**	The many symptoms of schizophrenia arise from a core cognitive deficit or set of deficits such as the capacity to use stored information about environmental regularities to filter out irrelevant incoming stimuli from relevant stimuli	Reduce arousal, reduce ambient stimulation and simplify important messages to take account of processing deficits
	Cognitive bias hypothesis	Emotional concomitants of positive symptoms, particularly delusions and hallucinations reflect the operation of cognitive biases and distortions in information processing	Challenge emotional biases associated with negative emotional states using cognitive therapy
	Prodromal hypothesis	The onset of an episode of psychosis is heralded by a clearly identifiable prodromal dysphoric syndrome	Prevent relapses or shorten psychotic episodes by learning relapse signature and responding with early intervention when the prodromal syndrome occurs
	Social class hypothesis	The stresses of low socioeconomic status contribute to schizophrenia but also schizophrenia leads to downward social mobility	Supportive interventions that reduce external stressors and skills training to manage external stresses
	Stressful life events hypothesis	Stressful life events precipitate psychotic episodes	
	Family environment hypothesis	Expressed emotion (EE), affective style (AS) and communication deviance (CD) affect the course of schizophrenia, particularly relapse rate	Family intervention to reduce emotional intensity of family interactions and increase the clarity of communication

| Integrative hypothesis | Diathesis–stress model | When faced with stressful life events, genetically vulnerable individuals or those whose vulnerabilities derive from intrauterine adversity, develop symptomatology which is maintained by ongoing arousal producing stressful interactions with family members. They are particularly sensitive to environmental stimulation because of problematic information-process-ing selectivity deficits and biases | Neuroleptic medication to reduce arousal and stimulation sensitivity. Family intervention to reduce family stress. Cognitive-behaviour therapy to manage positive symptomatology |

Biological theories

Genetic, neurophysiological and neuroanatomical factors have all been implicated in the aetiology of schizophrenia (Asarnow & Asarnow, 2003; Hollis, 2002; Remschmidt, 2001). These factors have been studied within the context of the theories outlined in this section. The biological theories provide a rationale for the pharmacological treatment of schizophrenia and also for psychoeducational or rehabilitative approaches.

Genetic hypothesis

The genetic hypothesis argues that a biological pre-disposition which is genetically inherited renders some individuals vulnerable to schizophrenia. The results of the most carefully controlled adult genetic studies, indicate that the lifetime risk for developing schizophrenia is proportional to the amount of shared genes. For monozygotic twins the risk is 48%; for the children of two parents with schizophrenia the risk is 46%; for dizygotic twins or children with one affected parent, the risk is 17%; for children of those affected the risk is 13%; for grandchildren the risk is 5%; and for members of the general population the risk is 1% (Owen, O'Donovan & Gottesman, 2002; Scourfield & McGuffin, 2001). In the scant literature on the genetics of childhood schizophrenia, the rate of the disorder in parents is almost double that found in studies of adults, suggesting that childhood schizophrenia may represent a condition with a higher genetic loading than adult-onset schizophrenia. The genetic mechanisms of transmission are unknown and a focus for current gene mapping and chromosomal research. Various neurobiological and psychological abnormalities associated with schizophrenia have been found in relatives of people with the disorder. These include enlarged cerebral ventricles, absence of normal cerebral lateralization, eye tracking abnormalities and integrative neurological abnormalities (Murray & Castle, 2000). These findings suggest that what is genetically transmitted is a set of vulnerabilities to schizophrenia. Many people who have a genetic pre-disposition to schizophrenia do not develop the syndrome. It is therefore likely that some intrauterine, social or physical environmental factors must also contribute to the development of the condition.

Neurodevelopmental hypothesis

The neurodevelopmental hypothesis argues that factors in the pre-natal intrauterine environment and peri-natal neurological insults lead to atypical neuroanatomical development, which contribute to the emergence of schizophrenia. The risk of this outcome is increased in genetically vulnerable individuals exposed to other environmental stresses, including psychosocial adversity, stressful life events, chronic stressful social relationships, drug abuse and so forth. A growing body of evidence offers some support for this position (Harrison, 2000; Hollis, 2002; McGrath, Feron, Burne, Mackay-Sim & Eyles, 2003; Murray, 1994; Murray & Castle, 2000). Obstetric complications resulting in hypoxic–ischaemic damage and intrauterine exposure to maternal flu virus during the second trimester are both associated with increased risk of schizophrenia. The following neuroanatomical abnormalities have consistently emerged in neuroimaging and post-mortem studies of schizophrenia: progressively decreasing cortical volume in adolescence with loss of grey matter and abnormal distribution of white matter; enlarged cerebral ventricles (particularly the left ventricle) associated with reduction in brain mass; reduced size of the frontal lobes and reduced levels of neurological functioning in the frontal lobes; disproportional progressive loss of volume during adolescence of the temporal lobe, including the amygdala and the hippocampus; disarray of hippocampal neurons; a decrease in thalamic volume and absence of full lateralization. In addition to these macroscopic structural abnormalities, there is evidence that, in schizophrenia, neurons at many sites are smaller than expected, more closely packed and characterized by a lower density of dendrites, all indicating deficient connectivity between neurons. This may arise due to excessive synaptic and dendritic pruning in late childhood or early adolescence, probably a developmental process under genetic control (McGlashen & Hoffman, 2000).

The dopamine hypothesis

The original dopamine hypothesis suggests that schizophrenia is caused by a dysfunction of the mesolimbic dopaminergic system (Asarnow & Karatekin, 2000; Kahn & Davis, 1995). There is continued controversy over the precise nature of this dysfunction. An excess of dopamine, an excess of dopamine receptors or a supersensitivity of post-synaptic dopamine receptors are the principal dysfunctional mechanisms for which there is some empirical support. The theory is supported by studies of pharmacological treatment of schizophrenia, which show that the neuroleptic medication blocks dopamine activity in people with schizophrenia. However, these drugs do not act immediately. They affect only positive symptoms (such as delusions and hallucinations) and have little impact on negative symptoms (such as inactivity or poverty of speech). They rarely completely eliminate positive symptoms; nor are they effective for all people with schizophrenia. About 25% of people with schizophrenia do not respond to anti-psychotic medication. In the neurophysiological domain, the dopamine hypothesis will ultimately be replaced by a far more complex hypothesis involving a number of neurotransmitter systems including serotonin and glutamate, which have been shown to be dysregulated in schizophrenia (Harrison, 2000). However, as yet such proposals are still in their infancy.

Two-syndrome hypothesis

The two-syndrome hypothesis argues that a distinction may be made between type 1 schizophrenia, which is a genetically inherited disease marked by a dysregulation of the mesolimbic dopaminergic system and characterized by positive symptoms such as delusions and hallucinations on the one hand, and type 2 schizophrenia, which is a neurodevelopmental disorder arising from pre- or peri-natal insults and marked by chronic negative symptoms including restricted activity, blunted affect and poverty of speech (Crow, 1985). Type 1 schizophrenia, it is suggested, has an acute onset, clear precipitants, a good response to anti-psychotic medication and good interepisode adjustment. Poor pre-morbid functioning, an insidious onset, a chronic course, neuropsychological deficits and a poor response to medication are thought to characterize type 2 schizophrenia. The two-syndrome hypothesis is an attempt to draw together and integrate the lines of research that have followed from the genetic hypothesis, the dopamine hypothesis and its derivatives on the one hand, and the neurodevelopmental hypothesis on the other. The two-syndrome hypothesis fits a good proportion of available data but is probably an over-simplification, since many cases show aspects of both syndromes. It was the conceptual forerunner of the three-dimension hypothesis.

Three-dimension hypothesis

In the three-dimension hypothesis it is proposed that characteristic symptoms of schizophrenia constitute three independent dimensions: (1) positive symptoms (also called reality distortion), including delusions and hallucinations; (2) negative symptoms (also called psychomotor poverty), including decreased spontaneous activity, blunted affect and poverty of speech; and (3) disorganization marked by a formal thought disorder (which presents as illogical thinking), inappropriate affect and bizarre behaviour (Liddle, 2000). The wide variability in symptom profiles shown by people with a diagnosis of schizophrenia according to this hypothesis reflects variation in the status of different cases on these three dimensions. The hypothesis is supported by many factor-analytic studies of psychotic symptoms (Liddle, 1999) and the embryonic body of evidence which suggests that each of the three factors is associated with specific neurobiological abnormalities (Liddle, 2001). Disorganization symptoms may be associated with increased dopaminergic transmission and abnormal connections between the ventral frontal cortex and other neocortical areas. Positive symptoms may be associated with increased dopaminergic transmission in association with abnormal connections from the neocortex to the hippocampus. Negative symptoms may be associated with impaired connectivity between the frontal lobes and other cerebral areas. It is probable that genetic factors render individuals vulnerable to environmental stresses that disrupt the development of the nervous system. Significant environmental stresses include both intrauterine and psychosocial adversity. Two main aspects of the development of the nervous system become disrupted: (1) the long-distance neural connections between cerebral regions; and (2) the dopamine system.

Psychosocial theories

Psychological theories have focused on the cognitive deficits and biases present in schizophrenia and on the impact of proximal and distal stresses on the course of the disorder. Psychological theories have provided the rationale for cognitive-behavioural and other psychological therapies.

Cognitive deficit hypotheses

Cognitive deficit theory argues that schizophrenia is characterized by a core cognitive deficit, which under-pins the many symptoms that define the disorder, including delusions, hallucinations, thought disorder, inactivity, poverty of speech and so forth. Cognitive theories fall within the tradition which began with the work of Bleuler (1911), who attempted to explain the symptoms of schizophrenia in terms of the breaking of associative threads. More recent cognitive deficit hypotheses have attempted to explain schizophrenia in terms of specific cognitive deficits. Available evidence from experimental and neuropsychological studies of children, adolescents and adults suggests that most cases show deficits in executive functioning (including attention, memory, speed of information procession, flexibility in changing set, and planning) and in a proportion of cases this is accompanied by a general cognitive deficit (lower pre-morbid full-scale IQ and a drop in full-scale IQ following the onset of psychosis) (Asarnow & Karatekin, 2001; Braff, 1999; Harrison, 2000). Executive functioning deficits probably precede the onset of psychotic episodes and may be a psychological risk factor for the development of psychosis.

A particularly sophisticated cognitive deficit hypothesis has been offered by Hemsley (1996), who proposes that the core difficulty in schizophrenia is a breakdown in the relationship between stored information and current sensory input. Usually, stored memories on regularities such as particular social situations (like entering a shop to buy groceries), influence which aspects of a situation are attended to and which are ignored. Such stored information also influences our expectancies and interpretation of the situation. This process normally occurs automatically and rapidly. According to Hemsley, for people with a diagnosis of schizophrenia, this rapid automatic orientation to a new context does not occur. The similarity of the new situation to other similar situations is not automatically recognized. There is no clarity about which internal or external stimuli to attend to and which to ignore.

The theory offers a useful framework for understanding the clinical features of schizophrenia. Auditory hallucinations, within this frame of reference, are a result of the sensory over-load that arises from this filtering problem. Internal events are misinterpreted as sensations arising from external stimulation. Inappropriate affect, such as giggling accompanied by unusual gesturing, may occur in response to such hallucinations.

Delusional belief systems, according to Hemsley's theory, reflect efforts to impose meaningful relationships on the barrage of highly confusing external and internal stimuli and hallucinations that enter consciousness without filtering. For example, tactile hallucinations may be interpreted as receiving messages from the TV. Early on in schizophrenia, such attempts may be sufficient to lead to the development of an internally consistent belief system, as in the case of paranoid schizophrenia. However, with time, it may become too difficult to retain internal consistency in the belief system and so there may be a later progression to non-paranoid schizophrenia. Impaired judgement and reality testing due to sensory over-load may prevent adolescents with schizophrenia from checking the validity of delusional beliefs against the facts.

Psychophysiological studies show that in the prodromal period before an acute psychotic episode, patients become hyperaroused by ambient environmental stress and also become hyper-reactive to certain social and environmental stimuli (Hemsley, 1996). This hyperarousal disrupts the perceptual and cognitive processes, which are already to some degree impaired. If habituation does not occur, and arousal increases beyond a critical threshold, then disruption of perceptual and cognitive processes continues and a florid psychotic episode will occur. The experience of sensory over-load entailed by the inability to select out the essential from the incidental may lead to a breakdown in the capacity for logical thinking. An inability to coherently give an account that follows logical progression occurs and this is referred to as formal thought disorder.

Negative symptoms such as impoverished or flattened affect, impoverished speech, impaired goal-directed behaviour and social withdrawal may all reflect attempts on the youngster's part to cope with the intense experience of sensory over-load and a complete breakdown in the attentional filter that is normally employed to orient us to different types of situation and screen-out irrelevant internal and external stimuli.

Anti-psychotic medication and the psychological therapies described below aim to restore the capacity to manage sensory input, reduce the complexity of this input, and re-establish routines of living.

Cognitive bias theory

The cognitive-behavioural approach to schizophrenia, rather than addressing the syndrome as a whole, offers discrete explanations for individual symptoms or discrete methods for conducting therapy to alter specific symptoms (Haddock & Slade, 1996). A tenet held by many cognitive-behavioural theorists is that psychotic symptoms do not form a syndrome which reflects an underlying disease or disorder. They also deny that alterations in psychological functioning which occur in people with a diagnosis of schizophrenia are discontinuous with normal psychological processes. Rather, psychotic experiences are viewed as being on a continuum with normal experiences. Thus delusions are not meaningless but are strongly held irrational beliefs, the formation of which has been influenced by cognitive biases in the same way, for example, as depressive beliefs are formed in mood disorders. Chadwick et al. (1996) have offered a clinically useful theoretical analysis of hallucinations and delusions in terms of an ABC framework: Activating events trigger Beliefs based on inferences and attributions and these ways of thinking about the activating events lead to emotional and behavioural Consequence. They argue that hallucinations (which are activating events) are loud thoughts that have been misattributed to other sources and about which inferences of power and need for compliance have been made, and that these beliefs lead to distressing emotions and behaviour, which are a consequence of the beliefs. The cognitive therapy of hallucinations involves challenging beliefs about the power of the voices and the importance of complying with the commands of the voices. When these are altered through collaborative empirical testing in therapy, then the emotional distress and related behaviour abate. Delusions are explained as beliefs or inferences, which have been constructed to make sense of particular activating events and lead to various negative consequences, including distressing emotions and behaviour. When these are altered through collaborative empirical testing in therapy, then the emotional distress and related behaviour abate. A growing body of evidence shows that treatment based on this type of analysis of psychotic symptoms ameliorates targeted symptoms (Haddock & Slade, 1996).

Prodromal hypothesis

The prodromal hypothesis argues that individuals with schizophrenia experience a prodromal set of symptoms, largely perceptual hypersensitivity and cognitive information-processing deficits, which herald the onset of a psychotic episode. These prodromal symptoms are exacerbated by inferences and attributions made by the adolescents about the controllability and origins of their unusual prodromal perceptual and cognitive experiences, and these attributions increase arousal and accelerate the onset of the relapse. Cognitive-behavioural interventions made during the prodromal period which target attributions, or pharmacological interventions which target alterations in perceptual and information-processing functions, should, according to the theory, prevent relapse or reduce the severity of the relapse (Birchwood, 1996; Birchwood, Spencer & McGovern, 2000).

Clinical studies have identified four stages in the development of a psychotic episode (Birchwood, 1996). In the first stage there is a feeling of a loss of control over cognitive and perceptual processes as a breakdown in perceptual selectivity occurs. This may be accompanied by a feeling of heightened awareness and mental efficiency and yet an inability to prevent internal and external events from invading consciousness. A sense of anxiety (a fear of going crazy) may occur at this point.

In the second stage, depression characterized by low mood, low self-esteem, social withdrawal, poor school performance and vegetative features such as sleep disruption occur in reaction to the deterioration of cognitive processes. Some youngsters try to cope with this deterioration by engaging in compulsive rituals that will give them a sense that they can impose order on what is an increasingly chaotic experience.

In the third stage, disinhibition occurs and youngsters act impulsively, giving free reign to aggression, self-destruction, sexual urges, wishes to travel and so forth. This impulsivity may lead adolescents, particularly, to create social situations in which they become exposed to high levels of stimulation, which in turn may precipitate the onset of florid psychotic symptoms. For example, becoming involved in fights, atypical sexual encounters or impulsively travelling a long distance may all lead to complex unpredictable and highly stressful experiences, which will be perceived as all the more stressful because of the breakdown in perceptual selectivity.

In the fourth stage, pre-psychotic thinking occurs, with frequent perceptual misinterpretations and delusional explanations given for them. Often, these delusional explanations involve ideas of reference or paranoid ideation. Thus, as perceptual processes become more dysfunctional, youngsters continue to try to make sense of their very unusual experiences by developing beliefs that are at variance with the culture and their usual belief systems.

It appears that each patient has his or her own unique 'relapse signature' with specific experiences occurring in a unique order, but following this broad four-stage model. Learning the pattern of this prodromal phase and developing a relapse drill to manage the escalation of psychotic symptoms can minimize deterioration and improve relapse management. Studies show that the shorter the duration of the untreated illness, the less likely the patient is to relapse in the subsequent two-year period (Birchwood, 1996; Birchwood et al., 2000).

Social class hypothesis

The social class hypothesis argues that stresses associated with low socioeconomic status probably contribute to the genesis of schizophrenia. The social drift hypothesis, in contrast, argues that people diagnosed as having schizophrenia are probably ill equipped to deal with the pressures associated with upward mobility and so drift into a lower socioeconomic bracket. This in turn may create stresses which exacerbate their coping problems. Available evidence supports both hypotheses. There is an inverse relationship between social class and schizophrenia and, following diagnosis, social drift occurs (Dohrenwend et al., 1992). However, the relationship between social class and schizophrenia is not a specific relationship. Many other psychological problems are more common in lower socioeconomic groups.

Stressful life events theory

That schizophrenia is a reaction to a build-up of life stress is the core tenet of this theory. A large body of evidence shows that stressful life events may precipitate a schizophrenic episode and contribute to variation in the severity of symptoms over time (Norman & Malla, 1993). However, people with schizophrenia do not report higher levels of stressful events than the general population or than those with other disorders. Bebbington et al. (1996) found a strong relationship between life events and the onset of psychotic episodes which was not influenced by social class, ethnicity or marital status.

Family environment theory

Recent theories about the role of the family in schizophrenia argue that regular intense, confusing or threatening interactions with family members may precipitate a relapse, increase the need for anti-psychotic medication or exacerbate symptomatology during a psychotic episode (Asarnow et al., 2001; Asarnow & Asarnow, 2003). The implication is that the impaired perceptual selectivity and cognitive information-processing deficits associated with schizophrenia make intense, confusing or threatening social stimuli very difficult to cope with. A further implication of this type of theory is that interventions which help family members to reduce the amount of intense, confusing or threatening interactions to which the youngster is exposed will reduce the relapse rate and need for medication.

Expressed emotion, a combined measure of criticism and over-involvement obtained in an individual interview with a parent have been shown to be related to the course of schizophrenia in adults and adolescents (Asarnow et al., 2001; Asarnow & Asarnow, 2003; Jablensky, 2000). While most current work on the family environment and schizophrenia focuses on the expressed emotion construct, the constructs of communication deviance and affective style have both been shown to be more prevalent in families with an adolescent member with a diagnosis of schizophrenia (Doane, West & Goldstein, 1981). Affective style is rated from transcripts of family interaction and more families containing a member with a diagnosis of schizophrenia show predominantly critical or intrusive interaction patterns. Communication deviance is assessed on the basis of parental responses to stimuli from the Rorschach test administered in a one-to-one context, but is interpreted as being reflective of family members' difficulties in maintaining a focus when engaged in joint problem solving. With communication deviance, an amorphous pattern of thinking may occur where there is little differentiation and communications are vague or a fragmented pattern where there is much differentiation by little integration of ideas. There is a growing consensus that expressed emotion and affective style probably reflect parental responses to the disorganized and bizarre behaviour characteristic of schizophrenia. There is also some consensus that communication deviance may reflect a genetic trait which finds expression as a sub-clinical thought disorder process in the parents.

The strongest evidence for the family environment hypothesis comes from intervention studies, which have shown that reducing the level of criticism and over-involvement in families with schizophrenic members reduces the need for medication, greatly prolongs the interepisode interval and significantly reduces the relapse rate (Tarrier, 1996).

Diathesis–stress theories

While early research on schizophrenia was guided by simple single-factor theories, since the publication of Zubin and Spring's paper *Vulnerability: a new view of schizophrenia*, in 1977, there have been increasingly numerous attempts to provide over-arching multi-factorial models of schizophrenia which provide a framework for integrating the results of research from a variety of biological and psychosocial perspectives (Nuechterlin & Dawson, 1984; Zubin & Ludwig, 1983). Typically, these have been termed diathesis–stress models. They argue that for the symptoms of schizophrenia to occur, a biologically vulnerable individual must be exposed to environmental stress. The interaction of the vulnerability factors with the stress factors leads to the occurrence of the symptomatology. This is subsequently maintained by ongoing exposure to environmental stress and by the way in which the person reacts to this stress and copes with the unusual experiences associated with schizophrenia. For clinicians and researchers alike, the challenge is to work out the vulnerabilities and stresses present in each case and the processes of interaction linking the two classes of factors. A diathesis–stress model of schizophrenia is presented in Figure 18.3. The model shows how genetic factors and intrauterine adversities may lead to a biological vulnerability to schizophrenia. This vulnerability may take the form of neurophysiological and neuroanatomical abnormalities. This biological vulnerability under-pins a psychological vulnerability, which includes perceptual and cognitive infor-mation-processing deficits. As part of the process of attempting to manage these unusual perceptual and cognitive experiences, cognitive distortions and misattributions may occur, which lead to a perception of internal stimuli (such as hallucinations) and external stimuli as threatening, as evidenced by anxiety-provoking delusions. The cognitive deficits and distortions lead to hyperarousal. With exposure to stressful life events, stresses associated with low socioeconomic status and stress associated with the family's response to pre-psychotic or psychotic symptomatology, hyperarousal and cognitive deficits and distortions may become exacerbated. This may lead in the first instance to the onset of a psychotic episode or subsequently to the main-tenance of psychotic experiences or relapse. This type of model has clear implications for intervention. Anti-psychotic medication may target the dys-regulation of the dopaminergic system. Family interventions may be used to reduce the stressfulness of family interactions. Cognitive-behavioural interventions may be employed to facilitate coping with positive symptoms. Contingency management may be used to increase activity levels and alter negative symptoms.

ASSESSMENT

In the management of cases of suspected childhood or adolescent psychosis, the first priority is to assess risk of self-harm or harm to others. Occasionally, prodromal impulsivity may lead to dangerous behaviour, and this requires management following the guidelines set out in the Chapter 16.

The next priority is to clarify symptomatology and exclude other conditions such as autism, drug-induced psychosis, mood problems and

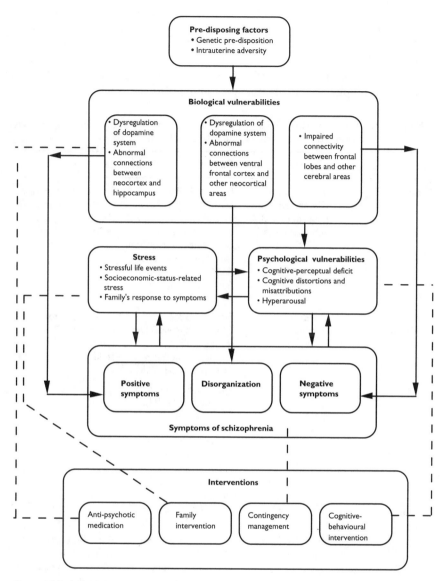

Figure 18.3 A diathesis–stress model of schizophrenia

obsessive-compulsive disorder. Careful interviewing using the diagnostic criteria set out in Table 18.1 is important here. Psychosis modules from structured interviews (listed in Table 3.11) may be used, especially the CAPA, CAS and KSADS. Standardized rating scales may also be useful is making a diagnosis. Rating scales for the full constellation of psychotic symptomatology and for specific symptoms are listed in Table 18.4. Careful observation, and a series of interviews with multiple informants over a number of sessions, will typically be necessary to assess symptomatology. Multi-disciplinary involvement is particularly important in cases where youngsters present with psychotic features. From the earliest stages in these cases, teamwork between clinical psychology and psychiatry is recommended.

Table 18.4 Psychometric instruments that may be used as an adjunct to clinical interviews in the assessment of psychosis and related constructs

Construct	Instrument	Publication	Comments
Diagnosis	Interview for Childhood Disorders and Schizophrenia	Russell, A., Bott, L. Sammons, C. (1989). The phenomenology of schizophrenia occurring in childhood. *Journal of the American Academy of Child and Adolescent Psychiatry*, 29, 399–407	Structured interview for the assessment of children's psychotic symptomatology
Change in psychiatric symptomatology	Children's Psychiatric Rating scale	Fish, B. (1985). Children's Psychiatric Rating scale. *Psychopharmacology Bulletin*, 21, 753–765	Rating scale for psychotic symptomatology in children
		Spencer, E., Alpert, M., & Pouget, E. (1994). Scales for the assessment of neuroleptic response in schizophrenic children. Specific measures derived from the CPRS. *Psychopharmacology Bulletin*, 30, 199–202	
	Brief Psychiatric Rating Scale	Overall, J. & Gorman, D. (1988). Brief Psychiatric Rating Scale: Recent developments in ascertainment and scaling. *Psychopharmacology Bulletin*, 24, 97–99	Assesses psychotic symptomatology on 24 seven-point scales and yields an overall index of psychopathology. This measure is sensitive to change and so good for measuring improvement, but poor for initial diagnosis

		Woerner, M., Mannuzza, S. & Kane, J. (1988). Anchoring the BPRS: An aid to improved reliability. *Psychopharmacology Bulletin*, 24, 112–117	
		Lukoff, D., Nuechterlein, K. Ventura, J. (1986). Manual for expanded Brief Psychiatric Rating Scale (BRS). *Schizophrenia Bulletin*, 12, 594–602	
	Present State Examination Change Rating Scale	Tres, K., Bellenis, C., Brownlow, J., Livinston, G. & Leff, J. (1987). Present State Examination Change Rating Scale. *British Journal of Psychiatry*, 150, 201–207	Assess short-term changes in symptomatology
Positive and negative symptoms in children	Positive and Negative Syndrome Scale for Children and Adolescents	Fields, J., Kay, S., Grosch, D., Alexander, G. et al (1991). *Positive and negative syndrome scale for children and adolescents (KIDDIE-PANSS) Interview Guide.* Toronto: Multi-Health Systems Inc	Rating scales for measuring positive and negative symptoms in children
Formal thought disorder in children	The Kiddie Formal Thought Disorder Rating Scales	Caplan,, R. Guthrie, D., Fish, B., Tanguay, P., & David-Lando, G. (1989). The Kiddie formal thought disorder rating scales: Clinical assessment, reliability and validity. *Journal of the American Academy of Child and Adolescent Psychiatry*, 28, 408–416	Rating scales for measuring thought disorder in children

Continued

Table 18.4 continued

Construct	Instrument	Publication	Comments
	Thought Disorder Index	Arboleda, C. & Holtzman, P. (1985). Thought disorder in children at risk for psychosis. *Archives of General Psychiatry*, 42, 1004–1013	Rating scales for measuring thought disorder in children
Delusional experiences in adolescents and adults	Dimensional Ratings	Brett-Jones, J., Garety, P. & Hemsley, D. (1987). Measuring delusional experiences: A method and its application. *British Journal of Clinical Psychology*, 26, 257–265	Beliefs are elicited and patients give ratings for level of conviction and pre-occupation. The interviewer rates degree of interference in everyday life and reaction to hypothetical contradiction
Hallucinations in adolescents and adults	Visual Analogue Scale	Hustig, H. & Hanfer, R. (1990). Persistent auditory hallucinations and their relationship to delusions and mood. *Journal of Nervous and Mental Disease*, 178, 264–267	Visual analogue scale for assessing loudness, clarity, distress and distractibility are described in this paper
Insight in adolescents and adults	Insight Scale	Birchwood, M., Smith, J., Drury, V., Healy, J. & Slade, M. (1994). A self-report insight scale for psychosis: reliability, validity and sensitivity to change. *Acta Psychiatrica Scandinavica*, 89, 62–67	Eight statements are scored on scales from 0 to 2. The items ask about need for medication; need for a doctor or hospitalization; acknowledgement of the illness; relabelling of psychotic experiences
Favourable attitude to medication and compliance	Drug Attitudes Inventory	Hogan, T., Awad, A. & Eastwood R. (1983). A self report scale predictive of drug compliance in schizophrenics: reliability and discriminative validity. *Psychological Medicine*, 13, 177–183	A 10-item self-report scale to measure attitudes to medication, predicative of compliance

Parents' knowledge of schizophrenia	Knowledge About Schizophrenia Interview (KASI)	Barrowclough, C., Tarrier, N., Watts, S., Vaughan, C., Bamrah, J. & Freeman, H. (1987). Assessing the functional value of relatives reported knowledge about schizophrenia. *British Journal of Psychiatry*, 151, 1–8	Assesses relatives' knowledge about diagnosis, symptomatology, aetiology, medication, prognosis, management
Parents' burden of care	Parental Stress	Fadden, G., Kupiers, I. & Bebbington, P. (1985). The burden of care: The impact of functional psychiatric illness on the patient's family. *British Journal of Psychiatry*, 150, 285–292	Assesses the impact of schizophrenia on carers
Family problems for adolescents and adults	Family Questionnaire	Barrowclough, C. & Tarrier, N. (1987). A behavioural family intervention with a schizophrenic patient: A case study. *Behavioural Psychotherapy*, 15, 252–271	A 50-item checklist of problems typically encountered in families with a psychotic member

Specific categories of pre-disposing, precipitating, maintaining and protective factors deserving assessment where psychotic features are the central concern are set out in Figure 18.4. These areas should be covered within the context of the assessment protocol set out in Chapter 4.

Pre-disposing factors

Both personal and contextual factors may pre-dispose youngsters to developing psychotic symptoms. At a personal level, a genetic vulnerability as indicated by a family history of disorders on the psychotic or schizophrenia spectrum may pre-dispose youngsters to developing schizophrenia. Youngsters may also develop a vulnerability to schizophrenia as a result of intrauterine adversity, as indicated by obstetric complications or maternal illness, particularly viral infection during pregnancy. Dysregulation of the dopaminergic mesolimbic system and neuroanatomical abnormalities, notably enlarged ventricles, may also pre-dispose adolescents to developing schizophrenia, although these biological factors are rarely assessed as a

PRE-DISPOSING FACTORS

PERSONAL PRE-DISPOSING FACTORS

Biological factors
- Genetic vulnerability
- Intrauterine adversity
- Dysregulation of dopaminergic mesolimbic system
- Neuroanatomical abnormalities
- Insidious onset

CONTEXTUAL PRE-DISPOSING FACTORS

Exposure to family problems in early life
- Social disadvantage
- Family disorganization

PERSONAL PROTECTIVE FACTORS

Biological factors
- Good physical health

Psychological factors
- Good pre-morbid functioning
- Acute onset
- Clear precipitant
- Positive symptoms
- Additional affective features
- Awareness of prodromal symptoms
- Female
- Older
- High IQ
- Easy temperament
- High self-esteem
- Internal locus of control
- High self-efficacy
- Optimistic attributional style
- Mature defence mechanisms
- Functional coping strategies

PERSONAL MAINTAINING FACTORS

Biological factors
- Dysregulation of dopaminergic mesolimbic system
- Hyperarousal

Psychological factors
- Lack of insight
- Cognitive distortions and misattributions
- Dysfunctional coping strategies

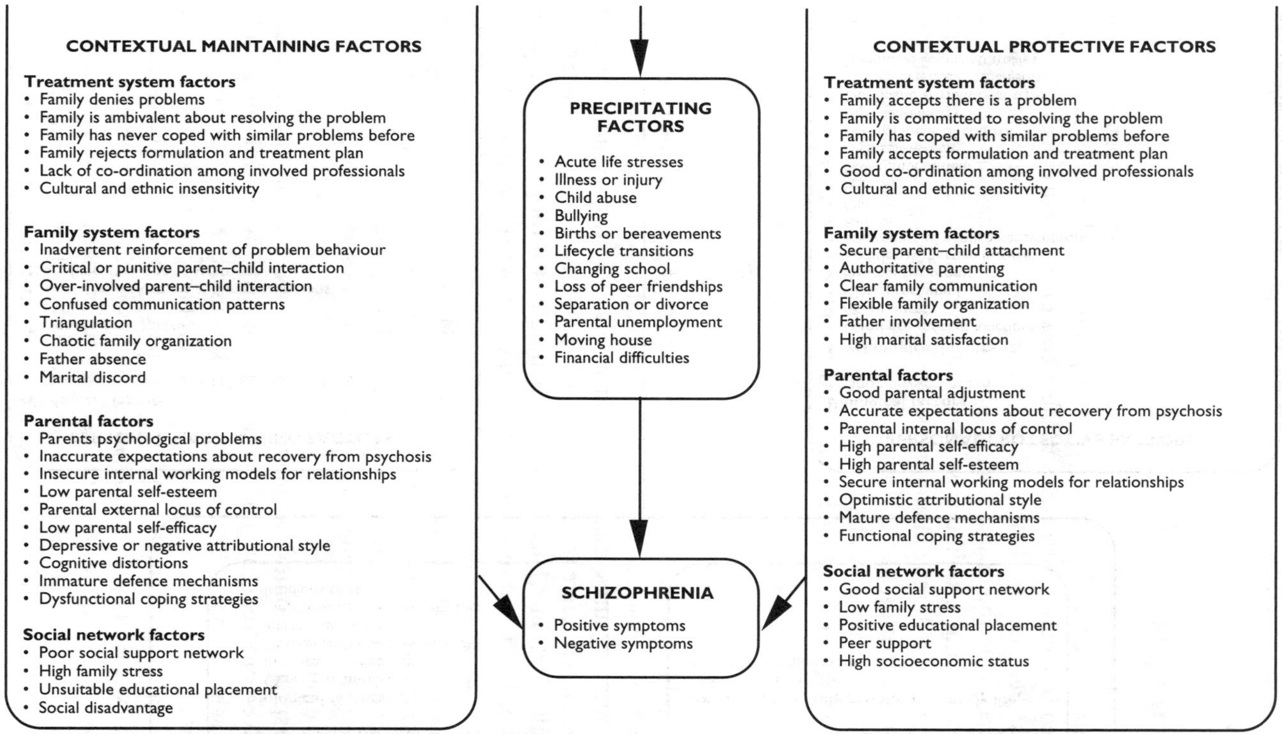

CONTEXTUAL MAINTAINING FACTORS

Treatment system factors
- Family denies problems
- Family is ambivalent about resolving the problem
- Family has never coped with similar problems before
- Family rejects formulation and treatment plan
- Lack of co-ordination among involved professionals
- Cultural and ethnic insensitivity

Family system factors
- Inadvertent reinforcement of problem behaviour
- Critical or punitive parent–child interaction
- Over-involved parent–child interaction
- Confused communication patterns
- Triangulation
- Chaotic family organization
- Father absence
- Marital discord

Parental factors
- Parents psychological problems
- Inaccurate expectations about recovery from psychosis
- Insecure internal working models for relationships
- Low parental self-esteem
- Parental external locus of control
- Low parental self-efficacy
- Depressive or negative attributional style
- Cognitive distortions
- Immature defence mechanisms
- Dysfunctional coping strategies

Social network factors
- Poor social support network
- High family stress
- Unsuitable educational placement
- Social disadvantage

CONTEXTUAL PROTECTIVE FACTORS

Treatment system factors
- Family accepts there is a problem
- Family is committed to resolving the problem
- Family has coped with similar problems before
- Family accepts formulation and treatment plan
- Good co-ordination among involved professionals
- Cultural and ethnic sensitivity

Family system factors
- Secure parent–child attachment
- Authoritative parenting
- Clear family communication
- Flexible family organization
- Father involvement
- High marital satisfaction

Parental factors
- Good parental adjustment
- Accurate expectations about recovery from psychosis
- Parental internal locus of control
- High parental self-efficacy
- High parental self-esteem
- Secure internal working models for relationships
- Optimistic attributional style
- Mature defence mechanisms
- Functional coping strategies

Social network factors
- Good social support network
- Low family stress
- Positive educational placement
- Peer support
- High socioeconomic status

PRECIPITATING FACTORS
- Acute life stresses
- Illness or injury
- Child abuse
- Bullying
- Births or bereavements
- Lifecycle transitions
- Changing school
- Loss of peer friendships
- Separation or divorce
- Parental unemployment
- Moving house
- Financial difficulties

SCHIZOPHRENIA
- Positive symptoms
- Negative symptoms

Figure 18.4 Factors to take into account in the assessment of schizophrenia

routine part of assessment. At a contextual level, a history of family dis-organization and social disadvantage may pre-dispose youngsters to develop-ing schizophrenia.

Precipitating factors

Schizophrenia may have an acute or an insidious onset; prognosis in the former case is better. The onset of an episode of schizophrenia may be precipitated by a build-up of stressful life events or the occurrence of lifecycle transitions. Personal or family illness or injury, child abuse or bullying may all precipitate the onset of schizophrenia. So too may the transition to adolescence, having a sibling leave home, the birth of a sibling or bereave-ments within the family. Parental separation, moving house, changing schools, losing friends, parental unemployment or increased financial hard-ship within the family may all precipitate the onset of a psychotic episode. All of these events place a sudden increase in demands on the youngster's coping resources.

Maintaining factors

Psychotic problems may be maintained by a range of personal and contextual factors. Delusions and related negative emotional experiences may be main-tained through cognitive distortions that involve selective misinterpretation of stimuli in a self-referent way, such as interpreting a car horn as an enemy signal. Hallucination-related distress is maintained through negative inter-pretations of hallucinations, for example interpreting voices as belonging to the devil and as having the power to force one to behave in distressing ways. Dysfunctional coping strategies, such as social withdrawal, may maintain negative symptoms, such as inactivity and poverty of speech. At a biological level, hyperarousal may maintain the condition by making it more likely that hallucinations and delusions will occur and more attractive to engage in negative symptoms.

With respect to contextual maintaining factors, patterns of interaction that involve confused communication, criticism or over-involvement may maintain schizophrenia by leading to a sustained level of stress-related hyperarousal. These types of interaction are probably more likely to occur in chaotically organized families, in families where there is marital discord and in families where the father is relatively uninvolved. Such communication may also occur in families where the adolescent is triangulated into parental conflict, with one parent taking an over-involved stance with respect to the adolescent and the other adopting a critical position. The symptoms of schizophrenia may be maintained, too, through inadvertent reinforcement by well-meaning family members who respond positively to the adolescent's symptoms.

Such patterns of parenting and family organization may be partially maintained by parents' personal experience of personal psychological difficulties. Where parents have insecure internal working models for relationships, low self-esteem, low self-efficacy, an external locus of control, immature defences and poor coping strategies, their resourcefulness in managing their children's difficulties may be compromised. Parents may also become involved in problem-maintaining interactions with their adolescents if they have inaccurate knowledge about schizophrenia and are unaware of the importance of the family in creating a low-stress environment to aid recovery and prevent relapse.

Psychotic symptoms may also be maintained by high levels of stress, limited support and social disadvantage within the family's wider social system, since these features may deplete parents' and siblings' personal resources for dealing constructively with the adolescent's condition. Educational placements which are poorly resourced and where teaching staff have little time to devote to home–school liaison meetings may also maintain psychotic symptoms, especially if teachers interact with the adolescent in critical or over-involved ways.

Within the treatment system, a lack of co-ordination and clear communication among involved professionals, including family physicians, paediatricians, psychiatrists, nurses, teachers, psychologists and so forth, may maintain psychotic problems. It is not unusual for various members of the professional network to offer conflicting opinions and advice on the nature and management of schizophrenia to adolescents and their families. These may range from viewing the child as ill and requiring medication only for the management of the illness to seeing the child as healthy but deviant and deserving punitive management. Where co-operation problems between families and treatment teams develop, and families deny the existence of the problems, the validity of the diagnosis and formulation, or the appropriateness of the treatment programme, then the child's difficulties may persist. Treatment systems that are not sensitive to the cultural and ethnic beliefs and values of the youngster's family system may maintain psychotic symptoms by inhibiting engagement or promoting drop-out from treatment and preventing the development of a good working alliance between the treamtent team, the youngster and his or her family. Parents' lack of experience in dealing with similar problems in the past is a further factor that may compromise their capacity to work co-operatively with the treatment team and so may contribute to the maintenance of the child's difficulties.

Protective factors

The probability that a treatment programme will be effective is influenced by a variety of personal and contextual protective factors. It is important that these be assessed and included in the later formulation, since it is protective factors that usually serve as the foundation for therapeutic change. Good pre-morbid functioning, an acute onset and a clear precipitant are all associated with a better outcome. In terms of good pre-morbid functioning, a high IQ, an easy temperament, high self-esteem, an internal locus of control, high self-efficacy, an optimistic attributional style and physical fitness are all important personal protective factors. Other important personal protective factors include mature defence mechanisms and functional coping strategies, particularly good problem-solving skills and a capacity to make and maintain friendships. A better outcome occurs for females rather than males and for adolescents rather than children. If there are additional affective features or a family history of affective disorders rather than schizophrenia there is a better prognosis.

Within the family, secure parent–child attachment and authoritative parenting are central protective factors, particularly if they occur within the context of a flexible family structure in which there is clear communication, high marital satisfaction and both parents share the day-to-day tasks of child care. Lower levels of family psychopathology are associated with better outcome.

Good parental adjustment is also a protective factor. Where parents have an internal locus of control, high self-efficacy, high self-esteem, internal working models for secure attachments, an optimistic attributional style, mature defences and functional coping strategies, then they are better resourced to manage their children's difficulties constructively. Accurate knowledge about schizophrenia is also a protective factor.

Within the broader social network, high levels of support, low levels of stress and membership of a high socioeconomic group are all protective factors for adolescents with schizophrenia. Where families are embedded in social networks that provide a high level of support and place few stressful demands on family members, then it is less likely that parents' and children's resources for dealing with schizophrenia will become depleted. A well-resourced educational placement may also be viewed as a protective factor. Educational placements where teachers have sufficient time and flexibility to attend home–school liaison meetings if invited to do so contribute to positive outcomes for adolescents with schizophrenia.

Within the treatment system, co-operative working relationships between the treatment team and the family, and good co-ordination of multi-professional input are protective factors. Treatment systems that are sensitive to the cultural and ethnic beliefs and values of the youngster's family are more likely to help families engage with, and remain in treatment, and foster the development of a good working alliance. Families are more likely to benefit from treatment when they accept the formulation of the problem given by the treatment team and are committed to working with the team to resolve it. Where families have successfully faced similar problems before, then they are more likely to benefit from treatment and in this sense previous experience with similar problems is a protective factor.

FORMULATION

The formulation should specify how specific precipitating factors triggered the onset of the psychosis and the pre-disposing factors that rendered the youngster vulnerable to developing the condition. The way in which the condition and its symptoms are maintained by patterns of interaction and intrapsychic factors, particularly cognitive distortions and attributions should be specified. Protective factors which have a bearing on prognosis should also be mentioned.

TREATMENT

The approach to management of schizophrenia set out here is based on a view of schizophrenia as a recurrent episodic condition, which is currently only partially understood and for which there is no cure or definitive solution. Pharmacological and psychological treatment aim to alter the course of the condition by shortening active periods and lengthening periods of remission so that children and adolescents with this condition may lead as normal a lifestyle as possible.

A diagnosis of schizophrenia according to ICD 10 criteria cannot be made for a month and, with DSM IV TR, a period of six months is required. In practice, with both first-episode cases and cases which are referred because of relapses, the best approach is to intervene immediately, with both pharmacological and psychosocial interventions, to ameliorate the psychotic symptoms and support the adolescent and family. Early intervention is important, since if left untreated youngsters may develop entrenched delusional belief systems and patterns of dysfunctional behaviour involving negative symptoms. Furthermore, patterns of family interaction may evolve which maintain these symptoms.

Treatment for adolescents and young adults with a diagnosis of schizophrenia should be multi-modal and multi-systemic and include the following components (American Academy of Child and Adolescent Psychiatry, 2001b; British Psychological Society Division of Clinical Psychology, 2000; McEvoy et al., 1999; National Collaborating Centre for Mental Health, 2003):

- Pharmacological therapy to control positive symptoms, including delusions, hallucinations and associated interventions to ensure adherence.
- Family intervention to help family members understand the concept of

schizophrenia and interact with the adolescent in a way that is maximally supportive and minimally stressful.

- Individual or group-based cognitive-behavioural therapy focused on helping the adolescent understand the disorder, cope with its symptoms and control environmental stress levels.
- Contingency management targeting negative symptoms.
- Group work for parents to provide them with education and support.

Unfortunately, most of the research on treatment, which informs the discussion below, has been conducted with adults. Until trials with children and adolescents have been reported, treatment of younger cases is guided by the results of studies conducted on adult populations.

Pharmacological treatment

Treatment with first-generation anti-psychotic drugs (such as chlorpromazine, haloperidol, flupenthixol) or second-generation anti-psychotic preparations (such as clozapine, risperidone, olanzapine and sertindome) are the main approaches to pharmacological intervention for psychotic conditions in children and adolescents (Fonagy et al., 2002; Perry, Alexander & Liskow, 1997). While these anti-psychotic agents control positive symptoms of schizophrenia, they have short-term side effects, such as parkinsonism, which is often controlled by an anti-parkinsonism agent such as cogentin. Tardive dyskinesia, an irreversible neurological condition, is one of the tragic long-term side effects of neuroleptic drug usage. For this reason, the lowest possible dose of neuroleptic medication should be used.

For a considerable proportion of people with a diagnosis of schizophrenia, residual positive symptoms including hallucinations and delusions persist. Many patients on medication, while not actively psychotic, develop negative symptoms, including restricted affect, limited speech and a lack of goal-directed behaviour. Despite pharmacological treatment, up to 80% of cases relapse within two to five years, especially if low dosages of medication are used to minimize side effects (Tarrier, 1994). For these reasons, individual and family-based psychological interventions are particularly important for people with a diagnosis of schizophrenia.

Family intervention

Over thirty randomized clinical trials with adolescents and adults with a diagnosis of schizophrenia have shown that multi-modal programmes involving anti-psychotic medication and family intervention are more effective than medication alone (McFarlane, Dixon, Lukens & Lucksted, 2003). Multi-modal programmes which include family intervention reduce relapse rates and improve both the youngster's recovery and the family's well-being. Such programmes aim to educate youngsters and families about schizophrenia and equip them to manage it as effectively as possible. Effective intervention combines family work with pharmacological treatment in an integrative and co-ordinated way, as described in treatment manuals (Falloon, Laporta, Fadden & Graham-Hole, 1993; Kuipers, Leff & Lam, 2002). Programmes typically span nine to twelve months and are usually offered in a phased format, with three months of weekly sessions, three months of fortnightly sessions, three months of monthly sessions and three-monthly reviews and crisis intervention as required. With respect to the content and process of treatment programmes, a number of core elements typify effective family-based interventions for schizophrenia. First, during the engagement phase an emphasis is placed on blame reduction, the positive role family members can play in the rehabilitation of the family member with schizophrenia and the degree to which the family intervention will alleviate some of the family's burden of care. Second, effective family intervention programmes for schizophrenia include psychoeducation, specifically targeting the unique difficulties that families face when coping with schizophrenia. Third, most programmes address medication adherence. Fourth, effective programmes include communication and problem-solving skills training. Fifth, most programmes incorporate, in addition, a variety of routine family therapy techniques such as externalizing the problem, re-framing and relapse prevention. Effective family intervention begins with a thorough assessment, and intervention plans are based on the formulation that arises from the assessment. Specific instruments for assessing family knowledge of schizophrenia, family problems associated with caring for a person with schizophrenia and burden of care for the family are listed in Table 18.4. Patterns of family interaction that have evolved around the youngster's symptoms, which may inadvertently be exacerbating the symptoms, should be assessed in particular detail.

Engagement

During the engagement phase, adopting a non-blaming stance with respect to the parents is particularly important since many parents inappropriately blame themselves for the occurrence of their child's symptoms. Following a thorough assessment of the teenager's symptoms over a period of weeks, a diagnosis of psychosis may be given, usually by the physician involved in the case. After six months, a DSM IV TR diagnosis of schizophrenia may be given. In either case, relatives are informed that the adolescent has a condition – either psychosis or schizophrenia – which is due to the interaction of a vulnerability towards the disorder with a build-up of life stress. Evidence for both the pre-disposition and the build-up of life stress should be drawn from the history constructed during the assessment phase. The teenager and the family are then invited to participate in a series of sessions at their home or in the clinic to help them understand the condition and how best to manage it and prevent relapse. This invitation may be met with resistance, since families may have had negative therapy experiences in the past, be suspicious of the therapist or fear being blamed or making things worse.

When faced with resistance, the three important strategies to adopt are first to be persistent and regularly represent the invitation to participate in therapy; second to be positive and concerned in all contacts with family members at which invitations to engage in therapy are offered; third to be flexible about the time and place where appointments are offered.

In conducting home-based family sessions, it is important to convey to the family that the sessions are occasions for working on methods for handling problems rather than social visits. The main dangers to be avoided are being so businesslike as to be rude on the one hand and allowing casual social conversation to take over the session on the other.

The rationale for family treatment should be that living with an adolescent who has schizophrenia is stressful, and implementing a home-based care plan for the adolescent is demanding and complex, and families may benefit from guidance with this. Also, adolescents with schizophrenia are sensitive to stress from others, for example the sort that is expressed when someone has had a hard day, and a family support programme may help the family member develop skills to shield the adolescent from this type of spill-over.

Working in a co-therapy team

Working with families where a teenager has a diagnosis of schizophrenia can be complex and tiring. The family's emotional response to the condition is often intense and communication and problem-solving routines may be very ineffective because of this. One way to cope with the demands of working with these families, without burning out, is to work with a co-therapist. For example, a clinical psychologist might work with a community-based psychiatric nurse. In selecting a co-therapist, try to choose someone with whom you can have a respectful, flexible and trusting working relationship. Before each session, jointly plan a set of aims to be achieved and arrange who is to do what during the session. One way of co-working is for one therapist to be the interviewer and the other to observe the interview and take notes if necessary. When the observer has an input to make it is useful if this is made by discussing it openly with the other therapist in front of the family. When both therapists have discussed the input, the observer withdraws into the role of observer again and the interviewing therapist asks the family for their views on the issue. A second style of co-therapy involves dividing the family into sub-systems and each therapist working with one sub-system. For example, one therapist may work with the parents and another with the symptomatic child. Or one therapist may work with the males in the family and another with the females. A vital part of co-therapy is debriefing after each session. Debriefing involves resolving any feelings of conflict that arose during the session between the therapists and also reflecting on progress that was made with the family during the session and possible avenues for future work with the family. The importance of resolving conflicts between the therapists cannot be over-emphasized. Often, deep-seated family conflicts become transmitted to the therapists, who adopt positions of different family members and feel an urge to act-out repetitive, unproductive patterns of interaction which characterize the family with which they have been working. Debriefing is one way to minimize this type of interaction-pattern-mirroring in the co-therapy team.

Psychoeducational sessions

In the early sessions, usually the first two or three, the main agenda is education. A number of key points need to be covered and these are set out in Figure 18.5, which may serve as a useful leaflet for parents and adolescents. This leaflet is based on the information sheet developed by the National Schizophrenia Fellowship. The parents and adolescent are given the leaflets to read before the meetings and the psychologist spends the sessions reading through each of the points, asking the family how they fit with their experience and discussing this with a view to helping the family develop a frame of reference into which they can incorporate their experience of the adolescent's condition. The educational sessions help the family to view schizophrenia as a condition to which the adolescent was vulnerable and the onset of which was precipitated by stress. This framing of the aetiology of the condition absolves the family from blame and guilt. The explanation of the positive symptoms (thought disorder, hallucinations and delusions) in concrete terms helps parents empathize with their symptomatic adolescent and so paves the way for a reduction in criticism. The explanation of the negative symptoms (flattened affect, withdrawal, lack of volition, hygiene problems) and their lack of response to medication helps the family avoid critical or hostile attempts to persuade the symptomatic teenager to instantly conform to parental expectations in these areas. The outline of the roles of medication, individual cognitive therapy and family intervention offer the family a clear rationale for taking steps to ensure that the adolescent takes medication and that therapy sessions are attended. The information on family treatment clarifies for family members that therapy will focus on helping the parents to reduce stress and increase support for their symptomatic family member. Finally, the information on prognosis offers the family hope by drawing an analogy between diabetes and schizophrenia as a chronic condition which, with proper management, can lead to an independent lifestyle.

**NOTES FOR FAMILIES WITH TEENAGERS OR YOUNG ADULTS
WHO HAVE A DIAGNOSIS OF SCHIZOPHRENIA**

Schizophrenia is an illness. The adolescent was born with the vulnerability to this illness. This vulnerability is genetically transmitted in some cases. In others it results from pre-natal exposure to infections. Symptoms occur when, during the teenage years, a build-up of life stress or conflict occurs. Details of where in the brain this vulnerability is located and how it works are not known and research is being done to answer these questions throughout the world.

Parents do not cause schizophrenia. However, they can help with treatment by being supportive; by reducing stress; and by making home life calm and predictable.

One in 100 people get schizophrenia over the course of the lifetime in all countries in the world.

One of the symptoms of schizophrenia is thought disorder. Adolescents may talk a great deal but appear to lose the thread of what they are saying so that it is hard to understand what they mean. This is because they have lost the ability to control the amount of thoughts that they think and to put their thoughts in a logical order. Other times they simply stop talking abruptly. This is because they have the experience of their mind going blank. The experience of thought disorder is very frightening and adolescents may worry a good deal about it and try to make sense of it in strange ways. Some times they may blame someone for putting thoughts into their head. Other times they may blame someone for robbing them of their thoughts because they experience their mind going blank.

Another symptom of schizophrenia is auditory hallucinations. Adolescents with schizophrenia may hear voices that sound like a running commentary or like two people conversing about them or like someone talking to them. This is a very frightening experience when it first happens and adolescents try to make sense of it by attributing the voices to a transmitter, the TV, god, aliens or some other source. Sometimes adolescents shout back at the voices to try to make them stop. Other times they feel compelled to follow instructions given by the voices.

A third symptom of schizophrenia is delusions. Adolescents with schizophrenia may hold strong beliefs which are implausible to members of their family community. For example, they may believe that they are being persecuted by hidden forces or family members or that they are on a mission from god who speaks to them. Usually delusions are an attempt to make sense of hallucinations or thought disorder. Adolescents with delusions usually refuse to change these even in the face of strong evidence that their position is implausible.

Problems with emotions may also occur when adolescents have schizophrenia. They often withdraw and show little affection or love. They may also have outbursts of laughter or anger which appear to be inexplicable. These outbursts are often in response to hallucinations and withdrawal may reflect a reoccupation with hallucinations or the intense experience of a high rate of uncontrollable thought. Occasionally adolescents with schizophrenia realize how the condition has damaged their lifestyle and relationships. This may result in depression. On other occasions they may deny that any changes have occurred and be overly excited and optimistic.

Problems with withdrawal, daily routines and hygiene may also occur. Adolescents with schizophrenia may have little energy, sleep a great deal, avoid the company of others and pay little attention to washing or personal hygiene. This is partly because the experiences of thought disorder and hallucinations and attempts to make sense of these experiences through delusions have left them exhausted and partly because of the realization that they no longer know how to fit in with other people. They may also have the feeling that they cannot control and direct their own behaviour. Because withdrawal, poor hygiene and a breakdown in daily routine are symptoms of an illness, it is almost impossible and probably harmful to try to persuade the adolescent to make major changes in these areas rapidly.

Some symptoms of schizophrenia are treatable with medication. Thought disorder, hallucinations and delusions may all become greatly reduced or disappear with medication. Some patients get their medication in pills and others get it by injection. Some patients want to stop taking medication because it has side effects such as shaking or feeling restless. It is important to take the pills or the injection according to the doctor's directions. Patients who stop taking their medication may feel fine for weeks or months but then relapse because they have not enough medication in their body to keep them from relapsing. Unfortunately, medication may have long-lasting side effects including a peculiar movement disorder called tardive dyskinesia involving strange facial movements and hand movements. These long-term side effects can be reduced if a lower dose of medication is taken.

Personal counselling may help your teenager to learn to control some symptoms and survive on a low dose of medication. For adolescents on low doses of medication, hallucinations, delusions and thought disorder can to some degree be brought under control by learning special skills in counselling. The social skills necessary to control the symptoms of withdrawal, poor hygiene and a breakdown in daily routines can also be learned through specialized individual or group counselling.

Family counselling may help you to support your teenager and reduce stress in his or her life. Family counselling helps you to help your teenager to feel supported and understood. It also helps you to learn how to reduce stress in his or her life. With high support and low stress, fewer relapses will occur and less medication will be needed. The key to high support is to avoid criticism of your adolescent and to avoid letting him or her know that you are worrying about him or her. One way to start doing this is to spend more time each day in separate rooms so that you do not get on each other's nerves or cause each other to worry. The key to low stress is to make small changes one at a time; to decide on all changes in a calm way; and to communicate clearly and simply about any changes; and to make home life predictable.

Most people with schizophrenia can live an independent life. Schizophrenia is a chronic condition like diabetes. Most diabetics, if they take their insulin, live relatively independent lives. The same is true for most people with a diagnosis of schizophrenia. One in four adolescents make a complete recovery from their first episode and do not relapse. The remaining three out of four live relatively independent lives but relapses occur at times of stress or when medication is stopped against medical advice. Between attacks, the adolescent is more withdrawn than he or she used to be before the onset of the condition.

Figure 18.5 Psychoeducational notes where a family member has a diagnosis of schizophrenia

Medication adherence

Where youngsters have difficulty adhering to medication, this is addressed in a supportive, non-confrontational way. Obstacles to medication adherence are identified and systematic problem-solving skills used to over-come these obstacles. Some obstacles require a practical solution, for example forgetting to take medication may be addressed by using personal memory aids. Other obstacles, such as not wanting to take medication because of the side effects, may involve more complex solutions, such as trying lower dosages, different anti-psychotic medications with fewer side effects, or weighing up the costs and benefits of living with and without medication and psychotic symptoms.

Aims of later sessions

After the psychoeducational sessions the family is invited to use the sessions to develop routines and solve problems that make family life predictable and calm so that the symptomatic adolescent will feel maximally supported in his or her attempts to cope with the illness and move towards independence and be minimally stressed while living in the family context.

At a structural level, the broad aims of these therapy sessions are to help parents in two-parent families to co-operate in their care of all of the children, but particularly the adolescent with a diagnosis of schizophrenia. Where one parent has been shouldering the burden of care, this may involve helping both parents share the load more equally. A second structural aim is to help the parents strengthen the boundary between themselves and the symptomatic adolescent, so that the youngster can move towards independence and the parents can spend more time with each other in a mutually supportive relationship. In single-parent families, the structural aim is to help the parent develop supportive links with members of the extended family and broader social network and strengthen the boundary between the single parent and the adolescent. This permits the youngster to move towards independence and the single parent to develop an alternative focus for his or her energies and interests.

Where there is a high level of over-involvement or enmeshment between one parent (usually the mother) and the symptomatic adolescent, the guilt that typically underlies the over-involvement may require considerable exploration and acknowledgement. However, the psychologist's message must be that parents don't cause schizophrenia, but can help youngsters make as good a recovery as possible by promoting independence, allowing the development of autonomy and respecting the adolescent's privacy.

Within these family sessions, broad structural aims are achieved by coaching family members in communication skills and problem-solving skills, and then helping them to use these skills to make structural changes.

Communication skills training

In communication skills training, family members are coached to follow the guidelines set out in Table 4.2 (p. 145). Family members may be invited to discuss a particular issue, such as how the next week-end should be spent, with a view to clarifying everyone's opinion about this. As they proceed, the therapist may periodically stop the conversation and point out the degree to which the family's typical communication style conforms to or contravenes the guidelines for good communication. All approximations to good communication should be acknowledged and praised. Alternatives to poor communication should be modelled by the therapist. Typically there are problems with everyone getting an equal share of talking time, with the symptomatic family member usually getting the least. Often messages are sent in a very unclear way and listeners rarely check-out that what they have understood is what the speaker intended. While two sessions should be exclusively devoted to explicitly training family members in using the guidelines set out in Table 4.2, coaching in communication skills occurs throughout most of the sessions that follow the preliminary psychoeducational sessions, insofar as from time to time the psychologist should acknowledge particularly good examples of clear communication and model alternatives when poor communication occurs.

Problem-solving skills training

In families where an adolescent has a diagnosis of schizophrenia, each member is able to identify particular problems associated with living with the symptomatic youngster that they would like solved. With problem-solving training, all such problems should be listed and prioritized as a series of goals. Big problems should be broken down into smaller problems and vague problems should be clarified before this prioritizing occurs. Families have a better chance of achieving goals if they are specific, visualizable and moderately challenging. In prioritizing goals it is important to explore the costs and benefits of goals for each family member, so that ultimately the list of high-priority goals meets the needs of as many family members as possible.

Common goals include: arranging exclusive time that the parents can spend together without their symptomatic adolescent; arranging ways in which adolescents can take on some age-appropriate responsibilities, such as meeting friends or cleaning their own clothes; managing money; ensuring that the adolescent has private living space free from parental intrusion; and taking medication regularly.

Once the list of target goals has been agreed, ways of achieving these goals are explored. This usually involves coaching family members in problem-solving skills. Both specific and general guidelines for problem solving are presented in Table 4.3 (p. 147). Family members should be asked to try to use these guidelines to solve a particular problem, and this attempt is observed by the treatment team. Feedback on problem-solving skills that were well used is given and alternatives to poor problem-solving skills are modelled by the therapists.

Common pitfalls for family members include vague problem definition, trying to solve more than one problem at a time and evaluating the pros and cons of solutions before all solutions have been listed. This is an important error to correct, since premature evaluating can stifle the production of creative solutions. Often, families need to be coached out of bad communication habits in problem-solving training, such as negative mind-reading where they attribute negative thoughts or feelings to others, blaming, sulking and abusing others. At the end of an episode of problem-solving coaching, family members typically identify a solution to the problem and they are invited to try-out this solution before the next session and a plan is made to review the impact of the solution on the problem in the next session. It is important to always review such tasks that clients have agreed to do between sessions.

Re-framing

Many parents believe that they are responsible for their adolescent's condition and feel intense guilt. This guilt may lead them to become either over-involved in their adolescent's life, to the point where they prevent the development of independence; many mothers show this response. For many fathers, guilt often fuels an angry response to the symptomatic adolescent and the father criticizes the youngster for his or her unusual behaviour. Often, the negative symptoms (such as social withdrawal or poor hygiene) are the focus of this criticism. All family members experience grief at the loss of the way their adolescent used to be before the onset of the symptoms and also a sense of loss concerning the hopes and expectations they had for their child and which must now be modified.

Part of the role of the psychologist is to help family members express these emotions, but in such a way that the critical, over-involved or despairing presentation of the emotions with respect to the symptomatic adolescent is minimized. By helping family members understand that much of the youngster's behaviour is not motivated by malicious intention, the psychoeducational sessions go some way to helping parents reduce criticism.

Re-framing statements about emotional states made by family members is a second technique that can be used to minimize the negative impact of intense emotional expression. For example, if a parent expresses criticism of the adolescent by saying:

I can't stand you. You're driving me crazy,

the psychologist may re-frame this as:

It sounds like you really miss the way Johnny used to be and sometimes these feelings of loss are very strong.

If a parent expresses over-involvement by saying:

I have to do everything for you because you can't manage alone,

the psychologist can re-frame this by saying:

It sounds like you find yourself worrying a lot about Johnny's future and wondering will he be able to fend for himself.

In response to parental statements like:

You make me so miserable with your silly carry-on. Sometimes I think what's the point.

A re-framing may be offered as follows:

When you see Johnny's symptoms, it reminds you of how he was before all this. Then you find your mood drops and this sadness and grief is hard to live with.

All of these re-framings involve labelling the emotional experience as arising out of underlying positive feelings that the parent has for the symptomatic adolescent. The re-framings also describe the emotions as arising from the way the parent is coping, rather than being caused exclusively by the symptomatic teenager. That is, they give the message that the parent *owns* the feeling, they are not *imposed* on the parent by the adolescent. Re-framing is a process that occurs throughout therapy rather than being covered in a couple of sessions.

Conflict management

Where parents and symptomatic youngsters become involved in escalating patterns of conflict that may result in violence, a structured approach to conflict management should be used. The co-therapy team should allow the parent and the adolescent an uninterrupted period of time each to outline how the conflict occurred or is occurring from their point of view. Once both viewpoints have been elicited, the co-therapists may then discuss possible ways that a compromise could be reached in a respectful manner in the presence of the family, thus modelling non-violent conflict management. If the conflict has escalated to an extreme degree, one co-therapist may meet with the parents to find out their viewpoint and another meet separately with the adolescent to find out his or her. Subsequently, both factions may meet with both co-therapists, who discuss the conflict in the presence of the family, with one co-therapist acting as an advocate for the adolescent and the other speaking as an advocate for the parents. When a successful resolution of the conflict is reached, therapists should help families plan ways in which conflicts at home may be managed in future. These may include avoiding specific situations that precipitate conflict, allowing a cooling-off period of a few minutes when angry exchanges occur, using turn-taking as each side presents their position and calling in the therapy team or the family doctor when a resolution cannot be reached.

Relapse prevention and disengagement

Signals that may herald relapse, such as the build-up of life stress or the occurrence of prodromal symptoms, may be discussed during the disengagement phase. Plans for reducing stress, increasing medication and avoiding catastrophic interpretation of symptoms may be made. Plans for booster sessions may also be discussed.

Cognitive-behavioural treatment

Multi-modal programmes which include cognitive-behaviour therapy (CBT) and anti-psychotic medication are more effective than medication alone (Turkington, Dudley, Warman & Beck, 2004). Within these programmes, CBT aims to help youngsters manage stressful situations that might exacerbate psychotic symptoms, to respond less intensely to hallucinations and other distressing psychotic experiences, and reduce the impact of delusional beliefs on their adaptation.

Cognitive and behavioural treatment methods require a thorough, fine-grained contextual assessment of each specific symptom, taking account of activating events (As), beliefs and associated cognitive distortions and misattributions (Bs) and resultant distressing emotions or maladaptive behavioural consequences (Cs) (Chadwick et al., 1996; Haddock & Slade, 1996) During this fine-grained cognitive-behavioural analysis, visual analogue scales are a particularly useful way to assess the magnitude of beliefs (Bs) and responses (Cs). Beliefs about voices heard as auditory hallucinations (which are, in cognitive-behavioural terms, defined as activating events) may be assessed as varying along a number of dimensions. Voices may be construed as benign or malevolent, controlling or impotent, all-knowing or knowing little about the person; and the person may feel compelled to do what the voice says or not. Delusions (which in cognitive-behavioural terms are defined as beliefs) may vary in the degree of conviction with which they are held (from great certainty to little certainty) and pre-occupation (the amount of time spent thinking about the belief). For both hallucinations and delusions, the amount of emotional distress they cause in terms of anxiety, depression, anger and so forth may be rated on visual analogue scales. So also may behavioural responses such as avoidance, level of activity or aggression.

Various cognitive and behavioural methods have been developed to help control certain aspects of schizophrenia and are well described in treatment manuals (Birchwood & Tarrier, 1994; Chadwick et al., 1996; Fowler, Garety & Kuipers, 1995; French & Morrison, 2004; Haddock & Slade, 1996; Kingdon & Turkington, 1991; Morrison, 2002; Nelson, 1997). These include stimulus control methods to alter situations that trigger symptoms, cognitive methods for addressing hallucinations and delusional belief systems, and coping skills training. It is useful in engaging adolescents to ask about the level of distress that they experience and offer to help exploring ways of changing that. An extended period of two to six sessions may be required to establish sufficient understanding and trust to introduce challenges to clients' belief systems. Psychoeducation about diathesis–stress models of schizophrenia tend to jeopardize the engagement process and this type of intervention is probably best left until later.

Stimulus control

Here the client and therapist identify specific situations where, for example, hallucinations occur and then isolate that aspect of the situation which precipitates the symptoms and work to change that. Where internal tension or a high state of arousal associated with external environmental pressures is associated with hallucinations, systematic desensitization may be used to eliminate the antecedent (arousal) which precipitates the hallucinations. Where high levels of auditory stimulation precipitate hallucinations, the use of earplugs or calming music listened to through headphones from a personal stereo may reduce this, thus reducing the frequency of the hallucinations.

Cognitive interventions

Cognitive interventions for voices and delusions are premised on the assumption that in both instances adolescents are distressed because they have made sense of internal stimuli (auditory hallucinations) or external stimuli (delusion-eliciting events) in ways that entail distressing beliefs. The thrust of therapy is to help youngsters weaken their faith in these beliefs by identifying the beliefs as inferences rather than facts and then testing the validity of these inferences within the context of the therapeutic relationship marked by collaborative empiricism.

Cognitive interventions for auditory hallucinations involve helping clients to test out their beliefs about their voices which lead to distress. Usually, beliefs that voices are powerful and that one must comply with them or face dire consequences are the most distressing. These beliefs about the power of voices and the necessity of complying with them should be tested-out first. Such interventions increase patients' sense of self-efficacy and promote an internal locus of control. Once the patient's belief in the power of the voice has been weakened, it becomes easier for him or her to challenge the identity or source of the voice. For example, it is easier to accept that the voice is not that of the devil if the voice cannot control your every move.

Cognitive intervention for changing delusional beliefs involves eliciting these beliefs and creating a hierarchy progressing from beliefs held with least conviction to those held with greatest conviction. A useful method for creating this hierarchy is to ask what the adolescent believes his or her response would be to a hypothetical contradiction. For example, 'How would you respond if the head of the TV station came in and assured us both that no special messages were being sent to you through your TV'. The therapist then invites the patient to begin by discussing the least strongly held delusional belief. The patient lists the supportive facts and observations for that belief. The therapist then invites the client to voice as many arguments as possible against the delusional belief. These may be expanded and reflected back by the therapist.

Coping skills training

One symptom at a time is selected as a focus for coping skills training. The selected symptom must be one for which the patient is currently using a positive coping strategy, such as those listed in Table 18.5. With appropriate

Table 18.5 Positive and negative coping strategies used to manage psychotic symptoms

Sensory strategies	+ Reducing sensory input, by for example, going somewhere less noisy and stimulating
Cognitive strategies	+ Distraction or attention switching
	+ Focusing or attention narrowing
	+ Self-instruction to act a particular way
	+ Self-instruction to reattribute the cause of a particular event
	− Engaging in conversation with hallucinated voices
Behaviour strategies	+ Increase physical activity levels by, for example, exercising
	+ Increase social activity level by, for example, talking to someone
	+ Modulating social activity level by temporary break from social interaction
	+ Testing out beliefs by checking if the facts fit with beliefs about causes or interpretations of events
	− Social isolation and withdrawal
	− Directing aggression towards self or others
Physiological strategies	+ Using relaxation skills to reduce tension
	− Abusing drugs or alcohol to reduce tension

Note: Adapted from Tarrier (1994).

planning and agreement, using the typical antecedent for the occurrence of the symptom, the patient is encouraged to demonstrate the symptom and the coping strategy to the therapist. The patient is then invited to rate the effectiveness of the strategy in controlling the symptom on a ten-point scale. This procedure is repeated until the patient can face the situation that elicits the symptom and cope with it, with ease. When a coping strategy is difficult to practise within a session, the patient may practise it in imagination and then practise it *in vivo* as homework. This may be done under parental supervision. Patients or their parents may be asked to keep a record of the use of strategy and its effectiveness as homework to be reviewed at the subsequent session. Where possible, two strategies should be worked on for each discretely identifiable symptom. For example, attention switching and relaxation could both be used to reduce auditory hallucinations.

CBT-based relapse prevention

In CBT, relapse prevention involves helping youngsters learn their cognitive, affective and behavioural relapse signatures and then develop relapse drills to manage potential relapse situations (Birchwood et al., 2000). Difficulty concentrating and planning, strange sensations, and thought content that verges on the delusional are common cognitive changes before a relapse. Increased negative mood states, such as anxiety, depression and irritability, or increased feelings of religiosity and powerfulness are common emotional precursors of a psychotic episode. Difficulty planning, following routines, sleeping, eating, managing personal hygiene and maintaining normal conversations are typical behavioural changes that occur before a relapse. To deal with relapses, youngsters may be invited to write down their relapse drill, which includes: (1) a detailed description of the cognitive, emotional and behavioural elements of their personal relapse signature; (2) the specific strategies that they will use to cope with prodromal symptoms; and (3) telephone numbers of key workers they can call to help them implement their strategy. Useful coping strategies include withdrawing from stressful situations, practising relaxation exercise, distracting oneself from upsetting thoughts by listening to music, challenging negative automatic thoughts, using problem-solving skills to reduce stress or obtaining support from a family member or key worker.

Lack of insight, lack of syndrome stability and a 'sealing over' recovery style may prevent youngsters from learning and using their relapse signatures to implement relapse drills to prevent relapses or minimize their impact (Birchwood et al., 2000). With lack of insight, the youngster does not conceptualize the psychotic episode as unreal. In these instances, it may be helpful to engage the family in learning the relapse signature and drill. With syndrome instability, there is great variability in the onset of each psychotic episode because of the person's emotional reaction to it or because of behavioural reactions such as engaging in co-morbid substance abuse. In these instances, each relapse is viewed as an opportunity to learn more about the relapse signature and to better manage emotional and behavioural reactions to it. With a 'sealing over' recovery style, the youngster views the psychotic experience as alien, and when it is over the youngster isolates the experience from his or her identity in a rigid uncompromising way. The clinical challenge is to form a strong enough therapeutic alliance in such cases to help youngsters develop a recovery style characterized by integration. Here youngsters see a continuity between their psychological functioning and identity before, during and after the psychotic episode. They assume personal responsibility for understanding and managing the changes that occur in psychological functioning at the onset of psychotic episodes, and adopt a flexible approach to recovery.

Contingency management

Contingency management, where specific target adaptive behaviours are reinforced and non-adaptive behaviours are not reinforced, may be used to help clients replace negative symptoms, such as lack of goal-directed behaviour, restricted expression of emotions and restricted or incoherent speech, with more adaptive alternatives. Contingency management approaches may also be used to help replace the behavioural manifestations of hallucinations or delusions with less bizarre behaviour. This treatment was developed within an institutional context in the form of token economy programmes. Patients received tokens for engaging in pro-social behaviours. Symptomatic behaviours were not reinforced and aggressive behaviour was reduced through the use of time-out. The token economy approach to contingency management is not feasible within the community. However, contingency contracts between the client and significant members of the family and professional network may form part of a community-based treatment approach. Within such contracts, there is an agreement that the attainment of certain target goals on the part of the client will lead to certain positive consequences. However, it is important to keep in mind that contingency treatment programmes for adults with diagnoses of schizophrenia have found that, for most cases, there is limited generalization of results beyond the treatment environment; for a proportion of patients there is a deterioration in behaviours not targeted by the contingency programme and another sub-group of patients shows no response to the programme whatsoever (Hemsley, 1994).

Group work for parents

Parent groups have been shown to reduce expressed emotion in families with a member with a diagnosis of schizophrenia and an approach to running such a group is given in Kuipers et al's (2002) treatment manual. Parent groups should ideally contain no more than twelve members and be of about ninety minutes duration with meetings occurring fortnightly over a period of about nine months. They may be open or closed and, ideally, should be run in the evenings in a convenient location to minimize temporal and geographic barriers to attendance. To recruit parents into a relatives' group it is useful to meet them at their homes for a couple of sessions of psychoeducation and then offer a place in the group as a place where they can discuss with other parents in similar circumstances how best to manage the process of living with an adolescent who has a diagnosis of schizophrenia. The specific aims of relatives' groups are to:

- help lower parental criticism and over-involvement
- help parents ventilate distressing feelings, such as sadness, anger and anxiety associated with the adolescent's condition
- provide a forum for group problem solving where parents can brainstorm solutions to the various difficulties that arise from living with an adolescent with a diagnosis of schizophrenia
- provide parents with a support network to counter feelings of isolation and stigmatization.

In the first meeting, the ground rules of turn-taking, support, respect, trust and a commitment to problem solving are established by the therapist inviting each person to briefly recount their story in about five to ten minutes, emphasizing things that they have done to keep going through difficult times. The therapist's role is to ensure that everyone gets a fair turn, with less forthcoming members being facilitated and the highly verbal being limited to ten minutes maximum. All subsequent meetings should open with a round, where each person has a turn to say what has happened since the previous meeting.

Initially, themes raised for discussion in the group are practical (e.g. how to deal with the adolescent's poor hygiene) or educational (e.g. what happens if medication is not taken). The therapist's role is to encourage the group to use its collective experience to solve these problems, and only offer expert information if the group lack this. If parents agree to try a particular solution as homework, this should be reviewed in the next group.

In later sessions, as trust develops, parents use the group to process distressing emotions, such as guilt for possibly causing their adolescent's condition, grief associated with the loss of their child's health, anger at their adolescent's unusual behaviour, fear that the adolescent will harm him- or herself or others, anxiety about who will care for the adolescent later in life when they are unable to and anger at service providers for their inadequacies. With emotional issues, the therapist's job is to facilitate emotional expression and processing on the one hand while encouraging the group to support members who are processing distressing emotions by acknowledging the value of them listening and empathizing on the other.

SUMMARY

Schizophrenia is a complex disorder or group of disorders which affects 1% of the population over eighteen years of age. It has its onset in late adolescence or early adulthood. The condition is marked by positive symptoms, such as delusions and hallucination, and negative symptoms such, as inactivity and poverty of speech. While in the past a broad definition of schizophrenia was used in North America and a narrow definition used in Europe, there is now considerable international agreement on a narrow-band definition of schizophrenia. In differential diagnosis, it should be distinguished from autism, affective conditions and adolescent precursors of adult personality disorders on the schizophrenia spectrum, particularly schizoid, schizotypal and paranoid personality disorder. In the biological domain, genetic factors, dopamine system dysregulation, and neuroanotomical abnormalities associated with pre- and peri-natal insults have all been implicated in the aetiology of schizophrenia. The two-syndrome hypothesis offers an integration of these findings. This hypothesis entails the view that a distinction may be made between type 1 schizophrenia, which is a genetically inherited disease marked by a dysregulation of the mesolimbic dopaminergic system and characterized by positive symptoms on the one hand, and type 2 schizophrenia, which is a neurodevelopmental disorder arising from pre- or perinatal insults marked by chronic negative symptoms, on the other. This has been supplanted by the three-dimension hypothesis in which the symptoms of schizophrenia are conceptualized as falling on three dimensions: positive symptoms, negative symptoms and disorganization. Each of these is subserved by a specific neurobiological structural or functional deficit. In the psychological domain, cognitive deficits, cognitive biases, management of prodromal symptoms and family- and community-based stresses have all been implicated in the genesis and maintenance of schizophrenia, and a variety of focal theories developed to explain the role of these specific factors. Diathesis–stress models of schizophrenia have also been developed, which argue that, for the symptoms of schizophrenia to occur, a biologically vulnerable individual must be exposed to environmental stress. The interaction of the vulnerability factors with the stress factors leads to the occurrence of the symptomatology. Symptoms are subsequently maintained by ongoing exposure to environmental stress and by the way in which the person reacts to this stress and copes with the unusual experiences associated with schizophrenia. Assessment premised on multi-factorial diathesis–stress models of schizophrenia address pre-disposing, precipitating and maintaining factors within the biological, psychological and contextual domains. Treatment programmes premised on diathesis–stress models involve anti-psychotic medication to address dysregulation of the dopamine system, family intervention to reduce family-based stress and individual intervention to enhance personal coping strategies.

EXERCISE 18.1

Re-read the case study presented in Box 18.1.

- Develop a plan for two sessions with Julian to help him begin to control his delusions and hallucinations.
- Develop a plan for the first two sessions with the family which aims to reduce the level of expressed emotion.

FURTHER READING

Birchwood, M. & Tarrier, N. (1994). *Psychological Management of Schizophrenia*. Chichester: Wiley.

Chadwick, P., Birchwood, M., & Trower, P. (1996). *Cognitive Therapy for Delusions, Voices and Paranoia*. Chichester: Wiley.

Falloon, I. Laporta, M., Fadden, G., & Graham-Hole, V. (1993). *Managing Stress in Families*. London: Routledge.

Fowler, D., Garety, P., & Kuipers, L. (1995). *Cognitive Behavioural Psychotherapy: A Rationale, Theory and Practice*. Chichester: John Wiley & Sons.

French, P. & Morrison, A. (2004). *Early Detection and Cognitive Therapy for People at High Risk of Developing Psychosis: A Treatment Approach*. Chichester: Wiley

Haddock, G. & Slade, P. (1996). *Cognitive-Behavioural Interventions with Psychotic Disorders*. London: Routledge.

Kingdon, D.G. & Turkington, D. (1991). *Cognitive-Behavioural Therapy of Schizophrenia*. Hove, UK: Lawrence Erlbaum Associates Ltd.

Kuipers, L., Leff, J., & Lam, D. (2002). *Family Work for Schizophrenia* (Second edition). London: Gaskell.

Nelson, H. (1997). *Cognitive Behavioural Therapy with Schizophrenia. A Practice Manual*. Cheltenham, UK: Thornes Publishers.

Perry, P., Alexander, B., & Liskow, B. (1997). *Psychotropic Drug Handbook* (Seventh edition). Washington, DC: APA Press.

FURTHER READING FOR FAMILIES

Bernheim, K., Lewine, R., & Beale, C. (1982). *The Caring Family: Living with Mental Illness*. New York: Random House.

Keefe, R. & Harvey, P. (1994). *Understanding Schizophrenia: A Guide to the New Research on Causes and Treatment*. New York: Free Press.

Marsh, D. & Dickens, R. (1998). *How to Cope with Mental Illness in Your Family: A Self-Care Guide for Siblings, Offspring and Parents*. New York: Tarcher/Putnam.

Mueser, K. & Gingerich, S. (1994). *Coping with Schizophrenia: A Guide for Families*. Oakland, CA: New Harbinger.

Sheehan, S. (1982). *Is There no Place on Earth for Me*. Boston, MA: Houghton Mifflin.

Torrey, E.F. (1995). *Surviving Schizophrenia: A Manual for Families, Consumers and Providers*. New York: Harper Perrenial.

Vine, P. (1982). *Families in Pain*. New York: Pantheon.

Wasow, M. (1982). *Coping with Schizophrenia*. Palo Alto, CA: Science and Behaviour Books.

WEBSITES

Mental Health Foundation: http://www.mentalhealth.org.uk
Mind: http://www.mind.org.uk
Omni Information page: http://omni.ac.uk/browse/mesh/C0036341L0036341.html
RETHINK: http://www.rethink.org/

Factsheets on schizophrenia and psychosis can be downloaded from the website for Rose, G. & York, A. (2004). *Mental Health and Growing Up. Fact sheets for Parents, Teachers and Young People* (Third edition). London: Gaskell: http://www.rcpsych.ac.uk

Section V

Child abuse

Chapter 19

Physical child abuse

Child abuse reflects the international consensus about what constitutes unacceptable child care and the violation of children's human rights. These rights are outlined in the United Nations' Convention on the Rights of the Child (1992). Physical abuse refers to deliberately inflicted injury and includes hitting, kicking, throwing, biting, burning, scalding, strangling, stabbing, suffocating, drowning and poisoning (American Academy of Child and Adolescent Psychiatry, 1999; Browne, 2002; Emery & Laumann-Billings, 2002; Jones, 2000; MacDonald, 2001; Myers & Stern, 2002). A typical case of physical child abuse is presented in Box 19.1. In some countries – such as the USA, Ireland and the UK – physical chastisement, by, for example, slapping or caning, is common. Here, punishment that leads to observable physical harm is defined as abuse and is legally distinguished from normal chastisement. The 'battered child syndrome', a particularly extreme outcome of physical abuse, refers to cases where young children present with multiple bruises, skeletal and head injuries, often accompanied by malnutrition and neglect and marked anxiety, and whose parents deny responsibility for these injuries (Kempe, Silverman, Steele, Droegemuller & Silver, 1962). Munchausen syndrome by proxy may sometimes involve physical abuse. With this syndrome, parents repeatedly bring their children for medical consultation for conditions that they have induced, or for fabricated symptoms. Usually, young mothers with pre-school children present with Munchausen's syndrome by proxy. Where physical abuse is involved, parents may induce symptoms by poisoning or partially suffocating their children (Jones, 2000). Physical abuse may be intrafamilial or institutional, and may occur alone or in conjunction with sexual abuse, neglect or emotional abuse. There is a high level of co-morbidity for physical abuse and neglect. This is probably because some common contextual risk factors are associated with both types of maltreatment. After discussing the epidemiology and effects of physical abuse, this chapter considers an approach to assessing risk and protective factors in cases where physical abuse has occurred and rehabilitation is being considered. One approach to treatment of such cases is then given; the final section of the chapter discusses prevention.

Box 19.1 A case of physical child abuse

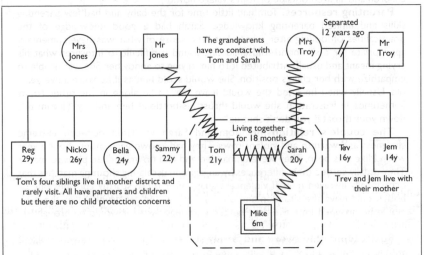

Referral. This case was referred to a child and family mental health team by social services following a non-accidental injury identified by the paediatrician in the district general hospital. The purpose of the referral was to see if Mike could be returned to the custody of his parents. At the time of the referral, Mike was in temporary foster care with the O'Sullivans. Mike had a torn frenulum, extensive facial bruising and burn marks from an electric heater on his arm. Sarah, the mother, brought the child to casualty after the child accidentally brushed against the heater. Sarah and Tom said the torn frenulum and bruising were due to two episodes of falling down. The paediatrician said the bruises and frenulum injuries were due to recent non-accidental injury (NAI). A place of safety order was taken and, after medical treatment, Mike was placed in foster care with the O'Sullivans. The parents were granted twice-weekly supervised access and these visits occurred at the O'Sullivan's house. The mother was charged by the police with grievous bodily harm, found guilty and put on probation. The team interviewed Tom and Sarah, observed family access visits and liaised with all involved professionals.

Assessment of the child. Mike was a difficult-temperament child who reacted strongly to all new stimuli by crying; he was difficult to soothe. He slept and ate at irregular times. He often vomited his food up. He did not look like a bonnie baby and probably bore little resemblance to Tom and Sarah's idea of a good baby. He had placed heavy demands on them since his birth and they were both exhausted from trying to care for him.

The mother's family history. Sarah, the mother, had a history of poor school performance. She had difficulty making and maintaining peer relationships. Her parents had a highly conflictual and violent marriage which ended when she was eight. She had a difficult relationship with her mother. Sarah experienced episodes of low mood that bordered on clinical depression and had poor frustration tolerance.

The father's family history. Tom, the father, had a history of truancy and was the youngest child in a conflictual and chaotic family. In particular he had a conflictual and violent relationship with his father. He also had limited skills for resolving conflicts and often resorted to violence when others disagreed with him. He had a chequered employment record. His parents disapproved of Sarah. Tom's three brothers and his sisters all had partners (either co-habitees or spouses) and children and all lived outside of Tom's village now.

Parenting resources. Tom had little time for the baby and had few parenting skills and limited parenting knowledge. Sarah had a good knowledge of the practicalities of looking after a baby but little sense of what was developmentally appropriate for a six-month-old child. She found it difficult to interpret what his crying meant and usually attributed it to him trying to annoy her. She was unable to empathize with her child's position. She would scold him as if he were a five-year-old. Usually when he cried she would leave him to lie alone in the other room. Sometimes, in frustration, she would thrust his bottle at him and say 'I'll ram this down your throat if you don't shut up'.

The couple's relationship. Tom and Sarah vacillated between extreme closeness and warmth and violent rows. They had known each other about a year when Mike was born. They were unmarried and had no immediate plans to marry. They usually settled their differences by engaging in escalating shouting matches that occasionally involved mutual violence. Usually after these stormy episodes one or both would leave the situation and one or both would get drunk. Later, the issue would be dropped until the next heated exchange, when it would be brought up again.

Social support network and family stresses. The Jones were very isolated with few friends. They were unsupported by the extended family and had no regular contact with either Tom's or Sarah's parents or siblings. They were financially stressed, since neither of them worked and they relied on welfare payments to support themselves. They lived in a two-room rented flat over a shop.

The abusive incident. The abusive incident involved the following sequence of events. Mike began to cry at 2.00 a.m. and would not stop. This was typical of him as a child with a difficult temperament. Sarah interpreted the crying as Mike trying to prove she was no good as a mother and as his attempt to punish her by stopping her from sleeping. When she expressed this view to Tom, he argued with her, which further upset Mike, and then Tom went back to sleep. Sarah's anger at the child escalated, and this was fuelled by her negative attributions concerning the child's motives, her lack of empathy for Mike, her anger at Tom, and her exhaustion. She took the child's bottle and shoved it into Mike's mouth and tore his frenulum. He tried to spit it out. She hit him twice, picked him up and then dropped him next to the heater, which he fell against. This act was influenced by her own punishment experiences as a child. Her mother had relied on corporal punishment as a routine method of control and often she was very severe. The act was also influenced by her habit of using a bottle to stop Mike from crying.

Capacity to co-operate with the team. Sarah accepted that the abuse was the result of her being unable to control her frustration in a stressful situation. She was committed to learning how to manage her child in stressful situations and to engaging in family work to learn child management skills. Sarah and Tom refused to accept that counselling for their personal or relationship difficulties would be of any benefit to them. Sarah was able to co-operate with the team and engaged well in the assessment. Tom found co-operation very difficult and only went along with the assessment procedures to placate Sarah.

Formulation. The Jones were a young single-child family in which physical child abuse had occurred. The violence of the mother towards the child was influenced by a number of factors, including the mother and father's difficulties in regulating anger and negative mood states; the parents' lack of childcare knowledge and skills; the couple's difficulty in sustaining a mutually supportive relationship; the lack of support from the extended family; and the multiple stresses on the couple, including financial difficulties and crowded accommodation. The main protective factor was the mother's acceptance of responsibility for the abuse and willingness to work with the team to develop parenting skills. However, an important related risk factor was the couple's refusal to acknowledge the contribution of personal and marital difficulties to the occurrence of the abuse, and the necessity of working to enhance mood regulation skills and marital communication.

Treatment. The treatment plan was to offer the parents parenting skills training and to offer the mother a place in a support group for mothers in which learning mood-regulation skills was central to the agenda. In addition, plans were made to help Sarah develop a more supportive relationship with her mother. However, the prognosis in this case was guarded because of the couple's refusal to acknowledge the role of marital factors and personal factors in the occurrence of the abuse.

EPIDEMIOLOGY

The overall prevalence of physical child abuse during childhood and adolescence is 10–25%, depending on the definition used, the population studied and the cut-off point for the end of adolescence (Wekerle & Wolfe, 2003). A review of international incidence studies confirms that physical abuse is a relatively common phenomenon (Creighton, 2004). Community surveys in the USA, the UK and other European countries in the 1990s found that the annual incidence of physical child abuse was 50–90 per 1000, or 5–9%. In these surveys, physical abuse was defined as being hit with an object, punched, bitten, kicked, beaten-up or attacked with a knife or gun. However, only a minority of such cases came to the attention of child protection services and were officially reported. Thus, the incidence of physical child abuse based on officially reported cases was far lower than that based on surveys. The annual incidence of physical abuse in the UK, Australia and North America, based on officially reported cases in the 1990s was between 0.5 and 2.5 per 1000. About a quarter of all reported cases of child maltreatment in these countries had suffered physical abuse, rather than sexual or emotional abuse or neglect.

EFFECTS OF PHYSICAL ABUSE

Physical child abuse has short- and long-term physical and psychological consequences (Cicchetti, 2004; Emery & Laumann-Billings, 2002; Jones, 2000; Kolko, 2002; Wekerle & Wolfe, 2003). The physical consequences of abuse include scarring, disfigurement, neurological damage, visual or auditory impairment and failure of growth. While the majority of these effects attenuate with time, most persist into adulthood.

The short-term psychological consequences include negative self-evaluative beliefs, problems with the development of linguistic and cognitive competencies, problems with affect regulation and associated excesses of internalizing and externalizing behaviour problems and relationship difficulties. Negative self-evaluative beliefs include low self-esteem and low self-efficacy. Cognitive and language deficits include developmental delays in the emergence of abilities and language usage; poor academic attainment; and lower levels of symbolic play. Affect regulation difficulties find expression in externalizing behaviour problems, such as uncontrolled anger and aggression. Affect regulation problems also find expression in internalizing behaviour problems, such as depression, anxiety, overly compliant behaviour in the face of authority and self-harm. Relationship difficulties, probably associated with the development of victim–abuser internal working models of caregiver relationships, are first evident in the abused children's anxious–avoidant or disorganized attachment to their primary caregivers (a fuller discussion of attachment problems is given in Chapter 20). The majority of children or teenagers who run away from home have been physically abused. Later, relationship difficulties occur with peers; abused children also have difficulty empathizing with others. The studies from which this list of consequences has been abstracted, for the most part, compared abused and non-abused children after the abuse occurred. It is, therefore, possible that some of the child characteristics found to typify abused children may represent the causes of abuse rather than the effects.

One of the central findings on the long-term effects of physical abuse is that individuals abused as children have a higher risk of externalizing and internalizing behaviour problems during adolescence and adulthood. Externalizing behaviour problems include teenage delinquency, aggression, domestic violence, child abuse and substance abuse. Internalizing behaviour problems include self-injury, suicide, anxiety, depression and somatization. Long-term adjustment difficulties in making and maintaining intimate relationships are also a possible outcome for individuals abused as children. The short-term cognitive and language delays which typify many abused children, in some cases lead to long-term educational and vocational problems.

While these long-term difficulties are more common among abused children than non-abused children, the majority of physically abused children do not develop serious long-term problems. For those that do, the difficulties seem to be related to characteristics of the abuse, characteristics of the child's family network and the way the placement and legal proceedings related to the abuse were managed. The frequency and severity of abuse, and the co-occurrence of neglect or emotional abuse are associated with a poorer outcome. The presence of a variety of contextual risk factors, including problems with parental adjustment, child adjustment and quality of the parent–child relationship; marital discord and high levels of family stress with low social support are all associated with poorer long-term adjustment. Details of these risk factors will be given in a later section. Poor long-term adjustment is also associated with multi-placement experiences and protracted legal proceedings associated with the abuse. Not all children develop serious long-term problems as a result of abuse. Children who are abused before the age of five and who do not sustain neurological damage tend to be more resilient, as do children with high ability levels, an easy temperament and the capacity and opportunity to form socially supportive relationships with adults in the extended family and elsewhere despite the abuse.

ASSESSMENT

There are no definitive procedures or criteria for diagnosing or validating cases of physical child abuse. Guidelines vary from country to country. However, the checklist set out in Table 19.1 contains items that raise suspicion of physical child abuse. If physical child abuse is suspected, it is vital to request consent from the parents to arrange a full medical examination of the child immediately and to request consent to contact other involved agencies. If the medical examination gives serious grounds for suspecting abuse, or if the parents refuse to permit a full medical examination, the primary concern should be the immediate protection of the child through hospitalization or placement of the child in substitutive care. These procedures will require the psychologist to follow local guidelines for liaising with the social services department and the paediatric medical service. At this stage, in areas where there is a policy or legislation requiring mandatory reporting of child abuse cases to the local law enforcement agency, such a report must be made. This may result in police enquiries that lead to charges being brought against the abusing parent.

It is usually the statutory responsibility of the social services department to arrange a case conference and plan a comprehensive assessment of the case with a view to long-term planning. In some districts, it is only at this stage that the clinical psychologist becomes involved. Clinical psychologists may be asked to contribute to the assessment of risk factors in the case and advise on, or contribute to, a programme which aims to reduce the risks of further abuse should the child be returned to the custody of the parents. It is in these two areas that clinical psychologists can make a significant contribution to the management of cases of physical child abuse. Such risk assessments and risk reduction programmes may be based on a thorough evaluation of the child, family and broader systemic context within which the abuse occurred (Kolko, 2002; MacDonald, 2001; Reder & Lucey, 1995; Wolfe & McEachran, 1997). It is useful, through interviewing, to reconstruct the abusive incident to understand the factors that contributed to the event. Such an understanding has clear implications for treatment and prevention of further abuse. In addition to this highly focused evaluation, it is also useful to construct a wide-ranging evaluation of known risk and protective factors associated with physical child abuse.

Table 19.1 Checklist of items that raise suspicion of physical child abuse

The injury	• Any bruises or fractures in a baby less than a year old • Multiple injuries at various stages of resolution • Bruises in the pattern of finger marks, strap marks or pinch marks • Burns from cigarettes • Scalding injuries • Bite marks • Bald spots from hair pulling • Injuries of the long bones such as spiral fractures • Tender or swollen joints • Multiple rib fractures caused by blows to the head or back • Head injuries (including subdural haematoma) from shaking or blows to the head • Whiplash from shaking • Black eyes • Torn frenulum • Poisoning
Previous injuries	• History of repeated injury • History of multiple attendances at different hospitals for children's injuries
Account of the recent injury	• The child says the parent intentionally injured him or her • Parent gives a vague account of an accident that led to injury • Parent gives an account of the accident which is incompatible with the injury • Contradictory accounts of the cause of the injury given by family members • Parents blame a third party (baby-sitter) • Parents say the injury was self-inflicted
Parents' relationship with assessment team	• A delay in seeking help • Greater self-concern than concern for the child • Defensiveness about responsibility for the injury • A wish to leave before the assessment is complete • Refusal to permit the team to contact other involved agencies • Co-operation problems with the assessment team and refusal to give information
Supporting evidence	• The child displays an ability to distinguish fact from fantasy • There are witnesses of the actual abusive acts • There are witnesses of some aspects of the child's account, such as the circumstances surrounding the abusive act, but not the acts themselves, and these are consistent with the child's account • The child's social context places him or her at risk for physical abuse • The child has personal characteristics which place him or her at risk for physical abuse

Reconstructing the abusive incident

An important part of a comprehensive assessment of a case where physical child abuse has occurred is the reconstruction of the abusive incident. To aid this assessment process, a sequential model of events which culminate in physical abuse is set out in Figure 19.1. The model is founded on an extensive empirical literature (Frude, 1990). Most abusive episodes occur in response to

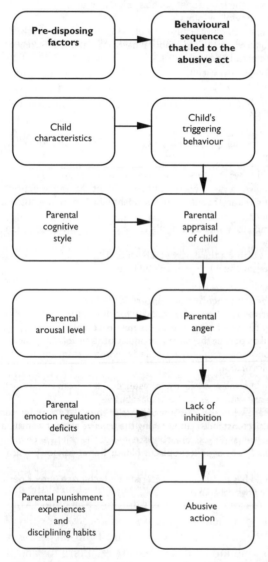

Figure 19.1 Model of the sequence of events leading to an abusive act

a triggering behaviour by the child which the parent experiences as aversive. Surveys show common triggers are:

- crying
- wetting
- refusing to eat
- stealing
- lying
- aggression.

Most abusive incidents are disciplinary encounters between parents and children, where parents use physical punishment in response to a child's trigger behaviour. The parent intends to punish the child for wrong-doing and uses physical punishment, since this is his or her typical method of disciplining children. However, the punishment is severe because of the high level of anger and the lack of inhibition. The high level of anger which fuels the parent's abusive act is determined by the parent's arousal level and appraisal of the child's trigger behaviour. If the parent's level of arousal or anger before the trigger behaviour is high, then this may be displaced on to the child. Parents who have been involved in a marital conflict or a stressful conflict with someone in their work situation, extended family or community may displace their arousal and anger into their punishment of the child. In other situations where the parent has been involved in a repetitive escalating cycle of stressful conflict with the child, the trigger behaviour may be the last straw in this escalating negative interaction pattern.

Prior to an abusive act, the parent typically appraises the child's behaviour as particularly negative and this appraisal (along with the parent's arousal level) leads to the high level of anger. Commonly, such appraisals involve attributing vindictive negative, global, stable intentions to the child as a motivation for the child's triggering behaviour. Parents who physically abuse their children fail to inhibit the extreme anger they experience in response to the child's trigger behaviour. Parents who do not abuse their children empathize with the child's position or use self-talk to control their tempers. Parents who abuse their children have difficulty empathizing with children and may use self-talk to increase their negative appraisal of their child and therefore their anger. The escalating severity of physical punishment which precedes abuse may desensitize parents to the dangerousness of their actions.

The nature of the abusive act may be determined by the form of punishment the parent received as a child, the typical type of punishment the parent uses with the child or the reason the parent is punishing the child. Abusive acts are often similar to those which the parent experienced as a child. The similarity may arise from the parent's internalization of the aggressive relationship as an internal working model for caregiving relationships and then the subsequent identification with the aggressor role rather than the victim role within this internal working model. Abusive acts can be an escalation of normal habits, for example hitting with a stick on the hand may become hitting the face with a stick. Where the nature of abusive acts are determined by the reason for the act, a distinction may be made between the following five reasons:

- instrumental: smothering a child to stop it crying
- symbolic/instrumental: washing out a child's mouth with caustic liquid following cursing or lying
- promise fulfilment: I told you I would put you in the fire
- retaliation: you pushed her so I'll pick you up and throw you and see how you like it
- opportunism: the parent uses what is to hand. Like stabbing a child with a fork for bad table manners.

Helping parents to construct a model of the abusive incident is a useful forum within which to assess the degree to which they accept responsibility for the abuse or continue to deny such responsibility.

Risk and protective factors

Arising out of the reconstruction of the abusive act, a wide range of hypotheses may emerge about particular features of the child, the parents and the broader social context that contributed to the risk for child abuse. Physical child abuse is not the result of any single risk factor. Rather, abuse occurs when there is an accumulation of risk factors that outweigh the beneficial influence of protective factors present in the case (Carr, 1997). Potential risk and protective factors, along with characteristics of the abuse discussed on pp. 902–904, determine the short- and long-term effects of the physical abuse on the child's adjustment and the risk of re-abuse. These various factors which have been included in the framework set out in Figure 19.2 are based on extensive empirical literature reviews (American Academy of Child and Adolescent Psychiatry, 1999; Browne, 2002; Cicchetti, 2004; Emery & Laumann-Billings, 2002; Jones, 2000; Kolko, 2002; MacDonald, 2001; Reder & Lucey, 1995; Wekerle & Wolfe, 2003; Wolfe & McEachran, 1997).

Child's personal characteristics

The personal characteristics of children may place them at risk for abuse and long-term adjustment problems. Physically abused children are typically young (up to five years) and both sexes are equally represented. This is different from sexual abuse, where older girls are the more common victims. Comparisons of abused and non-abused children show that many child attributes are often associated with abuse. Of course, such studies cannot identify which child characteristics are risk factors for abuse and which result from abuse. Examination of these factors suggests that the following child characteristics may be risk factors for abuse, since they place additional demands on parents: prematurity, low birth weight, developmental delays, frequent illness, difficult temperament and oppositional and aggressive behaviour.

In contrast, bright children of easy temperament who are physically healthy place fewer demands on their parents and so these attributes are protective factors. A variety of factors may be protective in terms of long-term adjustment. Children who are abused at a very early age and sustain no neurological damage have a better outcome. High self-esteem, an internal locus of control, high self-efficacy and an optimistic attributional style may all be important personal protective factors. Other potentially important personal protective factors for long-term adjustment include mature defence mechanisms and functional coping strategies, particularly good problem-solving skills and a capacity to make and maintain friendships.

Parental factors

Personal characteristics of the parents may place them at risk for physically abusing their children. Young parents are more likely to abuse their children than older parents. While many studies report that physical abuse is more commonly carried out by mothers, fathers may be more likely to abuse their children when the phenomenon is studied from the point of view of opportunities. That is, fathers may carry out more acts of physical abuse per hour of time they spend in the role of the child's primary caretaker. However, since mothers tend to spend far more hours in this role, overall, more acts of physical child abuse are carried out by mothers. This is different from sexual abuse where more perpetrators are male.

Parents from families with pro-aggressive attitudes are more likely to abuse their children. Better controlled studies indicate that about 30% of people abused as children go on to abuse their own children. The mechanisms of transmission probably involve the development of certain personality characteristics that make it likely that aggression will be used in stressful caregiving interactions and the introjection of internal working models for caregiving relationships that involve aggression. A variety of learning mechanisms are probably involved, including modelling, direct reinforcement of aggressive behaviour, coercion training and inconsistency training. With inconsistency training, the parent–child interactions are so unpredictable that the child actively initiates coercive interaction cycles because they are the only predictable types of interaction in the child's family life.

Psychological disorders, including depression, borderline personality disorder and substance abuse, are more common among parents who abuse their children than those that do not. All of these disorders are associated with low self-esteem, low self-efficacy, an external locus of control, immature defences

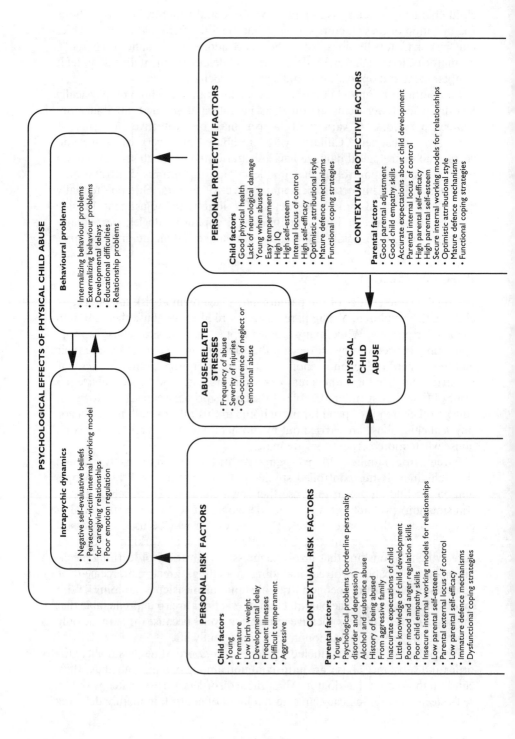

PSYCHOLOGICAL EFFECTS OF PHYSICAL CHILD ABUSE

Intrapsychic dynamics

- Negative self-evaluative beliefs
- Persecutor-victim internal working model for caregiving relationships
- Poor emotion regulation

Behavioural problems

- Internalizing behaviour problems
- Externalizing behaviour problems
- Developmental delays
- Educational difficulties
- Relationship problems

ABUSE-RELATED STRESSES

- Frequency of abuse
- Severity of injuries
- Co-occurence of neglect or emotional abuse

PHYSICAL CHILD ABUSE

PERSONAL RISK FACTORS

Child factors

- Young
- Premature
- Low birth weight
- Developmental delay
- Frequent illnesses
- Difficult temperament
- Aggressive

CONTEXTUAL RISK FACTORS

Parental factors

- Young
- Psychological problems (borderline personality disorder and depression)
- Alcohol and substance abuse
- History of being abused
- From aggressive family
- Inaccurate expectations of child
- Little knowledge of child development
- Poor mood and anger regulation skills
- Poor child empathy skills
- Insecure internal working models for relationships
- Low parental self-esteem
- Parental external locus of control
- Low parental self-efficacy
- Immature defence mechanisms
- Dysfunctional coping strategies

PERSONAL PROTECTIVE FACTORS

Child factors

- Good physical health
- Lack of neurological damage
- Young when abused
- Easy temperament
- High IQ
- High self-esteem
- Internal locus of control
- High self-efficacy
- Optimistic attributional style
- Mature defence mechanisms
- Functional coping strategies

CONTEXTUAL PROTECTIVE FACTORS

Parental factors

- Good parental adjustment
- Good child empathy skills
- Accurate expectations about child development
- Parental internal locus of control
- High parental self-efficacy
- High parental self-esteem
- Secure internal working models for relationships
- Optimistic attributional style
- Mature defence mechanisms
- Functional coping strategies

Parent–child relationship factors
- Attachment problems
- Parental negative cognitive set (negative bias and attributions)
- Coercive parent–child interaction
- Inconsistent parental discipline

Marital relationship
- Marital discord or violence
- Poor communication
- Poor problem-solving skills
- Based on insecure attachment
- Power and intimacy difficulties
- Negative cognitive set (negative bias and attributions)
- Negative interaction pattern
- Triangulation
- Father absence

Social network factors
- Poor social support network
- Poor relationship with extended family
- High family stress
- Social disadvantage
- Crowded living quarters
- Isolation

Treatment system factors
- Family denies problems and abuser does not accept responsibility for abuse
- Family rejects formulation and treatment plan
- Lack of co-ordination among involved professionals
- Cultural and ethnic insensitivity
- Multi-placement experience
- Protracted legal proceedings

Parent–child relationship factors
- Secure parent–child attachment
- Authoritative parenting

Marital relationship
- High marital satisfaction
- Good communication skills
- Good problem-solving skills
- Father involvement

Social network factors
- Good social support network
- Low family stress
- Positive educational placement
- High socioeconomic status

Treatment system factors
- Family accepts there is a problem and abusing parent accepts responsibility for abuse
- Family is committed to resolving the problem
- Family accepts formulation and treatment plan
- Good co-ordination among involved professionals
- Cultural and ethnic sensitivity

Figure 19.2 Risk and protective factors to consider in the assessment of physical child abuse

and poor coping strategies. However, poor emotional regulation (leading to depression, aggression and substance misuse) and poor empathy skills are two of the most important components of these broader psychological disorders from the point of view of increasing risk. It may be these characteristics which partially under-pin the intergenerational transmission of abuse. Poor empathy skills, are a particular handicap for parents since sensitive parenting necessitates reading the child's signals and inferring the child's emotional state. Poor personal emotional regulation is also a handicap because parents may have difficulty prioritizing the need to respond to the child in a way that regulates the child's emotional state since they are unable to carry out this function for themselves. Rather, they find themselves descending into a pit of depression or flying into a rage of anger and feel powerless to regulate these extreme emotional states. They also have difficulty reducing stresses associated with the wider social context in which they live. These include, crowding, social isolation and financial problems.

Good parental adjustment, in contrast, is a protective factor. Where parents have an internal locus of control, high self-efficacy, high self-esteem, internal working models for secure attachments, an optimistic attributional style, mature defences, functional coping strategies, and a capacity to empathize with their child then they are better resourced to manage the demands of childcare constructively. Accurate knowledge and expectations about child development is also a protective factor.

Parent–child relationship factors

The parent–child relationship in cases of physical abuse is typically conflictual. Research on attachment, social cognition and behavioural interaction offers a number of clinically useful insights into these conflictual parent–child relationships. The introjection of inadequate internal working models of attachment in caregiving relationships offers an over-arching framework for understanding the many difficulties that have been found to characterize unsatisfactory parent–child relationships associated with physical abuse. Many parents who physically abuse their children have not experienced parental sensitivity to their needs, nor have they experienced their parents as a secure base from which to explore the world. These parents therefore have no cognitive model to use as a basis for responding sensitively to their children's needs and to their children's requirement for a secure base.

Abusive parents' behaviour with their children is guided by a negative cognitive set. This cognitive set leads abusive parents to have unrealistically high standards for young children's behaviour and a negative bias in judging their children and so they experience many of their children's behaviours as negative. They attribute these negative behaviours to internal, global, stable factors, particularly the child's intentional defiance.

This negative cognitive set probably under-pins those behavioural patterns which have been found to uniquely characterize parents and children who have been involved in abuse. These patterns are typified by a lack of positive reciprocity, a high rate of negative reciprocity and a high rate of disciplinary encounters which escalate in severity. Parents who abuse their children control by punishment, not positive reinforcement, and the punishments, which are often severe, are out of all proportion to the child's transgression of the parent's rules for good conduct. In families where abuse occurs, children do not respond consistently to such parental control. Parents become frustrated by this ineffectiveness but have difficulty analysing why their approach to parenting is ineffective. They also have difficulty generating and testing-out alternative solutions.

In contrast to this negative parent–child interaction style, which places youngsters at risk for further abuse and long-term abuse-related adjustment difficulties, secure parent–child attachment and authoritative parenting are central protective factors, particularly if they occur within the context of a flexible family structure in which there is clear communication, high marital satisfaction and both parents share the day-to-day tasks of child care.

Marital factors

Conflict, instability, dissatisfaction, negative behaviour patterns, negative belief systems and poor communication and problem-solving skills are the main features of the marital relationship which place youngsters at risk for child abuse, recurrence of abuse and, later, abuse-related adjustment problems. Unresolved conflict is very common among parents who physically abuse their children. Conflict under-pins the structural instability characterized by a history of multiple separations and a low level of commitment which typifies these relationships. Low satisfaction is another feature of these relationships, because partners have difficulty meeting each other's needs for an acceptable level of intimacy and an equitable distribution of power. Conflict about intimacy often centres on the women in these relationships demanding more psychological intimacy and the men demanding more physical intimacy. Conflict about power may emerge in discussions about the division of labour within the household and about the way money is used.

These conflicts often remain unresolved because the couples lack the communication and joint problem-solving skills necessary for negotiation. Rather than using active listening skills to share information about how they would like their needs for power and intimacy met and then flexibly negotiating about these, they make inferences about this information based on those aspects of their partner's behaviour to which they selectively attend, and rigidly make demands based on the belief that in any negotiation there is a winner and a loser. These couples have difficulty conceptualizing a conflict being resolved to the satisfaction of both parties (i.e. a win–win resolution).

This process of inferring a partner's needs based on observations of his or her behaviour leads to further problems because such couples typically have negative cognitive styles. That is, both partners selectively attend to negative aspects of each other's behaviour and make personal attributions rather than situational attributions for negative behaviour. They attribute global, stable negative intentions to their partners. They also attribute all positive actions of their partners to external situational factors.

This negative cognitive style, along with the belief that in any negotiation there must be a winner and loser, in turn promotes negative patterns of interaction. These patterns of interaction are characterized by blaming rather than empathy, and escalating negative exchanges rather than positive exchanges. These negative exchanges may escalate into physical violence. Violent abusive marital relationships and violent parent–child relationships may be two aspects of a violent family culture. The negative cognitive sets and negative patterns of interaction that characterize these marriages lead to a situation where these couples work on a short-term quid pro quo system not a long-term goodwill system. Often, the child is triangulated into negative exchanges between the parents. For example, a father may refuse to feed or change the child, or to tolerate the child's crying, because the mother has not met the father's need for power or intimacy.

In contrast to these risk factors associated with the marital relationship, satisfying and structurally stable marriages in which the couple are able to use communication and problem-solving skills to resolve conflicts about power and intimacy may be viewed as protective factors. These marriages are protective because they offer a context within which parents are supported and buffered against the stressful demands of childcare.

Social network factors

We live in a culture that tolerates a high level of violence in media entertainment, sport, corporal punishment and the penal system. It is against this cultural back-drop that physical child abuse occurs. Low socioeconomic status, poverty, unemployment, poor housing, single parenthood and a low educational level are all risk factors for child abuse. Low socioeconomic status may lead to abuse because it is associated with greater overall life stress and fewer resources such as day-care programmes, crèches and nurseries. People with a low socioeconomic status may have less well-developed verbal skills for conflict resolution and this may lead to the use of violence as a way of resolving conflicts. A third alternative is that people of low socioeconomic status may hold pro-aggressive parenting beliefs that legitimize physical punishment.

Parental isolation and a low level of social support is associated with physical child abuse. It is the quality and not the number of supports that is crucial. Probably two mechanisms under-pin parental isolation. On the one hand, parents may live in neighbourhoods where there are few opportunities for social interaction and where they are distant from their families of origin and friends from school-going years. On the other hand, abusive parents may have a personal style that leads them to view others as threatening and so they do not initiate social interactions, or they may initiate interactions in a way that leads others to avoid them.

Parental isolation often includes isolation from the parents' families of origin. This isolation may be associated with unresolved conflicts between the parents and the grandparents of the abused child. So not only may the grandparents be unavailable as a source of support, they may also be perceived as a potential threat or source of stress.

A variety of environmental stressors, most notably crowding and inadequate housing, are associated with child abuse. Remaining with a crying child in cramped living quarters requires considerable frustration tolerance and so it is understandable that crowding is one of the factors that sets the stage for the occurrence of abuse.

In contrast to these risk factors, protective factors within the child's broader social network include high levels of support, low levels of stress and membership of a high socioeconomic group. Where families are embedded in social networks that provide a high level of support and place few stressful demands on family members, then it is less likely that parents' resources for dealing with childcare will become depleted and abuse will occur. The availability of a well-resourced pre-school placement may also be viewed as a protective factor.

Treatment-system factors

A number of features of the treatment system, which includes the family, the treatment team and involved professionals and agencies may place the child at risk for either repeated abuse, poor response to treatment or abuse-related adjustment difficulties. Denial of family problems, the abuser's refusal to accept responsibility for abuse, rejection of the treatment team's formulation and refusal to co-operate with the treatment plan may all be viewed as risk factors. Where there is a lack of co-ordination among involved professionals, this increases the risk of further abuse. Multi-placement experiences and protracted legal proceedings have a negative impact on long-term adjustment. A detailed discussion of problems associated with multi-placement experiences is given in Chapter 22. Treatment systems that are not sensitive to families' cultural and ethnic beliefs and values may put families at risk because they may inhibit engagement or promote drop-out from treatment and prevent the development of a good working alliance.

In contrast to these risk factors, certain features of the treatment system may be viewed as protective insofar as they reduce the risk of further abuse and enhance the possibility of positive changes within the child's psychosocial environment, which in turn reduce the risk of long-term abuse-related adjustment problems. Within the treatment system, co-operative working relationships between the treatment team and the family, and good co-ordination of multi-professional input are protective factors. Treatment systems that are sensitive to families' cultural and ethnic beliefs and values are more likely to help families engage with, and remain in, treatment, and foster the development of a good working alliance. Families are more likely to benefit from treatment when all family members accept that there is a problem and the abuser accepts responsibility for the abuse. Acceptance of the formulation of the problem given by the treatment team and a commitment to working with the team to resolve it are also protective factors.

Comprehensive assessment schedule

The over-arching aim of case management in cases of physical child abuse is to provide the child with a safe environment, which fosters development, and an opportunity to sustain relationships with both parents with a minimum of disruption and change in the child's environment, providing sustaining such a relationship with the parents does not place the child at risk for further episodes of abuse. In this context it is worth mentioning that surveys of abused children consistently show that the majority of abused children continue to feel loyalty to their abusing parents and to feel loved by them (Herzberger et al., 1981). Case management usually occurs within a statutory framework. The child is held in foster care under an appropriate statutory care order, or in the custody of the non-abusing parent, until a full assessment has been completed and a plan for long-term management developed. This is then presented to the case conference and a decision made on implementation of the plan.

The comprehensive assessment should cover all risk factors in the model set out in Figure 19.2, along with a reconstruction of the abusive incident following the sequential model set out in Figure 19.1. The reconstruction of the abusive incident will help to pin-point those factors that need to change in order for it to be safe for the child to return to the custody of both parents. Ideally, the comprehensive assessment should be carried out by a team rather than a single professional over a series of interview and observation sessions. A comprehensive child protection assessment schedule of interviews, and assessment procedures is presented in Table 19.2. This schedule is based on a number of principles. First, it is assumed that, to assess the wide variety of factors involved in child abuse cases, every significant family member or involved professional within the abused child's network should be interviewed to give their views on risk factors, the abusive incident and ways in which they might contribute to preventing future episodes of abuse. Second, it is assumed that specialist medical or psychological assessments of the child, and occasionally the parents, may be necessary. Third, it is assumed that it is necessary, in addition to interviewing, to observe interactions between key members of the network. For example, it is particularly important to observe

Table 19.2 Components of a comprehensive child-protection assessment package for use in cases of physical child abuse

Evaluation target	Evaluation methods and areas
Child	• Individual interview with child (if the child is old enough) to assess personal strengths and resources (including assertiveness) and his or her account of the abusive incident; perception of all relevant risk factors; and wishes for the future • Medical examination of the child's injuries • Assessment of weight and height compared to national norms for children of the same age • Psychometric assessment of the child's cognitive and language development (if appropriate) • Child-behaviour checklist to assess behavioural difficulties
Parents	• Individual interviews with parents to assess acceptance or denial or responsibility for abuse, parenting skills and deficits, personal resources and problems, reconstruction of the abusive incident and perception of all relevant risk factors • Psychometric assessment of specific parental characteristics (if appropriate) such as intelligence and psychopathology
Parent–child interaction	• Parent–child interaction observation sessions to assess positive aspects of parenting and risk factors associated with parent–child interactions • With physical abuse, emotional abuse and neglect, a brief trial (two sessions) of parent–child therapy to assess their responsiveness to behavioural coaching to increase the number of positive exchanges and decrease the number of negative exchanges
Marital couple	• Marital interview to assess marital risk factors, especially joint communication and problem-solving skills for dealing with child-care issues and conflict management • A brief trial (two sessions) of couple therapy to assess couple's responsiveness to coaching in joint communication and problem-solving skills for managing childcare issues • Psychometric assessment of each spouse's perception of marital relationship (if appropriate)
Family accommodation	• Visit to family residence to assess crowding, hygiene, safety of the home for the child and opportunities for age-appropriate cognitive stimulation and play
Role of extended family	• Individual interviews with other members of nuclear and extended family to assess their acceptance or denial of the abuse, their perception of risk factors, their reconstruction of the abusive incident (if appropriate), their childcare skills and deficits • Joint interviews with extended family and nuclear family to observe quality of their relationship to nuclear family and assess potential for support

Continued

Table 19.2 continued

Evaluation target	Evaluation methods and areas
Role of other involved professionals	• Individual interviews with other involved professionals from health, education, social services and justice to obtain their expert view of risks and resources within the family and their potential future involvement in supporting the family or providing services • Joint interviews with other community-based resource people, such as the foster parents with whom the child is temporarily based, home-help, befriender, leader of mother and toddler group, director of nursery or day-care facility, etc. to observe relationship to parents and assess potential for supporting the family in future

the primary caregiver and the child interacting to assess the quality of this parent–child relationship. This type of assessment may be conducted by observing parent–child interaction during access visits to the foster home where the child is placed. It is also important to observe the parents engage in joint problem solving about a childcare issue, such as how they should conduct themselves on access visits. Fourth, it is assumed that the capacity of the parents and the members of their network to engage in treatment must be assessed.

Judging treatability

The issue of treatability of cases deserves special attention because available evidence suggests that not all families in which child abuse has occurred can benefit from treatment. The checklist in Table 19.3 offers a framework for assessing a family's capacity to engage in treatment. It is based on the literature evaluating the efficacy of rehabilitation programmes in this area (Jones, 1987; Skuse & Bentovim, 1994). Where parents accept responsibility for the abuse, are committed to meeting their child's needs, are committed to improving their own psychological well-being and where they have the ability to change, the prognosis is good. In such cases it is worth allocating scarce resources to treatment. Where three out of four of these conditions are met, the prognosis is fair. Where less than three of these conditions are met, it is unlikely that even the most skilful professional team would be able to offer a viable treatment package. In such instances, foster care should seriously be considered as the least damaging option for the child.

TREATMENT

Where a family meet at least three of the conditions which suggest that they may respond positively to treatment, therapeutic plans may be developed

Table 19.3 Checklist of four conditions that predict positive treatment response in families where child abuse has occurred

1. Acceptance of responsibility for abuse	• Do the parents accept responsibility for abuse (or neglect)? • Do parents blame the child for provoking the abuse? • Do the parents deny that the abuse occurred?
2. Commitment to meeting their child's needs	• Do the parents accept that they have to change their parenting behaviour in order to meet their child's needs? • Are the parents committed to using available local resources (such as family-based parenting programmes or home-visiting programmes) to improve their parenting skills? • Can the parents place the child's needs ahead of their own needs?
3. Commitment to improving their own psychological well-being	• Do the parents accept that their own psychological problems (depression, substance abuse, anger management problems, marital discord) compromise their capacity to meet their child's needs? • Do the parents deny that they have psychological problems? • Are the parents committed to using available help (counselling, therapy or self-help group membership) to improve their psychological well-being?
4. Ability to change	• Do the parents have the cognitive ability to learn the skills necessary for meeting their child's needs? • Do the parents have the personal flexibility to change their parenting behaviour? • Do the parents have the emotional strength to follow through on parenting programmes, counselling programmes, home-visiting or self-help group programmes which require considerable tolerance for frustration? • Do the parents have the capacity to maintain a co-operative relationship with the local team of professionals who will offer the overall child-protection rehabilitation package?
Will definitely benefit from treatment	Four conditions are met
Will possibly benefit from treatment	Three conditions are met
Unlikely to benefit from treatment	Two or less conditions are met

which are clearly linked to achieving specific concrete goals identified in the assessment. Typical goals and related interventions are set out in Table 19.4.

In addition to having clearly defined goals, treatment for families where child abuse has occurred typically involves a multi-systemic intervention package including a number of the interventions listed in Table 19.4 (Azar & Wolfe, 1998; Browne, 2002; Brunk, Henggeler & Whelan, 1987; Cicchetti,

Table 19.4 Specific goals that may be targets for specific interventions in cases of child abuse and neglect

Locus	Goal	Intervention
Child	• Increasing the child's self-esteem • Increasing the child's cognitive and language skills	• Specialist nursery or pre-school placement • Training parents in age-appropriate cognitive stimulation for their children • Support group for physically abused children or adolescents
Parent	• Increasing parents' knowledge of child development • Increasing parents' capacities to control their anger and impulsivity • Help parents regulate their negative emotions particularly anxiety and depression • Help parents control drug and alcohol use	• Parent training, education and support groups • Anger control training • Cognitive or interpersonal therapy for depression • Treatment for alcohol or drug use
Parent–child relationship	• Improving parenting skills • Increasing frequency of positive parent–child interaction • Increasing the accuracy of the parents' expectations of the child • Helping the child develop regular eating and sleeping routines • Reducing child's behavioural problems	• Family-based treatment focusing on coaching parents in positive parent–child interaction skills and methods for managing eating and sleeping routines and behaviour problems
Couple	• Increasing positive exchanges • Increasing positive communication within the couple • Improving joint problem-solving skill • Increasing affective self-disclosure, empathy and insight into dysfunctional relational patterns	• Communications skills training • Problem-solving training • Behavioural exchange training
Wider social context	• Increasing social support from the extended family or the community for the parents • Reducing stress associated with poverty and the size of the family's living quarters	• Family-based treatment which aims to elicit support from the extended family • Arranging befriender or home-help home-visiting service

- Referral to parent support groups; mother and toddler groups; baby-sitting circle
- Arranging periodic relief foster care
- Arranging welfare payments, referral for career counselling
- Liaising with housing authority

2004; Dale, 1986; Donohue, Miller, Van Hasselt & Hersen, 1998; Edgeworth & Carr, 2000; Emery & Laumann-Billings, 2002; Jones, 2000; Kolko, 2002; MacDonald, 2001; Schuerman, Rzepmicki & Littem, 1994). However, it is important that these components are prioritized. Unless there is good reason to do otherwise, priority should always be given to intensive family-based treatment with the parents and the abused child. The central aim of this intervention should be preventing the occurrence of negative cycles of inter-action and promoting positive exchanges between the parents and child. Ideally, this should involve intensive contact of up to three sessions per week over a three-month period (Nicol et al., 1988). Interventions which target the parents and aim to increase their childcare knowledge and skills and manage their own personal difficulties are a second priority. Intensive input for the child in a specialist day care or nursery setting is a third priority. Marital work is a fourth priority, and intervention to the wider system including the extended family should be fifth in order of priority.

Around a central core of intensive family-based treatment, other com-ponents of the multi-systemic intervention package should be organized. The parents may work with a therapist or facilitator in an individual, couples or group format and the children may work with another professional, such as a teacher, speech therapist or play therapist in individual or group-based programmes.

When engaging these families in treatment, it is particularly important to have a clear treatment contract, with specific goals, a clear specification of the number of treatment sessions and the times and places at which these sessions will occur. Such contracts should be written and formally signed by the par-ents, the psychologist and the statutory social worker. Many families in which child abuse occurs have both financial problems and organizational difficul-ties. Non-attendance at therapy sessions associated with these problems can be significantly reduced by using a home-visiting format wherever possible, or organizing transportation if treatment must occur at a clinic. The following sections offer some guidelines for implementing different aspects of a multi-systemic intervention package.

Treatment focusing on parent–child interaction

The broad aim of treatment sessions targeting parent–child interaction is for the whole family to acknowledge that the parent abused the child, is no longer denying this, wishes to atone for this injustice and wishes to take concrete steps so no further abuse will occur. Effective family intervention programmes, while premised on a broad-based assessment and directed towards this overall goal, have focused on very specific parenting problems, with one target being tackled at a time using systematic behavioural principles (Brunk et al., 1987; Edgeworth & Carr, 2000; Nicol et al., 1988). The following principles are useful in guiding the development of such programmes. Psychologists should work with parents intensively (one to three sessions per week for three months). Wherever possible, sessions should occur in the home rather than the clinic. Within sessions, the therapist's role is that of a coach. The parents and child are coached in how to engage in positive exchanges and avoid negative exchanges. Between sessions, parents and children practise what has been learned in the sessions. As families successfully achieve targets, the frequency of the sessions is reduced.

Target behaviours should be highly specific and easy to count, so progress can be easily monitored by the parents using a simple recording system. Smaller targets should be tackled before larger targets are attempted. Typical targets for families with pre-schoolers include developing a positive parent–child play sequence like that described in Table 4.4 (p. 148) and engaging in it once a day, managing episodes of crying so that they end with the child being soothed by the parent, developing a pre-sleep routine like that described in Chapter 6 and managing feeding time routines without fights. For every target that involves reducing a negative behaviour or exchange (such as a parent shouting at a child or a child crying) a positive target should also be selected (such as the parent cuddling the child or the child playing).

For positive behavioural targets, there should be an emphasis on developing clear daily routines involving these targets. Thus, if the target is for the parent and child to play together without conflict for fifteen minutes per day using the skills for supportive play listed in Table 4.4, a routine needs to be evolved where the parent and child in preparation for this fifteen-minute period go to a particular room at a particular time each day and run through a particular sequence of anticipatory exchanges such as 'It's nearly playtime for Mummy and Billy. What is it? It's nearly playtime for Mummy and Billy. What is it? Yes it is' and so forth. This sequence is appropriate for a pre-schooler. Older children will require more age-appropriate exchanges.

Parents should be coached in how to neutralize the effects of negative cognitive sets or marital conflict before attempting to engage in anticipatory routines leading up to a target behaviour. Re-framing and re-labelling are the main skills parents need to be taught to break out of negative cognitive sets. Re-framing involves interpreting an ambiguous behavioural sequence in a positive or empathic way rather than by attributing negative intentions or qualities to the child. For example, in a situation where a child began crying when the mother answered the phone, the mother interpreted this ambiguous sequence to reflect 'the eight-month-old child's wish to prevent her from talking to her sister on the phone'. The mother was invited to re-frame this situation as one in which 'the child was startled by the phone ringing and disappointed at the loss of the mother's exclusive attention'.

Re-labelling involves using a positive adjective to label the child rather than a negative one, if the response that led to the labelling is sufficiently ambiguous to allow this. For example, a mother who labelled her four-month-old child as 'a brat' any time he cried, was encouraged to replace this internal, global, stable labelling with situational labels, like 'You sometimes cry when you're hungry, don't you?' Using re-framing and re-labelling is a skill parents who have abused their children must over-learn to correct their negative cognitive sets. Negative cognitive sets often interfere with setting-up positive routines.

Marital conflict can also interfere with setting-up positive parent–child routines. Methods for working with couples will be described in more detail below. However, here it is sufficient to say that the primary caregiver's partner (who is usually the father) must be given a specific role in the anticipatory routine that precedes episodes of positive caregiver–child interaction, otherwise there is a risk that the routine will be interrupted by conflict within the couple. This is often motivated by jealousy on the part of the father. This inclusion of both parents in the anticipatory routine, means that it is important for fathers to attend at least some of the parent–child sessions. In some instances, fathers may wish to take on the role of primary caretaker. In these cases mothers will require coaching in how to support the father in this role. (However, in my clinical experience, this type of situation is, unfortunately, not common.)

Shaping should be used as a central therapeutic method. That is, successive approximations to the target behaviours should be rewarded. The therapist should praise the parent and child for successive approximations to positive interaction. The parent should be coached in how to praise the child for successive approximations to age-appropriate positive behaviour.

The main emphasis should be on the use of rewards or positive reinforcement to shape behaviour and reach targets. Parents should be praised by therapists and parents should be trained in how to use rewards including praise, star charts and prizes for children who accumulate a certain number of stars.

Punishment should be avoided and parents should be coached in how to anticipate problem behaviour on the part of the child and attempt to avoid it by distracting the child or ignore it if problem behaviour occurs. Where parents are taught to use time-out routines, following the guidelines in Table 4.6 (p. 150), it is very important to frame these as brief episodes of no more than a couple of minutes in which the child has no access to positive interaction with the parent. Time-out periods should terminate when the child has been in time-out for three minutes or has stopped protesting about being in time-out for 30 seconds. Immediately after time-out, the parent must engage in a positive event with the child and re-establish positive parent–child interaction. There is always a danger that time-out will be used as an excuse to lock children in a room or closet for a couple of hours!

Parents should be encouraged to keep written records of progress and to celebrate success in reaching targets. There should also be an acceptance that relapses will occur and that therapists and parents will meet patches of resistance where co-operation problems occur from time to time; these should be managed in the ways suggested in Chapter 4.

Parent-focused interventions

Effective individual interventions for the parents fall into two broad categories (Edgeworth & Carr, 2000). In the first are those interventions which aim to improve parenting skills and knowledge about child development. In the second are those which aim to help parents with other psychological problems that are not exclusively associated with the parenting role, such as anger management, mood regulation and drug abuse.

Parent-craft and child-development classes are most effectively offered in a group format to as homogeneous a group of parents as possible. For example, it is useful if parents of pre-schoolers attend a different group to parents of primary-school-aged children. A structured curriculum covering the needs and competencies of children who fall into the same age-band as the group members' children should be covered. For example, where group members' children are pre-schoolers, the curriculum should cover child development up to the age of five. The curriculum should be organized in such a way that parents are given a conceptual understanding of a topic, followed by a practical exercise in which they plan in pairs how they will put this new knowledge into practice in caring for their child. Their success with this plan should be reviewed in the next session. This *plan–do–review* process under-pins all effective skill development. For example, with language development, some of the material in Chapter 1 could be presented in simplified form and parents could be asked to plan a fifteen-minute play session with their child in which they stimulate conversation about a topic of interest to the child. In the next session each parent could report on how these conversations went. With pre-schoolers, the range of topics should include attachment, the development of sleep, feeding and elimination routines, motor development and sensorimotor play routines, language development and parent–child language games, cognitive development with a particular emphasis on pre-operational egocentricism, the development of emotional control through using inner speech and children's friendships.

Individual or group work with parents to help develop anger- and mood-regulation skills should offer parents a way to conceptualize how in specific situations they are likely to become apparently uncontrollably angry, sad or anxious, and then provide them with a way of controlling their emotional states in these situations. Cognitive-behavioural frameworks are probably the most widely used in this type of work (Bowman-Edmondson & Cohen Conger, 1996; Carr & McNulty, in press a). Cognitive techniques allow parents to develop control over their emotional states by changing the thoughts they have that under-pin the negative mood states. Parents are trained first to identify antecedent situations that lead to negative emotional states such as anger, fear or sadness. Training then focuses on helping parents to listen to what they tell themselves in these situations and to notice how these stories they tell themselves (automatic thoughts) determine their emotional states. For example, with one mother, any time she received a compliment she felt very sad. This mood occurred because she told herself that the only reason she had received a compliment was because the other person saw just how pathetic she was and so was trying to cheer her up. In therapy, she was helped to look for alternatives to this interpretation and find evidence to support her alternatives. On one memorable occasion, she reported that she could accept a compliment as a reflection of her competence rather than people's pity for her. She had found a child wandering in the car-park outside the supermarket and returned her to her parents. She said that when she returned the child to the parents she understood their gratitude, because she knew what it was like to lose a child and have it returned. This experience allowed her to begin questioning how she misinterpreted many compliments she was paid so that they led to depression rather than joy.

Another mother said that her child's crying always led her to feel angry. She found that this occurred because she told herself that her child's crying was his way of saying that he didn't like the feed she gave him, or the way he played with him, or the way she dressed him and so on. These critical intentions she attributed to the child made her feel angry because she then felt unappreciated despite all she had done for her son. Part of her therapy focused on helping her to question these stories that she told herself about her five-month-old son's intentions each time he cried and to offer a more plausible and less-critical alternative, such as 'he might have wind because he's just had a feed'.

Behavioural interventions for anger, sadness and anxiety help parents by providing them with routines that break the behavioural pattern associated with the negative mood state. For example, with anger, parents may be trained to identify trigger situations and then to use some avoidance strategy when they encounter these trigger situations, such as leaving the room, counting to ten, or engaging in relaxation exercises. With sadness, daily pleasant events may be scheduled and graded activity schedules may be used where parents plan in a gradual way to increase their daily activity levels, especially the amount of exercise they take. With anxiety, a variety of behavioural methods such as relaxation training and systematic desensitization may be used to help parents control these negative emotional states.

Individual or group therapy for parents which aims to foster the regulation of negative mood states may focus on interpersonal themes as well as specific cognitive and behavioural emotion regulation techniques. Many parents who abuse their children have experienced abuse and internalized dysfunctional internal working models for caregiving relationships and indeed intimate marital relationships (Bateman & Holmes, 1995). Therapy may focus on articulating these internal working models and the abusive early experiences from which they have evolved. Common themes include difficulties managing power and negotiation without recourse to violence, problems with empathy and emotional self-disclosure, a tendency towards splitting and projection where people are seen as all good or all bad, feelings of engulfment or abandonment in intimate relationships and so forth. A clearer understanding of these themes and the dysfunctional relationship patterns in which they are embedded arise from this work.

Child-focused interventions

Child-focused interventions may aim to stimulate the child's cognitive and language development as well as fostering self-esteem, particularly in cases where physical abuse has occurred as part of a broader parent–child interaction pattern which includes neglect or emotional abuse (Edgeworth & Carr, 2000). These programmes are best run as pre-school group-based projects with a low teacher–pupil ratio and the cognitive and language curriculum geared to the child's developmental level. Parents should have maximum involvement in these projects and understand the rationale for the programme, the curriculum and the teaching methods and be given advice on how to extend the stimulation programme into the child's homelife.

With older children, the negative self-evaluative beliefs and beliefs about power and violence in relationships that evolve in response to the experience of abuse may be addressed in individual or group therapy. The aim of such therapy is to help children understand that the abuse was not caused by them, that they are not worthless, that they are not powerless and can be assertive with adults, that differences in relationships can be managed in non-violent assertive ways, that they can have mixed feelings of anger and loyalty towards their parents (and members of the treatment team including the foster parents) and that they can, in the long term, find a personal way to forgive their parents. Older children can benefit from assertiveness training where they learn assertive alternatives to aggression for managing interpersonal differences. They may also benefit from learning cognitive and behavioural anger control skills such as those described in the previous section.

Interventions focusing on the couple

Marital intervention may focus on helping couples solve conflicts without recourse to escalating angry exchanges which are displaced onto the child. Four components typify effective couples work (Carr & McNulty, in press b). These are communication skills training, problem-solving skills training, behavioural exchange training and coaching in affective self-disclosure, empathy and development of insight into relational patterns which under-pin discord, violence and dissatisfaction.

Guidelines for training in communication and problem solving are given in Table 4.2 (p. 145) and Table 4.3 (p. 147). However, they will be recapped here, with specific reference to working with couples. The overall strategy for training couples in refining these interpersonal skills is to explain the skills and point out how necessary they are for jointly handling stressful childcare tasks. Then couples are invited to demonstrate their current level of skill development by taking a non-emotive issue and communicating or problem solving around it. The therapist then gives feedback, first indicating the couple's competencies and then pin-pointing areas where improvements are required. Once the couple show competence in managing non-emotive issues, they are invited to progress to discussing emotive issues. The therapist interrupts them when they break the rules of good problem solving or communication and coaches them back on track. Homework assignments which involve practising these skills are also given.

In communication training, couples need to be trained in both listening to each other and in sending clear messages to each other. Listening skills include giving attention without interruption, summarizing key points made by their partner and checking that they have understood accurately. Skills required to send clear messages include discussing one problem at a time, being brief, deciding on specific key points, organizing them logically, saying them clearly, checking that they have been understood and allowing space for a reply. Couples are encouraged to make congruent 'I statements' such as 'I would like to watch *Into the West*' rather than 'you statements' such as 'You would love *Into the West*' or declarations such as 'Everyone knows that *Into the West* is a great film'. Couples are praised for avoiding negative mind-reading, blaming, sulking, name-calling or interruptions.

Problem solving involves defining large, vague and complex difficulties as a series of smaller and clearer problems, brainstorming options for solving these smaller problems one at a time, exploring pros and cons of each option, agreeing on a joint action plan; implementing the plan, reviewing progress, revising the original plan if it was unsuccessful and celebrating if it was successful.

Once couples have been coached in the basics of communication skills and problem-solving skills, they are invited to use them to try to solve emotive problems associated with joint childcare responsibilities, such as who should feed and change the baby on specific occasions and how personal time away from the responsibility of childcare should be organized for each person. The therapist should praise couples for using skills correctly and get them back on track if they fail to use problem-solving and communications skills correctly. With emotive problems, they should also be encouraged to declare that the problem (not their partner) makes them feel bad and to acknowledge their own share of the responsibility in causing the problem (rather than blaming their partner). They should be encouraged to anticipate obstacles when engaging in problem solving.

For families where child abuse has occurred, core beliefs about getting needs met are often a central obstacle to solving problems and reaching mutually acceptable agreements. Parents in these families tend to frame problems in terms of how they will get their own needs met, rather than how both members of the couple and the child can get as many needs met as possible. A common theme is that everyone cannot have their needs met, and if one person's needs are met, it must be at the expense of the needs of another not being met. A related idea is that in any negotiation about family members having their needs met there must be a winner and a loser. The idea that everyone can win if enough thought is given to solving a problem must constantly be re-introduced by the therapist.

Destructive behavioural routines are a second set of obstacles to solving problems and reaching mutually acceptable agreements. These routines may involve attributing negative intentions to one's partner without checking these out and then criticizing, nagging, blaming, name-calling or citing previous instances of the partner's misdemeanours on the one hand, or withdrawing, sulking or becoming intoxicated on the other. Often, anger from these types of exchanges is displaced onto the abused child.

Helping partners recognize these behavioural routines and patterns and the beliefs and feelings that under-pin them is a critical part of couples work. Once they are recognized, alternatives to them may be developed. Most of these routines are based on fears that needs related to personal power, esteem and intimacy will be thwarted, or a sense of being hurt when these needs have been thwarted. Alternative solutions to the escalating negative routines typically involve couples acknowledging and expressing feelings related to unmet needs and having their partner empathize with them about this. Therapists can help couples develop effective self-disclosure and empathy skills by interviewing them about these feelings and then empathizing with them. Couples may then be coached in how to interview each other about these feelings that are rarely articulated and how to empathize with each other.

Behavioural exchange offers a way to introduce greater positive reciprocity into a relationship marked by patterns of mutual punishment and conflict. It involves inviting both partners to list specific positive activities that their partner could carry out to show that they care for them. These items must be phrased positively rather than negatively and must not be the focus of a recent argument. The couple is invited to put the lists in a visible place in the house and to make a commitment to carry out some of the items on the list for their partner each day. However, quid pro quo arrangements are to be avoided. The idea is to increase the number of positive exchanges but within the context of a good-will ethic rather than a quid pro quo contract.

When couples engage in more positive exchanges, use communication and problem-solving skills and engage in affective self-disclosure and empathy, solving childcare problems becomes far less stressful and far less likely to result in domestic violence.

Intervention in the wider system

Interventions in the wider system aim to reduce stress and increase social support (Edgeworth & Carr, 2000). Such interventions must be tailored to the ecology of the family as mapped out during the assessment process. The following are common examples of interventions that fall into this category: work with members of the extended family to increase the amount of support they offer the child's primary caretaker, arranging a befriender, a home-help or a counsellor home-visiting service for an isolated parent, arranging participation in a local parent support self-help group, organizing a place for the child and caretaker in a local mother and toddler group, introducing the family to a baby-sitting circle, setting up periodic relief foster care, supporting an application for housing transfer to a less cramped residence and referring family members to medical or other professional services to solve problems requiring specialist input.

A specialized ecological approach to foster care is described in Chapter 22 (Minuchin, 1995). Within this approach, the foster parents with whom the child is placed during the comprehensive assessment are recruited as major sources of long-term support for the parents of the child. They effectively become like grandparents to the child and surrogate parents to the child's mother and father. As part of their role, during the assessment process they facilitate frequent access visits between parents and child. They also facilitate a gradual transition of responsibility for childcare from themselves to the parents when a decision is made that the child return home, with the child spending some nights at the parents' house and some at the foster parents' home. In the months that follow, they offer temporary respite care.

Countertransference reactions and polarization in therapy teams

Working with cases of child abuse evokes strong feelings in all of us (Carr, 1997). In cases of physical child abuse, the two most common countertransference reactions are *rescuing the child* and *rescuing the parents*. In the former reaction, the urge is to protect the child at all costs and to deny any loyalty that the child may have to the parents, or any competence or potential for therapeutic change on the part of the parents. In the latter reaction the urge is to protect the parents from criticism raised by other professionals, and to deny any parental shortcomings. Professionals within the same system adopting these two countertransference reactions tend to polarize and have difficulty co-operating with each other and the family with whom they are working. Recognizing this polarization process and discussing it openly is one way of preventing co-operation difficulties.

PREVENTION

Physical abuse occurs in families characterized by high levels of stress and low levels of support when children place demands on their parents which outstrip parental coping resources, and parents in frustration injure their children. Effective prevention programmes reduce stress, increase support, enhance parenting knowledge and skills, and promote child health so as to reduce demands children place on vulnerable parents (O'Riordan & Carr, 2002). In such programmes, families at risk for physical child abuse are screened pre-natally using the criteria listed in Table 19.5. They are then engaged by nurses or para-professionals in multi-modal community-based programmes which begin antenatally. These programmes include home visiting, behavioural parent training, stress management and life skills training, details of which are given in Table 19.5. The home-visiting element of such programmes is essential to maintain ongoing engagement and prevent drop-out. Clinical psychologists have an important role to play in setting up such multi-modal programmes, training, supervising staff and monitoring and evaluating programme effectiveness.

SUMMARY

Physical abuse refers to deliberately inflicted injury or deliberate attempts to poison a child. The overall prevalence of physical child abuse is between 10 and 25%. Child abuse has short- and long-term physical and psychological effects. Psychological effects include the development of negative self-evaluative beliefs, dysfunctional internal working models for relationships, emotion regulation problems, internalizing and externalizing behavioural problems, cognitive and attainment problems and relationship difficulties. The range, severity and duration of effects depend on the nature and extent of the abuse and the balance of risk and protective factors present in any given case. Risk and protective factors include features of the child, the parents, the parent–child relationship, the marriage, the wider social network and the treatment system. Multi-disciplinary validation of cases of physical child

Table 19.5 Components of physical child abuse prevention programmes

Screening	• *Child characteristics*: prematurity, low birth weight and difficult temperament • *Maternal characteristics:* teenage pregnancy, physical or mental health problems, substance abuse, chaotic lifestyle, personal adjustment difficulties, personal history of abuse or neglect, previously suspected of child abuse • *Family factors:* insecure mother–child attachment, being a single parent, lack of father involvement, lack of family support • *Social factors:* high levels of life stress, poverty, homelessness, and under-use of appropriate health and social services
Goals	• To increase parental knowledge of child development so as to modify unrealistic expectations • To help parents recognize and understand infants' signals when they require basic needs to be met • To help parents develop feeding, sleeping, cleaning, and playing/ stimulating routines with their infants • To help parents maintain socially supportive relationships with their partners and members of the extended family • To help parents maintain supportive relationships with health and social services professionals • To provide crisis intervention to help parents cope with psychosocial and economic crises that interfere with providing quality infant care • To help parents develop stress management skills so that stress-related anger will not lead parents to injure their children • To monitor children's health and development
Home visiting	• Professionals, para-professionals or trained volunteers visit mothers and infants frequently at the family home • Visiting, ideally begins before the birth of the child • The home visitor provides information about child development and childcare; helps with the development of parenting skills; and offers social support • The non-judgemental, supportive and empathic quality of the relationship that typifies the relationship between the home visitor and the mother are central to its effectiveness as a source of support for vulnerable or at-risk parents
Behavioural parent training	• The parent and child regularly visit an outpatient centre and the parent develops specific parenting skills by engaging in behavioural parent training with a professional • Behavioural parent training may be provided on a group or individual basis • The clear, precise procedures for developing feeding, sleeping, cleaning, and playing/stimulating routines which are based on well-established behavioural principles are central to the effectiveness of behavioural parent training
Life skills training	• In life skills training parents, through modelling, instruction and guided practice, acquire the skills necessary to manage certain psychosocial and economic life stresses that compromise their capacity to provide quality infant care

Continued

Table 19.5 Continued

	• These skills include money and household management; budgeting; dealing with health, social services, educational and financial agencies; enhancing problem-solving and communication skills
Stress management training	• In stress management training, parents through modelling, instruction and guided practice acquire the skills necessary to manage negative mood states such as anger, anxiety and depression that may compromise their capacity to provide quality infant care
	• These skills include recognizing the signs of stress early; challenging thoughts that maintain negative mood states; learning relaxation skills; changing potentially stressful situations so that they are less demanding; and using social support to reduce stress

Note: Adapted from O'Riordan & Carr (2002).

abuse typically involves medical examination and interviews to assess the degree to which the child's injuries are consistent with the parent and child's account of the injury, the history and other relevant factors. Comprehensive assessment following validation involves interviews with all members of the child system and should cover relevant risk and protective factors and a verbal reconstruction of the abusive incident. Where parents accept responsibility for the abuse, are committed to meeting their child's needs, are committed to improving their own psychological well-being and where they have the ability to change, the prognosis is good. Where less than three of these conditions are met, it is unlikely that a positive treatment response will occur. Treatment should be based on clear contracts to meet specific targets. Treatment and case management plans involve a central focus on improving parent–child interaction through direct work with parents and children together. This may be supplemented with individual work for parents focusing on parent-craft and the management of personal psychological difficulties such as mood and anger regulation. Children may receive input in therapeutic pre-school placements. Intervention may also focus on helping couples enhance their mutual supportiveness and the degree to which the extended family offer support. Effective prevention programmes reduce stress, increase support, enhance parenting knowledge and skills, and promote child health so as to reduce demands children place on vulnerable parents.

EXERCISE 19.1

Sally, aged nineteen years, and her child Ricky, aged eighteen months are referred to your team for assessment with a view to Ricky returning to the care of his mother, Sally. Ricky has been in foster care for a month following a non-accidental injury in which Sally hit him on the head with a tray because he wouldn't stay quiet. She was watching TV and drinking beer at 2.00 a.m. when this happened. She is very remorseful and says she will do anything to get him back except speak to his father. Jay, the father, left Sally when he found she was pregnant and hasn't been in touch since. Sally has four older sisters. She has no contact with them or her parents; they parted on poor terms. Sally lives in an almost derelict mansion, which she is caretaking for the owner, who lives abroad. The social worker in this case and the foster parents are in regular conflict. The foster parents do not want the child returned to Sally because they think that she is irresponsible and a poorly skilled parent. The social worker wants the child to be returned to the mother very soon. The referral for assessment was in part motivated by this difference in views.

- Offer a preliminary formulation of the case.
- Develop an assessment plan.
- On the basis of the available information, would you offer this family a treatment programme and what justification would you offer for your decision?
- If you think this case is treatable, ideally what type of programme would you offer?

EXERCISE 19.2

Role-play the first interviews with the mother, the social worker and the foster parents, and re-formulate the case on the basis of the information gained.

On the basis of the information arising from these interviews, would you offer this family a treatment programme and what justification would you offer for your decision?

FURTHER READING

Department of Health (2000). Department of Health Framework for the Assessment of Children in Need and their Families. London: Stationery Office. Available at: http://www.dh.gov.uk/PublicationsAndStatistics/Publications/PublicationsPolicy AndGuidance/PublicationsPolicyAndGuidanceArticle/fs/ en?CONTENT_ID=4008144&chk=CwTP%2Bc
Feindler, E., Rathus, J., & Silver, L. E. (2003). *Assessment of Family Violence. A*

Handbook for Researchers and Practitioners. Washington, DC: APA. (*Gives good description of a comprehensive catalogue of tests, but does not include the actual tests and measures.*)

MacDonald, G. (2001). *Effective Interventions for Child Abuse and Neglect. An Evidence-Based Approach to Planning and Evaluating Interventions*. Chichester: Wiley.

McNeish, D., Newman, T., & Roberts, H. (2002). *What Works for Children*. Buckingham: Open University Press.

Myers, J., Berliner, L., Briere, Hendrix, C., Jenny, C., & Reid, T. (2002). *APSAC Handbook on Child Maltreatment* (Second edition). Thousand Oaks, CA: Sage.

Rathus, J. & Feindler, E. (2004). *Assessment of Partner Violence. A Handbook for Researchers and Practitioners*. Washington, DC: APA. (*Gives good description of a comprehensive catalogue of tests, but does not include the actual tests and measures.*)

Reder, P. & Lucey, C. (1995). *Assessment of Parenting. Psychiatric and Psychological Contributions*. London: Routledge.

IRISH AND UK CHILD PROTECTION GUIDELINES

Children First National Guidelines for the Protection and Welfare of Children. A Summary (1999). Dublin, Ireland: Stationery Office. Available at: http://www.dohc.ie/publications/pdf/children_sum.pdf

Working Together to Safeguard Children (1999). London: The Stationery Office. Available at: http://www.dh.gov.uk/PublicationsAndStatistics/Publications/PublicationsPolicyAndGuidance/PublicationsPolicyAndGuidanceArticle/fs/en?CONTENT_ID=4007781&chk=BUYMa8

WEBSITES AND WEB RESOURCES

American Professional Society on the Abuse of Children (APSAC): http://www.apsac.org

BPS position paper on training in child protection: http://www.bps.org.uk/about/position_papers.cfm

Child abuse websites: http://www.childabuse.com/links.htm

International Society for Prevention of Child Abuse and Neglect (ISPCAN): http://www.ispcan.org

Irish Society for the Prevention of Cruelty to Children (ISPCC): http://www.ispcc.ie/

National Clearinghouse on Child Abuse and Neglect: http://nccanch.acf.hhs.gov

National Exchange Centre: http://www.preventchildabuse.com

National Society for the Prevention of Cruelty to Children NSPCC: http://www.nspcc.org.uk

UK Department of Health Framework for the Assessment of Children in Need and their Families: http://www.dh.gov.uk/PublicationsAndStatistics/Publications/PublicationsPolicyAndGuidance/PublicationsPolicyAndGuidanceArticle/fs/en?CONTENT_ID=4008144&chk=CwTP%2Bc

Factsheets on child abuse and neglect, domestic violence, parental mental illness and good parenting can be downloaded from the website for Rose, G. & York, A. (2004). *Mental Health and Growing Up. Fact sheets for Parents, Teachers and Young People* (Third edition). London: Gaskell: http://www.rcpsych.ac.uk

Chapter 20

Emotional abuse and neglect

Certain parenting or childcare styles entail passive neglect or active emotional abuse of infants and children (Browne, 2002; Dubowitz & Black, 2002; Erickson & Egeland, 2002; Glaser, 2002a; Hart, Brassard, Binggeli & Davidson, 2002; Hildyard & Wolfe, 2002; Iwaniec, 1995, 2004; Jones, 2000; MacDonald, 2001; Reder & Lucey, 1995; Smith & Fong, 2004; Wekerle & Wolfe, 2003). There is not an international consensus in this area. Some Eastern countries endorse institutional practices for orphans that are considered neglectful in the West. In contrast, some Western practices, such as infants sleeping in separate rooms from their parents, are considered neglectful in some Eastern cultures. Neglect and emotional abuse may lead to negative physical, cognitive and social outcomes for the child. Negative physical outcomes include non-organic failure to thrive and psychosocial dwarfism. Relationship difficulties and attachment problems are the principal negative social outcomes for children who suffer neglect or emotional abuse. Developmental delays are the principal cognitive sequelae of these aversive parenting practices. A typical case characterized by neglect, non-organic failure to thrive, developmental delay and attachment problems is presented in Box 20.1. After considering the definition of neglect, emotional abuse and related conditions, this chapter describes an approach to assessing risk and protective factors in these cases. Treatment and prevention are then discussed.

DEFINITIONS OF NEGLECT AND EMOTIONAL ABUSE

Considerable controversy surrounds the definition of emotional abuse and neglect. The working definitions set out in Table 20.1 are based on recent reviews of the area (Browne, 2002; Dubowitz & Black, 2002; Erickson & Egeland, 2002; Glaser, 2002a; Hart et al., 2002; Hildyard & Wolfe, 2002; Iwaniec, 1995, 2004; Jones, 2000; MacDonald, 2001; Smith & Fong, 2004; Wekerle & Wolfe, 2003). Emotional neglect and emotional abuse are two forms of child maltreatment in which particular parenting practices, usually

Box 20.1 A case of neglect, non-organic failure to thrive and inhibited reactive attachment disorder

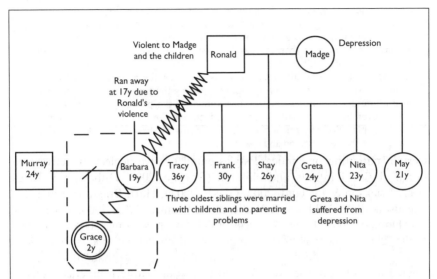

Referral. Grace, a two-year-old child, and her mother, Barbara, were referred for consultation to a multi-disciplinary paediatric team by the GP because Grace's weight fell below the 3rd centile. Her sensorimotor development, cognitive development and language were all delayed and there appeared to be problems with the mother–daughter relationship.

Family history. Barbara was one of seven children and had run away from home at seventeen because of her father's violence towards her. Her developmental history was marked by constant exposure to paternal violence and abuse. Ronald regularly hit all family members, including Barbara, her six siblings and her mother. Barbara's mother had been depressed throughout much of her up-bringing and Barbara was partly raised by her older siblings, who one-by-one left home to escape Ronald's aggression. Thus, neglect, physical abuse, and abandonment had been commonplace experiences for Barbara throughout her childhood.

Barbara's three older siblings were married to highly supportive partners and all three had children. There were, according to Barbara, no significant problems within these families. Two of the three remaining female siblings had, like their mother Madge, been treated for depression. The depression was related to the father, Ronald's, constant violence within the home.

Barbara, had met Grace's father, Murray, at a party shortly after she ran away from home and had become pregnant by mistake during the early stages of her brief relationship with Murray. Barbara had lived as a relatively isolated single parent since the birth of Grace and had no contact with Murray. She occasionally visited her eldest sister, Tracy. Her parents, Ronald and Madge, lived in another town and rarely visited, much to Barbara's relief. They disapproved of Barbara for keeping her illegitimate child and ruining the family's reputation.

Current living situation. In a preliminary home visit, it was noted that Barbara and Grace lived in a bedsit in a seaside resort. The room was sparsely furnished and there was no heating except for a single-bar electric fire, which was broken when we were visiting. There were few toys and no mobiles or children's pictures in the vicinity of the child's cot.

Observations of mother–child interaction. Grace was thin, with very dark circles under her eyes. She sat almost immobile in the corner of the room on the floor in dirty clothing. She responded to the psychologist's attempts to initiate a play sequence involving dolls and bricks with an unusual degree of familiarity and a lack of anxiety about the fact that the psychologist was a stranger. When her mother, Barbara, attempted to take over the role of the psychologist in this episode of play, Grace averted her gaze and ceased to show interest in the play materials. Barbara, in response, withdrew from the play sequence, telling the psychologist that this was a typical interaction and blaming the breakdown of the play sequence on the child. When, later, Barbara picked Grace up to feed her, she turned her head away and said 'No! No! No!' She refused a bottle and some mashed banana. And what little she did eat she regurgitated and spat out.

Assessment of the mother. In a later individual interview with Barbara it became apparent that she suffered from episodes of depression characterized by low mood, sleep problems and loss of appetite. Her score on the Beck Depression Inventory was in the clinical range. During Barbara's episodes of depression she rarely engaged in play or sustained feeding activities with Grace. Periodically, she drank excessively or used a variety of street drugs to alleviate her sense of depression and isolation. On a couple of occasions she had gone out to the pub and left Grace alone in the bedsit, strapped into her push-chair for up to two hours. Barbara had attended a mothers and toddlers group on a couple of occasions but felt rejected by the other mothers and so stopped going. She expressed little interest in personal counselling for her depression but wanted to be taught how to feed her child more effectively.

Formulation. Barbara and Grace had evolved a pattern of mother–child interaction characterized by attachment problems and neglect. A number of factors contributed to this. The primary factor was Barbara's difficulty in attuning herself to Grace's needs and Grace's despondency at not being able to elicit care from her mother. Barbara's difficulties had their roots in her own history of physical abuse and neglect and periodic episodes of depression and related drug abuse. Her depression was maintained by the lack of available social support from her extended family and peer group and the multiple economic and social stresses.

Treatment. The treatment plan was to offer Barbara coaching in interacting with her child in play and feeding situations. A second element of the plan was to offer her a place in a therapeutic mother and toddler group which offered social support, parenting skills training and a cognitive therapy approach to mood regulation.

spanning a substantial time period, lead to adverse consequences for the child, such as attachment difficulties and non-organic failure to thrive.

Neglect

With neglect, there is a passive ignoring of the child's needs. These include:

- physical needs for feeding, clothing and shelter
- safety needs for protection
- emotional needs for nurturance and a secure base

Table 20.1 Main features of neglect and emotional abuse

Neglect	Emotional abuse
There is a passive and **unintentional** ignoring of the child's needs. These include: • Physical needs for feeding, clothing and shelter • Safety needs for protection • Emotional needs for nurturance and a secure base • Intellectual needs for stimulation, social interaction and conversation • The need for age-appropriate limit setting and discipline • The need for age-appropriate opportunities for autonomy and independence	Emotional abuse involves **intentionally** carrying out some of the following actions with respect to the child: • Frequent punishment for minor misdemeanours • Frequent punishment for positive behaviours such as smiling, playing or solving problems • Frequent criticism, ridicule, humiliation and threats • Frequent rejection, discouragement of attachment and exclusion from family life • Frequent blocking the development of appropriate peer relationships • Frequent corruption through parents involving the child in drug use, prostitution, or theft • Frequent attitudinal corruption through encouraging prejudicial hatred of specific groups of people (on the basis of race, gender, religious beliefs, etc.)

Note: Adapted from Iwaniec (1995).

- intellectual needs for stimulation, social interaction and conversation
- the need for age-appropriate limit setting and discipline
- the need for age-appropriate opportunities for autonomy and independence.

Typically, parents who neglect their children do not do so intentionally. Rather, it arises through parents' lack of resources or lack of awareness of their children's needs. Physical neglect involves failing to meet the child's needs for food, clothing and shelter and failure to protect the child from harm, including environmental hazards, infections and illnesses. This is the most common form of neglect and is related to social disadvantage and poverty. With emotional neglect, parents fail to meet the child's needs for nurturance, stimulation, limits and independence. This is often related to a lack of knowledge, skills, emotional maturity and mental health. Parents may not know how important nurturance and stimulation are for child development. They may not have the skills for meeting the child's needs for stimulation and nurturance. They may not recognize illness or poor eating and growth patterns in their children. Or they may be unfamiliar with developmental milestones and so not recognize immaturity in their children. This ignorance may have its roots in a variety of personal and contextual factors.

These include a lack of exposure to good parenting models in childhood; personal experience of abuse or neglect; personal incapacities such as depression, impulsivity or alcohol and drug use; poor social problem-solving skills; marital discord or violence; a chaotic family lifestyle and a high level of life stress involving poverty and isolation.

Emotional abuse

In contrast to neglect, emotional abuse involves intentionally carrying out some of the following actions with respect to the child:

- frequent punishment for minor misdemeanours
- frequent punishment for positive behaviours such as smiling, playing or solving problems
- frequent criticism, ridicule, humiliation and threats
- frequent rejection, discouragement of attachment and exclusion from family life
- frequent blocking the development of appropriate peer relationships.
- frequent corruption through parents involving the child in drug use, prostitution or theft
- frequent attitudinal corruption through encouraging prejudicial hatred of specific groups of people or family members (on the basis of race, gender, religious beliefs, etc.).

Five dimensions of emotional abuse

Glaser (2002a) identifies five qualitative dimensions of parenting that underpin emotional abuse. These are:

- persistent negative mis-attributions to the child
- inaccurate developmental expectations
- emotional unavailability
- using the child to meet the parents' emotional needs
- deviant socialization.

Persistent punishment, criticism and rejection may be motivated by negative parental mis-attributions or inaccurate developmental expectations. The parents may inaccurately attribute negative intentions to the child, such as assuming that the child is not eating or crying to intentionally punish them. Alternatively, the parents may behave in a punitive or critical way towards the child because of a lack of accurate knowledge about child development. They may believe that criticism and punishment is character building or that very young children should be capable of a high degree of emotional and physical self-control. Rejection may reflect parental unavailability due to depression or drug abuse. The processes of mis-attribution and inaccurate expectations which lead to parental punishment, criticism and rejection lead the child to develop both negative self-evaluative beliefs and to internalize punitive internal models for caregiving relationships. Parents may use the child to meet their emotional needs by over-identifying with them and treating them as a confidant. This may include persistently confiding to the child their anger or hatred towards the child's other parent in cases of divorce or separation, or their intense anxiety about particular issues. In these instances, the child becomes triangulated between the over-involved parent and the other parent or adults in their lives, have difficulty developing a clear sense of autonomy and may internalize over-involved models of caregiving relationships. Deviant socialization processes under-pin parents' acts of corruption whereby they involve children in criminal activities and lead the child to develop internal standards that will foster the development of conduct disorders.

Four levels of severity of neglect and emotional abuse

Browne (2002) distinguishes between four levels of severity of neglect and emotional abuse: less severe, moderately severe, very severe and life-threatening. With less severe neglect, there is occasional withholding of love and affection, the child's weight is close to the third centile without organic cause, some developmental delay is present and the child is unwashed. With moderately severe neglect, there is frequent withholding of love and affection, non-organic failure to gain weight, poor hygiene and parental incapacitation due to significant mental health problems. With severe neglect, the parent is frequently unavailable to the child, the child is occasionally left alone, non-organic failure to thrive is present, severe nappy rash with skin lesions occurs and there are frequent significant episodes of parental mental illness. With life-threatening neglect, the parent is persistently absent, the child is frequently left alone, there is non-organic failure to thrive and the child is frequently ill and has infections due to poor hygiene.

According to Browne (2002), with less severe emotional abuse, there are occasional verbal assaults, denigration, humiliation, scapegoating and a confusing family atmosphere. With moderately severe emotional abuse, there are frequent verbal assaults, denigration, humiliation and occasional rejection. The child may also witness occasional family violence and parental intoxication. With severe emotional abuse, there is frequent rejection, occasional withholding of food and drink, enforced isolation and restriction of movement. The child frequently witnesses family violence and parental intoxication. With life-threatening emotional abuse, there is frequent rejection, failure to nurture, frequent withholding of food and drink, enforced isolation and restriction of movement. Parents terrorize and confine the child, and the child frequently witnesses parental psychotic episodes.

Treatment implications

The intentional nature of emotional abuse in contrast to the unintentional nature of neglect has important treatment implications. With neglect, one of the major goals of treatment is education and the provision of support. With emotional abuse, the personal and contextual factors that lead the parent to want to humiliate and reject their child must be addressed. Furthermore, cases of neglect often meet more of the criteria for treatability set out in Table 19.3 (p. 919) than cases of emotional abuse. Compared with cases of neglect, in cases of emotional abuse, it is less common for parents to accept responsibility for abuse and to be committed to meeting the child's needs.

Emotional abuse and neglect can lead to non-organic failure to thrive, psychosocial dwarfism, attachment disorders and developmental delays in the emergence of sensorimotor, cognitive and language skills.

EPIDEMIOLOGY

A review of international incidence studies confirms that neglect is the most common form of child maltreatment and that emotional abuse is less common (Creighton, 2004). The annual incidence of neglect in the UK, Australia and North America, based on officially reported cases in the 1990s, was between 1 and 10 per 1000. About half of all reported cases of child maltreatment in these countries had suffered neglect, rather than physical, sexual or emotional abuse or neglect. The annual incidence of emotional abuse in the UK, Australia and North America, based on officially reported cases in the 1990s was between 0.9 and 2.3 per 1000. About a fifth of all reported cases of child maltreatment in these countries had suffered emotional abuse, rather than physical or sexual abuse or neglect.

SHORT-TERM EFFECTS OF NEGLECT AND EMOTIONAL ABUSE

In the short term, neglect and emotional abuse can lead to parent–child attachment problems, non-organic failure to thrive, psychosocial dwarfism and developmental delays.

Attachment problems

Sixty per cent of children develop secure attachments; the remainder develop insecure attachments (Zennah, 1996). Two insecure attachment patterns are recognized in both ICD 10 and DSM IV TR and these are set out in Table 20.2 (O'Connor, 2002). The first, inhibited reactive attachment disorder,

Table 20.2 Reactive attachment disorder of infancy or early childhood

DSM IV TR	ICD 10
Reactive attachment disorder	**Reactive attachment disorder of childhood**

A. Markedly disturbed and developmentally inappropriate social relatedness in most contexts beginning before the age of five and as evidenced by either 1 or 2:

1. Persistent failure to initiate or respond in a developmentally appropriate fashion to most social interactions as manifested by excessively inhibited, hypervigilant or highly ambivalent and contradictory responses (e.g. response to caregiver with a mixture of approach/avoidance and resistance to comforting, or may exhibit frozen watchfulness)
2. Diffuse attachments as manifested by indiscriminate sociability with marked inability to exhibit appropriate selective attachments (e.g. excessive familiarity with relative strangers or lack of selectivity in choice of attachment figures)

B. The disturbance in criterion A is not accounted for by developmental delay or pervasive developmental disorder

C. Pathogenic care is evidenced by at least one of the following:
(1) persistent disregard of the child's basis emotional needs for comfort stimulation and affection
(2) persistent disregard of the child's basic physical needs
(3) repeated changes of primary caregiver that prevent formation of stable attachments (e.g. frequent changes of foster care)

D. There is a presumption that the care in criterion C is responsible for the disturbed behaviour in criterion A.

Specify **Inhibited type** if criterion A1 pre-dominates
Specify **disinhibited type** if criterion A2 pre-dominates

The key feature is an abnormal pattern of relationships with caregivers that developed before the age of five years, that involves maladaptive features not ordinarily seen in normal children, and that is persistent, yet reactive, to sufficiently marked changes in patterns of rearing. Young children with this syndrome show strongly contradictory or ambivalent social responses that may be most evident at time of partings or reunions. Thus infants may approach with averted look, gaze strongly away while being held, or respond to caregivers with a mixture of approach avoidance and resistance to comforting. The emotional disturbance may be evident in apparent misery, a lack of emotional responsiveness, withdrawal reactions such as huddling on the floor, and/or aggressive responses to their own or other's distress. Fearfulness and hypervigilance (frozen watchfulness), that are unresponsive to comforting, occur in some cases. In most cases, children show interest in peer interactions but play is impeded by negative emotional responses. The attachment disorder may be accompanied by a failure to thrive physically and by impaired physical growth. Reactive attachment disorders nearly always arise in relation to grossly inadequate childcare. This may take the form of psychological abuse or neglect or of physical abuse or neglect

Disinhibited attachment disorder of childhood

Diagnosis should be based on evidence that the child showed an unusual degree of diffuseness in selective attachments during the first five years and that this was associated with generally clinging behaviour in infancy and/or indiscriminately friendly, attention-seeking behaviour in early or middle childhood. Usually there is difficulty forming close confiding relationships with peers. There may or may not be associated emotional or behavioural disturbance. In most cases there will be a clear history of rearing in the first years that involved marked discontinuities in caregivers or multiple changes in family placements (as with multiple foster family placements)

Note: Adapted from DSM IV (APA, 2000a) and ICD 10 (WHO, 1992, 1996).

is associated with abuse and neglect. Specifically, it is associated with a rejecting or punitive parenting style or a parenting style where the parent is not promptly and appropriately responsive to the child's signals that it needs something from the parent. It is characterized by contradictory or ambivalent approach–avoidance social responses typically displayed during partings and reunions, emotional disturbance characterized by misery and withdrawal or aggression, and fearfulness and hypervigilance. The second disorder of attachment, disinhibited reactive attachment disorder, is associated with institutional upbringing or multi-placement experiences and is characterized by clinging behaviour in infancy, diffuseness of selective attachments in preschool years, indiscriminately friendly attention-seeking behaviour in middle childhood and a difficulty in forming confiding peer relationships in childhood and adolescence. Both types of attachment disorder are associated with difficult temperament and both may be precursors of conduct disorder and later personality disorders (Zennah, 1996).

Attachment disorders may be distinguished from pervasive developmental disorders. Children with attachment disorders have a normal capacity for social reciprocity, whereas those with pervasive developmental disorders do not. Children with reactive attachment disorder gradually develop more normal patterns of social interaction when placed in social context where their physical and psychological needs are met. In the case of pervasive developmental disorders, abnormal social behaviour persists despite environmental changes. Impaired intellectual and language development may characterize children with both disorders. However, those with pervasive developmental disorders show certain linguistic peculiarities, such as echolalia, and their intellectual deficits do not ameliorate markedly in response to environmental enrichment. Finally, stereotyped and ritualistic behaviour patterns characterize children with pervasive developmental disorders but not those with reactive attachment disorders.

Children do not need to be cared for by a single adult. However, multiple changing caregivers cannot meet a child's needs for secure attachment. Children need a small group of adults who provide consistent care over an extended period with whom to form a hierarchy of selective attachments. These adults should be responsive to their cues and available at times of tiredness or distress or in stressful, challenging circumstances. These principles should form the basis for both day-care services and residential childcare services (O'Connor, 2002).

Non-organic failure to thrive

While neglect and emotional abuse define parenting or caregiving problems, non-organic failure to thrive is a common outcome for the child who has received neglectful or emotionally abusive parenting. The clinical features of this condition are set out in Table 20.3 (Iwaniec, 1995, 2004; Smith & Fong,

Table 20.3 Main features of non-organic failure to thrive and psychosocial dwarfism

Non-organic failure to thrive	Psychosocial dwarfism
Growth retardation • Child falls below the 3rd centile in weight and often in height	**Growth retardation** • Child's weight, height, and head circumference falls below expected norms
Eating pattern • Refusal to take feeds • Vomiting • Diarrhoea	**Eating pattern** • Excessive eating • Gorging and vomiting • Scavenging food from waste-bins and begging food from strangers • Hoarding food and secretly searching for it at night • Eating non-food items
Developmental delay • Failure to achieve motor development milestones • Failure to reach language and intellectual milestones • Social and emotional immaturity	**Developmental delay** • Failure to achieve motor development milestones • Failure to reach language and intellectual milestones • Social and emotional immaturity
Attachment problems • Insecure attachment	**Attachment problems** • Insecure attachment, rejects mother, shows lack of stranger-anxiety
Physical features • Wasted body and thin arm and legs; large stomach • Red, cold, wet hands and feet • Thin, wispy, dull, falling hair • Dark circles around eyes • Frequent colds and infections	**Physical features** • Disproportionate body build with short legs and enlarged stomach • Small and thin • Reduced growth hormone levels
Psychological features • Lethargy and passivity • Little vocalization • Stares blankly and lack of exploratory behaviour • Sadness, tearfulness, frequent whining and little smiling • Withdrawal, detachment and lack of social responsivity or cuddliness	**Psychological features** • Depressed mood • Social withdrawal, detachment and lack of social responsivity or cuddliness • Mutism • Soiling, wetting and smearing • Aggressiveness and defiance • Self-harming behaviour • Short attention span • Insomnia

Note: Adapted from Iwaniec (1995).

2004). The syndrome was first identified by Spitz (1945) in a study of institutionalized infants who failed to grow despite adequate calorific intake. He attributed the condition to the fact that they received little stimulation and had multiple caretakers. Spitz coined the terms 'hospitalism' and 'anaclytic depression' to describe the clinical presentations of institutionalized children.

Recent studies of non-organic failure to thrive have pin-pointed the centrality of dysfunctional mother–child interaction patterns during feeding as the
main maintaining factor in non-organic failure to thrive. Four common patterns identified by Iwaniec (2004, 1995) are set out in Figure 20.1. With the
neglectful pattern, the mother fails to recognize the child's need for food and
the child become passive and withdrawn. With the aggressive feeding pattern,
the mother and child become embroiled in an aggressive feeding battle in
which the mother attempts to force-feed the child and the child refuses food
or vomits. In the non-persistent pattern, the mother becomes depressed and
filled with a sense of helplessness as she repeatedly fails to help her child to
feed. The final pattern involves the mother taking a flexible and tolerant
approach to coaxing her child to take food and to some degree this

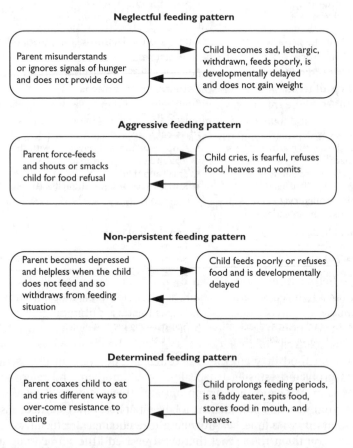

Figure 20.1. Four feeding patterns associated with non-organic failure to thrive

Note: Adapted from Iwaniec (1995).

adaptation is successful, although fadiness, spitting and retaining food in the mouth continue to occur.

For mothers to persist in the determined feeding pattern, they require low stress, high support, strong personal resources and the absence of problems such as depression. It is also important to acknowledge the role of children's temperament in initiating and maintaining these feeding patterns. Children's refusal to be fed by their mothers strikes at the heart of many mothers' identities. It may lead to definitions of the self as a failure and subsequent guilt and depression, or anger at the child and a wish to blame the child for bringing forth this view of the self as a failure. Non-organic failure to thrive, if treated in the first year, may have a good prognosis. Children who are not identified until they are two years or older continue to have long-term problems.

In DSM IV TR, non-organic failure to thrive is not listed as a diagnosis. However, three feeding disorders are mentioned, two of which may occur in non-organic failure to thrive. These are feeding disorder of infancy and early childhood and rumination disorder. The third disorder, pica, is probably not related to failure to thrive, but does occasionally occur with psychosocial dwarfism. Feeding disorder of infancy and early childhood is applied to infants who fail to eat adequately and do not gain weight over a period of at least a month. Where infants regurgitate their food regularly over a period of at least a month, a diagnosis of rumination disorder is given. Infants who eat non-nutritive substances regularly for a period of at least a month are given a diagnosis of pica.

In ICD 10, feeding disorder of infancy and childhood and pica are both listed. However, rumination disorder is subsumed into the feeding disorder of infancy and childhood and is not given a separate category of its own as in DSM IV.

Psychosocial dwarfism

Children suffering from psychosocial dwarfism are exceptionally short for their age, have reduced weight, a small head circumference despite normal calorific intake and no obvious organic basis for their failure to grow (Iwaniec, 1995). In addition to these growth problems, children with this condition show unusual patterns of eating behaviour, including gorging, scavenging, secretly seeking food at night and hoarding it. They also display serious attachment problems, refusing to speak to their mothers and referring to them as Miss or Mrs, and show inappropriate attachments to strangers. At home they are aggressive and defiant to their parents. They engage in self-injurious behaviour such as head-banging or inflicting superficial wounds and scratches on themselves. They frequently wet and soil. They may also urinate intentionally on their own or other's possessions, hide their stools in unusual places or smear them on the walls. These children also show physical, cognitive and social developmental delays. The home environment is typically characterized by extreme emotional abuse. When removed from the home environment, these youngsters show accelerated growth, which deteriorates when they are returned to their parents' care. It is not unusual for these youngsters to have difficult temperaments and to display problems of inattention and over-activity. A summary of these clinical features of psychosocial dwarfism is set out in Table 20.2.

Developmental delays and adjustment problems

Developmental delays and adjustment problems are common among emotionally abused and neglected children (MacDonald, 2001; Smith & Fong, 2004). In the short term, emotionally abused and neglected children show developmental delays in sensorimotor, cognitive development and language development, as indexed by poor performance on standardized tests and educational under-achievement. They also present with internalizing and externalizing behaviour problems and difficulties making and maintaining peer relationships. At an intrapsychic level these children also typically have low self-esteem and emotion regulation deficits, so they find it difficult to control negative mood states notably, anger, anxiety and depression. The attachment problems and peer relationship problems of emotionally abused and neglected children are often associated with victim–persecutor internal working models for relationships.

LONG-TERM EFFECTS OF NEGLECT AND EMOTIONAL ABUSE

Emotionally abused and neglected children show more serious long-term adjustment problems than physically abused children (Browne, 2002; Dubowitz & Black, 2002; Erickson & Egeland, 2002; Glaser, 2002a; Hart et al., 2002; Hildyard & Wolfe, 2002; Iwaniec, 1995, 2004; Jones, 2000; MacDonald, 2001; Smith & Fong, 2004; Wekerle & Wolfe, 2003). Internalizing behaviour problems include depression, social isolation and withdrawal, self-harm and suicide. Externalizing behaviour problems include impulsivity, aggression, domestic violence, child abuse and substance abuse. There are also very significant long-term difficulties making and maintaining intimate peer relationships, forming stable romantic attachments and, for those that form families, there are significant difficulties maintaining stable and viable marital and parent–child relationships. The short-term cognitive and language delays and educational difficulties of neglected and emotionally abused children can lead to vocational problems in adult life. Poor long-term adjustment is associated with the severity and duration of the neglect or emotional abuse, the co-occurrence of physical or sexual abuse, and multi-placement experiences.

ASSESSMENT

Unifactorial theories and research programmes that focus exclusively on characteristics of the child, the caregiver or the social context as causes of neglect, emotional abuse, non-organic failure to thrive, psychosocial dwarfism and attachment problems have now largely been supplanted by complex multi-factorial frameworks. One such framework, which draws on extensive literature reviews (Browne, 2002; Dubowitz & Black, 2002; Erickson & Egeland, 2002; Glaser, 2002a; Hart et al., 2002; Iwaniec, 1995, 2004; Hildyard & Wolfe, 2002; Jones, 2000; MacDonald, 2001; Reder & Lucey, 1995; Smith & Fong, 2004; Wekerle & Wolfe, 2003), is presented in Figure 20.2. There is obviously a considerable overlap between these risk factors and those outlined for physical child abuse considered in Chapter 19. To avoid repetition, details of the psychosocial processes that under-pin marital discord and certain aspects of negative parent–child exchanges (e.g. mis-attribution) will not be reiterated here and the reader is referred to the appropriate sections of Chapter 19. The framework presented in Figure 20.2 offers an outline of some of the more important issues to be covered in a comprehensive assessment of a child and family that presents with neglect, emotional abuse, non-organic failure to thrive, psychosocial dwarfism or attachment problems. Some structured assessment instruments that may be a useful adjunct to clinical interviewing and observation are presented in Table 20.4.

Personal child factors

In assessing the presenting problem in these cases, a multi-disciplinary approach is particularly important. A paediatric evaluation of the child should first be conducted to check the proximity of the child's weight and height to the third centile, which is one of the most important criteria for diagnosis of both psychosocial dwarfism and non-organic failure to thrive.

Any personal characteristics that make children difficult to care for put them at risk for neglect and emotional abuse. Difficult-temperament and slow-to-warm-up infants and infants who have had many illnesses or other difficulties are at particular risk for neglect, emotional abuse, non-organic failure to thrive, psychosocial dwarfism and attachment problems. Abused and neglected children typically show delays in sensorimotor, cognitive and language development. A thorough assessment of these functions should therefore routinely be conducted. Some psychometric tests for evaluating developmental status of pre-school children are described in Chapter 8.

Parental factors

Certain parental characteristics are particular risk factors in these cases and should be addressed during case evaluation. Of particular importance are

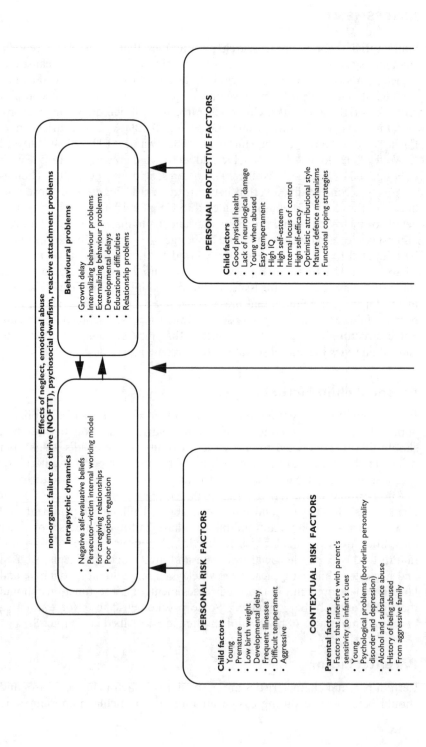

Effects of neglect, emotional abuse

non-organic failure to thrive (NOFTT), psychosocial dwarfism, reactive attachment problems

Intrapsychic dynamics

- Negative self-evaluative beliefs
- Persecutor–victim internal working model for caregiving relationships
- Poor emotion regulation

Behavioural problems

- Growth delay
- Internalizing behaviour problems
- Externalizing behaviour problems
- Developmental delays
- Educational difficulties
- Relationship problems

PERSONAL PROTECTIVE FACTORS

Child factors

- Good physical health
- Lack of neurological damage
- Young when abused
- Easy temperament
- High IQ
- High self-esteem
- Internal locus of control
- High self-efficacy
- Optimistic attributional style
- Mature defence mechanisms
- Functional coping strategies

PERSONAL RISK FACTORS

Child factors

- Young
- Premature
- Low birth weight
- Developmental delay
- Frequent illnesses
- Difficult temperament
- Aggressive

CONTEXTUAL RISK FACTORS

Parental factors

- Factors that interfere with parent's sensitivity to infant's cues
- Young
- Psychological problems (borderline personality disorder and depression)
- Alcohol and substance abuse
- History of being abused
- From aggressive family

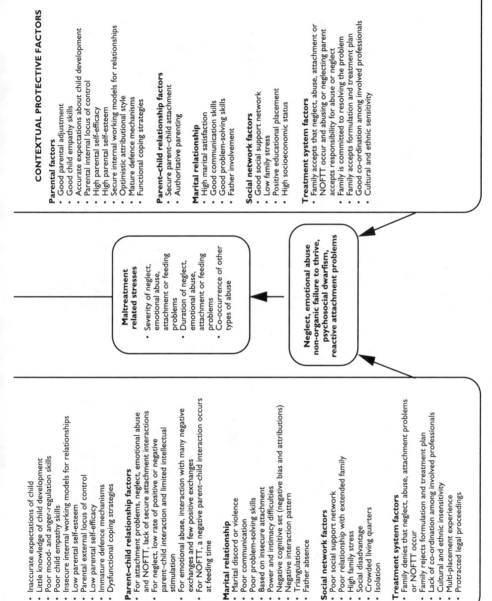

CONTEXTUAL PROTECTIVE FACTORS

Parental factors
- Good parental adjustment
- Good child empathy skills
- Accurate expectations about child development
- Parental internal locus of control
- High parental self-efficacy
- High parental self-esteem
- Secure internal working models for relationships
- Optimistic attributional style
- Mature defence mechanisms
- Functional coping strategies

Parent–child relationship factors
- Secure parent–child attachment
- Authoritative parenting

Marital relationship
- High marital satisfaction
- Good communication skills
- Good problem-solving skills
- Father involvement

Social network factors
- Good social support network
- Low family stress
- Positive educational placement
- High socioeconomic status

Treatment system factors
- Family accepts that neglect, abuse, attachment or NOFTT occur and abusing or neglecting parent accepts responsibility for abuse or neglect
- Family is committed to resolving the problem
- Family accepts formulation and treatment plan
- Good co-ordination among involved professionals
- Cultural and ethnic sensitivity

Maltreatment related stresses
- Severity of neglect, emotional abuse, attachment or feeding problems
- Duration of neglect, emotional abuse, attachment or feeding problems
- Co-occurrence of other types of abuse

Neglect, emotional abuse non-organic failure to thrive, psychosocial dwarfism, reactive attachment problems

- Inaccurate expectations of child
- Little knowledge of child development
- Poor mood- and anger-regulation skills
- Poor child empathy skills
- Insecure internal working models for relationships
- Low parental self-esteem
- Parental external locus of control
- Low parental self-efficacy
- Immature defence mechanisms
- Dysfunctional coping strategies

Parent–child relationship factors
- For attachment problems, neglect, emotional abuse and NOFTT, lack of secure attachment interactions
- For neglect, low rate of positive or negative parent–child interaction and limited intellectual stimulation
- For emotional abuse, interaction with many negative exchanges and few positive exchanges
- For NOFTT, a negative parent–child interaction occurs at feeding time

Marital relationship
- Marital discord or violence
- Poor communication
- Poor problem-solving skills
- Based on insecure attachment
- Power and intimacy difficulties
- Negative cognitive set (negative bias and attributions)
- Negative interaction pattern
- Triangulation
- Father absence

Social network factors
- Poor social support network
- Poor relationship with extended family
- High family stress
- Social disadvantage
- Crowded living quarters
- Isolation

Treatment system factors
- Family denies that neglect, abuse, attachment problems or NOFTT occur
- Family rejects formulation and treatment plan
- Lack of co-ordination among involved professionals
- Cultural and ethnic insensitivity
- Multi-placement experience
- Protracted legal proceedings

Figure 20.2. Risk and protective factors to consider in the assessment of neglect, emotional abuse and related problems

Table 20.4 Psychometric instruments that may be used as an adjunct to clinical interviews in the assessment of physical child abuse and neglect

Construct	Instrument	Publication	Comments
Parents' potential for child abuse	Child Abuse Potential Instrument	Milner, J. (1986). The Child Abuse Potential Inventory Manual (Revised). Webster, NC: Psytec Corporation	This 160-item inventory assesses parents' overall potential for child abuse and gives sub-scale scores on the following factors: distress, rigidity, child with problems, problems with family and others, unhappiness, loneliness, negative concept of child and self. In addition, the instrument contains a lie scale to assess the validity of responses. There are two response categories for all items and can be completed by parents with a reading age of 10 years
Parents' history of child abuse and neglect	Child Abuse and Trauma Scale	Saunders, B., Becker-Lausen, E. (1995). The measurement of psychological maltreatment: early data on the Child Abuse and Trauma Scale. Child Abuse and Neglect, 19, 315–323	A 38-item self-report scale for completion by parents gives information on their childhood experiences of abuse and neglect
Intrafamilial violence	Conflict Tactics Scale	Strauss, M. (1979). Measuring Intrafamilial conflict and violence: The Conflict Tactics (CT) Scale. Journal of Marriage and the Family, 41, 75–88.	This 18-item structured interview requires respondents to indicate the frequency with which they use various tactics for resolving intrafamilial conflicts. The tactics fall into three categories: reasoning, verbal hostility and physical aggression. Seven-point rating scales are provided for each item
Degree of neglect and extent to which child's needs are met by parents	Home Observation for Measurement of Environment (HOME)	Bradley, R. & Caldwell, B. (1979). Home Observation for Measurement of the Environment: A Revision of the Preschool Scale. American Journal of Mental Deficiency, 84, 235–244	This 45-item rating scale is completed on the basis of observations made during home visits and parental report. It gives scores on six sub-scales: emotional and verbal responsivity of the mother; avoidance of

			restriction and punishment; organization of the physical and temporal environment; provision of appropriate play materials; maternal involvement with the child; and opportunities for variety in daily stimulation
Abuse and neglect history	Checklist for Child Abuse	Petty, J. (1996). *Checklist for Child Abuse Evaluation.* Odessa: FL. Psychological Assessment Resources. http://www.parinc.com	264 items for evaluating child's historical and current status, emotional abuse, sexual abuse, physical abuse, neglect, child's psychological status, credibility and competence of the child

poor parental early attachment experiences and psychological difficulties such as depression, drug abuse, intellectual disability or ignorance of childcare skills, which compromise parents' sensitivity to their children's needs and their capacity to meet these. Of all of these parental characteristics, probably the sequelae of poor early attachment experiences are the most important to consider in cases of neglect or emotional abuse, where children go on to develop attachment problems, and so this issue deserves detailed comment.

Fonagy, Steele, Steele, Higgitt & Target (1994) explain disorders of attachment from a psychoanalytic perspective. They distinguish between the development of the physical (pre-reflective) self and the psychological (reflective self). Both aspects of self contain internal working models of relationships between self and others. The internal working models of relationships contained in the physical self are premised on physical attributes and concrete interpretations of actions. These models contain many inaccuracies because they fail to take account of the subjective states of others. By contrast, the internal working models of relationships contained in the psychological self incorporate an awareness of others' mental states. That is, they take account of feelings, perceptions, beliefs and intentions that others may hold. Internal working models of relationships contained in the psychological self are far more accurate than those of the physical self and so facilitate social adaptation.

The physical self evolves over the first six months of life and its development is facilitated through physical interaction. The psychological self, on the other hand, evolves more slowly and is probably not fully developed until adolescence. The child's primary caregiver has a critical role in the evolution of the psychological self. The responsive caregiver who maximally facilitates the evolution of the psychological self observes the child's actions and the context within which they occur, infers what the child feels or needs and responds to these inferred psychological states so as to meet the needs they entail. Through this process of inferring the child's mental state and responding to this as accurately as possible, the child develops the psychological self, which incorporates internal working models of relationships premised on a sensitivity to the mental states of others.

According to Fonagy's theory, responsive parenting is characterized primarily by the capacity of the parent to infer the mental state of the child and then to communicate with the child and meet the child's needs in the light of the inferred mental state. The coherence of the child's psychological self depends on the accuracy with which the caregiver infers the child's mental states.

If the caregiver has difficulty with inferring the child's psychological state, then the child is likely to adopt primitive defences, including avoidance or resistance and, in extreme cases, disorganization. The behavioural manifestations of these are typically seen in Ainsworth et al.'s (1978) 'strange situation' where infants have anxious–avoidant or anxious attachments; the defences protect the child's fragile psychological self. In more extreme situations where children are neglected, where the mother is chronically depressed or where the child is emotionally or physically abused, a variety of more extreme strategies may be adopted to preserve the psychological self. In some situations, a false self, dedicated to pleasing the caregiver, regardless of the personal costs, may develop (Winnicott, 1965). In others massive inhibition of the expression of emotions including aggression may occur. A third alternative is the continual expression of aggression.

Parents who have a poorly developed psychological self or reflective self are at risk of transmitting this to their own children by inaccurately inferring their own children's mental states. For example, by attributing negative intentions to the child's crying ('You're being a bad baby, trying to keep mummy awake' rather than 'Good baby telling mummy you have a wet nappy. We don't want to get nappy rash now do we?'). In Fonagy et al.'s (1994) series of studies, self-reflection was the single best predictor of secure attachment between mothers and infants. The capacity to accurately infer the psychological states of others and develop relationships within which this ability is used is an important protective factor because it permits the development of socially supportive relationships.

Parent–child interaction

Specific patterns of parent–child interaction are associated with neglect, emotional abuse, psychosocial dwarfism, non-organic failure to thrive and attachment problems. With neglect, a low rate of any exchanges, either positive or negative, is a central concern. With emotional abuse there is a high rate of negative exchanges compared with positive exchanges. In non-organic failure to thrive, the central interactional problem is with feeding routines. With attachment difficulties, the high rate of negative exchanges and lack of prompt and appropriate responses to the child's cues are important features of the interactional problems in which the child and the primary caregiver are engaged.

Direct observation of parent–child interaction, ideally, in the home, over a series of two or three ninety-minute sessions should be conducted. Parents should be invited to use some of the time to play with the child and some of the time to carry on doing household tasks, only interacting with the child when they think it necessary. It is a good idea to insist that the TV be turned off during these sessions. The observer should be as unintrusive as possible. Patterns of positive interaction should be noted, as should patterns of negative interaction. One crude index of the quality of the parent–child relationship is the ratio of positive interactions (involving intellectual stimulation or positive emotion) to negative interactions (involving lack of contact or aversive contact) during a one-hour period. In cases of neglect, the absolute number of interactions is fairly low. In cases of emotional abuse, a high ratio of negative to positive exchanges occurs. Where the central concern is non-organic failure to thrive it is important to observe a couple of episodes of feeding and to observe and describe the pattern of interaction between the parent and the child which under-pins the lack of calorific intake; four such patterns are described in Figure 20.1. Where the main concern is an attachment problem, the parent may be invited to leave the child in the room with the psychologist for a few minutes and then return and offer to comfort the child if he or she is distressed. The parent–child interaction may be observed and the degree to which the child's behaviour approximates the descriptions of inhibited and disinhibited reactive attachments disorders given earlier in this chapter may be determined.

Problematic parent–child interaction patterns may be under-pinned by negative cognitive sets and belief systems and inappropriate developmental expectations, such as those described in Chapter 19, in the discussion of parent–child interaction patterns and physical child abuse. That is, parents may attribute negative intentions to the child and view the child as deserving neglect or emotional abuse. These attributions typically involve an inaccurate understanding of the capabilities of children during early developmental stages. For example, it would be developmentally inaccurate to say that a four-month-old child would refuse to eat or cry to punish a mother.

Marital factors

Marital factors which increase the stress or reduce the support available to the child's primary caretakers (usually the mother) increase the risk of emotional abuse, neglect attachment problems, non-organic failure to thrive and psychosocial dwarfism. Such factors, which should be assessed, include marital discord or violence. These may be under-pinned by negative cognitive sets and belief systems, such as those described in Chapter 19 in the discussion of marital factors and physical child abuse.

Social network factors

Aspects of the wider social context that add to the stresses on the child's primary caretaker or fail to contribute to the primary caretaker's level of social support are risk factors for neglect, emotional abuse and related difficulties. Stresses such as low socioeconomic status, crowding and social isolation should be assessed along with levels of support available from family, friends and health and social welfare agencies.

Treatment system factors

Features of the treatment system, which includes the family, the treatment team and involved professionals and agencies may place the child at risk for either ongoing neglect or emotional abuse or poor response to treatment or abuse. Denial of the neglect or abuse, rejection of the treatment team's formulation and refusal to co-operate with the treatment plan may all be viewed as risk factors. Where there is a lack of co-ordination among involved professionals or unresolved disagreements about whether the case warrants a diagnosis of emotional abuse or neglect, this increases the risk of further abuse. Treatment systems that are not sensitive to the family's cultural and ethnic beliefs and values may be considered a risk factor, because they may be inhibiting engagement or promote drop-out from treatment and prevent the development of a good working alliance. As with all forms of abuse, multi-placement experiences and protracted legal proceedings have a negative impact on long-term adjustment. A detailed discussion of problems associated with multi-placement experiences is given in Chapter 22.

In contrast to these risk factors, certain features of the treatment system may be viewed as protective insofar as they reduce the risk of further abuse and enhance the possibility of positive changes within the child's psychosocial environment, which in turn reduce the risk of long-term adjustment problems. Within the treatment system, co-operative working relationships between the treatment team and the family and good co-ordination of multi-professional input are protective factors. Treatment systems that are sensitive to families' cultural and ethnic beliefs and values are more likely to help families engage with, and remain in, treatment and foster the development of a good working alliance. Families are more likely to benefit from treatment when all family members accept that there is a problem and the parents accept responsibility for the emotional abuse or neglect. Acceptance of the formulation of the problem given by the treatment team and a commitment to working with the team to resolve it are also protective factors.

Comprehensive assessment schedule

In cases of physical child abuse, typically comprehensive assessment and treatment occur within the context of a statutory framework, usually after a specific non-accidental injury has occurred. Often the child is in foster care, and the goal of assessment is to determine under what conditions it would be safe for the child to return home. With emotional abuse, neglect and the related problems of non-organic failure to thrive, psychosocial dwarfism and reactive attachment problems, it is less often the case that the child has been placed in foster care under a statutory childcare order. So comprehensive assessment and treatment is often carried out by psychologists at the request of social workers with a view to preventing statutory action occurring. In my experience, these families are often ambivalent about treatment and it may, therefore, be useful to ask the referring social worker to attend the first session in which the assessment contract is set up. If the family fails to attend later sessions, the referring social worker should be recontacted immediately and a further three-way meeting between the family, the psychologist and the referring agent should be conducted. A full account of these types of engagement and contracting difficulties is given in Chapter 4. When engaging these families in assessment and later in treatment, it is particularly important to have a clear contract, with specific goals, a clear specification of the number of sessions and the times and places at which these sessions will occur. Such contracts should be written and formally signed by the parents, the psychologist and the statutory social worker.

The aim of case management in cases of emotional abuse and neglect and related problems is to provide the child with a safe environment which fosters development and an opportunity to sustain relationships with both parents with a minimum of disruption and change in the child's environment, providing sustaining such a relationship with the parents does not place the child at risk for further episodes of neglect abuse. This aim takes account of the fact that most neglected and abused children continue to feel loyalty to their abusing parents and to feel loved by them (Herzberger, Potts & Dillon, 1981).

A comprehensive assessment should cover all risk factors in the model set out in Figure 20.2 and, ideally, should be carried out by a team rather than a single professional over a series of interview and observations sessions. A comprehensive child protection assessment schedule of interviews, and assessment procedures for use in cases of emotional abuse or neglect, is presented in Table 20.5. This schedule is based on the same principles as those outlined for cases of physical child abuse.

The issue of treatability of cases deserves special attention because available evidence suggests that not all families in which neglect or emotional abuse has occurred can benefit from treatment. The checklist in Table 19.3 (p. 919) offers a framework for assessing a family's capacity to engage in

Table 20.5 Components of a comprehensive child protection assessment package for cases of neglect or emotional abuse

Evaluation target	Evaluation method and areas
Child	• Individual interview with child (if the child is old enough) to assess personal strengths and resources (including assertiveness) and his or her account of the emotional abuse or neglect; perception of all relevant risk factors; and wishes for the future • Assessment of weight and height compared to national norms for children of the same age • Psychometric assessment of the child's cognitive and language development (if appropriate) • Child-behaviour checklist to assess behavioural difficulties
Parents	• Individual interviews with parents to assess acceptance or denial or responsibility for emotional abuse, wilful or unwitting nature of neglect, parenting skills and deficits, personal resources and problems, and perception of all relevant risk factors • Psychometric assessment of specific parental characteristics (if appropriate) such as intelligence and psychopathology
Parent–child interaction	• Parent–child interaction observation sessions to assess positive aspects of parenting; problems with feeding routines; problems with stimulating play sequences; and risk factors associated with parent–child interactions • A brief trial (2 sessions) of parent–child therapy to assess their responsiveness to behavioural coaching to improve feeding routines, increase parent's intellectual stimulation of the child; and increase the number of positive exchanges and decrease the number of negative exchanges between the parent and child
Marital couple	• Marital interview to assess marital risk factors especially joint communication and problem-solving skills for dealing with childcare issues and conflict management • A brief trial (2 sessions) of couples therapy, to assess couple's responsiveness to coaching in joint communication and problem-solving skills for managing childcare issues • Psychometric assessment of each spouse's perception of marital relationship (if appropriate)
Family accommodation	• Visit to family residence to assess crowding, hygiene, safety of the home for the child and opportunities for age-appropriate cognitive stimulation and play
Role of extended family	• Individual interviews with other members of nuclear and extended family to assess their acceptance or denial of the emotional abuse or neglect; their perception of risk factors, and their childcare skills and deficits • Joint interviews with extended family and nuclear family to observe quality of their relationship to nuclear family and assess potential for support

Role of other involved professionals	• Individual interviews with other involved professionals from health, education, social services and justice to obtain their expert view of risks and resources within the family and their potential future involvement in supporting the family or providing services • Joint interviews with other community-based resource people such as the foster parents with whom the child is temporarily based, home-help, befriender, leader of mother and toddler group, director of nursery or day-care facility etc. to observe relationship to parents and assess potential for supporting the family in future

treatment. At least three out of the following four conditions must be met for the family to be able to benefit from treatment:

- acceptance of responsibility for abuse
- commitment to meeting their child's needs
- commitment to improving their own psychological well-being
- ability to change.

TREATMENT

Where it is decided that a family could benefit from treatment, therapeutic plans must be clearly linked to achieving specific concrete goals identified in the assessment. Typical goals and related interventions for cases of physical and emotional abuse and neglect are set out in Table 19.4 (p. 920).

As with cases of physical abuse, treatment for families where emotional child abuse or neglect has occurred, in addition to having clearly defined goals, typically involves a multi-systemic intervention package including a number of the interventions listed in Table 19.4 (Azar & Wolfe, 1998; Browne, 2002; Brunk et al., 1987; Donohue et al., 1998; Jones, 2002; MacDonald, 2001; Schuerman et al., 1994). However, it is important that these components be prioritized. Unless there is good reason to do otherwise, priority should always be given to intensive family intervention with the parents and the abused or neglected child. The central aim is to prevent the occurrence of negative cycles of interaction and promote positive exchanges between the parents and child. Ideally, this should involve intensive contact of up to three sessions per week over an initial period of six to twelve weeks (Nicol et al., 1988). Interventions which target the parents, the individual child, the marriage and the wider community should be given lower priority.

Around a central core of intensive family intervention, other components of the multi-systemic intervention package should be organized. The parents may work with a therapist or facilitator in an individual, couples or group format and the children may work with another professional such as a teacher, speech therapist or play therapist in individual or group-based programmes.

Guidelines for intensive family intervention, individual interventions for children and parents, interventions which focus on the couple and interventions which target aspects of the wider social context are described in Chapter 19. All of these interventions may be appropriate elements to include in multi-systemic treatment packages for cases of neglect and emotional abuse. However, a specific type of family intervention is required to effectively deal with families containing a child who has developed non-organic failure to thrive.

Family-based treatment targeting non-organic failure to thrive

Iwaniec, Herbert and McNeish (1985) have developed an approach to working with families containing a child diagnosed as suffering from non-organic failure to thrive that was effective or moderately effective in over 80% of cases. This ten-month intensive family intervention programme was offered to seventeen families within the context of a broader multi-systemic intervention package involving child and parent support services and placement of children on an a statutory at-risk register. A series of twelve intensive twice-weekly home-based intervention sessions was offered over a six-week period, followed by twelve fortnightly follow-up sessions spread over a six- or seven-month period. The family sessions focused on the development of feeding routines and patterns of family functioning to support these, as well as enhancing mother–child attachment.

To develop more functional feeding routines, common feeding patterns were mapped out, in a manner similar to those patterns presented in Figure 20.1. Where meal-times had been chaotic or non-persistent, routines were developed so they became more predictable for the child and the parents. Where meal-times were rigid and aggressive, flexibility was introduced. The mothers were coached in how to relax before beginning a feeding session. Fathers were coached in how to support mothers before they engaged in feeding sessions. Food was decoratively arranged to look appetizing and preferred foods were used. Mothers were coached in how to use play and soothing speech to make feeding times relaxing and pleasant for their infants. In addition, routine information on nutrition was given to parents.

Concurrent with these feeding-focused interventions, there was also an attempt to improve mother–child attachment by coaching mothers and children in play sequences using guidelines similar to those set out in Table 4.4 (p. 148), within the therapy sessions and requiring mothers to schedule daily periods of special play time of ten minutes, increasing to thirty minutes over a four-week period. Within these sessions, mothers were prompted to initiate play and sustain it, while keeping negative exchanges to a minimum. Mothers were prompted to be sensitive to their child's wishes and respond to these promptly within the play session. They were encouraged to give the child wholehearted attention with frequent eye contact and cuddles. They were encouraged to anticipate negative exchanges and try to avoid these. After a month of this scheduled daily play, which typically occurred after the mother's partner returned from work in the evening, an intensive two-week period of sustained mother–child contact was scheduled, with considerable discussion, forethought and preparation on the part of the therapist and the family. The mother was encouraged to take the child everywhere with her for the two-week period and engage the child in frequent talk, to make a lot of eye contact, and to cuddle and hug the infant as much as possible.

After this intensive period, fortnightly contact with families over a six-month period was used to support the families in continuing the feeding routines and enhanced mother–child attachment. Less intensive interventions than this programme have been shown to have positive effects. However, Iwaniec's programme, which in total requires only 24 hours' contact per case, is a practice model worth emulating.

PREVENTION

Prevention programmes for physical abuse (described in Chapter 19) are, with minor modifications, appropriate for prevention of neglect and emotional abuse. Specific interventions have been developed to address mother–child attachment problems as a way of preventing neglect and abuse. In a review of sixteen studies of programmes for improving insecure attachment, Ijzen-doorn, Juffer and Duyvesteyn (1995) found that interventions were relatively effective in changing parental sensitivity but less effective in altering children's attachment insecurity. Brief, focused, preventive interventions that target parent sensitivity and behaviour were the most effective. In these programmes, mothers were given social support and both oral and written information about childcare during regular antenatal and post-natal home visits. During the post-natal home visits, mothers were coached to interpret and respond appropriately to their infant's cues. They learned to respond to different types of crying, energetic activity and passivity so as to meet their children's needs for the alleviation of distress and the provision of nurturance and stimulation. Mothers were also provided with baby carriers during the infants' first months of life so that they could carry their babies around with them and be more aware of and responsive to their infant's needs. Programmes involving these components should target families who are at risk as defined by the factors set out in the section on assessment.

SUMMARY

Intentional emotional abuse and inadvertent neglect have profound short- and long-term effects on children's physical, emotional, social and cognitive development. Particularly significant short-term effects include non-organic failure to thrive, psychosocial dwarfism, attachment disorders and developmental delays. Multi-disciplinary assessment is essential in these cases and should include evaluations of the child, parents, parent–child relationship, marital factors, and levels of stress and support in the wider social system. Where parents accept responsibility for the maltreatment, are committed to meeting their child's needs, are committed to improving their own psychological well-being and where they have the ability to change, the prognosis is good. Where less than three of these conditions are met, it is unlikely that a positive treatment response will occur. Treatment should be based on clear contracts to meet specific targets and involve a central focus on improving parent–child interaction through direct work with parents and children together. This may be supplemented with individual work for parents focusing on parent-craft and the management of personal psychological difficulties and children may receive input in therapeutic pre-school placements. Intervention may also focus on helping couples enhance their mutual supportiveness and the degree to which the extended family offer support. Brief, focused interventions that target parent sensitivity and behaviour are the most effective type of prevention programme.

EXERCISE 20.1

Helen and Mary are identical twins. They are referred to you for developmental assessment by a paediatrician in the district where you work. The paediatrician notes that over the past year they have both maintained heights and weights that place them just above the fourth percentile. Helen and Mary are now three years of age. They speak in short two- or three-word sentences and have very low activity levels. They sleep a lot during the day and wake at night regularly. Both were bottle-fed from the start and this was a big disappointment to Sarah, their mother. Sarah had no luck getting the twins to breast feed. Brian, her husband, thinks she fusses too much about the twins. Brian was married before and has a child by that marriage, who is grown up and gone to college. Brian is in his fifties and Sarah is twenty-eight years old. The twins are her first children. Sarah gave up her job when she had the twins and now finds she misses work a lot. Brian is on a disability pension, having retired early from the police force with an injury. Their vibrant relationship has deteriorated a lot since the birth of the twins and they go through spells where they don't talk to each other for days on end. However, they eventually overcome this and get back to a harmonious, if exhausting, lifestyle. The twins are due to start play-school soon.

- Offer a preliminary formulation of this case and an initial interview plan.
- From the information given, do you judge this case to be potentially treatable?
- What type of intervention package would you expect to consider in this case?

EXERCISE 20.2

Role-play a preliminary interview and reformulate the case on the basis of the information obtained.

FURTHER READING

Department of Health (2000). *Department of Health Framework for the Assessment of Children in Need and their Families*. London: Stationery Office. Available at: http://www.dh.gov.uk/PublicationsAndStatistics/Publications/PublicationsPolicyAndGuidance/PublicationsPolicyAndGuidanceArticle/fs/en?CONTENT_ID=4008144&chk=CwTP%2Bc

Feindler, E., Rathus, J., & Silver, L. E. (2003). *Assessment of Family Violence. A Handbook for Researchers and Practitioners*. Washington, DC: APA. (*Gives good description of a comprehensive catalogue of tests, but does not include the actual tests and measures.*)

Iwaniec, D. (2004). *Children Who Fail to Thrive: A Practice Guide*. Chichester: Wiley.

MacDonald, G. (2001). *Effective Interventions for Child Abuse and Neglect. An Evidence-Based Approach to Planning and Evaluating Interventions*. Chichester: Wiley.

McNeish, D., Newman, T., & Roberts, H. (2002). *What Works for Children*. Buckingham: Open University Press.

Myers, J., Berliner, L., Briere, Hendrix, C., Jenny, C., & Reid, T. (2002). *APSAC Handbook on Child Maltreatment* (Second Edition). Thousand Oaks, CA: Sage.

Rathus, J. & Feindler, E. (2004). *Assessment of Partner Violence. A Handbook for Researchers and Practitioners*. Washington, DC: APA. (*Gives good description of a comprehensive catalogue of tests, but does not include the actual tests and measures.*)

Reder, P. & Lucey, C. (1995). *Assessment of Parenting. Psychiatric and Psychological Contributions*. London: Routledge.

IRISH AND UK CHILD PROTECTION GUIDELINES

Children First National Guidelines for the Protection and Welfare of Children. A Summary (1999). Dublin, Ireland: Stationery Office. Available at: http://www.dohc.ie/publications/pdf/children_sum.pdf

Working Together to Safeguard Children (1999). London: The Stationery Office. Available at: http://www.dh.gov.uk/PublicationsAndStatistics/Publications/PublicationsPolicyAndGuidance/PublicationsPolicyAndGuidanceArticle/fs/en?CONTENT_ID=4007781&chk=BUYMa8

WEBSITES

American Professional Society on the Abuse of Children (APSAC): http://www.apsac.org

Association for the Treatment of Sexual Abusers: http://www.atsa.com

Child abuse websites: http://www.childabuse.com/links.htm

International Society for Prevention of Child Abuse and Neglect (ISPCAN): http://www.ispcan.org

Irish Society for the Prevention of Cruelty to Children (ISPCC): http://www.ispcc.ie/

National Clearing house on Child Abuse and Neglect: http://nccanch.acf.hhs.gov

National Exchange Centre: http://www.preventchildabuse.com

National Organisation for the Treatment of Abusers (NOTA): http://www.nota.co.uk/

National Society for the Prevention of Cruelty to Children NSPCC: http://www.nspcc.org.uk

Factsheets on child abuse and neglect, domestic violence, parental mental illness and good parenting can be downloaded from the website for Rose, G. & York, A. (2004). *Mental Health and Growing Up. Fact sheets for Parents, Teachers and Young People* (Third edition). London: Gaskell: http://www.rcpsych.ac.uk

Chapter 21

Sexual abuse

There is an international consensus that child sexual abuse represents unacceptable childcare and a violation of a child's human rights as outlined in the United Nations Convention on the Rights of the Child (1992). Child sexual abuse (CSA) refers to the use of a child for sexual gratification (American Academy of Child and Adolescent Psychiatry, 1997g, 1999b; Berliner & Elliott, 2002; Glaser, 2002b; Wekerle & Wolfe, 2003). Sexual abuse actions may vary in intrusiveness (from non-contact viewing or exposure to contact, ranging from touching to penetration) and frequency (from a single episode to frequent and chronic abuse). A distinction is made between intra-familial sexual abuse, the most common form of which is father–daughter incest, and extrafamilial sexual abuse where the abuser resides outside the family home. An example of a case of intrafamilial sexual abuse is presented in Box 21.1; a case of extrafamilial abuse is given in Box 21.2.

After considering the epidemiology of child sexual abuse, this chapter describes the cycle of sexual abuse and its effects. Factors affecting adjust-ment to abuse are then discussed. The management of cases in which child abuse is suspected is described, with a detailed account being given of assessment of the validity of allegations of sexual abuse and also of more general assessment procedures. Approaches to the treatment of both victims and offenders are then addressed. A discussion of issues to consider in legal proceedings in cases of child sexual abuse follows. The chapter closes with some comments on prevention.

EPIDEMIOLOGY

A review of the international epidemiological data on CSA allows the follow-ing conclusions to be drawn (Creighton, 2004). In community-based, random sample, self-report studies of CSA conducted in Europe, the USA and New Zealand from the 1980s up to the first decade of the twenty-first century, overall prevalence rates for contact and non-contact forms of sexual abuse were 3–25% for males and 8–42% for females. Prevalence rates for more

Box 21.1 A case of intrafamilial sexual abuse

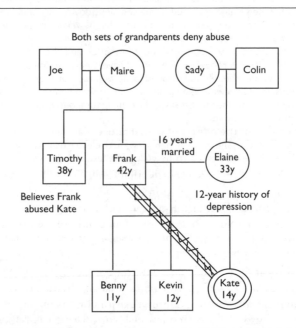

Both sets of grandparents deny abuse

Timothy 38y — Believes Frank abused Kate

Frank 42y — 16 years married — Elaine 33y — 12-year history of depression

Benny 11y   Kevin 12y   Kate 14y

Referral. Kate, aged fourteen, had been attending a child and family clinic because she had adjustment problems at school. She was falling behind in her academic work and was at the centre of a number of incidents that had occurred in the school grounds where two boys were fighting about their exclusive right to be her boyfriend. During the assessment of Kate and her family, which was conducted over a series of sessions, the school principal called the clinic one evening to say that Kate refused to go home because she was frightened of her father who she claimed had been sexually abusing her for over a year.

Preliminary assessment of allegations of abuse. In a subsequent evaluation of these allegations by a team including a police woman and a statutory social worker, Kate confirmed that oral and vaginal sex had been occurring weekly for about 15 months. Kate's mother suffered from clinical depression and was being treated by the GP and a member of the psychology department for this. Her two younger brothers apparently had no problems and were unaware of the sexual abuse.

History of the presenting problem from Kate's viewpoint. The abusive incidents had begun when Kate's mother, Elaine, had been hospitalized briefly following a car accident. The father, Frank, had crept into Kate's room on the second night after coming back from visiting Elaine in hospital. He did not usually drink, but had drunk some wine that evening to deal with his sadness concerning Elaine's condition. Both of Elaine's legs had been broken in the accident and this had occurred during a particularly debilitating episode of depression. Frank usually tucked Kate in and often stroked her hair to help her sleep. However, this night, which was warm, he extended the stroking to her buttocks and breasts. When she protested, he accused her of being ungrateful and said that it was soothing for him at this difficult time. He then began to masturbate and involved Kate in this. Over the subsequent months, these sessions recurred weekly, progressing from manual masturbation, to oral sex and vaginal intercourse. On some but not all occasions he drank alcohol. When Elaine returned home she slept downstairs, and Frank would initiate these episodes after he had said to Elaine that he was going upstairs to go to sleep. When Kate resisted, Frank said that if she told anyone about their secret, her mother would be unable to cope with the information and she would be guilty of preventing her mother's recovery. This would have a negative impact on the well-being of the boys and the whole family. Also, he pointed out that she enjoyed the secret sessions and had always liked physical contact with him since she was a little girl. He tried to convince her that this was just the natural outcome of such a special father–daughter relationship.

Kate's account of the effects of sexual abuse. Kate felt that there was little she could do because she had, in her view, actively participated in the sexual episodes and so believed herself to be guilty. She also did not want to upset her mother or brothers. And despite her anger at her father, she did not want him to leave the house, since the family could not cope without him. She was angry because she felt there was no way out and also because she felt like she was dirty. She also was angry because she felt like her father, who she had idolized, had let her down badly. These mixed feelings and worries about how to make things right again, made concentration at school difficult. She had always been a good student but her work had slowly begun to deteriorate. She had been popular in school, but now found that she fought with her girlfriends more and had fallen out with her best friend. She also found the attention she got from two older boys in the grade above her flattering. With each of them she had, without forethought or planning, found herself in situations coming home from school through the park where they had caressed and fondled her in a way that she felt was out of character for herself. She had laughed these incidents off and tried to avoid getting into similar situations again. However, these incidents appear to have led each of the boys to believe that they were Kate's exclusive boyfriend. It was this situation that led to the fight mentioned in the referral letter.

A television programme about sexual abuse along with the growing tension that Kate experienced led her to make the allegations, she said, at the time when she did.

Family assessment. The family evaluation showed that there was a partner-like relationship between Frank and Kate. Elaine, particularly when she was depressed, tended to fall into a daughter-like role. Both parents denied the occurrence of abuse. The maternal and paternal grandparents also refused to accept Kate's allegations. Only Frank's brother, Timothy, believed Kate's story.

Formulation. Kate was a fourteen-year-old girl who had been sexually abused over a period of 15 months by her father. The onset of the abuse had coincided with the mother's hospitalization. Thus she was not available to inhibit the father's abuse by protecting Kate. The father was probably motivated to abuse Kate because of limited sexual outlets. It is probable that his relationship with his wife Elaine was sexually unsatisfying because she had been episodically depressed over a number of years. The sexual abuse had led to Kate experiencing considerable emotional distress (including powerlessness, betrayal, and stigmatization), over-sexualized behaviour and academic problems. Frank's coercive threats about the negative impact of disclosure on the integrity of the family had prevented her from disclosing the abuse, but the TV programme on abuse, along with her growing distress and her trust in her teacher, precipitated the disclosure. The mother's depression and sense of helplessness probably prevented her from supporting her daughter.

Management. An application was made for a care order for the three children and arrangements were made for Kate to receive continued supportive counselling.

Box 21.2 A case of extrafamilial abuse

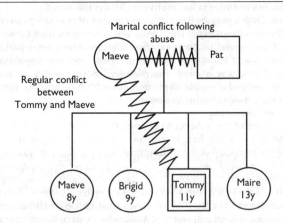

Referral. Tommy Muldoon, aged eleven, was referred for treatment at a child and family centre following an allegation that he had been sexually abused by Rudy, a nineteen-year-old baby-sitter over a period of eighteen months. During the six months preceding the allegations, Tommy had become involved in regular escalating battles with his parents, particularly his mother. These fights and arguments often occurred on Saturdays or Sundays, and it was usually on Saturday night that the baby-sitting episodes occurred. He sometimes refused to go into his bedroom and had smeared faeces on the wall at the end of his bed, and it was this incident that led to the conversation in which he made the allegations.

Family history. Prior to these episodes Tommy and his three sisters were all well-adjusted children with normal developmental histories. The parents, Maeve and Pat, were apparently a well-adjusted couple. The Muldoons lived in a council house and the children attended the local primary school.

Impact of the abuse on the family. Following the allegations, Tommy was interviewed by the police and charges were brought against Rudy, who pleaded guilty to a number of sexual assault charges but received suspended sentences and probation. This led to a situation where Tommy and his family regularly saw Rudy in the streets of the council housing estate every week. Tommy and his family found this very stressful. Tommy was frightened that the assaults would recur. He also felt dirty and guilty. He began to have night-mares and fantasized that he would be attacked by Rudy. Maeve and Pat wished to take revenge but knew that this could lead to them being charged with assault also. Maeve became clinically depressed and Pat distanced himself from family life. The marriage became far less satisfactory from both parents' viewpoints. After a number of weeks, Tommy refused to go into his room to sleep and spent many nights sleeping in his parents' bed, which compounded the marital difficulties. Pat objected to this behaviour but Maeve went along with it.

Formulation. The abuse of Tommy by Rudy, and Rudy's subsequent release on probation following Tommy's testimony, led Tommy to experience both internalizing and externalizing behaviour problems and a sense of powerlessness, betrayal and stigmatization. Concurrently, his parents experienced a sense of powerlessness, which led to the mother's depression and the father's withdrawal from family life. The parents' difficulties in coping with the situation exacerbated Tommy's difficulties.

> **Treatment.** The treatment plan in this case involved family work that focused on helping the parents support Tommy and individual work in which Tommy was helped to process the intense emotions concerning the abuse.
>
> **Outcome.** Over a period of months, the capacity of the parents to support each other and Tommy diminished. The family was also ostracized by some of their neighbours. They moved to another council estate. For a brief period Tommy's behaviour improved. He began to sleep alone and his aggression reduced considerably. There was a brief improvement in the quality of the marriage. However, eventually the couple separated, with Maeve retaining custody of the children and Pat seeing them on week-ends.

intrusive forms of sexual abuse involving contact were 1–16% for males and 6–20% for females. The annual incidence of CSA in the UK, Australia and North America, based on officially reported cases in the 1990s, was between 0.2 and 1.2 per 1000. About 10% of cases that came to the attention of child protection services had suffered CSA rather than neglect, or physical and emotional abuse. Other epidemiological trends based on extensive reviews deserve mention (Berliner & Elliott, 2002; Glaser, 2002b; Jones, 2000; Putnam, 2003; Sequeira & Hollis, 2003; Wekerle & Wolfe, 2003). More girls than boys are sexually abused. Most abusers are male. Less than a fifth of abusers are women. CSA occurs with children of all ages but there is a peak for girls at six to seven years and at the onset of adolescence. Compared with the normal population, rates of abuse are two to three times higher among children with physical and intellectual disabilities. Children in residential care are at higher risk of abuse. Estimates of the proportion of cases where CSA is intrafamilial range from about a third to three-quarters, depending on the sample and methodology. Intrafamilial cases are over-represented in clinical studies. Girls are more commonly abused intrafamilially and boys are more commonly abused extrafamilially. Intrafamilial sexual abuse is most commonly perpetrated by fathers, step-fathers and siblings. Extrafamilial sexual abuse is most commonly perpetrated by people whom the family trust, such as baby-sitters, club-leaders, teachers, residential care staff, neighbours and friends. While CSA usually entails threats of violence, co-morbidity with physical child abuse is only about 20%. Some sexual abuse occurs in isolation, but in a significant number of cases abuse is organized and may involve recruitment of children for paedophile rings, pornography, prostitution and sadistic or satanic practices.

THE CYCLE OF SEXUAL ABUSE

CSA cases referred for psychological consultation have typically involved repeated abuse. A simplified model of the cycle of repeated abuse is presented in Figure 21.1. The model attempts to integrate conclusions drawn from

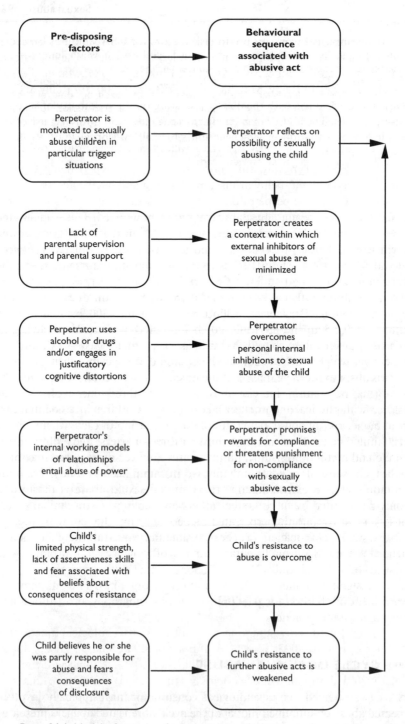

Figure 21.1 Model of pattern of interaction in which repeated sexual abuse may be embedded

reviews of empirical work on broad risk factors for CSA, findings on cycles of offending behaviour among sexual offenders and models of sexual offending (Chaffin, Letourneau & Silovsky, 2002; Finklehor, 1984; Marshall, Laws & Barbaree, 1990; O'Reilly, Marshall, Carr & Beckett, 2004; O'Reilly & Carr, 1998). The cycle starts with the abuser reflecting on the possibility of sexually abusing a child. The abuser may engage in such reflection both because of the specific trigger situation in which he finds himself and because of a general pre-disposition to be motivated to abuse children, such as that described by Finklehor (1984). Typically, this motivation involves experiencing CSA as emotionally congruent, being aroused by children and having access to adult partners blocked. The perpetrator then creates a situation in which external factors that may prevent abuse are removed or minimized. This is facilitated if the child has little parental supervision or support from a non-abusing parent and if the perpetrator and child are in a socially isolated situation. Once in a situation where there are few external inhibitors for CSA, the perpetrator overcomes personal inhibitions. He may minimize the impact of internal inhibitors, such as guilt or fear of being caught, through engaging in an internal dialogue in which the abuse in justified, its negative impact on the child is denied and the possibility of being detected is denied. Alcohol or drugs may also be used to reduce the inhibitory power of fear and guilt. The perpetrator may then coerce the child into sexual abuse by promising rewards for compliance and threatening punishment for non-compliance with the sexually abusive acts. This abuser may engage in this coercive behaviour because he has an internal working model for relationships with children that entail the abuse of power. Such internal working models may be based on early attachments that involved abuse. In response to the perpetrator's coercion, the child's resistance is overcome. The child may have difficulty resisting because of lack of strength, assertiveness skills or fears about the consequences of not engaging in abuse. Following the abusive acts, children's resistance to further abuse may be weakened because they believe they were partly responsible for the abuse and because they fear the consequences of disclosure. The cycle may repeat the next time the perpetrator finds himself in a trigger situation.

EFFECTS OF SEXUAL ABUSE

CSA has profound short- and long-term effects on psychological functioning (Berliner & Elliott, 2002; Browne & Finklehor, 1986; Glaser, 2002b; Jones, 2000; Kendall-Tackett, Williams & Finklehor, 1993; Paolucci, Genuis & Violato, 2001; Putnam, 2003; Sequeira & Hollis, 2003). About two-thirds of sexually abused children develop psychological symptoms. Behaviour problems shown by children who have experienced CSA typically include sexualized behaviour, excessive internalizing or externalizing behaviour problems and school-based attainment problems. However, a specific syndrome with a clearly defined cluster of behavioural difficulties unique to those who have experienced CSA has not been identified. Also, no single diagnostic category, such as post-traumatic stress disorder (PTSD), is present in all cases. Paolucci et al. (2001), in a meta-analysis of thirty-seven studies found unweighted effect sizes of .5 for PTSD, .6 for depression and suicide, .5 for sexual promiscuity, .4 for victim–perpetrator cycle and .2 for deterioration in academic performance. In the eighteen-month period following the cessation of abuse, behaviour problems abate in about two-thirds of cases. Up to a quarter of cases develop more severe problems and these may include those cases that were initially asymptomatic. About a fifth of cases show clinically significant long-term problems which persist into adulthood.

One of the most useful models for conceptualizing the intrapsychic processes that under-pin the behaviour problems or symptoms that arise from sexual abuse is Browne and Finklehor's (1986) traumagenic dynamics formulation. Within this formulation, traumatic sexualization, stigmatization, betrayal and powerlessness are identified as four distinct yet related dynamics that account for the wide variety of symptoms shown by children who have been sexually abused.

With traumatic sexualization, the perpetrator transmits misconceptions about normal sexual behaviour and morality to the child. The child is rewarded for sexual behaviour inappropriate to his or her developmental level and so sexual arousal becomes associated with rewards and the idea of receiving care, love and attention. In other instances, sexual activity becomes associated with negative emotions and memories. These experiences increase the salience of sexual issues for the child and lead to confusion about the relationship between sex and care giving. Confusion may also arise over sexual norms and sexual identity. These confused beliefs about sexual issues may lead to either over-sexualized behaviour or to avoidance of sex and difficulties in becoming sexually aroused.

With stigmatization, the perpetrator blames and denigrates the child and coerces the child into maintaining secrecy. Following disclosure, other members of the family or the network may blame the child for participating in the abuse. The child develops negative beliefs about the self, including the ideas of self-blame and self-denigration (the 'damaged goods' belief). These beliefs lead to self-destructive behaviours such as avoidance of relationships, drug abuse, self-harm and suicide. The child may also internalize the abuser's demand for secrecy and dissociate whole areas of experience from consciousness. These may occasionally intrude into consciousness as flashbacks.

The dynamics of betrayal begin when the trust the child has in the perpetrator is violated and the expectation that other adults will be protective is not met. These violations of trust and expectations of protection lead the child to believe that others are not trustworthy. This loss of a sense of trust in others may give rise to a variety of relationship problems, to delinquency and to intense feelings of sadness and anger.

The dynamics of powerlessness have their roots in the child's experience of being unable to prevent the abuse because of the perpetrator's use of physical force and psychological coercion. This may be compounded by the refusal of other members of the network to believe the child or take effective professional action. The child, as a result of this experience of being powerless, may develop beliefs about generalized personal ineffectiveness and develop an image of the self as a victim. These beliefs may lead to depression, anxiety and a variety of somatic presentations. The experience of powerlessness may also lead to the internalization of a victim–persecutor internal working model for relationships, which sows the seeds for the child later becoming a perpetrator when placed in a position where an opportunity to exert power over a vulnerable person arises.

FACTORS AFFECTING ADJUSTMENT TO ABUSE

The degree to which children develop the four traumagenic dynamics and associated behaviour problems following sexual abuse is determined by a wide range of factors. These include stresses associated with the abuse itself and the balance of risk and protective factors present in the child and the social context within which the abuse occurs (Furniss, 1991; Spaccarelli, 1994). Some of the more important factors deserving consideration as part of the assessment of cases of CSA are contained in Figure 21.2.

Abuse-related stresses

Aspects of the abuse, such as the frequency, invasiveness, amount of physical violence involved, amount of denigration involved and degree to which the child's trust in an adult was violated all have an impact on the level of abuse-related stress experienced (Carr & O'Reilly, 2004; Furniss, 1991; Spaccarelli, 1994). Whether the abuse was perpetrated by a family member or by someone outside the family is an important issue to consider when judging the degree to which trust was violated. In addition to features of the abuse, the child's personal attributes and the social context within which the sexual abuse occurs may affect the level of stress experienced by the child and the risk of re-abuse.

Risk and protective factors associated with the child

The risks of re-abuse or repeated abuse are enhanced by factors that prevent children resisting the abuser (Berliner & Elliott, 2002; Browne & Finklehor, 1986; Carr & O'Reilly, 2004; Glaser, 2002b; Jones, 2000; Kendall-Tackett

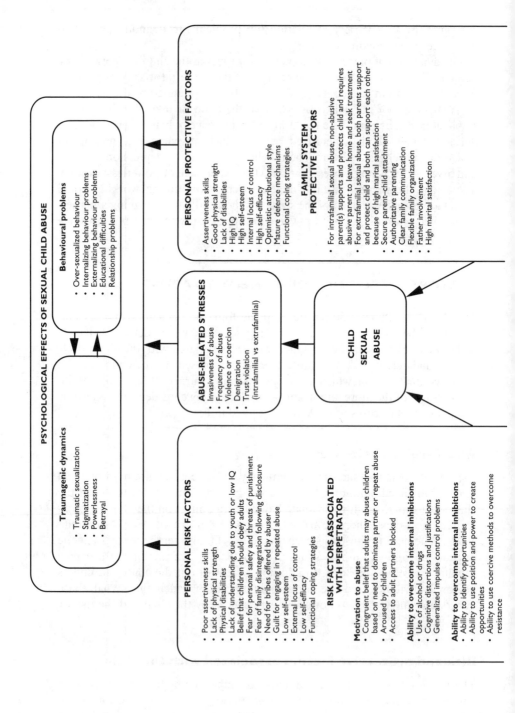

**RISK FACTORS ASSOCIATED
WITH FAMILY**

- Unprotective and unsupportive or punitive relationship between non-abusing parent(s) and child due to illness or depression (incest)
- Marital dissatisfaction, conflict-avoidance and lack of protection of child by non-abusing parent (incest)
- Chaotic family organization (all forms of abuse)
- Lax supervision (sibling abuse)
- Opportunities for trusted, powerful family friend to abuse (extrafamilial)

SOCIAL NETWORK RISK FACTORS

- Social network factors that prevent non-abusing parents and others from offering child protection and support
- Poor social support network
- Poor relationship with extended family
- High family stress
- Social disadvantage
- Crowded living quarters
- Isolation

TREATMENT SYSTEM RISK FACTORS

- Family deny that abuse occurred and fail to provide child with support and protection at disclosure
- Family reject formulation and treatment plan
- Lack of co-ordination among involved professionals and multiple investigative interviews
- Cultural and ethnic insensitivity
- Multi-placement experience
- Protracted non-child-centred legal proceedings

**SOCIAL NETWORK
PROTECTIVE FACTORS**

- Good social support network
- Low family stress
- Positive educational placement
- High socioeconomic status

**TREATMENT SYSTEM
PROTECTIVE FACTORS**

- Family accepts that abuse occurred
- Family is committed to supporting and protecting child
- Family has coped with major stresses before
- Family accepts formulation and treatment plan
- Good co-ordination among involved professionals and only a single disclosure interview used
- Cultural and ethnic sensitivity
- Brief child-centered legal proceedings occur
- Child remains with non-abusing parent(s) in family home while abuser lives elsewhere

Figure 21.2 Factors to consider in the comprehensive assessment of child sexual abuse

et al., 1993; Putnam, 2003; Spaccarelli, 1994). These include lack of assertiveness skills, lack of physical strength, physical disabilities, lack of understanding due to youthfulness or learning difficulties and a strongly held belief that children should obey adults in all circumstances. Once a pattern of abuse becomes entrenched it may continue because children fear that their own safety or the integrity of the family will be threatened if they disclose the abuse. Where children are relatively unsupported and have few positive relationships or resources, they may need the bribes or rewards they receive from the abuser. They may also fear reprisals from others and feel intense guilt associated with a belief that they were responsible for the abuse. Low self-esteem, low self-efficacy and an external locus of control all render children vulnerable to repeated abuse. The child may cope with abuse-related stress in a functional or a dysfunctional way. Dysfunctional coping strategies include accommodation to the abuser and the abuser's wishes, denial of the abuse, recanting and attempts to avoid disclosure and its consequences. These negative coping strategies are usually associated with certain appraisals of the outcome of disclosure. For example, abused children may blame themselves for the abuse and fear that disclosure will threaten the integrity of the whole family.

Functional coping strategies include seeking social support and using socially supportive relationships as opportunities for catharsis and re-evaluating beliefs associated with traumagenic dynamics, such as sexualization, stigmatization, powerlessness and betrayal. Functional coping strategies may be viewed as protective factors. So too are other personal characteristics that allow the child to resist repeated abuse. Such factors include assertiveness skills, physical strength, intelligence, high self-esteem, high self-efficacy, an internal locus of control, an optimistic attributional style and mature defences.

Risk factors associated with the abuser

Finklehor (1984) has argued that four pre-conditions must be met for child sexual abuse to occur, and there is considerable empirical support for the importance of all four pre-conditions as risk factors (Chaffin et al., 2002; Marshall et al., 1990; O'Reilly & Carr, 1998; O'Reilly et al., 2004):

- the abuser must be motivated to abuse the child
- he must over-come internal inhibitions
- he must over-come external inhibitions
- finally, he must over-come the child's resistance to the abuse.

Finklehor went on to offer a more detailed analysis of the initial motivation of the abuser and concluded that three main factors may under-pin the abuser's motivation to abuse children. First, abusers must feel some degree of emotional congruence about abusing children. Thus abuse must satisfy some emotional need, such as the need to feel a high level of control in a sexual relationship or the need to remediate early experiences of sexual abuse by re-enacting them. Second, abusers must find children particularly sexually arousing. Third, abusers' access to adult sexual relationships may be blocked. In cases of intrafamilial sexual abuse this may be due to the abuser's spouse being incapacitated by physical illness or depression or to marital discord. In extrafamilial sexual abuse or sibling abuse, lack of access to adult sexual partners may be due to poor social skills or social anxiety when meeting potential adult sexual partners.

The abuser motivation to abuse a child must be coupled with some way of over-coming internal inhibitions to abuse children. That is, the abuser must have a way to neutralize the belief that sexually abusing the child is illegal and may lead to negative consequences for the abuser and the child. Alcohol or drugs may be used to over-come inhibitions. So also may distorted justificatory cognitions, e.g. 'She provoked me'; 'I can't control myself'; 'We're in love'; 'It will do no harm because it's only a game'. Aspects of the abuser's personality may also pre-dispose him to easily over-coming internal inhibitions, especially generalized difficulties in controlling impulses associated with personality disorder, intellectual disability, psychotic illness or senility.

Even if potential perpetrators are motivated to abuse children and are capable of over-coming internal inhibitions, for abuse to occur they must also be able to over-come external factors that would prevent abuse. Lack of parental supervision, social isolation and crowded living conditions all create opportunities where the abuser may have little difficulty in over-coming external factors that might prevent the abuse. This is particularly true in situations where the abuser occupies a powerful social role with respect to the child and is able to use this position and power to create a secret context for abuse. The abuser must also be able to use coercive methods to over-come the child's resistance and prevent the child's disclosure. Bribes and rewards for compliance or threats and punishments for non-compliance are typically used.

Family risk and protective factors

While Finklehor's (1984) model of the four pre-conditions or sets of risk factors associated with CSA is a useful general framework for assessing cases of CSA, Bentovim, Elton, Hildebrand, Tranter and Vizard (1988; Bentovim, 1992) provide an important account of two patterns of family functioning which are commonly observed in cases of father–daughter incest. These are the disorganized and over-organized patterns of family functioning. In disorganized families, CSA occurs because the chaotic way the family functions entails few external inhibitors for the father's or older sibling's abuse of the children. The father typically abuses a number of children and this is partially acknowledged within the family but kept secret from the public. The father bullies the family into accepting his right to abuse the children, so the abuse serves to regulate conflict within the family. These families respond to the disclosure of abuse with less intensity than over-organized families and incorporate professionals into them like members of an extended family to help them manage their many problems, which often include social disadvantage, educational difficulties, physical child abuse, neglect and marital discord. These professionals often mirror the dysfunctional non-protective patterns of the family, unless members of the professional network agree on clear roles for all professionals. This problem of conflict-by-proxy will be discussed in a later section (Furniss, 1991).

Over-organized families apparently function in an ideal fashion with an idealized marriage and apparently adequate childcare. The father, typically abuses a single child and this is kept secret and remains unacknowledged within the family. Sexual dissatisfaction within the marital relationship, conflict avoidance within the marriage, and a non-supportive relationship between the abused child and the mother characterize these families. Physical illness or psychological problems, such as depression, may contribute to the mother's involvement in an unsatisfying relationship with her partner and an unsupportive relationship with her daughter. The father and daughter may take on parental roles with respect to the ill mother, or the father may take on the role of the bully to whom both his partner and daughter are subordinate. In other instances, sexual dissatisfaction within the marriage may be associated with the father viewing himself as subordinate to his partner. In these cases, the father and daughter may both adopt child-like roles with respect to the mother.

Following disclosure, mothers in these families may immediately file for divorce and fathers attempt suicide because of the discrepancy between the reality and the idealized family image. Eventually, these families can make changes and benefit from treatment if they deal with the underlying issues of conflict avoidance within the marriage, sexual dissatisfaction and the mother's need to develop protection skills.

In both over-organized and under-organized families, a central risk factor is the absence of a supportive and protective relationship between the non-abusing parent and the child. With intrafamilial sexual abuse, where the non-abusing parent offers the child support, and for extrafamilial abuse, where both parents offer the child support, these relationships are protective factors. Secure parent–child attachment and authoritative parenting within the context of a flexibly organized family in which there is clear communication create a protective context for youngsters who have been sexually abused by someone outside the family. With intrafamilial abuse, a central protective factor is the insistence, by the non-abusing parent, that the abusing parent leaves the home, engages in treatment and has no unsupervised contact with the child.

Social network risk and protective factors

Features of the child's broader social context may influence their adjustment to CSA (Berliner & Elliott, 2002; Browne & Finklehor, 1986; Carr & O'Reilly, 2004; Glaser, 2002b; Jones, 2000; Kendall-Tackett et al., 1993; Putnam, 2003; Spaccarelli, 1994). Social contexts in which the child and abuser are relatively isolated create opportunities for abuse and re-abuse and so isolation is an important risk factor. High levels of stress coupled with low support in the wake of disclosure, particularly, may compromise the child's ability to cope adequately with this stressful period. In contrast, children who are offered high levels of support tend to show better adjustment.

Treatment system factors

Features of the treatment system, which includes the family, the treatment team and involved professionals and agencies may place the child at risk for either ongoing sexual abuse, a poor response to treatment or long-term adjustment problems. Denial of the abuse, rejection of the treatment team's formulation and refusal to co-operate with the treatment plan may all be viewed as risk factors. Where there is a lack of co-ordination among involved professionals or unresolved disagreements about whether the case warrants a diagnosis of sexual abuse, this increases the risk of further abuse. Factors associated with child protection processes, including a lack of support at disclosure, multiple investigative interviews, multi-placement experiences, extended legal proceedings and proceedings that are not child centred or child friendly all contribute to the amount of stress experienced by the child. Treatment systems that are not sensitive to the family's cultural and ethnic beliefs and values may place children at risk because they may inhibit engagement in, or promote drop-out from, treatment and prevent the development of a good working alliance.

In contrast to these risk factors, certain features of the treatment system may be viewed as protective insofar as they reduce the risk of further abuse and enhance the possibility of positive changes within the child's psycho-social environment, which in turn reduce the risk of long-term adjustment problems. Within the treatment system, co-operative working relationships between the treatment team and the family and good co-ordination of multi-professional input are protective factors. Treatment systems that are sensitive to the family's cultural and ethnic beliefs and values are more likely to help family members engage with, and remain in, treatment and foster the development of a good working alliance. Families are more likely to benefit from treatment when all family members accept that there is a problem and the parent accepts responsibility for the abuse. Acceptance of the formulation of the problem given by the treatment team and a commitment to working with the team to resolve it are also protective factors.

TAKING ACTION WHEN THERE IS A FIRST-LINE SUSPICION OF CHILD SEXUAL ABUSE

Assessment in cases of CSA is ideally conducted by a multi-disciplinary team, which includes members from law enforcement agencies, statutory child welfare agencies and child health agencies. All action taken in cases of CSA must be taken in the best interests of the child. In some instances these interests may conflict with those of the parents. Different courses of action will be required depending on the relationship of the child to the alleged abuser and the level of suspicion that abuse has occurred.

With extrafamilial abuse, where the alleged abuser lives outside of the child's home, immediate action may be taken in almost all cases to interview the child and family without placing the child at risk for further abuse or intimidation. The only complicating factor in these cases is where both of the parents have a particularly close relationship with the alleged abuser and are likely to disbelieve the child. In these cases, and in cases of sibling abuse, however, it is often possible to arrange for parents to put protective measures in place to prevent further abuse, without them fully accepting the reality of the abuse, since the alternative may be for the child to be placed in care. Dealing with disbelief may then be a focus for subsequent family-based intervention.

In cases of intrafamilial parent–child sexual abuse, a rapid response to allegations of abuse may do more harm than good. It is useful in these cases to draw a distinction between vague first-line suspicions and well-founded, well-documented second-line suspicions (Furniss, 1991). With vague first-line suspicions little information on the factors listed in Figure 21.2 or Table 21.1 (see pp. 985–987) is available. A problem with arranging a full assessment without considerable forethought and planning is that, if sufficient information cannot be gathered to determine whether or not abuse occurred, the child may return to a situation in which he or she is intimidated into retracting his or her statement.

So, with first-line suspicions the main course of action is to convene a meeting of all involved professionals to pool information and plan further information-gathering strategies, such as a review of contacts with the family doctor or a behaviour monitoring programme at school. Junior staff should always involve senior staff in these cases from the outset. This professional network meeting should include the *trusted person*, if such exists, to whom the child made a complete or partial disclosure, the child's teacher, the family doctor, health professionals or professionals from other services, such as probation, who have had significant contact with the family, the local law enforcement or child protection personnel who have responsibility for child abuse cases and other relevant professionals. It is vital that a case co-ordinator is appointed to take responsibility for directing this process of information gathering and arranging periodic reviews with the professional network to determine if the vague first-line suspicion has developed into a clear and well-documented second-line suspicion. In jurisdictions where there is mandatory reporting of all cases of suspected child abuse, such a report must be made at this early stage unless there is a stipulation in the mandatory reporting policy about the amount of supporting evidence that must be available before reporting suspected child sexual abuse.

Central to this process is ongoing contact between the trusted person and the child. The trusted person may be a teacher, a school counsellor, a psychotherapist or an adult involved in the child's leisure or sports activities. The trusted person should continue to have regular contact with the child and monitor the child's willingness to make a full disclosure in a videotaped interview. The trusted person must let the child know in realistic terms what may happen following disclosure. One possible outcome is that the non-abusing parent may take a protective stance with respect to the child and demand that the abuser leave the house temporarily or permanently, and that contact between the child and the abuser would always be supervised. A second option is that the non-abusing parent disbelieves the child and the child would then be placed in residential care, foster care or with relatives temporarily or for a long-term placement. Other possibilities should also be discussed with the child. The process of sustaining ongoing contact with a child undergoing chronic abuse is highly stressful. It is important for all members of the professional network to support the trusted person during this work. If the trusted person feels fully supported by the professional network, that person will convey confidence and support to the abused child who, in turn, will be more likely to feel free to engage in a videotaped disclosure interview.

There is an argument that holding strategy meetings without the consent of the child or the involved family (in cases of suspected intrafamilial abuse) is unethical insofar as client confidentiality is being breached. The main argument against this position is that informing families that intrafamilial child abuse is suspected on the basis of a vague first-line suspicion may lead to a situation where the child is coercively silenced by the family member who is abusing him or her and subjected to long-term abuse under threat of violence. In many jurisdictions there is agreement that breaching confidentiality in professional network strategy meetings is ethically acceptable because it is done in the best interests of the child. The ethics of conducting pre-assessment network meetings and breaching client confidentiality must be discussed by professionals in child protection networks sufficiently to permit professionals to develop local working procedures with which they feel ethically comfortable. If these issues are not discussed and clarified at a local level, the professional network will have co-ordination difficulties that will inevitably lead to problems in protecting abused children.

Different countries have different approaches to reporting child sexual abuse. At one extreme, in the USA and Canada there is a legal requirement for psychologists to report all suspected cases of child abuse. At the other extreme, in contrast to mandatory reporting, in Holland and Belgium the emphasis is on referring cases for family support services. The UK and Ireland fall between these extremes and there are strict education, health and social service guidelines which psychologists must follow in cases where child abuse is suspected.

In some jurisdictions where there is mandatory reporting, such reports may not be required until the stage when a well-documented, second-line suspicion of sexual abuse has been developed. Once a decision has been made to investigate a case of suspected child sexual abuse, all professionals should work together and take account of the traumatizing effects of repeated interviews, repeated physical examinations and insensitively conducted interviews and medical examinations. It is also vital that arrangements be made for taking the child into care immediately following the preliminary assessment session, in case the child alleges abuse and a protective environment within the child's home cannot be agreed by family members. For example, in cases where children allege that they have been repeatedly abused by the father and threatened with violence if they disclose, and both father and mother deny the abuse, it is vital that the child be taken into care immediately. If the child is returned home, inevitably the child will be intimidated, threatened with violence and the child in response will retract his or her statement. The abuse will continue and the child will be unlikely to make further allegations because of the threats of violence from the abuser and the ineffectiveness of the professional network in providing protection. Where children do not make a clear allegation in an investigative interview, then contact with the trusted person may continue with periodic feedback to meetings of the professional network until the child is prepared to make a clear statement in an investigative interview. Where the non-abusing parent believes the child and agrees to protect the child, the child may return home provided the abuser leaves the household. A flow-chart of the process of taking action following an allegation of child sexual abuse is presented in Figure 21.3. Once it has been decided to conduct an assessment, a contract for this may be offered to the family in a courteous way, but obviously a long delay between offering an appointment and conducting the assessment will place the child at risk of further intimidation. Parents should be asked to give written consent for the assessment to be conducted, and this should include clauses concerning recording of interviews and medical examination. Refusal to give consent for the child to be assessed in conjunction with other information may be grounds for pursuing child protection proceedings.

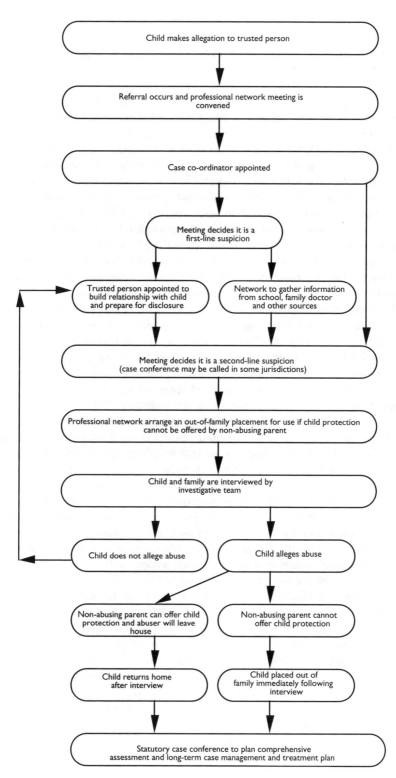

Figure 21.3 Taking action following an allegation of child sexual abuse

ASSESSING THE VALIDITY OF CHILDREN'S ALLEGATIONS OF SEXUAL ABUSE

Cases of suspected child sexual abuse may be referred as new cases for assessment or, in other instances, while working with cases referred for some other problem, such as recurrent abdominal pain or anorexia, the possibility of sexual abuse as an explanation for the original referral problems emerges. In a study of over 500 consecutive referrals of allegations of sexual abuse, Jones and McGraw (1987) concluded that less than 10% of allegations were fictitious and that in most of these cases the fictitious allegations were part of a conflictual process in families where separation or divorce had occurred. Factors which raise suspicion of child abuse are set out in Table 21.1. These factors, which have been identified in comprehensive literature reviews (Glaser, 2002b; Heiman, 1992; Wolfe & Birt, 1997), have been divided into those related to the child's behaviour, those focusing specifically on the child's account of the sexual abuse, those related to the child's medical conditions and, finally, those related to the child's social context. Sexualized behaviour and avoidance of possible abuse-related situations, and stimuli occurring in conjunction with other difficulties, such as conduct problems, emotional problems or attainment difficulties, are the main features of children's behaviour which raise suspicion of child sexual abuse.

Various aspects of the content and form of the child's account lend support to the view that sexual abuse has occurred. These include sexual knowledge that is not age appropriate, the use of age-inappropriate language, the account being given from the child's perspective, the account being con-textually detailed and internally consistent and the account being given in an emotive way and describing attempts by the abuser to silence the child through the use of coercion or bribery. If children give their accounts spon-taneously in response to an open non-leading question, if the answer does not sound like a rehearsed story and if the account is consistent for major details with repeated telling but has a different sentence structure, this lends support to the view that the allegations are true. Accounts given using anatomically correct dolls or drawings must also be consistent with the verbal account given by the child.

Increased confidence may be placed in the truth of the child's allegations if the child's medical condition is consistent with the verbal account given of the abuse. Some of the physical correlates of various types of sexual abuse have been listed in Table 21.1.

Certain features of the context of the disclosure lend support to allegations of abuse. An account that is given some time after the abuse has occurred, one that occurs against a history of allegations and retractions by the child, and one that contradicts accounts given by the alleged perpetrator and those that sympathize with him is more likely to be true than an account that does not have these features. Allegations are more likely to be true if it can be

Table 21.1 A framework of factors indicative of child sexual abuse

The child's behaviour	Sexualized behaviour	• Change in routine behaviour patterns so that the child displays more sexualized behaviour than usual • Excessive and age-inappropriate sexual play or conversation, either solitary or with others • Excessive, age-inappropriate and often relatively public sexual self-stimulation • Attempts to engage others in sexual activities through exposing sex parts to others, rubbing sex-parts against others, inappropriate kissing, request to engage others in sexual acts
	Non-sexualized conduct and emotional problems	• Change in the child's behaviour so that the child shows increased conduct and emotional problems • Increased externalizing behaviour problems and related emotions and beliefs (aggressive behaviour, destructiveness, hyperactivity, running away, illegal behaviour, substance abuse, anger, frustration, suspicion and lack of trust of others) • Increased internalizing behaviour and related negative emotions and beliefs (social withdrawal, somatic complaints, self-injurious behaviour; anxiety, depression, low self-esteem)
	Academic problems	• Deterioration in academic performance at school
	Response to abuse-related stimuli	• The child avoids persons or situations associated with the abuse • The child avoids persons or situations symbolic of the abuse (e.g. refusal to go to bedroom if abuse happened in a bedroom; refusal to undress for swimming; avoidance of older men if the perpetrator was a man) • The child responds to persons or situations associated with the abuse or symbolic of the abuse with distress and intensification of emotional and conduct problems • The child responds to persons or situations associated with the abuse or symbolic of the abuse by showing regressive attachment behaviour towards the mother or primary caregiver (e.g. clinging and refusing to be left alone)
The child's account	Content of the account of the sexual abuse	• The child says a person within or outside the family sexually abused him or her • The description of the abusive events may entail sexual knowledge that is beyond that usually displayed by children of the same age • Within the account the child describes attempts by the perpetrator to conceal the sexual abuse through bribery or coercive threats

Continued

Table 21.1 continued

	Form of the account of sexual abuse	• The child's account is given spontaneously or in response to a non-leading question • The account is given in age-appropriate language • The account is given from a child's point of view rather than from an adult's perspective • The account is contextually detailed and internally consistent • The account is given in an emotive way and the emotions (anger, fear, distress, sadness) are congruent with the events described • The account does not sound like a rehearsed story which the child has been coached to tell by an adult
	Form of repeated accounts	• The same sentence structure is not used in a retelling of the account (as would occur if the account were a rehearsed story) • On repeated telling, the account is consistent for major details but may be inconsistent for minor details
	Anatomically correct dolls and drawings in giving the account	• Accounts of the abusive events enacted using anatomically correct dolls or portrayed with drawings are consistent with verbal accounts
The child's medical condition		• The child's medical condition is consistent with the account of the abuse • Overt or covert trauma to genital or rectal areas • Infections of the genital or rectal areas • Sexually transmitted disease • Foreign bodies in genital, urethral or anal openings • Abnormal dilatation of the urethral, anal or vaginal openings • Torn or blood-stained underclothing • Pregnancy
The child's context	**Context of the disclosure**	• The disclosure is given some time after the abuse occurred • There may have been a pattern of previous allegations and retractions • Contradictory accounts of circumstances surrounding the abuse are given by the alleged perpetrator (and those sympathetic to the perpetrator) • The alleged perpetrator (and sympathizers) blame a third party (e.g. baby-sitter)
	Supporting evidence	• The child displays an ability to distinguish fact from fantasy • There are witnesses of the actual abusive acts • There are witnesses of some aspects of the child's account, such as the circumstances surrounding the abusive act, but not the acts themselves, and these are consistent with the child's account

- The child's social context places him or her at risk for sexual abuse (the alleged abuser is motivated to abuse the child; the alleged abuser is capable of overcoming internal inhibitions which might prevent him or her abusing the child; the abuser has access to child in the absence of other adults; the abuser occupies a position of social power with respect to the child and those who support the child; the child has a low level of parental support, vis-a-vis the abuser; the child lives in sociocultural context in which he or she believes that disclosure will not be believed by other adults)
- The child has personal characteristics which place him or her at risk for sexual abuse (lack of assertiveness to adults; highly compliant with a strong need to please; intellectual disability)

demonstrated that the child has the ability to distinguish between fact and fantasy and if there are witnesses for the abusive acts or events surrounding these which are consistent with the child's account.

If the child's social context contains risk factors that have been shown empirically to be associated with CSA, then it is more likely that the child's allegations are true. Some of the more important risk factors have been discussed above and are listed in Figure 21.2.

ASSESSMENT

With cases of sexual abuse, assessment progresses through two main phases (Glaser, 2002b; Heiman, 1992; Wolfe & Birt, 1997). The first phase is concerned with the question: 'Has this child been sexually abused?' If this question is answered in the affirmative, the second assessment question is 'What impact has the abuse had on the child and family and what elements should be included in a multi-systemic treatment package for the child and family?' A complicating factor in the assessment of cases of child sexual abuse is that the data used to answer the first question may be required for use as evidence in legal proceedings to ensure the child's protection or to prosecute the abuser.

Of course, the abuser, the abused child, some members of the family and some members of the professional network are aware of this, and this has an impact on their co-operation with the assessment process. Usually, the abused child and those who sympathize with the child's position want the assessment to proceed but fear that if the child's position is not believed or supported by the results of the assessment then the child will be punished by the abuser. Typically, the abuser does not want the assessment to proceed but may co-operate superficially, since refusal to co-operate may be interpreted as an admission of guilt. Throughout the process of assessment, the abuser may attempt to intimidate the abused child into retracting the allegations of abuse.

Therefore it is vital that the first phase of the assessment be brief, provide an opportunity for the child and other family members to give detailed accurate information on the abuse if it occurred, and do so within a social context where the child is protected from intimidation by the abuser. The child and family must also be informed of the probable short-, medium- and long-term consequences if the assessment indicates that abuse occurred and, indeed, if the assessment fails to answer this question.

The information gathered in the assessment must throw light on a complex range of factors listed in Figures 21.1 and 21.2 and Table 21.1 and, for legal proceedings, this information must meet certain criteria (Lanning, 2002; Myers, 2002; Myers & Stern, 2002; Saywitz, Goodman & Lyon, 2002). For child protection legal proceedings, there must be sufficient evidence to state that, *in the balance of probabilities*, child abuse has occurred. However, it must be shown *beyond reasonable doubt* that child abuse occurred in criminal legal proceedings, where the alleged abuser is charged with a sexual offence.

Comprehensive assessment schedule

The components for a comprehensive assessment of cases of child sexual abuse is presented in Table 21.2. The table outlines the members of the child's family and professional network who should be interviewed and important areas to cover in these interviews, and there is reference to special assessment procedures such as forensic medical examination of the child. However, the cornerstone of the assessment procedure is the interview (or series of interviews) with the child, since it is the child's account of the abuse which is the main basis for deciding whether abuse occurred. In many cases, following the interview with the child and each of the parents, a decision can be made about a change of residence for the abuser and the abused child and the remainder of the comprehensive assessment may occur some time later.

Interviewing children

The principal aim of the individual interviews with the child is to obtain the child's account of the abusive incidents (if such occurred) in response to non-leading questions (Jones, 2003; Saywitz et al., 2002). A second aim of the individual interviews with the child is to assess the impact of the abuse on the child. In particular, it is important to assess any abnormal behavioural patterns and the traumagenic dynamics of sexual traumatization, stigmatization, betrayal and powerlessness. A third aim of the child interviews is to assess the child's perception of risk and protective factors within the family. In particular, an account of the child's perception of the non-abusing parent's capacity to be protective is required. A fourth aim of the child interviews is to establish the ways in which the child has coped with the abuse and his or her personal strengths and resources, particularly assertiveness and

Table 21.2 Components of a comprehensive child protection assessment package for use in cases of child sexual abuse

Evaluation target	Evaluation methods and areas
Child	• Child's spontaneous account of the abusive incidents • The location of the abuse • The frequency and duration of the abuse • The use of violence or threats • The presence of other people during the abuse • The use of drugs or alcohol by the perpetrator or the child • Whether photographs or recordings of the abuse were made • Impact of the abuse on the child and traumagenic dynamics of sexual traumatization, stigmatization, betrayal and powerlessness • Child's perception of risk factors • Child's perception of the non-abusing parent's capacity to be protective • Coping strategies and personal strengths and resources, particularly assertiveness • Child's wishes for the future • Medical examination of the child • Sexual behaviour checklists to assess sexualized behaviour • General child-behaviour checklist to assess internalizing and externalizing behaviour problems • Assessment of cognitive abilities and attainment levels if disability or school-related problems are present
The non-abusing parent(s)	• The degree to which the parent believes the child's allegations • The degree to which the parent aids the child's disclosure • The degree to which the parent emotionally supports and empathizes with the child • The degree to which the parent views the abuser and not the child as solely responsible for the abuse • The degree to which the parent pursues options that will separate the abuser from the child and protect the child • The degree to which the parent co-operates with statutory agencies such as social services • The degree to which the parent is prepared to discuss the abuse with other family members such as siblings or grandparents • The degree to which the parent has protected him- or herself from sexual abuse • The degree to which the parent can enlist other supports to help • Relevant risk factors (abuser's motivation and over-coming internal and external inhibitions) • Reconstruction of an account of factors surrounding the abusive incidents • Personal resources and problems (particularly history of personal abuse) • Parenting skills and deficits
Abuser	• Denial of the abuse • Denial of the frequency or severity of the abuse • Denial of the abuser's addiction to the abusive acts

Continued

Table 21.2 continued

Evaluation target	Evaluation methods and areas
	• Denial of the effects of the abusive acts • Denial of the abuser's responsibility for the abuse • Relevant risk factors (motivation and over-coming internal and external inhibitions) • Reconstruction of an account of the abusive incidents • Personal resources and problems (particularly history of personal abuse) • Parenting skills and deficits
Marital couple	• In father–daughter incest – the non-abusing parent's ability to confront the denial of the abusing parent • In father–daughter incest – dependence of non-abusing parent on the abusing parent • In extrafamilial and sibling abuse – degree to which parents can jointly support child • In sibling abuse – degree to which parents can set limits on abuser without scapegoating
Siblings	• Possibility that they may also have been abused • Perception of risk factors • Perception of the non-abusing parent's capacity to be protective • Wishes for the future • Perception of routines of family life
Role of extended family	• Acceptance or denial of the abuse • Perception of risk factors • Perception of the non-abusing parent's capacity to be protective • Wishes for the future • Perception of routines of family life • Childcare skills and deficits • Potential for contributing to a long-term child protection plan
Role of other involved professionals	• Health, education, social services and justice professionals' expert view of risks and resources within the family • Potential future involvement in supporting the family and protecting the child in future • Community-resource people's potential for supporting the family and protecting the child in future

self-protective skills. It is also important to obtain a clear account of the child's wishes for the future.

Interviews may be conducted in any setting where an uninterrupted meeting can occur for about an hour and where there is sufficient space and lighting to record the interview. Drawing materials and anatomically correct dolls are useful aids to interviewing. Ideally, the child should be interviewed alone. If the non-abusing parent or trusted person insists on being present, he or she should sit outside of the child's visual field and remain silent, or view the interview from behind a one-way screen if this facility is available, to minimize their impact on the child's account.

The interview may begin with rapport-building questions about school and hobbies, and move from there to open questions that may elicit information about abusive events:

> I have spoken to Mrs Duffy, and she said that you were worried about some things that were happening recently. Can you tell me a bit about that?

> Your Mum told me that someone has being doing things with you that are upsetting. Can you tell me the stuff you told her last week?

If these open enquiries do not lead to a spontaneous account, closed questions may be asked:

> Has anyone ever touched your private parts that your swimming suit covers so it made you feel bad? . . . Can you tell me about that?

Leading questions, that suggest who did what, should be avoided. For example:

> Did daddy touch you on your Mary Anne?

If the child gives a verbal account and some clarification is required, some things should be avoided. Do not use any other words for body parts other than those used by the child, so it is good practice to ask:

> Where did he put his willy?

and incorrect to ask:

> Where did he put his penis?

Avoid asking questions about the alleged perpetrator which uses a pronoun rather than the child's name for the person. Ask:

> What did Daddy do then?

not:

> What did he do then?

Avoid lecturing the child about the rights and wrongs of child abuse or asking questions that might make the child feel guilty such as: 'Why did you do that?'

Drawings or anatomically correct dolls should be used as an aid to factual interviewing, not as a projective test. Research on anatomically correct dolls

(Koocher et al., 1995) shows that children who have not been sexually abused inspect and touch sexual body parts but do not enact sexual activities such as oral, anal or genital intercourse with the dolls. Neither do anatomically correct dolls lead to undue distress or traumatization. Anatomically correct dolls are a useful aid to communication. They allow the interviewer to find out the child's idiosyncratic terms for body parts and to provide a medium through which to communicate about sexually abusive acts. With pre-school children, caution is required because of the suggestibility of younger children and anatomically correct dolls should probably only be used after an allegation of abuse has been made rather than beforehand. It is also critical with younger children to avoid leading questions.

In view of these conclusions from the research on anatomically correct dolls, the following practice guidelines are offered. First, the child may be shown the dolls clothed and asked to identify a doll that represents herself and one that represents the alleged abuser. The child may wish to name other dolls as representing other family members. Second, the child may be asked to undress the dolls representing herself and the alleged abuser, inspect them and name the private parts of the dolls using his or her own terms. Third, the child may be invited to enact, with the dolls, the abusive events that occurred between herself and the abuser. A similar procedure may be used with drawings, where the child draws herself and the abuser, fills in their private parts and then points to what went where.

Once the child has given a spontaneous general account of the abuse, information about specific details should be obtained. Important areas to cover are:

- the location of the abuse
- the frequency and duration of the abuse
- the use of violence or threats
- the presence of other people during the abuse
- the use of drugs or alcohol by the perpetrator or the child
- whether photographs or recordings of the abuse were made
- the child's psychological reactions to the abuse.

With younger children it is important to ask for this information in terms of yardsticks that are meaningful to the child. For example, in obtaining information about the duration of the abuse, select significant annual events in the child's life such as Christmas or summer holidays as the basis for questions:

Did this first happen before Christmas or after Christmas?

Wolfe, Gentile, Nichienzi, Sas and Wolfe's (1991) Child Impact of Traumatic Events Scale may be used to evaluate some of the effects of the abuse on the child in a relatively structured way. This structured interview is described in Table 21.3.

Table 21.3 Psychometric instruments that may be used as an adjunct to clinical interviews in the assessment of child sexual abuse

Construct	Instrument	Publication	Comments
Behaviour problems arising from sexual abuse	Child Sexual Behaviour Inventory	Friedrich, W., Grambsch, P., Damon, L. et al. (1992). Child Sexual Behaviour Inventory. *Psychological Assessment*, 4, 303–311. Available from http://www.parinc.com	35-item parent report form checklist which discriminates between CSA and non-CSA children
PTSD symptoms and belief systems about self and others arising from sexual abuse	Child Impact of Traumatic Events Scale (Revised)	Wolfe, V. et al. (1991). Child Impact of Traumatic Events Scale. A measure of post-sexual-abuse PTSD symptoms. *Behavioural Assessment*, 13, 359–383	This 78-item structured interview for children yields scores on the following sub-scales: intrusive thoughts, avoidance, hyperarousal, sexual anxiety, negative reactions by others, social support, self-blame, guilt, personal vulnerability, dangerous world; empowerment, eroticism
Trauma reactions	Trauma Symptom Checklist for Children (TSCC)	Briere, J. (2004). *Trauma Symptom Checklist for Children (TSCC)*. Odessa, FL: PAR. Available at http://www.parinc.com/product.cfm?ProductID=150	This 54-item self-report questionnaire for 8- to 16-year-olds yields scores for anger, anxiety, depression, dissociation, post-traumatic stress, and sexual concerns
Dissociative states following PTSD	Child Dissociation Checklist	Putnam, F., Helmers, K., & Trickett, P. (1993). Development, reliability and validity of a child dissociation scale. *Child Abuse and Neglect*, 17, 731–742	A scale to measure dissociative responses to trauma
Sexual abuse of boys	Structure Interview of Symptoms Associated with Sexual Abuse (SASA)	Wells, S., McCann, J., Adams, J., Voris, J. & Duhl, D. (1997). A validation study of the Structure Interview of	A 26-item structured questionnaire for parents of sexually abused boys

Continued

Table 21.3 continued

Construct	Instrument	Publication	Comments
		Symptoms Associated with Sexual Abuse (SASA) using three samples of sexually abused, allegedly abused and nonabused boys. *Child Abuse and Neglect*, 21, 1159–1167	
Exposure to sexual stressors	Checklist of Sexual Abuse and Related Stressors (C-SARS)	Spaccarelli, S. & Fuchs, L. (1997). Variability in symptom expression among sexually abused girls: Developing multivariate models. *Journal of Clinical Child Psychology*, 26, 25–35	This checklist of 70 events yields scores for three sub-scales: abuse-specific events, abuse-related events, and public disclosure events
Reactions to anatomically detailed dolls	Anatomical Doll Questionnaire	Levy, H., Markovic, J., Kalinowski, M., Ahart, S., & Torres, H. (1995). Child sexual abuse interviews. The use of anatomical dolls and the reliability of information. *Journal of Interpersonal Violence*, 10, 334–353	The interview offers a reliable and structured way to code response to anatomically detailed dolls

Most abused children have been threatened that disclosure will be punished and so it is not unusual for children to show signs of fear and ask the interviewer not to tell anyone about the abuse. It is important to empathize with the child's discomfort but to avoid re-assuring the child that everything will be fine and no one will be told about the interview, since these assurances are untrue. The period following disclosure is usually very stressful and the child's account of the abuse will be reported to the professional network, the family and possibly the court. So empathic and supportive responses like this should be used:

I know it's a bit hard to talk about this stuff. But you are doing very well.

There is also a temptation to cuddle children when they look fearful and distressed. This should be avoided because physical cuddling may have sexual connotations for a sexually abused child.

Because of the stressful nature of disclosure, periods of questioning may be interspersed with periods of free play. Therefore it may be useful to have other play materials available in the interviewing room.

At the end of the disclosure interview or interviews, it is important for the child and the non-abusing parent to meet with the interviewer and for the interviewer to summarize the information the child disclosed. This should be done even if the mother was in the interview room but out of the field of vision of the child or behind a one-way screen if this facility was available. This hand-over meeting marks the beginning of helping the non-abusing parent develop a protective relationship with the child. The non-abusing parent will be torn between disbelief and the wish to protect the child, and so this meeting is stressful for the parent. If, at the end of this meeting, the non-abusing parent can agree to protect the child, then a member of the professional network, ideally a law enforcement officer, should confront the abuser before the child and the non-abusing parent have had time to meet with the alleged abuser. This is important, since the alleged abuser may intimidate and coerce the child and the non-abusing parent into retracting the allegations of abuse. Ideally, the abuser should move out of the home under a court-ordered injunction until the assessment is completed and sufficient progress has been made in subsequent therapy for it to be safe for the abuser to have unsupervised access with to child. These issues are discussed in more detail in the section on treatment, below.

If the non-abusing parent is unable to believe the child's disclosure and unable to make a commitment to protect the child, then an immediate, emergency out-of-home placement under a child protection order should be made. It is important that the foster parents or childcare key worker for the abused child meet with the child, the non-abusing parent and the interviewer for a hand-over meeting in which the interviewer explains the allegations and the reason for the out-of-home placement in front of the child and the non-abusing parent. It is important to clarify visiting arrangements at this point and to maximize contact between the child and the non-abusing parent, since in some cases after a brief period the non-abusing parent decides to believe the child's account of the abuse and to offer protection. In these instances, the child can return home after a brief out-of-home placement. In other instances, family sessions aimed at a hypothetical exploration of how the family would organize itself if in fact everyone believed the child's account of the abuse may lead to a shift in the non-abusing parent's disbelief.

The importance of planning and co-ordination within the professional network prior to conducting a disclosure interview or series of interviews is critical for maximizing the protection of the child. Failure to set up an emergency out-of-home placement for use in case the non-abusing parent cannot protect the child, or failure to arrange for a law enforcement officer to be available to confront the abuser after the disclosure interview, may lead to situations where the child is exposed to further intimidation, coercion and ultimately more severe abuse.

Other aspects of the assessment of the child

A full physical and medical forensic examination of the child should be conducted as part of a comprehensive assessment following guidelines for good practice. Parents and teachers may be asked to complete both the Child Behaviour Checklist (Achenbach & Rescorla, 2000, 2001) and the Child Sexual Behaviour Inventory (Friedrich et al., 1992) to obtain information of internalizing, externalizing and sexualized behaviour problems. Other instruments listed in Table 21.3 may be used as required. PTSD can be evaluated using the structured interviews and self-report scales in Table 12.10 (pp. 498–501). Where intellectual disability may be a risk factor in CSA, or where attainment problems have occurred in response to CSA, a psychometric assessment of the child's abilities and attainments may be conducted following the guidelines in Chapter 8.

Evaluation of the non-abusing parent

Individual interviews with non-abusing parents and conjoint interviews with the non-abusing parent and the abused child should be conducted to assess their capacity to protect the child. Smith's (1995) framework for assessing protectiveness includes the following items:

- the degree to which the parent believes the child's allegations
- the degree to which the parent aids the child's disclosure
- the degree to which the parent emotionally supports and empathizes with the child
- the degree to which the parent views the abuser and not the child as solely responsible for the abuse
- the degree to which the parent identifies and pursues options that will separate the abuser from the child and protect the child
- the degree to which the parent co-operates with statutory agencies, such as social services
- the degree to which the parent is prepared to discus the abuse with other family members, such as siblings or grandparents
- the degree to which the parent has protected him- or herself from sexual abuse
- the degree to which the parent can enlist other supports to help deal with vulnerabilities such as physical or intellectual disability.

In addition to assessing these items, non-abusing parents' childcare skills and deficits, their reconstruction of the abusive incidents or events surrounding them; and their perception of all relevant risk factors should be evaluated. In some instances, psychological assessment of specific parental characteristics (e.g. intelligence) and psychopathology (e.g. depression) may be required, especially in cases where personal deficits of a non-abusing parent created opportunities for the other parent to abuse the child.

Evaluation of the abusing parent

When the abusing parent is confronted with the allegations of abuse, and his or her impact on the child and family, the following aspects of denial are assessed:

- denial of the abuse ('It never happened')
- denial of the frequency or severity of the abuse ('It only happened once or twice and all I did was touch her once or twice')
- denial of the abuser's addiction to the abusive acts ('I didn't feel compelled to do it', 'It was a casual thing')
- denial of the effects of the abusive acts ('It will not do any harm')
- denial of the abuser's responsibility for the abuse ('She provoked me', 'She was asking for it').

The process of confrontation may be conducted in different ways. Some professionals confront the abuser themselves in individual interviews; others show the abuser a videotape or transcript of the child's account of the abuse; others favour family confrontation sessions in which the abused child, supported by the whole family, confronts the abuser. Whatever method is used, the aim of this procedure is to determine the openness of the abuser to giving up denial and to do this without unduly distressing the abused child.

Abusers engage in denial because giving it up may entail leaving the family home, prosecution, social stigmatization and personal admission of guilt. It is important to empathize with the alleged abuser about his reasons for engaging in denial, and to preface this with the statistic that in less than 10% of cases do children make false allegations (Jones & McGraw, 1987).

Furniss (1991) has developed a hypothetical interviewing style that he uses in family interviews where one or both parents deny the abuse. He explores who within the family is best and worst at bottling-up secrets (such as birthday surprises). He asks each family member what they believe would happen if the abuse had occurred and the abuser admitted to it. Who would be responsible for the abuse? Who would be responsible for protection? What would be the consequences for those who failed to protect the child? What would be the consequences for each family member of lack of trust?

In addition to assessing level of denial, risk factors associated with motivation to abuse and ways of over-coming internal and external inhibitions, discussed earlier, should also be assessed. Where perpetrators admit to abuse, they should be helped to reconstruct a model of the abusive cycle. Personal resources and problems, particularly a history of personal abuse and parenting skills and deficits, should be evaluated.

Evaluation of the marital couple

Conjoint interviews with the parents of the abused child may be used to assess the quality of their relationship. In cases of parent–child incest, the evaluation of the marital couple must address the degree to which the non-abusing parent can confront the denial of the abusing parent and the degree to which the non-abusing parent is dependent on the abusing parent. For eventual partial or complete family re-unification, the non-abusing parent must be able to confront the abusing parent, ask him to leave the house and then later decide whether to work towards permanent separation or family re-unification, whichever is the preferable option. To be able to follow this route there must be sufficient differentiation within the marriage, at the time of disclosure, for the non-abusing parent to be able to confront the abuser. In cases of extrafamilial abuse, the evaluation of the marital couple focuses on the degree to which parents can work together in supporting the abused child. In cases of sibling abuse, there is the additional issue of the capacity of the parents to work as a team in confronting the abuser's denial, setting limits on his behaviour and yet not scapegoating him or ostracizing him from family life.

Evaluation of the siblings

Interviews with the siblings should focus on the possibility that they may also have been abused. In addition, they may have information about risk factors, events surrounding the abusive episodes and other important aspects of family life.

Evaluation of the role of the extended family

Interviews with other members of the nuclear and extended family may be conducted to assess their acceptance or denial of the abuse, their perception of risk factors, their knowledge about the abusive episodes, their childcare skills and deficits and potential for contributing to a long-term child-protection plan. In some situations it may be possible for the abuser to stay with members of the extended family, provided this does not put other children at risk for abuse. In situations where both parents deny the abuse, the abused child may be placed with relatives who do not deny the abuse. A court-ordered injunction may be obtained to prevent the abuser from entering the relatives' house where the child is placed. However, this type of extended family placement may create family conflicts that are difficult to resolve in the long term.

Evaluation of the role of other involved professionals

Individual interviews with other involved professionals from health, education, social services and justice agencies may be conducted to obtain their expert views of risks and resources within the family and their potential future involvement in supporting the family, protecting the child or providing services. Interviews with other people in community-based resource settings may be conducted to obtain information relevant to the case and the protection plan. These people may include the foster parents with whom the child is temporarily based, home-helpers, befrienders, leaders of mother and toddler groups and nursery or day-care facility staff.

Children abused in care

The assessment package set out in Table 21.2 is appropriate for most cases of intrafamilial sexual abuse and cases of extrafamilial abuse where the child is living with his or her parents. It may, however, be adapted for use in cases where the child alleges that abuse has occurred while living in foster care or a residential childcare institution. The guidelines for interviewing the child and the abuser may be followed with little alteration. However, there are typically a great deal more non-abusing parties available as potential allies for the child in cases where children are in residential institutional care. Of these, the director of the unit and the staff member who has the best working relationship with the child are the most important to interview, and both should be encouraged to play a protective and supportive role with respect to the child. With foster care, the child's natural parents, the child's statutory social worker and the non-abusing foster parent all are potential child protectors and their capacity to support and protect the child requires assessment.

TREATMENT

In cases of intrafamilial sexual abuse, an important question is whether treatment aimed at partial or complete family re-unification should be offered. A checklist to aid assessment of the family's suitability for treatment is presented in Table 19.3 (p. 919). Bentovim et al. (1988), in a two- to six-year follow-up study of 120 cases treated at Great Ormond Street Hospital, found that only 14% of abused children remained with both parents; 38% remained with one parent and 28% went to foster or residential care or relatives; the remainder left home. So treatment must be offered with an awareness that family re-unification is probably an appropriate treatment goal for only a minority of cases.

Where family treatment aimed at partial or complete family re-unification cannot be offered, and the child is placed in long-term foster care, individual child therapy, along the lines described below, may be offered in conjunction with a programme of support and consultation for the foster parents. Foster parents need prognostic information, such as that set out earlier in this chapter when discussing the effects of CSA, on the probable course of the child's behaviour problems over the short, medium and long term. They also need to understand the traumagenic dynamics of child sexual abuse (discussed above) and how they relate to the formulation of the child's unique situation, so that they can interpret the child's behaviour problems, particularly their aggression and inappropriate sexual behaviour. Finally, they need support in developing behaviour management programmes to achieve particular goals derived from the formulation where age-appropriate behaviour and relationships are encouraged and rewarded and aggressive and inappropriate sexualized behaviour is extinguished. Reward programmes coupled with time-out may be used with younger children, and contingency contracts with teenagers.

Where families (or sub-systems of families, such as the non-abusing parent and the children) meet three of the four criteria in Table 19.3, a treatment contract for achieving specific goals may be offered. The goals should be based on a formulation derived from the assessment. The treatment contract should be designed to help family members meet these specific goals and progress should be reviewed periodically. Treatment goals for abused children include:

- developing assertive self-protective skills
- developing a protective relationship with the non-abusing parent or carer
- learning to control internalizing, externalizing and sexualized behaviour problems
- processing intense emotions associated with the abuse and related coercion
- developing positive self-evaluative beliefs
- being open to negotiating a relationship with the abuser that has appropriate boundaries.

Typical goals for non-abusing parents or carers are:

- learning how to offer the abused child a protective and supportive relationship
- working through the mixed feelings arising from the abuse.

Typical treatment goals for perpetrators include:

- giving up denial and accepting full responsibility for the abuse
- developing a lifestyle that does not involve sexual abuse

- demonstrating remorse and offering a full statement of responsibility and apology to the abused child and other family members.

The Great Ormond Street Group ran a complex programme for cases of intrafamilial father–daughter abuse where the father agreed to live outside the family for the duration of therapy (Bentovim et al, 1988; Furniss, 1991). Group therapy was offered to the abused girls together, the abusing fathers together, the mothers together and the siblings together. Concurrent mother–daughter sessions and spouse sessions were held. Once the father had accepted responsibility fully and the daughter felt adequately supported by the mother, a daughter–father confrontation session was held. The model is based on Giaretto's (1982) work in the USA. Giaretto conducted his programme in a probation department as an alternative to incarceration. While the group work in these multi-systemic intervention programmes is critical for therapeutic progress, a systemic formulation of the problem, concurrent family treatment for various dyads and for the whole family is central to the approach. Members of the professional network with statutory responsibility for child protection orders may be invited to some family sessions, particularly the sessions in which the contract for family-based treatment is offered, to negotiate about issues of access of the perpetrator to the abused child and related issues. A very similar model for working with families (one family at a time) has been described in Trepper's step-by-step manual (Trepper & Barrett, 1989). An outline of the principles for family-based treatment with CSA cases and individual or group work with abused children, non-abusing parents and perpetrators follows.

Family-based treatment

In the following discussion, the description of family-based treatment given is appropriate for cases of father–daughter incest; family-based treatment in cases of sibling abuse and extrafamilial abuse will be dealt with at the end of the section. Family-based treatment may be offered with the goal of helping family members negotiate a protective and supportive living environment for the abused child (Bentovim et al., 1988; Furniss, 1991; Trepper & Barrett, 1989), that is, an environment in which abuse will not recur. Periodically, whole-family meetings may be interspersed with a series of sessions attended by critical dyads within the family. The abuser must live outside the family for the duration of the therapy, until the family develops protective patterns of interaction to prevent re-abuse. This may require at least a year of work. In many cases of father–daughter sexual abuse, family re-unification may not be possible and therapy may aim to negotiate a protective home environment in which it is safe for the father to have periodic supervised access to the children.

The timing of whole-family meetings needs to be sensitively matched to the emotional state of family members. The whole-family meetings are a forum in which the reality of sexual abuse is shared by all family members. The pattern of family interaction in which the abuse was embedded may be elaborated. Conflict-avoiding or conflict-regulating patterns entailing weak intergenerational boundaries may be identified and the dangers associated with them noted. Avoidance of these patterns will emerge as a feature of the protective family environment that the non-abusing parent, the siblings and the abused child wish to create. Each time a family meeting occurs and the reality of the abuse is acknowledged by all family members, the processes of denial, secrecy and coercion that accompanied the abuse are further weakened. Family meetings provide a forum where siblings can contribute to supporting a family ethos that undermines the secrecy of abuse. Where siblings have been abused or have been in danger of abuse, this may emerge in whole-family meetings. However, to hold family meetings in situations where the abuser is still strongly locked into denial and the non-abusing parent has not yet taken a protective stance towards the abused child may compound the abused child's distress. In these situations, it may be more fruitful to postpone whole-family meetings until the mother has developed a more protective stance and the father has begun to let go of denial.

The development of a more protective relationship between the non-abusing parent and the abused child may be identified as a particular focus for work to prevent the recurrence of the abuse. This work may require the child to express her anger and disappointment to the non-abusing parent and the non-abusing parent to express regret and guilt. Mothers, in cases of father–daughter incest, face many obstacles in reaching a position where they can wholeheartedly support their abused daughters. Many mothers view supporting their daughter as synonymous with leaving their husband, and in many cases where husbands are locked into denial this is true. Some mothers also have feelings of jealousy towards their daughter for displacing them from their role of being their husband's sexual partner. If mothers in these situations are unable to give up denial, it is unlikely that family-based treatment will lead to partial or complete family re-unification.

When the abused child and the non-abusing parent have expressed their views about the past and their roles in the abuse-maintaining system, the focus moves to ways in which the abused child and the non-abusing parent may spend time together to develop a supportive relationship. Often this will involve closing the emotional gap that has developed during the period of the abuse.

A difficulty with this type of work is that while the non-abusing parent is trying to develop this supportive relationship with the abused child, the abused child will typically be showing a range of internalizing, externalizing and sexualized behaviour problems. Behavioural family work on these using contingency contracts and reward systems for appropriate behaviour will be required. This work will help non-abusing parents draw a clear generational boundary between themselves and the abused child. The struggle around these issues of behavioural control may span a considerable period of time, since a lack of appropriate generational boundaries is an integral aspect of child sexual abuse. Non-abusing parents may use the forum of group therapy to seek support during these difficult struggles. Abused children may use individual or group therapy as a forum for developing self-control skills also.

Once the relationship between the abused child and the non-abusing parent has become protective and a firm intergenerational boundary has been drawn, and once the abusing parent's denial has begun to decrease markedly as a result of group therapy for abusers, a series of sessions in which the abused child and the protective parent meet with the abuser may be convened. In these sessions, the abused child, supported by the protective parent, confronts the abuser with her experience of the abuse and forcefully expresses the anger and distress associated with abuse, the coercion and the secrecy, and requests that the abuser give up denial. It is important that, in these sessions, the full impact of the abuse on the child is made clear to the abuser. When the abuser says that he wishes to give up denial, apologizes and makes a commitment that he will not re-abuse the child again, the more family members that are a witness to this the better. It may be appropriate to involve all siblings and members of the extended family in this apology session. However, it is important that the abused child feel no pressure to forgive the abuser. Abused children may say that they hope they will be able to forgive the abuser when he has consistently shown over a period of years that he can be true to his word.

At this stage, a series of sessions for the mother and father may be held. These sessions may be used to help the couple work through the feelings that they have for each other arising from the abuse. Abusers may use these sessions to express guilt and remorse. Non-abusing parents may use the sessions to express anger and disappointment. There may then be a shift in focus to the present and to planning either the gradual re-introduction of the abuser into family life or separation. In either situation the therapist coaches the couple in conflict management skills, since problems in conflict management or negotiation skills is a central difficulty for many families in which abuse occurs. Over-organized families tend to avoid conflict, and often abuse is part of a conflict-avoidance behaviour pattern. Under-organized families tend to use acting-out sexually or aggressively as a way of regulating conflict.

Bentovim et al. (1988) found that 46% of their series of 120 families engaged in a full course of family therapy and 36% partially completed the family therapy programme. In a two- to six-year follow-up, positive changes in the family structure were evident in 70% of cases. In 19% of cases no change occurred and in 3% of cases deterioration occurred, with other children being abused or other serious family problems developing (such as suicide). However, it is important to mention that the 70% improvement rate does not mean that all of these families were re-united. In 50% of families, divorce or separation occurred and only 14% of children remained with both parents.

Elements of the approach to family work outlined here may be used in cases of sibling abuse where the offender is an adolescent. However, in such cases the abused child is helped to form a protective relationship with both parents rather than just the mother. Also, the re-introduction of the abuser into the household as he gives up denial and develops strategies for identifying and avoiding trigger situations requires sessions in which parents negotiate a set of limits to which the abuser must adhere so as to avoid re-offending (Borduin, Henggeler, Blaske & Stein, 1990).

With extrafamilial abuse, in many cases the abuser is a trusted friend or relative from outside the nuclear family. Family work focuses on helping the parents support and protect the abused child and managing the behaviour problems that accompany abuse, particularly the sexualized behaviour. If the abuser gives up denial and wishes to help the abused child recover, a confrontation session may be arranged similar to that described above for father–daughter incest cases.

Therapy for abused children

Therapy for abused children should facilitate processing intense and often complex mixed feelings arising from the abuse. It should promote positive changes in the inaccurate and debilitating self-evaluative cognitions of sexually abused children. It should promote the development of protective and supportive relationships with non-abusing parents, carers and treatment staff, which are characterized by appropriate intergenerational boundaries. It should also provide the abused child with the assertiveness skills required to prevent further abuse (Friedrich, 2002).

A combination of individual, group and family-based treatment modalities may be used to achieve these over-arching treatment goals (Bentovim et al, 1988; Furniss, 1991; Friedrich, 2002; Tonge & King, 2005). Individual therapy may be used as a forum for helping abused children ventilate feelings, process traumatic abuse-related memories, examine self-perceptions and learn assertiveness skills. Play, drawing and other media may be used to help the child articulate his or her feelings and beliefs about sexual traumatization. Children may be helped to articulate their confusion about relationships and sexuality, and to explore beliefs and related feelings of guilt, depression and anger about being dirty and responsible for the abuse, and about having lost valued aspects of their life and relationships. Psychoeducation and the CTR (challenge, test, reward) routine for challenging dysfunctional beliefs (described in Chapters 12 and 16) may be used to help children develop more adaptive belief systems. Key positive themes include the idea that the child was not responsible for the abuse, but is responsible in future for learning and using self-protections skills; abusive sex is distressing and destructive, but sex can be fulfilling and constructive within the context of age-appropriate relationships characterized by strong romantic attachment; care and attachment can occur in the absence of sex; not all adults (or men) are untrustworthy, so we must learn the skills required for distinguishing between those who are and are not. To manage anxiety- and abuse-related PTSD symptoms, youngsters may be coached in relaxation and cognitive coping skills, and then invited to use these to manage the anxiety associated with graded exposure to traumatic abuse-related memories, as outlined in Chapter 12 on anxiety disorders. Role-play and rehearsal may be used to develop skills for managing disclosure-related situations where the youngster has to talk to others about the abuse, and self-protective assertiveness skills to prevent further abuse. The therapeutic relationship may also provide the child with an alternative model for appropriate parent–child interaction to that experienced in the abusive situation.

However, it is important to keep in mind that, in individual therapy, the exclusivity and privacy surrounding the relationship between the child and the therapist mirror some features of the abusive relationship for which the child is receiving therapy. For this reason, children often transfer sexual, aggressive or anxiety-related feelings from the abusive situation into the individual therapy situation and act these out by becoming fearful of the therapist, aggressive towards the therapist or openly attempting to sexually seduce the therapist and accusing the therapist of rape if he or she does not accommodate to the child's wishes. Needless to say, psychotherapy supervision is particularly important when working with these cases.

Group work has the advantage of avoiding replicating the secrecy element of the abusive relationship and also offers both social support and an opportunity for interpersonal peer feedback unavailable in individual therapy. A useful model for such group work has been developed at Great Ormond Street Hospital in London (Bentovim et al., 1988; Furniss, 1991). Group therapy is typically conducted as a short-term (twelve session) programme with five to eight group members in a closed group. For these groups to work well it is useful if they are fairly homogeneous, with participants being the same age and having suffered either intrafamilial or extrafamilial abuse. Ideally, such groups are run by a male and a female therapist, who offer the children an alternative model of parenting to that offered by their own parents, marked by openness, clear communication and respect. Group work for abused children provides a forum in which they can recount and remember the traumatic abusive events and ventilate their intense mixed feelings about the abuse. These feelings include anger, sadness, anxiety, loyalty, sexual feelings and confusion. Often, these intense feelings and related memories have been split-off from awareness and have not been integrated into the children's views of themselves. Through recounting and remembering, this material may be integrated into the view of the self. Gradually, children may reach a situation where they explicitly recall the abuse and the feelings, both negative and positive associated with it. They must be helped to clarify that it was the abuser who was guilty and not them, although things that the abuser said may have made them feel guilty, as may the pleasurable aspects of sexual arousal that they may have felt. They may be offered an opportunity to experience their anger towards the abuser, their fear of him, their sadness at the loss of the type of relationship they would have liked to have had, their anxiety that the family may split up for ever, and their continued loyalty to the abuser and guilt about disclosure which conflicts with their feelings of loyalty to the abuser. Anger at the non-protective parent may also be explored, and sadness that the non-protective parent was unable to help.

A second function of the group is to learn to distinguish between needs for affection and care on the one hand and sexual needs on the other. Abused children may have difficulty making this distinction and may therefore signal to peers or carers that they require sexual gratification when they actually want emotional support. In this context, information about normal sexual development and the normal way people's sexual needs are met may be given. Normal heterosexual and homosexual development may be discussed. For children who have been abused by a same-sex parent, beliefs that this will affect their sexual orientation need to be addressed. Where children or teenagers engage in sexual acting-out behaviour, a behaviour modification programme in which the child is rewarded for appropriate rather than sexualized attempts to get emotional needs met may be used. This type of programme may be run in the group and at home, with the non-abusing parent monitoring the child and giving the rewards for appropriate behaviour. With teenage children, a self-control and self-reinforcement system may be used.

A third function of the group is to provide the children with peer-based social support. In this context it is important that groups be narrowly age-banded since during childhood and adolescence children find it easier to gain social support from peers of about the same age.

A fourth function of the group is to learn to identify situations in which abuse might occur and how to manage these assertively. Role-play and rehearsal or video feedback are useful methods for learning assertiveness skills.

A fifth function of the group is to help abused children work out what they would like to achieve in their relationships with their parents. Usually, this involves finding a way to speak to the parents, particularly about intense negative feeling, so that the abused child feels heard rather than silenced or coerced into secrecy. Children can use the group to rehearse what they want to say to the family in family sessions about their anger and disappointment, their sense of betrayal, their sense of being worthless and powerless, their wish to forgive and to trust but their difficulty in doing so.

A final function of the group is to help abused children develop a view of the self as good, worthwhile and powerful rather than powerless.

Bentovim et al. (1988), in their study of 120 abused children at two- to six-year follow-up, found that 73% showed no sign of sexualized behaviour problems and 43% showed no other emotional problems; 61% were judged by their statutory social workers to be improved. However, in 16% of cases further sexual abuse occurred.

Therapy for non-abusing carers

Individual, group and family treatment formats may be used to provide therapy for non-abusing carers (Bentovim et al., 1988; Furniss, 1991; Trepper & Barrett, 1989). Ideally, therapy for non-abusing carers should be conducted in homogeneous groups coupled with family sessions. So, for example, with extrafamilial abuse or sibling abuse, such groups may include mothers and fathers; with father–daughter incest these groups should include mothers of abused children only. Group therapy has a number of advantages over individual therapy, including providing members with peer support, additional problem-solving resources and an effective format within which to let go of residual disbelief or denial.

Group work should allow members to ventilate feelings of remorse and guilt and to receive support from other group members. Non-abusing carers may receive information on how to establish a protective relationship with their children and support each other during the difficult process of recovery within the group. The group may be used as a forum for exploring how non-abusing carers may manage their relationship with abusers. In cases of father–daughter incest, this will involve a focus on how wives may re-negotiate their relationships with their husbands. With sibling abuse, the issue will be on balancing supervision and control with age-appropriate autonomy and privacy. The group is also a forum in which non-abusing carers may brainstorm methods for effectively protecting their abused children in future. A final function of group work for non-abusing carers is to provide a place for dealing with issues arising from non-abusing carers' own experiences of intrafamilial sexual abuse. Their children's disclosure may re-awaken memories and feelings associated with this abuse which may be processed within the group.

Therapy for abusers

Therapy with abusers has two main goals. The primary goal is to let go of denial and own up to the sexual abuse. The second goal is to accept the addictive nature of sexual abuse and to develop a lifestyle that includes strategies for managing potential relapses (Marshall et al., 1990; O'Reilly et al., 2004; Vizard, Monck & Misch, 1995). While therapy may be offered on an individual basis, the group treatment context is particularly well suited to achieving these aims because abusers are able to offer each other a more potent combination of confrontation and support required to achieve these goals than would be available in individual therapy. However, once progress has been made with letting go of denial, for intrafamilial parent–child or sibling abuse, family therapy sessions are a useful forum within which to negotiate aspects of the abuser's new lifestyle with other family members (Bentovim et al, 1988; Borduin et al., 1990; Trepper & Barrett, 1989).

A high level of persistent confrontation coupled with empathy and support is required to help abusers give up denial because of the many important functions fulfilled by this defence. Denial wards off a sense of guilt for having hurt the abused child and allows the abuser to preserve a view of the self as good. Denial removes the fear of prosecution, punishment and loss of family relationships. Denial may also allow abusers to avoid recognition of their own abusive childhood experiences. Finally, denial allows the abuser to continue to engage in a psychologically addictive process.

For abusers to construct a lifestyle that includes strategies for avoiding relapsing into abuse, the combined problem-solving resources of a group are particularly useful, both in generating ideas and options and in critically evaluating group members' attempts to implement these experiments in new ways of living.

To achieve the goals of letting go of denial and developing a new lifestyle, a number of therapeutic approaches are useful. In the early stages of the group treatment programme, members may begin by describing to the group, the sequence of events that commonly occur in their episodes of abuse. These cycles typically begin with a specific triggering event or build-up of stresses that leads the abuser to feel tension. This in turn leads the abuser to engage in a sexual fantasy, which often involves images of abusing the child. The fantasy leads on to active planning about how to arrange the next episode of abuse. Here sexual arousal may become more intense and be the precursor of the abusive actions. The abusive act may lead to a sense of relief for the abuser and may be followed by coercive threats or bribes to retain a veil of secrecy around the abuse. Putting the abusive cycle into words is an important first step in letting go of denial.

These patterns of interaction that surround abusive episodes may occur within the context of wider patterns of interaction that involve attempts to control the abuse. From time to time abusers may feel guilt because they recognize that the abuse is damaging the child and so they attempt to stop. Anxiety, irritability and restlessness may then be experienced, particularly when trigger events occur and so the abuser relapses into the original pattern of abusive behaviour.

Abusers' behaviour in these cycles of interaction is often under-pinned by dysfunctional internal working models of intimate or care-giving relationships, which in turn may often have their basis in pre-disposing early life experiences of physical or sexual abuse. Making these links between the pattern of interaction in which the abuse is embedded, the beliefs and expectations concerning relationships and abusive early life experiences is an important part of therapy. Some abusers may find that this work re-awakens traumatic memories and so they may show PTSD-like symptoms. In such instances, abusers may be offered some individual sessions in which they learn relaxation and cognitive coping skills and then use these to cope with the anxiety associated with gradual exposure to abuse-related memories in the manner outlined in Chapter 12.

Typically, abusers pepper their accounts of these abusive cycles with cognitive distortions that reflect their denial of their responsibility and culpability. They may deny that the abuse happened at all, minimize the number of times it happened, minimize the degree of coercion or violence involved, minimize the effects of the abuse by claiming it will probably do little harm in the long term and minimize the degree of their wrong-doing by pointing to more severe cases of abuse. They may also attempt to reduce their guilt by maximizing or exaggerating their virtues. Thus they may point out ways in which they have been helpful or caring to the abused child or behave like a perfect group member, showing pseudo-remorse and supporting the therapist in his or her attempts to help other group members show remorse. Denial may also find expression in projecting blame. The abused child may be blamed for provoking the abuse. Abusers may also blame outside factors for their abusive actions. For parents who sexually abuse their children, these factors may include drug or alcohol use or the sexual difficulties that they have with their partners. For adolescent offenders, stresses may include conflictual relationships with parents, social isolation or boredom. This projection of blame involves defining the self as powerless to control the addictive abusive behaviour. The therapist's role is to encourage the group to confront all of these expressions of denial, while also inviting the group to support the group member and empathize with his need to engage in the denial process. Ultimately, abusers must develop the skill of self-confrontation, and recognize their own attempts to use denial as a way of warding off abuse-related guilt or avoiding the negative consequences of abusive behaviour. Towards the end of this phase of group therapy, the abuser may use a number of concurrent family therapy sessions to acknowledge the abuse to the whole family, to acknowledge the impact of the abuse on the abused child and other family members; to apologize for the abuse and make a commitment not to re-offend.

When abusers have made marked progress in giving up denial and developed some self-confrontational skills, the focus of the group work shifts to developing lifestyles that include strategies for reducing the chances of relapses. Group members may develop profiles of high-risk situations and related fantasies and brainstorm methods for avoiding the situations and terminating the fantasies. This may require decisions to avoid being alone with the abused child or other potential victims. In concurrent family therapy sessions, abusers may negotiate with the non-abusing family members how best to use the resources of the family to avoid re-abusing the child. For fathers who have abused their children, this may lead on to exploring ways in which they may appropriately take on a parental role in the future. That is, how they can meet their children's needs for affection, control, increasing autonomy, intellectual stimulation and so forth without sexualizing the interactions and without introducing secrecy. For adolescents who have abused their siblings, the task is to develop a way to have a supportive non-threatening relationship with the abused child.

During this part of therapy, some abusers may acknowledge the impact of early abusive experiences on themselves and identify how trigger situations re-activate internal working models of abuser–victim relationships. When these internal working models are articulated, abusers may make a pact with the group, with themselves and with their families not to re-enact the abuse they experienced.

As abusers explore ways to restructure their lifestyle within the family so as to avoid future sexual abuse, the focus shifts to ways of managing their own sexual and emotional needs. With father–daughter sexual abuse, this often involves addressing marital issues within marital therapy. The central concern is to help couples develop communication and problem-solving skills and facilitate them in using these skills to address the way in which they address their mutual needs for intimacy and power sharing within the marriage.

With extrafamilial abuse, or where the abuser is an older sibling, at this stage in group therapy the focus may move to learning social skills required for developing socially acceptable types of relationships, for meeting intimacy needs and for ways of managing depression, boredom or anxiety.

Long-term membership of a self-help support group may be a useful way for abusers to avoid relapse. If this option is unavailable, booster sessions offered at widely spaced intervals is an alternative for managing the long-term difficulties associated with sexual offending.

In Bentovim et al.'s (1988) study of 120 cases, only 29% of abusers gave up denial and admitted to sexual abuse; 61% of the 120 cases were tried and, of this group, only two-thirds (48 cases) served a prison sentence, which in the majority of cases was between one and five years.

Adolescent abusers

While there are many similarities in the treatment of juvenile and adult per-petrators, there are a sufficient number of differences to warrant the separate consideration of their assessment and treatment (American Academy of Child and Adolescent Psychiatry, 1999b; Becker & Kaplan, 1993; Borduin et al., 1990; Carr & O'Reilly, 2004; O'Reilly & Carr, 1998; O'Reilly et al., 2004). Fifty per cent of adult offenders commit their first acts of sexual abuse in adolescence. The majority of their victims are children, who may reside both inside and outside the family, and the majority of young offenders have been abused either sexually, physically or emotionally as children. Assessment should be thorough and cover the relevant factors listed in Figures 21.1, 21.2

and Table 21.2. The framework for assessing children with conduct disorders (described in Chapter 10) may also be used. Treatment should be contractually based and involve a contract dawn up between the offender, the treatment team, the offender's family and the probation or juvenile liaison officer. A primary aim of treatment should be to protect the victim, and so intrafamilial perpetrators should be placed outside the home and extrafamilial perpetrators should be denied access to the victim until satisfactory progress in treatment has been made.

In the USA, the prevailing view is that juvenile perpetrators should be charged within the justice system, with the penalty matching the severity of the crime. Taking a lenient view with juveniles and channelling perpetrators into diversion programmes may strengthen denial and minimization and so compromise the youngster's capacity to benefit from treatment. Within treatment, it is the responsibility of the treatment team to notify the justice system if there is a change in the status of the risk the perpetrator poses to the community. Thus, if the perpetrator discloses other episodes of abuse that suggest he poses a more serious risk than was originally suspected, or if he does not comply with treatment, the justice department should be notified.

Borduin et al. (1990) have shown that multi-systemic treatment involving the child, parents, school and other agencies is particularly effective. Family work may focus on helping parents give up denial of their child's abuse while at the same time offering support to the juvenile abuser. Work with the school may address attainment problems, supervision so that abusive episodes do not occur in school and prevention of deviant peer-group membership. Close links with juvenile justice agencies should be maintained. Group treatment is an important element of a multi-systemic programme. The growing literature on juvenile sex offenders suggest that, ideally, treatment programmes should include the following components (O'Reilly et al., 2004):

- confronting denial and building empathy
- tracking the cycle of abuse
- coaching in relapse-prevention skills
- developing a supportive network
- developing social skills
- working through personal victimization issues
- developing a healthy sexuality
- changing deviant arousal patterns.

Confronting denial and building empathy

In the first stage of treatment, the central tasks are confrontation of denial and minimization and fostering empathy in the perpetrator for the victim. However, this process should continue throughout treatment, since denial and minimization may continue to operate, albeit at reduced levels, throughout the perpetrator's life. Denial is extreme and categorical, whereas minimization is graded. Perpetrators may deny that any interaction occurred, the sexual nature of the act or the fact that the act was one of abuse by insisting that the sexual interaction was non-coercive. Perpetrators may attempt to minimize their responsibility for the action, the extent of sexual abuse or the impact of the abuse. In denying responsibility, perpetrators may blame the victim for initiating the sexual interaction by being provocative. Alternatively, they may claim they were not responsible for their actions because of external stresses (such as lack of sexual outlets) or internal factors (such as intoxication). With respect to the extent of the abuse, perpetrators may minimize the frequency of the abuse, the number of victims, the amount of violence or coercion used or the intrusiveness of the sexual acts. Finally, perpetrators may minimize the impact of the abuse on the victim or highlight its educational features. Young abusers may identify their denial process through role-playing abusive episodes in group treatment while prompting group members to verbalize their cognitive distortions. Youngsters may also be invited to write down the justifications that they used for their abusive actions. These may be discussed in the group and group members may be invited to confront each other's distortions. Writing an apology letter is an important part of breaking down the denial process and learning empathy skills. Whether this apology letter is sent depends on the context of the abuse. With extrafamilial abuse it may be inappropriate to send the letter, while with intrafamilial abuse the apology letter may be used as the focus for a family-based apology session in which the abuser reads the apology letter to the victim, with the rest of the family as witnesses.

Tracking the cycle of abuse

In the second stage, the perpetrator is helped to closely track those circumstances that have led to abuse. This includes the situational triggers, the deviant fantasies and use of pornography, the behavioural routines, the negative and positive feelings, the distorted cognitions and the decision-making processes that under-pin abuse. Role-play is a useful way to track the cycle of abuse in a group setting.

Coaching in relapse-prevention skills

When a clear understanding of the cycle of abuse has been achieved, treatment focuses on coaching perpetrators to develop strategies for identifying and avoiding high-risk situations that precipitated episodes of abuse. Group exercises where perpetrators list external situational factors and internal thoughts and feelings that act as triggers may be used. Lists of triggers can be put up on a flip-chart and common features highlighted. Where such situations cannot be avoided, strategies for coping with these situations may be explored through group brainstorming or coaching in specific skills, such as managing negative mood states (including depression and anger), self-confrontation of cognitive distortions which involve denial or minimization and taking control of the decision-making processes that may lead to abuse.

For anger management, Becker and Kaplan (1993) use the RETHINK protocol:

- **R**ecognize when you feel angry
- **E**mpathize with the other's viewpoint
- **T**hink about the situation in a new way
- **H**ear what the other person is saying
- **I**nclude respect into what you say when you are angry
- **N**otice how you can calm yourself through relaxation
- **K**eep your attention on solving the problem.

Specific situations that elicit anger are role-played and youngsters are trained to use the RETHINK protocol to reduce their anger and avoid acting it out.

Becker and Kaplan (1993) use covert sensitization, in which young perpetrators imagine negative consequences following on from a trigger situation. For example, perpetrators imagine situations where they are looking at a potential victim playing alone in a secluded place and they approach them with the intention to abuse the child; they follow this by imagining themselves in jail. These risk–consequence scenarios are put on audiotape and perpetrators are required to listen to them repeatedly as homework, as well as during treatment sessions.

Developing a supportive network

For treatment to be successful, the family of the perpetrator must both confront the youngster's denial and minimization but also support the teenager in his attempts to control his sexually abusive behaviour. Thus group work for young perpetrators must occur within the context of ongoing family work. This therapy aims to help parents to give up denial and yet provide support for the young perpetrator. It is also important for the youngster to disengage from deviant peers if the abuse occurred as part of a deviant peer-group culture.

Developing social skills

Some juvenile offenders lack the skills necessary for making and maintaining heterosexual friendships. Social skills training in this area may therefore be necessary for some cases. Assertiveness training in peer-group situations and developing dating skills are key elements of this part of a treatment programme, and role-playing is the most useful training technique.

Working through personal victimization issues

Many young offenders have been abused or neglected, and their abuse of others is premised on internal working models that entail the roles of victim and abuser. Working through or processing feelings related to abusive experiences, recognizing the presence of these deviant internal working models and developing alternative healthy models for relationships is an important treatment process. That is, models that do not entail the abuse of power and that permit the development of empathy and intimacy.

Developing a healthy sexuality

Counselling on the role of sexuality in intimate relationships is required by many young perpetrators, since they have a distorted conception of the place of sex in friendship. Becker and Kaplan (1993) use educational films on the anatomy and physiology of male and female reproductive organs, birth control, sexual hygiene and sexually transmitted diseases to supplement group discussion on the place of sex in relationships. Useful group activities include breaking into teams and competing for the longest list of reasons for having sex or engaging in a quiz on sexual myths.

Changing deviant arousal patterns

To help perpetrators alter deviant patterns of arousal, Becker and Kaplan (1993) have developed verbal satiation therapy. Here the youngster is shown a series of slides (usually one in each of eight to ten thirty-minute sessions). The slides depict the type of victim that the perpetrator finds sexually arousing, for example, a young naked girl. The perpetrator is then asked to focus on the slide and repeat for thirty minutes a statement describing the sexual act of abuse they would most like to engage in with the person depicted on the slide. For example, 'I want her to touch my willie'. Becker and Kaplan (1993), using plethismographic measurements of arousal, have found that this procedure leads to habituation and, after this treatment, sexual arousal is not elicited by the types of sexual stimuli depicted on the slides.

Unhelpful interventions and their management

In cases of parent–child incest, a high degree of co-operation between many professionals in child protection, law enforcement and the therapeutic professions is required so that a multi-systemic therapeutic package may be offered to families within a statutory framework. This type of work is fraught with pitfalls. Three common pitfalls are to try to deal with intrafamilial CSA by only prosecuting the father, by only removing the child under a child protection order or by conducting therapy without involving child protection or law enforcement agencies (Furniss, 1991). These pitfalls deserve some elaboration.

Removing the abuser from the household allows those who intervene (the mother and law enforcement agencies) to feel satisfied that they have solved the problem decisively by identifying and eliminating what is perceived to be the single cause of the abuse. However, they have not had to look at the complex nature of the problem. In the longer term, this intervention alone may be ineffective because it fails to take account of a number of powerful forces. These are:

- the child's loyalty to the abuser
- the child and the mother's guilt for extruding the father
- the mother and abused daughter's sexual competitiveness
- the child's anger and disappointment at the mother's failure to protect her.

When this type of primary punitive intervention is ineffective and the abuser is not convicted, the abuse of the child continues but with a greater level of coercion and a greater degree of hopelessness on the child's part, since she is aware that the abuser can evade the law.

Placing the child in substitutive care allows those who intervene (child protection agencies) to feel satisfied that they have solved the problem decisively by identifying and eliminating what are perceived to be the two main causes of the abuse. That is, the abusing parent and the parent who failed to protect the child, without having to look at the complex nature of the problem. In the longer term, this intervention alone may be ineffective because it fails to take account of a number of powerful forces. These are:

- the child's loyalty to both parents
- the child's attachment to siblings
- the social support available from the peer group and the school in the child's neighbourhood
- the secondary victimization that may occur when the family scapegoat the removed child and label him or her negatively
- the difficulties that foster parents or childcare staff may have in offering a good-enough parenting environment, especially in cases where the abused child engages in extreme internalizing, externalizing or sexualized behaviour problems
- the parents' denial of their own marital difficulties.

When this type of intervention is ineffective and the child is returned from substitutive care to the custody of the family, the abuse of the child usually continues but with a greater level of coercion and a greater degree of hope-lessness on the child's part since the child is aware that the abuser can evade the law and she now lives in a home where all family members scapegoat her.

Attempting to conduct individual or family therapy aimed at rehabilitating the abuser or the abused child or reorganizing family relationships without involving law enforcement or child protection agencies allows therapists to feel that they are dealing sensitively with the problem and preventing secondary traumatization associated with legal proceedings. However, these interventions amount to a collusion with the family's secrecy about the abuse. This may lead to further abuse and threats or punishments for attempting to make the disclosure of abuse public.

Unhelpful interventions are typically instigated when members of the network engage in conflict by proxy (Furniss, 1991). Network members identify with particular family members and act-out the same pattern of conflict as the family within the professional network (Carr, 1997). The extraordinary capacity of CSA cases to lead reasonable, level-headed professionals into these types of conflicts, if acknowledged and discussed openly, can be resolved. To resolve this conflict by proxy, network members must state their positions and give reasons why they passionately believe, for example, that the father should be punished, the child removed or the family offered therapy outside a statutory framework. When these positions have been heard and the advantages of each identified, the network members may then attempt to negotiate a course of action which is based on an understanding of all of the extreme positions. This process of conflict resolution by proxy, provides the network with a potential solution to managing the case and also with valuable information about the types of conflict-resolution processes that the family will have to go through to become protective of the child and prevent further abuse.

CSA work, particularly managing countertransference and conflict by proxy, can result in rapid burn-out. The importance of personal supervision and carrying a balanced case-load cannot be over-emphasized as methods for avoiding burn-out. Psychologists who see CSA cases as part of a mixed case-load should attempt to keep a fair balance between CSA cases and other types of work. The greater the amount of CSA work on their case-load, the greater the requirement for personal supervision. Psychologists who specialize in CSA work require a high level of ongoing supervision and team support. My own view is that this type of clinical work in specialist teams must be balanced with research, teaching or other duties, and with occasional career breaks where clinical work is conducted in other areas.

LEGAL PROCEEDINGS

Two types of legal proceedings may occur in CSA cases: civil law proceedings, where the focus is obtaining a child protection order, and criminal law proceedings, where the concern is prosecution of the perpetrator. In both types of proceedings, clinical psychologists may be required to act as expert witnesses and the abused child may be required to testify. In civil law proceedings, the psychologist's testimony and the child's testimony may be required to support a case which argues that the parents are unable to meet the child's need for safety and so the child should be placed under the care of the State. In criminal law proceedings, the child's testimony and the psychologist's testimony may be required to support a case which argues that the perpetrator committed a criminal offence involving the sexual assault of the child.

The admissibility of videotaped evidence, and indeed of child testimony, varies from country to country. From a legal perspective, four key questions must be addressed by the assessment team when conducting investigative interviews with a view to using these as videotaped evidence in court (Flin & Spencer, 1995). The answers to these will depend on the rules and laws governing child testimony in civil and criminal courts in the jurisdiction in question:

- Must the child give all evidence in person?
- Are children recognized as competent to give evidence?
- Are children (if they give evidence) treated in the same way as adults (or are there protective measures)?
- What weight does the court put on children's evidence?

Each of these questions will be addressed below.

Must the child give all evidence in person? In certain jurisdictions, video recordings are considered to be hearsay evidence when presented alone and, when presented in conjunction with a child's verbal testimony in court, they are considered to represent a violation of the *rule against narrative*. Guidelines on good practice for videorecording children's interviews are given in the UK Memorandum on Good Practice, which is based on psychological research (Davies & Westcott, 1999; HMSO, 1992; Westcott, Davies & Bull, 2002).

Are children recognized as competent to give evidence? People are judged by a court to be competent to give evidence if they can demonstrate that they understand the nature of the oath under which they give evidence. In some jurisdictions, certain age limits are specified. However, psychologists may present evidence, for example the results of psychometric evaluations, to testify to children's competence to give an intelligible account of the abuse they have suffered.

Are children (if they give evidence) treated in the same way as adults (or are measures taken to take account of their vulnerability)? Witnesses are usually required to give evidence in a formal court-room. The use of less formal rooms and dress, a screen to separate the child from the perpetrator, a video link or a single, neutral cross-examiner are some of the special protective measures recommended for use with children in certain jurisdictions.

What weight does the court put on children's evidence? Traditionally, in

criminal law but not civil law, children's evidence has always required corroboration, although rules governing this have now been abolished in most
countries. However, some judges still act as if corroboration were required.

From a psychological perspective, as distinct from a legal perspective, there
is now a consensus about the conditions under which children can give reliable
testimony (Ceci, 2002; Ceci & Bruck, 1993):

> If the child's disclosure was made in a non-threatening, non-suggestible
> atmosphere, if the disclosure was not made after repeated interviews, if
> the adults who had access to the child prior to his or her testimony are
> not motivated to distort the child's recollections through relentless and
> potent suggestions and outright coaching, and if the child's original
> report remains highly consistent over a period of time, then the young
> child would be judged to be capable of providing much that is forensic-
> ally relevant. The absence of any of these conditions would not, in and of
> itself, invalidate a child's testimony but it ought to raise cautions in the
> mind of the court.
>
> (Ceci & Bruck, 1993, p. 433)

Children may be helped to present accurate testimony in court and to
reduce the anxiety caused by the experience through pre-trial preparation.
Such programmes should help children develop five critical competencies
(Flin & Spencer, 1995):

- recalling information accurately
- understanding questions and indicating non-comprehension
- resisting complying with leading questions
- coping with anxiety
- understanding trial procedures.

Information packs and videos (such as those produced by the NSPCC, 1998,
2000), coupled with communication training and anxiety management
training, are the optimal procedures for preparing child witnesses for giving
testimony in court.

PREVENTION

Clinical psychologists have an important role to play in supporting the
implementation of primary prevention programmes for child sexual abuse.
In an extensive review of evaluation studies of such programmes, Duane and
Carr (2002) concluded that they can lead to significant gains in children's
safety knowledge and skills and an increase in CSA disclosure rates. They
recommended that validated prevention programmes, covering the curriculum in Table 21.4, which equip pre-adolescent children with the skills

Table 21.4 Core concepts in curricula of CSA school-based prevention programmes

Body ownership	• The child's body belongs to her or him and the child has a right to control access to her or his body
Touch	• A distinction may be made between 'good', 'bad' and 'confusing' touches • A child may permit a good touch and reject a bad or confusing touch from an adult or another child
Saying 'NO'	• A child has the right to say 'No' when approached or touched inappropriately and the skill of saying 'No' should be practised
Escape	• It is important to escape from potential perpetrators, and skills for escaping must be practised so the child will be prepared if the need to escape arises
Secrecy	• A distinction may be made between appropriate surprises (which are fun) and inappropriate secrets (which are scary) • A child should talk about any touch he or she is asked to keep a secret
Intuition	• A child should trust his or her own feelings when he or she feels something is not quite right
Support systems	• Children should identify adults that they can turn to for help when they wish to make a disclosure of abuse or attempted abuse • A child should seek help from another adult if the first adult does not listen or believe his or her disclosure
Blame	• A child is not to blame if he or she is abused or victimized
Bullying	• Bullying is unfair and wrong • Be assertive with bullies and tell trusted adults about them • Support your friends if they are bullied

necessary for preventing CSA should be routinely included in primary school curricula. Such programmes should be developmentally staged, with different programme materials for younger and older children; be of relatively long duration spanning a school term; be taught using multi-media materials and active skills training methods; and be multi-systemic. That is, programmes should include components which target not only children but also parents, teachers and members of the local health, social and law enforcement services.

SUMMARY

CSA is a relatively common problem. Most abusers are male. About two-thirds of all victims develop psychological symptoms and for a fifth these problems remain into adulthood. Children who have been sexually abused show a range of conduct and emotional problems coupled with over-sexualized behaviour. Traumatic sexualization, stigmatization, betrayal and powerlessness are four distinct yet related dynamics that account for the wide variety of symptoms shown by children who have been sexually abused. The degree to which children develop the four traumagenic dynamics and associated behaviour problems following sexual abuse is determined by stresses associated with the abuse itself and the balance of risk and protective factors present in the child and the social context within which the abuse occurs. A distinction is made between first- and second-line suspicions of CSA. With first-line suspicions, the main course of action is to convene a meeting of all involved professionals to pool information and plan further information-gathering strategies. With second-line suspicions, a thorough assessment is required and this should be preceded by preparation of a place of safety to which the child can be taken if abuse is disclosed and the non-abusing parent disbelieves the child. Factors related to the child's behaviour, features in the child's account of the sexual abuse, the child's medical conditions and the presence of contextual risk factors should be taken into account when judging the validity of the child's statement. Assessment involves interviews with the child, relevant members of the family and the wider network. Case management requires the separation of the child and the abuser to prevent further abuse. A programme of therapeutic intervention should be put in place to help the child process the trauma of the abuse, develop a protective relationship with the non-abusing parent and develop assertiveness skills to prevent further abuse. For the abuser, therapy focuses on letting go of denial and developing an abuse-free lifestyle. Primary prevention programmes should be a routine part of the primary school curriculum.

EXERCISE 21.1

Look again at Box 21.1.

1   What types of behaviour problems and traumagenic dynamics were present for Kate's case and on what parts of the account do you base your professional opinion?
2   How were Finklehor's four pre-conditions for child sexual abuse met in Kate's case?
3   Which of the family types described by Bentovim's group did Kate's family most closely resemble?
4   How would you proceed in the management of Kate's case?

EXERCISE 21.2

Look again at Box 21.2.

1　How were Finklehor's four pre-conditions for sexual abuse met in the Muldoon case and which traumagenic dynamics were present?

2　What family process led to the separation and why did the separation happen when it did, in your professional opinion?

3　What types of interventions might have prevented the Muldoons from separation and why?

FURTHER READING

Deblinger, A. & Heflinger, A. (1996). *Treating Sexually Abused Children and their Non-offending Parents: A Cognitive Behavioural Approach.* Thousand Oaks, CA: Sage.

Department of Health (2000). *Department of Health Framework for the Assessment of Children in Need and their Families.* London: Stationery Office. Available at: http://www.dh.gov.uk/PublicationsAndStatistics/Publications/PublicationsPolicyAnd Guidance/PublicationsPolicyAndGuidanceArticle/fs/ en?CONTENT_ID=4008144&chk=CwTP%2Bc

Furniss, T. (1991). *The Multiprofessional Handbook of Child Sexual Abuse: Integrated Management, Therapy and Legal Intervention.* London: Routledge.

Jones, D. (2003). *Interviewing Vulnerable Children. A Guide for Practitioners.* London: Gaskell.

Myers, J., Berliner, L., Briere, J., Hendrix, C., Jenny, C., & Reid, T. (2002). *APSAC Handbook on Child Maltreatment* (Second edition). Thousand Oaks, CA: Sage.

O' Reilly, G., Marshall, W., Beckett, R. & Carr, A (2004). *The Handbook of Clinical Intervention with Adolescents who Sexually Abuse.* London: Brunner-Routledge.

Trepper, T. & Barrett, M. (1989). *Systemic Treatment of Incest. A Therapeutic Handbook.* New York: Brunner-Mazel.

FURTHER READING FOR CLIENTS

NSPCC (1998). *Young Witness Pack.* NSPCC, 42 Curtain Road, London EC2A 3NH, UK. Available at: http://www.nspcc.org.uk/

NSPCC (2000). Giving Evidence – what's it really like? Video. NSPCC, 42 Curtain Road, London EC2A 3NH, UK. Available at: http://www.nspcc.org.uk/

IRISH AND UK CHILD PROTECTION GUIDELINES

Children First National Guidelines for the Protection and Welfare of Children. A Summary (1999). Dublin, Ireland: Stationery Office. Available at: http://www.dohc.ie/publications/pdf/children_sum.pdf

Working Together to Safeguard Children (1999). London: The Stationery Office. Available at: http://www.dh.gov.uk/PublicationsAndStatistics/Publications/Publications PolicyAndGuidance/PublicationsPolicyAndGuidanceArticle/fs/ en?CONTENT_ID=4007781&chk=BUYMa8

WEBSITES

American Professional Society on the Abuse of Children (APSAC): http://www.apsac.org

Association for the Treatment of Sexual Abusers: http://www.atsa.com

Child abuse websites: http://www.childabuse.com/links.htm

International Society for Prevention of Child Abuse and Neglect (ISPCAN): http://www.ispcan.org

Irish Society for the Prevention of Cruelty to Children (ISPCC): http://www.ispcc.ie/

National Clearinghouse on Child Abuse and Neglect: http://nccanch.acf.hhs.gov

National Exchange Centre: http://www.preventchildabuse.com

National Society for the Prevention of Cruelty to Children NSPCC: http://www.nspcc.org.uk

The National Organisation for the Treatment of Abusers (NOTA): http://www.nota.co.uk/

Factsheets on child abuse and neglect, domestic violence and good parenting can be downloaded from the website for Rose, G. & York, A. (2004). *Mental Health and Growing Up. Fact sheets for Parents, Teachers and Young People* (Third edition). London: Gaskell: http://www.rcpsych.ac.uk The factsheets contain links to websites for parents and professional support and interest groups.

Section VI

Adjustment to major life transitions

Chapter 22

Foster care

Children are considered for placement in care when their parents are unavailable or unable to meet their needs for safety, care and control (Chamberlain, 2003; Kluger, Alexander & Curtis, 2000; McNeish et al., 2002; Reder & Lucey, 1995; Rushton & Minnis, 2002; Steinhauer, 1991; Thoburn, 2000). An example of such a case is presented in Box 22.1. These cases fall into four categories. First, a small number of children are placed in foster care because their parents die or are unable to meet the children's needs due to parental physical illness or disability following an accident. Second, arrangements for temporary, voluntary, respite care are often made for children with intellectual or physical disabilities. This type of foster care allows parents some respite from the constant stressful demands of caring for their disabled offspring. Third, foster-care placements may be made in situations where parents are having difficulties meeting children's needs for safety or adequate care and nurturance. In these cases child abuse or neglect may have occurred or the risk of abuse or neglect may be present. Fourth, foster placements may be made where parents have difficulty meeting children's needs for control, clear limits and a structured approach to managing conduct problems. In these situations, the demands of managing the child's conduct problems effectively outweigh the parents' capacity to cope with these parenting challenges.

In the routine practice of child and adolescent clinical psychology, these latter two categories of cases (those where child protection or conduct problems are the central concerns) more commonly require consultation. For this reason, these types of cases will be a central concern in this chapter. Of related interest are Chapters 10, 19, 20, and 21, which deal with conduct problems, abuse and neglect.

Within the field of foster care, distinctions are made between voluntary and statutory placement. With voluntary placements, parents request that their child to be placed in care and retain parental rights over their children. With statutory placements, the child is usually placed in care following a court order and responsibility for the child is transferred from the parents to a State agency, such as a court, a social services department or a health

Box 22.1 The Rogers: A case of foster care

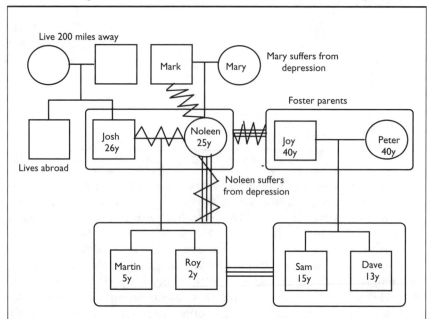

Martin (five years) and Roy (two years) and their parents Josh (26 years) and Noleen (25 years) Rogers were referred because the social worker, Terry Denny, was concerned that the boys should be re-placed with foster parents Joy (40 years) and Peter (40 years). Noleen had been at her wits' end trying to manage Martin, who she describes as wilful, and Roy, who is a poor sleeper. Roy had also been crying incessantly in recent weeks. The situation was particularly stressful for the family since Josh changed from a day job to shift work at the local canning factory.

Martin and Roy had spent three months in foster care about a year prior to the current referral. The placement was made when Noleen was in an episode of depression. At that time she was unable to cope and asked that the children be taken into voluntary care. This was arranged and Josh and Noleen visited the boys regularly while Noleen was treated for depression on an outpatient basis. It was a reasonably successful placement, although from time to time Josh and Noleen became involved in conflicts with Joy and Peter over the management of the children. A positive feature of the placement were the good relationships that Sam (15 years) and Dave (13 years), the foster parents' children, made with Martin and Roy.

Josh's parents live over 200 miles away and his brother lives abroad, so little immediate support was available from the extended family. Noleen, an only child, had a moderately good relationship with her mother, who also suffered from depression. However, Noleen had a highly conflictual relationship with her father. For this reason she was adamant that she would not allow her boys to stay with her parents when she felt she could not cope.

A worrying development in the case when it was referred was that Noleen had shaken Roy quite severely one night when he would not stop crying and in response Josh had hit her across the face with his hand. The couple were contrite about this and admitted it readily but were frightened that this might lead to statutory child protection proceedings.

board. Distinctions are also made between family foster care and institutional foster care. In the former case, the child is cared for by parents who usually have minimal training in their own home; in the latter, the child is typically cared for by professionally trained childcare workers in a building owned by the childcare agency. With family foster care, further distinctions are made between kinship fostering, where the foster parents are part of the child's extended family, and regular family foster care, where the child and foster parents are not biologically related. Permanent or long-term foster care is distinguished from short-term foster care. With permanent foster care there is a plan for children to remain with their foster families until they reach adulthood, whereas with short-term foster care, re-unification with the biological family within a given time-frame is part of the overall care plan. Finally, a distinction is made between custodial foster care and treatment foster care, where foster parents are specially trained and supported to work as para-professional members of a foster-care team to achieve specific treatment goals with children and families.

After considering epidemiological issues, this chapter describes the process of attachment disruption entailed by foster care. A framework for conceptualizing statutory childcare systems is then given and against this backdrop, decision-making about foster placement is discussed. Issues central to the transition to foster care and adjustment during foster care will be addressed before the principles of assessment in cases where foster placement may be required are highlighted. Two approaches to the use of foster care as a therapeutic intervention are then outlined. The chapter closes with a discussion of permanency planning.

EPIDEMIOLOGY

About 50 per 10,000 children are in out-of-home placements in the UK, and about 75 per 10,000 in the USA (Rushton & Minnis, 2002). These span the pre-school, school-age and teenager developmental periods. In addition to disruption of attachment through placement in foster care, children in care have typically been exposed to a variety of other stresses and present with a wide range of health problems and adjustment difficulties (Rushton & Minnis, 2002; Thoburn, 2000). They are typically from disadvantaged families with young parents and most are admitted to care voluntarily. It is more common for children from ethnic minorities to be admitted to care. Many children admitted to care have experienced abuse or neglect. It is therefore not surprising that many suffer from health problems, including growth deficiencies, sensory problems, dental abnormalities and developmental delays. Allergies, asthma, digestive disorders and skin problems are more common among foster children. Children of parents with drug problems and children born with HIV infection are probably over-represented among children in care. Mental health difficulties and behavioural and emotional problems are far more common among children in foster care, as are learning difficulties. In teenagers admitted to care, delinquency is commonplace. Rejection and abandonment are the most consistent psychological themes that pre-occupy children in care.

ATTACHMENT DISRUPTION

While placement in foster care may protect children from exposure to the risk of abuse or neglect, it disrupts parent–child attachment and so should be considered only when all other options have been excluded. Bowlby (1980) identified three stages of mourning following separation from an attachment figure, and this three-stage model provides a useful framework for conceptualizing children's responses to placement in care. In the protest stage, the child cries, pleads, bargains and aggresses in an attempt to force the absent parent to return. In the stage of despair, the child appears listless; having given up hope of forcing a re-union with the parents, he or she continues to pine. However, at this stage the child is not ready to form a new selective attachment. In the third stage of detachment, the child can re-attach to a substitute parent. However, if an adequate substitute parent is unavailable during a brief window of opportunity, the child may fail to re-attach and enter a state of permanent detachment. Unfortunately, this sometimes happens when children enter the foster care system and experience multiple placements. Such multiple placements normally occur because foster parents are untrained to deal with behavioural problems that arise as part of the child's protest against separation from parents.

As toddlers, detached children are indiscriminately friendly. When they mature they appear cold, aloof, shallow, demanding and manipulative. The detached child shows selective inattention to stimuli in the self or others that elicit attachment-seeking behaviour. These children can neither love others nor experience being loved. Within relationships, intimacy is avoided and others are used only for personal gratification (Steinhauer, 1991). This adaptation makes it difficult for such people to form stable marriages and provide adequate care for their own children in later life. Detached children may engage in self-soothing behaviours, such as thumb sucking, masturbation and rocking and idealization of their lost attachment figures. The experience of abandonment and unmet dependency needs may lead to self-blame for causing the abandonment, helplessness, hopelessness, low self-esteem, chronic depression, and self-harm. It may also lead to persistent and diffuse rage at the parent for abandoning the child. Multi-placement children typically show some or all of these behaviours and pose a profound challenge for even the most skilful foster parent.

Steinhauer (1991) has drawn the following conclusions from a review of the attachment literature relevant to foster placement. Children are particularly sensitive to separation between the ages of six months and four years. Those with a history of separations tend to interpret out-of-home placements as rejections and develop conduct problems that provoke future rejections from even the most resilient foster parents. Separation from parents has a particularly detrimental effect on children with insecure attachments to their parents and children with difficult temperaments. Children who have not formed selective attachments before four years of age have difficulty forming attachments to foster parents. They also have difficulty making and maintaining peer relationships in childhood and later life. The ill effects of separation from parents may be modified by making the new environment as familiar as possible. This may be achieved by, for example, placing siblings together in the same foster home and by providing the child with a supportive relationship with a foster parent as soon as possible. The transitional period between leaving the biological family and placement in a stable foster family should be as brief as possible. Temporary emergency placements in hospital or residential institutions prior to placement in a foster family should be as brief as possible.

Longer separations are more detrimental than brief separations (Steinhauer, 1991). Reviews of empirical studies have pin-pointed risk factors associated with multi-placement experiences and longer placements away from home associated with extensive attachment disruption as well as protective factors associated with placement stability and shorter placements associated with minimal attachment disruption (Berridge, 2002; Davis & Ellis-MacLeod, 1994; Jackson, 2002). Longer-term placements and multi-placement experiences are more common among older children from ethnic minorities with more severe behaviour problems, more disorganized and disadvantaged families in which parents have psychological problems. Multi-placement experiences are also more common among infants admitted to care. Placement stability is associated with an agency philosophy of empowering families to care for their children, arranging frequent high-quality parent–child contact while the child is in care, helping children maintain contact with important people in their social networks while in care, involvement of parents in placement planning, placement with relatives or people known to the family, placement in smaller caring (rather than larger controlling) residential care institutions, placement in a residential care setting with strong leadership, staff stability and training rather than in residential settings without these features, placement of siblings together in the same setting, regular school attendance and higher rates of payment for foster carers.

STATUTORY CHILDCARE SYSTEMS

Statutory childcare systems are complex and involve at least six distinct elements (Steinhauer, 1991). First, there are children at risk who live in families where their needs for safety, care and control are not being met. Second, there is the court, which decides whether these children's needs for safety, care and control can be adequately met within their biological families. Third, there is the childcare agency, often staffed by social workers or childcare workers, with the statutory responsibility of protecting children at risk, arranging foster care and co-ordinating support services to the families of children in care or at risk. Fourth, there is a panel of foster parents who are recruited, trained and paid by the childcare agency or, in other instances, a panel of childcare staff that work in residential institutions. Fifth, there are the biological parents of the children in care or at risk who participate in programmes co-ordinated by the childcare agency which aim to help them provide a safe home environment to which their children can return after foster care. Finally, there is a panel of consultants who may be contracted to consult to the childcare agency to select, support and train agency staff and foster parents. Members of this panel may also contribute to the management of specific cases, particularly complex cases involving issues such as violence and child abuse. It is usually in this role that clinical psychologists work with substitutive care systems.

THE DECISION TO MAKE A FOSTER PLACEMENT

Foster placements are typically considered by parents and professionals at times of extreme stress. For example, following the birth of a second child, parents with crowding problems, financial difficulties and depression may see placement as the only option. Or social workers in an agency where a child on an at-risk register dies and a colleague is disciplined or dismissed as a result, may consider foster placement as the first option in working with any multi-problem family. The tendency to view placement in care or remaining at home as the only two available options is a reflection of a black-and-white approach to problem solving which occurs under stress; often, other options are available. Part of the clinical psychologist's role in consulting to such cases is to facilitate the exploration of other options, following comprehensive family assessment. A general family assessment framework is presented in Chapter 4 and specific frameworks for cases of neglect and abuse are presented in Chapters 19, 20 and 21. Options which represent alternatives to foster placement may include providing ongoing family support services for the parents, providing day placements for the children in nurseries or other facilities, providing boarding school placements for older children, arranging financial help or alternative housing for the family and enlisting the aid of the extended family.

Foster placement may be considered if there is a danger of repeated severe abuse or neglect and the parents are unable to create a safe home environment even with input from the professional network or the extended family. A system for assessing parents responsivity to treatment has been presented in Table 19.3 (p. 919). Where parents do not meet two of the four criteria listed, foster care should be considered.

The benefits to the child of foster placements must outweigh the cost to the child of remaining with the biological parents. The possible benefits of staying with parents may include avoiding multiple disruptions of parent–child attachment, avoiding violation of loyalty to the natural family, avoiding being placed in an unfamiliar foster environment, maintaining positive relationships with peers, maintaining a positive and supportive educational placement, and avoidance of being blamed or scapegoated by the family for breaking up the family unit. The costs of remaining in an abusive or neglectful family situation may include impairment of physical growth in the case of neglect, psychological traumatization due to abuse and illness, injury or death due to abuse.

In conducting the cost–benefit analysis associated with decision making about foster care, account should be taken of the vulnerability or resilience of the child to remaining in a sub-optimal home environment or to managing the transition to foster care; the capacity for the natural family to meet the child's needs for safety, care and control; and the capacity of the foster placement to meet the child's needs. Older, resilient children with easy temperaments and secure attachment to one parent, who can tolerate abuse or criticism from another parent, may fare better at home than being placed with inexperienced, poorly trained or burnt-out foster parents (Steinhauer, 1991).

THE TRANSITION TO FOSTER CARE

The decision to place a child in care should form part of an integrated plan. The placement should have particular goals in addition to protecting the child. With long-term foster placement, the goal of placement is permanency planning. Children must detach themselves psychologically from their biological parents, mourn this loss and attach themselves to their new foster parents. Long-term foster parents require continual support to be able to cope effectively with these grief-related issues.

With short-term foster care, the foster parents must support regular contact between the child and the biological parents. This may involve building a relationship with often hostile biological parents and also managing the child's grief reaction to separations following regular visits.

Where children are in danger of abuse or neglect, the short-term placement should form part of a family intervention programme that aims to empower the family to care safely for the child. One such approach to fostering, with its roots in structural family therapy, is described below. Where short-term placements are made because children are beyond parental control, the placement agenda may be helping the child to develop internal controls.

Treatment foster care, an approach to using foster placements to help young-sters with conduct problems, will be described later in this chapter.

Up to 35% of long-term and 10% of short-term placements break down due to child behaviour problems and a mismatch between children's problems on the one hand and foster parents' expectations and child management skills on the other (Rushton & Minnis, 2002). Transference problems may contri-bute to placement breakdown. With both long- and short-term foster place-ments, children in care experience transference towards their foster parents and so unconsciously and repeatedly re-enact the relationships that they had with their biological parents in the foster-care situation, with the expectation that the foster parents will respond in the same way as their natural parents (Steinhauer, 1991). With children who have been abused, neglected or cared for in a chaotic way, this unconscious testing-out process poses a serious challenge to foster parents. Supporting foster parents during this testing-out process, and helping them understand and manage it, is an important part of facilitating the transition into a successful foster-care placement. Failure to provide foster parents with sufficient support during this process may lead to placement breakdown, and the greater the number of placement breakdowns a child experiences, the worse the child's prognosis. Fortunately, it is often at this point that clinical psychologists are asked to consult to foster-care cases and an important contribution may be made by helping the foster parents and social worker understand and manage this testing-out period, during which the children need warmth and acceptance on the one hand and consist-ent management of their conduct problems with behavioural programming on the other.

ADJUSTMENT TO FOSTER CARE

Adjustment to foster care follows a number of trajectories and is influenced by a variety of factors (Horan et al., 1993; Pecora & Maluccio, 2000; Rushton & Minnis, 2002). The course of adjustment in foster care involves deterior-ation first and then improvement. Problems get worse before they get better over a period of up to five years. The impact foster placement has on the child will depend on the way in which the childcare system is organized. With co-operative childcare systems, there is good communication, realistic expectations, an agreed agenda, an agreed plan and mechanisms for trouble-shooting difficulties. Conflictual systems result in placement breakdown and multi-placement cases. They lack the characteristics of co-operative systems. Specific child characteristics, characteristics of the foster placement and characteristics of the natural parents are associated with particular outcomes. Children with fewer behaviour problems and better initial adjustment in school have a better prognosis. Multi-placement children who have been in care for more than three years have a worse outcome than children on their first placement who have only spent a short time in care. The abuse of children in care is now well documented and this is associated with a poorer outcome. Placement in foster families with young parents, many children, multiple supports, a lack of juvenile court involvement, and a good relationship with the foster agency is associated with better outcome. When the biological family is well supported, is unencumbered by financial difficulties and where the natural parents visit their child frequently while in foster care, a better outcome occurs.

ASSESSMENT

The frameworks for assessment presented in Chapters 4, 19, 20 and 21 may be supplemented with the following agenda, which is based on Reder and Lucey's (1995) approach to the assessment of parenting. They argue that in assessing the child's need for foster care, the parents' capacity to take on a parenting role, the parents' capacity to form a positive attachment to the child, the impact of the child's personal characteristics on the parent and the impact of family relationships on the child's parenting environment, the parents' relationships with the wider social and professional network, including the capacity to benefit from professional input, all require assessment. In each of these areas a number of key questions must be answered.

With respect to the parents' ability to take on the parenting role, the central questions to be addressed are:

- Can the parents meet children's needs for safety or are children expected to be responsible for their own protection?
- Can the parents meet children's physical needs for food, clothing, housing arrangements and hygiene?
- Can the parents meet the children's needs for age-appropriate emotional care?
- Can the parents meet children's needs for age-appropriate supervision and control?
- Have the parents insight into the impact of their own childhood experiences of parenting on their performance as a parent?
- Do the parents accept that they are responsible for their behaviour as parents?
- If there are parenting problems, do they acknowledge them?

The answers to these questions will, to some degree, depend on the parents' current and past physical and psychological health. Thus, a full evaluation of the parents' psychological and physical well-being is an essential part of the assessment process.

In assessing the parent–child relationship, a number of important questions deserve inquiry. These are:

- Do the parents promote the development of a secure attachment between themselves and their child?
- Can the parents empathize with their children and understand how they feel?
- Can the parents view the child a separate person deserving age-appropriate autonomy?
- Can the parents give children's needs primacy over their own desires, by, for example, acknowledging that to protect their child they must leave their abusive spouse?

Characteristics of the child, particularly those that increase the demands that the child places on the parents, should be taken into account when assessing the adequacy of the parenting environment. Important questions here are:

- Do the children have difficulties in forming predictable sleeping and eating routines?
- Do the children respond to change with strong negative emotions?
- Do the children have disabilities, developmental delays or illnesses that increase the demands of care they place on parents?
- Have the children conduct problems that make them difficult to control?
- Do the children have particular characteristics that evoke negative emotional reactions from their parents by, for example, reminding them of people or events that they have found particularly stressful?

For the assessment of the impact of family circumstances on the child's parenting environment, key questions to be addressed are the following:

- Are the parents able to be mutually supportive?
- Are the parents able to manage conflict without resort to violence?
- Are the parents able to manage conflict without triangulating the child by, for example, pressuring the child to take sides with one or other parent or using the child as a go-between to carry messages from one parent to another?
- Are the parents able to agree on a joint approach to meeting children's needs?

The parents' relationships with the wider family and professional network have a bearing on their parenting capacity. These relationships may be assessed by pursuing the following inquiries:

- Have the parents socially supportive relationships with members of their extended family and peer group?
- In the past, have the parents been able to form good working relationships with healthcare and social service professionals?
- Can the obstacles to forming relationships that will enhance parenting capacity within the family, peer and professional networks be clearly identified?
- Can these obstacles be overcome?

All of these questions, which must be addressed in a parenting assessment, may be answered using a variety of assessment techniques, including individual, dyadic and family interviews; observation sessions; psychometric assessment sessions; brief trials of parental responsiveness to therapy or parent training; and reviews of available reports and correspondence from other involved professionals. Parenting assessments should invariably be conduced over a series of meetings spanning a sufficient period of time to determine the temporal consistency of parental behaviour and the consistency of the reports of involved parties.

PRINCIPLES OF PRACTICE

Foster-care placements should be made following comprehensive assessment and as part of an overall plan with specific goals. Where an emergency interim placement is made prior to such a planned placement, it should be as brief as possible.

Throughout the assessment and subsequent follow-up period, a key worker for the case should be maintained. This continuity is important, since the success of foster care rests on the quality of the working alliances developed between the parents, the foster parents, the case workers and the child. A problem faced by social workers in managing these cases is carrying the dual role of being responsible for presenting court evidence to obtain a care order on the one hand, and of co-ordinating a therapeutic plan that includes foster care and other components on the other. Parents and children may have difficulty accepting that a single person may take on these dual roles, particularly if they think in black and white terms. They may see the social worker as 'the person who took our child away' and be unable to integrate this with the a view of the social worker as 'the person who will help up provide a safe home for our child'. There are a number of solutions to this problem. One option is to divide the functions between two workers. Whatever the solution chosen, from the child's perspective, it is important that there is continuity in the person with whom he or she has contact.

When parents are unable to meet their children's needs for safety, care and control, rather than looking at their own shortcomings, or at the *poorness of fit* between themselves and their child, they usually blame the child for all the difficulties. Exposure to blaming and criticism, and lack of warmth and acceptance, inevitably leads the child to present with internalizing or external-izing behaviour problems. The presence of these problems may then be used by parents as justification for their blaming and criticism. A central tenet of good practice in consulting to foster-care systems is never, under any circumstances, to collude in this scapegoating process. It is also useful to acknowledge that the child's natural parents and members of the extended family or the professional network who sympathize with their position will invariably create emotional pressure for everyone involved in the case to col-lude with this scapegoating, since this will help the parents avoid accepting responsibility for being unable to meet their children's needs.

By the same token, it is also a tenet of good practice to avoid blaming or scapegoating parents for their shortcomings in meeting their children's needs. It is not unusual for involved professionals, foster parents or members of the extended family to scapegoat the parents. While it is important to acknow-ledge that the parents have been unable to meet their children's needs, and that they may have difficulty accepting responsibility for this, it is difficult to facilitate the development of a co-operative foster-care system which includes the child, the biological parents, the foster parents and the involved profes-sionals if a focus on parents' shortcomings is over-emphasized. A useful position to adopt is acknowledging that there is a poor match between the child's needs and the parents' personal resources. Assessment should focus on specifying ways that this mismatch may be improved. Foster-care placement may be construed as one aspect of a plan to improve this mismatch.

Whenever possible, voluntary foster care should be arranged rather than statutory placements, since this places less strain on the social worker's alli-ance with the family. It is easier for natural parents to co-operate with an overall care and treatment plan if they are not coerced by law to place their child in foster care. Wherever possible, short-term care should be the arrangement of choice rather than long-term care. When other factors are equal, a kinship foster placement is preferable to a foster placement with a family that is unrelated to or unknown to the child. Unless there are extenuat-ing circumstances, siblings should be placed in foster care together. It is also preferable that children be placed with families that share their culture, race, ethnicity, religion and values.

Ideally, a series of pre-foster-placement visits should be arranged to allow the child, the biological parents and the foster parents to become familiar with each other and to form good working relationships.

A highly structured routine should be developed for parental visits, parti-cularly when children are in short-term foster placements, and these visits should be frequent so that the child maintains and evolves a more positive relationship with the natural parents. Foster parents may be supported and coached in managing the difficult behaviour which typically follows returns from these visits. Where foster parents oppose frequent visits and argue that these disturb the child, the critical point to make is that continued contact with the natural parents is the single factor that makes the most difference to long-term adjustment following a short-term foster placement. Therefore, the central role of the foster parents is in developing an alliance with the biological parents and working co-operatively to contain the difficult behaviour the child shows around these visits.

A supportive forum within which foster parents may meet with other foster parents should be provided. Some portion of the time may be devoted to task-centred training in child management skills and communication skills for working with biological parents. However, it is valuable to set aside some time for foster parents to reflect on the personal issues (or countertransference reactions) that the foster children evoke in them (through their transferentially based behaviour) (Carr, 1997). Children who have been physically abused or exposed to violence may alternately evoke protective and violent sentiments in foster parents. Initially out of sympathy, parents may be moved to nurture them, but later they may become punitive when they experience the foster child's continual attempts to unconsciously provoke similar treatment from them as they received from their abusive parents. Children who have been sexually abused evoke sexual tension in foster parents through their over-sexualized behaviour. Marital tensions may emerge in response to children who have been exposed to chronic marital discord and triangulation in their biological families. These children may consciously or unconsciously play one foster parent off against the other, just as their biological parents involved them in triangulation. This countertransferential material requires acknowledgement. Unless such acknowledgement occurs, productive management of the child in foster care may become problematic and rifts may occur in the working relationship between the foster parents and the biological parents.

Maps of two extreme patterns of foster-care system organization are presented in Figures 22.1 and 22.2. Figure 22.1 is the co-operative ideal to be striven for. Within this system the biological and foster parents have a strong working alliance with each other. They are supported by the statutory social worker, who has a good working alliance with them, and all three adult sub-systems have strong positive relationships with the child. Figure 22.2 represents a common pattern for conflictual foster-care systems. Within this system there is conflict between the biological and foster-parent sub-systems. These two groups of parents have difficulty working co-operatively to provide a joint parenting environment for the child. Furthermore, within each of the couples (the foster-parent couple and the biological-parent couple) conflict is present. The tension between these two factions is exacerbated by the difficulty the statutory social worker has in remaining impartial, finding him- or herself working co-operatively with the foster family but unable to develop a co-operative relationship with the biological parents. Within this conflictual

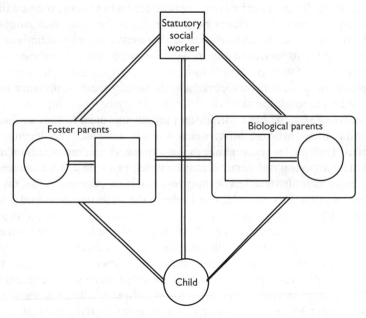

Figure 22.1 A co-operative foster-care system

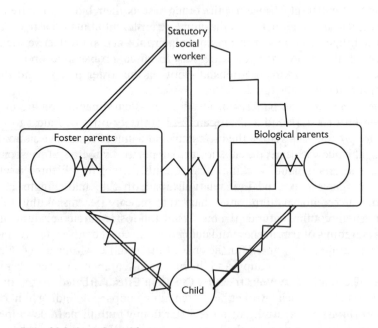

Figure 22.2 A conflictual foster-care system

system, the child finds herself having ambivalent feelings and intense conflictual relationships with both her natural parents and her foster parents. These co-operative and, conflictual systems represent extreme positions and, probably, most fostering systems fall somewhere between these two extremities.

The role of the clinical psychologist consulting conflictual foster-care systems is to help the adult parties (social worker, foster parents and biological parents) acknowledge the child's need for a united approach to the provision of care and contract with both natural and foster parents and to negotiate such a plan. For the management of behaviour problems, a shared understanding of behavioural programmes may be developed within joint meetings involving both the biological and the foster parents. Alongside this task-focused agenda there is a role in acknowledging the potential stress and grief associated with the fostering process.

The management of transitions of the child from the natural family to the foster family, and, in the case of short-term foster care, back again to the natural family, in addition to being productive and protective, is also stressful; it may evoke a deep sense of grief. For the child there is potentially the sense of being rejected at both transition points. For the natural parent there is the loss of the child and the loss of self-esteem associated with admitting that one is unable to care for one's child. For the foster parents, the motivation to care for foster children is often some complex mixture of altruism and a desire for appreciation from the fostered child. Such appreciation is rarely offered by the child in the short term. Indeed, aggressive and difficult behaviour devoid of gratitude is the norm among children in foster care. Facilitating the ventilation of this grief is an important aspect of the role of the psychologist consulting to conflictual foster-care systems, since it is usually these unprocessed grief-related emotions that prevent co-operative problem solving in conflictual foster-care systems.

The ecological approach to foster care, developed by Minuchin (1995), and Chamberlain's (2003) treatment foster care, both offer ways of framing the foster-care process to privilege the productive potential of foster placements. That is, they allow natural parents, foster parents and children to construe foster care as an opportunity to work co-operatively to solve problems, rather than as a sign that a child is intrinsically bad or sick, that parents are inadequate irremediable failures and that foster parents are intrinsically better and different from natural parents. What follows is a brief account of these two exemplary approaches to foster care.

AN ECOLOGICAL APPROACH TO FOSTER CARE

Minuchin (1995) has argued that an ecological approach to practice in the area of foster care should address the system that contains the biological and the foster families, the child and the involved professionals. The thrust of the work should aim to create an extended kinship system in which members of the biological family and foster family are united by their mutual involvement in care for children, and this is facilitated by the social worker or foster-care staff member. Within this approach, the foster-care parents and social work staff work as co-operative members of a team, with the social worker taking responsibility for facilitating contact and co-operation between the foster parents and biological parents and the foster parents working as para-professionals in both caring for the children and empowering the biological parents. The approach has been used with both regular foster parents and with kinship fostering, where the foster parents are biologically related to the child.

The approach is guided by the following principles. First, attempts should be made to symbolically preserve the integrity of the child's biological family by, for example, arranging regular contact between the child and the biological parents. If this symbolic unity of the family can be maintained throughout the placement, then it is more likely that the child may eventually be re-united with the biological family. Second, an attempt should be made throughout the consultation process to empower the biological parents to become more resourceful and capable of providing an adequate parenting environment for their child. They should be involved in decision making, given responsibility and respected rather than blamed and instructed. Third, attempts should be made to involve the extended family as a resource in the process of reuniting the child with the family. Foster parents may be a useful bridge to the extended family and may be able to contact them in an informal and non-threatening way. Fourth, an awareness of the impact of the transitions, the stress they entail, and the resultant need to provide support to family members to manage this stress should be maintained throughout the consultation process. For children, the transition to living in a foster family environment and, later, the return home may lead to emotional and behavioural problems and both foster and biological parents may require considerable support and training to be empowered to manage these problems. Fifth, the developmental stage of the child and the lifecycle stages of the biological and foster families should be borne in mind when consulting to foster-care systems. For example, separation and re-union with the biological family may be more difficult for a pre-school child than for an adolescent. Managing the adjustment reactions of children may be easier for foster parents who have reared three children who are now in their teens than for a young couple whose first child is in care.

Foster parents may be trained to use four key sets of skills in their relationships with biological parents and their participation in the fostering system. These skills, which have been developed within the field of family therapy, are joining, mapping, searching for strengths and working with complementarity. Joining involves conveying interest, respect and acceptance by listening and accommodating to the viewpoint of the other person without forcefully imposing one's own viewpoint on the other. Mapping is the skill required for drawing genograms of both biological and foster families and indicating on these the lifecycle stages, strengths and stresses faced by family members. Searching for strengths requires the foster parents to acknowledge the fact that the biological parents are experts on the child's developmental history and characteristics and on particular child management practices that were effective in the past. Searching for strength is the skill that foster parents must develop to allow them to avoid blaming the biological parents and defining the biological parents as wholly inadequate. In working with complementarity, foster parents are coached in recognizing that in any interaction with the biological parents, the more the foster parents do in the way of competent parenting the less space there is for the biological parents to demonstrate parenting competence. With this awareness, foster parents may gradually and consciously hold back from parenting the child in certain situations, thus opening up space within which the biological parents can exercise their emerging parenting competencies.

TREATMENT FOSTER CARE

Many youngsters who present with extreme externalizing or internalizing behavioural problems are unsuitable for routine foster care. Their extreme behavioural difficulties pose too great a challenge for untrained foster parents to manage. Treatment foster care is a specialized form of foster care in which foster parents are trained to manage child behaviour problems and use psychological treatment principles to help youngsters normalize deviant behaviour (Chamberlain, 1994, 2003; Chamberlin & Mihalic, 1998; Chamberlain & Smith, 2003).

Treatment foster care gives youngsters aged eleven to eighteen years opportunities to live successfully in the community by providing them with intensive supervision, support and skills training and separation from deviant peers in a programme where foster care by well-trained foster parents is a key element. In addition, treatment foster care concurrently offers youngsters' biological parents intensive parenting training to prepare them to re-integrate their deviant child back into the family. Treatment foster care placements typically span six to nine months. These programmes are offered by teams that include a range of professionals with clearly defined roles:

- Service directors manage the overall service, accepting referrals, allocating cases to specific programme teams and supporting programme supervisors in weekly meetings and other staff as required.
- Foster-family recruiters and trainers usually are experienced foster parents who have been trained in the principles and practices of behavioural

parent training and social learning theory, and have used these successfully with a number of cases. They work with the director to recruit and train new foster parents in behavioural parenting skills, and also in the overall approach to working with staff, referred youngsters and their families in the treatment foster-care system.

- Programme supervisors, usually masters' level therapists, carry a caseload of about ten and co-ordinate all work for these ten cases. This includes daily telephone contact with all ten foster families to complete the Parent Daily Report points system (Chamberlain & Reid, 1987) and weekly meetings with all foster families and other involved team members, as well as frequent liaison with youngsters' probation officers, schools and other involved community agencies.

- Family therapists work with referred youngsters' biological families in weekly clinic-based sessions and regular home visits. Family therapy involves alliance building with the parents; coaching parents in behavioural parenting skills for managing all of their children, not just the referred child and life skills for reducing family disorganization. Gradually, over the course of the programme, as parenting skills improve, increasingly longer contacts between biological parents and their referred children are scheduled. Initial contacts are brief, clinic-based supervised meetings. Later contacts are longer and occur in the biological parents' home.

- Individual therapists have weekly sessions with referred youngsters. These sessions provide youngsters with support and advocacy, as well as training in social problem solving and anger management skills, and an opportunity to address educational and vocational issues.

- Behaviour support specialists have twice-weekly contact with referred youngsters in community settings such as restaurants, libraries and sports facilities. In these 'real-life' settings they support and coach the youngster in developing life skills and provide a bridge between clinical and foster-home-based therapy and life out in the community.

- Consulting psychiatrists link closely with programme supervisors and monitor and manage medication for symptoms of DSM IV diagnoses for youngsters with conditions such as ADHD or major depression.

The development of treatment foster care programmes depends on careful planning and the development of a good infrastructure. Recruitment of parents into treatment foster programmes is a major challenge. The winter and spring are the best months for recruitment and a planned and co-ordinated campaign spanning a designated time period of at least a week using multiple media such as TV, radio, newspapers and billboards aid recruitment. It is better to stress the professional challenge and opportunities for personal and professional development associated with being a professional foster parent than to appeal to people's sympathy for disadvantaged children. This may be done by stressing the need for commitment and problem-solving skills when faced with extreme externalizing behaviour problems. Reference to case vignettes may be made in advertisements or radio broadcasts. Foster parents who join treatment foster programmes with a sympathy motive often drop out when faced with the challenges of applying behavioural programmes to modify extreme internalizing and externalizing behaviour problems. A structure for managing ongoing inquiries from potential foster parents, and for following these up, should be put in place, along with levels of remuneration equal to those that would be provided by a second part-time income. The principal criteria for selection are the parenting skills of the couple, the character and reputation of the couple and the suitability of the couple's physical residence.

Placement should be based on an assessment of the child's needs, the ability of the family to meet these and the acceptability of the arrangement to the child, the foster parents and the biological parents. A thorough assessment of the child's needs and the family's resourcefulness as a treatment foster placement require assessment. A series of pre-placement visits to examine the fit between the child and the foster parents is essential, and this should involve at least one overnight stay.

To prevent burn-out, treatment foster parents require ongoing training and support. Core skills taught in a twenty-hour pre-placement module include analysing antecedents and consequences of problem behaviours, agreeing on house rules with youngsters, systematically using positive reinforcement to increase the rate of appropriate behaviour, rarely using punishment to control bad behaviour, nurturing and accepting the child, giving age-appropriate responsibilities and modelling appropriate behaviour. Treatment foster parents should attend up to 20 hours ongoing training per annum in a group setting and regular monthly consultations about children in their care. Outstanding treatment foster care parents may be recruited onto the training team.

Programme supervisors carry small case-loads of no more than ten to permit intensive contact. Staff are provided with regular supervision, which is problem-solving focused. Twenty-four hour, on-call emergency back-up is provided for crisis management.

Youngsters placed in treatment foster care are those who traditionally would have been placed in institutional residential care. Treatment foster care offers three main advantages over institutional residential treatment (Meadowcroft & Trout, 1990). Treatment foster care offers children a stable and relatively normal (rather than institutional) residence and reference group. In contrast with an institutional placement, the negative influence of deviant peers is absent and the routines are those of family life rather than institutional life. Second, within treatment foster care, the foster parents alone implement behavioural programmes and so offer far more consistency than may be possible in an institutional setting, where a variety of staff may be involved in implementing the treatment programme. Third, treatment foster parents can develop strong and lasting links with youngsters' natural parents and facilitate transfer of routines used in treatment foster care homes to the child's natural home. Concurrently with treatment foster care, family therapy is offered to the youngster and his or her parents to help them prepare for family reunification.

Evaluations of treatment foster care show that it is more effective than residential group home treatment (Chamberlain & Smith, 2003). It leads to lower rates of offending and incarceration. Programme effectiveness is mediated by the improvements in biological parents' parenting skills and the reduction in contact with deviant peers. Costs of treatment foster care are one-third less than treatment in a residential group setting. Treatment foster care was developed in North America, it is currently under evaluation in the UK (Jones, Roberts & Scott, 2005).

PERMANENCY PLANNING

Where parents are unwilling or unable to co-operate with a treatment plan that includes short-term foster placement and eventual return of the child to their care, other options must be included in the long-term permanency plan. These include adoption and long-term fostering. A number of factors have consistently been found to lead to a poor outcome for adopted children. These are severe deprivation in the first two years of life, multi-placment experiences, conduct disorder prior to placement, removal from a well-established, long-term foster family situation, removal from a situation where there was a well-established relationship with a biological parent or sibling and entrenched behaviour patterns that are at variance with the adoptive parents' expectations (Steinhauer, 1991). In light of these findings, adoption may be the option of choice if the child is under four years of age and free to form a primary attachment with the adoptive parents; if the child is over four and the adoptive parents can accept that the child may take a long time to form a primary attachment to them and if the child and the adoptive family can survive the period of testing-out that will inevitably happen with an older child. A full discussion of adoption is beyond the scope of this chapter (Cohen, 2002).

Planned permanent foster care may be the permanence arrangement of choice for a child who has formed a strong attachment to a foster family, for an older child with conduct problems that can be accommodated within a foster family and for a child who remains attached to the natural parent and who has established a visiting routine that can be accommodated by the foster family.

Where children's lives have been disrupted through multiple placements and they enter an adoptive home or long-term foster placement, life-story book work may help them achieve some sense of autobiographical coherence, which in turn may help them adjust to their permanent placement. Life-story book work involves helping the child to construct a biographical account using words, photographs and pictures which makes sense of, and sequences, the event of their lives (Ryan & Walker, 2003).

SUMMARY

About 5 per 1000 children are placed in foster care in the UK and about 7.5 per 1000 in the USA. Children are considered for placement in care when their parents are unavailable or unable to met their needs for safety, care and control due to illness, death, family disorganization or parenting-skills deficits. While placement in foster care may protect children from exposure to the risk of abuse or neglect, it disrupts parent–child attachment and so should only be considered when all other options have been excluded. In conducting the cost–benefit analysis associated with decision making about foster care, account should be taken of the vulnerability or resilience of the child to remaining in a sub-optimal home environment or to managing the transition to foster care; the capacity for the natural family to meet the child's needs for safety, care and control; and the capacity of the foster placement to meet the child's needs. The decision to place a child in care should form part of an integrated plan, so the placement will have particular goals in addition to protecting the child. With long-term foster placement, the goal of placement is permanency planning, whereas with short-term foster care the goal is to empower the biological parents to improve the parenting environment they provide for their child and for the child to alter difficult behavioural patterns so he or she can return home. The ecological approach to foster care and treatment foster care are two specific approaches to short-term fostering that have been found to be particularly effective in facilitating an improvement in the fit between the child's needs and the parents' capacity to meet them. Up to 35% of long-term and 10% of short-term placements break down due to child behaviour problems and a mismatch between children's problems on the one hand and foster parents' expectations and child management skills on the other. Placement breakdown is more common among multi-placement children who have been in care for more than three years and who have many behaviour problems. Placement in foster families with young parents, multiple supports and a good relationship with the biological family and the foster agency is associated with better outcome. When evaluating the child's need for foster care, the parents' capacity to take on a parenting role, parent–child attachment, the impact of the child's personal characteristics on the parent, the impact of family relationships on the child's parenting environment, the parents' relationships with the wider social and professional network, including the capacity to benefit from professional input, all require assessment. Throughout the assessment and subsequent follow-up period, a key worker for the case should be maintained. Regular structured schedules of visits for the biological parents and professional support for both biological and foster families should be provided. The role of the clinical psychologist consulting to conflictual foster-care systems is to help the adult parties (social worker, foster parents and biological parents) acknowledge the child's need for a united approach to the provision of care and contract with both natural and foster parents and to negotiate such a plan. Alongside this task-focused agenda there is a role in acknowledging the potential stress and grief associated with the fostering process.

EXERCISE 22.1

Ricky, a six-year-old boy and his mother, Bev (aged twenty-four), are referred to you for comprehensive family assessment by the social worker, Gail, who needs to make a decision about foster placement in this case.

Ricky is Bev's only child. He is described by Gail as being completely out of control. On three occasions he has been found wandering around town at night looking for his father, Nobby (aged thirty), who lives nearby. On each of these occasions Ricky climbed out his bedroom window unknown to Bev. It is suspected that Bev may have a drug problem and may on these occasions have been unaware of her son's exit from the house, having taken some drugs.

Ricky attends junior infants in the local primary school and prior to that attended play-school. In both contexts, it was noted that he has a language delay and severe behaviour problems. Ricky was a low-birth-weight baby and is currently small for his age (below the third percentile for height and weight).

Ricky and his mother have an intense relationship and have rarely been apart over the past six years. They vacillate between clinging to each other like two lost children and, at other times, not speaking to each other after major rows. Bev has smacked Ricky hard from time to time in fits of temper but afterwards has been remorseful.

Bev and Nobby never lived together; Ricky was conceived during a casual encounter. Nobby visits Ricky and takes him on week-end outings erratically. He also provides occasional financial support, which is badly needed by Bev, who lives on welfare payments.

Bev's mother, Martha, lives nearby and has offered to foster Ricky on two occasions but Bev has objected to this. Bev and Martha have a highly conflictual relationship and Martha may have physically abused Bev when she was a child.

- Draw a genogram of the case.
- What factors suggest that Bev is providing an adequate parenting environment for Ricky?
- What factors suggest that Bev is not meeting Ricky's needs?
- Draw up a schedule of assessment meetings to evaluate this case so as to answer these questions. Indicate who you would invite to each meeting and the areas you would cover.

EXERCISE 22.2

A year after your assessment, Ricky's case is re-referred to you. He is in voluntary foster care with Kate and Larry (who have a fourteen-year-old daughter, Kelly) and visits his mother for two days every week-end. You advised that Ricky would benefit from short-term foster care, during which time the foster parents would use an intensive behavioural programme to help Ricky develop pro-social behaviour, particularly how to control his temper and follow rules at home and at school. The programme included the use of reward systems and time-out. You also advised that Bev be trained in how to use this behavioural programme to manage Ricky when he visits her for week-ends.

The case is re-referred to you because Kate and Larry want the visits to Bev to be made less frequent. They find that the visits disrupt their family life and that Ricky is always more aggressive and defiant when he returns from visits with Bev on Sunday night. They believe that Bev is not implementing the behavioural programme as advised. Bev has asked Gail the social worker if she can take Ricky out of care because she feels attacked and undermined by Kate and Larry. Gail believes that Ricky has improved dramatically over the past year. He is doing better in school and his behaviour is dramatically improved. His Child Behaviour Checklist scores are all within the normal range. Gail thinks that Ricky needs to spend at least another six months in care for these changes to be consolidated and has referred the case to you to see if you can facilitate this.

- Draw a genogram of the case indicating alliances and conflictual relationships.
- What would your consultation goals be in this case?
- List a schedule of meetings you would hold to achieve these goals.
- Role-play one of these meetings with members of your training group.
- For the person playing the role of the psychologist, note what aims you achieved in the role-play meeting.
- For the people playing family members (or the social worker), describe the things that the psychologist did that helped you to feel like your interests were being served by the meeting.

FURTHER READING

Chamberlain, P. (1994). *Family Connections: A Treatment Foster Care Model for Adolescents With Delinquency*. Eugene, OR: Northwest Media Inc. Available at http://www.northwestmedia.com/foster/connect.html

Chamberlain, P. (2003). *Treating Chronic Juvenile Offenders: Advances Made Through the Oregon Multidimensional Treatment Foster Care Model*. Washington, DC: American Psychological Association.

Reder, P. & Lucey, C. (1995). *Assessment of Parenting. Psychiatric and Psychological Contributions*. London: Routledge.

Ryan, T. & Walker, R. (2003). *Life Story Work*. London: British Association of Adoption and Fostering.

Steinhauer, P. (1991). *The Least Detrimental Alternative. A Systematic Guide to Case Planning and Decision Making for Children in Care*. Toronto: University of Toronto Press.

Thoburn, J. (1994). *Child Placement: Principles and Practice* (Second edition). Hants., UK: Arena.

WEBSITES

British Association for Adoption and Fostering: http://www.baaf.org.uk/

International Foster Care Organization: http://www.ifco.info/ (*contains links to many national fostering organizations*)

Irish Foster Care Association: http://www.ifca.ie/info.html

Professor June Thoburn's UK website: http://www.uea.ac.uk/swk/people/faculty/JT.htm

Treatment Foster Care Consultants: http://www.mtfc.com/

USA Family Preservation and Child Welfare Network: http://www.familypreservation.com/

Factsheets on good parenting, parental mental illness and domestic violence can be downloaded from the website for Rose, G. & York, A. (2004). *Mental Health and Growing Up. Fact sheets for Parents, Teachers and Young People* (Third edition). London: Gaskell: http://www.rcpsych.ac.uk

Chapter 23

Separation and divorce

Children and families where separation or divorce has occurred may be referred for psychological consultation when help is required with the management of separation-related adjustment difficulties or where expert advice on child custody arrangements following separation is needed. An example of a case referred for post-separation adjustment problems is presented in Box 23.1. This chapter describes guidelines for dealing with these types of referrals and custody evaluations, following a cursory account of some of the more clinically relevant findings concerning the psychology of family separation. First, relevant epidemiological issues will be discussed. Factors which contribute to divorce are then outlined. This is followed by a discussion of the demographic correlates of divorce and the impact of divorce on parental well-being. Factors that mediate parental adjustment to divorce are then considered and the immediate impact of divorce on parenting is outlined. The short-, medium- and long-term effects of divorce on children and the important personal and contextual factors that mediate these effects are then described. A developmental model of family transformation following separation and re-marriage is then given. A discussion of the characteristics of step-families and children's adjustment following re-marriage is outlined before guidelines for assessment and treatment of children's post-divorce adjustment difficulties are presented. After considering the central features of child custody evaluations, the chapter closes with a brief discussion of mediation.

EPIDEMIOLOGY

Divorce is no longer considered to be an aberration in the normal family lifecycle but a normative transition for a substantial minority of families (Greene, Anderson, Hetherington, Forgatch & DeGarmo, 2003; Haskey, 1999). In the US and the UK, between a third and a half of marriages end in divorce. Most divorces happen in first ten years of marriage. About half of divorces involve children. Between 80 and 90% of cases culminate in the child

Box 23.1 Case example of adjustment problems following separation

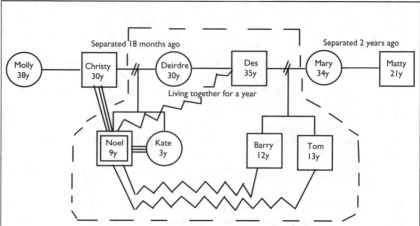

Separated 18 months ago

Separated 2 years ago

Living together for a year

Referral. Noel was referred because of conduct problems. Over the preceding year since he and his mother, Deirdre, and sister, Kate, moved in with Des and his two sons (Barry and Tom), the conduct problems had become worse. He had stolen and destroyed a number of toys belonging to Barry and Tom. He had scratched Des's car with a Stanley knife and recently exploded fireworks in his dark-room, destroying about £500-worth of equipment. It was also suspected that he had stolen up to £100 over the preceding year in small amounts from Des's wallet. He usually denied his misdeeds. At the time of referral, Deirdre and Des were considering moving into separate houses because of the strain that Noel's conduct problems were putting on their relationship. On the CBCL completed by Deirdre, Noel's internalizing and externalizing scores were in the clinical range. On the CBCL completed by Christy, his father, and the school, his scores were within the normal range.

Family background. Deirdre and Christy had separated about eighteen months prior to the referral, after Deirdre discovered that Christy was having an affair with Molly, an older single woman whom he had met in the course of his work as an estate agent. The separation had occurred suddenly, without a long period of overt conflict. Noel and Kate (the baby) visited Christy's house every second week-end and occasionally during the week. These visits were uneventful. Noel liked Molly and idolized his father. Des and Mary had separated under very similar circumstances, but in Des's case his wife Mary openly declared that she was leaving the marriage to live with a college student, Matty, whom she had met at night school. Des ran his business from home and, for various reasons including this, an arrangement was reached where the boys spent three or four days with Des and three or four days with Mary each week.

Within both families, the development of all four children had been broadly within normal limits. Barry and Tom were in secondary school and were doing well at their studies. Both shared an interest in photography with their father. Both tolerated Noel and only occasionally became involved in open conflict with him, but they doted on Kate. They also both liked Deirdre. Barry and Tom got on well with their mother, Mary, and paid little attention to Matty. He spent little time with them. Both co-parental couples (Deirdre and Christy and Des and Mary) contained their anger and disappointment with their ex-partners and did not let it greatly interfere in the childcare arrangements to any great degree. However, there were marked differences in parenting style.

Deirdre, Des and Mary were all fairly consistent in their insistence on clear daily routines and clear sanctions for misbehaviour; Matty played little part in parenting. Christy, on the other hand took a more chaotic approach. Most of the time he was very lax and only occasionally reprimanded or sanctioned Noel for rule-breaking. However, when he did so, he usually became extremely angry, imposed a severe penalty and later, in a fit of remorse, bought Noel a treat. Usually, Molly went along with whatever Christy thought best and took a fairly lax approach with Noel. In the instances where Barry, Tom and Des's belongings were damaged or stolen by Noel, Christy took the view that it was down to Des and Deirdre to manage these misdemeanours, which he saw as minor and blown out of all proportion. He did not think it appropriate to use the limited access time he had with his son to engage in punitive interactions.

In individual interviews Noel, expressed his admiration for his father and his anger at Des, Barry and Tom who he felt ganged up on him and didn't want him in their house. He denied all misdemeanours except the fireworks incident which he claimed was an accident. He said that he felt as if he had done something to cause his parents' separation and wanted them to re-unite. If they did not he feared that he would be left with nowhere to turn because he did not fit into his mother's household and knew that his father's business commitments prevented him from living with him.

Formulation. Noel's conduct problems in this case were precipitated by parental separation and maintained by the lack of co-parental consistent management on the one hand and a lack of co-parental support on the other.

Treatment. Intervention in this case involved working with Dierdre, Christy and Noel, initially to increase co-parental support for Noel. In these sessions, both parents jointly explained to Noel that the separation arose from marital dissatisfaction and not problems in the parent-child relationship. They then made separate commitments to Noel for weekly episodes of special time. In later sessions, a consistent set of house rules for both houses were agreed, along with a reward programme and sanctions for rule-breaking that applied to both houses. In the final set of sessions, Des and Deirdre and the boys attended. Noel admitted to some of the misdemeanours and apologized. Des and the boys accepted the apology and said they understood that Noel felt like the odd-man-out and they wanted to change this. Tension in the house decreased, as did Noel's conduct problems.

---

living with the mother. About three-quarters of divorced men and women co-habit or re-marry, although slightly more men re-marry than women. A proportion of these co-habiting relationships are relatively transient. Thus, the majority of children of divorced parents experience transient or stable step-family situations, with the stresses and challenges that these sorts of family configurations entail.

REASONS FOR DIVORCE

Difficulties with communication and intimacy on the one hand, and the power balance or role structure of the marriage on the other, are the two major reasons given in major US surveys for divorce (Greene et al., 2003; Kitson & Sussman, 1982). Both men and women identify lack of communication and understanding on the part of their partner as the main reason for divorce. These communication problems are typically part of the wider difficulty of establishing and maintaining a satisfactory level of psychological intimacy. Disagreement over roles and power relationships is the second most common reason for divorce. Men complain of their wives being too authoritarian and too ready to engage in nagging and fault-finding. Women complain of the constraints that the marriage places on them fulfilling their needs for personal autonomy and independence. Other prominent reasons for divorce are infidelity, immaturity, alcohol abuse and lack of sexual satisfaction. With sex, women complain about the quality; men complain about the quantity.

Observational studies (e.g. Driver, Tabares, Shapiro, Young-Nahm & Gottman, 2003) of distressed couples who subsequently separate show that they gradually engage in more negative interactions than positive interactions. This escalation of a negative interactional style includes four linked behaviours: criticism, contempt, defensiveness and stone-walling. As the ratio of negative to positive interaction increases, both partners attend selectively to their spouses' negative behaviours while ignoring positive behaviours. Partners in distressed marriages also consistently attribute global, stable, negative intentions to their spouses for negative or ambiguous behaviour but attribute their spouses' positive behaviour to situational factors. This negative cognitive style, coupled with the increase in negative interactions, leads to growing feelings for both partners of hurt or fear on the one hand and anger on the other. Both of these emotional states exacerbate the negative interaction patterns and negative cognitive styles. As these negative cognitive, emotional and interactional processes become stronger, members of the couple perceive the marital problems as more severe and engage in more solitary rather than shared problem solving. At this stage, partners become isolated from each other and begin to live parallel lives. Eventually, usually following some critical incident, the whole history of the marriage is reconstrued in a negative way, which gives a rationale for the decision to divorce.

Men and women differ in their stress responses to the process of separation and divorce (Amato, 2000; Bray & Hetherington, 1993; Faust & McKibben, 1999). Women are unhappy in their marriages for longer than men. Economic difficulties are a primary reason for women not divorcing while men give primacy to the fear of separation from their children. Women's most stressful period is that just before the divorce. For men it is the period which follows the divorce that is most stressful. This is evidenced by the low level at which the immune system functions in women and men during the pre- and post-divorce periods, respectively. Immune-system functioning improves as attachment to the ex-spouse decreases.

CORRELATES OF DIVORCE

Socioeconomic status, urban/rural geographical location, age at marriage, pre-marital pregnancy, psychological adjustment and parental divorce have all been associated with divorce (Faust & McKibben, 1999; Raschke, 1987). Divorce is more common among those from lower socioeconomic groups with psychological problems who live in urban areas and who have married before the age of twenty. It is also common where pre-marital pregnancy has occurred and where parental divorce has occurred. Divorce is less common among those from higher socioeconomic groupings without psychological problems who live in rural areas and who have married after the age of thirty. Where pre-marital pregnancy has not occurred and where the couple's parents are still in their first marriage divorce is also less common. The economic resources associated with high socioeconomic status, the community integration associated with rural living, the psychological resources associated with maturity and the model of marital stability offered by non-divorced parents are the more common explanations given for the associations among these factors associated with divorce. It is important to note that the relationship between these various factors and divorce, while consistent, are moderate to weak. That is, there are significant sub-groups of people who show some or all of these risk factors but do not divorce.

EFFECTS OF DIVORCE ON PARENTS

Divorce leads to multiple life changes which affect parental well-being, and the impact of these changes on parental well-being is mediated by a range of personal and contextual factors, which are described below (Amato, 2000; Anderson, 2003; Bray & Hetherington, 1993; Faust & McKibben, 1999; Greene et al., 2003; Hetherington & Kelly, 2002; Raschke, 1987).

Life changes

Divorce leads custodial parents to experience major changes in their lives, including a change in residential arrangements, economic disadvantage, loneliness associated with social network changes and role-strain associated with the task over-load that results from having to care for children and work outside the home. Non-custodial parents experience all of these changes with the exception of role-strain. For custodial fathers, role-strain and task over-load are less extreme than for women for two reasons. First, members of men's networks are more likely to see them as incompetent home-makers and so offer help with cooking and cleaning. Second, men are more economically advantaged and so are better able to afford child-minders or domestic help. Also, the impact of economic disadvantage is less for divorced men than women. In American surveys, non-custodial fathers have been shown to suffer few long-term economic difficulties as a result of divorce. After three years, their post-divorce income is only marginally below their pre-divorce income in the majority of cases. Women suffer major economic problems following divorce. About half are below the poverty line during the first two years post-divorce and, during this period, they suffer a 35% drop in income.

Health

Changes in divorced couples' residential arrangements, economic status, social networks and role demands lead to a deterioration in physical and mental health for the majority of individuals immediately following separation. However, for most people these health problems abate within two years of the divorce.

Mood swings

Both men and women suffer extreme emotional lability in the period leading up to separation and for two years post-separation. An awareness of the opportunities for a new way of life and escape from the emotional pain of chronic marital discord both lead to periods of elation. The loss of a familiar way of life, the loss of a long-standing partner and a fear that alone one may not meet the extraordinary challenges that go with being a single person or a single parent commonly are associated with episodes of depressed mood.

Identity problems

For women in particular, separation is associated with a crisis of identity. Prior to separation, many women define themselves in terms of their husbands or their children. Also, women may rely on their husbands to develop a social network of friends. After separation, women who have relied on their husbands for self-definition find that they experience confusion about their identity. They have to re-define their self-concept in terms of their own role and develop their own social network. Women who have jobs outside the home experience fewer identity problems in the aftermath of divorce.

RISK AND PROTECTIVE FACTORS FOR PARENTAL POST-DIVORCE ADJUSTMENT

The following factors affect parental adjustment to divorce: the way the divorce decision was made, age, length of marriage, income, occupational status, social supports, and personal psychological resources (Amato, 2000;

Amato & Keith, 1991; Anderson, 2003; Bray & Hetherington, 1993; Faust & McKibben, 1999; Greene et al., 2003; Hetherington & Kelly, 2002; Raschke, 1987). Better adjustment following divorce occurs when individuals are young, have been married for a brief period and have either initiated the divorce or mutually agreed to divorce. A good income and having a job before the divorce occurred leads to good post-divorce adjustment, particularly for women. A belief in one's personal effectiveness, high self-esteem and a high tolerance for change are associated with good post-divorce adjustment, as are an egalitarian gender-role orientation, diminished attachment to the ex-spouse and the availability of social support from friends and the extended family. Poorer adjustment following divorce occurs when individuals are older, have been married for a long period and have had little input to the decision to divorce. A low income and the absence of a job outside the home before the divorce leads to poor post-divorce adjustment, particularly for women. A sense of personal powerlessness, low self-esteem and a low tolerance for change are associated with post-divorce maladjustment, as are a traditional gender-role orientation and a sustained attachment to the ex-spouse.

IMMEDIATE IMPACT OF DIVORCE ON PARENTING

The stresses and strains of residential changes, economic hardship, role changes and consequent physical and psychological difficulties associated with the immediate aftermath of separation and divorce may compromise parents' capacity to co-operate in meeting their children's needs for safety, care, control, education and relationships with each parent (Amato, 1993, 2000; Amato & Gilbreth, 1999; Anderson, 2003; Bray & Hetherington, 1993; Faust & McKibben, 1999; Greene et al., 2003; Hetherington & Kelly, 2002). Authoritarian–punitive parenting, lax, *laissez-faire* or neglectful parenting, and chaotic parenting, which involves oscillating between both of these extreme styles, are not uncommon among both custodial and non-custodial parents who have divorced. Some parents manage to develop a supportive authoritative parenting style, especially if there are many protective factors present. Three distinct co-parenting styles have been identified in studies of divorced families. These are described below and their impact on children's adjustment given.

Co-operative parenting

Parents here develop a unified and integrated set of rules and routines about managing the children in both households. This is the optimal arrangement but occurs only in about one in five cases.

Parallel parenting

Here, each parent has his or her own set of rules for the children and only limited attempts are made to integrate these. Fortunately, such separate sets of rules typically hold much in common. The greater the degree of over-lap between parents' separate rule systems and the greater the degree of respect parents hold for each other's sets of parenting standards, the better their children's adjustment. Where parallel parenting systems are not too discrepant and parents do not undermine each other's parenting practices unduly, most children in the medium and long term show few major adjustment problems. This is the most common pattern.

Conflictual parenting

In this situation the couple do not communicate directly with each other; all messages are passed through the child. This leads to major adjustment problems for the child. The go-between role, forced on the child, is highly stressful.

A summary of factors contributing to parental post-separation adjustment and parenting abilities is presented in Figure 23.1 and is based on the information presented in preceding sections.

EFFECTS OF DIVORCE ON CHILDREN

A distinction may be made between the short-, medium- and long-term effects of divorce, which are described below (Amato, 2000, 2001; Amato & Gilbreth, 1999; Kelly, 2000; Leon, 2003; Reifman, Villa, Amans, Rethinam & Telesca, 2001; Rogers, 2004; Wallerstein, 1991).

Short-term effects

For the two-year period immediately following divorce, most children show some adjustment problems. Boys tend to display conduct or externalizing behaviour problems and girls tend to experience emotional or internalizing behaviour problems. Both boys and girls may experience educational problems and relationship difficulties within the family, school and peer group.

Medium-term effects

The impact of divorce on children between the third and tenth year following divorce may be statistically expressed in two ways: (1) as differences between the average or mean level of well-being or maladjustment of children of divorce compared with the mean level of well-being or maladjustment in

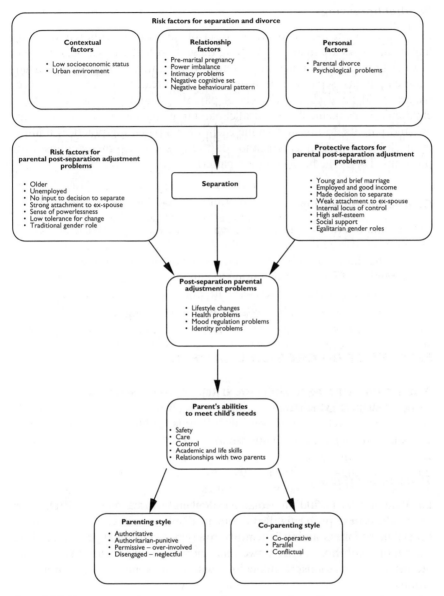

Figure 23.1 Factors contributing to parental post-separation adjustment and parenting abilities

intact families; (2) as the percentage of children of divorce who show adjustment difficulties.

The mean level of maladjustment has consistently been found to be worse for children of divorce in comparison with those from intact families on a variety of measures of adjustment including conduct difficulties, emotional problems, academic performance, self-esteem and relationships with parents. This has led to the erroneous conclusion by some interpreters of the literature that divorce always has a negative effect on children.

When the impact of divorce on children is expressed in terms of the percentages of maladjusted children, it is clear that divorce leads to maladjustment for only a minority of youngsters. Between 20 and 25% of children of divorced parents show serious long-term psychological problems. By comparison, 4–23% of children from intact marriages show serious long-term psychological problems, as can be seen from the results of epidemiological surveys reviewed in Table 3.8 (p. 96).

Long-term effects

In adult life, a small proportion of individuals from families where divorce has occurred have difficulty making and maintaining stable marital relationships, have psychological adjustment difficulties and attain a lower socioeconomic level than adults who have grown up in intact families.

FACTORS RELATED TO CHILDREN'S ADJUSTMENT FOLLOWING DIVORCE

Certain characteristics of children and certain features of their social contexts mediate the effects of parental divorce on their adjustment (Amato, 2000, 2001; Amato & Gilbreth, 1999; Anderson, 2003; Faust & McKibben, 1999; Hetherington & Kelly, 2002; Greene et al., 2003; Kelly, 2000; Leon, 2003; Reifman et al., 2001; Rogers, 2004; Visher, Visher & Pasley, 2003; Walker, 1993; Wallerstein, 1991). These factors have been classified as pre-disposing, protective and maintaining factors and are summarized in Figure 23.2. These factors probably have a cumulative effect, with more pre-disposing and maintaining factors being associated with worse adjustment and more protective factors being associated with better adjustment.

Pre-disposing personal factors

Males between the ages of three and eighteen are particularly at risk for post-divorce adjustment problems, especially if they have biological vulnerabilities associated with genetic factors, pre-natal and peri-natal difficulties, or a history of serious illness or injury. Children with low intelligence, a difficult temperament, low self-esteem, an external locus of control, and a history of psychological difficulties are also pre-disposed to developing post-separation problems.

Pre-disposing contextual factors

Children are more likely to develop post-separation difficulties if there have been serious difficulties with the parent–child relationship prior to the separation. Included here are insecure attachment, inconsistent discipline and authoritarian, permissive or neglectful parenting. Exposure to chronic family problems, including parental adjustment problems, marital discord, domestic violence, family disorganization, and a history of previous separations and re-unions also place children at risk for post-separation adjustment problems. Early life stresses, such as abuse or bereavement, may also compromise children's capacity to deal with stresses entailed by parental separation.

Personal maintaining factors

Adjustment problems may be maintained by rigid sets of negative beliefs related to parental separation. These beliefs may include a view that the child caused the separation and has the power to influence parental reunification, or a belief that abandonment by parents and rejection by peers is inevitable. Low self-efficacy beliefs, a dysfunctional attributional style, dysfunctional coping strategies and immature defences may also maintain post-separation adjustment problems.

Contextual maintaining factors

Adjustment problems following separation may be maintained by certain features of the child's social context. Poorer adjustment occurs in the first two years following divorce when there is little parental co-operation and parental conflict is channelled through the children. The use of non-optimal parenting styles, a lack of consistency in parental rules and routines across custodial and non-custodial households, a lack of clarity about new family roles and routines within each household and confused family communication may all maintain children's post-separation adjustment problems. Those parenting and co-parenting problems which maintain children's adjustment difficulties are in turn often a spin-off from parents' personal post-separation adjustment problems, which have been described above. The degree to which parental post-separation problems compromise their capacity to provide a co-parenting environment that minimizes rather than maintains their children's adjustment reactions is partially determined by the stresses parents face in the aftermath of separation. These include the loss of support, financial hardship and social disadvantage. The challenges that parents face in

PRE-DISPOSING FACTORS

PERSONAL PRE-DISPOSING FACTORS

Demographic factors
- Male gender
- Aged 3–18 years

Biological factors
- Genetic vulnerabilities
- Pre- and peri-natal complications
- Early insults, injuries and illnesses

Psychological factors
- Previous psychological problems
- Low intelligence
- Difficult temperament
- Low self-esteem
- External locus of control

CONTEXTUAL PRE-DISPOSING FACTORS

Parent–child factors in early life
- Attachment problems
- Lack of intellectual stimulation
- Authoritarian parenting
- Permissive parenting
- Neglectful parenting
- Inconsistent parental discipline

Exposure to family problems in early life
- Parental psychological problems
- Parental alcohol and substance abuse
- Parental criminality
- Marital discord or violence
- Family disorganization
- Previous parental separation and reunification

Stresses in early life
- Bereavements
- Separations
- Child abuse
- Social disadvantage

PERSONAL MAINTAINING FACTORS

Psychological factors
- Guilt beliefs for causing separation
- Beliefs that child can cause reunification
- Fear of abandonment by parents
- Fear of rejection by peers
- Low self-efficacy
- Dysfunctional attributional style
- Negative cognitive distortions
- Immature defence mechanisms
- Dysfunctional coping strategies

PERSONAL PROTECTIVE FACTORS

Demographic factors
- Female gender
- Under 3 and over 18 years

Psychological factors
- High IQ
- Easy temperament
- High self-esteem
- Internal locus of control
- High self-efficacy
- Optimistic attributional style
- Mature defence mechanisms
- Functional coping strategies

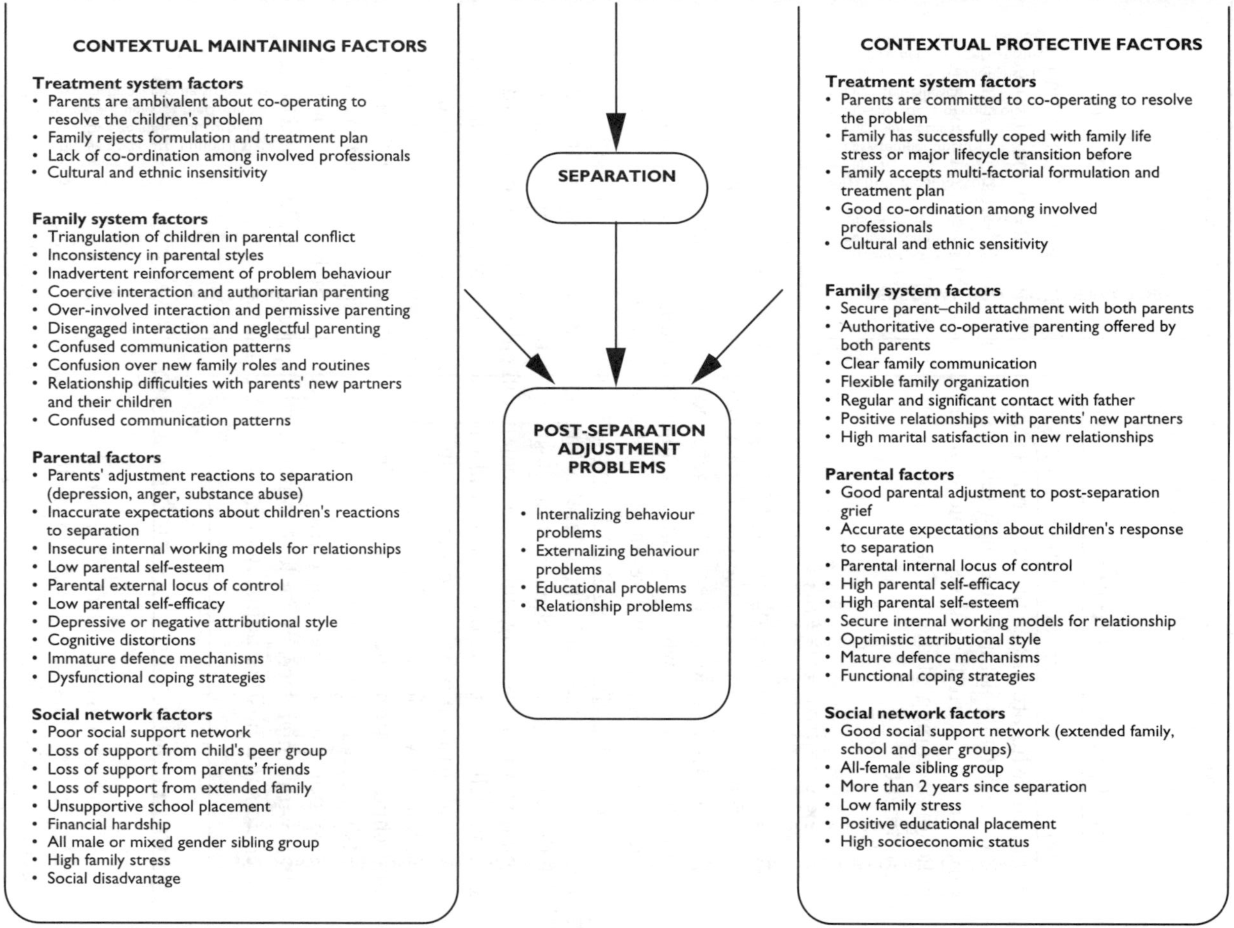

CONTEXTUAL MAINTAINING FACTORS

Treatment system factors
- Parents are ambivalent about co-operating to resolve the children's problem
- Family rejects formulation and treatment plan
- Lack of co-ordination among involved professionals
- Cultural and ethnic insensitivity

Family system factors
- Triangulation of children in parental conflict
- Inconsistency in parental styles
- Inadvertent reinforcement of problem behaviour
- Coercive interaction and authoritarian parenting
- Over-involved interaction and permissive parenting
- Disengaged interaction and neglectful parenting
- Confused communication patterns
- Confusion over new family roles and routines
- Relationship difficulties with parents' new partners and their children
- Confused communication patterns

Parental factors
- Parents' adjustment reactions to separation (depression, anger, substance abuse)
- Inaccurate expectations about children's reactions to separation
- Insecure internal working models for relationships
- Low parental self-esteem
- Parental external locus of control
- Low parental self-efficacy
- Depressive or negative attributional style
- Cognitive distortions
- Immature defence mechanisms
- Dysfunctional coping strategies

Social network factors
- Poor social support network
- Loss of support from child's peer group
- Loss of support from parents' friends
- Loss of support from extended family
- Unsupportive school placement
- Financial hardship
- All male or mixed gender sibling group
- High family stress
- Social disadvantage

SEPARATION

POST-SEPARATION ADJUSTMENT PROBLEMS
- Internalizing behaviour problems
- Externalizing behaviour problems
- Educational problems
- Relationship problems

CONTEXTUAL PROTECTIVE FACTORS

Treatment system factors
- Parents are committed to co-operating to resolve the problem
- Family has successfully coped with family life stress or major lifecycle transition before
- Family accepts multi-factorial formulation and treatment plan
- Good co-ordination among involved professionals
- Cultural and ethnic sensitivity

Family system factors
- Secure parent–child attachment with both parents
- Authoritative co-operative parenting offered by both parents
- Clear family communication
- Flexible family organization
- Regular and significant contact with father
- Positive relationships with parents' new partners
- High marital satisfaction in new relationships

Parental factors
- Good parental adjustment to post-separation grief
- Accurate expectations about children's response to separation
- Parental internal locus of control
- High parental self-efficacy
- High parental self-esteem
- Secure internal working models for relationship
- Optimistic attributional style
- Mature defence mechanisms
- Functional coping strategies

Social network factors
- Good social support network (extended family, school and peer groups)
- All-female sibling group
- More than 2 years since separation
- Low family stress
- Positive educational placement
- High socioeconomic status

Figure 23.2 Factors contributing to children's adjustment following separation or divorce

managing children's post-separation adjustment problems are greatest where the sibling group is all male or contains boys and girls. These types of sibling group, in comparison with all-female sibling groups, tend to become involved in problem-maintaining interaction patterns.

Personal protective factors

Better post-separation adjustment occurs in intelligent girls of easy temperament who are either in their infancy or late adolescence when divorce occurs, especially if they have high self-esteem, an internal locus of control, an optimistic attributional style and high self-efficacy. Mature defences and functional coping strategies may also contribute to positive post-divorce adjustment.

Contextual protective factors

Certain characteristics of the child's family, social network and school environment may protect the child from developing adjustment problems following separation. Better adjustment occurs usually after a two-year period has elapsed, where parental conflict is minimal and not channelled through the child, and where an authoritative parenting style is employed. Where parents cope well with post-separation grief, have good personal psychological resources and a high level of marital satisfaction within their new relationships, children show better post-separation adjustment. Parental commitment to resolving child-management difficulties and a track-record of coping well with transitions in family life may be viewed as protective factors. Fewer adjustment problems occur in families where the sibling group is composed entirely of females. The availability of social support, for both parents and children, from the extended family; peers and the absence of financial hardship are also protective factors for post-separation adjustment. Where the school provides a concerned, student-centred, achievement-oriented ethos with a high level of student contact and supervision, children are more likely to show positive adjustment following separation.

DEVELOPMENTAL STAGES OF FAMILY TRANSFORMATION

Family transformation through separation, divorce and re-marriage may be conceptualized as a process involving a series of stages. Carter and McGoldrick's (1999) model of the stages of adjustment to divorce is presented in Table 23.1. This model outlines tasks that must be completed during various stages of the transformation process that involves separation and re-marriage. Failure to complete tasks at one stage may lead to adjustment problems for family members at later stages.

Table 23.1 Extra stages in the family lifecycle entailed by separation or divorce and re-marriage

Stage	Task
1. **Decision to divorce**	• Accepting one's own part in marital failure
2. **Planning separation**	• Co-operatively developing a plan for custody of the children, visitation and finances • Dealing with the families of origin's response to the plan to separate
3. **Separation**	• Mourning the loss of the intact family • Adjusting to the change in parent–child and parent–parent relationships • Avoiding letting marital arguments interfere with parent-to-parent co-operation • Staying connected to the extended family • Managing doubts about separation and becoming committed to divorce
4. **Post-divorce period**	• Maintaining flexible arrangements about custody, access and finances without detouring conflict through the children • Ensuring both parents retain strong relationships with the children • Re-establishing peer relationships and a social network
5. **Entering a new relationship**	• Completing emotional divorce from the previous relationship • Developing commitment to a new marriage
6. **Planning a new marriage**	• Planning for co-operative co-parental relationships with ex-spouses • Planning to deal with children's loyalty conflicts involving natural and step-parents • Adjust to widening of extended family
7. **Establishing a new family**	• Re-aligning relationships within the family to allow space for new members • Sharing memories and histories to allow for integration of all new members

Note: Adapted from Carter and McGoldrick (1999).

In the first stage, the decision to divorce occurs and accepting one's own part in marital failure is the central task. In the second stage, plans for separation are made. A co-operative plan for custody of the children, visitation, finances and dealing with the wider family's response to the plan to separate must be made if positive adjustment is to occur. The third stage of the model is separation. Mourning the loss of the intact family, adjusting to the change in parent–child and parent–parent relationships, preventing marital arguments from interfering with interparental co-operation, staying connected to the extended family and managing doubts about separation are the principal tasks at this stage. The fourth stage is the post-divorce period. Here, couples must maintain flexible arrangements about custody, access and finances without detouring conflict through the children; they must retain strong relationships with the children and re-establish peer relationships. Establishing a new relationship occurs in the fifth stage. For this to occur, emotional divorce from the previous relationship must be completed and a commitment to a new marriage must be developed. The sixth stage of the model is planning a new marriage. This entails planning for co-operative co-parental relationships with ex-spouses and planning to deal with children's loyalty conflicts involving natural and step-parents. It is also important to adjust to the widening of the extended family. In the final stage of the model, establishing a new family is the central theme. Re-aligning relationships within the family to allow space for new members and sharing memories and histories to allow for integration of all new members are the principal tasks of this stage.

CHARACTERISTICS OF STEP-FAMILIES

The majority of divorced people re-marry and these step-families have unique characteristics, which are, in part, affected by the conditions under which they are formed (Hetherington & Kelly 2002; Raschke, 1987; Visher et al., 2003). On the positive side, surveys of step-families have found them to be more open in communication, more willing to deal with conflict, more pragmatic and less romantic, and more egalitarian with respect to childcare and housekeeping tasks. On the negative side, compared with intact first marriages, step-families are less cohesive and more stressful. Step-parent–child relationships on average tend to be more conflictual than parent–child relationships in intact families. This is particularly true of step-father–daughter relationships and may be due to the daughter's perception of the step-father encroaching on a close mother–daughter relationship.

CHILDREN'S ADJUSTMENT FOLLOWING RE-MARRIAGE

Children's adjustment following re-marriage is associated with age, gender and parents' satisfaction with the new marriage (Greene et al., 2003; Hetherington & Kelly, 2002; Visher et al., 2003). Good adjustment occurs when the custodial parent re-marries while children are pre-adolescent or in their late adolescence or early adulthood. All children in divorced families resist the entry of a step-parent, but during the early teenage years (ten to fifteen) this resistance is at a maximum. Divorced adults with children in middle childhood and early adolescence who wish to re-marry should try to wait until the children have reached about sixteen to eighteen years if they want their new relationship to have a fair chance of survival. Re-marriage is more disruptive for girls than for boys. Marital satisfaction in the new relationship has a protective effect for young boys and it is a risk factor for preadolescent girls. Young boys benefit from their custodial mothers forming a satisfying relationship with a new partner. Such satisfying relationships lead step-fathers to behave in a warm, child-centred way towards their step-sons and to help them learn sports and academic skills. These skills help young boys become psychologically robust. Pre-adolescent girls feel that the close supportive relationship they have with their divorced mothers is threatened by development of a new and satisfying marital relationship. They usually respond with increased conduct problems and psychological difficulties. In adolescence, when the re-marriage has occurred while the children were preadolescent, a high level of marital satisfaction is associated with good adjustment and a high level of acceptance of the step-parent for both boys and girls.

ASSESSMENT AND FORMULATION

Where youngsters present with adjustment difficulties associated with separation, a thorough assessment of child and family functioning should be conducted. The assessment protocol set out in Chapter 4 may be supplemented with the frameworks given in Figures 23.1, 23.2 and Table 23.3. Some psychometric instruments that may be useful in the assessment of cases where separation has occurred are set out in Table 23.2. Salient points from the assessment should be integrated into a coherent formulation that specifies key pre-disposing, maintaining and protective factors present in the case. A management plan based on the formulation should then be given.

THERAPY PROGRAMMES FOR ADJUSTMENT PROBLEMS

Reviews of therapy programmes for adjustment problems following separation and divorce show that group-based child-focused and adult-focused interventions can lead to significant improvements in children's adjustment (Herbert, 2005; O'Halloran & Carr, 2000; Stathakos & Roehrle, 2003). There is also a broad clinical literature which advocates the use of family-therapy-based interventions following separation and divorce to help family members deal with the transitions entailed by divorce, adjust to their new role demands and address various adjustment difficulties (Dowling & Gorell-Barnes, 1999; Emery & Sbarra, 2002; Kaslow, 1995; Robinson, 1997; Visher et al., 2003; Walker, 1993; Walsh, 1991). The guidelines for practice, set out below, have been drawn from this literature.

Table 23.2 Structured assessment instruments for use in cases of separation or divorce

Construct	Instrument	Author & Date of Publication	Comments
Children's perception of divorce and separation	Children's Beliefs about Parental Divorce Scale	Kurdek, L. (1987). Children's beliefs about parental divorce scale. Psychometric characteristics and concurrent validity. *Journal of Consulting and Clinical Psychology*, 55, 712–718	This 36-item self-report scale yields scores on beliefs about peer ridicule, paternal blame, maternal blame, self-blame, fear of abandonment, hope of reunification
	Divorce Events Schedule for Children	Wolchik, S., Sandler, I., Braver, S. & Fogas, B. (1985). Events of parental divorce: Stressfulness ratings by children, parents and clinicians. *American Journal of Community Psychology*, 14, 59–74	This 62-item live events inventory allows children to rate how stressful various divorce-related life events are for them
	Child Adjustment Inventory	Portes, P. R., Lehman, A. J., & Brown, J. H. (1999). The child adjustment inventory: Assessing transition in child divorce adjustment. *Journal of Divorce & Remarriage*, 30 (1/2), 37–45. Available at: http://www.twu.ca/cpsy/Documents/Theses/Grace%20Dent%20Thesis.pdf	This 23-item instrument assesses the child's feelings and thoughts about the divorce
Parents' perceptions of co-parenting and conflict following separation	Divorce Adjustment Inventory-Revised	Portes, P. R., Smith, T. L., & Brown, J. H. (2000). The divorce adjustment inventory-revised: Validation of a parental report concerning children's post-custody adjustment. Unpublished manuscript,	This 36-item parent-completed scale yields scores for family conflict and dysfunction, favourable divorce conditions and child coping ability, positive divorce resolution, external support systems and divorce transition

		University of Louisville. Available at http://www.twu.ca/ cpsy/Documents/ Theses/ Grace%20Dent% 20Thesis.pdf	
	Co-parenting Scale	Camplair, C. & Stolberg, L. (1987). Post-divorce custody arrangements: decision influences and consequent environmental change. *Journal of Divorce*, 10, 43–56	This 12-item parent self-report scale measures frequency of co-parenting behaviours in separated families and differentiates between co-operative and non-co-operative couples
	Acrimony Scale	Emery, R. (1982). Interparental conflict and the children of discord and divorce. *Psychological Bulletin*, 92, 310–330	This 25-item scale measures interparental conflict
Child's perception of parents	Bricklin Scales	Bricklin, B. (1990). *The Bricklin Perceptual Scales: Child Perception of Parent Series (revised)*. Doylestown, PA: Village http:// www.custody-vp.com	This 64-item scale (32 for perceptions of mother and 32 for perceptions of father) systematically obtains information from children 6 years and older about the child's overall perceptions of each parent in four critical areas: competency, supportiveness, consistency, and admirable traits. Computer and hand scoring systems are available
	Perception-of-Relationships Test	Bricklin, B. (1990). *Perception of Relationships Test*. Doylestown, PA: Village. http:// www.custody-vp.com	The test, for under 5s, contains seven tasks (mostly drawings) that measure the degree to which a child seeks to be

Continued

Table 23.2 continued

Construct	Instrument	Author & Date of Publication	Comments
			psychologically 'close' to each parent, and the strengths and weaknesses developed as a result of interacting with each parent. Computer and hand scoring systems are available
	Discipline Index	Lampel, A., Bricklin, D. & Elliot, G. (2005). *Discipline Index.* Doylestown, PA: Village http:// www.custody-vp.com	This 64-item scale (32 for perceptions of mother and 32 for perceptions of father) systematically obtains information from children 6 years and older about the child's overall perceptions of each parent's discipline style and practices. The six areas covered are clear expectations, effectively monitors behaviour, consistent enforcement, fairness, attunement, moderates anger. Computer and hand scoring systems are available
Parenting	The Parent Awareness Skills Survey	Bricklin, D. (2005). *The Parent Awareness Skills Survey.* Doylestown, PA: Village http:// www.custody-vp.com	Measures the sensitivity and effectiveness with which a parent responds to typical childcare situations and yields scores for parental awareness of critical issues in a given situation; adequate solutions; the need to communicate in terms understandable to a child; the

			desirability of acknowledging a child's feelings; the importance of the child's own past history in the present circumstance; and the need to pay attention to how the child is responding in order to fine-tune one's own response
	Co-Parenting Behavior Questionnaire	Macie, K. & Stolberg, A. (2003). Assessing parenting after divorce: The Co-Parenting Behavior Questionnaire. *Journal of Divorce & Remarriage*, 39(1–2), 89–107	This 86-item questionnaire assesses co-parenting interactions and parenting skills of divorced parents from the viewpoint of the child
Custody evaluation	Custody Evaluation Questionnaires, Interviews and Observations and Home Visiting kits	Lampel, A., Bricklin, D. & Elliot, G. (2005). *Custody Evaluation Questionnaires Interviews and Observations and Home Visiting Kits.* Doylestown, PA: Village. http://www.custody-vp.com	Comprehensive custody evaluation kits containing questionnaires, interviews and observation systems for gathering and collating data from families and involved professionals in families requiring custody and access assessments
	Uniform Child Custody Evaluation System	Munsinger, H. & Karlson, K. (1996). *Uniform Child Custody Evaluation System.* Odessa Florida: Psychological Assessment Resources. http://www.parinc.com	This system contains a series of interviewing and observation forms covering all areas important for custody evaluation including: • characteristics of the parents • parent–child relationships • suitability of parents for joint custody

Continued

Table 23.2 continued

Construct	Instrument	Author & Date of Publication	Comments
			In addition the forms cover the administration of the case and allow the professional to keep a tally of contacts with the case. There is also a manual describing step-by-step how to conduct a custody evaluation
Parent's suitability for mediation	Mediation Readiness Inventory	Fuhr, J. (1989). *Mediation readiness. Family and Conciliation Court Review*, 27, 71–74	This 30-item self-report scale yields scores on trust, communication and conflict management sub-scales
	Mediation Obstacle Scale	Fuhr, J. (1989). *Mediation readiness. Family and Conciliation Court Review*, 27, 71–74	A set of six rating scales for use by mediators to rate on the dimensions of co-operation, communication, negotiation, benevolent attitude, separate issues and motivation
Parent's post-separation adjustment as an individual	Fisher Divorce Adjustment Scale	Fisher, B. (1976). *Fisher Divorce Adjustment Scale.* Available at: http://www. fisherseminars.com/ MiniQuiz.htm	This 100-item self-report inventory assesses parental adjustment to divorce and yields scores on self-worth, investment in past love relationship, anger at former partner, grieving loss of relationship, fear of social intimacy, and an overall adjustment to end of relationship

Acceptance of Marriage Termination Scale	Thompson, L & Spanier, G. (1983). The end of marriage and acceptance of marriage termination. *Journal of Marriage and the Family*, 45, 103–113	This 15-item self-report scale measures lack of commitment to the marriage and acceptance that it has ended

When families present with post-separation adjustment difficulties, a multi-systemic intervention package based on a thorough assessment and formulation is probably the best course of action to take. Such multi-systemic intervention programmes may include work with the entire system, including the original family and the new partners and their children. It may also include work with a variety of sub-systems, including individual family members or various groupings of family members. Multi-systemic programmes may include one or more of the following elements:

- psychoeducation
- clarifying family routines and roles
- arranging cross-household consistency in rule systems and parenting styles
- parenting skills training
- facilitating support for the child from the school and the extended family
- providing support and skills training for parents and children
- facilitating grief work.

Psychoeducation

Psychoeducational interventions provide parents with information about legal and financial issues related to separation or direct them to appropriate sources for such information. Both parents and children also require information on what we currently know about the psychology of separation and divorce. Begin by noting that while separation feels like an extremely unusual event for almost everyone, it has become a routine experience for one in three families in most Western cultures. All family members should be given information about the stages of transition, set out in Table 23.1, that occur when a family is transformed through separation. It is important to stress that the process of transformation and the adjustment problems that follow tend to be quite intense for a year and that, after two years, the majority of families and children will have completed making the more important aspects of their adjustment to the separation. Thus, most children's conduct problems abate after two years.

For children, it is important to highlight that the separation reflects a problem with the marital relationship rather than a problem with the parent–child relationship, and so children cannot be blamed for parental divorce, nor is there typically anything that they can do to re-unite their parents.

The importance of maintaining as much stability as possible in the children's routines should be emphasized. Thus, ideally, children should remain in the same house, attend the same school, engage in the same peer activities and so forth.

The importance of avoiding triangulation or attempting to persuade the children to take sides with one or other parent should be stressed. Parents and children should be helped to clearly distinguish between the marital relationship, which is dissolved through separation, and the co-parental relationship, which continues despite the fact that parents live in different houses. It is important to emphasize that parents must prevent negative feelings associated with the marital relationship from interfering with interparental co-operation in caring for the children, since failure to do so will have a negative effect on the children.

Separation inevitably involves grieving, and the intense and painful experiences of loss, denial, sadness, anger, anxiety and eventually acceptance. At times, these emotional experiences are almost unbearable but most people work through them successfully and emerge from the grieving process hurt but strengthened by the experience.

Clarifying family routines and roles

When parents separate and establish separate households, with or without new partners and with or without other children, new routines need to be clarified. Thus, new daily routines for getting up and going to work or school, meal-times, leisure activities, cleaning, transportation and so forth need to be developed. There are also new weekly routines for visiting with both parents now that they live in separate households. Annual routines for managing holidays, birthdays, Christmas and other special events all require clarification. One role of the clinician is to facilitate the negotiation of these new routines and roles with appropriate family sub-systems.

Where parents have new partners, with or without children, the role relationships between family members who have not lived together before need to be worked out. This process of negotiating role relationships typically involves a practical aspect and an emotional aspect. At a practical level, there are negotiations such as who does what chores around the house; who sleeps where; who gets priority in using the car, the TV or any other resource; and the hierarchy in the household. That is, who can tell who what to do. At an emotional level, the attachments between family member need to evolve and each member needs to find a way to feel that they are adequately supported at an emotional level.

Where families have difficulty evolving new routines and role relationships, meetings may be held with the whole family or with various sub-systems to facilitate this process. Typically, this work involves brainstorming options and selecting the option that seems most viable; inviting relevant family members to try apparently viable options and reviewing and revising these options in follow-up meetings.

Within such meetings, the clinician's function is to slow the pace of communication and introduce a fair system of turn-taking, since often intense emotions are aroused by issues such as where children should spend Christmas or who should have the right to use the car! One system that I find helpful is to make a rule that only one person may speak at a time in these sessions and that person must be holding a token (such as a pen or a flag), which all agree is a symbol for permission to speak. Without some system for turn-taking, these meetings degenerate into chaotic free-for-alls or silent, tension-ridden sessions.

Arranging cross-household consistency in rule systems

One particularly important set of role relationships are those associated with the family hierarchy. Prior to separation this is usually fairly clear. Both parents are in charge of all of the children and the children therefore adopt a subordinate role, particularly with respect to house rules about education, time keeping, safety, aggression, sex, drug usage and so forth. Following separation, a variety of common problems occur. First, parents may have difficulty agreeing on one set of rules and one set of sanctions for both households. One parent may consciously or unconsciously undermine the other's rule system. Second, within one or both households, parents may find that the stress associated with separation has compromised their capacity to set clear rules and follow through on consequences. A third common problem is that there may be a lack of clarity about whether or not step-parents may set and enforce house rules.

During the transitional period following separation, many children, but particularly boys, respond to the stress with aggression and conduct problems. Often under-pinning this aggression is guilt about causing the separation and a fear of abandonment. What is required in such instances is, first, family work that aims to increase the child's sense of security with both parents. A useful way to achieve this is to help families set up weekly episodes of special time for the youngster with each parent.

The second important way to manage conduct problems is to maximize consistency of the rule systems used across both households and arrange for all parents and step-parents to participate in implementing this system. In some cases it is possible to hold family meetings in which all parents meet with the psychologist at the same time and agree on a set of rules, rewards and sanctions applicable in both households and then subsequently meet with the child and explain these as a group. However, often the interparental conflict is too intense to permit this type of ideal intervention and the same agreement is negotiated separately with the adults in each household and then explained to the child by each set of parents in separate meetings.

Parenting skills training

In some instances where attempts to arrange cross-household consistency in rule systems is unsuccessful, it becomes apparent that one or more parents or step-parents lacks parenting skills. In such instances they may be trained to track positive and negative target behaviours, no more than three at a time. They may then be trained to use reward programmes and star charts to increase positive behaviours and time-out to decease negative behaviours. With adolescents, training in negotiation skills and contingency contracting may be used. Parenting skills training is discussed more fully in Chapter 10, where conduct problems are the central concern. Once all parents are proficient in basic behavioural parenting skills, family work should focus on arranging cross-household consistency in rule systems and the rule systems should be implemented using behavioural parenting methods.

Some children present with elimination problems, sleep difficulties, anxiety states, mood problems and substance abuse as part of an adjustment reaction to separation. In such instances, guidelines for managing these problems set out elsewhere in this text should be followed. However, for all of these problems, it is vital to ensure that cross-household consistency is arranged in the understanding and management of the youngsters' difficulties.

Facilitating support for the child from the school and the extended family

The school and extended family are important potential sources of support for youngsters with adjustment problems following separation. However, these potential sources of support may become sources of stress if teachers, grandparents and others misunderstand youngsters' adjustment problems. One role for the psychologist is to empower parents to explain the youngster's situation to teachers or to facilitate meetings between parents, children and teachers in which the child's situation may be explained. The core agenda for such meetings is to clarify that the child is coping with family transformation and that this is very stressful. Sometimes children respond to this stress by failing to concentrate, becoming angry or becoming sad. These problems are transitory. The school may help the child cope by understanding these difficulties and agreeing on a joint management plan with the parents and the child.

With extended families, separation often leads to a decrease in the amount of supportive contact that the child has with grandparents, aunts and uncles, particularly in the non-custodial parent's family. This is unfortunate, since during stressful life transitions children require an increase rather than a decrease in such contacts. Thus, an important role of the psychologist is to increase the frequency of supportive contracts between the child and members of the extended family.

Providing support

Many parents require ongoing support to deal with the sense of isolation, failure and rejection which often accompanies divorce. They require a regular opportunity to ventilate their feelings and process the intense emotions that occur as part of family transformation. This type of support may be provided within individual sessions, in sessions where parents attend with their new partners or in groups for separated parents. In most districts there is a self-help support group for separated parents, and it is useful to make information about such groups available as early as possible in the consultation process, since most parents find them extraordinarily supportive. Common themes that emerge in such groups include the sense of isolation, the sense of being overwhelmed by the life transition, the loss of the spouse role, parenting difficulties, managing co-parenting, dealing with the possibilities of dating and sex, grieving and letting go of the marriage and managing the extended family.

For children, such support groups are less readily available. It is therefore not surprising that clinical psychologists have developed a number of proto-cols for running such groups. Most of these provide children with informa-tion of the type mentioned in the section above on psychoeducation, and provide children with an opportunity to express their intense feelings about the separation process using verbal or artistic media. Common themes which emerge in such expressive sessions are a fear of abandonment by one or both parents, a wish to re-unite the family, guilt for having caused the separation, splitting parents into the wholly good parent and the wholly bad parent and directing anger at the bad parent while idealizing the good parent, anger at parents' new partners; a fear of peer rejection because of the separation, a sense of loss and sadness and a sense of helplessness and confusion.

Grief work and letting go

Parental separation and divorce involve loss. One set of relationships and one pattern of family organization is lost and replaced by another. For children whose father or mother moves out of the family home, this may be experienced as losing their daddy or mummy. For parents, the loss is of a partner, a role and a way of life. In response to these losses, family members typically experience some of the following grief processes over an extended period of time, which may last up to about two years in their most intense form:

- shock at first hearing of the separation
- denial or disbelief
- bargaining about making changes so that the family may be re-united
- anger at others for causing the separation
- guilt for having caused the separation
- yearning and searching for the person who has left or the old form of family organization
- depression and sadness about the loss
- anxiety about abandonment by family members
- anxiety about the reaction of others (peers and extended family) to the separation
- despair and hopelessness about surviving without the family as it was
- relief that the separation has put an end to the constant conflict
- acceptance that the separation has occurred.

These grief processes typically begin with shock and end with acceptance, but beyond that there is marked variability in the patterning of these reactions. A fuller description of grief and loss is given in Chapter 24.

Grief work involves acknowledging the reality of the loss of the family as it was and modifying one's world views so that it takes account of the loss. These aims may be achieved by reviewing, repeatedly and in detail, life as it was before the separation and life as it is now and will be following the separation, and experiencing in full all of the intense and painful emotions that are aroused by this. The role of the clinician is to help family members do this grief work at their own pace and within a context that they find most supportive. For example, many adults prefer to do this work within the context of an individual counselling relationship or with a group of peers who are going through the same loss experience. Some children may find that they can work through these issues best with their siblings and custodial parent; others find that an individual counselling or support group context is more suitable.

Anniversary grief reactions are common-place in families where separation has occurred. Family members may need to be alerted to this possibility and also provided with invitations to return for additional sessions at anniversaries if further grief counselling is desired at these times.

CHILD CUSTODY EVALUATIONS

In child custody evaluations, the central question typically concerns the best parenting environment for the child (American Academy of Child and Adolescent Psychiatry, 1997h; American Psychiatric Association, 1988; American Psychological Association, 1994; Gardner, 1989; Stahl, 1994). The aim of assessment in these cases is to establish what custody arrangements the parents and child want and, ultimately, what is in the best interests of the child. Child custody evaluations typically begin with a contracting meeting in which a schedule of appointments and fees is agreed. Contracting in child custody cases is particularly important, since adherence to the assessment contract is one indicator of parents' capacity to meet their children's need for a co-operative parenting environment. Contracting is also important where court fees are involved (as is often the case) and the American Psychological Association (1994) recommends that financial arrangements be clarified from the outset. One common practice is for involved parties to pay a fixed fee, or retainer, before the evaluation begins. Another is to make the financial contract with the clients' legal representatives.

A child custody evaluation should typically include individual and conjoint interviews with both parents, the involved children, and relevant members of the extended family. Home visits and observation of parent–child interaction may be appropriate to intensively assess some aspects of parenting capacity. Where appropriate, school reports and reports from other involved professionals should be obtained. It is critical in child custody cases to obtain written consent to contact the school, other family members and other involved professionals such as psychiatrists or probation officers. It is also important to keep detailed notes of all contacts and to list these in the final court report. A useful set of standard contracting and information-collecting forms for conducting custody evaluations has been developed by Munsinger and Karlson (1996) and by Lampel, Bricklin and Elliot (2005) (described in Table 23.2). Helpful guides to conducting such assessments have been developed by the American Academy of Child and Adolescent Psychiatry (1997h), the American Psychiatric Association (1988), American Psychological Association (1994), Gardner (1989) and Stahl (1994).

In assessing the custody arrangement that would be in the best interests of the child, the areas listed in the assessment framework presented in Table 23.3 should be covered, at a minimum. First, the child's wishes and the wishes of each parent concerning custody requires assessment. In light of this, the degree of agreement between parties and the level of parental conflict may be assessed. At one extreme there are situations where each parent wants sole custody. At the other extreme, there are situations where considerable agreement about custody and childcare is present. In some such instances, joint custody may be the best alternative. For this type of recommendation to be made, the parents must display the psychological skills necessary to prevent their negative feelings about each other, as marital partners, from interfering with their effective joint parental care of their children. Thus they must make a conceptual distinction between the marital relationship and the co-parental relationship. Making this distinction allows them to control their anger towards their spouse, as a marital partner who has let them down, so that they may work co-operatively with their ex-spouse to care for the children. This involves the parents giving priority to the child's needs for a co-operative parental environment over their own needs to engage in

Table 23.3 Areas requiring assessment for custody evaluation

Adherence to contract	Degree of agreement with initial contract for custody evaluation (including appointment schedule, conditions, and fees where appropriate)
	Degree to which parents complied with contract
Expressed wishes	Child's wishes
	Parents' wishes
Joint custody criteria	Degree of parental agreement about current and future custody arrangements and capacity to negotiate about this
	Parental capacity to give child's needs priority and co-operate with spouse
Parenting abilities	Parent's ability to meet child's need for safety
	Parent's ability to meet child's need for care (food and shelter, attachment, empathy, understanding and emotional support); the child's attachment to the parent; and the parent's goodness-of-fit with child
	Parent's ability to meet child's need for control (clear limits, supervision and appropriate rewards and sanction) and to manage conduct problems without violence. This covers parent's discipline style and conflict resolution style
	Parent's ability to meet child's need to learn academic and life skills (age-appropriate intellectual stimulation, schooling, age-appropriate responsibilities and a clear role model) and to avoid neglect
	Parent's ability to meet child's need to maintain relationships with both parents (and to negotiate about access visits, etc.), i.e. continuity of attachments
	Parent's ability to meet any special needs the child has arising from sensory, motor or intellectual disabilities or illnesses
Child's adjustment	Child's current, past and projected behavioural adjustment in each parent's house and neighbourhood
	Child's current, past and projected future adjustment at school
	Current, past and potential future relationships with siblings
	Current, past and potential future relationships with extended family
Parental adjustment	Parental history of violence, child or spouse abuse or potential for future violence
	Parent's psychological or physical adjustment problems (including immaturity, substance abuse, depression, serious illness) that may compromise capacity to meet child's needs and parental strengths (problem solving, planning, endurance)
	Parent's financial situation and work schedule, which impact on the capacity to meet physical needs and the needs the child has for the parent to be available
	Opportunities for children to have access to religious practices without becoming triangulated into parental conflicts over religion
	Opportunities for children to have access to ethnic and cultural practices without becoming triangulated into parental conflicts over these

continued conflict with each other. Where parents are capable of this, they typically show in joint interviews that, despite their mixed feelings or anger towards each other, they can communicate and negotiate once the focus of concern is the children's welfare. They also demonstrate that they can make flexible arrangements about shared childcare responsibilities and follow through on these without the child being triangulated. A summary of the criteria for making decisions about joint custody is set out in Table 23.4.

Where there is disagreement between parents about custody arrangement then the decision about what is in the child's best interests must be based on evaluation of each of the parent's capacities to meet the child's needs for safety, care, control and education; factors that may have a bearing on these capacities are set out in Table 23.5. With respect to safety, a central concern is whether the parent is at risk for abusing the child. A history of violence, spouse abuse or any form of child abuse is a strong indicator that the parent may have difficulty meeting the child's needs for safety. Where there is a suspicion of child abuse, a thorough assessment following the sets of guide-lines set out in Chapters 19, 20 and 21 should be conducted. Where parents are clearly unable to meet their children's needs for safety, then it should be recommended that the other party be given custody. However, in any case where the child construes one parent as 'all good' and the other as 'all bad', with no suggestion of any attachment or loyalty to that parent, parent alien-ation syndrome (Gardner, 1998; described in the next section), should be considered.

Table 23.4 Criteria for deciding for or against joint custody

Criteria for recommending joint custody	Criteria for recommending against joint custody
The parents want a joint custody arrangement	One or both parents do not want a joint custody arrangement
The parents have the psychological skills necessary to prevent their negative feelings about each other as marital partners from interfering with their effective joint care of the children	One or both parents lack the psychological skills necessary to prevent their negative feelings about each other as marital partners from interfering with their effective joint care of the children
The parents give priority to the child's needs for a co-operative parental environment over their own needs to engage in continued conflict with each other	One or both parents are intensely angry and give priority to their need to express this anger over their child's needs for a co-operative parental environment
The parents can communicate and negotiate with each other	The parents disagree about childrearing
The parents can make flexible arrangements about shared childcare responsibilities	The parents live 100 miles or more apart

Note: Based on Munsinger and Karlson (1996).

Table 23.5 Criteria for deciding for or against custody as being in the best interests of the child

Criteria for recommending custody	Criteria for recommending against custody
The parents agree on the custody arrangement	The parent has engaged in child or spouse abuse and/or poses a threat of physical, emotional or sexual abuse or neglect to the child
The parent can meet the child's needs for • safety • care • control • education	The parent is unable to meet the child's needs for • safety • care • control • education
The child prefers to live with the parent	
The custody arrangement allows the child a minimum of disruption and a maximum of continuity in their living arrangements	There is a lack of attachment between the parent and child which prevents the parent from meeting the child's needs
The custody arrangements permits children to remain in their present school and with their present peer-group (except where their school or peer-group environment is problematic)	There is a lack of goodness-of-fit between the parent and the child which prevents the parent from meeting the child's needs
The parent is the child's primary caretaker	The parent, as a result of immaturity, psychological problems, substance abuse, or physical health problems is unable to meet the child's needs
The parent can meet the child's special needs associated with youthfulness or disability	
Siblings remain together	
Support from the extended family is available	
The child has previously shown good adjustment within the custodial parent's home	

Note: Based on Munsinger and Karlson (1996).

Parents' ability to meet the child's need for care should include a consideration of their capacity to plan sufficiently well to provide basic food and shelter. It should also address the degree of attachment between the parent and the child, the goodness-of-fit between the child's temperament and the parents' expectations and abilities to cope with the child's demands, and the capacity of the parent to empathize with children and understand their point of view. In particular, it is important to assess the degree to which parents know how difficult it is for children to feel divided loyalties.

With respect to children's need for control, parental capacities to set clear limits and rules of conduct, monitor and supervise the degree to which children conform to these expectations, and to offer appropriate rewards and sanctions should be assessed. Extremely lax or neglectful parenting and highly punitive parenting are both detrimental to child development. Between these extremes, a range of approaches to parenting may meet the children's needs for control.

Parents' ability to meet the child's need to learn academic and life skills also requires assessment. With infants and toddlers this involves providing age-appropriate intellectual stimulation. With school-going children it involves requiring children to meet age-appropriate responsibilities within the home, the school and the community. Providing children with a clear role model is another important aspect of meeting the child's need to learn life skills.

A variety of factors that may compromise parents' capacities to meet their children's needs deserve assessment also, especially psychological adjustment problems and physical illness. Common psychological adjustment difficulties requiring routine screening include excessive impulsivity (associated with borderline personality disorder), conduct problems (associated with anti-social personality disorder), substance abuse, mood disorders and anxiety disorders.

Where parents are equally placed with respect to parenting skills, other factors may be taken into account when making custody recommendations. Custody arrangements that take account of children's preferences, arrangements that entail a minimum of disruption and a maximum of continuity in children's home and school placement and routines, arrangements that permit siblings to stay together and arrangements that maximize support from the extended family, the school and the peer group are preferable. Where the child has previously shown good adjustment within the custodial parent's home, where a parent is the child's primary caretaker, and where a parent is particularly well equipped to meet a child's special needs associated with youthfulness or disability, then custody with that parent is preferable.

In writing a court report outlining the results of a child custody evaluation, the following structure may be used:

- name, qualifications and experience of clinical psychologist conducting the assessment
- names, dates of birth and addresses of children and parents
- date on which the report was written
- sources on which the report is based (list of interviews conducted indicating dates and people interviewed and list of other reports reviewed)
- circumstances of referral
- relevant family history
- mother's adjustment, adherence to assessment contract and parenting skills
- father's adjustment, adherence to assessment contract and parenting skills
- children's adjustment and custody preferences
- factors for and against joint custody

- factors for and against paternal custody
- factors for and against maternal custody
- recommendations.

Guidelines on testifying in court in child custody cases are presented in Munsinger and Karlson (1996). A developing witness skills pack is available from the British Psychological Society and gives guidance on presenting expert testimony in court and managing cross-examination (BPsS, 1996).

PARENTAL ALIENATION SYNDROME

The parental alienation syndrome (PAS) is a construct over which there is considerable controversy. It will be some time before the scientific community reaches a consensus on PAS but in the mean time it is important for clinical psychologists in training to be aware of the construct. Gardner (1998) argues that PAS is a psychological disorder which children develop in the course of child-custody disputes (Gardner, 1998). With PAS, the child denigrates the alienated parent without justification, in response to programming, brainwashing and indoctrination by the other parent. This denigration may range from mild animosity, through moderate disrespect, to severe violence and fabrication of accusations of abuse and neglect against the target parent. The alienating parent's reason for brainwashing the child to denigrate the target parent is to gain leverage in court. The child is motivated to denigrate the target parent by a fear of being rejected by the other parent for not doing so. Children with PAS meet the following criteria: (1) they engage in a campaign of denigration; (2) they may offer weak, frivolous or absurd rationalizations for the deprecation; (3) they show a lack of ambivalence in their relationships with their parents, viewing one as 'all good' and the other as 'all bad'; (4) they insist that they have not been brainwashed by the other parent but have developed their hatred of one parent independently; (5) they show reflexive support for the alienating parent in the parental conflict; (6) they show an absence of guilt over cruelty to, and exploitation of, the alienated parent; (7) they use age-inappropriate language and scenarios repeated almost verbatim, borrowed from the alienating parent in his or her campaign of denigration against the targeted parent; (8) they spread their animosity to friends and extended family members. An important clinical issue is to determine whether allegations of mistreatment of the child by the targeted parent reflect actual child abuse or a fabricated account reflective of PAS. To make this differential diagnosis it is important to assess youngsters for abuse and neglect. Children who have been abused or neglected report the experience in age-appropriate language. In cases of actual abuse or neglect there is usually evidence of personal and contextual pre-disposing risk factors, triggering factors for each episode and maintaining factors for the duration of the abuse, as outlined in Chapters 19, 20 and 21. It is probably difficult to establish the presence or absence of such factors in cases of PAS.

MEDIATION AND CONCILIATION

While conducting custody evaluations and providing therapy for children's post-separation adjustment problems are the principal services that clinical psychologists typically offer to families where separation has occurred, increasingly, psychologists are becoming involved in mediation. Mediation (or conciliation as it is often called in the UK) is a structured approach to negotiating agreements about childcare and financial issues where marital partners are separating (Benjamin & Irving, 1995; Emery & Wyre, 1987; Folberg & Milne, 1988; Walker, 1989). Mediation is a co-operative alternative to adversarial litigation and, in most instances, mediation is far less stressful for children. It may be conducted by a clinical psychologist (with special mediation training) or by a psychologist and lawyer team. When mediation and litigation are compared, mediation is more efficient and effective in leading to initial agreements about childcare arrangements and finances. It is also far less costly to the family and the State. Mediation may also lead to better long-term co-operation between partners in managing children. However, mediation does not ameliorate short-term psychological distress and adjustment problems associated with divorce. Guidelines on how to conduct mediation are presented in Folberg and Milne (1988).

SUMMARY

Separation and divorce are no longer considered to be aberrations in the normal family lifecycle but normative transitions for between a third and a half of all families. Difficulties with communication and intimacy on the one hand and the power balance or role structure of the marriage on the other are the two major reasons for separation. Prior to separation, a negative cognitive style coupled with an increase in negative interactions lead to growing negative feelings for both partners. Partners become isolated from each other and begin to live parallel lives. Economic difficulties are a primary reason for women not divorcing, while men give primacy to the fear of separation from their children. Parental adjustment to divorce is influenced by a range of risk and protective factors. The stresses and strains of residential changes, economic hardship, role changes and consequent physical and psychological difficulties associated with the immediate aftermath of separation and divorce may compromise parents' capacity to co-operate in meeting their children's needs for supportive relationships with each parent and clear, consistent discipline from both parents. For the two-year period immediately following divorce, most children show some adjustment problems; 20–25% of children of divorced parents show serious long-term psychological problems. Such children typically have a profile characterized by many risk factors and few protective factors. Family transformation through separation, divorce and re-marriage may be conceptualized as a process involving a series of stages. Failure to complete tasks at one stage may lead to adjustment problems for family members at later stages. When families present with post-separation adjustment difficulties, a multi-systemic intervention package based on a thorough assessment and formulation is the management approach of choice. Such intervention programmes should contain some of the following elements: psychoeducation, clarifying family routines and roles, arranging cross-household consistency in parenting, parenting skills training, facilitating support for the child from the school and the extended family, providing support for parents and children and facilitating grieving. In child custody evaluations, the central question typically concerns the best parenting environment for the child. A child custody evaluation should typically include individual and conjoint interviews with both parents, the involved children, and relevant members of the extended family, along with home visits, observation of parent–child interaction and reviews of other relevant professional reports. The decision about what is in the child's best interests must be based on evaluation of each of the parent's capacities to meet the child's needs for safety, care, control and education and factors that have a bearing on these capacities.

EXERCISE 23.1

Laura (aged 9) and Betty (aged 12) are referred for psychological consultation because they are both very tearful at school and are not sleeping well. They also refuse to speak to their mother's new partner, John. The mother, Nancy, has been seeing John regularly for six months. He lives in his own apartment but sleeps over at Nancy' house about 50% of the time. The children stay with their father, Louis, on three days (Friday, Saturday and Sunday) one week and four days the next (Monday, Tuesday, Wednesday and Thursday). Nancy and Louis are still very angry at each other. Louis blames Nancy for the separation. He says she did not support his career in building construction. He makes his views known to the girls regularly. Nancy blames Louis for never being available to help with the children and for infidelity. She lets the children know her views regularly. The children have remained at the same school which has a primary and secondary section since the separation two and a half years ago.

- Write a formulation for this case, a plan for assessment and speculate on what components might be included in a treatment programme.
- Role-play preliminary interviews with: (1) the children; (2) Nancy and John; and (3) Louis.

FURTHER READING FOR CLINICIANS

Dowling, E. & Gorell-Barnes, G. (1999). *Working with Children and Parents Through Separation and Divorce: The Changing Lives of Children.* Basingstoke, UK: Macmillan Press.

Folberg, J. & Milne, A. (1988). *Divorce Mediation: Theory and Practice.* New York: Guilford.

Gardner, R. (1989). *Family Evaluation In Child Custody Mediation, Arbitration, And Litigation.* Cresskill, NJ: Creative Therapeutics.

Stahl, P. (1994). *Conducting Child Custody Evaluations: A Comprehensive Guide.* Thousand Oaks, CA: Sage.

Visher, E. & Visher, J. (1988). *Old Loyalties, New Ties: Therapeutic Strategies With Step-Families.* New York; Brunner Mazel.

FURTHER READING FOR CLIENTS

Althea, A. (1980). *I Have Two Homes.* Cambridge: Dinosaur Publications.

Benedek, E. & Brown, C. (1995). *Helping Your Child Through Divorce.* Washington, DC: APPI Press.

Bernet, W (1995). *Children of Divorce.* New York: Vantage Press.

Cohen, J. (1994). *Helping Your Grandchildren Through Their Parents' Divorce.* New York: Walker and Company.

Herbert, M. (1996). *Separation and Divorce: Helping Children Cope.* Leicester: British Psychological Society.

Hetherington, E. & Kelly, J. (2002). *For Better or for Worse: Divorce Reconsidered.* New York: Norton.

Hildebrand, J. (1988). *Surviving Marital Breakdown. Emotional and Behavioural Problems in Adolescents: A Multidisciplinary Approach to Identification and Management.* Windsor, Berkshire: NFER Nelson.

Ives, S. & Fassler, D. (1985). *Changing Families: A Guide for Kids and Grown-ups.* Burlington, VT: Waterfront Books.

Ives, S. & Fassler, D. (1985). *The Divorce Workbook: A Guide for Kids and Families.* Burlington, VT: Waterfront Books.

Ives, S., Fassler, D., & Lash, M. (1994). *The Divorce Workbook.* Burlington, VT: Waterfront Books.

Krashny, L. & Brown, M. (1988). *Dinosaurs Divorce: A Guide for Changing Families.* Boston, MA: Little Brown.

Lansky, V. (1996). *Vicki Lansky's Divorce Book for Parents – Helping Your Children Cope with Divorce and Its Aftermath* (Third edition). New York: Book Peddlers.

LeShan, E. (1986). *What's Going to Happen to Me: When Parents Separate or Divorce* (Revised edition). New York: MacMillan.

Neuman, G. & Romanowski, P. (1998). *Helping your Kids Cope with Divorce*. New York: Times Books.

Sharry, J., Reid, P., & Donohoe, E. (2001). *When Parents Separate: Helping Your Children Cope*. Dublin: Veritas.

Stolberg, A., Zacharias, M., & Complair, C.W. (1991). *Children of Divorce: Leaders Guide, Kids Book and Parents Book*. Circle Pines, MN: American Guidance Service.

Visher, E. & Visher, J. (1982). *How to Win as a Step-Family*. New York: Dembner.

Wallerstein, J. & Blakeslee, S. (1989). *Second Chances*. New York: Ticknor and Fields.

Wallerstein, J. & Kelly, J. (1980). *Surviving the Break-up: How Children and Parents Cope with Divorce*. New York: Basic Books.

WEBSITES

Divorce source website: http://www.divorcesource.com
Mediation website: http://www.mediate.com/

Factsheets on divorce and parental separation can be downloaded from the website for Rose, G. & York, A. (2004). *Mental Health and Growing Up. Fact sheets for Parents, Teachers and Young People* (Third edition). London: Gaskell: http://www.rcpsych.ac.uk

Chapter 24

Grief and bereavement

Psychological consultation to children and families where the child's adjustment to bereavement or a life-threatening condition is the central concern, is examined in this chapter. Bereavement is an inevitable part of the lifecycle. During childhood and adolescence most children experience the death of a family member or friend and manage the process of grieving satisfactorily. However, in some circumstances bereavement impairs the child's adjustment to a marked degree or the youngster's grief reactions do not conform to the expectations of significant members of their social network, particularly their parents (Black, 2000, 2002; Corr & Balk, 1996; Kissane & Block, 2002; Smith & Pennell, 1996; Stroebe, Hansson, Stroebe & Schut, 2001; Walsh & McGoldrick, 2004; Webb, 2002; Worden, 2002). Such expectations may be coloured by the parents' or network members' own grief reactions and also by popular misconceptions about grief propagated by the media. Thus, both the child's behavioural reactions following bereavement and expectations of significant others may prompt a referral for psychological consultation. An example of such a routine referral is presented in Box 24.1. Children may also be referred for psychological consultation when they have been diagnosed as having a life-threatening illness or injury (Abu-Saad, 2001; Black, 1994; Hurwitz, Duncan & Wolfe, 2004). Children's adjustment to bereavement or life-threatening medical conditions is in part dependent on their understanding of the concept of death. This chapter begins, therefore, with a discussion of the development, through childhood and adolescence, of the concept of death. This is followed by a description of grief processes, a review of theoretical explanations for these processes and a summary of the available evidence on types of grief reactions. A framework for conceptualizing the wide variety of factors that influence grief reactions is then given. The assessment and management of cases where grief is a central issue is then presented.

Box 24.1 Case study on bereavement

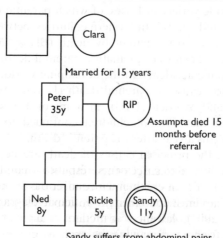

Married for 15 years

Assumpta died 15
months before
referral

Sandy suffers from abdominal pains,
sleeplessness and school problems

Sandy was an eleven-year-old girl referred in February because of abdominal pains,
sleeplessness and school problems. She was falling behind in her schoolwork and
had become increasingly isolated from her peer group over the preceding few
months. A paediatric examination showed that the abdominal pains were not due to
clearly identifiable organic factors. Sandy lived with her father, Peter, and two
younger brothers, Ned (8 years) and Rickie (5 years). Sandy's mother, Assumpta, had
died about 15 months previously following a lengthy battle with cancer. Assumpta
had died peacefully in her husband's arms. The children attended the funeral and
Peter's mother, Clara, who lived nearby had helped to care for the three children in
the wake of Assumpta's death. Over the next year, Sandy was the best adjusted of the
three children. The two boys became defiant and aggressive and posed a great
challenge for Peter and his mother to manage. Sandy, however had been tearful and
sad for some months but never troublesome. Peter, had buried himself in his work
for much of the year but recently on the advice of the GP had begun to play tennis
regularly and had begun to socialize again. The whole family, who were Roman
Catholics, had attended the anniversary Mass, three months prior to the referral
and following this, Sandy had become very tearful and despairing. Over the
subsequent three months, she had distanced herself from her peers at school and
left the hockey team. She criticized her father for his attempts at developing a social
life. Periodically, she developed stomachaches for which no organic cause could be
found and, on occasion, her father had been recalled from work or tennis to take
Sandy to the family doctor. Sandy occasionally had dreams in which she and her
mother were together again.

EPIDEMIOLOGICAL ISSUES

Children suffer a wide variety of losses, of which parental death is probably the most traumatic and painful. In Western countries, between 1.5 and 4% of children under 18 have lost a parent by death (Black, 2002). In Western countries, the principal causes of premature parental death are cancer, heart disease and road traffic accidents; in the developing world, HIV/AIDS is an increasingly common cause of parental death (Havens, Mellins & Hunter, 2002). Silverman and Worden (1993), in a major US study of parental bereavement, found that 19% of children continued to show significant psychological problems a year after the parent's death.

Among children, the principal causes of death are peri-natal complications, congenital abnormalities, accidents, respiratory conditions and cancer (Black, 1994). About 25% of children with cancer die of their disease and so they and their families must cope with the anticipatory grief of this eventuality (Hurwitz et al., 2004). Advances in modern medicine have increased the survival rate for life-threatening illnesses such as cancer or renal failure. While many children survive into adulthood, for a significant minority the prolongation of life through intensive medical care takes its toll. Before the advent of modern sophisticated medical techniques, these children and their families would have been exposed to the acute trauma of a relatively sudden childhood death. Now, they are exposed to the chronic stress of living in the shadow of death. In many instances, children die not from a disease process but from complications associated with their medical treatment. Where children survive, they and their families must find a way to live with the side effects of treatment, which may include disfigurement, frailty, limited autonomy and sterility. It is therefore not surprising that about 30–40% of children with severe paediatric illness develop significant psychological problems (Mrazek, 2002).

DEVELOPMENT OF DEATH CONCEPT

Much of the work on the development of the concept of death has been guided by Piagetian theory, which argues that the child's concept of death is constrained by the availability of certain cognitive skills (Kenyon, 2001; Spence & Brent, 1984; Stambrook & Parker, 1987). According to Piagetian theory, the pre-operational child (under seven years) should not be able to understand the irreversibility of death and may confuse it with sleep. Also, the inability of pre-operational children to distinguish thought and action may lead them to hold beliefs such as their anger towards someone caused that person to die. Once children reach the concrete operational stage, according to Piagetian theory, they understand the irreversibility of death but they may have difficulty accepting its universality and so may not be able to conceptualize death as something that will happen to them. Rather, they may view it as being confined to the old, the frail and those in apparent danger. With the onset of the formal operational period in early adolescence, the universality of death comes to be fully appreciated. That is, according to Piaget, young teenagers realize that they will die.

Empirical studies reviewed by Kenyon (2001) and Spence and Brent (1984) show that the evolution of the concept of death follows the broad pattern suggested by Piaget but that there are many exceptions because children's concept of death evolves not only as cognitive maturation occurs but also as experience of death broadens. The key features of death may be appreciated by children during the pre-operational stage, provided they have been exposed to particular death-related experiences, such as having a terminal illness or having experienced multiple bereavements. These key features include the irreversibility of death, which entails the view that the dead cannot return to life; the universality of death, which entails the view that all creatures die; and the functionality of death, which entails the view that all functions cease at death. While most adolescents recognize the inevitability of their own death at a cognitive level, the full emotional significance of this is not apprehended until adulthood, unless multiple bereavements or other traumatic events occur. Kalish and Reynolds (1976), in a survey of over 400 adults, found that the number of people who emotionally accepted the inevitability of their own death increased as a function of age. In early adulthood, 36% of respondents accepted that they would inevitably die. In middle adulthood the figure rose to 52% and in later adulthood 71% accepted the inevitability of their own death.

GRIEF PROCESSES, RESPONSE PATTERNS AND ADJUSTMENT PROBLEMS

For children, following bereavement or during the course of a life-threatening illness, there is considerable variability in grief processes, response patterns and related adjustment difficulties (Black, 2000, 2002; Silverman & Worden, 1993; Wortman & Silver, 1989, 2001). Some children manage the death of significant members of their network or their own impending death with considerable courage and resilience; others do not. Within Western culture, the normative expectation is for people facing a serious loss to show extreme initial distress, which declines with time. However, this is just one of three common patterns. In the second pattern, extreme protracted distress occurs and the third pattern is characterized by little distress initially or later. These latter two grief response patterns are also referred to as morbid grief and absent grief, respectively. Both of these grief response patterns may lead to referral because they are outside our cultural expectations. There is also some evidence that children adjust to bereavement and life-threatening illness more quickly than adults, so in some instances, children who have completed their grief work more rapidly than their parents may be referred for assessment because of their apparent failure to grieve.

Following bereavement, or during adjustment to life-threatening illness, children may be referred for psychological consultation because they display one or more highly salient adjustment difficulties. These include internalizing or externalizing behaviour problems, somatic complaints such as stomach-aches, poor adherence to medical regimes, school problems and relationship difficulties within the family or peer group. All of these types of problems typically reflect the child's involvement in one or more of the following grief processes:

- shock
- denial or disbelief
- yearning and searching
- sadness
- anger
- anxiety
- guilt and bargaining
- acceptance.

There is not a clear-cut progression through these processes from one to the next (Black, 1994, 2000, 2002; Corr & Balk, 1996; Kissane & Block, 2002; Smith & Pennell, 1996; Stroebe et al., 2001; Walsh & McGoldrick, 2004; Webb, 2002; Worden, 2002). Rather, at different points in time one or other process pre-dominates when a child has experienced a loss or faces death, and there may be movement back and forth between processes.

Shock is the most common initial reaction, it can take the form of physical pain, numbness, apathy or withdrawal. The child may appear to be stunned and unable to think clearly. This may be accompanied by denial, disbelief or avoidance of the reality of the bereavement, a process that can last minutes, days or even months. During denial, children may behave as if the dead person is still living, albeit elsewhere. Thus, the child may speak about future plans that involve the deceased. Terminally ill children may talk about them-selves and their future as if they were going to live through until old age.

A yearning to be with the deceased, coupled with disbelief about their death, may lead the child to engage in frantic searches for the dead person, wandering or running away from the home in a quest for the person who has died. The child may telephone relatives or friends trying to trace the person who has died. During this process, children who have lost family members or very close friends report seeing them or being visited by them. Some children carry on full conversations with what presumably are hallucinations of the deceased person. Mistaking other people for the deceased is also a com-mon experience during the denial process. Children may be referred for psychological assessment because of denial-related behaviours such as running away or insisting that they can see and hear the dead person. With terminally ill children, the yearning for health may lead to a frantic search for a miracle cure and to involvement in alternative medicine.

When denial gives way to a realization of the irreversibility of the death, the child may experience profound sadness, despair, hopelessness and depression. The experience of sadness may be accompanied by low energy, sleep disruption, a disturbance of appetite, tearfulness, an inability to concentrate and a retreat from social interaction. The child's experience is expressed in the sentiment 'I am lost and lonely without you'. Young children experiencing the despair process may regress and begin to behave as if they were babies again, wetting their beds and sucking their thumbs, hoping that, by becoming a baby, the dead person may return to comfort them. This type of wish reflects the magical thinking of the pre-operational child. Regressed behaviour or depressed mood may precipitate a referral for psychological consultation. With children who are terminally ill, despair, hopelessness and depression find expression in an unwillingness to fight the illness.

Complementing the despair process, there is also an anger process, which, for bereaved children, may be expressed in the sentiment 'I am angry because you abandoned me forever'. Temper tantrums, misbehaviour, defiance, delinquency, drug and alcohol abuse, refusal to go to school or to complete school work are some of the common ways that grief-related anger finds expression in children and teenagers. All of these troublesome behaviours may lead the youngster to be referred for psychological assessment. With children who are suffering from terminal illness, the anger may be projected onto family members, members of the medical team, friends or teachers and conflicts in these relationships, in which intense anger is expressed, may occur. This often involves an angry refusal to adhere to medical regimes, to take medication or to participate in physiotherapy.

The expression of such anger may often be followed by remorse or fear of retribution. Young children may fear that the deceased person will punish them for their anger and so it is not surprising that they may want to leave the light on at night and may be afraid to go to bed alone. In older children and adolescents, anxiety is attached to reality-based threats. So, children who have lost a friend or family member through illness or an accident may worry that they too will die from similar causes. This can lead to a belief that one is seriously ill and to a variety of somatic complaints such as stomachaches and headaches. It may also lead to a refusal to leave home lest a fatal accident occur. Referral for assessment of separation anxiety, recurrent abdominal pain, headaches, hypochondriasis and agoraphobia may occur in these cases. The guilt process is marked by self-blame for causing or not preventing the death of the deceased. There may also be thoughts that if the surviving child died this might magically bring back the deceased. Thus, the guilt process may under-pin suicidal ideation or self-injury, which invariably leads to referral for mental health assessment. With children who are terminally ill, the illness may be experienced as a punishment for having done something wrong. This sense of guilt under-pins the bargaining process in which many youngsters facing death engage. The bargaining process is reflected in the following sentiment 'If you let me live, I promise to be good'.

The final grief process is acceptance. With bereavement, the child reconstructs their view of the world so that the deceased person is construed as no longer living in this world, but a benign and accessible representation of them is constructed, which is consistent with the family's belief system. For example, a Christian child may imagine that their parent is in heaven and looking down on them in a protective way. Most children maintain a relationship with this representation of the deceased through the use of symbols and rituals. So children may regularly look at photographs, gifts, and belongings of the deceased. They may regularly visit the grave or a place of special significance and carry on imaginary dialogues with the deceased. For terminally ill children, the acceptance involves a modification of the world view so that the future is foreshortened and therefore the time remaining is highly valued and is spent living life to the full rather than searching in vain for a miracle cure.

For the bereaved child, new lifestyle routines are evolved as part of the process of accepting the death and the child's family system and broader social network is re-organized to take account of the absence of the deceased person. If children have been well supported during the early stages of grief, they may show increased maturity and psychological strength once they take steps towards acceptance. Children who lose friends or siblings through death may become more compassionate and understanding. Those that lose a parent may become more responsible and helpful in the management of the household. For terminally ill children, once the child and family accept the inevitability of the child's immanent death, routines which enhance the quality of life of the dying child may be evolved.

A summary of the grief processes and related adjustment problems that may lead to referral is presented in Table 24.1.

GRIEF THEORIES

Many theories have been developed to offer a coherent explanation for these grief-related processes. Some of the more important conceptualizations have been grouped here under six headings: biological theories, psychoanalytic theories, behavioural theories, family systems theories, stage theories and psychosocial transition theories.

Table 24.1 Behavioural expressions of themes underlying children's grief processes following bereavement or facing terminal illness that may lead to referral

Grief process	Bereavement Underlying theme	Behavioural expressions of grief processes that may lead to referral	Terminal illness Underlying theme	Behavioural expressions of grief processes that may lead to referral
Shock	• I am stunned by the loss of this person	• Complete lack of affect and difficulty engaging emotionally with others • Poor concentration and poor schoolwork	• I am stunned by my prognosis and loss of health	• Complete lack of affect and difficulty engaging emotionally with others • Poor concentration and poor schoolwork
Denial	• The person is not dead	• Reporting seeing or hearing the deceased • Carrying on conversations with the deceased	• I am not terminally ill	• Non-compliance with medical regime
Yearning and searching	• I must find the deceased	• Wandering or running away • Phoning relatives	• I will find a miracle cure	• Experimentation with alternative medicine
Sadness	• I am sad, hopeless and lonely because I have lost someone on whom I depended	• Persistent low mood, tearfulness, low energy and lack of activity • Appetite and sleep disruption • Poor concentration and poor schoolwork	• I am sad and hopeless because I know I will die	• Giving up the fight against illness • Persistent low mood, tearfulness, low energy and lack of activity • Appetite and sleep disruption • Poor concentration and poor schoolwork

Anger	• I am angry because the person I needed has abandoned me	• Aggression, tantrums, defiance, delinquency • Conflict with parents, siblings, teachers and peers • Drug or alcohol abuse • Poor concentration and poor schoolwork	• I am angry because it's not fair. I should be allowed to live	• Non-compliance with medical regime • Aggression, tantrums, defiance, delinquency • Conflict with medical staff, parents, siblings, teachers and peers • Drug or alcohol abuse • Poor concentration and poor schoolwork
Anxiety	• I am frightened that the deceased will punish me for causing their death or being angry at them. I am afraid that I too may die of an illness or fatal accident	• Separation anxiety, school refusal, regressed behaviour, bedwetting • Somatic complaints, hypochondriasis and agoraphobia associated with a fear of accidents • Poor concentration and poor schoolwork	• I am frightened that death will be painful or terrifying	• Separation anxiety and regressed behaviour
Guilt and bargaining	• It is my fault that the person died so I should die	• Suicidal behaviour	• I will be good if I am allowed to live	• Over-compliance with medical regime
Acceptance	• I loved and lost the person who died and now I must carry on without them while cherishing their memory	• Return to normal behavioural routines	• I know that I have only a short time left to live	• Attempts to live life to the full for the remaining time

Biological theories

Biological conceptualization of the grief process focuses on the impact of loss on physiological functioning. In its broadest form, the biological hypothesis concerning grief is that individuals faced with the stress of bereavement or a life-threatening illness react with a variety of physiological responses, notably immunosuppression, and this in turn leads to greater mortality and morbidity. Available epidemiological evidence, largely from studies of adults, supports this, as does the limited body of evidence from studies of immunological process of adults and animals following bereavement (Hall & Irwin, 2001; Segerstrom & Miller, 2004).

Psychoanalytic theory

Freud (1917) argued that, following loss of a loved one, there is a tendency to psychologically prolong the existence of the loved one by fantasizing that they continue to live. However, this tendency is combated by the process of reality testing. Where this does not occur, Freud believed that morbid grief reactions may develop and that psychotherapy, which facilitates grief work, is necessary. Each memory and expectation concerning the loved one has to be brought into consciousness, confronted, worked through and tested against the reality of the deceased's absence. Eventually, this grief work leads to detachment from the loved one and the bereaved person is free to become attached to others. Following Freud, Lindeman (1944, 1979), also working within the psychoanalytic tradition, argued that the process of remembering the deceased and working through feelings of loss was optimally achieved gradually, by a process not unlike desensitization. At each step, increasingly more painful memories are recalled and processed, until all have been confronted and endured. Results of a small handful of treatment outcome studies show that brief psychodynamic psychotherapy can lead to improved functioning in bereaved adults, but data for children are unavailable (Raphael, Minkov & Dobson, 2001).

Cognitive-behavioural theories

Cognitive-behavioural formulations of pathological grief reactions argue that memories of the deceased and specific environmental cues that remind the person of the deceased are perceived as highly aversive stimuli, since they evoke negative grief-related emotions (Fleming & Robinson, 2001; Malkinson, 2001). These internal and external aversive stimuli are avoided by the cognitive processes of distraction or suppression or behavioural avoidance. These cognitive and behavioural avoidance responses are negatively reinforced because they bring relief by distancing the person from the aversive stimuli. However, the behavioural avoidance responses lead to a constricted lifestyle and the cognitive avoidance responses lead to a failure to emotionally process memories of the deceased, which continue to intrude into consciousness and cause distress. Behavioural treatment involves gradual or sudden exposure to the internal and external grief-eliciting stimuli within the context of a supportive therapeutic relationship. Treatment of morbid grief with desensitization to grief-related material or flooding with grief stimuli has been shown to be effective with adults, but controlled studies with children have not been conducted (Malkinson, 2001).

Family systems theories

Family systems conceptualizations of grief focus on the social context within which bereavement and grief reactions occur (Walsh & McGoldrick, 2004). Bereavement is viewed as a normative event in the family lifecycle that requires members of the family to complete two specific tasks. First, to acknowledge the shared experience of loss, and second to reorganize roles, routines, rules and relationships within the family to take account of the deceased. Family adaptation to loss is influenced by the unique circumstances of the death or loss; the family structure, functioning and lifecycle stage; and the family's sociocultural context. Where children face grief-related difficulties, family therapy facilitates acknowledgement of the shared loss experience and reorganization of the family system to take account of the loss. Family therapy has been shown to help children adjust to bereavement (Kissane & Bloch, 2002). In one controlled study, the morbidity was reduced from 40% to 20% in a group of children who had lost a parent (Black & Urbanowicz, 1987).

Stage theories

Various theorists have argued that grief following bereavement, and anticipatory grief prior to death, may be conceptualized as a sequence of stages through which the individual passes from initial shock towards an end-point of resolution. Bowlby (1969, 1973, 1980, 1988) conceptualized loss and bereavement within the framework of attachment theory and argued that the function of grief was to motivate the person to seek proximity with a primary attachment figure. Thus, immediately following bereavement there is a period of protesting against separation, characterized by shock, pining and anger. This is followed by a period of despair when the reality of the separation is acknowledged and the internal representational models of self in relation to significant others are modified. In this modified representational model, the deceased exists in the past but not the present as a significant attachment figure. Once this cognitive restructuring is complete, detachment occurs and the bereaved person is free to form other attachments. Thus progression through the stages of protest, despair and detachment are central to Bowlby's conceptualization of grief.

Kübler-Ross (1969, 1974, 1982, 1983) conceptualized the anticipatory grieving of people facing death as involving a progression through the stages of denial, anger, bargaining for extra time, depression and acceptance. The first three of these stages (denial, anger and bargaining) bear a remarkable resemblance to Bowlby's protest stage. Kübler-Ross' stages of depression and acceptance closely resemble Bowlby's stages of despair and detachment, respectively.

Longitudinal research has shown that there is wide variability in the temporal patterning grief reactions, which cannot be accounted for by simplistic stage models (Wortman & Silver, 1989, 2001). Many people do not experience distress and do not require a period to work through their grief. From a clinical perspective, it is accurate to assume that some children will experience some of the types of processes described by stage theorists, but not necessarily in an invariant order.

Psychosocial transition theories

Parkes (1993) conceptualized bereavement and life-threatening illness as psychosocial transitions where the central task is modification of the assumptive world, so that the loss is coherently accommodated into the person's world view. This task of modifying the assumptive world is achieved by identifying discrepancies between the external world and the assumptive world. This entails reviewing routines of daily life and the old assumptions about how one's life and relationships were organized before bereavement or the diagnosis of terminal illness occurred. This process is emotionally painful. People cope with this pain and anxiety by using denial-based defences or distraction-based coping strategies, which regulate the pace at which grief-related material is processed.

The modification of the assumptive world is important, since an accurate assumptive world is vital for safety and survival. Without an accurate assumptive world, many events are experienced as unpredictable, and people feel unsafe, anxious and disorganized. Common strategies for coping with this sense of anxiety include avoidance of demanding social situations and confiding in a small number of trusted people.

People's assumptive worlds are shaped by a variety of personal and contextual factors, such as significant life experiences, family system characteristics and wider cultural and religious beliefs and practices. The ease with which bereavement or loss experiences can be incorporated into one's world view varies, depending on the content and flexibility of the world view, the type of loss experience and the availability of personal and contextual coping resources to aid the incorporation of the loss into the world view. Wortman and Silver (2001) have shown that, with adults, the wide variability in adult grief reactions can be largely accounted for by the ease with which the loss experience can be incorporated into the world view. Where this accommodation process happens relatively easily, grief may be quickly resolved. However, where, the loss requires major revisions to the person's world view, then a protracted grieving process may occur. Thus, adults who have a strong sense of self-efficacy, an internal locus of control and a history of achievement are particularly vulnerable to untimely bereavement, since they find such uncontrollable loss requires a major revision of their view of themselves and the degree of control they have over significant life events. In contrast, Silverman and Worden (1993) found that children with an internal locus of control showed more rapid recovery following bereavement.

Self-help groups are the treatment interventions most closely aligned with psychosocial transition theories of bereavement. Self-help groups provide a supportive forum within which to review one's world view and receive credible feedback from people in similar circumstances. Unfortunately, data on the efficacy of such groups for children and adolescents are unavailable (Lieberman, 1993).

A summary of the key principles of each of the types of grief theory reviewed in this section is presented in Table 24.2.

EMPIRICAL FINDINGS CONCERNING GRIEF REACTIONS

Reviews of empirical studies of bereavement and loss allow a number of conclusions to be drawn which are of particular relevance to clinical practice (Black, 2000, 2002; Corr & Balk, 1996; Kissane & Block, 2002; Smith & Pennell, 1996; Stroebe et al., 2001; Walsh & McGoldrick, 2004; Webb, 2002; Worden, 2002). First, grief processes either anticipatory or grief following loss, do not occur as an ordered and invariant sequence of stages as suggested by Bowlby and Kübler-Ross. There is a progression from shock through a variety of emotional reactions including anger, depression, anxiety and guilt to acceptance. However, there is wide variability in the way this progression occurs and not everyone experiences all processes. Second, depression following bereavement is not universal; only about a third of people suffer depression following bereavement. Third, failure to show emotional distress initially does not necessarily mean that later adjustment problems are inevitable. It appears that different people use different coping strategies to cope with loss. Some use distraction or avoidance, while others use confrontation of the grief experience and working through. Those who effectively use the former coping strategy may not show emotional distress. Fourth, extreme distress following bereavement commonly occurs in those who show protracted grief reactions. Fifth, not everyone needs to work through their sense of loss by immediate intensive conversation about it. Many people who work through their sense of loss early have later problems. Sixth, a return to normal functioning does not always occur rapidly. While the majority of people approximate normal functioning within two years, a substantial minority of bereaved people

Table 24.2 Theories of grief

Theories	Hypothesis
Biological theories	The stress of bereavement leads to immunosuppression and this in turn leads to greater mortality and morbidity following bereavement
Psychoanalytic theories	Grief work involves subjecting the fantasy of the deceased's continued existence to reality testing and working through the related painful emotions
Cognitive-behavioural theories	Grief work involves desensitization to memories and cues that provoke distress associated with loss
Family systems theory	Bereavement is a normative event in the family lifecycle that requires members of the family to acknowledge the shared experience of loss and to re-organize roles, routines, rules and relationships within the family to take account of the loss. Family adaptation to loss is influenced by the circumstances of the death or loss; the family structure, functioning and lifecycle stage; and the sociocultural context
Stage theories	Anticipatory grief work (in the case of life-threatening illness) or grief work following bereavement involves movement through a series of invariantly ordered stages. These include an initial stage where denial and anger are central themes; a midstage where despair is the core theme; and a final stage where acceptance of the loss occurs
Psychosocial transition theories	Bereavement is a psychosocial transition, where a central task is the modification of the world views by reviewing discrepancies between the external world and the assumptive world. Defences and coping strategies are used to pace this process. The ease with which bereavement or loss experiences can be incorporated into one's world view varies, depending on the world view itself; the type of loss experience and the availability of personal and contextual coping resources that can aid the incorporation of the loss into the world view

continue to show adjustment difficulties even seven years after bereavement. Seventh, resolution and acceptance of death does not always occur. For example, parents who lose children or those who lose a loved one in an untimely fatal accident show protracted patterns of grief. Eighth, detachment, as described by Bowlby, often does not occur as part of children's grief processes. Rather, an internal representation of the deceased is constructed and the child continues to have a relationship with the deceased. Ninth, grief may have a marked effect on physical functioning. Infections and other illnesses are more common among bereaved children and this is probably due to the effect of loss-related stress on the functioning of the immune system. However, with the passage of time immune system functioning returns to normal. Tenth, children's grief reactions tend to be similar in form to those of adults but to be briefer and less intense, probably because in comparison with adults, children do not tend to focus for a protracted time period on memories or lost possibilities concerning the bereaved person. Children's anticipatory grief reactions to their own life-threatening illness are less intense than those found in adults with chronic illness. Also, parents of children with life-threatening illness tend to show more profound adjustment reactions to the condition than their children. The quality of the parents' marriage may change in response to childhood chronic illness, with discordant marriages becoming more discordant as the illness progresses and stable marriages remaining so as the child approaches death. Finally, bereavement, particularly loss of a parent, leaves children vulnerable to depression in adult life. Adults bereaved as children have double the risk of developing depression when faced with a loss experience in adult life compared with their non-bereaved counterparts. Bereaved children most at risk for depression in adulthood are girls who were young when their parents died a violent or sudden death and who subsequently received inadequate care associated with the surviving parent experiencing a prolonged grief reaction.

FACTORS THAT CONTRIBUTE TO ADJUSTMENT AFTER LOSS

The variability in children's grief reactions mentioned in the previous section may probably be accounted for by differences in loss-related stresses and differences in personal and contextual pre-disposing factors, problem maintaining factors and protective factors (Black, 2000, 2002; Corr & Balk, 1996; Kissane & Block, 2002; Smith & Pennell, 1996; Stroebe et al., 2001; Walsh & McGoldrick, 2004; Webb, 2002; Worden, 2002). A framework within which to conceptualize important variables in each of these categories is presented in Figure 24.1. This framework is a variation on Figure 2.1 (p. 42). To avoid repetition, in the following discussion only those variables which have been added to Figure 2.1 to give the framework contained in Figure 24.1 will be considered in detail.

Loss-related stresses

Unique features of loss experiences have an impact on children's adjustment. In the case of bereavement, the significance of the deceased to the child affects the course of the grieving process. The most profound grief occurs when a child loses a primary carer. Not only do such children lose a primary attachment relationship, but they are usually also exposed, over an extended time period, to the remaining parent's grief and may, in addition, suffer stresses associated with the financial hardship incurred by the loss of the

PRE-DISPOSING FACTORS

PERSONAL PRE-DISPOSING FACTORS

Biological factors
- History of life-threatening illness
- Age (between over 2 and 16)
- Genetic vulnerabilities

Psychological factors
- Low intelligence
- Difficult temperament
- Low self-esteem
- External locus of control

CONTEXTUAL PRE-DISPOSING FACTORS

Parent–child factors in early life
- Attachment problems
- Lack of intellectual stimulation
- Authoritarian parenting
- Permissive parenting
- Neglectful parenting
- Inconsistent parental discipline

Exposure to family problems in early life
- Parental psychological problems
- Parental alcohol and substance abuse
- Parental criminality
- Marital discord or violence
- Family disorganization
- Deviant siblings

Stresses in early life
- Bereavements
- Separations
- Child abuse
- Social disadvantage
- Institutional upbringing

PERSONAL PROTECTIVE FACTORS

Biological factors
- Under 2 or over 16
- Robust physical condition (if facing life-threatening illness)

Psychological factors
- High IQ
- Easy temperament

PERSONAL MAINTAINING FACTORS

Protracted shock
- Extreme denial
- Depressive cognition and self-defeating behaviour
- Extreme anger and blaming
- Anxiety, threat-related cognition and avoidance behaviour
- Guilt, self-blaming and self-harming behaviour

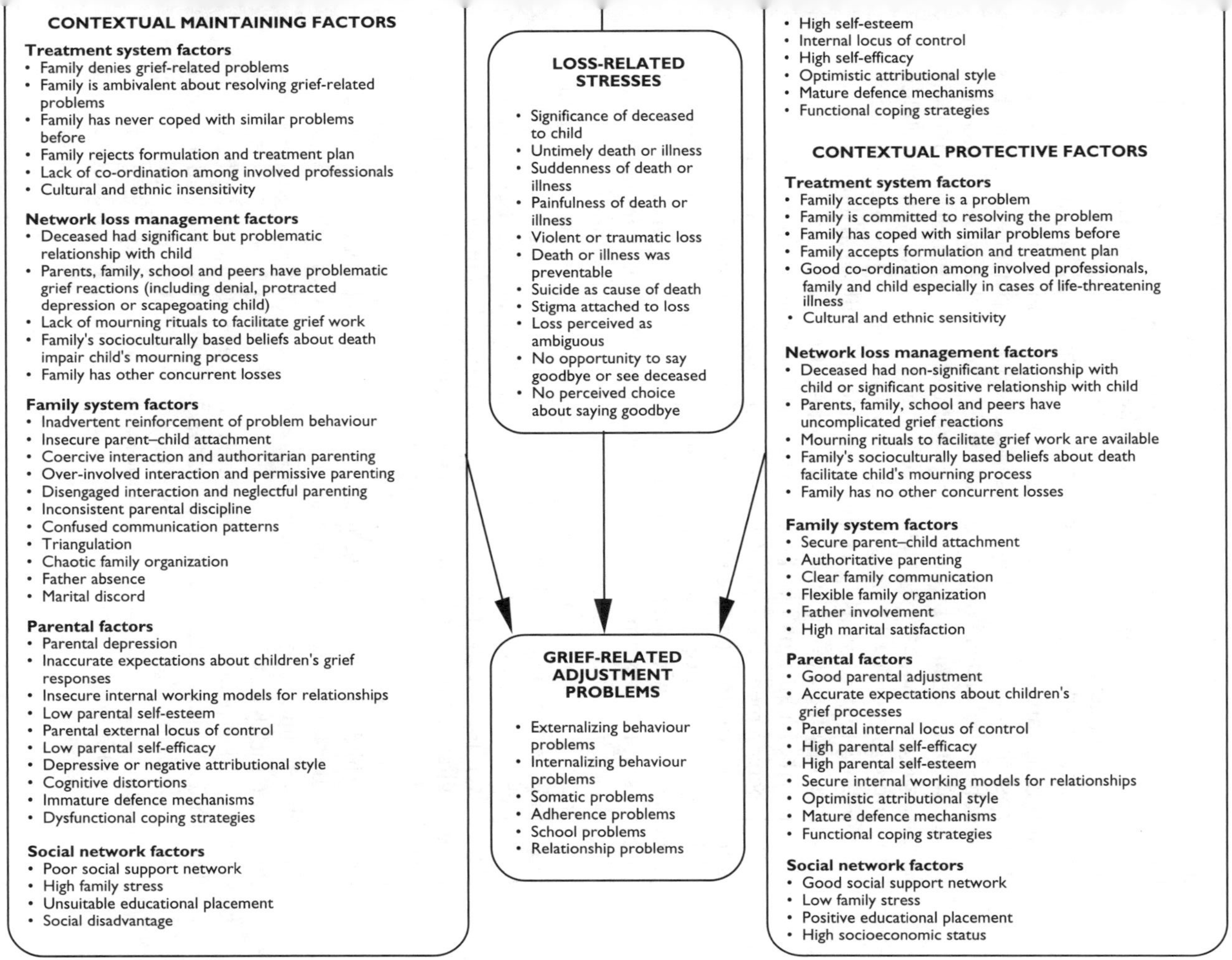

CONTEXTUAL MAINTAINING FACTORS

Treatment system factors
- Family denies grief-related problems
- Family is ambivalent about resolving grief-related problems
- Family has never coped with similar problems before
- Family rejects formulation and treatment plan
- Lack of co-ordination among involved professionals
- Cultural and ethnic insensitivity

Network loss management factors
- Deceased had significant but problematic relationship with child
- Parents, family, school and peers have problematic grief reactions (including denial, protracted depression or scapegoating child)
- Lack of mourning rituals to facilitate grief work
- Family's socioculturally based beliefs about death impair child's mourning process
- Family has other concurrent losses

Family system factors
- Inadvertent reinforcement of problem behaviour
- Insecure parent–child attachment
- Coercive interaction and authoritarian parenting
- Over-involved interaction and permissive parenting
- Disengaged interaction and neglectful parenting
- Inconsistent parental discipline
- Triangulation
- Chaotic family organization
- Father absence
- Marital discord
- Confused communication patterns

Parental factors
- Parental depression
- Inaccurate expectations about children's grief responses
- Insecure internal working models for relationships
- Low parental self-esteem
- Parental external locus of control
- Low parental self-efficacy
- Depressive or negative attributional style
- Cognitive distortions
- Immature defence mechanisms
- Dysfunctional coping strategies

Social network factors
- Poor social support network
- High family stress
- Unsuitable educational placement
- Social disadvantage

LOSS-RELATED STRESSES

- Significance of deceased to child
- Untimely death or illness
- Suddenness of death or illness
- Painfulness of death or illness
- Violent or traumatic loss
- Death or illness was preventable
- Suicide as cause of death
- Stigma attached to loss
- Loss perceived as ambiguous
- No opportunity to say goodbye or see deceased
- No perceived choice about saying goodbye

GRIEF-RELATED ADJUSTMENT PROBLEMS

- Externalizing behaviour problems
- Internalizing behaviour problems
- Somatic problems
- Adherence problems
- School problems
- Relationship problems

- High self-esteem
- Internal locus of control
- High self-efficacy
- Optimistic attributional style
- Mature defence mechanisms
- Functional coping strategies

CONTEXTUAL PROTECTIVE FACTORS

Treatment system factors
- Family accepts there is a problem
- Family is committed to resolving the problem
- Family has coped with similar problems before
- Family accepts formulation and treatment plan
- Good co-ordination among involved professionals, family and child especially in cases of life-threatening illness
- Cultural and ethnic sensitivity

Network loss management factors
- Deceased had non-significant relationship with child or significant positive relationship with child
- Parents, family, school and peers have uncomplicated grief reactions
- Mourning rituals to facilitate grief work are available
- Family's socioculturally based beliefs about death facilitate child's mourning process
- Family has no other concurrent losses

Family system factors
- Secure parent–child attachment
- Authoritative parenting
- Clear family communication
- Flexible family organization
- Father involvement
- High marital satisfaction

Parental factors
- Good parental adjustment
- Accurate expectations about children's grief processes
- Parental internal locus of control
- High parental self-efficacy
- High parental self-esteem
- Secure internal working models for relationships
- Optimistic attributional style
- Mature defence mechanisms
- Functional coping strategies

Social network factors
- Good social support network
- Low family stress
- Positive educational placement
- High socioeconomic status

Figure 24.1 Factors to consider in the assessment of children's grief reactions

parent, if he or she was a financial provider for the family. Where children have very ambivalent feelings about the attachment figure, this 'unfinished business' may exacerbate the grief reaction. That is, youngsters may feel they cannot lay their parent to rest because they still feel intense anger over unresolved conflicts.

Untimely deaths, for example when a child loses a young parent unexpectedly through a sudden accident, may have a more profound impact than those that occur in a timely way, such as when the parent is older and has undergone a protracted illness and is expected to die. When children face life-threatening illness, this is by definition an untimely loss in which the child and family's original hopes, expectations and plans associated with the child's future must be replaced with a more limited agenda to live life to the full for the time that remains. The more flexible the child and family are in reconstructing their world view to take account of the child's untimely death, the better the child's quality of life will be for his or her remaining days.

With bereavement, the suddenness of death, the painfulness and the degree of trauma or violence involved may all contribute to the intensity and quality of the grief experience, since sudden, painful and traumatic events require a greater degree of emotional processing and are less easily accommodated into the child's world view. Similarly, when children face life-threatening illness or injury following an accident, the more unexpected the diagnosis and prognosis, the painfulness of the condition and the trauma entailed by the condition and its treatment all have an impact on the child's adjustment. Unexpected diagnostic and prognostic information may be better processed if it is given repeatedly (for example, by permitting the family to audiotape the consultation) and in circumstances that allow the child and family to assimilate it gradually (such as in an extended consultation). The availability of psychological or pharmacological methods for pain control may make it easier for children to manage the grief of coping with their condition. Understanding the rationale for chemotherapy, radiotherapy or other treatments that have traumatic or unpleasant side effects may reduce their negative impact on the child.

With bereavement, particularly bereavement due to suicide and where children suffer certain illnesses such as AIDS or accidents that lead to fatal injury, children's views on the preventability of the loss may affect their adjustment. In all of these circumstances, the children may ask if they or others could have prevented the death, illness or injury. Where children and families become preoccupied with such issues, self-directed anger and guilt or anger at others may become central organizing themes in their grieving processes. This pre-occupation with preventability (and attributing culpability) may in some instances prevent assimilation of the loss into the world view and resolution of the loss. Where litigation occurs, for example for medical malpractice, following bereavement, this type of protraction of the grieving process may occur.

Where suicide is the cause of death, or in other instances where there is a stigma attached to the cause of death, as in the case of AIDS, adjustment to the loss may be compromised when families prevent the child from discussing the death by defining it as a taboo subject or insisting on secrecy. Where ambiguity surrounds a loss, this too makes grief work problematic. For example, in cases where family members have dementia or are in a protracted coma for a number of years, it is difficult for children and surviving family members to view these family members as absent. This is because although they are psychologically absent, they continue to be physically present. It is difficult for children and surviving family members to modify their world view to accommodate such losses when there continues to be ambiguity about them. Ambiguity about diagnostic and prognostic information poses similar problems for children facing life-threatening illness. They require clear, accurate information about their condition if they are to adjust to it.

This process of modifying one's world view following bereavement is greatly facilitated if there are opportunities to perceive the concrete reality of death and to acknowledge the transition in the relationship with the deceased by saying farewell. Being present at the death, viewing the body, attending the funeral or ceremony, visiting the grave or place of rest, and formally or informally saying farewell are rituals that promote the grieving process. Children's perception of choice about the way they engage in these leave-taking rituals may affect their subsequent grief work. Allowing some latitude for children to decide how they will engage in such processes gives children a sense of control over the rate at which they will confront grief-related information, cues and stimuli. Children who do not have opportunities to process the reality of the death and who are given inaccurate information have more difficulty adjusting to loss. In some instances, parents may believe that they gave children a choice about viewing the body or attending the funeral because they verbally asked their children to make a decision about these issues. However, children may have perceived little choice because, for example, they felt that the parents' non-verbal signals indicated that to view the body or attend the funeral would have negative consequences.

For children with life-threatening illness, there is also the need to arrange leave-taking rituals. First, there is the need for the child and family to acknowledge that the child's life-span of three score and ten years, as they originally thought of it, has been lost. Second, there is the need to plan a goodbye ritual for the child's last day of life. These two loss rituals help children and families to modify their world views so that they accurately reflect the child's state of health, and this maximizes the chance that the child and their family will live life to the full for their remaining days.

Pre-disposing factors

Children's adjustment to bereavement may be influenced by background pre-disposing factors within both the personal and contextual domains.

Personal pre-disposing factors

The child's past mental health and developmental level, both cognitive and emotional, their overall ability level and their temperament may affect the way in which they respond to bereavement and to life-threatening illness. Between the ages of two and sixteen years, children are particularly vulnerable to major loss experiences. They are past the age where lack of comprehension protects them from an awareness of the implications of major losses and have not yet developed adult coping strategies and defences. Children with lower ability levels who have temperaments associated with slow adjustment to new situations are more likely to become fixed in the denial process and find the bereavement or illness experience confusing and difficult to cope with. Children with an external locus of control and low self-esteem may find bereavement and life-threatening illness more difficult to cope with, probably because they view themselves as ill equipped to cope with the overwhelming nature of these experiences. Where children have had a stressful previous experience of a life-threatening illness or know that they have a vulnerability to serious illness, they may find that these background stresses compromise their capacity to cope with a current episode of life-threatening illness.

Contextual pre-disposing factors

Children who have grown up in families where their relationships with their parents were problematic, where they were exposed to chronic internal family stresses such as parental psychological problems and where they experienced multiple stressful life events, such as abuse or separations, may be pre-disposed to developing adjustment problems when faced with bereavement or life-threatening illness. These contextual pre-disposing factors may prevent the child from viewing the family as a source of much-needed social support when faced with loss. They may also leave the child with ambivalent relationships to resolve when a parent dies, and grief associated with such relationships, in which there is *unfinished business*, is more stressful than grief associated with the loss of a cherished parent.

Maintaining factors

When children develop adjustment problems following bereavement or during life-threatening illness, these may be maintained by the way the child copes at a personal level with loss-related stresses. These adjustment difficulties may also be maintained by the way in which members of the child's family and network manage the situation.

Personal maintaining factors

Adjustment difficulties may be maintained by excessive entrenchment in a single aspect of the grief process. So, protracted shock, extreme denial, excessive despair, sustained intense anger and blaming, intense anxiety and avoidance, or guilt-related self-injury may all maintain loss-related adjustment problems. For example, externalizing behavioural problems involving aggression towards others, or non-compliance with medical regimes, may be maintained by displacing sustained intense anger toward the deceased, or the child's own life-threatening illness onto others. Internalizing behaviour problems, such as social withdrawal and self-injury, may be maintained through protracted depressive rumination associated with despair, threat-related rumination associated with anxiety and self-blame associated with guilt.

Contextual maintaining factors

Features of the treatment system, the family system, the social network and characteristics of the child's parents may maintain adjustment problems associated with bereavement or life-threatening illness. Many of these, listed in Figure 24.1, have been described in detail in Chapter 2, so the focus here will be on contextual maintaining factors unique to loss-related adjustment problems. Adjustment problems following bereavement or associated with life-threatening illness may be maintained by members of the child's network if the membership of the network is unstable and the child experiences frequent changes in primary carers, through, for example, multiple placements. Adjustment problems following bereavement or associated with life-threatening illness may also be maintained by members of the child's network if these people have inadequate loss-management resources. Thus, if parents, family members, peers, teachers or involved professionals are ill equipped to manage loss, then the way they treat the child may maintain the child's loss-related adjustment difficulties.

Children are likely to show poorer adjustment when parents and other network members have problematic grief reactions and where the bereavement occurs within the context of multiple life stresses. Problematic parental grief reactions often occur when the family has had difficulty resolving losses in the past and where there are clear parallels between the current loss and previous losses within the nuclear family or losses in previous generations. Parents, professionals or other network members may become entrenched in denial and this may inhibit the child from moving beyond denial. With life-threatening illness, this type of parental reaction may under-pin poor compliance with treatment regimes, since the child may deny the reality of the illness and the need for treatment. Where parents or others become entrenched in anger, the bereaved or ill child may be scapegoated and this may maintain aggressive or depressive reactions on the child's part. When network members suffer ongoing deep despair, children may find that the inability of these network members to offer social support maintains their adjustment problems.

The roles of the referred child and the deceased within the overall social network and the relationship between the bereaved child and the deceased have an impact on the way in which the child manages the grief process. It has already been mentioned that, where the deceased occupied a central role for the child within the family network, then poorer adjustment may be expected than if the deceased occupied a more peripheral role. Thus, death of a parent, particularly the untimely death of the mother or primary caregiver, is probably one of the most painful losses for a child to endure. Where children have an ambivalent or unduly dependent relationship with the bereaved person, adjustment tends to be poorer because the complexity of the mixed emotions felt by the child complicates and protracts the grieving process. The child has to address the 'unfinished business' of the dependent or ambivalent relationship with the deceased, modify their assumptive world to accommodate the loss and negotiate a new set of relationships within the family with members who may have conflicting loyalties to the child and the deceased.

Confused communication within the family and wider social and professional network may maintain loss-related adjustment problems. Secrecy, myths and taboos about death, loss or life-threatening illness prevent children from modifying their world view and altering their roles accordingly. Lack of co-ordination among professionals dealing with children who have life-threatening illness may under-pin confused communication between the medical team and the family, which in turn may maintain children's problems adjusting to their illness. With both bereavement and life-threatening illness, the lack of availability of mourning rituals and the absence of facilitative sociocultural or religious belief systems may compromise children's capacity to manage loss experiences. Treatment systems that are not sensitive to the cultural and ethnic beliefs and values of the youngster's family system may maintain grief-related problems by inhibiting engagement or promoting drop-out from treatment and preventing the development of a good working alliance between the treatment team, the youngster and his or her family.

Protective factors

Children's personal characteristics and certain aspects of their social network may facilitate their adjustment to bereavement and life-threatening illness.

Personal protective factors

Children show better adjustment to loss experiences either before the age of two, when they are unable to appreciate the significance of major losses, or in late adolescence when they have developed sophisticated coping strategies for dealing with loss. With life-threatening illness such as cancer, physical fitness is a protective factor. Intelligent children with easy temperaments, an internal locus of control and high self-esteem may adjust better to bereavement, and probably adjust better to chronic illness than children who lack these assets. A range of coping strategies for eliciting social support from others, mature defence mechanisms, an optimistic attributional style and high self-efficacy may also lead to better adjustment in the face of significant loss experiences.

Contextual protective factors

Good adjustment following bereavement or during life-threatening illness is more likely where the child's family has experienced previous losses but acknowledged and processed these and developed support networks for working through loss. Better adjustment may also occur when family members have ways of incorporating loss into personal and family world views, and strategies for re-organizing the family to accommodate losses. In such situations, parents typically have uncomplicated grief reactions and so are better able to offer their children the support they require.

Where the child's role prior to the bereavement or illness was one where much support was available from family members, peers and school staff, the child may be better equipped to manage grief work, particularly if this network support persists. Where children are permitted the free expression of vulnerability and grief-related emotions, then good adjustment may be expected. Clear communication and flexibility within the family, school and peer group probably lead to good adjustment. This type of support, communication and flexibility tends to occur where a strong marital relationship is present, where family relationships are positive and where the family has good relationships with the school, the medical team and other involved agencies. Where bereaved children or those with terminal illness feel well supported, and where family roles, routines, rules, responsibilities and relationships can be re-negotiated with limited difficulty, then adjustment will probably be better than where such events do not occur. Open communication between parents and children about bereavement or a child's terminal illness and impending death, offered in a supportive and realistic yet hopeful way, is probably associated with better adjustment. This requirement for clear communication is important for the medical team also. Families and children adjust better to childhood terminal illness when members of the treatment team offer clear, unambiguous information in a supportive way and involve the child in decision making about his or her medical care. A sensitivity to the parents' needs for support and to the whole family's need for an opportunity to say goodbye in the terminal phase of the illness when further medical intervention is futile may contribute to better family adjustment in the long term. Long-term family adjustment to the death of a child following terminal illness may also be better when children die at home rather than in a hospital setting.

In families where members model an appropriate grieving process, this may help children manage their own grief. Of particular importance is the way in which parents (or other primary carers) manage this process. Parents who acknowledge the loss and express their grief-related feelings in a culturally appropriate way show their child how the process of grieving is to be conducted. With both bereavement and life-threatening illness, the availability of mourning rituals along with sociocultural and religious beliefs that facilitate the grieving process contribute to the child's adjustment. Treatment systems that are sensitive to the cultural and ethnic beliefs and values of the youngster's family are more likely to help families engage with, and remain in, treatment, and foster the development of a good working alliance.

ASSESSMENT AND FORMULATION

The management of cases where children have been bereaved or face life-threatening illness should be based on a thorough evaluation and formulation of the child's grief-related problems. In addition to the routine assessment procedures set out in Chapter 4, the framework presented in Figure 24.1 may be used to encapsulate clinically relevant information and develop a formulation. This formulation should explain how loss-related stresses, pre-disposing factors and maintaining factors under-pin adjustment difficulties. However, it is critical to also identify personal and contextual factors that have the potential to contribute to the child's better management of the loss experience.

In some instances, children are referred for consultation following bereavement or when facing life-threatening illness, and their adjustment is well within normal limits but parents or other involved professionals are concerned that there may be loss-related adjustment difficulties. In these instances, highlighting the many protective factors present in the case is a central part of case management.

Some children, when dealing with loss, develop problems which meet the diagnostic criteria for childhood depression, post-traumatic stress disorder, somatization disorder, oppositional defiant disorder or drug abuse. It may, therefore, be useful to review the chapters dealing with these problem areas when formulating cases in which loss is the core theme but where one or more of these problems occur as part of the grieving process. Principles for managing specific symptoms outlined in these chapters may also be usefully incorporated into treatment programmes for children involved in the grieving process.

Some psychometric instruments that may be a useful adjunct to the assessment of grief-related phenomena in adolescents are listed in Table 24.3.

INTERVENTION WITH BEREAVED CHILDREN

Intervention with children and adolescents who have experienced bereavement aims to help the child and family acknowledge the loss, incorporate it into their world view and re-organize their lives to take account of the loss. In

Table 24.3 Psychometric instruments that may be used as an adjunct to clinical interviews in the assessment of grief and related constructs

Construct	Instrument	Publication	Comments
Adolescent grief reactions	Grief Assessment Protocol	Jimerson Grief Assessment Protocol. Available at: http://www.education.ucsb.edu/jimerson/griefassessment.htm	This protocol contains a battery of multi-informant instruments for assessing grief reactions in adolescents which are being used in Project Loss – an ongoing treatment programme evaluation study
Adult grief following bereavement	Texas Revised Inventory of Grief (TRIG)	Faschingbauer, T. (1981). *Texas Revised Inventory of Grief (TRIG)*. Houston, TX: Honeycomb	This 21-item inventory yields scores on two sub-scales: feelings and actions at the time of the death; and present feelings and actions. It may be useful with older adolescents
	Grief Experiences Inventory	Sanders, C., Maugher, P. & Strong, P. (1985). *Grief Experiences Inventory*. Palo Alto: CA. Consulting Psychologists Press	This 135-item inventory yields scores on 9 sub-scales: despair, anger, guilt, social isolation, loss of control, rumination, depersonalization, somatization and death anxiety. It may be useful with older adolescents

Continued

Table 24.3 continued

Construct	Instrument	Publication	Comments
	Hogan Grief Reaction Checklist	Hogan, N., Greenfield, D. & Schmidt L. (2001). Development and validation of the Hogan Grief Reaction Checklist. *Death Studies*, 25(1), 1–32	This inventory yields scores for despair, panic behaviour, blame and anger, detachment, disorganization, and personal growth
Quality of life	The Minneapolis-Manchester Quality of Life Instrument	Bhatia, S., Jenney, M., Bogue, M., Rockwood, T., Feusner, J., Friedman, D., Robison, L. & Kan, R. (2002). The Minneapolis-Manchester Quality of Life Instrument: Reliability and Validity of the Adolescent Form. *Journal of Clinical Oncology*, 20, 4692–4698	This is a standardized child self-report instrument designed to assess quality of life in adolescent survivors of childhood cancer
	Paediatric Oncology Quality of Life Scale	Bijttebier, P., Vercruysse, T., Vertommen, H., Van Gool, S., Uyttebroeck, A. & Brock, P. (2001). New evidence on the reliability and validity of the Paediatric Oncology Quality of Life Scale. *Psychology & Health*, 16, 461–469	This is a standardized child self-report instrument designed to assess quality of life in survivors of childhood cancer

working towards these goals, account should be taken of personal and contextual factors identified in the formulation that maintain adjustment problems, and of those that have the potential to facilitate future adjustment. Family, individual and group-based interventions may be appropriate, depending on the unique features of the case. Webb (2002) argues that in the early stage of grief work, family-based work is the most appropriate, since it allows family members to develop a shared acknowledgement of the loss. Later, individual or group work may be offered concurrently with family sessions.

Family-based grief work

Family-based work in cases of bereavement has three central goals (Black & Urbanowicz, 1987; Kissane & Bloch, 2002; Walsh & McGoldrick, 2004; Webb, 2002). These are:

- acknowledging the reality of the death
- modifying the family's world view so that it incorporates the loss
- re-organizing the family system and moving on.

All three goals may be addressed at all stages of the consultation process. However, in the opening phase of therapy, acknowledgement of reality of the death tends to be the central focus and, in later therapy sessions, the emphasis tends to be on family re-organization. Modification of the family's world view so that it incorporates the loss is addressed throughout therapy and for some time afterwards, but is given particular attention in the middle phase of family therapy for bereavement. Three issues which deserve special attention when working with bereaved children are:

- the use of rituals
- managing unfinished business
- psychoeducation about the grief process.

Each of these will be discussed below following a consideration of the three main tasks of family-based grief work.

Acknowledgement of loss

In the opening sessions, the core task is helping the child and family to construct a shared understanding of the events surrounding the loss, while at the same time inviting them to employ sufficient defences to prevent being overwhelmed by the emotional impact of the loss. During this phase, the psychologist invites each family member to give a detailed account of their understanding of the events before, during and after the death up to the present time. If hospitalization occurred, memories of this may be reviewed. Each person's recollection of the deceased's final hours and their reflections on these may be recalled. Details of the funeral, cremation or other rituals may be covered. This stage is concluded when there is agreement that everyone has been given an opportunity to acknowledge that the death occurred and the sequence of events that led to and followed this event.

Incorporating the loss into the world view

In the second phase of therapy the child and family are invited to expose themselves to the full implications of the loss for the whole family and bear the emotional pain that accompanies this. By responding to this invitation and examining the discrepancies between the world as it is now and as it was before the loss, the family's world view is modified so that it can incorporate the loss. Family members are invited to remember the dead person and acknowledge that they had an important place in the child and family's life but are no longer present in this world and this causes all family members great pain. Opportunities for full expression of the wide range of emotions associated with the grief process may be given. Opportunities to modify the family's assumptive world so that it can accommodate the loss may be created by reviewing how the absence of the bereaved person will affect all aspects of family life. This review may begin with an exploration of how daily, weekly, monthly and annual routines will be different now from the way they were in the past. The more vividly the past can be remembered and compared with the present, the more effective this process will be. Children and family members may be invited to bring photographs, family videotapes, clothing, favourite pieces of music, perfume, personal effects and memorabilia associated with the deceased into the therapy sessions to facilitate this review process. The place of the deceased in the wider extended family and community network may also be explored and the implications of the death for changes in routines involving the extended family and community may be discussed. Finally, it is useful to fully review the current death within a multigenerational perspective, and explore the role of the dead person in the family as a system that runs through time for many generations. Similarities and differences between the current loss and other losses may be reviewed. Genograms and lifelines, described in Chapter 4, are particularly useful tools for exploring and tracking the impact of loss on the wider family context.

The second phase of therapy is complete when the family's world view has shown signs of beginning to change so as to incorporate the reality of the loss. Such signs include talking about the deceased in the past tense, accepting that painful reminders of the loss will have to be encountered regularly rather than avoided, acknowledging that the pace with which parents come to terms with loss has an effect on the pace at which children can progress through the grieving process and acknowledging that coming to terms with death for some family members may take a long time.

Re-organization

In the third phase of therapy, the main focus is on helping the child and family to re-organize their roles, routines, rules, responsibilities and relationships so that energy is directed into moving on and completing other tasks within the family lifecycle, while allowing a place for the memory of the deceased in this new organizational arrangement. For example, following the death of a parent, the caregiving, breadwinning and leadership responsibilities of the parent have to be re-allocated to other family members, including the surviving parents, grandparents, aunts, uncles and older siblings. The place accorded to the memory of the dead family member should be congruent with the family's sociocultural and religious beliefs and with the individual developmental stages of family members. Thus, young children who believe in an after-life may imagine that the deceased continues to look down on the family from heaven. Those without a belief in the after-life may think of the deceased surviving in the memory of all family members and in the photographs or memorabilia left behind. Families show that they are moving on when there are signs that it may be possible for them to invest their energy in future projects in a way that is clearly not a frenetic attempt to distract them from the loss they have experienced in the past.

An episode of time-limited family-based therapy for bereaved children may be concluded when there are signs that the child can fulfil his or her role within the family, school and peer group without showing excessive internalizing or externalizing behaviour problems or somatic symptoms.

Rituals

Throughout the therapy process, children and families may be invited to use or develop rituals to help them manage the grieving process (Imber-Black, Roberts, Whiting & Whiting, 2003). Rituals may be used by families to acknowledge loss, to modify their world view so that it now incorporates a symbol of the person who has died in a meaningful way and to symbolize that the family is moving on through the lifecycle despite the death that has occurred. Where families find that their cultural or religious beliefs and practices do not provide adequate ready-made rituals for managing loss, they may be invited to develop their own and embed these into their family traditions. The main requirements for such rituals are that they be meaningful to the family, that they are congruent with family tradition, that they are stylized symbolic transactions as distinct from routine conversations and that they occur at times and places which have significance with respect to the loss. For example, an extra place may be set at the dinner table on the anniversary of a dead family member to acknowledge loss but show that the person is remembered. In another instance, to mark the fact that the family has moved on despite loss, children and other family members may write a letter to the deceased a year after his or her death outlining how each person in the family has managed the twelve months that have elapsed since the funeral.

Unfinished business

Where children or other family members had ambivalent or dependent relationships with the deceased, or where the family is divided in its loyalty to the deceased, this unfinished business may need to be resolved before the family can re-organize itself and move on. Unfinished business may be resolved through a written or spoken monologue with a symbolic representation of the deceased and by representing one's position to other family members. The central process in resolving unfinished business is having a forum within which the mixed feelings are expressed, processed, acknowledged and reflected on.

In family-based therapy, children who feel intensely ambivalent or dependent on a deceased parent or relative may be invited to write them a series of letters in which they outline how they feel, what events led them to feel that way and how they would like to feel. They may be subsequently invited to read these out in an appropriate place, such as at the graveside, in the family sessions or in individual sessions. In other instances, an empty chair may be included in family sessions to symbolically represent the deceased and the child may be invited to address their mixed feelings to this symbolic representation of the deceased. Throughout such work, parents and other family members may be invited to support the child who is attempting to resolve the unfinished business.

Psychoeducation

Parents and children may require psychoeducation about the nature and range of possible grief reactions that they may expect to experience. This has to be offered supportively so that they do not feel objectified or misunderstood. The conceptualization of grief processes given earlier in this chapter may be given verbally to the family. A second option is to offer books to families, such as those listed at the end of this chapter. Another option is to invite the family to watch a film that dramatizes a bereavement similar to their own and then discuss, in the family sessions, the ways in which different people within the film managed the grief process. For example, in a family where a mother had died and the boys were presenting with behavioural problems, the boys and their father watched *Into the West*, which was about a travelling family in Ireland going through the same type of bereavement.

Individual sessions for PTSD

Individual sessions are particularly appropriate where children have suffered traumatic bereavement and develop PTSD. This may occur where children witness violent death, for example, within the context of suicide, an armed robbery, a car crash or a natural disaster. In such instances, assessment of PTSD using procedures outlined in Chapter 12 is appropriate. Where children meet the criteria for PTSD, they require coaching in anxiety management skills and an opportunity to use these to regulate their anxiety during gradual and prolonged exposure to traumatic memories, following the procedures outlined in Chapter 12.

Group work for isolated children

Where children have experienced loss, and their parents are physically or psychologically unavailable to go through the grieving process with them, group therapy may be used as a forum for grief work. With group work, children benefit from peer support and the experience of seeing how other children are learning to cope with death. With group work, various expressive media such as drawings, paintings, sculpture, music, scrapbooks, drama and so forth may be used as vehicles for the telling and re-telling of bereaved children's experiences of loss, so that they can modify their world view and accommodate the reality of their losses. A number of useful workbooks are listed at the end of the chapter.

PRE-BEREAVEMENT COUNSELLING

Children referred prior to bereavement where, for example, a parent is terminally ill or injured, may be helped through pre-bereavement counselling to prepare to manage the immanent loss. During this preparation process they can write a letter or rehearse what they wish to say to their dying or dead parent as part of a leave-taking ritual. They may then be briefed about what they may expect to experience when they are with their dying or dead parent. For example, if the parent is dead or in a coma, the way the parents will appear, the parent's skin temperature and so forth may be explained so the child will not be surprised when they enter the room in which the parent is dying or laid out. During the leave-taking ritual, arrangements should be made for the child to be accompanied by a supporting adult. This may be the surviving parent, an older sibling or an aunt. The most important issued here is that the supporting person be able to focus on the child's need for support; in some instances, the surviving parent may be so involved in his or her own grief experience that they are unable to be sensitive to their child's needs. After the leave-taking ritual, the supporting person should be available to the child to help them process their grief-related emotions by talking through their reaction to the ritual.

INTERVENTION WITH DYING CHILDREN

Clinical accounts of good practice in the management of terminally ill children permit certain core principles for case management to be identified, and these are described below (American Academy of Paediatrics Committee on Bioethics and Committee on Hospital Care, 2000; Black, 1994; Herbert, 1996).

Family-oriented care for terminally ill children is ideally offered by an entire multi-disciplinary team involved with the child's care, including physicians, nurses, chaplains, social workers and psychologists who share a common approach to care. Within this team, clinical psychologists may take responsibility for convening family consultation sessions. All significant members of the child's nuclear and extended family may be invited to some of these sessions.

Children and their families should be informed of the diagnosis and prognosis in age-appropriate language and in a factual way, with the name of the disease and the fact that some people with the disease die. However, the information should be given so that it provides the child with an opportunity to be hopeful, insofar as that is possible, and in a socially supportive context. Failure to communicate honestly may lead to a sense of isolation and distrust. However, such information should probably be given repeatedly since acceptance of the fatality of illness dawns on children gradually and progresses through the following levels (Herbert, 1996):

- 'I am very ill'
- 'I have an illness that can kill people'
- 'I have an illness that can kill children'
- 'I may not get better'
- 'I am dying'

Dying involves three distinct types of loss. First, there is the loss of comfort. Terminal illness often entails pain, discomfort and loss of control over bodily functions such as sleeping and elimination. Second, there is the loss of lifestyle routines such as engaging in exercise, being mobile, playing sports and so forth. Finally, there is the anticipated loss of intimate relationships. Children know that they will not have the same type of relationship with their parents and siblings once they die and they sense the family's grief and attempts to avoid acknowledging their own impending death. However, in order to enjoy the remainder of their life to the full, the reality of immanent death must be openly acknowledged by the family.

Once this acknowledgement has begun, the family may be encouraged to maximize the child's quality of life for his or her remaining days. So, for example, if there is only one Christmas left, making the most of it becomes a priority. The family is helped to use the remaining time in a way that will not leave the parents or other family members with regrets. Thus, while the treatment team must make it clear that they are offering the family support in managing the child's last weeks or days of life, and that the child's death is immanent, they should encourage the expression of hope; specifically, hope that particular events (such as a family picnic) may occur before the child dies.

Acknowledging the reality for the child's immanent death and attempting to incorporate this fact into the family's world view, precipitates anticipatory grief processes. Intense feelings of anger, sadness, anxiety and guilt are experienced. These profound emotional experiences may be explored and contained within family consultations. In anticipating life after the child's death, for most parents the idea of 'coming to terms with a child's death' has been found to be less accurate and useful than the idea of 'living with the death of the child'.

Certain key messages should be woven into consultations with dying children and their families and, wherever possible, the parents or primary caregivers should be empowered to communicate these messages to the child (Spinetta, 1980). First, children should be informed that they will not be alone when they face death and after they die. Second, they should be told that they have done all that they could do with their lives and that their lives had a good purpose. Third, children should be given permission to fully express their sadness, anger and confusion about death and dying. Fourth, they should be told that their parents and all members of the family probably have similar feelings of sadness, anger and confusion about death and dying and so they may see their parents crying because they do not want their children to die. Fifth, children should be told that adults (including parents and the medical team) will do everything to prevent death but that there are some diseases or injuries that cannot be healed. Sixth, children may be assured that there will be no pain after death. Seventh, the fact that there will be an opportunity for them to say goodbye to their family and friends should be clarified. Eighth, children may be told that they will continue to have a link with their family and friends beyond death. This link should be expressed within the context of the family's belief system. So, for families that believe in the after-life, the promise of a re-union may be mentioned. For families that do not hold such beliefs, the fact that the family will always remember the child and the good times that were shared may be discussed. Where children are dying, life-story book work may help them achieve some sense of auto-biographical coherence and may make accepting their death less painful. Life-story book work involves helping the child to construct a biographical account using words, photographs and pictures which make sense of, and sequences, the event of his or her life (Ryan & Walker, 2003).

The context within which people die can have a profound effect on the quality of the dying process for themselves and their families. For children, where possible, it is preferable to spend the final days at home with their families. If the demands associated with this exceed parental coping resources, a hospice offers an alternative to a hospital setting. The hospice movement provides family-centred care and helps people die with a minimum of pain and discomfort and a maximum of dignity and integrity.

Following the death of a child, families continue to require support, and this may be most usefully provided by the many self-help groups that have been established for bereaved parents. Such groups include Friends and the Candlelighter's Foundation.

SUMMARY

Children's adjustment to bereavement or life-threatening medical conditions in part depends on their understanding of the concept of death. Empirical

studies show that the concept of death evolves not only as cognitive maturation occurs but also as experience of death broadens. The irreversibility,
universality and functionality of death may be appreciated by children during
the pre-operational stage provided they have been exposed to particular
death-related experiences, such as having a terminal illness or have experienced multiple bereavements. Within Western culture, the normative expectation is for people facing a serious loss to show extreme initial distress, which
declines with time. However, this is just one of three common patterns. In the
second pattern, extreme protracted distress occurs and the third pattern is
characterized by little distress initially or later. Shock, denial, sadness, anger,
anxiety, guilt and acceptance are the principal grief processes. These do not
occur in an invariant order, nor do they occur in all cases (as stage theories
suggest) and this idiosyncratic patterning of grief responses is probably most
comprehensively accommodated within multi-systemic theories that conceptualize loss as a psychosocial transition. Theoretical accounts of grief
have also been put forward within the biopsychological, psychodynamic,
behavioural, and family systems traditions and treatment programmes based
on behavioural, psychodynamic and family systems principles have been
developed. For children, family-based treatment is probably the intervention
of choice to help them adjust to loss experiences. Such treatment should be
based on a comprehensive formulation, which takes account of the particular
adjustment problems or grief response patterns presented by the child, the
child's characteristics, the relevant contextual factors and the loss-related
factors that under-pin the adjustment problems. However, it is crucial to
consider personal and contextual factors that have the potential to contribute
to the child's better management of the loss experience.

EXERCISE 24.1

Develop a preliminary formulation for the case presented in Box 24.1 and
develop a plan for an intake assessment interview that would allow you to
refine your formulation.

FURTHER READING

Herbert, M. (1996). *Supporting Bereaved and Dying Children and Their Parents.*
   Leicester: British Psychological Society Books.
Kissane, D. & Bloch, S. (2002). *Family Focused Grief Therapy: A Model of Family-
   centred Care during Palliative Care and Bereavement.* Buckingham, UK: Open
   University Press.
Walsh, F. & McGoldrick, M. (2004). *Living Beyond Loss: Death in the Family* (Second
   edition). New York: Norton.

Webb, N. (2002). *Helping Bereaved Children: A Handbook for Practitioners* (Second edition). New York: Guilford.

Worden, J. (2002). *Grief Counselling and Grief Therapy: A Handbook for the Mental Health Practitioner* (Third edition). New York: Springer.

RESOURCES FOR CLIENTS

Krementz, J. (1981). *How it Feels When a Parent Dies*. New York: Knopf.

Mallon, B. (1998). *Helping Children to Manage Loss. Positive Strategies for Renewal and Growth*. London: Jessica Kingsley.

Rando, T. (1991). *How to Go on Living When Someone You Love Dies*. New York: Bantam.

Schaefer, D. & Lyons, C. (1986). *How Do We Tell the Children*. New York: Newmarket.

Turner, M. (1998). *Talking with Children and Young People about Death and Dying. A Workbook*. London: Jessica Kingsley.

Ward, B. (1995). *Good Grief: Exploring Feelings Loss and Death* (Second edition: volume 1 for under elevens; volume 2 for over elevens and adults).

WEBSITES

Cruse Bereavement Care: http://www.crusebereavementcare.org.uk/

Jessica Kingsley's webpage on bereavement resources: http://www.jkp.com/catalogue/index.php/cat/bereavement

Speechmark Publishing: http://www.speechmark.net/

The Child Bereavement Trust: http://www.childbereavement.org.uk/

Winston's Wish: http:// www.winstonswish.org.uk

Factsheets on bereavement can be downloaded from the website for Rose, G. & York, A. (2004). *Mental Health and Growing Up. Fact sheets for Parents, Teachers and Young People* (Third edition). London: Gaskell: http://www.rcpsych.ac.uk

References

AA. (1986). *The Little Red Book*. City Centre, MN: Halelden.

Abramson, L., Seligman, M. & Teasdale, J. (1978). Learned helplessness in humans: Critique and reformulation. *Journal of Abnormal Psychology*, 87, 49–74.

Abu-Arefeh, I. & Russell, G. (1994). Prevalence of headache and migraine in school-children. *British Medical Journal*, 309, 765–769.

Abu-Saad, H. (2001). *Evidence-Based Palliative Care Across the Lifespan*. Oxford: Blackwell Science.

Achenbach, T. (1991). *Integrative Guide for the 1991 CBCL/4–18, YSR and TRF profiles*. Burlington, VT: University of Vermont Department of Psychiatry.

Achenbach, T. M. & Rescorla, L. A. (2000). *Manual for ASEBA Preschool Forms & Profiles*. Burlington, VT: University of Vermont, Research Centre for Children, Youth, & Families. http://www.aseba.org/

Achenbach, T. M. & Rescorla, L. A. (2001). *Manual for ASEBA School-Age Forms & Profiles*. Burlington, VT: University of Vermont, Research Centre for Children, Youth, & Families. http://www.aseba.org/

Adams, G. (1999). *Comprehensive Test of Adaptive Behaviour – Revised*. Seattle, WA: Educational Achievement Systems. http://www.edresearch.com

Aichorn, A. (1935). *Wayward Youth*. New York: Viking Press.

Ainsworth, M., Blehar, M., Waters, E. & Wass, S. (1978). *Patterns of Attachment: A Psychological Study of the Strange Situation*. Hillsdale, NJ: Lawrence Erlbaum Associates Inc.

Aldred, C., Green, J. & Adams, C. (2004). A new social communication intervention for children with autism: Pilot randomized controlled treatment study suggesting effectiveness. *Journal of Child Psychology and Psychiatry*, 45, 1420–1430.

Alexander, F. (1950). *Psychosomatic Medicine: Its Principles and Applications*. New York: Norton.

Allen, J. & Rapee, R. (2005). Anxiety disorders. In P. Graham (ed.), *Cognitive Behaviour Therapy for Children and Families* (Second edition, pp. 300–319). Cambridge: Cambridge University Press.

Alsaker, F. (1996). The impact of puberty. *Journal of Child Psychology and Psychiatry*, 37, 249–258.

Altschuler, J. (1997). *Working with Chronic Illness: A Family Approach*. London: Macmillan.

Amato, P. (1993). Children's adjustment to divorce. Theories, hypotheses and empirical support. *Journal of Marriage and the Family*, 55, 23–38.

Amato, P. (2000). The consequences of divorce for adults and children. *Journal of Marriage and the Family*, 62, 1269–1287.

Amato, P. (2001). Children of divorce in the 1990s: An update of the Amato and Keith (1991) meta-analysis. *Journal of Family Psychology*, 15, 355–370.

Amato, P. & Gilbreth, J. G. (1999). Non-resident fathers and children's well-being: A meta-analysis. *Journal of Marriage and the Family*, 61, 557–573.

Amato, P. & Keith, B. (1991). Consequences of parental divorce for adult well-being: A meta-analysis. *Journal of Marriage and the Family*, 53, 43–58.

Ambrosini, P. (2000). Historical development and present status of the Schedule for Affective Disorders and Schizophrenia for School-Age Children (K-SADS). *Journal of the American Academy of Child and Adolescent Psychiatry*, 39, 49–58.

American Academy of Child and Adolescent Psychiatry (1997a). Practice parameters for the assessment and treatment of children and adolescents with conduct disorder. *Journal of the American Academy of Child and Adolescent Psychiatry*, 36 (Supplement). http://www.aacap.org/clinical/parameters/

American Academy of Child and Adolescent Psychiatry (1997b). Practice parameters for the assessment and treatment of children, adolescents, and adults with attention-deficit/hyperactivity disorder. *Journal of the American Academy of Child and Adolescent Psychiatry*, 36 (Supplement 10). http://www.aacap.org/clinical/parameters/

American Academy of Child and Adolescent Psychiatry (1997c), Practice parameters for the assessment and treatment of children and adolescents with anxiety disorders. *Journal of the American Academy of Child and Adolescent Psychiatry*, 36 (Supplement). http://www.aacap.org/clinical/parameters/

American Academy of Child and Adolescent Psychiatry (1997d). Practice parameters for the assessment and treatment of children and adolescents with obsessive compulsive disorder. *Journal of the American Academy of Child and Adolescent Psychiatry*, 37 (Supplement 10). http://www.aacap.org/clinical/parameters/

American Academy of Child and Adolescent Psychiatry (1997e). Practice parameters for the assessment and treatment of children and adolescents with substance use disorders. *American Academy of Child and Adolescent Psychiatry*, 36 (Supplement). http://www.aacap.org/clinical/parameters/

American Academy of Child and Adolescent Psychiatry (1997f), Practice parameters for the assessment and treatment of children and adolescents with bipolar disorder. *Journal of the American Academy of Child and Adolescent Psychiatry*, 36 (Supplement). http://www.aacap.org/clinical/parameters/

American Academy of Child and Adolescent Psychiatry (1997g). Practice parameters for the forensic evaluation of children and adolescents who may have been physically or sexually abused. *Journal of the American Academy of Child and Adolescent Psychiatry*, 36 (Supplement). http://www.aacap.org/clinical/parameters/

American Academy of Child and Adolescent Psychiatry (1997h). Practice parameters for child custody evaluation. *Journal of the American Academy of Child and Adolescent Psychiatry*, 36 (10 Supplement). http://www.aacap.org/clinical/parameters/

American Academy of Child and Adolescent Psychiatry (1998a). Practice parameters for the assessment and treatment of children and adolescents with language and learning disorders. *Journal of the American Academy of Child and Adolescent Psychiatry* 37(Supplement). http://www.aacap.org/clinical/parameters/

American Academy of Child and Adolescent Psychiatry (1998b). Practice parameters for the assessment and treatment of children and adolescents with posttraumatic stress disorder. *Journal of the American Academy of Child and Adolescent Psychiatry*, 37(Supplement). http://www.aacap.org/clinical/parameters/

American Academy of Child and Adolescent Psychiatry (1998c). Practice parameters for the assessment and treatment of children and adolescents with depressive disorders. *Journal of the American Academy of Child and Adolescent Psychiatry*, 37 (Supplement). http://www.aacap.org/clinical/parameters/

American Academy of Child and Adolescent Psychiatry (1999a). Practice parameter for the assessment and treatment of children, adolescents, and adults with autism and other pervasive developmental disorders. *Journal of the American Academy of Child and Adolescent Psychiatry*, 38 (Supplement). http://www.aacap.org/clinical/parameters/

American Academy of Child and Adolescent Psychiatry (1999b). Practice parameter for the assessment and treatment of children and adolescents who are sexually abusive of others. *Journal of the American Academy of Child and Adolescent Psychiatry*, 38 (Supplement). http://www.aacap.org/clinical/parameters/

American Academy Of Child and Adolescent Psychiatry (2001a). Practice parameter for the assessment and treatment of children and adolescents with suicidal behaviour. *Journal of the American Academy of Child and Adolescent Psychiatry*, 40 (Supplement). http://www.aacap.org/clinical/parameters/

American Academy of Child and Adolescent Psychiatry (2001b). Practice parameters for the assessment and treatment of children and adolescents with schizophrenia. *Journal of the American Academy of Child and Adolescent Psychiatry*, 40 (Supplement). http://www.aacap.org/clinical/parameters/

American Academy of Child And Adolescent Psychiatry (2002). Practice parameter for the prevention and management of aggressive behaviour in child and adolescent psychiatric institutions with special reference to seclusion and restraint. *Journal of the American Academy of Child and Adolescent Psychiatry*, 41 (Supplement). http://www.aacap.org/clinical/parameters/

American Academy of Paediatrics Committee on Bioethics and Committee on Hospital Care (2000). Palliative Care for Children. *Paediatrics*, 106, 351–357.

American Psychiatric Association (1988). *Child Custody Consultation: Report of the Task Force on Clinical Assessment in Child Custody*. Washington, DC: American Psychiatric Association.

American Psychiatric Association (2000a). *Diagnostic and Statistical Manual of the Mental Disorders (Fourth Edition-Text Revision, DSM–IV-TR)*. Washington, DC: APA.

American Psychiatric Association (2000b). Practice guidelines for the treatment of eating disorders (revision). American Psychiatric Association Work Group on Eating Disorders. *American Journal of Psychiatry*, 157, 1–39.

American Psychological Association (1994). Guidelines for child custody evaluations in divorce proceedings. *American Psychologist*, 49, 677–680. Available at: http://www.apa.org/practice/childcustody.html

American Sleep Disorders Association (1997). *International Classification of Sleep Disorders, Revised: Diagnostic and Coding Manual*. Rochester, MN: American Sleep Disorders Association.

Anastopoulos, A., Barkley, R. & Shelton, T. (1996). Family based treatment: Psychosocial intervention for children and adolescents with attention deficit hyperactivity disorder. In E. Hibbs & P. Jensen (eds.), *Psychosocial Treatments for*

Child and Adolescent Disorders. Empirically Based Strategies for Clinical Practice (pp. 267–284). Washington, DC: APA.

Anastopoulos, A. & Farley, S. (2003). A cognitive-behavioural training programme for parents of children with attention-deficit/hyperactivity disorder. In A. Kazdin, & J. Weisz (eds.), *Evidence Based Psychotherapies for Children and Adolescents* (pp. 187–203). New York: Guilford.

Anderson, C. (2003). The diversity, strengths and challenges of single-parent households. In F. Walsh (ed.), *Normal Family Processes* (Third edition, pp. 121–151). New York: Guilford.

Anderson, C. & Stewart, S. (1983). *Mastering Resistance*. New York: Guilford.

Anderson, J., Williams, S., McGee, R. & Silva, P. (1987). DSM III disorders in preadolescent children. *Archives of General Psychiatry*, 44, 69–76.

Anderson, V., Northam, E., Hendy, J. & Wrennall, J. (2001). *Developmental Neuropsychology: A Clinical Approach*. Philadelphia, PA: Psychology Press.

Andrasik, F. (1986). Relaxation and biofeedback for chronic headaches. In A. Holzman & D. Turk (eds.). *Pain Management: A Handbook of Psychological Treatment Approaches*. New York: Pergamon.

Angold, A. (2002). Diagnostic interviews with parents and children. In M. Rutter, E. & Taylor (eds.), *Child and Adolescent Psychiatry* (Fourth edition, pp. 32–51). Oxford: Blackwell.

Angold, A. & Costello, E. (2000). The Child and Adolescent Psychiatric Assessment (CAPA). *Journal of the American Academy of Child & Adolescent Psychiatry*, 39, 39–48.

Angold, A. & Costello, E. (2001). The epidemiology of depression in children and adolescents. In I. Goodyer (ed.), *The Depressed Child and Adolescent* (Second edition, pp. 143–178). Cambridge: Cambridge University Press.

Annett, R. & Bender, B. (1994). Neuropsychological dysfunction in asthmatic children. *Neuropsychology Review*, 4, 91–115.

Anthony, E. (1957). An experimental approach to the psychopathology of childhood: encopresis. *British Journal of Medical Psychology*, 30, 146–175.

Armitage, R., Hoffmann, R., Emslie, G., Weinberg, W., Mayes, T. & Rush, J. (2002). Sleep microarchitecture as a predictor of recurrence in children and adolescents with depression. *International Journal of Neuropsychopharmacology*, 5, 217–228.

Asarnow, J. & Asarnow, R. (2003). Childhood-onset schizophrenia. In J. Mash & R. Barkley (eds.), *Child Psychopathology* (Second edition, pp. 455–485). New York: Guilford.

Asarnow, J., Thompson, M. & Goldstein, M. (2001). Psychosocial factors: The social context of child and adolescent onset schizophrenia. In H. Remschmidt (ed), *Schizophrenia in Children and Adolescents* (pp. 168–191). Cambridge: Cambridge University Press.

Asarnow, J., Thompson, M. & McGrath, E. (2004). Annotation: Childhood-onset schizophrenia: Clinical and treatment issues. *Journal of Child Psychology and Psychiatry*, 45, 180–194.

Asarnow, R. & Karatekin, C. (2001). Children with schizophrenia: A neurobehavioral perspective. In H. Remschmidt (ed), *Schizophrenia in Children and Adolescents* (pp. 135–167). Cambridge: Cambridge University Press.

Asendorpf, J. (1993). Abnormal shyness in children. *Journal of Child Psychology and Psychiatry*, 34, 1069–1081.

Asperger, H. (1944/1991). Die 'autistischen psychopathen' in kind esalter. Arc hive fur Psychiatrie nnd Nervenkrankheiten, 117, 76–136. Translated by U. Frith (ed.), *Autism and Asperger Syndrome* (1991, pp. 37–92). Cambridge: Cambridge University.

Aubrey, C., Eaves, J., Hicks, C. & Newton, M. (1982). *Aston Portfolio*. Wisbech, UK: Learning Development Aids.

Azar, S. & Wolfe, D. (1998). Child physical abuse and neglect. In E. Mash & R. Barkley (eds.), *Treatment of Childhood Disorders* (Second edition, pp. 501–544). New York: Guilford.

Azrin, N. & Besalel, V. (1979). *A Parent's Guide to Bedwetting Control*. New York: Simon & Schuster.

Azrin, N. & Nunn, R. (1973). Habit reversal: A method of eliminating nervous habits and tics. *Behaviour Research and Therapy*, 11, 619–628.

Azrin, N. & Peterson, A. (1990). Treatment of Tourette syndrome by habit reversal. A waiting list control group comparison. *Behaviour Therapy*, 21, 305–318.

Azrin, N., Sneed, T., & Fox, R. (1974). Dry bed training: Rapid elimination of childhood enuresis. *Behaviour Research and Therapy*, 12, 147–156.

Bailey, A., Phillips, W. & Rutter, M. (1996). Autism: Towards an integration of clinical genetic neuropsychological and neurobiological perspectives. *Journal of Child Psychology and Psychiatry*, 37, 89–126.

Bailey, N. (1993). *Bailey's Scales II*. San Antonio, TX: Psychological Corporation.

Bailey, S. (2002). Treatment of delinquents. In M. Rutter, E. & Taylor (eds.), *Child and Adolescent Psychiatry* (Fourth edition, pp. 1019–1037). Oxford: Blackwell.

Baker, L. & Cantwell, D. (1982). Psychiatric disorder in children with different types of communication disorder. *Journal of Communication Disorders*, 15, 113–126.

Bandura, A. (1997). *Self-Efficacy*. New York: Freeman.

Bandura, A. & Walters, R. (1959). *Adolescent Aggression*. New York: Ronald Press.

Banez, G. & Cunningham, C. (2003). Paediatric gastrointestinal disorders: Recurrent abdominal pain, inflammatory bowel disease and rumination disorder/cyclic vomiting. In M. Roberts (ed.), *Handbook of Paediatric Psychology* (Third edition, pp. 462–480). New York: Guilford.

Barclay, D. & Houts, A. (1995). Childhood enuresis. In C. Schaefer (ed.), *Clinical Handbook of Sleep Disorders in Children* (pp. 223–252). Northvale, NJ: Jason Aronson.

Barkley, R. (1997). *Defiant Children: A Clinician's Manual for Parent Training* (Second edition). New York: Guilford Press.

Barkley, R. (1998a). *Attention Deficit Hyperactivity Disorder: A Handbook for Diagnosis and Treatment* (Second edition). New York. Guilford.

Barkley, R. (1998b). Attention deficit hyperactivity disorder. In E. Mash & R. Barkley (eds.), *Treatment of Childhood Disorders* (Third edition, pp. 55–110). New York: Guildfod.

Barkley, R. (2003). Attention deficit hyperactivity disorder. In E. Mash & R. Barkley (eds.), *Child Psychopathology* (Second edition, pp. 75–143). New York: Guildford.

Barkley, R., Guevremont, A., Anastopoulas, A. & Fletcher, K. (1992). A comparison of three family therapy programs for treating family conflicts in adolescents with attention deficit hyperactivity disorder. *Journal of Consulting and Clinical Psychology*, 60, 450–462.

Barlow, D. (2002). *Anxiety and its Disorders* (Second edition). New York: Guilford.

Barlow, D. & Cerny, J. (1988). *Psychological Treatment Of Panic.* New York: Guilford.

Bar-On, R. & Parker, J. (2000). *The Handbook of Emotional Intelligence.* San Francisco, CA: Jossey-Bass.

Baron-Cohen, S., Mortimore, C. Moriarity, J. Izaguirre, J. & Roberson, M. (1999). The prevalence of Gilles de la Tourette's syndrome in children and adolescents with autism. *Journal of Child Psychology and Psychiatry,* 40, 213–218.

Baron-Cohen, S., Tager-Flusberg, H, & Cohen, D. (2000). *Understanding Other Minds: Perspectives from Developmental Neuroscience* (Second edition). Oxford: Oxford University Press.

Barrett, P., Healy-Farrell, L., Piacentini, J. & March, J. (2004). Obsessive-compulsive disorder in childhood and adolescence: Description and treatment. In P. Barrett & T. Ollendick (eds.), *Handbook of Interventions that Work with Children and Adolescents: Prevention and Treatment* (pp. 187–216). Chichester: Wiley.

Barrett, P. & Shortt, A. (2003). Parental involvement in the treatment of anxious children. In A. Kazdin, & J. Weisz (eds.), *Evidence-Based Psychotherapies for Children and Adolescents* (pp. 101–119). New York: Guilford.

Bates, E., Bretherton, I. & Snyder, L. (1988). *From First Words to Grammar: Individual Differences and Dissociable Mechanisms.* New York: Cambridge University Press.

Battle, J. (2002). *Culture-Free Self-Esteem Inventories. Examiner's Manual* (Third edition). Austin, TX: Pro-ed. http://www.jamesbattle.com/cfsei.htm

Bebbington, P., Wilkins, S., Sham, P., Jones P., van Os, J., Murray, R., Toone B. & Lewis, S. (1996). Life events before psychotic episodes: Do clinical and social variables affect the relationship? *Social Psychiatry Psychiatric Epidemiology,* 31, 122–128.

Beck, A. (1976). *Cognitive Therapy and the Emotional Disorders.* New York: International Universities Press.

Beck, A. & Clark, D. (1997). An information processing model of anxiety: Automatic and strategic processes. *Behaviour Research and Therapy,* 35, 49–58.

Beck, A., Emery, G. & Greenberg, R. (1985). *Anxiety Disorders and Phobias.* New York: Guilford.

Becker, J. & Kaplan, M. (1993). Cognitive behavioural treatment of the juvenile sex offender. In H. Barbaree, W. Marshall & S. Hudson (eds.), *The Juvenile Sex Offender* (pp. 264–277). New York: Guilford.

Beer, D., Karitani, M., Leonard, H., March, J. & Swedo, S. (2002). Obsessive-compulsive disorder. In S. Kutcher (ed.), *Practical Child and Adolescent Psychopharmacology* (pp. 159–186). Cambridge: Cambridge University Press.

Behan, J. & Carr, A. (2000). Oppositional defiant disorder. In A. Carr (ed.), *What Works With Children And Adolescents? A Critical Review Of Psychological Interventions With Children, Adolescents And Their Families* (pp. 102–130). London: Routledge.

Beidel, E., Morris, T. & Turner M., (2004). Social phobia. In T. Morris & J. March (2004). *Anxiety Disorders in Children and Adolescents* (Second edition, pp. 141–163). New York: Guilford.

Benjamin, M & Irving, H. (1995). Research in family mediation: Review and implications. *Mediation Quarterly,* 13, 53–82.

Bentall, R. (2004). *Madness Explained.* London: Penguin.

Bentovim, A. (1992). *Trauma-Organized Systems: Physical and Sexual Abuse in Families.* London: Karnac.

Bentovim, A., Elton, A., Hildebrand, J., Tranter, M. & Vizard, E. (1988). *Child Sexual Abuse within the Family: Assessment and Treatment.* London: Wright.

Berger, M. (1996). Outcomes and Effectiveness in Clinical Psychology Practice. *Division of Clinical Psychology Occasional Paper No 1.* Leicester: British Psychological Society.

Berger, M., Hill, P., Sein, E., Thompson, M. & Verduyn, C. (1993). *A Proposed Core Data Set for Child and Adolescent Psychology and Psychiatry Services.* London: Association for Child Psychology and Psychiatry.

Berliner, L. & Elliott, D. (2002). Sexual abuse of children. In J. Myers, L. Berliner, J. Briere, C. Hendrix, C. Jenny & T. Reid (eds.), *APSAC Handbook on Child Maltreatment* (Second edition, pp. 55–78). Thousand Oaks, CA: Sage.

Berman, A. & Jobes, D. (1996) *Adolescent Suicide: Assessment and Intervention.* Washington DC: APA.

Berridge, D. (2002). Residential care. In D. McNeish, T. Newman, & H. Roberts (eds.), *What Works for Children* (pp. 83–104). Buckingham: Open University Press.

Bettelheim, B. (1967). *The Empty Fortress.* New York: Free Press.

Beutler, L., Machado, P. & Neufeldt, S, (1994). Therapist variables. In A. Bergin & S. Garfield (eds.), *Handbook of Psychotherapy and Behaviour Change* (Fourth edition, pp. 229–269). Chichester: Wiley.

Bibace, R. (1981). *Children's Conceptions of Health, Illness and Bodily Functions.* San Francisco: Jossey Bass.

Bibace, R. & Walsh, M. (1979). Developmental stages in children's conceptions of illness. In G. Stone, F. Cohen & N. Adler (eds.), *Health Psychology: A Handbook.* San Francisco: Jossey Bass.

Bibring, E. (1965). The mechanism of depression. In P. Greenacre (ed.), *Affective Disorders* (pp.13–48). New York: International Universities Press.

Biederman, J., Faraone, S., Doyle, A., Krifcher-Lehman, B., Kraus, I., Perrin, J. & Tsuang, M. (1993). Convergence of the Child Behaviour Checklist with structured interview-based psychiatric diagnoses of ADHD children with and without co-morbidity. *Journal of Child Psychology and Psychiatry*, 34, 1241–1251.

Bieri, D., Reeve, R., Champion, G. & Addicoat, L. (1990). The faces pain scale for the self-assessment of the severity of pain experienced by children: Development, initial validation and preliminary investigation for ratio scale properties. *Pain*, 41, 139–150.

Birchwood, M. (1996). Early intervention in psychotic relapse. Cognitive approaches to detection and management. In G. Haddock & P. Slade (eds.), *Cognitive-behavioural Interventions with Psychotic Disorders.* (pp. 171–211). London: Routledge.

Birchwood, M., Spencer, E. & McGovern, D. (2000). Schizophrenia: Early warning signs. *Advances in Psychiatric Treatment*, 6, 93–101.

Birchwood, M. & Tarrier, N. (1994). *Psychological Management of Schizophrenia.* Chichester: Wiley.

Bird, H., Canino, G., Rubio-Stipec, M., Gould, M., Ribera., J. Sesman, M., Woodbury, M., S. Huertas-Goldman, S., Pagan, A. & Sanchez-Lacay, A. (1988). Estimates of the prevalence of childhood maladjustment in a community survey in Puerto Rico. *Archives of General Psychiatry*, 45, 1120–1126.

Bishop, D. (1992). The underlying nature of specific language impairment. *Journal of Child Psychology and Psychiatry*, 33, 3–66.

Bishop, D. (2002). Developmental disorders of speech and language. In M. Rutter & E. Taylor (eds.) *Child and Adolescent Psychiatry* (Fourth edition, pp. 664–681). Oxford: Blackwell.

Bishop, D. & Adams, C. (1990). A prospective study of the relationship between specific language impairment, phonological disorders and reading retardation. *Journal of Child Psychology and Psychiatry*, 31, 1027–1050.

Black, D. (1994). Psychological reactions to life-threatening and terminal illness and bereavement. In M. Rutter, E. Taylor & L. Hersov (eds.), *Child and Adolescent Psychiatry: Modern Approaches* (Third edition, pp. 77–793). London: Blackwell.

Black, D. (2000). The effects of bereavement in childhood. In. M. Gelder, J. Lopez-Ibor & N. Andreasen (eds.), *New Oxford Textbook of Psychiatry* (volume 2, section 9.3.5, pp.1855–1858). Oxford: Oxford University Press.

Black, D. (2002). Bereavement. In M. Rutter & E. Taylor (eds.), *Child and Adolescent Psychiatry: Modern Approaches* (Fourth edition, pp. 299–308). London: Blackwell.

Black, D., Harris-Hendricks, J. & Wolkind, S. (1998). *Child Psychiatry and the Law* (Third edition). London: Gaskell and Royal College of Psychiatrists.

Black, D. & Urbanowicz, M. (1987). Family intervention with bereaved children. *Journal of Child Psychology and Psychiatry*, 28, 467–476.

Blagg, N. (1987). *School Phobia and its Treatment*. London: Croom Helm.

Blancher, J. & Kraemer, B. (2005). Supporting families who have children with disabilities. In G. O'Reilly, G. P. Walsh, A. Carr, & J. McEvoy (eds.), *Handbook of Intellectual Disability and Clinical Psychology Practice*. London: Brunner-Routledge.

Blatt, S. (2004). *Experiences of Depression. Theoretical, Clinical and Research Perspectives*. Washington, DC: APA.

Bleuler, E. (1911). *Dementia Praecox or the Group of Schizophrenias*. New York: International University Press.

Blount, R., Piira, T. & Cohen, L. (2003). Management of paediatric pain and distress due to medical procedures. In M. Roberts (ed.), *Handbook of Paediatric Psychology* (Third edition, pp. 216–233). New York: Guilford.

Boer, B. & Lindhout, I. (2001). Family and genetic influences: Is anxiety 'all in the family'? In W. Silverman & P. Treffers (eds.) *Anxiety Disorders in Children and Adolescents. Research Assessment and Intervention* (pp. 235–254). Cambridge: Cambridge University Press.

Bolton, P. & Holland, A. (1994). Chromosomal abnormalities. In M. Rutter, E. Taylor & L. Hersov (eds.) *Child and Adolescent Psychiatry: Modern Approaches* (Third edition, pp. 152–171). Oxford: Blackwell.

Bondy, A. & Frost, L. (1994) The Picture Exchange Communication System. *Focus on Autistic Behaviour*, 9, 1–19.

Borduin, C., Henggeler, S., Blaske, D. & Stein, R. (1990). Multisystemic treatment of adolescent sex offenders. *International Journal of Offender Therapy and Comparative Criminology*, 34, 105–113.

Bornstein, M. & Sigman, M. (1986). Continuity in mental development from infancy. *Child Development*, 57, 251–274.

Bowlby, J. (1944). Forty-four juvenile lives: Their characters and homelife. *International Journal of Psychoanalysis*, 25, 1–57.

Bowlby, J. (1969). *Attachment and loss. Volume 1*. London: Hogarth Press.

Bowlby, J. (1973). *Attachment and Loss. Volume 2*. London: Hogarth Press.

Bowlby, J. (1980). *Attachment and Loss. Volume 3*. London: Hogarth Press.

Bowlby, J. (1988). *A Secure Base: Clinical Applications of Attachment Theory*. London: Hogarth Press.

Bowman-Edmondson, C. & Cohen Conger, J. (1996). A review of treatment efficacy for individuals with anger problems: Conceptual, assessment and methodological issues. *Clinical Psychology Review*, 16, 251–275.

Boyle, M. (2002). *Schizophrenia. A Scientific Delusion* (Second edition). London: Routledge.

Bradley, C. (1937). The behaviour of children receiving benzedrine. *American Journal of Psychiatry*, 94, 577–585.

Bradley, C. (1994a). Contributions of psychology to diabetes management. *British Journal of Clinical Psychology*, 33, 11–21.

Bradley, R. (1994b). The HOME Inventory: Review and reflections. In H. Reese (ed.), *Advances in Child Development and Behaviour* (pp. 241–288). San Diego, CA; Academic Press.

Bradley, R., Caldwell, B., Rock, S. & Ramey, C. (1989). Home environment and cognitive development in the first three years of life: A collaborative study involving six sites and three ethnic groups in North America. *Developmental Psychology*, 25, 217–235.

Braff, D. (1999). Psychophysiological and information processing approaches to schizophrenia. In D., Charney, E. Nestler & B. Bunney (eds.), *Neurobiological Foundations of Mental Illness* (pp. 258–271). New York: Oxford University Press.

Bray, J. & Hetherington, M. (1993). Special section: Families in transition. *Journal of Family Psychology*, 7, 3–103.

Bregman, J. & Gerdtz, J. (1997). Behavioural interventions. In D. Cohen & F. Volkmar, (eds.), *Handbook of Autism and Pervasive Developmental Disorders* (Second edition, pp. 606–631). New York: Wiley.

Brent, D. (1997). The aftercare of adolescents with deliberate self-harm. *Journal of Child Psychology and Psychiatry*, 38, 277–286.

Brent, D., Gaynor, S. & Weersing, V. (2002). Cognitive behavioural approaches to the treatment of depression and anxiety. In M. Rutter, E. & Taylor (eds.), *Child and Adolescent Psychiatry* (Fourth edition, pp. 921–937). Oxford: Blackwell.

Brewin, C. (2001). A cognitive neuroscience account of post-traumatic stress disorder and its treatment. *Behaviour Research and Therapy*, 39, 373–393.

Brinkley, A., Cullen, R. & Carr, A. (2002). Prevention of adjustment problems in children with asthma. In A. Carr (ed.), *Prevention: What Works with Children and Adolescents? A Critical Review of Psychological Prevention Programmes for Children, Adolescents and their Families* (pp. 222–248). London: Routledge.

Brinkmeyer, M. & Eyberg, S. (2003). Parent–child interaction therapy for oppositional children. In A. Kazdin, & J. Weisz (eds.), *Evidence Based Psychotherapies for Children and Adolescents* (pp. 204–223). New York: Guilford.

British Psychological Society (BPsS) (1995). *Professional Practice Guidelines 1995*. Leicester, UK: BPsS.

British Psychological Society (BPsS) (1996). *Expert Testimony: Developing Witness Skills*. Leicester, UK: BPsS.

British Psychological Society, Division of Clinical Psychology (2000). *Recent*

Advances in Understanding Mental Illness and Psychotic Experiences. Leicester, UK: BPsS.

Bronfenbrenner, U. (1986). Ecology of the family as a context for human development: Research perspectives. *Developmental Psychology*, 22, 723–742.

Brook, J., Brook, D., Gordon, A., Whiteman, M. & Cohen, P. (1990). The psychosocial aetiology of adolescent drug abuse: A family interactional approach. *Genetic, Social and General Psychology Monographs*, 116, 111–267.

Brooks-Gunn, J., Auth, J., Petersen, A. & Compas, B. (2001). Physiological processes and the development of childhood and adolescent depression. In I. Goodyer (ed.). *The Depressed Child and Adolescent* (Second edition, pp. 79–118). Cambridge: Cambridge University Press.

Brosnan, R. & Carr, A. (2000). Adolescent conduct problems. In A. Carr (ed.), *What Works With Children And Adolescents? A Critical Review Of Psychological Interventions With Children, Adolescents And Their Families* (pp. 131–154). London: Routledge.

Browne, A. & Finklehor, D. (1986). The impact of child sexual abuse: A review of the research. *Psychological Bulletin*, 99, 66–77.

Browne, K. (2002). Child protection. In M. Rutter, E. & Taylor (eds.), *Child and Adolescent Psychiatry* (Fourth edition, pp. 1158–1174). Oxford: Blackwell.

Bruch, H. (1973). *Eating Disorders.* New York: Basic Books.

Bruininks, R., Woodcock, R., Weatherman, R. & Hill, B. (1996). *Scales of Independent Behaviour – Revised.* Ithaca, IL: Riverside.

Bruner, J. (1983). *Child's Talk: Learning to use Language.* New York: Norton.

Bruni, O., Ottaviano, S., Guidetti, V., Romoli M., Innocenzi, M., Cortesi, F. & Giannotti, F. (1996). The Sleep Disturbance Scale for Children (SDSC). Construction and validation of an instrument to evaluate sleep disturbances in childhood and adolescence. *Journal of Sleep Research*, 5, 251–61.

Brunk, M., Henggeler, S. & Whelan, J. (1987). Comparison of multisystemic therapy and parent training in the brief treatment of child abuse and neglect. *Journal of Consulting and Clinical Psychology*, 55, 171–178.

Bryant-Waugh, R. (2000). Overview of the eating disorders. In B. Lask & R. Bryant-Waugh (eds.), *Anorexia Nervosa and Related Eating Disorders in Childhood and Adolescence* (Second edition, pp. 27–40). London: Brunner-Routledge.

Bryant-Waugh, R. & Lask, B. (1999). *Eating Disorders: A Parent's Guide.* London: Penguin.

Buchanan, A. (1992). *Children Who Soil. Assessment and Treatment.* Chichester: Wiley.

Burke, J., Loeber, R. & Birmaher, B. (2002). Oppositional defiant disorder and conduct disorder: A review of the past 10 years, part II. *Journal of the American Academy of Child & Adolescent Psychiatry*, 41(11), 1275–1293.

Caldwell, B. & Bradley, R. (2001). *Home Observation for Measurement of the Environment-HOME Inventory and Administration Manual.* Little Rock, AR: University of Arkansas at Little Rock. http://www.ualr.edu/~crtldept/home4.htm

Campo, J. & Fritsch, S. (1994). Somatization in children and adolescents. *Journal of the American Academy of Child and Adolescent Psychiatry*, 33, 1223–1235.

Cantwell, D. & Rutter, M. (1994). Classification: Conceptual issues and substantive findings. In M. Rutter, E. Taylor & L. Hersov (eds.), *Child and Adolescent Psychiatry: Modern Approaches* (Third edition, pp. 3–21). Oxford: Blackwell.

Carr, A. (1993). Epidemiology of psychological disorders in Irish children. *Irish Journal of Psychology*, 14, 4, 546–560.

Carr, A. (1995). *Positive Practice: A Step-by-Step Approach to Family Therapy.* Reading, UK: Harwood.

Carr, A. (1997). *Family Therapy and Systemic Consultation.* Lanham, MD: University Press of America.

Carr, A. (2000a). *What Works with Children and Adolescents? A Critical Review of Psychological Interventions with Children, Adolescents and Their Families.* London: Routledge.

Carr, A. (2000b). *Family Therapy: Concepts, Process and Practice.* Chichester: Wiley.

Carr, A. (2002a). *Prevention: What Works? A Critical Review of Research on Psychological Prevention Programmes with Children, Adolescents and their Families.* London: Brunner-Routledge.

Carr, A. (2002b). *Depression and Attempted Suicide in Adolescence.* Oxford: Blackwell.

Carr, A. (2004a). *Positive Psychology. The Science of Happiness and Human Strengths.* London: Brunner-Routledge.

Carr, A. (2004b). Interventions for post-traumatic stress disorder in children and adolescents. *Paediatric Rehabilitation*, 7, 1–14.

Carr, A., McDonnell, D. & Owen, P. (1994). Audit and family systems consultation: Evaluation of practice at a child and family centre. *Journal of Family Therapy*, 16, 143–157.

Carr, A. & McNulty, M. (in press a). Cognitive behavioural approaches. In A. Carr & M. McNulty (eds.), *Handbook of Adult Clinical Psychology: An Evidence-Based Practice Approach.* London: Brunner-Routledge.

Carr, A. & McNulty, M. (in press b). Interpersonal and systemic approaches. In A. Carr & M. McNulty (eds.), *Handbook of Adult Clinical Psychology: An Evidence-Based Practice Approach.* London: Brunner-Routledge.

Carr, A. & McNulty, M. (in press c). Depression. In A. Carr & M. McNulty (eds.), *Handbook of Adult Clinical Psychology. An Evidence-Based Practice Approach.* London: Brunner-Routledge.

Carr, A. & O'Reilly, G. (2004). *Clinical Psychology in Ireland, Volume 5: Empirical Studies of Child Sexual Abuse.* Wales: Edwin Mellen Press.

Carr, A. & O'Reilly, G. (2005). Diagnosis, classification and epidemiology of disabilities. In G. O'Reilly, P. Walsh, A. Carr, & J. McEvoy (eds.), *Handbook of Intellectual Disability and Clinical Psychology Practice.* London: Brunner-Routledge.

Carter, B. & McGoldrick, M. (1999). *The Expanded Family Lifecycle. Individual, Family and Social Perspectives* (Third edition). Boston: Allyn & Bacon.

Cassidy, J. & Shaver, P. (1999). *Handbook of Attachment.* New York: Guilford.

Cattell, R. (1963). Theory of fluid and crystallized intelligence: A critical experiment. *Journal of Educational Psychology*, 54, 1–22.

Cecchin, G. (1987). Hypothesizing, circularity and neutrality revisited: An invitation to curiosity. *Family Process*, 26, 405–413.

Ceci, S. (2002). *Expert Witnesses in Child Abuse Cases: What Can and Should Be Said in Court?* Washington, DC: American Psychological Association.

Ceci, S. & Bruck, M. (1993). Suggestibility of the child witness: A historical review and synthesis. *Psychological Bulletin*, 113, 403–439.

Celano, M. & Geller, R. (1993). Learning, school performance, and children with asthma: How much at risk? *Journal of Learning Disabilities*, 26, 23–32.

Chadwick, P., Birchwood, M. & Trower, P. (1996). *Cognitive Therapy for Delusions, Voices and Paranoia*. Chichester: Wiley.

Chaffin, M., Letourneau, E. & Silovsky, J. (2002). Adults, adolescents, and children who sexually abuse children: A developmental perspective. In J. Myers, L. Berliner, J. Briere, C. Hendrix, C. Jenny & T. Reid (eds.), *APSAC Handbook on Child Maltreatment* (Second edition, pp. 205–232). Thousand Oaks, CA: Sage.

Chalder T. (1995). *Coping with Chronic Fatigue Syndrome*. London: Sheldon.

Chalder, T. (2005). Chronic fatigue syndrome. In P. Graham (ed.), *Cognitive Behaviour Therapy for Children and Families* (Second edition, pp. 385–401). Cambridge: Cambridge University Press.

Chalder T. & Hussain, K. (2002). *Self-help for Chronic Fatigue Syndrome: A Guide for Young People*. Oxford: Blue Stallion.

Chamberlain, P. (1994). *Family Connections: A treatment foster care model for adolescents with delinquency*. Eugene, OR: Castalia.

Chamberlain, P. (2003). *Treating Chronic Juvenile Offenders: Advances Made Through the Oregon Multidimensional Treatment Foster Care Model*. Washington, DC: American Psychological Association.

Chamberlin, P. & Mihalic, S. (1998). *Blueprints for Violence Prevention, Book Eight: Multidimensional Treatment Foster Care (MTFC)*. Boulder, CO: Center for the Study and Prevention of Violence. http://www.colorado.edu/cspv/publications/blueprints.html

Chamberlain, P. & Reid J. (1987). Parent observation and report of child symptoms. *Behavioural Assessment*, 9, 97–109.

Chamberlain, P. & Smith, D. (2003). Antisocial behaviour in children and adolescents. The Oregon multidimensional treatment foster care model. In A. Kazdin, & J. Weisz (eds.), *Evidence-Based Psychotherapies for Children and Adolescents* (pp. 281–300). New York: Guilford.

Chambers, W., Puigh-Antich, J., Hirsch, M., Paez, P., Ambrosini, P., Tabrizi, M. & Davies, M. (1985). The assessment of affective disorders in children and adolescents by semistructured interview: Test-retest reliability of the Schedule for Affective Disorders and Schizophrenia for school age children. Present episode version. *Archives of General Psychiatry*, 42, 696–702.

Charman, T. & Baird, G. (2002). Practitioner review: Diagnosis of autism spectrum disorder in 2- and 3-year-old children. *Journal of Child Psychology and Psychiatry*, 43, 289–306.

Chassin, L., Ritter, J. Trim, R., & King, K. (2003). Adolescent substance use disorders. In E. Mash & R. Barkley (eds.), *Child Psychopathology* (Second edition, pp. 199–230). New York: Guilford.

Chervin, R., Hedger, K., Dillon, J. & Pituch, K. (2000). Paediatric Sleep Questionnaire (PSQ): Validity and reliability of scales for sleep-disordered breathing, snoring, sleepiness and behavioural problems. *Sleep Medicine*, 1, 21–32.

Chess, S. & Thomas, A. (1995). *Temperament in Clinical Practice*. New York: Guilford.

Chiauzzi, E. & Liljegren, S. (1993). Taboo topics in addiction treatment: An empirical review of clinical folklore. *Journal of Substance Abuse Treatment*, 10, 303–316.

Chiavaroli, T. (1992). Rehabilitation from substance abuse in individuals with a history of sexual abuse. *Journal of Substance Abuse Treatment*, 9, 349–354.

Chowdhury, U. (2004). *Tics and Tourette Syndrome. A Handbook for Parents and Professionals*. London: Jessica Kingsley.

Chowdhury, U., Frampton, I. & Heyman, I. (2004). Clinical characteristics of young people referred to an obsessive compulsive disorder clinic in the United Kingdom. *Clinical Child Psychology & Psychiatry*, 9, 395–401.

Cicchetti, D. (1991). Fractures in the crystal: Developmental psychopathology and the emergence of self. *Developmental Review*, 11, 271–287.

Cicchetti, D. (2004). Odyssey of discovery: Lessons learned through three decades of research on child maltreatment. *American Psychologist. Special Awards Issue 2004*, 59, 731–741.

Clark, A. (2001). Proposed treatment for adolescent psychosis. 2. Bipolar illness. *Advances in Psychiatric Treatment*, 7, 143–149.

Clark, D. (1986). A cognitive approach to panic. *Behaviour Research and Therapy*, 24, 461–470.

Clark, D. & Wells, A. (1995). Cognitive model of social phobias. In R. Heinberg, D. Liebowitz, D. Hope & F. Schneier (eds.), *Social Phobia: Diagnosis, Assessment and Treatment* (pp. 69–93). New York: Guilford.

Clark, L., Watson, D. & Reynolds, S. (1995). Diagnosis and classification of psychopathology: Challenges to the current system and future directions. *Annual Review of Psychology*, 46, 121–153.

Clarke, G., DeBar, L. & Lewinsohn, P. (2003). Cognitive-behavioural group treatment for adolescent depression. In A. Kazdin, & J. Weisz (eds.), *Evidence-Based Psychotherapies for Children and Adolescents* (pp. 120–134). New York: Guilford.

Clayden, G., Taylor, E., Loader, P., Borztskowski, M. & Edwards, M. (2002). Wetting and soiling in childhood. In M. Rutter, & E. Taylor (eds.), *Child and Adolescent Psychiatry* (Fourth edition, pp. 793–810). Oxford: Blackwell.

Cloward, R. & Ohlin, L. (1960). *Delinquency and Opportunity*. Glencoe, IL: Free Press.

Cohen, D., & Volkmar, F. (1997). *Handbook of Autism and Pervasive Developmental Disorders* (Second edition). New York: Wiley.

Cohen, N. (2002). Adoption. In M. Rutter, & E. Taylor (eds.), *Child and Adolescent Psychiatry* (Fourth edition, pp. 373–381). Oxford: Blackwell.

Cohen, P., Cohen, J., Kasen, S., Velez, C., Hartmark, C., Johnson, J., Rojas, M., Brook, J. & Streuning, E. (1993). An epidemiological study of disorders in late childhood and adolescence. 1. Age- and gender-specific prevalence. *Journal of Child Psychology and Psychiatry*, 34, 851–867.

Colapinto, J. (1991). Structural family therapy. In A. Gurman & D. Kniskern (eds.), *Handbook of Family Therapy. Volume II* (pp. 417–443). New York: Brunner Mazel.

Colby, A. & Kohlberg, L. (1987). *The Measurement of Moral Judgement Volumes 1 and 2*. Cambridge: Cambridge University Press.

Cole, T., Freeman, J. & Preece, M. (1995). Body mass index reference curves for the UK, 1990. *Archives of Disease in Childhood*, 73, 25–29.

Coleman, J. (1995). *Teenagers and Sexuality*. London: Hodder and Stoughton.

Coleman, R. & Cassell, D. (1995). Parents who misuse drugs and alcohol. In P. Reder & C. Lucey (eds.), *Assessment of Parenting: Psychiatric and Psychological Contributions* (pp. 182–193). London: Routledge.

Collier, D. & Treasure, J. (2004). The aetiology of eating disorders. *British Journal of Psychiatry*, 185, 363–365.

Commission on Classification and Terminology of the International League Against Epilepsy (1989). Proposal for revised classification of epilepsies and epileptic syndromes. *Epilepsia*, 30, 389–399.

Compton, S., March, J., Brent, D., Albano, A. Weersing, V. & Curry, J. (2004). Cognitive-behavioural psychotherapy for anxiety and depressive disorders in children and adolescents: An evidence-based medicine review. *Journal of the American Academy of Child & Adolescent Psychiatry*, 43, 930–959.

Connelly, M. (2003). Recurrent paediatric headache: A comprehensive review. *Children's Health Care*, 32, 153–189.

Conners, C. (1997). *Connors Rating Scales. Revised Technical Manual.* North Tonawanda, NY: Multihealth Systems.

Conte, H. & Plutchik, R. (1995). *Ego Defences: Theory and Measurement.* New York: Wiley.

Cooper, P. (1995). *Bulimia Nervosa: A Guide to Recovery.* London: Robinson Publishing.

Corcoran, K. & Fischer, J. (2000). *Measures for Clinical Practice: A Sourcebook: Volume 1: Couples, Families, and Children* (Third edition). New York: Free Press.

Cormack, C. & Carr, A. (2000). Drug abuse. In A. Carr (ed.), *What Works with Children and Adolescents? A Critical Review of Psychological Interventions with Children, Adolescents and their Families* (pp. 155–177). London: Routledge.

Corr, C. & Balk, D. (1996). *Handbook of Adolescent Death and Bereavement.* New York: Springer.

Costello, A., Edelbrock, C., Dulcan, M., Kalas, R. & Klaric, S. (1984). *Report on the Diagnostic Interview Schedule for Children (DISC).* Pittsburgh, PA: Department of Psychiatry, University of Pittsburgh.

Cottrell, D. (2003). Outcome studies of family therapy in child and adolescent depression. *Journal of Family Therapy*, 25, 406–416.

Coughlan, B., Doyle, M. & Carr, A. (2002). Prevention of teenage smoking, alcohol use and drug abuse. In A. Carr (ed.), *Prevention: What Works with Children and Adolescents? A Critical Review of Psychological Prevention Programmes for Children, Adolescents and their Families* (pp. 267–286). London: Routledge.

Coyle, K. (2005). Person-centred planning and intellectual disability. In G. O'Reilly, P. Walsh, A. Carr, & J. McEvoy (eds.), *Handbook of Intellectual Disability and Clinical Psychology Practice.* London: Brunner-Routledge.

Creighton, S. (2004). *Prevalence and Incidence of Child Abuse: International Comparisons.* NSPCC Information Briefings. UK: NSPCC Research Department. http://www.nspcc.org.uk/inform

Crick, N. & Dodge, K. (1994). A review and reformulation of social information processing mechanisms in children's social adjustment. *Psychological Bulletin*, 115, 74–101.

Crisp, A. (1983). Anorexia nervosa. *British Medical Journal*, 287, 855–858.

Crome, I., Ghodse, H., Gilvarry, E. & McArdle, P. (2004). *Young People and Substance Misuse.* London: Gaskell.

Crome, I. & McArdle, P. (2004). Prevention programmes. In I. Crome, H. Ghodse, E. Gilvarry & P. McArdle (eds.), *Young People and Substance Misuse* (pp. 15–30). London: Gaskell.

Crow, T. (1985). The two syndrome concept: Origins and current status. *Schizophrenia Bulletin*, 9, 471–486.

Cull, C. & Goldstein, L. (1997). *The Clinical Psychologist's Handbook of Epilepsy*. London: Routledge.

Cullen, J. & Carr, A. (1999). Co-dependency: An empirical study from a systemic perspective. *Contemporary Family Therapy*, 21, 505–526.

Cunningham, C., Bremmer, R. & Boyle, M. (1995). Large group community based parenting programmes for families of preschoolers at risk for disruptive behaviour disorders: Utilisation, cost effectiveness and outcome. *Journal of Child Psychology and Psychiatry*, 36, 1141–1160.

Dahlem, N. W., Zimet, S. G. & Walker, R. (1991) The Multidimensional Scale of Perceived Social support: A Confirmation Study. *Journal of Clinical Psychology*, 47, 756–761.

Dale, P. (1986). *Dangerous Families: Assessment and Treatment of Child Abuse*. London: Tavistock.

Dalton, P. (1983). Family treatment of an obsessive compulsive child: A case report. *Family Process*, 22, 99–108.

Damon, W. & Hart, D. (1988). *Self-understanding in Childhood and Adolescence*. New York: Cambridge University Press.

Dare, C. (1985). The family therapy of anorexia nervosa. *Journal of Psychiatric Research*, 19, 435–453.

Dare, C. & Crowther, C. (1995a). Living dangerously: Psychoanalytic psychotherapy of anorexia nervosa. In G. Szmukler, C. Dare & J. Treasure (eds.), *Handbook of Eating Disorders* (pp. 293–308). Chichester: Wiley.

Dare, C. & Crowther, C. (1995b). Psychodynamic models of eating disorders. In G. Szmukler, C. Dare & J. Treasure (eds.), *Handbook of Eating Disorders* (pp. 125–140). Chichester: Wiley.

Darling, N, & Steinberg, L. (1993). Parenting styles as context: An integrative model. *Psychological Bulletin*, 113, 487–496.

Dausch, B. M., Miklowitz, D. J. & Richards, J. A. (1996). Global assessment of relational functioning scale (GARF): II. Reliability and validity in a sample of families of bipolar patients. *Family Process*, 35(2), 175–189.

Davies, G. & Westcott, H. (1999). *Interviewing Child Witnesses under the Memorandum of Good Practice: A Research Review*. London, UK: Home Office Policing and Reducing Crime Unit. http://www.homeoffice.gov.uk/rds/prgpdfs/fprs115.pdf

Davis, C. (1980). *Perkins–Binet Tests of Intelligence for the Blind*. Watertown, MA: Perkins School for the Blind.

Davis, I. & Ellis-MacLeod, E. (1994). Temporary foster care. In J. Blancher (ed.), *When There's no Place Like Home* (pp. 123–161). Baltimore, MD: Brookes.

de Wilde, E., Kienhorst, I. & Diekstra, R. (2001). Suicidal behaviour in adolescents. In I. Goodyer (ed.), *The Depressed Child and Adolescent* (Second edition, pp.267–291). Cambridge: Cambridge University Press.

Deary, I. (2000). *Looking Down on Human Intelligence. From Psychometrics to the Brain*. Oxford: Oxford University Press.

DeSilva, P. Rachman, S. & Seligman, M. (1977). Prepared phobias and obsessions: Therapeutic outcome. *Behaviour Research and Therapy*, 15, 65–77.

Doane, J., West, K. & Goldstein, M. (1981). Parental communication deviance and affective style: Predictors of subsequent schizophrenia spectrum disorders in vulnerable adolescents. *Archives of General Psychiatry*, 38, 670–685.

Dodge, E., Hodes, M., Eisler, I. & Dare, C. (1995). Family therapy for bulimia nervosa in adolescents: An exploratory study. *Journal of Family Therapy*, 17, 59–77.

Dohrenwend, B., Levav, I. Shrout, P., Schwartz, S., Naveh, G., Link, B., Skodol, A. & Stueve, A. (1992). Socio-economic status and psychiatric disorders: The causation-selection issue. *Science*, 255, 946–952.

Donohue, B., Miller, E. Van Hasselt, V. & Hersen, M. (1998). An ecobehavioural approach to child maltreatment. In E. Van Hasselt & M. Hersen (eds.), *Handbook of Psychological Treatment Protocols for Children and Adolescents* (pp. 279–356). Mahwah, NJ: Lawrence Erlbaum Associates Inc.

Dosen, A. & Day, K. (2001). Epidemiology, aetiology and presentation of mental illness and behaviour disorders in persons with mental retardation. In A. Dosen & K. Day (eds.), *Treating Mental Illness and Behaviour Disorders in Children and Adults with Mental Retardation* (pp. 3–26). Washington,DC: American Psychiatric Association.

Dougherty, E. (1996). *Report Writer: Children's Intellectual and Achievement Tests*. Odessa: FL: Psychological Assessment Resources.

Douglas, J. (1989). Training parents to mange their child's sleep problem. In C. Schaefer & J. Briesmeister (eds.), *Handbook of Parent Training* (pp.13–37). New York: Wiley.

Douglas, J. (2005). Behavioural approaches to eating and sleeping problems in young children. In P. Graham (ed.), *Cognitive Behaviour Therapy for Children and Families* (Second edition, pp. 187–206) Cambridge: Cambridge University Press.

Douglas, J. & Richman, N. (1985). *Sleep Management Manual*. London: Institute of Child Health, Hospital for Sick Children, Great Ormond Street.

Douglas, V. (1983). Attention and cognitive problems. In M. Rutter (ed.), *Developmental Neuropsychiatry* (pp. 280–329). New York: Guilford.

Dowden, C. & Andrews. D. (1999). What Works in Young Offender Treatment: A Meta-Analysis. *Forum on Corrections Research*, 11 (2), 21–24.

Dowling, E. & Gorell- Barnes, G. (1999). *Working with Children and Parents Through Separation and Divorce: The Changing Lives of Children*. Basingstoke, UK: Macmillan Press.

Dowling, E. & Osborne, E. (1994). *The Family and The School. A Joint Systems approach to Problems with Children* (Second edition). London: Routledge.

Doyle, J. & Bryant-Waugh, R. (2000). Epidemiology. In B. Lask & R. Bryant-Waugh (ed.), *Anorexia Nervosa and Related Eating Disorders in Childhood and Adolescence* (Second edition, pp. 41–62). London: Brunner-Routledge.

Driver, J., Tabares, A., Shapiro, A., Young-Nahm, E. & Gottman, J. (2003). Interactional patterns in marital success or failure. Gottman laboratory Studies. In F. Walsh (ed.), *Normal Family Processes* (Third edition, pp. 493–513). New York: Guilford.

Drummond, D. & Fitzpatrick, G. (2000). Children of substance misusing parents. In P. Reder, M. McLure & A. Jolley (eds.), *Family Matters. Interfaces Between Child and Adult Mental Health* (pp. 135–149). London: Routledge.

Duane, Y. & Carr, A. (2002). Prevention of sexual abuse. In A. Carr (ed.), *Prevention: What Works with Children and Adolescents? A Critical Review of Psychological*

Prevention Programmes for Children, Adolescents and their Families (pp. 181–204). London: Routledge.

Dubowitz, H. & Black, M. (2002). Neglect of children's health. In J. Myers, L. Berliner, J. Briere, C. Hendrix, C. Jenny & T. Reid (eds.), *APSAC Handbook on Child Maltreatment* (Second edition, pp. 269–292). Thousand Oaks, CA: Sage.

Dunn, J. & McGuire, S. (1992). Sibling and peer relationships in childhood. *Journal of Child Psychology and Psychiatry*, 33, 67–105.

Dunn, L. & Dunn, L. (1981). *Peabody Picture Vocabulary Test-Revised*. Circle Pines: MN: American Guidance Service.

Dweck, C. (1975). The role of expectations and attributions in the alleviation of learned helplessness. *Journal of Personality and Social Psychology*, 31, 674–685.

Earls, F. & Mezzacappa, E. (2002). Conduct and oppositional disorders. In M. Rutter, & E. Taylor (Eds.), *Child and Adolescent Psychiatry* (Fourth edition, pp. 419–436). Oxford: Blackwell.

Edgeworth, J. & Carr, A. (2000). Child abuse. In A. Carr (ed.), *What Works with Children and Adolescents? A Critical Review of Psychological Interventions with Children, Adolescents and their Families* (pp. 17–48). London: Routledge.

Edwards, S., Fletcher, M., Garman, A. Hughes, A., Letts, C. & I. Sinka (1997). *Reynell Developmental Language Scales. III*. Windsor: NFER-Nelson.

Egger, H. & Angold, A. (2004). The Preschool Age Psychiatric Assessment (PAPA): A structured parent interview for diagnosing psychiatric disorders in preschool children. In R. Delcarmen-Wiggens & A Carter (eds.), *Handbook of Infant and Toddler Mental Health Assessment* (pp. 223–246). New York: Oxford University Press.

Egger, J., Carter, C., Graham, P., Gumley, D. & Soothill, J. (1985). Controlled trial of oligoantigenic treatment in the hyperkinetic syndrome. *Lancet*, i, 540–545.

Ehlers, A. & Clark, D. (2000). A cognitive model of post-traumatic stress disorder. *Behaviour Research and Therapy*, 38, 319–336.

Eisler, I. (1995). Family models of eating disorders. In G. Szmukler, C. Dare & J. Treasure (eds.), *Handbook of Eating Disorders* (pp. 155–176). Chichester: Wiley.

Eisler, I., Le Grange, D. & Aisen, A. (2003). Family Interventions. In J. Treasure, U. Schmidt & E. van Furth (eds.), *Handbook of Eating Disorders* (Second edition, pp. 291–310). Chichester: Wiley.

Eley, T., Collier, D. & McGuffin, P. (2002). Anxiety and eating disorders. In P. McGuffin, M. Owen & I. Gottesman (eds.), *Psychiatric Genetics and Genomics* (pp. 303–340). Oxford: Oxford University Press.

Eley, T. & Gregory, A. (2004). Behavioral Genetics. In T. Morris & J. March (eds.), *Anxiety Disorders in Children and Adolescents* (Second edition, pp. 71–97). New York: Guilford.

Elliott, C. (1996). *British Ability Scales. Second edition. (BAS II)*. Windsor: NFER-Nelson.

Ellis, N., Upton, D. & Thompson, P. (2000). Epilepsy and the family: A review of current literature. *Seizure*, 9, 22–30.

Emerson, E. (2001). *Challenging behaviour. Analysis and Intervention in People with Severe Intellectual Disabilities* (Second edition). Cambridge: Cambridge University Press.

Emery, R. & Laumann-Billings, L. (2002). Child abuse. In M. Rutter, & E. Taylor (eds.), *Child and Adolescent Psychiatry* (Fourth edition, pp. 325–339). Oxford: Blackwell.

Emery, R. & Sbarra, D. (2002). Addressing separation and divorce during and after couple therapy. In A. Gurman & N. Jacobson (eds.), *Clinical Handbook of Couple Therapy* (Third edition, pp. 508–530). New York: Guilford Press.

Emery, R. & Wyre, M. (1987). Divorce mediation. *American Psychologist*, 42, 472–480.

Eminson, M., Benjamin, S., Shortall, A. & Woods, T. (1996). Physical symptoms and illness attitudes in adolescents: An epidemiological Study. *Journal of Child Psychology and Psychiatry*, 37, 519–528.

Endler, N. and Parker, J. (1996). *Coping Inventory for Stressful Situations* (Second edition). Toronto, Canada: Multi Health Systems.

Enright, S. & Carr, A. (2002). Chapter 15. Prevention of post-traumatic adjustment problems in children and adolescents. In A. Carr (ed.), *Prevention: What Works with Children and Adolescents? A Critical Review of Psychological Prevention Programmes for Children, Adolescents and their Families* (pp. 314–335). London: Routledge.

Erickson, M. & Egeland, B. (2002). Child neglect. In J. Myers, L. Berliner, J. Briere, C. Hendrix, C. Jenny & T. Reid (eds.), *APSAC Handbook on Child Maltreatment* (Second edition, pp. 3–20). Thousand Oaks, CA: Sage.

Erikson, E. (1968). *Identity, Youth and Crisis*. New York: Norton.

Essau, C. (2004). Prevention of substance abuse in children and adolescents. In P. Barrett & T. Ollendick (eds.), *Handbook of Interventions that Work with Children and Adolescents: Prevention and Treatment* (pp. 517–540). Chichester: Wiley.

Ewing-Cobbs, L., Levin, H., Fletcher, J., Miner, M. & Eisenberg, H. (1990). The Children's Orientation and Amnesia Test: Relationship to severity of acute head injury and to recovery of memory. *Neurosurgery*, 27, 683–691.

Eysenck, H. (1967). *The Biological Basis for Personality*. Baltimore, MD: University Park Press.

Fagan, J. (1988). *The Social Organization of Drug Use and Drug Dealing Among Urban Gangs*. New York: Jay College of Criminal Justice.

Fairburn, C. (1995). *Overcoming Binge Eating*. New York: Guilford.

Fairburn, C. (1997). Eating disorders. In D. Clark & C. Fairburn (eds.), *The Science and Practice of Cognitive Behaviour Therapy* (pp. 209–241). Oxford: Oxford University Press.

Fairburn, C.G., Marcus, M.D. & Wilson, G.T. (1993). Cognitive behaviour therapy for binge eating and bulimia nervosa: A comprehensive treatment manual. In C.G. Fairburn & G.T. Wilson (eds.), *Binge Eating: Nature, Assessment, and Treatment* (pp. 361–404). New York: Guilford Press.

Falloon, I., Laporta, M., Fadden, G. & Graham-Hole, V. (1993). *Managing Stress in Families*. London: Routledge.

Faraone, S., Biederman, J., Weber, W. & Russell, R. (1998). Psychiatric, neuro-psychological, and psychosocial features of DSM IV subtypes of attention deficit hyperactivity disorder: Results from a clinically referred sample. *Journal of the American Academy of Child and Adolescent Psychiatry*, 37, 185–193.

Farmer, A. & McGuffin, P. (1989). The classification of depressions: Contemporary confusions revisited. *British Journal of Psychiatry*, 155, 437–443.

Farrell, E., Cullen, R. & Carr, A. (2002). Prevention of adjustment problems in children with diabetes. In A. Carr (ed.), *Prevention: What Works with Children and*

Adolescents? A Critical Review of Psychological Prevention Programmes for Children, Adolescents and their Families (pp. 249–266). London: Routledge.

Farrington, D. (1995). The twelfth Jack Tizard Memorial Lecture. The development of offending and antisocial behaviour from childhood: Key findings of the Cambridge Study of Delinquent Development. *Journal of Child Psychology and Psychiatry*, 36, 929–964.

Faust, K. & McKibben, J. (1999). Marital dissolution: Divorce, separation, annulment, and widowhood. In M. Sussman, S. Steinmetz, & G. Peterson, (eds.), *Handbook of Marriage and the Family* (Second edition). New York: Kluwer-Plenum.

Fawcett, A. & Nicolson, R. (1996). *Dyslexia Screening Test (DST)*. London: Psychology Corporation.

Fawcett, A. & Nicolson, R. (1997). *Dyslexia Early Screening Test (DEST)*. London: Psychology Corporation.

Feindler, E. & Ecton, R. (1985). *Adolescent Anger Control: Cognitive-Behavioural Techniques*. New York: Pergamon.

Feingold, B. (1975). Hyperkinesis and learning difficulties linked to artificial food flavours and colours. *American Journal of Nursing*, 75, 797–803.

Feinman, S. (1992). *Social Referencing and the Social Construction of Reality In Infancy*. New York: Plenum.

Feldman, W., McGrath, P., Hodgson, C., Ritter, H. & Shipman, R. (1985). The use of dietary fibre in the management of simple childhood recurrent abdominal pain: Results in a prospective double blind randomized controlled trial. *American Journal of Diseases in Childhood*, 139, 1216–1218.

Ferber, R. (1985). *Solve Your Child's Sleep Problems*. London: Dorling Kindersley.

Ferber, R. & Kryger, M. (1995). *Principles and Practice of Sleep Medicine in the Child*. Philadelphia, PA: Saunders.

Fergusson, D. & Lynskey, M. (1996). Adolescent resiliency to family adversity. *Journal of Child Psychology and Psychiatry*, 37, 281–292.

Field, T., Healy, B., Goldstein, S. & Guthertz, M. (1990). Behaviour-state matching and synchrony in mother–infant interactions of nondepressed versus depressed dyads. *Developmental Psychology*, 26, 7–14.

Fielding, D. & Doleys, D. (1988). Elimination problems. Enuresis and encopresis. In E. Mash & L. Terdal (eds.), *Behavioural Assessment of Childhood Disorders* (Second edition, pp. 586–526). New York: Guilford.

Findling, R. L., Kowatch, R. A. & Post, R. M. (2003). *Paediatric Bipolar Disorder: A Handbook for Clinicians*. London: Cromwell Press.

Finklehor, D. (1984). *Child Sexual Abuse: New Theory and Research*. New York: Free Press.

Finnegan, L. & Carr, A. (2002). Prevention of adjustment problems in children with autism. In A. Carr (ed.), *Prevention: What Works with Children and Adolescents? A Critical Review of Psychological Prevention Programmes for Children, Adolescents and their Families* (pp. 107–128). London: Routledge.

Fisman, S. (2002). Pervasive development disorder. In S. Kutcher (ed.), *Practical Child and Adolescent Psychopharmacology* (pp. 265–304). Cambridge: Cambridge University Press.

Fitzpatrick, C. (2004). *Coping with Depression in Young People. A Guide for Parents*. Chichester: Wiley.

Flannery-Schroeder, E. (2004). Generalized anxiety disorder. In T. Morris & J. March

Anxiety Disorders in Children and Adolescents (Second edition, pp. 125–140). New York: Guilford.

Fleming, S. & Robinson, P. (2001). Grief and cognitive-behavioural therapy: The reconstruction of meaning. In M. Stroebe, R. Hansson, W. Stroebe & H. Schut (eds.), *Handbook of Bereavement Research: Consequences, Coping, and Care* (pp. 647–669). Washington, DC: American Psychological Association.

Fletcher, J. (1988). Brain-injured children. In E Mash & L. Terdal (eds.), *Behavioural Assessment of Childhood Disorders* (Second edition, pp. 451–488). New York Guilford.

Flin, R. & Spencer, J. (1995). Annotation: Children as witnesses: Legal and psychological perceptive. *Journal of Child Psychology and Psychiatry*, 36, 171–189.

Folberg, J. & Milne, A. (1988). *Divorce Mediation: Theory and Practice*. New York: Guilford.

Fombonne, E. (2003). Epidemiological survey of autism and other pervasive developmental disorders: An update. *Journal of Autism and Developmental Disorders*, 33, 365–382.

Fonagy, P. & Kurtz, A. (2002). Disturbance of conduct. In P. Fonagy, M. Target, D. Cottrell, J. Phillips & A. Kurtz (eds.), *What Works for Whom. A Critical Review of Treatments for Children and Adolescents* (pp. 106–192). New York: Guilford.

Fonagy, P. & Moran, G. (1990). Studies of the efficacy of child psychoanalysis. *Journal of Consulting and Clinical Psychology*, 58, 684–695.

Fonagy, P., Steele, M., Steele, H., Higgitt, A. & Target, M. (1994). The Emmanuel Miller Memorial Lecture, 1992. The theory and practice of resilience. *Journal of Child Psychology and Psychiatry*, 35, 231–257.

Fonagy, P., Target, M., Cottrell, D. Phillips, J. & Kurtz, A. (2002). *What Works for Whom. A Critical Review of Treatments for Children and Adolescents*. New York: Guilford.

Fordyce, M. (1977). Development of a programme to increase personal happiness. *Journal of Counseling Psychology*, 24, 511–520.

Fordyce, W. (1976). *Behavioural Methods for Chronic Pain and Illness*. St Louis: Mosby.

Försterling, F. (1985). Attributional retraining: A review. *Psychological Bulletin*, 98, 495–512.

Fowler, D., Garety, P. & Kuipers, L. (1995). *Cognitive Behavioural Psychotherapy: A Rationale, Theory and Practice*. Chichester: Wiley.

Freeman, J., Garcia, A., Miller, Dow, S. & Leonard, H. (2004). Selective mutism. In T. Morris & J. March (eds.), *Anxiety Disorders in Children and Adolescents* (Second edition, pp. 280–304). New York: Guilford.

French, P. & Morrison, A. (2004). *Early Detection and Cognitive Therapy for People at High Risk of Developing Psychosis: A Treatment Approach*. Chichester: Wiley.

Freud, S. (1894). The psychoneuroses of defence. In J. Strachey (ed. and trans.), *The Standard Edition of the Complete Works of Sigmund Freud* (Volume 3). London: Hogarth Press.

Freud, S. (1905). Three essays on the theory of sexuality. In J. Strachey (ed. and trans.), *The Standard Edition of the Complete Works of Sigmund Freud* (Volume 7). London: Hogarth Press.

Freud, S. (1909a). The analysis of a phobia in a five year old boy. In J. Stratchey (ed. and trans.), *The Standard Edition of the Complete Works of Sigmund Freud* (Volume 10). London: Hogarth Press.

Freud, S. (1909b). Notes upon a case of obsessional neurosis. In J. Stratchey (ed. and trans.), *The Standard Edition of the Complete Works of Sigmund Freud* (Volume 10). London: Hogarth Press.

Freud, S. (1917). Mourning and melancholia. In J. Stratchey (ed. and trans.), *The Standard Edition of the Complete Works of Sigmund Freud. Collected Papers* (Volume 4, pp. 142–170) London: Hogarth Press.

Frichter, M. & Pirke, K. (1995). Starvation models and eating disorders. In G. Szmukler, C. Dare & J. Treasure (eds.), *Handbook of Eating Disorders* (pp. 83–108). Chichester: Wiley.

Friedberg, R. & McClure, J. (2002). *Clinical Practice of Cognitive Therapy with Children and Adolescents.* New York: Guilford.

Friedman, H. & Boothby-Kewley, S. (1987). The disease-prone personality: A meta-analytic view of the construct. *American Psychologist*, 42, 539–555.

Friedman, R. & Chase-Lansdale, P. (2002). Chronic adversities. In M. Rutter, & E. Taylor (eds.), *Child and Adolescent Psychiatry* (Fourth edition, pp. 261–276). Oxford: Blackwell.

Friedrich, W. (2002). An integrated model of psychotherapy for abused children. In J. Myers, L. Berliner, J. Briere, C. Hendrix, C. Jenny & T. Reid (eds.), *APSAC Handbook on Child Maltreatment* (Second edition, pp. 141–158). Thousand Oaks, CA: Sage.

Friedrich, W. Grambsch, P., Damon, L. & Hewitt, S. (1992). Child sexual behaviour inventory. *Psychological Assessment*, 4, 303–311.

Frischer, M., McArdle, P. & Crome, I. (2004). The epidemiology of substance misuse in young people. In I. Crome, H. Ghodse, E. Gilvarry & P. McArdle (eds.), *Young People and Substance Misuse* (pp. 31–50). London: Gaskell.

Fristad, M., Weller, E. & Weller, R. (1992), The Mania Rating Scale: Can it be used in children? A preliminary report. *Journal of the American Academy of Child and Adolescent Psychiatry*, 31, 252–257.

Frith, U. (2004). Emanuel Miller Lecture. Confusions and controversies about Asperger's syndrome. *Journal of Child Psychology and Psychiatry*, 45, 672–686.

Frude, N. (1990). *Understanding Family Problems.* Chichester: Wiley.

Fryers, T. (2000). Epidemiology of mental retardation. In. M. Gelder, J. Lopez-Ibor & N. Andreasen (eds.), *New Oxford Textbook of Psychiatry* (volume 2, section 10.2, pp. 1941–1945). Oxford: Oxford University Press.

Furniss, T. (1991). *The Multiprofessional Handbook of Child Sexual Abuse: Integrated Management, Therapy and Legal Intervention.* London: Routledge.

Gaines, R., Sandgrund, A., Green, A., & Power, E. (1978). Etiological factors in child maltreatment: A multivariate study of abusing, neglecting and normal mothers. *Journal of Abnormal Psychology*, 87, 531–540.

GAP (1996). Global Assessment of Relational Functioning Scale (GARF): 1. Background and rationale. *Family Process*, 35, 155–172.

Gardner, H. (2000). *Intelligence Reframed: Multiple Intelligences for the 21st Century.* New York: Basic.

Gardner, R. (1989). *Family Evaluation iIn Child Custody Mediation, Arbitration, and Litigation.* Cresskill, NJ: Creative Therapeutics.

Gardner, R. (1998). *The Parental Alienation Syndrome* (Second edition). Cresskill, NJ: Creative Therapeutics.

Garland, E. (2002). Anxiety disorders. In S. Kutcher (ed.), *Practical Child and Adolescent Psychopharmacology* (pp. 187–229). Cambridge: Cambridge University Press.

Garmezy, N. & Masten, A. (1994). Chronic adversities. In M. Rutter, E. Taylor & L. Hersov (eds.), *Child and Adolescent Psychiatry: Modern Approaches* (Third edition, pp. 191–208). London: Blackwell.

Garralda, M. (1992). A selective review of child psychiatric syndromes with a somatic presentation. *British Journal of Psychiatry*, 161, 759–773.

Garralda, M. (1999). Practitioner review: Assessment and management of somatisation in childhood and adolescence: A practice perspective. *Journal of Child Psychology and Psychiatry*, 40, 1159–1167.

Garralda, E. & Rangel, L. (2002). Annotation: Chronic fatigue syndrome in children and adolescents. *Journal of Child Psychology & Psychiatry*, 43, 169–176.

Geller, B. & DelBello, M. (2003). *Bipolar Disorder in Childhood and Early Adolescence*. New York: Guilford Press.

Gelles, R. (1995). *Contemporary Families: A Sociological View*. Thousand Oaks, CA: Sage.

Gergen, K. (1994). *Realities and Relationships*. Cambridge, MA: Harvard University Press.

Giaretto, H. (1982). A comprehensive child sexual abuse treatment programme. *Child Abuse and Neglect*, 6, 263–278.

Gillberg, C. (2000). Epidemiology of early onset schizophrenia. In H, Remschmidt (ed.), *Schizophrenia in Children and Adolescents* (pp. 43–59). Cambridge: Cambridge University Press.

Gillberg, C. (2003). ADHD and DAMP: A general health perspective. *Child & Adolescent Mental Health*, 8, 106–113.

Gillberg, C. & Coleman, M. (2000). *The Biology of the Autistic Syndromes* (Third edition). London: McKeith Press.

Gilles de la Tourette, G. (1885). Étude sur une affection nerveuse caracterisée par de l'incoordination motorice accompagnee d'echolalie et de coprolalie. *Archives de Neurologie*, 9 (19–42), 1310–1315.

Gilliam, J. (1991). *Gilliam Autism Rating Scale*. Odessa, FL: Psychological Assessment Resources. http://www.parinc.com

Gilligan, C. (1982). *In a Different Voice: Psychological Theory and Women's Development*. Cambridge, MA: Harvard University Press.

Girolametto, L., Weitzman, E. & Pearce, P. (1996). Interactive focused stimulation for toddlers with expressive vocabulary delays. *Journal of Speech and Hearing Research*, 39, 1274–1283.

Glaros, A. & Epkins, C. (2003). Habit disorders: Bruxism, trichotillomania, and tics. In M. Roberts (ed.), *Handbook of Paediatric Psychology* (Third edition, pp. 561–577). New York: Guilford.

Glaser, D. (2002a). Emotional abuse and neglect (psychological maltreatment): A conceptual framework. *Child Abuse & Neglect*, 26, 697–714.

Glaser, D. (2002b). Child sexual abuse. In M. Rutter, & E. Taylor (eds.), *Child and Adolescent Psychiatry* (Fourth edition, pp. 314–358). Oxford: Blackwell.

Gledhill, J. & Garralda, E. (2000). The relationship between physical and mental health in children and adolescents. In. M. Gelder, J. Lopez-Ibor & N. Andreasen (eds.), *New Oxford Textbook of Psychiatry* (volume 2, section 9.3.2, pp. 1834–1843). Oxford: Oxford University Press.

Goldberg, D. (1978). *The General Health Questionnaire.* Windsor: NFER-NELSON. http://www.nfer-nelson.co.uk/

Goldberg, D., Magrill, L., Hale, J., Damaskinidou, Paul, J. & Tham, S. (1995). Protection and loss: Working with learning-disabled adults and their families. *Journal of Family Therapy,* 17, 263–280.

Goldstein, A. & Glick, B. (1987). *Anger Replacement Training. A Comprehensive Intervention for Aggressive Youth.* Champaign, IL: Research Press.

Goleman, D. (1995). *Emotional Intelligence.* London: Bloomsbury.

Goodlin-Jones, B. & Anders, T. (2004). Sleep disorders. In R. Delcarmen-Wiggens & A. Carter (eds.), *Handbook of Infant and Toddler Mental Health Assessment* (pp. 271–288). New York: Oxford University Press.

Goodman, K. (1976). Reading: A psycholinguistic guessing game. In H. Singer & R. Ruddell (eds.), *Theoretical Models and Processes of Reading* (Second edition, pp. 497–508). Newark, DE: International Reading Association.

Goodman, R. (2001). Psychometric properties of the Strengths and Difficulties Questionnaire (SDQ). *Journal of the American Academy of Child and Adolescent Psychiatry,* 40, 1337–1345. http://www.sdqinfo.com/

Goodman, R. (2002). Brain disorders. In M. Rutter & E. Taylor (eds.), *Child and Adolescent Psychiatry* (Fourth edition, pp. 241–260). Oxford: Blackwell.

Goodman, R., Ford, T., Richards, H., Gatward, R. & Meltzer, H. (2000). The Development and Well-Being Assessment: Description and initial validation of an integrated assessment of child and adolescent psychopathology. *Journal of Child Psychology and Psychiatry,* 41, 645–655. http://www.dawba.com/

Goodyer, I. (2001a). *The Depressed Child and Adolescent* (Second edition). Cambridge: Cambridge University Press.

Goodyer, I. (2001b). Life events: Their nature and effects. In I. Goodyer (ed.), *The Depressed Child and Adolescent* (Second edition, pp. 204–232). Cambridge: Cambridge University Press.

Gopnik, A. & Meltzoff, A. (1987). Early semantic developments and their relationship to object permanence, means-ends understanding and categorization. In K. Nelson & A. Van Kleek (eds.), *Children's Language* (Volume 6). Hillsdale, NJ: Lawrence Erlbaum Associates Inc.

Gordon, D. & Rolland-Stanar, C. (2003). Lessons learned from the dissemination of Parenting Wisely, A Parent Training CD-ROM. *Cognitive and Behavioral Practice,* 10, 312–323.

Gowers, S. & Bryant-Waugh, R. (2004). Management of child and adolescent eating disorders: The current evidence base and future directions. *Journal of Child Psychology and Psychiatry,* 45, 63–83.

Gowers, S.G., Harrington, R.C. & Whitton, A. (1998). *HoNOSCA Report on Research and Development.* London CRU. http://www.liv.ac.uk/honosca/Home.htm

Greene, S., Anderson, E., Hetherington, E., Forgatch, M. & DeGarmo, D. (2003). Risk and resilience after divorce. In F. Walsh (ed.), *Normal Family Processes* (Third edition, pp. 96–120). New York: Guilford.

Griffiths, R. (1970). *Griffiths Mental Development Scales.* High Wycombe, UK: Test Agency.

Guevara, J., Wolf, F., Grum, C. & Clark, N. (2003). Effects of educational interventions for self-management of asthma in children and adolescents: Systematic review and meta-analysis. *British Medical Journal*, 326, 1308–1309.

Guilleminault, C. (1987). *Sleep and its Disorders in Children*. New York: Raven Press.

Guilleminault, C. & Pelayo, R. (2000). Narcolepsy in prepubertal children. *Annals of Neurology*, 43, 135–142.

Haddock, G. & Slade, P. (1996). *Cognitive-behavioural Interventions with Psychotic Disorders*. London: Routledge.

Haggerty, R., Sherrod, L., Garmezy, N. & Rutter, M. (1994). *Stress, Risk and Resilience in Children and Adolescents: Processes, Mechanisms and Interventions*. Cambridge: Cambridge University Press.

Haley, J. (1967). Towards a theory of pathological Systems. In G. Zuk & I. Boszormenyi Nagi (eds.), *Family Therapy and Disturbed Families*. Palo Alto, CA: Science and Behaviour.

Hall, M. & Irwin, M. (2001). Physiological indices of functioning in bereavement. In M. Stroebe, R. Hansson, W. Stroebe & H. Schut (eds.), *Handbook of Bereavement Research: Consequences, Coping, and Care* (pp. 473–492). Washington, DC: American Psychological Association.

Halpern, D. (2000). *Sex Differences in Cognitive Abilities (Third edition)*. Hillsdale, NJ: Lawrence Erlbaum Associates Inc.

Hammen, C. & Rudolph, K. (2003). Childhood mood disorders. In E. Mash & R. Barkley (eds.), *Child Psychopathology* (Second edition, pp. 233–278). New York: Guilford.

Hands, M. & Dear, G. (1994). Co-dependency: A critical review. *Drug and Alcohol Review*, 13, 437–445.

Happé, F. & Frith, U. (1996). The neuropsychology of autism. *Brain*, 119, 1377–1400.

Harrington, R. (1993). *Depressive Disorder in Childhood and Adolescence*. Chichester: Wiley.

Harrington, R. (1998). Tourette Syndrome. In L. Phelps (ed.), *Health-related Disorders in Children and Adolescents: A Guidebook for Understanding and Educating* (pp. 641–651). Washington, DC: American Psychological Association.

Harrington, R. (2002). Affective disorders. In M. Rutter, & E. Taylor (eds.), *Child and Adolescent Psychiatry* (Fourth edition, pp. 463–485). Oxford: Blackwell.

Harrington, R., Whittaker, J., & Shoebridge, P. (1998). Psychological treatment of depression in children and adolescents. A review of treatment research. *British Journal of Psychiatry*, 173, 281–298.

Harris, S. & Handleman, J. (1997). Helping children with autism enter the mainstream. In D. Cohen & F. Volkmar (eds.), *Handbook of Autism and Pervasive Developmental Disorders* (Second edition, pp. 665–676). New York: Wiley.

Harrison, P. (2000). The neurobiology of schizophrenia. In. M. Gelder, J. Lopez-Ibor & N. Andreasen (eds.), *New Oxford Textbook of Psychiatry* (Volume 1, Section 4.3.5.2, pp. 605–612). Oxford: Oxford University Press.

Harrison, P. & Oakland, T. (2000). *ABAS. Adaptive Behaviour Assessment System*. San Antonio, TX: Psychological Corporation.

Hart, C. & Hart, B. (1996). The use of hypnosis with children and adolescents. *The Psychologist*, 9 (11), 506–509.

Hart, S., Brassard, M., Binggeli, N. & Davidson, H. (2002). Psychological maltreatment. In J. Myers, L. Berliner, J. Briere, C. Hendrix, C. Jenny & T. Reid (eds.),

APSAC Handbook on Child Maltreatment (Second edition, pp. 79–104). Thousand Oaks, CA: Sage.

Harter, S. (1999). *The Cognitive and Social Construction of the Developing Self*. New York: Guilford Press.

Haskey, J. (1999). Divorce and remarriage in England and Wales. *Population Trends*, 95. 18–22.

Hauser, P., Zametkin, A., Martinez, P., Vitietllo, B., Matochik, J., Mixon, A. & Weintraub, B. (1993). Attention deficit hyperactivity disorder in people with generalized resistance to thyroid hormone. *New England Journal of Medicine*, 328, 997–1001.

Havens, J., Mellins, C. & Hunter, J. (2002). Psychiatric aspects of HIV/AIDS in childhood and adolescence. In M. Rutter & E. Taylor (eds.), *Child and Adolescent Psychiatry: Modern Approaches* (Fourth edition, pp. 829–841). London: Blackwell.

Hawkins, J., Catalano, R. & Miller, J. (1992). Risk and protective factors for alcohol and other drug problems in adolescence and early adulthood: Implications for substance use prevention. *Psychological Bulletin*, 112, 64–105.

Haley, J. (1980). *Leaving Home*. New York: McGraw Hill.

Heiman, M. (1992). Annotation: Putting the puzzle together: Validating allegations of child sexual abuse. *Journal of Child Psychology and Psychiatry*, 33, 311–329.

Hemsley, D. (1994). Schizophrenia: Treatment. In S. Lindsay & G. Powell (eds.), *The Handbook of Clinical Adult Psychology* (Second edition, pp. 309–328). London: Routledge.

Hemsley, D. (1996). Schizophrenia: A cognitive model and its implications for psychological intervention. *Behaviour Modification*, 20, 139–169.

Henggeler, S. & Lee, S. (2003). Multisystemic treatment of serious clinical problems. In A. Kazdin, & J. Weisz (eds.), *Evidence-Based Psychotherapies for Children and Adolescents* (pp. 301–324). New York: Guilford.

Henggeler, S. & Sheidow, A. (2003). Conduct disorder and delinquency. *Journal of Marital and Family Therapy*, 29, 505–522.

Henggeler, S., Schoenwald, S., Bordin, C., Rowland, M, & Cunningham, P. (1998). *Multisystemic Treatment of Antisocial Behaviour in Children and Adolescents*. New York: Guilford.

Herbert, M. (1996). *Supporting Bereaved and Dying Children and Their Parents*. Leicester, UK: British Psychological Society.

Herbert, M. (2002). Behavioural therapies. In M. Rutter, & E. Taylor (eds.), *Child and Adolescent Psychiatry* (Fourth edition, pp. 900–920). Oxford: Blackwell.

Herbert, M. (2005). Adjustment to separation and divorce. In P. Graham (ed.), *Cognitive Behaviour Therapy for Children and Families* (Second edition, pp. 170–186). Cambridge: Cambridge University Press.

Herjanic, B. & Reich, W. (1982). Development of a structured psychiatric interview for children. *Journal of Abnormal Child Psychology*, 10, 307–324.

Hermelin, B. & O'Connor, N. (1970). *Psychological Experiments with Autistic Children*. London: Pergamon Press.

Herzberger, S., Potts, D., & Dillon, M. (1981). Abusive and non-abusive parental treatment from the child's perspective. *Journal of Consulting and Clinical Psychology*, 49, 81–90.

Hester, N., Foster, R. & Kristensen, K. (1990). Measurement of pain in children:

Generalizability and validity of the pain ladder and the poker chip tool. In D. Tyler & E. Krane (eds.), *Paediatric Pain. Advances in Pain Research and Therapy* (volume 15, pp. 79–84). New York: Raven.

Hetherington, E. & Kelly, J. (2002). *For Better or for Worse: Divorce Reconsidered.* New York: Norton.

Hewison, J. (1988). The long term effectiveness of parent involvement in reading: A follow up to the Harringey reading project. *British Journal of Educational Psychology*, 58, 184–190.

Heyman, I., Fombonne, E., Simmons, H., Ford, T., Meltzer, H. & Goodman, R. (2001). Prevalence of obsessive compulsive disorder in the British nationwide survey of child mental health. *British Journal of Psychiatry*, 179, 324–329.

Heyne, D., & King, N. (2004). Treatment of school refusal. In P. Barrett & T. Ollendick (eds.), *Handbook of Interventions that Work with Children and Adolescents: Prevention and Treatment* (pp. 243–272). Chichester: Wiley.

Heyne, D. King, N. & Ollendick, T. (2005). School refusal. In P. Graham (ed.), *Cognitive Behaviour Therapy for Children and Families* (Second edition, pp. 320–341). Cambridge: Cambridge University Press.

Heyne, D. & Rollings, S. (2002). *School Refusal.* Oxford: Blackwell.

Hibbs, E., Hamburger, S., Lenane, M., Rapoport, J., Kruesi, M., Keysor, C. & Goldstein, M. (1991). Determinants of expressed emotion in families of disturbed and normal children. *Journal of Child Psychology and Psychiatry*, 32, 757–770.

Hickey, D. & Carr, A. (2002). Prevention of suicide in adolescence. In A. Carr (ed.), *Prevention: What Works with Children and Adolescents? A Critical Review of Psychological Prevention Programmes for Children, Adolescents and their Families* (pp. 336–358). London: Routledge.

Hildyard, K. & Wolfe, D. (2002). Child neglect: Developmental issues and outcomes. *Child Abuse & Neglect*, 26, 679–695.

Hill, J. (2002). Biological, psychological and social processes in the conduct disorders. *Journal of Child Psychology and Psychiatry*, 43, 133–165.

Hinshaw, S. (1994). *Attention Deficits and Hyperactivity in Children.* Thousand Oaks, CA: Sage.

Hinshaw, S. (1996). Enhancing social competence: Integrating self-management strategies with behavioural procedures for children with ADHD. In E. Hibbs & P. Jensen (eds.), *Psychosocial Treatments for Child and Adolescent Disorders. Empirically Based Strategies for Clinical Practice* (pp. 285–309). Washington, DC: APA.

Hirshfeld-Becker, D., Biederman, J. & Rosenbaum, J. (2004). Behavioral Inhibition. In T. Morris & J. March (2004). *Anxiety Disorders in Children and Adolescents* (Second edition, pp. 27–58). New York: Guilford.

HMSO (1992). *Memorandum of Good Practice on Videorecorded Interviews with Child Witnesses for Criminal Proceedings.* London: HMSO.

Hobson, R. (1993). *Autism and the Development of Mind.* Hillsdale, NJ. Lawrence Erlbaum Associates Inc.

Hodges, K. (1993). Structured interviews for assessing children. *Journal of Child Psychology and Psychiatry*, 34, 49–68.

Hodges, K., Cools, J. & McKnew, D. (1989). Test-retest reliability of a clinical research interview for children: The Child Assessment Schedule (CAS). *Psychological Assessment: Journal of Consulting and Clinical Psychology*, 1, 317–322.

Hodges, K., Gordon, Y. & Lennon, M. (1990). Parent–child agreement on symptoms assessed via a clinical research interview for children: The Child Assessment (CAS). *Journal of Child Psychology and Psychiatry*, 31, 427–436.

Hoffman, M. (1970). Moral development. In P. Mussen (ed.), *Carmichael's Manual of Child Psychology*. Chichester: Wiley.

Hollis, C. (2002). Schizophrenia and allied disorders. In M. Rutter & E. Taylor (eds.), *Child and Adolescent Psychiatry* (Fourth edition, pp. 612–636). Oxford: Blackwell.

Horan, S. Kang, G., Levine, M., Duax, C., Luntz, B. & Tasa, C. (1993). Empirical studies on foster care: Review and assessment. *Journal of Sociology and Social Welfare*, 20, 131–154.

Horne, J. (1992). Annotation: Sleep and its disorders in children. *Journal of Child Psychology and Psychiatry*, 33, 473–487.

Houts, A. (2003). Behavioural treatment for enuresis. In A. Kazdin & J. Weisz (eds.), *Evidence-Based Psychotherapies for Children and Adolescents* (pp. 389–406). New York: Guilford Press.

Houts, A. & Liebert, R. (1984). *Bedwetting: A guide for Parents and Children*. Springfield, IL: Charles C Thomas.

Howlin, P., Baron-Cohen, S. & Hadwin, J. (1999). *Teaching Children with Autism to Mind-read: A Practical Guide*. Chichester: Wiley.

Hudson, J., Hughes, A. & Kendall, P. (2004). Treatment of generalized anxiety disorder in children and adolescents. In P. Barrett & T. Ollendick (eds.), *Handbook of Interventions that Work with Children and Adolescents: Prevention and Treatment* (pp. 115–144). Chichester: Wiley.

Hunt, S. & Adams, M. (1989). Bibliotherapy based dry bed training: A pilot study. *Behavioural Psychotherapy*, 17, 290–302.

Huntley, M., (1996). *Griffiths Mental Development Scales from Birth to Two Years*. London: Test Agency.

Hurwitz, C., Duncan, J. & Wolfe, J. (2004). Caring for the Child with Cancer at the Close of Life: 'There Are People Who Make It, and I'm Hoping I'm One of Them'. *Journal of the American Medical Association*, 292, 2141–2149.

Ijzendoorn, M., Juffer, F. & Duyvesteyn, M. (1995). Breaking the intergenerational cycle of insecure attachment: A review of the effects of attachment-based interventions on maternal sensitivity and infant security. *Journal of Child Psychology and Psychiatry*, 36, 225–248.

Illingworth, R. (1987). *The Development of the Infant and Young Child* (Ninth edition). New York: Livingstone.

Imber-Black, E. (1991). A family-larger-system-perspective. In A. Gurman & D. Kniskern (eds.), *Handbook of Family Therapy* (volume 2, pp. 583–605). New York: Brunner/Mazel.

Imber-Black, E., Roberts, J., Whiting, R. & Whiting, R. (2003). *Rituals in Families and Family Therapy* (Revised edition). New York: Norton.

Ioannou, C. (1991). Acute pain in children. In M. Herbert (ed.), *Clinical Child Psychology* (pp. 331–339). Chichester: Wiley.

Isenberg, S., Lehrer, P. & Hochron, S. (1992). The effects of suggestion and emotional arousal on pulmonary functions in asthma: A review and a hypothesis regarding vagal mediation. *Psychosomatic Medicine*, 54, 192–216.

Iwaniec, D. (1995). *The Emotionally Abused and Neglected Child: Identification, Assessment and Intervention*. Chichester: Wiley.

Iwaniec, D. (2004). *Children who fail to Thrive: A Practice Guide*. Chichester: Wiley.

Iwaniec, D., Herbert, M. & McNeish, A. (1985). Social work with failure to thrive children and their families. Part II: Behavioural social work intervention. *British Journal of Social Work*, 15, 375–389.

Jablensky, A. (2000). Course and outcome of schizophrenia and their prediction. In. M. Gelder, J. Lopez-Ibor & N. Andreasen (eds.), *New Oxford Textbook of Psychiatry* (Volume 1, Section 4.3.6, pp. 621–621). Oxford: Oxford University Press.

Jackson, S. (2002). Promoting stability and continuity in care away from home. In D. McNeish, T. Newman, & H. Roberts (eds.), *What Works for Children* (pp. 37–58). Buckingham: Open University Press.

James, A. & Javaloyes, A. (2001). The treatment of bipolar disorders in children and adolescents. *Journal of Child Psychology and Psychiatry*, 42, 439–449.

James, D. E., Schumm, W. R., Kennedy, C. E., Grigsby, C. C., Shectman, K. L. & Nichols, C. W. (1985). Characteristics of the Kansas Parental Satisfaction Scale among two samples of married parents. *Psychological Reports*, 57, 163–169.

Jampala, V., Sierles, F., & Taylor, M. (1986). Consumers' views of DSM III. Attitudes and practices of US psychiatrists and 1984 graduate residents. *American Journal of Psychiatry*, 143, 148–153.

Jenkins, J. & Smith, M. (1990). Factors protecting children living in disharmonious homes: Maternal reports. *Journal of the American Academy of Child and Adolescent Psychiatry*, 29, 60–69.

Jensen, P., Roper, M., Fisher, P. Piacentini, J., Canino, G., Richters, J., Rubio-Stipec, M., Dulcan, M., Goodman, S. & Davies, M. (1995). Test-retest reliability of the Diagnostic Interview Schedule for Children (DISC 2.1). *Archives of General Psychiatry*, 52, 61–71.

Jessor, R. & Jessor, S. (1977). *Problem Behaviour and Psychosocial Development*. New York: Academic Press.

Johns, M. (1991). A new method for measuring daytime sleepiness: The Epworth Sleepiness Scale. *Sleep*, 14, 540–545.

Johnson, M. & Wintgens, A. (2001). *The Selective Mutism Resource Manual*. Bicester, UK: Speechmark.

Johnson, S. & Denton, W. (2002). Emotionally focused couple therapy: Creating secure connections. In A. Gurman & N. Jacobson (eds.), *Clinical Handbook of Couple Therapy* (Third edition, pp. 221–250). New York: Guilford.

Johnstone, E. & MRC Autism Review Group (2001). *Medical Research Council Review of Autism Research: Epidemiology and Causes*. London: Medical Research Council.

Jones, D. (1987). The untreatable family. *Child Abuse and Neglect*, 11, 409–420.

Jones, D. (2000). Child abuse and neglect. In. M. Gelder, J. Lopez-Ibor & N. Andreasen (eds.), *New Oxford Textbook of Psychiatry* (Volume 2, Section 9.3.1, pp. 1825–1834). Oxford: Oxford University Press.

Jones, D. (2003). *Communicating with Vulnerable Children. A Guide for Practitioners*. London: Gaskell.

Jones, D. & McGraw, J. (1987). Reliable and fictitious accounts of sexual abuse to children. *Journal of Interpersonal Violence*, 2, 27–45.

Jones, H., Roberts, R. & Scott, S. (2005). Treatment foster care in England. In A. Wheal (ed.), *RHP Companion to Foster Care* (Second edition). Lyme Regis, UK: Russell House Publishing.

Jones, I., Kent, L. & Cradock, N. (2002). Genetics of affective disorders. In

P. McGuffin, M. Owen & I. Gottesman (eds.), *Psychiatric Genetics and Genomics* (pp. 211–246). Oxford: Oxford University Press.

Jordan, R. (2005). Autistic spectrum disorders. In G. O'Reilly, P. Walsh, A. Carr & J. McEvoy (eds.), *Handbook of Intellectual Disability and Clinical Psychology Practice*. London: Brunner-Routledge.

Jordan, R. & Powell, S. (1995). *Understanding and Teaching Children with Autism*. New York: Wiley.

Kabacoff, R. Miller, I., Bishop, D., Epstein, N. & Keitner, G. (1990). A psychometric study of the McMaster Family Assessment Device. *Journal of Family Psychology*, 3, 431–439.

Kagan, J. & Lamb, S. (1987). *The Emergence of Moral Concepts in Young Children*. Chicago: University of Chicago Press.

Kagan, J., Reznick, M. & Gibbons, J. (1989). Inhibited and uninhibited types of children. *Child Development*, 60, 838–845.

Kahn, A., Mozin, M., Rebuffat, E., Sottiaux, M. & Muller, M. (1989). Milk intolerance in children with persistent sleeplessness: A prospective double-blind crossover evaluation. *Paediatrics*, 84, 595–603.

Kahn, R. & Davis, K. (1995). New developments in dopamine and schizophrenia. In E. Bloom & D. Kupfer (eds.), *Psychopharmacology: The Fourth Generation of Progress* (pp. 1193–1203). New York: Raven.

Kalish, R. & Reynolds, D. (1976). *An Overview of Death and Ethnicity*. Farmingdale, NY: Baywood.

Kandel, D. & Andrews, K. (1987). Processes of adolescent socialization by parents and peers. *International Journal of the Addictions*, 22, 319–342.

Kanner, L. (1943). Autistic disturbances of affective contact. *Nervous Child*, 2, 217–250.

Kaplan, S. & Busner, J. (1993). Treatment of nocturnal enuresis. In T. Giles (ed.), *Handbook of Effective Psychotherapy* (pp. 135–150). New York: Plenum.

Karpman, S. (1968). Fairy tales and script drama analysis. *Transactional Analysis Bulletin*, 7 (26), 39–44.

Kashani, J., Beck., N., Hoeper, E., Fallahi, C., Corcoran, C., McAllister, J., Rosenberg, T. & Reid, J. (1987). Psychiatric disorders in a community sample of adolescents. *American Journal of Psychiatry*, 144, 584–589.

Kasius, M., Ferdinand, R., van den Berg, H. & Verhulst, F. (1997). Associations between different diagnostic approaches for child and adolescent psychopathology. *Journal of Child Psychology and Psychiatry*, 38, 625–632.

Kaski, M. (2000). Aetiology of mental retardation: General issues and prevention. In. M. Gelder, J. Lopez-Ibor & N. Andreasen (eds.), *New Oxford Textbook of Psychiatry* (Volume 2, Section 10.3, pp. 1948–1952). Oxford: Oxford University Press.

Kaslow, F. (1995). The dynamics of divorce therapy. In R. Mikesell, D. Lusterman & S. McDaniel (eds.), *Integrating Family Therapy. Handbook of Family Psychology and Systems Theory* (pp. 271–284). Washington, DC: APA.

Kaslow, N., Morris, M. & Rehm, L. (1998). Childhood depression. In R. Morris, & T. Kratochwill (eds.), *The Practice of Child Therapy* (Third edition, pp. 48–90). Needham Heights, MA: Allyn & Bacon.

Kaufman, A. & Kaufman, N. (2004). *Kaufman Assessment Battery for Children. Second Edition (KABC-II)*. Circle Pines, MN: American Guidance Service.

Kaye, K. (1982). *The Mental and Social Life of Babies*. Chicago: University of Chicago Press.

Kazak, A., Rourke, M. & Crump, T. (2003). Families and other systems in paediatric psychology. In M. Roberts (ed.), *Handbook of Paediatric Psychology* (Third edition, pp. 159–175). New York: Guilford.

Kazdin, A. (1995). *Conduct Disorders in Childhood and Adolescence* (Second edition). Thousand Oaks, CA: Sage.

Kazdin, A. (1997). Psychosocial treatments for conduct disorder in children. *Journal of Child Psychology and Psychiatry*, 38, 161–178.

Kazdin, A. (2003). Problem-solving skills training and parent management training for conduct problems. In A. Kazdin, & J. Weisz (eds.), *Evidence-Based Psychotherapies for Children and Adolescents* (pp. 241–262). New York: Guilford.

Kazdin A. & Weisz, J. (2003). *Evidence-Based Psychotherapies for Children and Adolescents*. New York: Guilford Press.

Kelly, C. (1996). Chronic constipation and soiling in children: A review of the psychological and family literature. *Child Psychology and Psychiatry Review*, 1, 59–66.

Kelly, G. (1955). *The Psychology of Personal Constructs. Volumes 1 and 2*. New York: Norton.

Kelly, J. (2000). Children's adjustment in conflicted marriage and divorce: A decade review of research. *Journal of the American Academy of Child & Adolescent Psychiatry*, 39(8), 963–973.

Kempe, H., Silverman, E., Steele, B., Droegemuller, W. & Silver, H. (1962). The battered child syndrome. *Journal of the American Medical Association*, 181, 17–24.

Kendall, P., Aschenbrand, S. & Hudson, J. (2003). Child-focused treatment of anxiety. In A. Kazdin, & J. Weisz (eds.), *Evidence-Based Psychotherapies for Children and Adolescents* (pp. 81–100). New York: Guilford.

Kendall-Tackett, K., Williams, L. & Finklehor, D. (1993). Impact of sexual abuse on children. *Psychological Bulletin*, 113, 164–180.

Kendell, R. (1976). The classification of depressions: A review of contemporary confusion. *British Journal of Psychiatry*, 129, 15–88.

Kennedy, B. & Carr, A. (2002). Prevention of challenging behaviour in children with intellectual disabilities. In A. Carr (ed.), *Prevention: What Works with Children and Adolescents? A Critical Review of Psychological Prevention Programmes for Children, Adolescents and their Families* (pp. 129–153). London: Routledge.

Kenyon, B. (2001). Current research in children's conceptions of death: A critical review. *Omega: Journal of Death & Dying*, 43, 63.

Kerr, A. (2002). Annotation: Rett syndrome: recent progress and implications for research and clinical practice. *Journal of Child Psychology and Psychiatry*, 43, 277–288.

Khantzian, E. (1985). The self-medication hypothesis of addictive disorders: Focus on heroin and cocaine dependence. *American Journal of Psychiatry*, 142, 1259–1264.

Kiecolt-Glaser, J. & Glaser, R. (2002). Depression and immune function: Central pathways to morbidity and mortality. *Journal of Psychosomatic Research*, 53, 873–876.

King, N., Muris, P. & Ollendick, T. (2004). Specific phobias. In T. Morris & J. March. *Anxiety Disorders in Children and Adolescents* (Second edition, pp. 263–279). New York: Guilford.

Kingdon, D. & Turkington, D. (1994). *Cognitive-Behavioural Therapy of Schizophrenia*. Hillsdale, NJ: Lawrence Erlbaum Associates Inc.

Kirk, S., & Kutchins, H. (1992). *The Selling of DSM: The Rhetoric of Science in Psychiatry*. New York: Aldine de Gruyter.

Kissane, D. & Bloch, S. (2002). *Family Focused Grief Therapy: A Model of Family-centred Care during Palliative Care and Bereavement*. Buckingham, UK: Open University Press.

Kitson, G. & Sussman, M. (1982). Marital complaints, demographic characteristics and symptoms of mental distress in divorce. *Journal of Marriage and the Family*, 44, 87–101.

Klaus, M. & Kennell, J. (1976). *Maternal-infant bonding*. St Louis: Mosby.

Klein, R. & Pine, D. (2002). Anxiety disorders. In M. Rutter & E. Taylor (eds.), *Child and Adolescent Psychiatry* (Fourth edition, pp. 486–509). Oxford: Blackwell.

Kluger, M., Alexander, G. & Curtis, P. (2000). *What Works in Child Welfare*. Washington, DC: Child Welfare League of America.

Kochanska, G. (1993). Towards a synthesis of parental socialization and child temperament in the early development of conscience. *Child Development*, 64, 325–347.

Koegel, L. & Koegel, R. (1996). The child with autism as an active communicative partner. In E. Hibbs & P. Jensen (eds.), *Psychosocial Treatments for Child and Adolescent Disorders: Empirically Based Strategies for Clinical Practice* (pp. 553–572). Washington, DC: American Psychological Association.

Koegel, R., Schreibman, L., O'Neill, R. & Burke, J. (1983). The personality and family interaction characteristics of parents of autistic children. *Journal of Consulting and Clinical Psychology*, 51, 683–692.

Kolko, D. (2002). Child physical abuse. In J. Myers, L. Berliner, J. Briere, C. Hendrix, C. Jenny & T. Reid (eds.), *APSAC Handbook on Child Maltreatment* (Second edition, pp. 21–54). Thousand Oaks, CA: Sage.

Kolvin, I. & Hartwin-Sadowski, H. (2001). Childhood depression: Clinical phenomenology and classification. In I. Goodyer (ed.), *The Depressed Child and Adolescent* (Second edition, pp. 119–142). Cambridge: Cambridge University Press.

Koocher, G., Goodman, G., White, S., Friedrich, W., Sivan, A. & Reynolds, C. (1995). Psychological science and the use of anatomically detailed dolls in child sexual-abuse assessments. *Psychological Bulletin*, 118, 199–222.

Kovacs, M. & Sherrill, J. (2001). The psychotherapeutic management of major depressive and dysthymic disorders in childhood and adolescence: Issues and prospects. In I. Goodyer (ed.), *The Depressed Child and Adolescent* (Second edition, pp. 325–352). Cambridge: Cambridge University Press.

Kraepelin, E. (1896). *Psychiatrie*. (Fifth edition). Leipzig: Barth.

Kronfol, Z. (2002). Immune dysregulation in major depression: A critical review of existing evidence. *International Journal of Neuropsychopharmacology*, 5, 333–343.

Krug, D., Arick, J. & Almond, P. (1980). Behaviour checklist for identifying severely handicapped children with high levels of autistic behaviour. *Journal of Child Psychology and Psychiatry*, 21, 221–229.

Krug, D., Arick, J. & Almond, P. (1996). *Autism Screening Instrument for Educational Planning* (Second edition). Odessa, FL: Psychological Assessment Resources.

Kübler-Ross, E. (1969). *On Death and Dying*. New York: Macmillan.

Kübler-Ross, E. (1974). *Questions and Answers on Death and Dying*. New York: Macmillan.

Kübler-Ross, E. (1982). *Living with Death and Dying*. New York: Souvenir.

Kübler-Ross, E. (1983). *On Children and Death*. New York: Macmillan.

Kuipers, E., Peters, E. & Bebbington, P. (in press). Schizophrenia. In A. Carr & M. McNulty (eds.), *Handbook of Adult Clinical Psychology. An Evidence-Based Practice Approach*. London: Brunner-Routledge.

Kuipers, L., Leff, J. & Lam, D. (2002). *Family Work for Schizophrenia* (Second edition). London: Gaskell.

Kupfer, D. & Reynolds, C. (1992). Sleep and affective disorders. In E. Paykel (ed.), *Handbook of Affective Disorders* (Second edition, pp. 311–323). Edinburgh: Churchill Livingstone.

Kusumakar, V., Lazier, L., MacMaster, F. & Santor, D. (2002). Bipolar mood disorders: Diagnosis, aetiology and treatment. In S. Kutcher (ed.), *Practical Child and Adolescent Psychopharmacology* (pp. 106–133). Cambridge: Cambridge University Press.

Kutcher, S., Aman, M., Brooks, S., Buitelaar, J., VanDaalen, E., Fegert, J., Findling, R., Fisman, S., Greenhill, L., Huss, M., Kusumakar, V., Pine, D., Taylor, E. & Tyano, S. (2004). International consensus statement on attention-deficit/hyperactivity disorder (ADHD) and disruptive behaviour disorders (DBDs): Clinical implications and treatment practice suggestions. *European Neuropsychopharmacology*, 14(1), 11–28.

Labbé, E., Williamson, D. & Southard, D. (1985). Reliability and validity of children's reports of migraine headache symptoms. *Journal of Psychopathology and Behavioural Assessment*, 7, 375–383.

Lacro, J., Dunn, L. Dolder, C., Leckband, S. & Jeste, D. (2002). Prevalence of and risk factors for medication nonadherence in patients with schizophrenia: A comprehensive review of recent literature. *Journal of Clinical Psychiatry*, 63(10), 892–909.

Laird, J. & Green, R. (1996). *Lesbians and Gays in Couples and Families: A Handbook for Therapists*. San Francisco: Jossey-Bass.

Lam, D. & Jones, S. (in press). Bipolar disorder. In A. Carr & M. McNulty (eds.), *Handbook of Adult Clinical Psychology. An Evidence-Based Practice Approach*. London: Brunner-Routledge.

Lamb, M. (2004). *The Role of the Father in Child Development* (Fourth edition). Chichester: Wiley.

Lambert, M. (2003). *Bergin and Garfield's Handbook of Psychotherapy and Behaviour Change* (Fifth edition). Chichester: Wiley.

Lambert, N., Nihira, K. & Leyland, H. (1993). *Adaptive Behaviour Scale-School Version Second Edition*. Washington, DC: AAMR.

Lampel, A., Bricklin, D. & Elliot, G. (2005). *Custody Evaluation Questionnaires Interviews and Observations and Home Visiting Kits*. Doylestown, PA: Village.

Lange, G. & Carr, A. (2002). Prevention of cognitive delays in socially disadvantaged children. In A. Carr (ed.), *Prevention: What Works with Children and Adolescents? A Critical Review of Psychological Prevention Programmes for Children, Adolescents and their Families*. London: Routledge.

Lange, G., Sheerin, D., Carr, A., Dooley, B., Barton, V., Marshall, D., Mulligan, A., Lawlor, M., Belton, M. & Doyle, M. (2005). Family factors associated with attention deficit hyperactivity disorder and emotional disorders in children. *Journal of Family Therapy*, 27, 76–96.

Lanning, K. (2002). Criminal investigation of sexual victimization of children. In J. Myers, L. Berliner, J. Briere, C. Hendrix, C. Jenny & T. Reid (eds.), *APSAC Handbook on Child Maltreatment* (Second edition, pp. 329–347). Thousand Oaks, CA: Sage.

Lansdown, R. & Sokel, B. (1993). Approaches to pain management in children. *ACCP Review*, 15 (May), 105–111.

Larsen, D., Attkinson, C., Hargreaves, W. & Nguyen, T. (1979). Assessment of client/patient satisfaction: Development of a general scale. *Evaluation and Programme Planning*, 2, 197–207.

Lask, B. (1995). Night terrors. In C. Schaefer (ed.), *Clinical Handbook of Sleep Disorders in Children* (pp. 125–134). Northvale, NJ: Jason Aronson.

Lask, B. (2000). Aetiology. In B. Lask & R. Bryant-Waugh (eds.), *Anorexia Nervosa and Related Eating Disorders in Childhood and Adolescence* (Second edition, pp. 63–75). London: Brunner-Routledge.

Lask, B. & Bryant-Waugh, R. (1993). *Childhood Onset Anorexia Nervosa and Related Disorders*. Hove UK: Lawrence Erlbaum Associates Ltd.

Lask, B. & Bryant-Waugh, R. (2000). *Anorexia Nervosa and Related Eating Disorders in Childhood and Adolescence* (Second edition). London: Brunner-Routledge.

Lask, B. & Fosson, A. (1989). *Childhood Illness: The Psychosomatic Approach*. Chichester: Wiley.

Last, C. (1987). Developmental considerations. In G. Last and M. Hersen (eds.), *Issues in Diagnostic Research* (pp. 201–216). New York: Plenum.

Leckman, J. & Cohen, D. (2002). Tic disorders. In M. Rutter & E. Taylor (eds.), *Child and Adolescent Psychiatry* (Fourth Edition, pp. 593–611). Oxford: Blackwell.

LeCoutier, A., Lord, C. & Rutter, M. (2003). *Autistic Diagnostic Interview-Revised* (ADI-R). Los Angeles, CA: Western Psychological Services.

Leon, K. (2003). Risk and protective factors in young children's adjustment in parental divorce: A review of the research. *Family Relations: Interdisciplinary Journal of Applied Family Studies*, 52, 58–270.

Lerner, M. & Clum, G. (1990). Treatment of suicide ideators: A problem-solving approach. *Behaviour Therapy*, 21, 403–411.

Levine, D. (1994). Utility of suggestion induced spells in diagnosis of pseudoseizures. *Annals of Neurology*, 36, 450.

Levine, F. & Ramirez, R. (1989). Contingent negative practice as a home based treatment of tics and stuttering. In C. Schaefer & J. Briesmeister (eds.), *Handbook of Parent Training* (pp. 38–59). New York: Wiley.

Levy, G. & Fivush, R. (1993). Scripts and gender: A new approach for examining gender role development. *Developmental Psychology*, 13, 126–146.

Lewinsohn, P., Clarke, G., Hops, H. & Andrews, J. (1990). Cognitive behavioural treatment for depressed adolescents. *Behaviour Therapy*, 21, 385–401.

Lewinsohn, P., Clarke, G. & Rohde, P. (1994). *Psychological Approaches to the Treatment of Depression in Adolescents*. New York: Plenum.

Lewis, C., Hitch, G. & Walker, P. (1994). The prevalence of specific arithmetic difficulties and specific reading difficulties in 9 to 10 year old boys and girls. *Journal of Child Psychology and Psychiatry*, 35, 283–292.

Liddle, H. & Hogue, A. (2001). Multidimensional family therapy for adolescent substance abuse. In E. F. Wagner & H. B. Waldron (eds.), *Innovations in Adolescent Substance Abuse Interventions* (pp. 229–261). London: Elsevier.

Liddle, P. (1999). The multidimensional phenotype of schizophrenia. In C. Taminga (ed.), *Schizophrenia in a Molecular Age* (pp. 1–28). Washington, DC: American Psychiatric Press.

Liddle, P. (2000). Descriptive clinical features of schizophrenia. In M. Gelder, J. Lopez-Ibor & N. Andreasen (eds.), *New Oxford Textbook of Psychiatry* (Volume 1, Section 4.3.2, pp. 571–576). Oxford: Oxford University Press.

Liddle, P. (2001). *Disordered Mind and Brain*. London: Gaskell.

Lieberman, M. (1993). Bereavement self-help groups: A review of conceptual and methodological issues. In M. Stroebe, W. Stroebe, & R. Hansson (eds.), *Handbook of Bereavement: Theory, Research, and Intervention* (pp. 411–426). New York: Cambridge University Press.

Lindemann, E. (1944). Symptomatology and management of acute grief. *American Journal of Psychiatry*, 101, 141–148.

Lindemann, E. (1979). *Beyond Grief*. New York: Aronson.

Lines, S. (2004). Chronic Fatigue: A survey, outcome study and proposals. *Child & Adolescent Mental Health*, 9, 168–176.

Lipowski, Z. (1987). Somatization: Medicine's unsolved problem. *Psychosomatics: Journal of Consultation Liaison Psychiatry*, 28, 294–297.

Lipsitt, L. (1992). Discussion: The Bayley Infant Scales of Development: Issues of prediction and outcome revisited. In C. Rovee-Collier & L. Lipsitt (eds.), *Advances in Infancy Research* (volume 7, pp. 239–245). Norwood, NJ: Ablex.

Llewelyn, S. & Kennedy, P. (2003). *Handbook of Clinical Health Psychology*. Chichester: Wiley.

Lochman, J., Barry, T. & Pardini, D. (2003). Anger control training for aggressive youth. In A. Kazdin, & J. Weisz (eds.), *Evidence Based Psychotherapies for Children and Adolescents* (pp. 263–281). New York: Guilford.

Lochman, J., Phillips, N., McElroy, H. & Pardini, D. (2005). Conduct disorders in adolescence. In P. Graham (ed.), *Cognitive Behaviour Therapy for Children and Families* (Second edition, pp. 443–458). Cambridge: Cambridge University Press.

Lock, J. J. & Le Grange, D. (2004). *Help Your Teenager Beat an Eating Disorder*. London: Brunner-Routledge.

Lock, J., LeGrange, D., Agras, W. & Dare, C. (2001). *Treatment Manual for Anorexia Nervosa. A Family Based Approach*. New York: Guilford.

Loeber, R., Burke, J., Lahey, B., Winters, A. & Zera, M. (2000). Oppositional defiant and conduct disorder : A review of the past 10 years, Part I. *Journal of the American Academy of Child & Adolescent Psychiatry*, 39(12), 1468–1484.

Lofthouse, N. & Fristad, M. A. (2004). Psychosocial interventions for children with bipolar disorder. *Clinical Child and Family Psychology Review*, 7, 71–88.

Lord, C. & Bailey, A. (2002). Autism spectrum disorders. In M. Rutter & E. Taylor (eds.), *Child and Adolescent Psychiatry* (Fourth edition, pp. 636–663). Oxford: Blackwell.

Lord, C. & National Research Council (2001). *Educating Children with Autism*. Washington, DC: National Academy Press.

Lord, C., Rutter, M. & DiLavore, P (1997). *Autism Diagnostic Observation Schedule-Generic (ADOS-G)*. New York: The Psychological Corporation.

Lovaas, O. (1987). Behavioural treatment and normal educational and intellectual functioning in young autistic children. *Journal of Consulting and Clinical Psychology*, 55, 3–9.

Lovaas, O. & Smith, T. (2003). Early and intensive behavioural intervention for autism. In A. Kazdin, & J. Weisz (eds.), *Evidence Based Psychotherapies for Children and Adolescents* (pp. 325–340). New York: Guilford.

Luckasson, R., Borthwick-Duffy, S., Buntinx, W., Coulter, D., Craig, E., Reeve, A., Schalock, R., Snell, M., Spitalnik, D., Spreat, S. & Tasse, M. (2002). *Mental Retardation: Definition, Classification, and Systems of Supports* (Tenth edition). Washington, DC: American Association on Mental Retardation.

Luthar, S. (2003). *Resilience and Vulnerability: Adaptation in the Context of Childhood Adversities*. Cambridge: Cambridge University Press.

Lynn, D. & King, B. (2002). Aggressive behaviour. In S. Kutcher (ed.), *Practical Child and Adolescent Psychopharmacology* (pp. 305–327). Cambridge: Cambridge University Press.

MacDonald, G. (2001). *Effective Interventions for Child Abuse and Neglect. An Evidence-based Approach to Planning and Evaluating Interventions*. Chichester: Wiley.

Macintosh, K. & Dissanayake, C. (2004). Annotation: The similarities and differences between autistic disorder and Aperger's disorder. *Journal of Child Psychology and Psychiatry*, 45, 421–434.

Madanes, C. (1991) Strategic family therapy. In A. Gurman & D. Kniskern (eds.), *Handbook of Family Therapy* (volume 2, pp. 396–416). New York: Brunner/Mazel.

Malan, D. (1995). *Individual Psychotherapy and the Science of Psychodynamics* (Second edition). London: Butterworth-Heinemann.

Malik, N. & Furman, W. (1993). Practitioner review: Problem in children's peer relations: What can the clinician do? *Journal of Child Psychology and Psychiatry*, 34, 1303–1326.

Malkinson, R. (2001). Cognitive-behavioural therapy of grief: A review and application. *Research on Social Work Practice*, 11, 671–698.

Maloney, M., McGuire, J. & Daniels, S. (1988). Reliability testing of the Children's Version of the Eating Attitudes Test. *Journal of the American Academy of Child and Adolescent Psychiatry*, 27, 541–543.

Manor, O. (1991). Assessing the work of a family centre. Services offered and referrers' perceptions: A pilot study. *Journal of Family Therapy*, 13, 285–294.

March, J., Frances, A., Carpenter, D. & Kahn, D. (1997). The expert consensus guidelines series: Treatment of obsessive compulsive disorder. *Journal of Clinical Psychiatry*, 58 (Supplement 4), 2–72.

March, J., Franklin, M., Leonard, H. & Foa, E. (2004). Obsessive-compulsive disorder. In T. Morris & J. March, *Anxiety Disorders in Children and Adolescents* (Second edition, pp. 212–240). New York: Guilford.

March, J. & Mulle, K. (1998). *OCD in Children and Adolescents: A Cognitive Behavioural Treatment Manual*. New York: Guilford.

Marcia, J. (1981). Identity and self-development. In R. Lerner, A. Petersen & J. Brooks-Gunn (eds.), *Encyclopaedia of Adolescence* (Volume 1). New York: Garland.

Marcus, L., Kunce, L. & Schopler, E. (1997). Working with families. In D. Cohen & F. Volkmar (eds.), *Handbook of Autism and Pervasive Developmental Disorders* (Second edition, pp. 631–649). New York: Wiley.

Marlatt, G. & Gordon, J. (1985). *Relapse Prevention*. New York: Guilford.

Marshall, W., Laws, D. & Barbaree, H. (1990). *Handbook of Sexual Assault: Issues, Theories, and Treatment of the Offender*. New York: Kluwer/Plenum.

Matthews, G., Deary, J. & Whiteman, M. (2003). *Personality Traits* (Second edition). Cambridge: Cambridge University Press.

Mattis, S. & Pincus, D. (2004). Treatment of SAD and panic disorder in children and adolescents. In P. Barrett & T. Ollendick (eds.), *Handbook of Interventions that Work with Children and Adolescents: Prevention and Treatment* (pp. 145–170). Chichester: Wiley.

Mattison, R., Cantweell, D., Russell, D. & Will, L. (1979). A comparison on DSM-11 and DSM-111 in the diagnosis of childhood psychiatric disorders-11. Interrater agreement. *Archives of General Psychiatry*, 36, 1217–1222.

Maughan, B. (1995). Annotation: Long term outcomes of developmental reading problems. *Journal of Child Psychology and Psychiatry*, 36, 357–371.

Maurice, C. (1993). *Let me Hear Your Voice*. New York: Knopf.

McArdle, P., O'Brien, G. & Kolvin, I. (1995). Hyperactivity: Prevalence and relationship with conduct disorder. *Journal of Child Psychology and Psychiatry*, 36, 279–304.

McCarthy, D. (1972). *McCarthy Scales of Children's Abilities*. San Antonio, TX: Psychological Corporation.

McCarthy, O. & Carr, A. (2002). Prevention of bullying. In A. Carr (ed.), *Prevention: What Works with Children and Adolescents? A Critical Review of Psychological Prevention Programmes for Children, Adolescents and their Families* (pp. 205–221). London: Routledge.

McCauley, E., Pavlidis, K. & Kendall, K. (2001). Developmental precursors of depression: the child and the social environment. In I. Goodyer (ed.), *The Depressed Child and Adolescent* (Second edition, pp. 46–78). Cambridge: Cambridge University Press.

McConaughy, S. & Achenbach, T. (1994). Comorbidity of empirically based syndromes in matched general population and clinical samples. *Journal of Child Psychology and Psychiatry*, 35, 1141–1157.

McCubbin, H., Patterson, J. & Wilson, L. (1982). Family Inventory of Life Events and changes: FILE. In D. Olson, H. McCubbin, H. Barnes, A. Larsen, M. Muxen & M. Wilson (eds.), *Family Inventories* (pp. 69–88). St Paul, MN: University of Minnesota.

McCullough-Vaillant, L. (1997). *Changing Character: Short-Term Anxiety Regulating Psychotherapy for Restructuring Defences, Affects and Attachments*. New York: Basic Books.

McEachin, J., Smith, T. & Lovaas, O. (1993). Long term outcome for children with autism who received early intensive behavioural treatment. *American Journal of Mental Retardation*, 97, 359–372.

McEvoy, J., Scheifler, P. & Frances, A. (1999). The Expert Consensus Guideline Series: Treatment of Schizophrenia 1999. *Journal of Clinical Psychiatry*, 60 (Supplement 11). http://www.psychguides.com/gl-treatment_of_schizophrenia_1999.html

McFarlane, W., Dixon, L., Lukens, E. & Lucksted, A. (2003). Family psychoeducation and schizophrenia: A review of the literature. *Journal of Marital and Family Therapy*, 29: 223–246.

McGee, R., Feehan, M., Williams, S., Partridge, F., Silva, P. & Kelly, J. (1990). DSM III disorders in a large sample of adolescents. *Journal of the American Academy of Child and Adolescent Psychiatry*, 29, 611–619.

McGlashen, T. & Hoffman, R. (2000). Schizophrenia as a disorder of developmentally reduced synaptic connectivity. *Archives of General Psychiatry*, 57, 637–648.

McGoldrick, M., Gerson, R., & Shellenberger, S. (1999). *Genograms: Assessment and Intervention* (Second edition). New York: Norton.

McGrath, J., Feron, F., Burne, T., Mackay-Sim, A. & Eyles, D. (2003). The neurodevelopmental hypothesis of schizophrenia: A review of recent developments. *Annals of Medicine*, 35(2), 86–93.

McGrath, P. (1995). Aspects of pain in children and adolescents. *Journal of Child Psychology and Psychiatry*, 36, 717–731.

McGrath, P. & Goodman, J. (2005). Pain in childhood. In P. Graham (ed.), *Cognitive Behaviour Therapy for Children and Families* (Second edition, pp. 426–443). Cambridge: Cambridge University Press.

McGrath, P. & Hiller, L. (1999). Controlling children's pain. In R. Gatchel & D. Turk (eds.), *Psychological Approaches to Pain Management. A Practitioner's Handbook* (pp. 331–370). New York: Guilford.

McGrath, P., Johnson, G., Goodamn, J., Schillinger, J., Dunn, J. & Chapman, J. (1985). CHEOPS: A behavioural scale for rating post operative pain in children. In H. Fields, R. Dubner & F. Cerveero (eds.), *Advances in Pain Research and Therapy* (volume 9, pp. 395–401). New York: Raven.

McGuffin, P., Owen, M. & Gottesman, I. (2002). *Psychiatric Genetics and Genomics*. Oxford: Oxford University Press.

McGurk, H., Caplan, M., Hennessy, E. & Moss, P. (1993). Controversy, theory and social context in contemporary day care research. *Journal of Child Psychology and Psychiatry*, 34, 3–23.

McKnight, C., Compton, S. & March, J. (2004). Posttraumatic Stress Disorder. In T. Morris & J. March, *Anxiety Disorders in Children and Adolescents* (Second edition, pp. 241–262). New York: Guilford.

McNeish, D., Newman, T. & Roberts, H. (2002). *What Works for Children*. Buckingham: Open University Press.

McQuaid, E. & Walders, N. (2003). Paediatric asthma. In M. Roberts (ed.), *Handbook of Paediatric Psychology* (Third edition, pp. 269–285). New York: Guilford.

Meadowcroft, P. & Trout, B. (1990). *Troubled Youth in Treatment Homes: A Handbook of Therapeutic Foster Care*. Washington, DC: Child Welfare League of America.

Meichenbaum, D. (1977). *Cognitive-Behaviour Modification: An Integrative Approach*. New York: Plenum Press.

Meltzer, H., Gatward, R. Goodman, R. & Ford, T. (2000). *The Mental Health of Children and Adolescents in Great Britain: The report of a survey carried out in 1999 by Social Survey Division of the Office for National Statistics on behalf of the Department of Health, the Scottish Health Executive and the National Assembly for Wales*. London: The Stationery Office.

Melzak, R. & Wall, P. (1989). *Textbook of Pain*. London: Churchill Livingstone.

Menkes, J. (1990). *Textbook of Child Neurology* (Fourth edition). Philadelphia: Lea & Febiger.

Merry, S. & Werry, J. (2001). Course and prognosis. In H. Remschmidt (ed.), *Schizophrenia in Children and Adolescents* (pp. 268–297). Cambridge: Cambridge University Press.

Mesibov, G., Schopler, E. & Caison, W. (1989). *Adolescent and Adult Psycho-Educational Profile* (AAPEP). Austin, TX: Pro-ed.

Middleton, J. (2001). Practitioner review: Psychological sequelae of head injury in children and adolescents. *Journal of Child Psychology & Psychiatry*, 42, 165–180.

Mikulas, W. & Coffman, M. (1989). Home-based treatment of children's fear of the dark. In C. Schaefer & J. Briesmeister (eds.), *Handbook of Parent Training* (pp. 179–202). New York: Wiley.

Milby, J. & Weber, A. (1991). Obsessive compulsive disorders. In T. Kratochwill & R. Morris (eds.), *The Practice of Child Therapy* (Second edition, pp. 9–42). New York: Pergamon Press.

Miller, B. & Wood, B. (1991). Childhood asthma in interaction with family, school and peer systems: A developmental model of primary care. *Journal of Asthma*, 28, 405–414.

Miller, W. & Rollnick, S. (2002). *Motivational Interviewing. Preparing People for Change* (Second edition). New York: Guilford.

Minde, K., Popiel, K., Leos, N., Faulkner, S., Parker, K. & Handley-Derry, M. (1993). The evaluation and treatment of sleep disturbances in young children. *Journal of Child Psychology and Psychiatry*, 34, 521–533.

Mindell, J. & Andrasik, F. (1987). Headache classification and factor analysis with a paediatric population. *Headache*, 27, 96–101.

Mindell, J. & Owens, J. (2003). *A Clinical Guide to Paediatric Sleep: Diagnosis and Management of Sleep Problems*. Philadelphia: Lippincott Williams & Wilkins. http://www.rch.org.au/clinicalguide/pages/sleep_handouts.html

Minuchin, P. (1995). Foster and natural families. Forming a co-operative network. In L. Combrinck-Graham (ed.), *Children in Families at Risk. Making the Connections* (pp. 251–274). New York: Guilford.

Minuchin, S. (1974). *Families and Family Therapy*. Cambridge, MA: Harvard University Press.

Minuchin, S., Rosman, B. & Baker, L. (1978). *Psychosomatic Families: Anorexia Nervosa in Context*. Cambridge, MA: Harvard University Press.

Mirza, K. (2002). Adolescent substance use disorder. In S. Kutcher (ed.), *Practical Child and Adolescent Psychopharmacology* (pp. 328–381). Cambridge: Cambridge University Press.

Mitchell, K. & Carr, A. (2000). Anorexia and bulimia. In A. Carr (ed.), *What Works with Children and Adolescents? A Critical Review of Psychological Interventions with Children, Adolescents and their Families* (pp. 233–257). London: Routledge.

Moffit, T. (1993). The neuropsychology of conduct disorder. *Development and Psychopathology*, 5, 135–151.

Moffit, T. & Caspi, A. (1998). The implications of violence between partners for child psychologists and psychiatrists. *Journal of Child Psychology and Psychiatry*, 39, 137–144.

Mooney, K. (1985). Children's night-time fears: Ratings of content and coping behaviours. *Cognitive Therapy and Research*, 9, 309–319.

Mooney, K. & Sobocinski, M. (1995). The treatment of night-time fears: A cognitive-developmental approach. In C. Schaefer (ed.), *Clinical Handbook of Sleep Disorders in Children* (pp. 69–102). Northvale, NJ: Jason Aronson.

Moore, M. & Carr, A. (2000). Depression and grief. In A. Carr (ed.), *What Works with*

Children and Adolescents? A Critical Review of Psychological Interventions with Children, Adolescents and their Families (pp. 203–232). London: Routledge.

Morgan, A. & Hilgard, J. (1979). Stanford Hypnotic Scale for Children. *American Journal of Clinical Hypnosis*, 21, 155–169.

Morgan, R. & Young, G. (1975). Parental attitudes and the conditioning treatment of childhood enuresis. *Behaviour Research and Therapy*, 13, 197–199.

Morris, R. (1988). Classification of learning disabilities: Old problems and new approaches. *Journal of Consulting and Clinical Psychology*, 56, 789–794.

Morris, T. (2004). Treatment of social phobia in children and adolescents. In P. Barrett & T. Ollendick (eds.), *Handbook of Interventions that Work with Children and Adolescents: Prevention and Treatment* (pp. 171–186). Chichester: Wiley.

Morris, T. & March, J. (2004). *Anxiety Disorders in Children and Adolescents* (Second edition). New York: Guilford.

Morrison, A. (2002). *A Casebook of Cognitive Therapy for Psychosis*. Hove, UK: Brunner-Routledge.

Mowrer, O. (1960). *Learning Theory and Behaviour*. New York: Wiley.

Mrazek, D. (2002). Psychiatric aspects of somatic disease and disorders. In M. Rutter & E. Taylor (eds.), *Child and Adolescent Psychiatry* (Fourth edition, pp. 810–827). Oxford: Blackwell.

MTA Cooperative Group (1999). A 14 month randomized clinical trial of treatment strategies for attention deficit hyperactivity disorder. *Archives of General Psychiatry*, 56, 1073–1086.

Mufson, L., Dorta, K., Moreau, D. & Weissman, M. (2004). *Interpersonal Psychotherapy for Depressed Adolescents* (Second edition). New York: Guilford.

Mufson, L. & Pollack, K. (2003). Interpersonal psychotherapy for depressed adolescents. In A. Kazdin, & J. Weisz (eds.), *Evidence Based Psychotherapies for Children and Adolescents* (pp. 148–164). New York: Guilford.

Mulvaney, F. (2000). *Annual Report of the National Intellectual Disability Database Committee*. Dublin: Health Research Board.

Mundy, P. & Neale, A. (2001). Neural plasticity, joint attention and a transactional social-orienting of autism. In L. Glidden (ed.), *International Review of Research in Mental Retardation. Autism* (volume 23, pp. 139–168). San Diego, CA: Academic Press.

Munsinger, H. & Karlson, K. (1996). *Uniform Child Custody Evaluation System*. Odessa FL: Psychological Assessment Resources.

Murphy, E. & Carr, A. (2000a). Enuresis and encopresis. In A. Carr (ed.), *What Works with Children and Adolescents? A Critical Review of Psychological Interventions with Children, Adolescents and their Families* (pp. 49–64). London: Routledge.

Murphy, E. & Carr, A. (2000b). Paediatric pain problems. In A. Carr (ed.), *What Works with Children and Adolescents? A Critical Review of Psychological Interventions with Children, Adolescents and their Families* (pp. 258–279). London: Routledge.

Murray, R. (1994). Neurodevelopmental schizophrenia: The rediscovery of dementia praecox. *British Journal of Psychiatry*, 25, 6–12.

Murray, R. & Castle, D. (2000). Genetic and environmental risk factors for schizophrenia. In M. Gelder, J. Lopez-Ibor & N. Andreasen (eds.), *New Oxford Textbook of Psychiatry* (Volume 1, Section 4.3.5.1, pp. 599–605). Oxford: Oxford University Press.

Myers, J. (2002). The legal system and child protection. In J. Myers, L. Berliner, J. Briere, C. Hendrix, C. Jenny & T. Reid (eds.), *APSAC Handbook on Child Maltreatment* (Second edition, pp. 305–327). Thousand Oaks, CA: Sage.

Myers, J., Berliner, L., Briere, J., Hendrix, C., Jenny, C. & Reid, T. (2002). *APSAC Handbook on Child Maltreatment* (Second edition). Thousand Oaks, CA: Sage.

Myers, J. & Stern, P. (2002). Expert testimony. In J. Myers, L. Berliner, J. Briere, C. Hendrix, C. Jenny & T. Reid (eds.), *APSAC Handbook on Child Maltreatment* (Second edition, pp. 379–402). Thousand Oaks, CA: Sage.

Myers, M., Brown, S. & Vik, P. (1998). Adolescent substance use problems. In E. Mash & L. Terdal (eds.), *Treatment of Childhood Disorders* (Second edition, pp. 692–730). New York: Guilford.

Nasser, M. & Katzman, N. (2003). Sociocultural theories of eating disorders. In J. Treasure, U. Schmidt & E. van Furth (eds.), *Handbook of Eating Disorders* (Second edition, pp.139–150). Chichester: Wiley.

National Advisory Committee on Drugs and the Drug and Alcohol Information and Research Unit (2004). Drug use in Ireland and Northern Ireland. 2003/2003 Drug Prevalence Survey. Health Board (Ireland) and Social Service Board (Northern Ireland) Results. *Bulletin 1.* http://www.nacd.ie and http://www.dhsspsni.gov.uk

National Centre for Social Research and the National Foundation for Educational Research (2002). Drug use, smoking and drinking among young people in England in 2001. http://www.official-documents.co.uk/document/deps/doh/sddyp02/dsd–01.htm

National Collaborating Centre for Mental Health (2003). *Schizophrenia: Full National Clinical Guideline on Core Interventions in Primary and Secondary Care.* London: Gaskell and the British Psychological Society.

Neiderman, M. (2000). Prognosis and outcome. In B. Lask & R. Bryant-Waugh (eds.), *Anorexia Nervosa and Related Eating Disorders in Childhood and Adolescence* (Second edition, pp. 81–97). London: Brunner-Routledge.

Nelson, H. (1997). *Cognitive Behavioural Therapy with Schizophrenia. A Practice Manual.* Cheltenham, UK: Thornes Publishers.

NESS Research Team (2004). The national evaluation of Sure Start local programmes in England. *Child and Adolescent Mental Health*, 9 (1), 2–8.

Newland, T. (1971). *Blind Learning Aptitude Test.* Champaign, IL: University of Illinois Press.

Newman, B. & Newman, P. (2003). *Development Through Life* (Eighth edition). Pacific Grove, CA: Brooks/Cole.

NICE (2004). *Eating Disorders: Core Interventions in the Treatment and Management of Anorexia Nervosa, Bulimia Nervosa and Related Disorders. A National Clinical Practice Guideline.* London: National Institute for Clinical Excellence. http://www.nice.org.uk/page.aspx?o=101243

NICE (2005). *Depression in Children and Young People. Identification and management in Primary, Community and Secondary Care. National Clinical Practice Guideline Number 28.* London: British Psychological Society and Royal College of Psychiatrists.

Nicol, A., Smith, J., Kay, B., Hall, D., Barlow, J. & Williams, B. (1988). A focused casework approach to the treatment of child abuse: A controlled comparison. *Journal of Child Psychology and Psychiatry*, 29, 703–711.

Nielsen, S. & Bará-Carril, N. (2003). Family, burden of care and social consequences. In J. Treasure, U. Schmidt & E. van Furth (eds.), *Handbook of Eating Disorders* (Second edition, pp. 191–217). Chichester: Wiley.

Nigg, J. (2001). Is ADHD an inhibitory disorder? *Psychological Bulletin*. 125, 571–596.

Nihira, K., Leyland, H. & Lambert, N. (1993). *Adaptive Behaviour Scale-Residential and Community Version* (Second edition). Austin, TX: Pro-ed.

Nikapota, A. (2002). Culture and ethnic issues in service provision. In M. Rutter, & E. Taylor (eds.), *Child and Adolescent Psychiatry* (Fourth edition, pp. 1148–1157). Oxford: Blackwell.

NíNualláin, M., O'Hare, A. & Walsh, D. (1990). The prevalence of schizophrenia in three counties in Ireland. *Acta Psychiatrica Scandinavica*, 82, 136–140.

Nolan, M. & Carr, A. (2000). Attention deficit hyperactivity disorder. In A. Carr (ed.), *What Works with Children and Adolescents? A Critical Review of Psychological Interventions with Children, Adolescents and their Families* (pp. 65–102). London: Routledge.

Noll, R. & Kazak, A. (1997). Standards for psychosocial care. In A. Ablin (ed.), *Supportive Care of Children with Cancer* (pp. 263–273). Baltimore, MD: Johns Hopkins University Press.

Norman, R. & Malla, A. (1993). Stressful life events and schizophrenia: I. A review of the research. *British Journal of Psychiatry*, 162, 161–166.

Novaco, R. (1975). *Anger Control: The Development and Evaluation of an Experimental Treatment*. Lexington, MA: Heath & Co.

Nowicki, S. & Strickland, B. (1973). A locus of control scale for children. *Journal of Consulting and Clinical Psychology*, 40, 148–155.

NSPCC (1998). *Young Witness Pack*. NSPCC, 42 Curtain Road, London EC2A 3NH. http://www.nspcc.org.uk/

NSPCC (2000). Giving evidence – what's it really like? Video. NSPCC, 42 Curtain Road, London EC2A 3NH. http://www.nspcc.org.uk/

Nuechterlin, K. & Dawson, M. (1984). A heuristic vulnerability-stress model of schizophrenic episodes. *Schizophrenia Bulletin*, 10, 200–312.

O'Connor, J. (1983). Why can't I get hives: brief strategic therapy with an obsessional child. *Family Process*, 22, 201–209.

O'Connor, T. (2002). Attachment disorders of infancy and childhood. In M. Rutter & E. Taylor (eds.), *Child and Adolescent Psychiatry* (Fourth edition, pp. 776–792). Oxford: Blackwell.

O'Halloran, M. & Carr, A. (2000). Adjustment to parental separation and divorce. In A. Carr (ed.), *What Works with Children and Adolescents? A Critical Review of Psychological Interventions with Children, Adolescents and their Families* (pp. 280–299). London: Routledge.

O'Reilly, G. & Carr, A. (eds.) (1998). Understanding, assessing and treating juvenile and adult sex offenders. Special guest-edited issue of the *Irish Journal of Psychology*, 19(1). Dublin: PSI.

O'Reilly, G., Marshall, W., Carr, A. & Beckett, R. (eds.) (2004). *The Handbook of Clinical Intervention with Young People who Sexually Abuse*. London: Brunner-Routledge.

O'Reilly, G., Walsh, P., Carr, A. & McEvoy, J. (2005a). *Handbook of Intellectual Disability and Clinical Psychology Practice*. London: Brunner-Routledge.

O'Reilly, M., Sigafoos, J., Lancioni, G., Green, V., Olive, M., Lacey, C. & Cannella, H. (2005b). Applied Behavior Analysis. In G. O'Reilly, P. Walsh, A. Carr & J. McEvoy (eds.), *Handbook of Intellectual Disability and Clinical Psychology Practice*. London: Brunner-Routledge.

O'Riordan, D. & Carr, A. (2002). Prevention of physical abuse. In A. Carr (ed.), *Prevention: What Works with Children and Adolescents? A Critical Review of Psychological Prevention Programmes for Children, Adolescents and their Families* (pp. 154–180). London: Routledge.

O'Sullivan, A. & Carr, A. (2002). Prevention of developmental delay in low birth weight infants. In A. Carr (ed.), *Prevention: What Works with Children and Adolescents? A Critical Review of Psychological Prevention Programmes for Children, Adolescents and their Families* (pp.17–40). London: Routledge.

Oliver, C. (1995). Annotation: Self-injurious behaviour in children with learning disabilities: Recent advances in assessment and intervention. *Journal of Child Psychology and Psychiatry*, 30, 909–927.

Ollendick, T., Davis, T & Muris, P. (2004). Treatment of specific phobia in children and adolescents. In P. Barrett & T. Ollendick (eds.), *Handbook Interventions that Work with Children and Adolescents: Prevention and Treatment* (pp. 273–300). Chichester: Wiley.

Ollendick, T., King, N. & Yule, W. (1994). *International Handbook of Phobic and Anxiety Disorders in Children and Adolescents*. New York: Plenum.

Ollendick, T. & March, J. (2003). *Phobic and Anxiety Disorders in Children and Adolescents: A Clinical Guide to Effective Psychosocial and Pharmacological Interventions*. Oxford: Oxford University Press.

Olness, K. & Gardner, G. (1988). *Hypnosis and Hypnotherapy with Children*. Philadelphia: Grune and Stratton.

Olness, K., McFarland, F. & Piper, J. (1980). Biofeedback: A new modality in the management of children with faecal soiling. *Journal of Paediatrics*, 96, 505–509.

Olson, D. (1993). Circumplex model of marital and family systems: Assessing family functioning. In F. Walsh (ed.), *Normal Family Processes* (Second edition, pp. 104–1137). New York: Guilford.

Olweus, D. (1993). *Bullying at School: What we Know and What we can Do*. Oxford: Blackwell.

Oosterlaan, J. (2001). Behavioural inhibition and the development of childhood anxiety disorders. In W. Silverman & P. Treffers (eds.), *Anxiety Disorders in Children and Adolescents. Research Assessment and Intervention* (pp. 45–71). Cambridge: Cambridge University Press.

Öst, L. & Treffers, P. (2001). Onset, course, and outcome for anxiety disorders in children. In W. Silverman & P. Treffers (eds.), *Anxiety Disorders in Children and Adolescents. Research Assessment and Intervention* (pp. 293–312). Cambridge: Cambridge University Press.

Owen, M., O'Donovan, M. & Gottesman, I. (2002). Schizophrenia. In P. McGuffin, M. Owen, & I. Gottesman (eds.), *Psychiatric Genetics and Genomics* (pp. 247–266). Oxford: Oxford University Press.

Owens, J., Spirito, A. & McGuinn, M. (2000). The Children's Sleep Habits Questionnaire (CSHQ): Psychometric properties of a survey instrument for school-aged children. *Sleep,* 23, 1043–1051.

Ozonoff, S. (1997). Components of executive function deficits in autism and other disorders. In J. Russell (ed.), *Autism as an Executive Disorder* (pp. 179–211). Oxford: Oxford University Press.

Pagliaro, A. & Pagliaro, L. (1996). *Substance Use Among Children and Adolescents*. New York: Wiley.

Palasti, S. & Potsic, W. (1995). Managing the child with obstructive sleep apnoea. In C. Schaefer (ed.), *Clinical Handbook of Sleep Disorders in Children* (pp. 253–266). Northvale, NJ: Jason Aronson.

Paolucci, E., Genuis, M. & Violato, C. (2001). A meta-analysis of the published research on the effects of child sexual abuse. *Journal of Psychology*, 135, 17–36.

Papolos, D. & Papolos, J. (2002). *The Bipolar Child: The Definitive and Reassuring Guide to Childhood's Most Misunderstood Disorder* (Second edition). New York: Broadway.

Park, R. & Goodyer, I. (2000). Clinical guidelines for depressive disorders in childhood and adolescence. *European Journal of Child and Adolescent Psychiatry*, 9, 147–161.

Parkes, C. (1993). Bereavement as a psychosocial transition: Processes of adaptation to change. In M. Stroebe, W. Stroebe, & R. Hansson (eds.), *Handbook of Bereavement: Theory, Research, and Intervention* (pp. 91–101). New York: Cambridge University Press.

Parmenter, T. (2001). Intellectual disabilities – quo vadis? In G. Albrecht, K. Seelman & M. Bury (eds.), *Handbook of Disability Studies* (pp. 267–296). Thousand Oaks, CA: Sage.

Patterson, G. (1982). *Coercive Family Process*. Eugene, OR: Castalia.

Patterson, G., Reid, J. & Dishion, T. (1992). *Antisocial Boys*. Eugene, OR: Castalia.

Pecora, P. & Maluccio, A. (2000). What works in family foster care. In M. Kluger, G. Alexander & P. Curtis (eds.), *What Works in Child Welfare* (pp. 139–155). Washington, DC: Child Welfare League of America.

Pehlivantuerk, B. & Unal, F. (2002). Conversion disorder in children and adolescents: A 4-year follow-up study. *Journal of Psychosomatic Research*, 52, 187–191.

Pelham, W. & Hinshaw, S. (1992). Behavioural intervention for attention deficit disorder. In S. Turner, K. Calhoun & H. Adams (eds.), *Handbook of Clinical Behaviour Therapy* (volume 2, pp. 259–283). New York: Wiley.

Pelham, W. & Walker, K. (2005). Attention deficit hyperactivity disorder. In P. Graham (ed.), *Cognitive Behaviour Therapy for Children and Families* (Second edition, pp. 225–243). Cambridge: Cambridge University Press.

Perfetti, C. (1985). *Reading Ability*. New York: Oxford University Press.

Perrin, S., Smith, P. & Yule, W. (2004). Treatment of PTSD in children and adolescents. In P. Barrett & T. Ollendick (eds.), *Handbook of Interventions that Work with Children and Adolescents: Prevention and Treatment* (pp. 317–242). Chichester: Wiley.

Perry, P., Alexander, B., & Liskow, B. (1997). *Psychotropic Drug Handbook* (Seventh edition). Washington, DC: APA Press.

Piaget, J. (1932). *The Moral Judgement of the Child*. New York: Free Press.

Platt, S. (1992). Parasuicide in Europe. The WHO/EURO multicentre study on parasuicide. *Acta Psychiatrica Scandanavia*, 85, 97–104.

Prinz, R. & Dumas, J. (2004). Prevention of oppositional defiant disorder and conduct disorder in children and adolescents. In P. Barrett & T. Ollendick (eds.),

Handbook of Interventions that Work with Children and Adolescents: Prevention and Treatment (pp. 475–488). Chichester: Wiley.

Prizant, B., Schuler, A., Wetherby, A. & Rydell, P. (1997). Enhancing language and communication development: Language based approaches. In D. Cohen & F. Volkmar (eds.), *Handbook of Autism and Pervasive Developmental Disorders* (Second edition, pp. 572–605). New York: Wiley.

Prochaska, J. DiClement, C. & Norcross, J. (1992). In search of how people change. *American Psychologist*, 47, 1102–1114.

Putnam, F. (2003). Ten-year research update review: Child sexual abuse. *Journal of the American Academy of Child and Adolescent Psychiatry*, 42, 269–278.

Quay, H. (1983). A dimensional approach to children's behaviour disorder: Revised Behaviour Problem Checklist. *School Psychology Review*, 12, 244–249.

Quay, H. (1997). Inhibition and attention deficit hyperactivity disorder. *Journal of Abnormal Child Psychology*, 25, 7–13.

Quine, L. & Rutter, D. (1994). First diagnosis of severe mental and physical disability. *Journal of Child Psychology and Psychiatry*, 35, 1273–1289.

Quinn, P, Stern, J. & Russell, N. (1998). *The 'Putting on the Brakes' Activity Book for Young People with ADHD*. Washington, DC: Magination Press.

Quinn, P, Stern, J. & Russell, N. (2001). *Putting on the Brakes: Young People's Guide to Understanding Attention Deficit Hyperactivity Disorder*. Washington, DC: Magination Press.

Rachman, S. (2002). *Anxiety* (Second edition). Hove, UK: Psychology Press.

Raine A. (1993). *The Psychopathology of Crime: Criminal Behaviors as a Clinical Disorder*. San Diego, CA: Academic Press.

Raine, A. (2002). The role of prefrontal deficits, low autonomic arousal, and early health factors in the development of antisocial and aggressive behaviour. *Journal of Child Psychology and Psychiatry*, 43, 417–434.

Ramchandani, P., Wiggs, L., Webb, V. & Stores, G. (2000). A systematic review of treatments for settling problems and night waking in young children. *British Medical Journal*, 320, 209–213.

Rapee, R., Spense, S., Cobham, V. & Wignal, A. (2000). *Helping Your Anxious Child: A Step-By-Step Guide for Parents*. San Francisco: New Harbinger.

Raphael, B., Minkov, C. & Dobson, M. (2001). Psychotherapeutic and pharmacological intervention for bereaved persons. In M. Stroebe, R. Hansson, W. Stroebe & H. Schut (eds.), *Handbook of Bereavement Research: Consequences, Coping, and Care* (pp. 587–612). Washington, DC: American Psychological Association.

Rapin, I. (1996). Practitioner review: Developmental language disorders: A clinical update. *Journal of Child Psychology and Psychiatry*, 37, 643–655.

Rapoport, J. & Inoff-Germain, G. (2000). Practitioner review: Treatment of obsessive compulsive disorder in children and adolescents. *Journal of Child Psychology and Psychiatry*, 41, 419–431.

Rapoport, J. & Swedo, S. (2002). Obsessive compulsive disorder. In M. Rutter & E. Taylor (eds.), *Child and Adolescent Psychiatry* (Fourth edition, pp. 571–592). Oxford: Blackwell.

Raschke, H. (1987). Divorce. In M. Sussman & S. Steinmetz (eds.), *Handbook of Marriage and the Family* (pp. 348–399). New York: Plenum.

Rauch, S. & Baxter, L. (1998). Neuroimaging of OCD and related disorders. In

M. Jenike, L. Baer, & W. Minichiello (eds.), *Obsessive Compulsive Disorders: Practical Management* (pp. 222–253). Boston, MA: Mosby.

Rechtschaffen, A. & Kales, A. (1968). *A Manual of Standardized Terminology, Techniques, and Scoring System for Sleep Stages of Human Subjects.* Los Angeles, CA: UCLA Brain Information Service, Brain Research Institute.

Reder, P., Duncan, S. & Lucey, S. (2004). *Studies in the Assessment of Parenting.* London: Routledge.

Reder, P. & Lucey, C. (1995). *Assessment of Parenting. Psychiatric and Psychological Contributions.* London: Routledge.

Reder, P., McClure, M. & Jolley, A. (2000). *Family Matters. Interfaces between Child and Adult Mental Health.* London: Routledge.

Reich, W. (2000). Diagnostic Interview for Children and Adolescents (DICA). *Journal of the American Academy of Child and Adolescent Psychiatry*, 39, 59–66.

Reid, G. (2003). *Dyslexia: A Practitioner's Handbook* (Third edition). Chichester: Wiley.

Reifman, A., Villa, L., Amans, J., Rethinam, V. & Telesca, T. (2001). Children of divorce in the 1990s: A meta-analysis. *Journal of Divorce and Remarriage*, 36, 27–36.

Remschmidt, H. (2001). Definition and classification. In H. Remschmidt (ed.), *Schizophrenia in Children and Adolescents* (pp. 24–42). Cambridge: Cambridge University Press.

Reynolds, C. & Ray, I. (1997). *Handbook of Clinical Child Neuropsychology* (Second edition). New York: Plenum.

Rice, F., Harold, G. & Thapar, A. (2002). The genetic aetiology of childhood depression: A review. *Journal of Child Psychology and Psychiatry*, 43, 65–79.

Richards, J. (2000). Chronic fatigue syndrome in children and adolescents. *Clinical Child Psychology and Psychiatry*, 5, 31–51.

Richardson, J. & Joughin, C. (2002). *Parent Training Programmes for the Management of Young Children with Conduct Disorders.* London: Gaskell.

Richman, J. (1984). The family therapy of suicidal adolescents. In H. Saudak, A. Ford & N. Rushforth (eds.), *Suicide in the Young* (pp 393–406). Little, MA: John Wright PSG.

Richman, N. (1981). A community survey of characteristics of one to two year olds with sleep disruptions. *Journal of the American Academy of Child Psychiatry*, 20, 281–291.

Richman, N. (1983). Choosing treatments for encopresis. *Newsletter of the Association of Child Psychology and Psychiatry*, 16, 34.

Riegel, K. (1973). Dialectic operations: The final period of cognitive development. *Human Development*, 16, 346–70.

Roberts, M. (2003). *Handbook of Paediatric Psychology* (Third edition). New York: Guilford.

Robin, A. & Foster, S. (1989). *Negotiating Parent–Adolescent Conflict.* New York: Guilford Press.

Robins, L. (1999). A 70 year history of conduct disorder. Variations in definition, prevalence and correlates. In P. Cohen (ed.), *Historical and Geographical Influence on Psychopathology* (pp. 37–56). Mahwah, NJ: Lawrence Erlbaum Associates Inc.

Robinson, M. (1997). *Divorce as Family Transition.* London: Karnac.

Roelofs, K., Hoogduin, K., Keijsers, G., Naering, G., Moene, F. & Sandijck, P. (2002a). Hypnotic susceptibility in patients with conversion disorder. *Journal of Abnormal Psychology*, 11, 390–395.

Roelofs, K., Keijsers, G., Hoogduin, K., Naering, G. & Moene, F. (2002b). Childhood abuse in patients with conversion disorder. *American Journal of Psychiatry*, 159, 1908–1913.

Roffwarg, H., Muzio, J. & Dement, W. (1966). Ontogenetic development of the human sleep-dream cycle. *Science*, 152, 604–619.

Rogers, K. (2004). A theoretical review of risk and protective factors related to post-divorce adjustment in young children. *Journal of Divorce and Remarriage*, 40(3–4), 135–147.

Rogers, S. & Benneto, L. (2000). Intersubjectivity in autism: The roles of imitation and executive function. In A. Wetherby & B. Brizant (eds.), *Autism Spectrum Disorders: A Transactional Developmental Perspective* (pp. 79–107). Baltimore, MD: Paul H. Brookes.

Roid, G. (2003). *Stanford–Binet Intelligence Scales, fifth edition (SB-V)*. Itasca, IL: Riverside Publishing. http://www.riverpub.com/products/clinical/sbis/home.html

Roid, G. & Miller, L. (1997). *Leiter International Performance Scale-Revised*. Odessa, FL: Psychological Assessment Resources.

Rolf, J., Masten, A., Cicchetti, D., Nuchterlein, K. & Weintraub, S. (1990). *Risk And Protective Factors In The Development of Psychopathology*. New York: Cambridge University Press.

Rolland, J. (2003). Mastering family challenges in illness and disability. In F. Walsh (ed.), *Normal Family Process* (Third edition, pp. 460–492). New York: Guilford.

Rose, G. & York, A. (2004). *Mental Health and Growing Up. Factsheets for Parents, Teachers and Young People* (Third edition). London: Gaskell.

Rosenbaum Asarnow, J., Tompson, M., Woo, S. & Cantwell, D. (2001). Is expressed emotion a specific risk factor for depression or a non-specific correlate of psycho-pathology? *Journal of Abnormal Child Psychology*, 29, 573–583.

Rosenberg, S. (1993). Chomsky's theory of language: Some recent observations. *Psychological Science*, 4, 15–19.

Rotherham-Borus, M., Piancentini, J., Miller, S., Grase, F. & Castro-Blanco, D. (1994). Brief cognitive behavioural treatment for adolescent suicide attempters and their families. *Journal of the American Academy of Child and Adolescent Psychiatry*, 33, 508–517.

Rotherham-Borus, M., Piancentini, J., Van Rossem, R., Grace, F., Cantwell, C., Castro-Blanco, D., Miller, S. & Feldman, J. (1996). Enhancing treatment adherence with a specialized emergency room programme for adolescent suicide attempters. *Journal of the American Academy of Child and Adolescent Psychiatry*, 35, 654–663.

Rotter, J. (1966). Generalised expectancies for internal versus external control of reinforcement. *Psychological Monographs*, 90, 1–28. (*Contains the original Locus of Control Scale.*)

Routh, C., Hill, J., Steele, H., Elliott, C. & Dewey, M. (1995). Maternal attachment status, psychosocial stressors and problem behaviour: Follow-up after parent training courses for conduct disorder. *Journal of Child Psychology and Psychiatry*, 36, 1179–1198.

Rowe, C. & Liddle, H. (2003). Substance abuse. *Journal of Marital and Family Therapy*, 29, 86–120.

Royal College of Psychiatrists (2002). *Guidelines for the Nutritional Management of Anorexia Nervosa. A report of the Eating Disorders Special Interest Group*. London: Royal College of Psychiatrists.

Rumball, D. & Crome, I. (2004). Social influences. In I. Crome, H. Ghodse, E. Gilvarry & P. McArdle (eds.), *Young People and Substance Misuse* (pp. 62–71). London: Gaskell.

Rushton, A. & Minnis, H. (2002). Residential and foster family care. In M. Rutter & E. Taylor (eds.), *Child and Adolescent Psychiatry* (Fourth edition, pp. 359–372). Oxford: Blackwell.

Rutter, M. (1967). A children's behaviour questionnaire for completion by teachers: Preliminary findings. *Journal of Child Psychology and Psychiatry*, 8, 1–11.

Rutter, M. (1985a). Family and school influences on cognitive development. *Journal of Child Psychology and Psychiatry*, 26, 683–704.

Rutter, M. (1985b). Family and school influences on behavioural development. *Journal of Child Psychology and Psychiatry*, 26, 349–368.

Rutter, M. (1985c). The treatment of autistic children. *Journal of Child Psychology and Psychiatry*, 26, 193–214.

Rutter, M. (2002a). Development and psychopathology. In M. Rutter & E. Taylor (eds.), *Child and Adolescent Psychiatry* (Fourth edition, pp. 309–324). Oxford: Blackwell.

Rutter, M. (2002b). Substance use and abuse: Causal pathways considerations. In M. Rutter & E. Taylor (eds.), *Child and Adolescent Psychiatry* (Fourth edition, pp. 455–462). Oxford: Blackwell.

Rutter, M., Bailey, A., Lord, C. & Berument, S. (2003). *Social Communication Questionnaire*. Los Angeles, CA: Western Psychological Services.

Rutter, M. & Casaer, P. (1991). *Biological Risk Factors for Psychosocial Disorders*. Cambridge: Cambridge University Press.

Rutter, M., Giller, H. & Hagell, A. (1998). *Antisocial Behavior by Young People: A Major New Review*. Cambridge: Cambridge University Press.

Rutter, M., Maughan, N., Mortimore, P. & Ouston, J. (1979). *Fifteen Thousand Hours*. London: Open Books.

Rutter, M. & Nikapota, A. (2002). Culture, ethnicity, society and psychopathology. In M. Rutter & E. Taylor (eds.), *Child and Adolescent Psychiatry* (Fourth edition, pp. 277–286). Oxford: Blackwell.

Rutter, M. & Rutter, M. (1993). *Developing Minds: Challenge and Continuity across the Lifespan*. London: Penguin.

Rutter, M., Shaffer, D. & Shepherd, M. (1975). *A Guide to a Multiaxial Classification Scheme for Psychiatric Disorders in Childhood and Adolescence*. Geneva: WHO.

Rutter, M. & Yule, W. (1975). The concept of specific reading retardation. *Journal of Child Psychology and Psychiatry*, 16, 181–197.

Ryan, N. (2002). Depression. In S. Kutcher (ed.), *Practical Child and Adolescent Psychopharmacology* (pp. 91–105). Cambridge: Cambridge University Press.

Ryan, T. & Walker, R. (2003). *Life Story Work*. London: British Associatioan of Adoption and Fostering.

Saarni, C. (1999). *Developing Emotional Competence*. New York: Guilford.

Sage, R. & Sluckin, A. (2004). *Silent Children: Approaches to Selective Mutism*. Leicester: University of Leicester.

Salkovski, P., Forrester, E. & Richards, C. (1998). Cognitive behavioural approach to understanding obsessional thinking. *British Journal of Psychiatry*, 173 (Suppl. 35), 53–63.

Sandberg, S. & Rutter, M. (2002). The role of acute life stresses. In M. Rutter & E. Taylor (eds.), *Child and Adolescent Psychiatry* (Fourth edition, pp. 287–294). Oxford: Blackwell.

Sanders, M., Markie-Dadds, C., Turner, K. & Ralph, A. (2004). Using the Triple P system of intervention to prevent behavioural problems in children and adolescents. In P. Barrett & T. Ollendick (eds.), *Handbook of Interventions that Work with Children and Adolescents: Prevention and Treatment* (pp. 489–516). Chichester: Wiley.

Sanders, M., Shepard, R., Cleghorn, G. & Woolford, H. (1994). The treatment of recurrent abdominal pain in children: A controlled comparison of cognitive behavioural family intervention and standard paediatric care. *Journal of Consulting and Clinical Psychology*, 62, 306–314.

Sarafino, E. (2001). *Health Psychology* (Fourth edition). New York: Wiley.

Sattler, J. (1992). *Assessment of Children. Revised and Updated Third Edition*. San Diego, CA: Sattler.

Sattler, J. (2001a). *Assessment of Children. Cognitive Applications* (Fourth edition). San Diego, CA: Sattler. http://www.sattlerpublisher.com/

Sattler, J. (2001b). *Assessment of Children. Behavioural and Clinical Applications* (Fourth edition). San Diego, CA: Sattler. http://www.sattlerpublisher.com/

Sattler, J. & Dumont, R. (2004). *Assessment of Children with the WISC IV and WPPSI III Supplement*. SanDiego: Sattler. http://www.sattlerpublisher.com/

Saywitz, K., Goodman, G. & Lyon, T. (2002). Interviewing children in and out of court: Current research and practice implications. In J. Myers, L. Berliner, J. Briere, C. Hendrix, C. Jenny & T. Reid (eds.), *APSAC Handbook on Child Maltreatment* (Second edition, pp. 349–378). Thousand Oaks, CA: Sage.

Schachar, R. (1991). Childhood hyperactivity. *Journal of Child Psychology and Psychiatry*, 32, 155–191.

Schachar, R. & Ickowitcz, A. (2000). Attention deficit hyperkinetic disorders in childhood and adolescence. In. M. Gelder, J. Lopez-Ibor & N. Andreasen (eds.), *New Oxford Textbook of Psychiatry* (Volume 2, Section 9.2.3, pp. 1734–1750). Oxford: Oxford University Press.

Schachar, R. & Tannock, R. (2002). Syndromes of hyperactivity and attention deficit. In M. Rutter & E. Taylor (eds.), *Child and Adolescent Psychiatry* (Fourth edition, pp. 399–418). Oxford: Blackwell.

Schaefer, C. (1995). *Clinical Handbook of Sleep Disorders in Children*. Northvale, NJ: Jason Aronson.

Schinke, S., Botvin, G. & Orlandi, M. (1991). *Substance Abuse in Children and Adolescents: Evaluation and Intervention*. Thousand Oaks, CA: Sage.

Schmidt, U. (2005). Motivational interviewing. In P. Graham (ed.), *Cognitive Behaviour Therapy for Children and Families* (Second edition, pp. 67–83). Cambridge: Cambridge University Press.

Schopler, E. (1997). Implementation of TEACHH philosophy. In D. Cohen & F. Volkmar, (eds.), *Handbook of Autism and Pervasive Developmental Disorders* (Second edition, pp. 767–795). New York: Wiley.

Schopler, E. Richler, R. & Renner, B. (1986). *The Childhood Autism Rating Scale*

(CARS) for Diagnostic Screening and Classification of Autism. New York: Irvington.

Schopler, E., Reichler, R., Bashford, A., Lashing, M. & Marcus, L. (1990). *Psychoeducational Profile Revised (PEP-R).* Austin, TX: Pro-ed.

Schreibman, L. & Koegel, R. (1996). Fostering self-management: Parent-delivered pivotal response training for children with autistic disorder. In E. Hibbs & P. Jensen (eds.), *Psychosocial Treatments for Child and Adolescent Disorders: Empirically Based Strategies for Clinical Practice* (pp. 525–552). Washington, DC: American Psychological Association.

Schuckit, M. (1994). Low level of response to alcohol as a predictor of future alcoholism. *American Journal of Psychiatry,* 151, 184–189.

Schuerman, J., Rzepmicki, T. & Littem J. (1994). *Putting Families First. An Experiment in Family Preservation.* New York: Aldine de Gruytner.

Schuler, A., Prizant, B. & Wetherby, A. (1997). Enhancing language and communication development: Prelinguistic approaches. In D. Cohen & F. Volkmar (eds.), *Handbook of Autism and Pervasive Developmental Disorders* (Second edition, pp. 539–571). New York: Wiley.

Schulz, E. & Remschmidt, H. (2001). Pharmacology of depressive states in childhood and adolescence. In I. Goodyer (ed.), *The Depressed Child and Adolescent* (Second edition, pp. 292–324). Cambridge: Cambridge University Press.

Schumm, W.R., Paff-Bergen, L.A., Hatch, R.C., Obiorah, F.C., Copeland, J.M., Meens, L.D. & Bugaighis, M.A. (1986). Concurrent and discriminant validity of the Kansas Marital Satisfaction Scale. *Journal of Marriage and the Family,* 48, 381–387.

Schwartz, L. (1996). *Brain Lock.* New York: Harper Collins.

Scott, S. (1994). Mental retardation. In M. Rutter, E. Taylor & L. Hersov (eds.), *Child and Adolescent Psychiatry: Modern Approaches* (Third edition, pp. 616–646). London: Blackwell.

Scourfield, J. & McGuffin, P. (2001). Genetic aspects. In H. Remschmidt (ed.), *Schizophrenia in Children and Adolescents* (pp. 119–134). Cambridge: Cambridge University Press.

Segal, L. (1991). Brief therapy: The MRI approach. In A. Gurman & D. Kniskern (eds.), *Handbook of Family Therapy* (volume 2, pp. 17–199). New York: Brunner/Mazel.

Segerstrom, S. & Miller, G. (2004). Psychological stress and the human immune system: A meta-analytic study of 30 years of inquiry. *Psychological Bulletin.* 130, 601–630.

Selvini Palazzoli, S. (1988). *The Work of Mara Selvini Palazzoli.* New York: Jason Aronson.

Selye, H. (1976). *Stress in Health and Disease.* Reading, MA: Butterworth.

Sequeira, H. & Hollis, S. (2003). Clinical effects of sexual abuse on people with learning difficulty. *British Journal of Psychiatry,* 182, 13–19.

Serbin, L., Powlishta, K. & Gulko, J. (1993). The development of sex typing in middle childhood. *Monographs for the Society for Research in Child Development* (Volume 58, Serial No. 232, pp. 1–74). Oxford: Blackwell.

Serpell, L. & Troup, N. (2003). Sociocultural theories of eating disorders. In J. Treasure, U. Schmidt & E. van Furth (eds.), *Handbook of Eating Disorders* (Second edition, pp.151–167). Chichester: Wiley.

Sexton, T. & Alexander, J. (2003). Functional family therapy. A mature clinical model for working with at-risk adolescents and their families. In T. Sexton, G. Weeks & M. Robbins (eds.), *Handbook of Family Therapy* (pp. 323–350). New York: Brunner-Routledge.

Sexton, T., Weeks, G. & Robbins, M. (2003). *Handbook of Family Therapy*. New York: Brunner-Routledge.

Shaffer, D. (1994). Enuresis. In M. Rutter, E. Taylor & L. Hersov (eds.), *Child and Adolescent Psychiatry: Modern Approaches* (Third edition, pp. 505–519). Oxford: Blackwell.

Shaffer, D., Fisher, P., Lucas, C., Dulcan, M. & Schwab-Stone, M. (2000). NIMH Diagnostic Interview Schedule for Children version IV (NIMH DISC-IV): Description, differences from previous versions, and reliability of some common diagnoses. *Journal of the American Academy of Child and Adolescent Psychiatry*, 39, 28–38.

Shaffer, D., Gould., M., Brasis, J., Ambrosini, P., Fisher, P., Bird, H. & Aluwahlia, S. (1983). A children's global assessment scale (C-GAS). *Archives of General Psychiatry*, 40, 1228–1231. http://depts.washington.edu/wimirt/Index.htm

Shaffer, D. & Gutstein, J. (2002). Suicide and attempted suicide. In M. Rutter & E. Taylor (eds.), *Child and Adolescent Psychiatry* (Fourth edition, pp. 529–554). Oxford: Blackwell.

Shaffer, D., Schwab-Stone, M., Fisher, P., Davies, M., Piacentini, J. & Gioia, P. (1988). *A Revised version of the Diagnostic Interview Schedule for Children (DISC-R) – Results of a field trial and proposal for a new instrument (DISC–2)*. Report Submitted to the Division of Epidemiology and Biometrics at the National Institute of Mental Health, Washington DC.

Shafran, R. (2001). Obsessive compulsive disorder in children and adolescents. *Child Psychology and Psychiatry Review*, 6, 50–58.

Sharry, J. & Fitzpatrick, C. (2000). *Parenting Plus Programme*. Mater Hospital, Dublin: Parenting Plus.

Sherrill, J. & Kovacs, M. (2000). Interview schedule for children and adolescents (ISCA). *Journal of the American Academy of Child & Adolescent Psychiatry*, 39, 67–75.

Sheslow, D. & Adams, W. (2004). *Wide Range Assessment of Memory and Learning, Second Edition (WRAML2)*. Odessa FL: Psychological Assessment Resources.

Shields, J. (2001). NAS Early Bird programme: Partnership with parents in early intervention. *Autism: the International Journal of Research and Practice*, 5, 1, 49–56.

Shure, M. (1992). *I Can Problem Solve (CPS): An Interpersonal Cognitive Problem Solving Program*. Champaign, IL: Research Press.

Sigafoos, J., O'Reilly, M. & Green, V. (2005). Communication Difficulties & Promotion of Communication Skills. In G. O'Reilly, P. Walsh, A. Carr, & J. McEvoy (2005). *Handbook of Intellectual Disability and Clinical Psychology Practice*. London: Brunner-Routledge.

Silverman, P. & Worden, J. (1993). Children's reaction to the death of a parent. In M. Stroebe, W. Stroebe, & R. Hansson (eds.), *Handbook of Bereavement: Theory, Research, and Intervention* (pp. 300–316). New York: Cambridge University Press.

Silverman, W. & Dick-Niederhauser, A. (2004). Separation Anxiety Disorder. In

T, Morris & J. March, *Anxiety Disorders in Children and Adolescents* (Second Edition, pp. 164–188). New York: Guilford.

Silverman, W., Fleisig, W., Rabian, B. & Peterson, R. (1991). Childhood anxiety sensitivity index. *Journal of Clinical Child Psychology*, 20, 162–168.

Silverman, W. & Treffers, P. (2001). *Anxiety Disorders in Children and Adolescents. Research Assessment and Intervention.* Cambridge: Cambridge University Press.

Simmonds, J. & Parraga, H. (1982). Prevalence of sleep disorder and sleep behaviours in children and adolescents. *Journal of the American Academy of Child Psychiatry*, 21, 383–388.

Simonoff, E. (2001). Genetic influences on conduct disorders. In J. Hill & B. Maughan (eds.), *Conduct Disorder in Childhood and Adolescence* (pp. 202–234). Cambridge: Cambridge University Press.

Simpson, R. (2005). *Autism Spectrum Disorders: Interventions and Treatments for Children and Youth.* Thousand Oaks, CA: Corwin.

Skuse, D. (1984). Extreme deprivation in early childhood. II. Theoretical issues and a comparative review. *Journal of Child Psychology and Psychiatry*, 25, 543–572.

Skuse, D. & Bentovim, A. (1994). Physical and emotional maltreatment. In M. Rutter, E. Taylor & E. Hersov (eds.), *Child & Adolescent Psychiatry: Modern Approaches* (Third edition, pp. 209–229). Oxford: Blackwell.

Skynner, R. & Cleese, J. (1983). *Families and how to Survive Them.* London: Metheun.

Slade, P. (1995). Prospects for prevention. In G. Szmukler, C. Dare & J. Treasure (eds.), *Handbook of Eating Disorders* (pp. 385–400). Chichester: Wiley.

Slade, P. & Dewey, M. (1986). Development and preliminary validation of SCANS: A screening instrument for identifying individuals at risk of developing anorexia and bulimia nervosa. *International Journal of Eating Disorders*, 5, 517–538.

Slade, P., Dewey, M., Kiemle, G. & Newton, T. (1990). Update on SCANS: A screening instrument for identifying individuals at risk of developing an eating disorder. *International Journal of Eating Disorders*, 9, 583–584.

Sluckin, A. (1981). Behavioural social work with encopretic children, their families and the school. *Child Care, Health and Development*, 7, 67–80.

Sluckin, W., Herbert, M. & Sluckin, A. (1983). *Maternal Bonding.* Oxford: Basil Blackwell.

Smith, G. (1995). Assessing protectiveness in cases of child sexual abuse. In P. Reder & C. Lucey (eds.), *Assessment of Parenting: Psychiatric and Psychological Contributions* (pp. 87–101). London: Routledge.

Smith, M. & Fong, R. (2004). *The Children of Neglect.* London: Brunner-Routledge.

Smith, P., Cowie, H. & Blades, M. (2003). *Understanding Children's Development* (Fourth edition). Oxford: Blackwell.

Smith, S. & Pennell, M. (1996). *Interventions With Bereaved Children.* London: Jessica Kingsley.

Snider, L. & Swedo, S. (2003). Childhood-onset obsessive-compulsive disorder and tic disorders: Case report and literature review. *Journal of Child and Adolescent Psychopharmacology. Special Issue: Obsessive-compulsive disorder*, 13(2), 81–88.

Snow, C. & Ferguson, C. (1977). *Talking to Children: Language Input and Acquisition.* Cambridge: Cambridge University Press.

Snow, J. & Hooper, S. (1994). *Paediatric Traumatic Brain Injury.* Thousand Oaks, CA: Sage.

Snowling, M. (1996). Annotation: Contemporary approaches to the teaching of reading. *Journal of Child Psychology and Psychiatry*, 37, 139–148.

Snowling, M. (2002). Reading and other learning difficulties. In M. Rutter & E. Taylor (eds.), *Child and Adolescent Psychiatry* (Fourth edition, pp. 682–696). Oxford: Blackwell.

Solokov, S. & Kutcher, S. (2001). Adolescent depression: neuroendocrine aspects. In I. Goodyer (ed.). *The Depressed Child and Adolescent* (Second edition, pp. 233–266). Cambridge: Cambridge University Press.

Solomon, R. (1980). The opponent process theory of motivation: The costs of pleasure and the benefits of pain. *American Psychologist*, 35, 691–712.

Sonuga-Barke, E. (1998). Categorical models of childhood disorder: A conceptual and empirical analysis. *Journal of Child Psychology and Psychiatry*, 39, 115–133.

Spaccarelli, S. (1994). Stress, appraisal and coping in child sexual abuse: A theoretical and empirical review. *Psychological Bulletin*, 116, 340–362.

Sparrow, S., Balla, D. & Cicchetti, D. (1984). *Vineland Adaptive Behaviour Scales*. Pine Circles, MN: American Guidance Service.

Spence, M. & Brent, S. (1984). Children's understanding of death: A review of three components of a death concept. *Child Development*, 55, 1671–1686.

Spencer, T., Biederman, J. & Wilens, T. (2002). Attention deficit hyperactivity disorder. In S. Kutcher (ed.), *Practical Child and Adolescent Psychopharmacology* (pp. 230–264). Cambridge: Cambridge University Press.

Spielberger, C. (1973). *Manual For The State Trait Anxiety Inventory For Children*. Palo Alto, CA. Consulting Psychologists Press.

Spinetta, J. (1980). Disease-related communication: How to tell. In J. Kellerman (ed.), *Psychological Aspects of Childhood Cancer* (pp. 257–269). Springfield, IL: Thomas.

Spitz, R. (1945). Hospitalism: An inquiry into the genesis of psychiatric conditions in early childhood. *Psychoanalytic Study of the Child*, 1, 53–74.

Spitzer, R. & Fleiss, J. (1974). A re-analysis of the reliability of psychiatric diagnosis. *British Journal of Psychiatry*, 125, 341–347.

Spivac, G. & Shure, M. (1982). The cognition of social adjustment: Interpersonal cognitive problem-solving thinking. In B. Lahey & A. Kazdin (eds.), *Advances in Clinical Child Pychology* (volume 5, pp. 323–372). New York: Plenum.

Sprenkle, D. (2002). *Effectiveness Research in Marriage and Family Therapy*. Alexandria, VA: American Association for Marital and Family Therapy.

Stahl, P. (1994). *Conducting Child Custody Evaluations: A Comprehensive Guide*. Thousand Oaks, CA: Sage.

Stallard, P. (2002). *Think Good – Feel Good. A Cognitive Behaviour Therapy Workbook for Children and Young People*. Chichester: Wiley.

Stambrook, M. & Parker, K. (1987). The development of the concept of death in childhood. A review of the literature. *Merrill-Palmer Quarterly*, 33, 133–157.

Stanton, D. & Heath, A. (1995). Family treatment of alcohol and drug abuse. In R. Mikeselle, D. Lusterman & S. McDaniel (eds.), *Integrating Family Therapy: Handbook of Family Therapy and Systems Theory* (pp. 529–541). Washington, DC: APA.

Stanton, M. & Todd, T. (1982). *The Family Therapy of Drug Abuse and Addiction*. New York: Guilford.

Stathakos, P. & Roehrle, B. (2003). The effectiveness of intervention programmes for children of divorce – a meta-analysis. *International Journal of Mental Health Promotion*, 5, 31–37.

Steiger, H., Leung, F. & Houle, L. (1992). Relationships among borderline features, body dissatisfactions and bulimic symptoms in nonclinical families. *Addicitive Behaviours*, 17, 397–406.

Stein, A. & Barnes, J. (2002). Feeding and sleep disorders. In M. Rutter & E. Taylor (eds.), *Child and Adolescent Psychiatry* (Fourth edition, pp. 754–775). Oxford: Blackwell.

Stein, M. & Seedat, S. (2004). Pharmacotherapy. In T. Morris & J. March (eds.), *Anxiety Disorders in Children and Adolescents* (Second edition, pp. 329–354). New York: Guilford.

Steinhauer, P. (1991). *The Least Detrimental Alternative. A Systematic Guide to Case Planning and Decision Making for Children in Care.* Toronto: University of Toronto Press.

Steinhausen, H., Williams, J. & Spohr, H. (1994). Correlates of psychopathology and intelligence in children with fetal alcohol syndrome. *Journal of Child Psychology and Psychiatry*, 35, 323–331.

Steinhausen, J. (2002a). Anorexia and bulimia nervosa. In M. Rutter & E. Taylor (eds.), *Child and Adolescent Psychiatry* (Fourth edition, pp. 555–570). Oxford: Blackwell.

Steinhausen, J. (2002b). The outcome of anorexia nervosa in the 20th century. *American Journal of Psychiatry*, 159, 1284–1293.

Sternberg, R. (2000). *Handbook of Intelligence.* Cambridge: Cambridge University Press.

Stewart, A. (2005). Disorders of eating control. In P. Graham (ed.), *Cognitive Behaviour Therapy for Children and Families* (Second edition, pp. 359–384). Cambridge: Cambridge University Press.

Stice, E. (2002). Risk and maintainance factors for eating pathology. A meta-analytic review. *Psychological Bulletin*, 128, 825–848.

Stice, E., Agras, S. & Hammer, L. (1999). Risk factors for the development of childhood eating disturbances: A five year prospective study. *International Journal of Eating Disorders*, 25, 375–387.

Still, G. (1902). The Coulstonian lectures on some abnormal physical conditions in children. *Lancet*, i, 1008–1012, 1077–1082, 1163–1169.

Stores, G. (2001). *A Clinical Guide to Sleep Disorders in Children and Adolescents.* Oxford: Oxford University Press.

Stores G. & Wiggs, L. (2001). *Sleep Disturbance in Children and Adolescence with Disorders of Development; Its Significance and Management.* London: MacKeith Press.

Stradling, J., Thomas, G., Warley, A., Williams, P. & Freeland, A. (1990). Effect of adenotosillectomy on nocturnal hypoxaemia, sleep disturbance, and symptoms of snoring in children. *The Lancet*, 335, 249–253.

Strober, M. (2001). Family-genetic aspects of juvenile affective disorders. In I. Goodyer (ed.). *The Depressed Child and Adolescent* (Second edition, pp. 179–203). Cambridge: Cambridge University Press.

Stroebe, M., Hansson, R., Stroebe, W. & Schut, H. (2001). *Handbook of Bereavement Research: Consequences, Coping, and Care.* Washington, DC: American Psychological Association.

Sullivan, H. (1953). *The Interpersonal Theory of Psychiatry.* New York: Norton.

Sussman, F. (1999). *More than Words: A Revised HANEN Programme*. New Brunswick: The Hanen Centre.

Svoboda, W. (2004). *Childhood Epilepsy: Language Learning and Behavioural Complications*. Cambridge: Cambridge University Press.

Swanson, J., Sergeant, J., Taylor, E. Sonuga-Barke, E., Jensen, P. & Cantwell, D. (1998). Attention deficit hyperactivity disorder and hyperkinetic disorder. *Lancet*, 351, 429–433.

Swedo, S., Allen, A., Glod, C., Clark, C., Teicher, M., Richter, D., Hoffman, C., Hamburger, S., Dow, S., Brown, C. & Rosenthal, N. (1997). A controlled trial of light therapy for the treatment of paediatric seasonal affective disorder. *Journal of the American Academy of Child and Adolescent Psychiatry*, 36, 816–821.

Swedo, S., Leonard, H., Garvey, M. Mittleman, B., Allen, A., Perlmutter, S., Dow, S., Zamkoff, J., Dubbert, B. & Lougee, L. (1998). Paediatric autoimmune neuropsychiatric disorders associated with streptococcal infections (PANDAS): A clinical description of the first fifty cases. *American Journal of Psychiatry*, 155, 264–271.

Sylva, K. (1994). School influences on children's development. *Journal of Child Psychology and Psychiatry*, 35, 135–170.

Szapocznik, J. & Kurtines, W. (1989). *Breakthroughs In Family Therapy With Drug Abusing Problem Youth*. New York: Springer.

Szmukler, G. & Dare, C. (1991). The Maudsley Hospital study of family therapy in anorexia nervosa and bulimia nervosa. In B. Woodside & L. Shekter-Wolfson (eds.), *Family Approaches in Treatment of Eating Disorders*. Washington, DC: APA Press.

Szmukler, G. & Patton, G. (1995). Sociocultural models of eating disorder. In G. Szmukler, C. Dare & J. Treasure (eds.), *Handbook of Eating Disorders* (pp. 177–194). Chichester: Wiley.

Tallal, P., Miller, S. & Bedi, G. (1996). Language comprehension in language-learning impaired children improved with acoustically modified speech. *Science*, 271, 81–84.

Tannock, R. (1998). Attention deficit hyperactivity disorder: Advances in cognitive, neurobiological and genetic research. *Journal of Child Psychology and Psychiatry*, 39, 65–100.

Target, M. & Fonagy, P. (1994). The efficacy of psychoanalysis for children: Developmental considerations. *Journal of the American Academy of Child & Adolescent Psychiatry*, 33, 1134–1144.

Tarrier, N. (1994). Management and modification of residual positive psychotic symptoms. In M. Birchwood & N. Tarrier (eds.), *Psychological Management of Schizophrenia* (pp. 109–132). Chichester: Wiley.

Tarrier, N. (1996). Family interventions and schizophrenia. In G. Haddock & P. Slade (eds.), *Cognitive-behavioural Interventions with Psychotic Disorders* (pp. 212–234). London: Routledge.

Taylor, E. (1994). Syndromes of attention deficit and overactivity. In M. Rutter, E. Taylor & L. Hersov (eds.), *Child and Adolescent Psychiatry: Modern Approaches* (Third edition, pp. 285–307). London: Blackwell.

Taylor, E. & Rutter, M. (2002). Classification: Conceptual issues and substantive findings. In M. Rutter & E. Taylor (eds.), *Child and Adolescent Psychiatry* (Fourth edition, pp. 3–17). Oxford: Blackwell.

Taylor, E., Sergeant, J. & Doepfner, M. (1998). European guidelines: Clinical guidelines for ADHD. *European Journal of Child and Adolescent Psychiatry*, 7, 194–200.

Teasdale, G. & Jennett, B. (1974). Assessment of coma and impaired consciousness: A practical scale. *Lancet*, 2, 81–84.

Tharper, A. & Scourfield, J. (2002). Childhood disorders. In P. McGuffin, M. Owen & I. Gottesman (eds.), *Psychiatric Genetics and Genomics* (pp. 147–180). Oxford: Oxford University Press.

Thoburn, J. (2000). The effects on child mental health of adoption and foster care. In. M. Gelder, J. Lopez-Ibor & N. Andreasen (eds.), *New Oxford Textbook of Psychiatry* (Volume 2, Section 9.3.3, pp. 1843–1848). Oxford: Oxford University Press.

Thompsen, P. (1998). Obsessive compulsive disorder in children and adolescents. Clinical Guidelines. *European Child and Adolescent Psychiatry*, 7, 1–11.

Thompson, M. (1990). *Developmental Dyslexia* (Third edition). London: Whurr.

Tonge, B. & King, N. (2005). Cognitive behavioural treatment of the emotional and behavioural consequences of sexual abuse. In P. Graham (ed.), *Cognitive Behaviour Therapy for Children and Families* (Second edition, pp. 157–169). Cambridge: Cambridge University Press.

Topping, K. (1986). *Parents as Educators: Training Parents to Teach Their Children*. London: Croom Helm.

Tourette Syndrome Classification Study Group (1993). Definition and classification of tic disorders. *Archives of Neurology*, 50, 1013–1016.

Treasure, J. (1997). *Anorexia Nervosa. A Survival Guide for Families Friends and Sufferers*. Hove, UK: Psychology Press.

Treasure, J. & Schmidt, U. (1993). *Getting Better Bit(e) by Bit(e): A Survival Kit for Sufferers of Bulimia Nervosa and Binge Eating*. Hove, UK: Lawrence Erlbaum Associates Ltd.

Trepper, T. & Barrett, M. (1989). *Systemic Treatment of Incest. A Therapeutic Handbook*. New York: Brunner-Mazel.

Turk, D., Meichenbaum, D. & Genest, M. (1983). *Pain and Behavioural Medicine: A Cognitive Behavioural Perspective*. New York: Guilford.

Turkington, D., Dudley, R. Warman, D. & Beck, A. (2004). Cognitive-behavioural therapy for schizophrenia: A review. *Journal of Psychiatric Practice*, 10, 5–16.

Turner, A. & Finkelhor, D. (1996). Corporal punishment as a stressor among youth. *Journal of Marriage and the Family*, 58, 155–166.

Uchino, B., Cacioppo, J. & Kiecolt-Glaser, J. (1996). The relationship between social support and physiological processes: A review with emphasis on underlying mechanisms and implications for health. *Psychological Bulletin*, 119, 488–531.

United Nations Convention on the Rights of the Child (1992). London: HMSO.

US-UK Team (1974). The diagnosis and psychopathology of schizophrenia in New York and London. *Schizophrenia Bulletin*, 1, 80–102.

Vaillant, G. (1977). *Adaptation to life: How the Best and Brightest Came of Age*. Boston: Little Brown.

Valliant, G. (2000). Adaptive mental mechanisms. Their role in positive psychology. *American Psychologist*, 55, 89–98.

Van Acker, R. (1997). Rett's syndrome: A pervasive developmental disorder. In

D. Cohen & F. Volkmar (eds.), *Handbook of Autism and Pervasive Developmental Disorders* (Second edition, pp. 60–93). New York: Wiley.

Vandereycken, W., Kog, E. & Vanderlinden, J. (1989). *The Family Approach to Disorders: Assessment and Treatment of Anorexia Nervosa and Bulimia.* New York: PMA.

Vannatta, K. & Gerhardt, C. (2003). Paediatric oncology: Psychosocial outcomes for children and families. In M. Roberts (ed.), *Handbook of Paediatric Psychology* (Third edition, pp. 342–358). New York: Guilford.

Varni, J., Katz, E., Colegrove, R. & Dolgin, M. (1996). Family functioning predictors of adjustment in children with newly diagnosed cancer: A prospective analysis. *Journal of Child Psychology and Psychiatry*, 37, 321–328.

Varni, J., Thompson, K. & Hanson, V. (1987). The Varni-Thompson Paediatric Pain Questionnaire: 1. Chronic musculo-skeletal pain in juvenile rheumatoid arthritis. *Pain*, 28, 27–38.

Vasta, R., Haith, M. & Miller, S. (2003). *Child Psychology: The Modern Science* (Fourth edition). New York: Wiley.

Vellutino, F., Fletcher, J., Snowling, M. & Scanlon, D. (2004). Specific reading disability (dyslexia): What have we learned in the past four decades. *Journal of Child Psychology and Psychiatry*, 45, 2–40.

Verhulst, F. (2001). Community and epidemiological aspects of anxiety disorders in children. In W. Silverman & P. Treffers (eds.), *Anxiety Disorders in Children and Adolescents. Research Assessment and Intervention* (pp. 273–292). Cambridge: Cambridge University Press.

Vik, P., Brown, S. & Myers, M. (1997). Adolescent substance use problems. In E. Mash & R. Barkley (eds.), *Assessment of Childhood Disorders* (Third edition, pp. 717–748). New York: Guilford.

Visher, E., Visher, J. & Pasley, C. (2003). Remarriage families and step parenting. In F. Walsh (ed.), *Normal Family Processes* (Third edition, pp. 121–151). New York: Guilford.

Vitulano, L., King, R., Scahill, L. & Cohen, D. (1992). Behavioural treatment of children and adolescents with trichotillomania. *Journal of the American Academy of Child and Adolescent Psychiatry*, 31, 139–146.

Vizard, E., Monck, E. & Misch, P. (1995). Child and adolescent sex abuse perpetrators: A review of the research literature. *Journal of Child Psychology and Psychiatry*, 36, 731–756.

Volkmar, F. & Dykens, E. (2002). Mental retardation. In Rutter, M. & Taylor, E. (eds.), *Child and Adolescent Psychiatry* (Fourth edition, pp. 697–710). Oxford: Blackwell.

Volkmar, F., Lord, C., Bailey, A., Schultz, R. & Klin, A. (2004). Autism and pervasive developmental disorders. *Journal of Child Psychology and Psychiatry*, 45, 135–170.

Volkmar, F., Klin, A. & Cohen, D. (1997a). Diagnosis and classification of autism and related conditions: Consensus and issues. In D. Cohen & F. Volkmar (eds.), *Handbook of Autism and Pervasive Developmental Disorders* (Second edition, pp. 5–40). New York: Wiley.

Volkmar, F., Klin, A., Marans, W. & Cohen, D. (1997b). Childhood disintegrative disorder. In D. Cohen & F. Volkmar (eds.), *Handbook of Autism and Pervasive Developmental Disorders* (Second edition, pp. 47–59). New York: Wiley.

Volkmar, F. & Schwabe-Stone, M. (1996). Annotation: Childhood disorders in DSM-IV. *Journal of Child Psychology and Psychiatry*, 37, 779–784.

Vygotsky, L. (1934/1962). *Thought and Language*. Cambridge, MA: MIT Press (originally published in 1934).

Walker, C. (2003). Elimination disorders. In M. Roberts (ed.), *Handbook of Paediatric Psychology* (Second edition, pp. 544–560). New York: Guilford.

Walker, J. (1989). Family conciliation in Great Britain: From research to practice to research. *Mediation Quarterly*, 24, 29–54.

Walker, J. (1993). Co-operative parenting post-divorce: Possibility or pipe dream? *Journal of Family Therapy*, 15, 273–292.

Walkup, J. (2002). Tic disorders and Tourette syndrome. In S. Kutcher (ed.), *Practical Child and Adolescent Psychopharmacology* (pp. 382–409). Cambridge: Cambridge University Press.

Wall, L. (2004). *Autism and Early Years Practice*. London: Paul Chapman Publishing.

Wallander, J., Thompson, R. & Alriksson-Schmidt, A. (2003). Psychosocial adjustment of children with chronic physical conditions. In M. Roberts (ed.), *Handbook of Paediatric Psychology* (Third edition, pp. 141–158). New York: Guilford.

Wallander, J. & Varni, J. (1992). Adjustment in children with chronic physical disorders: Programmatic research on a disability-stress-coping model. In A. LaGreca, L. Siegel, J. Wallander & C. Walker (eds.), *Stress and Coping in Child Health* (pp. 279–298). New York: Guilford.

Wallander, J. & Varni, J. (1998). Effects of paediatric chronic physical disorders on child and family adjustment. *Journal of Child Psychology and Psychiatry*, 39, 29–48.

Wallerstein, J. (1991). The long term effects of divorce on children: A review. *Journal of the American Academy of Child and Adolescent Psychiatry*, 30, 349–360.

Walsh, F. (1991). Promoting healthy functioning in divorced and remarried families. In A. Gurman & D. Kniskern (eds.), *Handbook of Family Therapy* (volume 2, pp. 525–545). New York: Brunner/Mazel.

Walsh, F. (2003). *Normal Family Processes* (Third edition). New York: Guilford.

Walsh, F. & McGoldrick, M. (2004). *Living Beyond Loss: Death in the Family* (Second edition). New York: Norton.

Warner-Rogers, J. (2002). Attention deficit hyperactivity disorder. In P. Howlin & O. Udwin (eds.), *Outcomes in Neurodevelopmental and Genetic Disorders* (pp. 1–25). Cambridge: Cambridge University Press.

Warr, P. (1987). *Work, Unemployment and Mental Health*. Oxford: Clarendon Press.

Webb, N. (2002). *Helping Bereaved Children. A Handbook for Practitioners* (Second edition). New York: Guilford Press (*contains lists of materials and practical advice*).

Weber, G. & Stierlin, H. (1981). Familiendynamik und Famlientherapie der Anroresxia Nervosa Familie. In R. Merman (ed.), *Anorexia Nervosa* (pp. 108–122). Wurzburg, Germany: Ferdinand Enke.

Webster, C., Douglas, K., Eaves, D. & Hart, S. (1997). *HCR-20. Assessing Risk of Violence (Version 2)*. Vancouver, Canada: Mental Health Law and Policy Institute, Simon Fraser University.

Webster-Stratton, C. & Reid, M. (2003). The Incredible Years parents, teachers and children training series: A multifaceted treatment approach for young children with conduct problems. In A. Kazdin, & J. Weisz (eds.), *Evidence Based Psychotherapies for Children and Adolescents* (pp. 224–262). New York: Guilford.

Wechsler, D. (1991). *Wechsler Intelligence Scale for Children. Third Edition (WISC-III)*. San Antonio, TX: Psychological Corporation.

Wechsler, D. (1992). *Wechsler Intelligence Scale for Children. Third Edition UK (WISC-III^uk)*. San Antonio, TX: Psychological Corporation.

Wechsler, D. (1999). *Wechsler Adult Intelligence Scale – Third Edition (WAIS-III)*. San Antonio, TX: Psychological Corporation.

Wechsler, D. (1999a). *Wechsler Adult Intelligence Scale – Third Edition UK (WAIS-III^uk)*. San Antonio, TX: Psychological Corporation.

Weschler, D. (1999b). *Wechsler Abbreviated Scale of Intelligence. (WASI)*. San Antonio, TX. Psychological Corporation.

Wechsler, D. (2001). *Wechsler Individual Achievement Tests II (WIAT-II)*. San Antonio, TX. Psychological Corporation.

Wechsler, D. (2003a). *Wechsler Preschool and Primary Scale of Intelligence – Third Edition (WPPSI-III)*. San Antonio, TX: Psychological Corporation.

Wechsler, D. (2003b). *Wechsler Intelligence Scale for Children. Fourth Edition (WISC-IV)*. San Antonio, TX: Psychological Corporation.

Wechsler, D. (2004a). *Wechsler Intelligence Scale for Children. Fourth Edition UK (WISC-IV^uk)*. San Antonio, TX: Psychological Corporation.

Wechsler, D. (2004b). *Wechsler Preschool and Primary Scale of Intelligence – Third Edition UK (WPPSI-III^uk)*. San Antonio, TX: Psychological Corporation.

Wechsler, D. (2005). *Wechsler Individual Achievement Test – II UK (WIAT-II^uk)*. San Antonio, TX: Psychological Corporation.

Weersing, V. & Brent, D. (2003). Cognitive-behavioural therapy for adolescent depression. Comparative efficacy, mediation, moderation and effectiveness. In A. Kazdin, & J. Weisz (eds.), *Evidence Based Psychotherapies for Children and Adolescents* (pp. 135–147). New York: Guilford.

Wehmeyer, M. & Lee, S. (2005). Educating children with intellectual disabilities. In G. O'Reilly, P. Walsh, A. Carr, & J. McEvoy (eds.), *Handbook of Intellectual Disability and Clinical Psychology Practice*. London: Brunner-Routledge.

Wehr, T. and Rosenthal, N. (1989). Seasonality and affective illness. *American Journal of Psychiatry*, 146, 829–839.

Weinberg, W., Harper, C. & Brumback, R. (2002). Substance use and abuse: Epidemiology, pharmacological considerations, identification and suggestions towards management. In M. Rutter & E. Taylor (eds.), *Child and Adolescent Psychiatry* (Fourth edition, pp. 437–454). Oxford: Blackwell.

Weiss, B. (1992). Trends in bicycle helmet use by children: 1985–1990. *Paediatrics*, 89, 78–80.

Weisz, J. & Kazdin A. (2003). Concluding thoughts. Present and future of evidence-based psychotherapies for children and adolescents. In A. Kazdin & J. Weisz (eds.), *Evidence-Based Psychotherapies for Children and Adolescents* (pp. 439–451). New York: Guilford Press.

Weisz, J., Southam-Gerow, M. Gordis, E. & Connor-Smith, J. (2003). Primary and secondary control enhancement training for youth depression. Applying the deployment-focused model to treatment development and testing. In A. Kazdin, & J. Weisz (eds.), *Evidence Based Psychotherapies for Children and Adolescents* (pp. 165–186). New York: Guilford.

Weisz, J. & Weiss, B. (1993). *Effects of Psychotherapy with Children and Adolescents*. London: Sage.

Wekerle, C. & Wolfe, D. (2003). Child maltreatment. In E. Mash & R. Barkley (eds.), *Child Psychopathology* (Second edition, pp. 632–684). New York: Guilford.

Wells, A. (2005). Generalized anxiety disorder. In A. Carr & M. McNulty (eds.), *Handbook of Adult Clinical Psychology: An Evidence Based Approach*. London: Brunner Mazel.

Wells, K. (2004). Treatment of ADHD in children and adolescents. In P. Barrett & T. Ollendick (eds.), *Handbook of Interventions that Work with Children and Adolescents: Prevention and Treatment* (pp. 343–369). Chichester: Wiley.

Welner, Z., Reich, W., Herjanic, B., Jung, K. & Amado, H. (1987). Reliability, validity and parent-child agreement studies of the Diagnostic Interview for Children and Adolescents (DICA). *Journal of the American Academy of Child and Adolescent Psychiatry*, 26, 649–653.

Westcott, H., Davies, G. & Bull, R. (2002). *Children's Testimony: A Handbook of Psychological Research and Forensic Practice*. Chichester: Wiley.

Westenberg, P., Siebelink, B. & Treffers, P. (2001). Psychosocial developmental theory in relation to anxiety and its disorders. In W. Silverman & P. Treffers (eds.) *Anxiety Disorders in Children and Adolescents. Research Assessment and Intervention* (pp. 72–89). Cambridge: Cambridge University Press.

White, M. (1984). Pseudo-encopresis: From avalanche to victory, from vicious to virtuous circles. *Family Systems Medicine*, 2, 150–160.

White, M. & Epston, D. (1990). *Narrative Means to Therapeutic Ends*. New York: Norton.

Whitehurst, G. & Fischel, J. (1994). Practitioner review: Early developmental language delay: What, if anything should the clinician do about it? *Journal of Child Psychology and Psychiatry*, 35, 613–648.

Wieder, H. & Kaplan, E. (1969). Drug use in adolescents: Psychodynamic meaning and pharmacological effect. *Psychoanalytic Study of the Child*, 24, 399.

Wikler, A. (1973). Dynamics of drug dependence. *Archives of General Psychiatry*, 28, 611–616.

Wilkinson, G. (1993). *Wide Range Achievement Test – 3 (WRAT–3)*. Wide Range Inc, 15 Ashley Place, Suite 1a, Wilminton Delaware 19804–1314, USA. Phone 302–652–4990.

Williams, B. & Gilmore, J. (1994). Annotation: Sociometry and peer relationships. *Journal of Child Psychology and Psychiatry*, 35, 997–1013.

Williamson, D. (1993). Advances in paediatric headache research. In T. Ollendick & R. Prinz (eds.), *Advances in Clinical Child Psychology* (volume 15, pp. 275–304). New York: Plenum Press.

Wills, T. & Filer, M. (1996). Stress-coping model of adolescent substance use. In T. Ollendick & R. Prinz (eds.), *Advances in Clinical Child Psychology* (pp. 91–132). New York: Plenum.

Wilson, T., Black-Becker, C. & Heffernan, K. (2003). Eating disorders. In E. Mash & R. Barkley (eds.), *Child Psychopathology* (Second edition, pp. 687–715). New York: Guilford.

Wilson, T. & Fairburn, C. (2002). Treatments for eating disorder. In P. Nathan & J. Gorman (eds.), *A Guide to Treatments that Work* (Second edition, pp. 559–592). New York: Oxford University Press.

Wilson, T. & Pike, M. (2001). Eating disorders. In D. Barlow (ed.), *Clinical Handbook of Psychological Disorders. A Step-by-Step Treatment Manual* (Third edition, pp. 332–375). New York: Guilford.

Wing, L. (1996). *The Autistic Spectrum: A Guide for Parents and Professionals.* London: Constable.

Wing, L., Leekham, S.R., Libby, S.J., Gould, J. & Larcombe, M. (2002). The diagnostic interview for social and communication disorders: background, inter-rater reliability and clinical use. *Journal of Child Psychology and Psychiatry*, 43, 307–325.

Winick, C. (1962). Maturing out of narcotic addiction. *United Nations Bulletin on Narcotics*, 14, 1–10.

Winnicott, D. (1965). *The Maturational Processes and the Facilitating Environment.* London: Hogarth.

Wolfe, D. & McEachran, A. (1997). Child physical abuse and neglect. In E. Mash & L. Teirdal (eds.), *Assessment of Childhood Disorders* (Third edition, pp. 523–568). New York: Guilford.

Wolfe, V. & Birt, A. (1997). Child sexual abuse. In E. Mash & L. Teirdal (eds.), *Assessment of Childhood Disorders* (Third edition, pp. 569–623). New York: Guilford.

Wolfe, V., Gentile, C., Nichienzi, T., Sas, L. & Wolfe, D. (1991). The children's impact of traumatic events scale: A measure of post-sexual-abuse PTSD symptoms. *Behavioural Assessment*, 13, 359–383.

Wood, B. (1994). One articulation of the structural family therapy model: A biobehavioural family model of chronic illness in children. *Journal of Family Therapy*, 16, 53–72.

Wood, B. (1996). A developmental biopsychosocial approach to the treatment of chronic illness in children and adolescent. In R. Mikesell, D. Lusterman & S. McDaniel (eds.), *Integrating Family Therapy. Handbook of Family Psychology and Systems Theory* (pp. 437–458). Washington, DC: American Psychological Association.

Wood, B. & Miller, B. (2003). A biopsychosocial approach to child health. In F. Kaslow (ed.), *Comprehensive Handbook of Psychotherapy: Integrative/Eclectic* (volume 4, pp. 59–80). New York: Wiley.

Worden, J. (2002). *Grief Counselling and Grief Therapy: A Handbook for the Mental Health Practitioner* (Third edition). New York: Springer.

World Health Organization (1992). *The ICD-10 Classification of Mental and Behavioural Disorders.* Geneva: WHO.

World Health Organization (1996). *Multi-axial Classification of Child and Adolescent Psychiatric Disorders: ICD 10 Classification of Mental and Behavioural Disorders in Children and Adolescents.* Cambridge: Cambridge University Press.

World Health Organization (1997–1999). *World Health Statistics Annual.* Geneva: WHO. http://www.who.int/whois

World Health Organization (2001). *The International Classification of Functioning, Disability and Health (ICF).* Geneva: WHO.

Wortman, C. & Silver, R. (1989). The myths of coping with loss. *Journal of Consulting and Clinical Psychology*, 57, 349–357.

Wortman, C. & Silver, R. (2001). The myths of coping with loss revisited. In M. Stroebe, R. Hansson, W. Stroebe & H. Schut (eds.), *Handbook of Bereavement Research: Consequences, Coping, and Care* (pp. 405–429). Washington, DC: American Psychological Association.

Wright, P., McLeod, H. & Cooper, M. (1983). Waking at night. The effect of early feeding experience. *Child Care Health and Development*, 9, 309–319.

Wysocki, T., Greco, P. & Buchloh, L. (2003). Childhood diabetes in psychological context. In M. Roberts (ed.), *Handbook of Paediatric Psychology* (Third edition, pp. 304–320). New York: Guilford.

Yamada, J. (1990). *Laura: A Case For The Modularity of Language*. MA, MIT Press.

Yeates, K., Ris, M. & Taylor, H. (1999). *Paediatric Neuropsychology: Research, Theory, and Practice*. New York: Guilford.

Zeider, M. & Endler, N. (1996). *Handbook of Coping: Theory, Research, Applications*. New York: Wiley.

Zennah, C. (1996). Beyond insecurity: A reconceptualization of attachment disorders of infancy. *Journal of Consulting and Clinical Psychology*, 64, 42–52.

Zero to Three (1994). Diagnostic Classification: 0–3: Diagnostic Classification of Mental Health and Developmental Disorders of Infancy and Early Childhood. Arlington, VA: National Centre for Clinical Infant Programs.

Zubin, J. & Ludwig, A. (1983). What is schizophrenia? *Schizophrenia Bulletin*, 9, 331–334.

Zubin, J. & Spring, B. (1977). Vulnerability: A new view of schizophrenia. *Journal of Abnormal Psychology*, 86, 103–126.

Index